Handbook of Venous Disorders
2nd Edition

Handbook of Venous Disorders 2nd Edition

Guidelines of the American Venous Forum

Edited by

Peter Gloviczki, MD
Professor of Surgery, Mayo Medical School and Chair, Division of Vascular Surgery, Mayo Clinic and Mayo Foundation, Rochester, MN, USA

and

James S T Yao, MD PhD
Magerstadt Professor of Surgery, Division of Vascular Surgery, Northwestern University Medical School, Chicago, IL, USA

ARNOLD
A member of the Hodder Headline Group
LONDON • NEW YORK • NEW DELHI

First edition published in 1996 by Chapman & Hall
Second edition published in Great Britain in 2001 by
Arnold, a member of the Hodder Headline Group,
338 Euston Road, London NW1 3BH

http://www.arnoldpublishers.com

Distributed in the United States of America by
Oxford University Press Inc.,
198 Madison Avenue, New York, NY10016
Oxford is a registered trademark of Oxford University Press

British Library Cataloguing in Publication Data
A catalogue record for this book is available from the British Library

Library of Congress Cataloging-in-Publication Data
A catalog record for this book is available from the Library of Congress

ISBN 0 340 76130 X

1 2 3 4 5 6 7 8 9 10

Commissioning Editor: Nick Dunton
Development Editor: Michael Lax
Project Manager: Susan Parmentier
Production Editor: James Rabson
Production Controller: Iain McWilliams
Cover Design: Terry Griffiths

Typeset in 10 on 12 pt Minion by Phoenix Photosetting, Chatham, Kent
Printed and bound in Great Britain by The Bath Press, Bath

Contents

Contributors

Frederick A Anderson, Jr PhD
Research Professor, Department of Surgery, University of Massachusetts Medical Center, Worcester, MA

Clifford T Araki PhD
Assistant Professor of Surgery, Technical Director, Noninvasive Vascular Laboratory, UMDNJ-New Jersey Medical School, Newark, NJ

Berndt Arfvidsson MD
Straub Clinic and Hospital, Honolulu, HI

Enrico Ascher MD
Professor of Surgery, Director, Division of Vascular Surgery, Maimonides Medical Center, Brooklyn, NY

Hugh G Beebe MD
Clinical Professor of Surgery, University of Michigan Medical School, Director, Jobst Vascular Center, Toledo, OH

Claire E Bender MD
Professor of Radiology, Mayo Medical School, Consultant in Radiology, Department of Radiology, Mayo Clinic And Foundation, Rochester, MN, and University of New York Health Center, Brooklyn, NY

John J Bergan MD, FACS, FRCS Hon(Eng)
Professor of Surgery, University of California, San Diego, Attending Surgeon, Scripps Memorial Hospital, La Jolla, CA

Amardip S Bhuller MD
Department of Surgery, Division of Vascular Surgery, Indiana University School of Medicine, Indianapolis, IN

Thomas C Bower MD
Professor of Surgery, Mayo Medical School, Division of Vascular Surgery, Mayo Clinic and Foundation, Rochester, MN

Andrew Bradbury BSc, MB, MD, FRCSEd
Professor of Vascular Surgery, University of Birmingham, Heartlands Hospital, Birmingham, UK

Jerome F Breen MD
Assistant Professor of Radiology, Mayo Medical School, Consultant, Department of Diagnostic Radiology, Mayo Clinic and Foundation, Rochester, MN

Kellie R Brown MD
Medical College of Wisconsin, Milwaukee, WI

Kevin G Burnand MS, FRCS
Professor of Vascular Surgery, Academic Department of Surgery, St. Thomas Hospital, London, UK

Robert A Cambria MD
Associate Professor of Surgery, Medical College of Wisconsin, Chief, Section of Vascular Surgery, Clement J. Zablocki VAMC, Milwaukee, WI

Linda C Canton RN, BSN
Division of Vascular Surgery, Mayo Clinic and Foundation, Rochester, MN

Stephen W Carmicheal PhD, DSc
Professor and Chair, Department of Anatomy, Mayo Medical School, Consultant, Department of Radiology, Mayo Clinic and Foundation, Rochester, MN

Kenneth J Cherry, Jr MD
Professor of Surgery, Mayo Medical School, Consultant, Division of Vascular Surgery, Mayo Clinic and Foundation, Rochester, MN

Jae-Sung Cho MD
Senior Staff Surgeon, Henry Ford Hospital, Detroit, MI

Philip D Coleridge Smith DM, MA, BCH, FRCS
Department of Surgery, University College London Medical School, Middlesex Hospital, London, UK

Anthony J Comerota MD, FASC
Professor of Surgery, Temple University School of Medicine, Chief of Vascular Surgery, Department of Surgery, Temple University Hospital, Philadelphia, PA

Robert Cranley MD, FACS
Good Samaritan Hospital, Co-Director, Kachelmacher Memorial Clinic, Cincinnati, OH

Michael C Dalsing MD
Professor of Surgery, Department of Surgery, Division of Vascular Surgery, Indiana University School of Medicine, Indianapolis, IN

Hai P. Dang MD
Northeast Medical Center, Humble, TX

Gail de Imus MD
Chief Resident, Boston University School of Medicine, Department of Dermatology and Skin Surgery, Roger Williams Medical Center Providence, RI

Ralph G DePalma MD, FACS
Professor of Surgery and Vice Chair, Department of Surgery, University of Nevada School of Medicine, Chief Surgical Services, VA Sierra Nevada Healthcare System, Reno, NV

James A DeWeese MD
Professor of Surgery, Chair Emeritus Division Cardiothoracic Surgery, Section of Vascular Surgery, University of Rochester, Rochester, NY

Walter N Durán MD
Professor of Physiology and Surgery, Director, Research Program in Vascular Biology, UMDNJ-New Jersey Medical School, Newark, NJ

Bo Eklof MD, PhD
Clinical Professor of Surgery, University of Hawaii, John A. Burns School of Medicine, Vascular Surgeon, Straub Clinic and Hospital, Honolulu, HI

Vincent Falanga MD, FACP
Professor of Dermatology and Biochemistry, Boston University School of Medicine, Chairman, Department of Dermatology and Skin Surgery, Roger Williams Medical Center, Providence, RI

Cindy Felty RN, MSN, C-ANP
Director, Vascular Ulcer/Wound Healing Center, Mayo Clinic and Foundation, Rochester, MN

David L Gillespie MD
Associate Professor of Surgery, Chief, Division of Vascular Surgery, Uniformed Services University of the Health Sciences, F Edward Herbert School of Medicine, Bethesda, MD

Peter Gloviczki MD
Professor of Surgery, Mayo Medical School, and Chair, Division of Vascular Surgery, Mayo Medical School, Mayo Clinic and Foundation, Rochester, MN

Mitchel P Goldman MD
Associate Clinical Professor of Medicine (Dermatology), University of California, San Diego, La Jolla, CA

Richard Green MD
Professor of Surgery, Chief, Division of Vascular Surgery, University of Rochester Medical Center, Rochester, NY

Lazar J Greenfield MD
Frederick A Coller Distinguished Professor and Chairman, Department of Surgery, University of Michigan, Ann Arbor, MI

Edmund J. Harris, Jr MD
Stanford University Medical School, Stanford, CA

Mary F Hauser MD
Assistant Professor of Radiology, Mayo Medical School, Consultant in Nuclear Medicine, Department of Radiology, Mayo Foundation, Rochester, MN

John A Heit MD
Associate Professor of Medicine, Mayo Medical School, Director, Thrombohilia Center, Mayo Clinic and Foundation, Rochester, MN

Anil Hingorami MD
Divison of Vascular Surgery, Maimonides Medical Center, Brooklyn, NY

Robert W Hobson II MD
Professor of Surgery and Physiology, UMDNJ-New Jersey Medical School, Director, Division of Vascular Surgery, UMDNJ-University Hospital, Newark, NJ

Russell D Hull MBBs, MSc
Professor, Department of Medicine, University of Calgary, Director, Thrombosis Research Unit, FootHills Hospital, Calgary, Canada

Karl A Illig MD
Associate Professor of Surgery, University of Rochester, Rochester, NY

C Michael Johnson MD
Consultant in Diagnostic Radiology, Mayo Clinic and Foundation, Rochester, MN

Corey Jost MD
Fellow, Division of Vascular Surgery, Mayo Clinic and Foundation, Rochester, MN

Manju Kalra BBS
Fellow, Division of Vascular Surgery, Mayo Clinic and Foundation, Rochester, MN

Curtis B Kamida MD
Clinical Assistant Professor of Radiology, University of Hawaii, John A. Burns School of Medicine, Interventional Radiologist, Straub Clinic and Hospital, Honolulu, HI

Robert L Kistner MD
Clinical Professor of Surgery, University of Hawaii, John A. Burns School of Medicine, Vascular Surgeon, Straub Clinic and Hospital, Honolulu, HI

Stephen G Lalka MD
Professor of Surgery, Division of Vascular Surgery, Indiana University School of Medicine, Indianapolis, IN

Joan M Lohr MD FACS
Good Samaritan Hospital, Medical Director, John J. Cranley Vascular Lab, Cincinnati, OH

Thomas Lynch
Associate Professor of Surgery, Department of Surgery, University of Nebraska Medical Center, Omaha, NE

Elna Masuda MD
Assistant Professor of Surgery, Surgical Residency Program, University of Hawaii, John A. Burns Medical School, Vascular Surgeon, Straub Clinic and Hospital, Honolulu, HI

Mark A Mattos MD
Associate Professor of Surgery, Department of Surgery, Section of Peripheral Vascular Surgery, Southern Illinois University School of Medicine, Springfield, IL

Michael A McKusick MD
Assistant Professor of Radiology, Department of Diagnostic Radiology, Mayo Clinic and Foundation, Rochester, MN

Mark H Meissner MD
Associate Professor of Surgery, Department of Surgery, University of Washington School of Medicine, Seattle, WA

Gregory L Moneta MD
Professor of Surgery, Chair, Department of Surgery, Division of Vascular Surgery, Oregon Health and Sciences University, Veterans Affairs Medical Center, Portland, OR

Géza Mózes MD, PhD
Resident in Surgery, Department of Surgery, Mayo Clinic and Foundation, Rochester, MN

Ryan D Nachreiner MD
Department of Surgery, Division of Vascular Surgery, Indiana University School of Medicine, Indianapolis, IN

Alexander D Nicoloff MD
Department of Surgery, Division of Vascular Surgery, Oregon Health and Sciences University, Portland, OR

Audra A Noel MD
Assistant Professor of Surgery, Mayo Medical School, Division of Vascular Surgery, Mayo Clinic and Foundation, Rochester, MN

Thomas F O'Donnell, Jr MD, FACS
Andrews Professor of Surgery, Tufts University School of Medicine, CEO & President, New England Medical Center, Boston, MA

Francisco J Osse, MD
Santa Casa De Sao Paulo – Brazil, Coordinator of Venous Disorders Services, Sao Paulo, Brazil

Kenneth Ouriel MD
Professor of Surgery, Chairman, Department of Vascular Surgery, The Cleveland Clinic and Foundation, Cleveland, OH

Frank Padberg, Jr MD
Professor of Surgery, UMDNJ – New Jersey Medical School, Chief, Section of Vascular Surgery, Center for Vascular Disease, Doctor's Office Center, UMNJ Healthcare System, Newark, NJ

Peter C Pairolero MD
Division of Vascular Surgery, Mayo Clinic and Foundation, Rochester, MN

Peter J Pappas MD
Associate Professor of Surgery, UMDNJ – New Jersey Medical School, Attending Surgeon, UMDNJ – University Hospital, Newark, NJ

William H Pearce MD, FACS
Professor of Surgery, Northwestern University Medical School, Chief, Division of Vascular Surgery, Northwestern Memorial Hospital, Chicago, IL

John R Pfeifer MD
Professor of Surgery, University of Michigan, Director of Venous Disease Center, Livonia, MI

Graham Pineo MD
Professor, Departments of Medicine and Oncology, University of Calgary, Director, Thrombosis Research Unit, Foothills Hospital, Calgary, Canada

The late John M Porter MD
Formerly Professor of Surgery, Department of Surgery, Division of Vascular Surgery, Oregon Health and Sciences University, Veterans Affairs Medical Center, Portland, OR

Mary C Proctor MS
University of Michigan, Ann Arbor, MI

Elizabeth Rachael MD
Endovascular Fellow, Baptist Hospital, Louisville, KY

Robert Y Rhee MD
Assistant Professor of Surgery, University of Pittsburgh, Presbyterian-University Hospital, Pittsburgh, PA

Jeffrey M Rhodes MD
Assistant Professor of Surgery, University of Rochester Medical Center, Rochester, NY

Norman M Rich MD
Chief, Department of Surgery, Uniformed Services University of the Health Sciences, F Edward Herbert School of Medicine, Bethesda, MD

Thom W Rooke MD
Professor of Surgery, Mayo Medical School, Mayo Clinic, Director of Goudré Vascular Center, Mayo Clinic and Foundation, Rochester, MN

C Vaughan Ruckley ChM, FRCSEd, CBE
Emeritus Professor of Vascular Surgery, University of Edinburgh, Royal Infirmary, Edinburgh, UK

Robert B Rutherford MD, FACS, FRCS(Glasg)
Emeritus Professor of Surgery, University of Colorado, School of Medicine, Denver, CO

Sergio X Salles-Cunha PhD
Clinical Research Director, Jobst Vascular Center, Toledo, OH

Nancy Schindler MD
Assistant Professor of Surgery, Northwestern University Medical School, Evanston Northwestern Hospital, Evanston, IL

Richard K Spence MD
Director of Surgery, Staten Island University Hospital, Staten Island, NY

Anthony W Stanson MD
Associate Professor of Surgery, Mayo Medical School, Consultant, Department of Diagnostic Radiology, Mayo Clinic and Foundation, Rochester, MN

Yaron Sternbach MD, CM
Assistant Professor, Vascular Surgery, University of Rochester, Director, Endovascular Surgery, Strong Memorial Hospital, Rochester, NY

D Eugene Strandness, Jr MD
Professor of Surgery, Department of Surgery, University of Washington School of Medicine, Seattle, WA

David S Sumner MD
Distinguished Professor of Surgery Emeritus, Southern Illinois School of Medicine, Springfield, IL

Patricia E Thorpe MD
Director of Venous Disorders, Heart & Vascular Institute of New York, Lenox Hospital, New York City, NY

Jonathan B Towne MD
Professor of Surgery, Medical College of Wisconsin, Chairman, Vascular Surgery, Froedtert Memorial Lutheran Hospital, Milwaukee, WI

J Leonel Villavicencio MD, FACS
Professor of Surgery, Uniformed Services University of the Health Sciences, F Edward Herbert School of Medicine, Bethesda, MD

Robert L Vogelzang MD
Professor of Radiology, Northwestern University Medical School, Chief of Vascular and Interventional Radilogy, Northwestern Memorial Hospital, Chicago, IL

Thomas W Wakefield MD
Professor of Surgery, University of Michigan, Ann Arbor, MI

Robert A Weiss MD
Assistant Professor of Dermatology, Johns Hopkins University School of Medicine, Baltimore, MD

Margaret Weiss MD
Assistant Professor of Dermatology, Johns Hopkins University School of Medicine, Baltimore, MD

H Brownell Wheeler MD
Harry M Haidak Distinquished Professor Emeritus, University of Massachusetts Medical Center, Worcester, MA

James S T Yao MD, PhD
Magerstadt Professor of Surgery, Division of Vascular Surgery, Northwestern University Medical School, Northwestern Memorial Hospital, Chicago, IL

Preface

Reasons to publish a new, second edition of the *Handbook of Venous Disorders* are legion. In the past five years, substantial new information has emerged in many areas of acute and chronic venous disease, on venous malformations and lymphatic disorders. Our knowledge has advanced in molecular biology and cellular physiology, and we understand better the basic pathomechanisms of both acute venous thromboembolism and chronic venous insufficiency. We also have more data on the epidemiology and the natural history of venous diseases. Experience has accumulated with the use of new classification systems, and the diagnosis of venous disease has become more accurate and less invasive. Evaluation of venous function has been perfected and duplex scanning is now widely available. There is a need, therefore, to provide the latest practical guidelines for the use of duplex ultrasonography in the diagnosis of acute venous thrombosis, chronic valvular incompetence and venous occlusion. Fast computed tomography has emerged as a diagnostic tool of pulmonary embolism, magnetic resonance imaging has progressed and contrast venography has been used more selectively; their roles and advantages are discussed in detail.

Out-patient therapy of acute deep venous thrombosis by low-molecular weight heparin has been approved in the United States by the Food and Drug Administration in 1998 and this treatment is now widely prescribed in the office practice and in thrombophilia clinics. Endovascular techniques have rapidly progressed, catheter-directed thrombolytic treatment has become more popular and venous stents have been placed percutaneously with increasing frequency with good early results. Published data on new technology, including minimally invasive techniques used for primary varicosity, need critical analysis and recommendations using new therapy should be given by leaders of the American Venous Forum. Surgical treatments for both acute and chronic venous diseases have evolved, and new series with reconstructions for both venous incompetence and obstruction have been published. Endoscopic venous surgery has advanced and results of large single center series and those of the North American Subfascial Endoscopic Perforator Surgery (NASEPS) Registry have been published. Further studies are needed but experience supports surgical treatment to correct abnormal venous hemodynamics in patients with venous ulcers. Drugs to improve the venous circulation have shown promise in experimental and initial clinical studies and the care of venous ulcer has progressed. Substantial new knowledge has accumulated on wound healing, including the use of growth factors and human fibroblasts to accelerate epidermal growths. Lymphedema clinics have emerged and provide the latest therapy for this disabling condition. Reviews of the latest information on lymphatic and chylous disorders are included in this volume.

The new edition of the *Handbook* also includes summaries and complete texts of consensus documents on classification, evaluation and management of venous diseases. New chapters on reporting standards and outcome analysis, and a new report of the American Venous Forum Research Committee on basic and clinical research in venous and lymphatic disease are included.

Similar to the first edition, it is the purpose of the new edition to provide comprehensive and up-to-date information on acute and chronic venous and lymphatic diseases and malformations and to discuss the latest knowledge on epidemiology, pathophysiology, clinical evaluation, diagnostic imaging, medical, endovascular and surgical management.

The book is authored by leaders and founding members of the American Venous Forum, a society of increasing recognition within the US and abroad, dedicated to research, education and clinical practice of venous and lymphatic diseases. The second edition will also include several international authors, all experts in venous disease, most being regular or honorary members of the American Venous Forum.

The manual is intended for medical students, house officers, residents and fellows in vascular surgery, interventional radiology, vascular and internal medicine and cardiology, and to all physicians, surgeons, vascular laboratory technologists and vascular nurses who are involved in the investigation, evaluation or management of venous and lymphatic diseases or malformations.

The first edition, published in 1996, was very successful and reviews ranked it to be one of the most important and comprehensive textbooks on venous disease. The authors and editors are hopeful that this new edition of the *Handbook of Venous Disorders* will equally be useful and popular and become the essential reference source on the diagnosis and treatment of venous and lymphatic diseases. Those who purchase this volume will also be pleased to learn that they contribute to a noble cause: all royalties made on this Handbook will be offered to the American Venous Forum Foundation to support basic and clinical research in venous and lymphatic disease.

Peter Gloviczki, MD
James S T Yao, MD

PART I

Basic considerations

1

Venous and lymphatic disease: an historical review

KARL A ILLIG AND JAMES A DEWEESE

Venous disease is among the most common medical condition to affect mankind – approximately 1–3% of the population of the Western world is estimated to have severe venous problems at some point in their lives.[1] Venous problems have been recognized since antiquity, being mentioned in one form or another in the Old Testament (Isaiah I:6), the Ebers papyrus in 1550 BC, and by Hippocrates five centuries before Christ.[2–4]

A chapter of this length can only be a brief overview of the important historical highlights of venous and lymphatic problems. The reader is directed to several excellent collections of original sources relating to the history of the venous and lymphatic systems by Bergan[2,5] and Gloviczki,[6] respectively.

ANATOMY AND PATHOPHYSIOLOGY

Interestingly, the true anatomy of the veins was relatively accurately understood before the basic concept of circulation of the blood was known, although each contributor in this sequence was a student of the former. Vesalius published the first accurate description of human anatomy, *De Humani Corporis Fabrica* (1543). Fabricus, his student, elaborated (1603) by describing the venous valves and their locations, and decided they were there to prevent reflux (Fig. 1.1). Finally, William Harvey, who in turn studied under Fabricus, published his preliminary observations in 1616 and definitive work (*Exercitatio Anatomica De Moto Cordis et Sanguinis*) describing the circulatory system in 1628.[2,3]

The basic pathophysiology of venous disorders seems to have been fairly accurately understood by the ancients, then lost in the dark ages of Galen's humoral theories. It was Hippocrates who said 'it was better not to stand in the case of an ulcer on the leg',[7] whilst Marianus Sanctus felt that the cause of varicose veins and ulceration was 'standing too much before kings'.[8] Unfortunately, Galen felt that venous ulcers were caused by an excess of black bile, and that whilst excluding this black bile from the ulcer and varicosities was worthy, espoused the theory that tight compression would express these evil humors into the general circulation, making the patient critically ill.[2] Luckily, by the fifteenth century, perhaps sparked by the works of Vesalius and Harvey, medicine and treatment of venous disease became grounded on more rational, empiric information and theories.

DEEP VENOUS THROMBOSIS

Elucidation of the pathophysiology of clotting, of course, dates from more 'modern' times. Virchow, in the mid-1800s, recognized and described the three contributing factors for thrombosis: stasis, endothelial injury and hypercoagulability.[9] Despite a century and a half of research and refinement, this classic triad remains

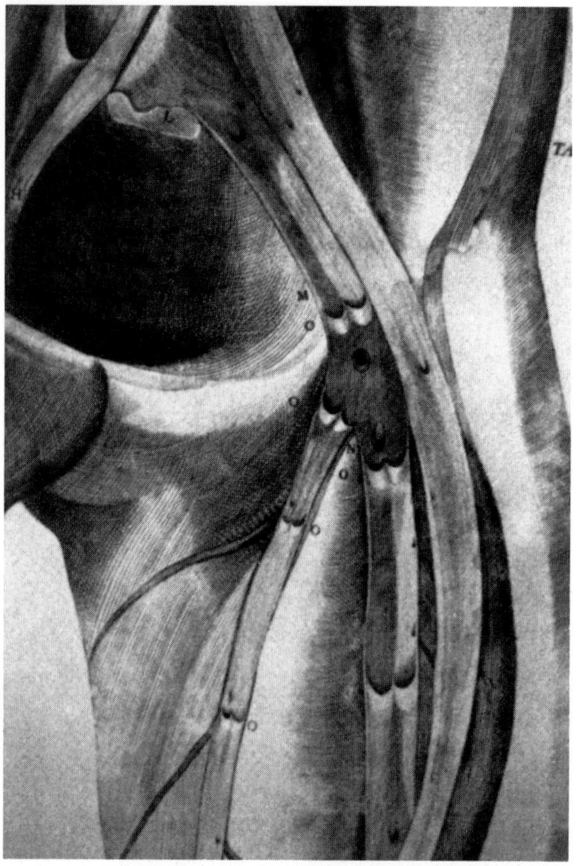

Figure 1.1 *Illustration from Fabricus' atlas (1603), clearly showing the presence of valves in the veins of the lower extremity. (Reproduced with permission from Bergan JJ. Historical highlights. In Bergan JJ, Yao JST.* Venous Disorders. *Philadelphia: WB Saunders, 1991: 5)*

the simplest and best way of approaching any thrombotic process, and is almost literally mentioned every day in every teaching hospital in the world.

John Homans' contributions were critical in understanding all facets of venous disease, especially the causes, effects and sequela of deep venous thrombosis (DVT). He produced some of the earliest 'modern' descriptions of historical and physical findings in patients with DVT, recognized and emphasized such classic risk factors as the operation, bed rest, and dehydration, and pointed out the ability of popliteal clot to fatally embolize.[10,11] It is, of course, his description in the late 1930s of pain with foot dorsiflexion in the presence of DVT that is best remembered today, at least to the casual student in this field.[11,12] The fact that he was quite specifically referring to calf vein thrombosis only is unknown to many who refer to and use 'Homans' sign', as is the fact that he and others later questioned its value and accuracy.[13]

Unfortunately, even after Homans' contributions, history and physical examination remained unreliable methods for the diagnosis of DVT, and it soon became apparent that more objective testing was needed. Although phlebography was first described in humans in 1923, it was not until the 1930s that its use became common.[14] Because of its low morbidity and high accuracy, and, of course, for want of a better test, it has been regarded as the 'gold standard' for diagnosis of venous disorders in general and DVT specifically for decades. Because it is not entirely innocuous, however, noninvasive diagnostic testing was pursued. Although venous occlusion plethysmography was first used in 1905 to measure arterial blood flow,[15] it seems to have been first applied for evaluation of venous problems and the diagnosis of DVT in the late 1960s and early 1970s.[16,17] Gomez first described the administration of radioactive (^{125}I-labeled) fibrinogen to identify venous thrombosis in 1963, although this test was limited to actively forming thrombus.[18] Both plethysmography and radioisotope scanning continue to be used for specific special cases (such as air- and photoplethysmography for the evaluation of valvular incompetence), but neither has displaced phlebography for the assessment of DVT.

Soon after Satomura's original description of the measurement of arterial blood flow using Doppler ultrasound in 1959,[19] clinicians, notably Strandness, applied this technique to the arterial and venous circulation, beginning in the late 1960s.[20,21] Initial continuous-wave devices relied, of course, on indirect evidence of obstruction and reflux, but with the advent of duplex technology in the 1970s and 80s the benefit of ultrasound became apparent. Extensive work and clinical experience has resulted in a refinement of this technique to the point where it has displaced phlebography as the procedure of choice for diagnosis of DVT at most institutions.

Prior to the 1930s, treatment of venous thrombosis was limited to bed rest and elevation, with the only interventional methods attempted being operative clot extraction or venous ligation.[22,23] John (Jay) McLean discovered heparin in 1916 when he was a 24-year-old medical student at Johns Hopkins, but never followed up on this line of work. Howell and Holt and Best, at the University of Toronto, expanded his results, purifying and characterizing it, whereas Murray, also at Toronto, conducted the first large-scale clinical trials.[4] Coumadin was discovered after a veterinary observation that blood failed to clot in cattle that had eaten moldy sweet clover hay. Dicoumarol was isolated and synthesized by Stahmann in 1941, and clinical results were published in 1942.[24]

PULMONARY EMBOLUS

Ligation of the inferior vena cava was apparently first performed by Trendelenburg in 1906 as part of the treatment of a woman with puerperal sepsis, but routine femoral venous ligation was first generally advocated as a specific treatment for prevention of pulmonary embolus in patients with deep venous thrombosis by Homans in 1934.[10] Because venous ligation was associated with a high incidence of severe venous stasis and recurrent, often fatal, embolization, Dale suggested temporary caval ligation, but this never proved practical. Because of these problems, solutions were proposed that involved partial caval interruption, allowing flow of liquid blood but entrapment of larger emboli in the late 1950s and early 1960s. Marion 'Bill' DeWeese developed a technique whereby interrupted silk sutures were placed but not tightened, producing an intraluminal 'harp-grid' network to trap emboli, and thus performed the first intravascular partial venous interruption. Spencer suggested plicating the cava with interrupted sutures, while Moretz and Miles both developed plastic clips to narrow the vena cava. Subsequently, Adams and DeWeese combined the best elements of both to arrive at what became the most widely used such device.[25]

First described in 1969, the Mobin-Uddin umbrella, a plastic disc with small holes allowing blood flow, was the first practical method of caval interruption able to be introduced through a remote access site without the need for major operation.[26] Although complete caval occlusion frequently occurred, the development of modern devices, pioneered by Greenfield's original steel Greenfield filter and now joined by multiple similar devices, has almost eliminated this problem.[27] In recent years, systemic and catheter-directed thrombolysis has been added in an effort to quickly reduce clot burden and ameliorate postphlebitic problems,[28] but this has yet to gain a secure foothold in this arena.

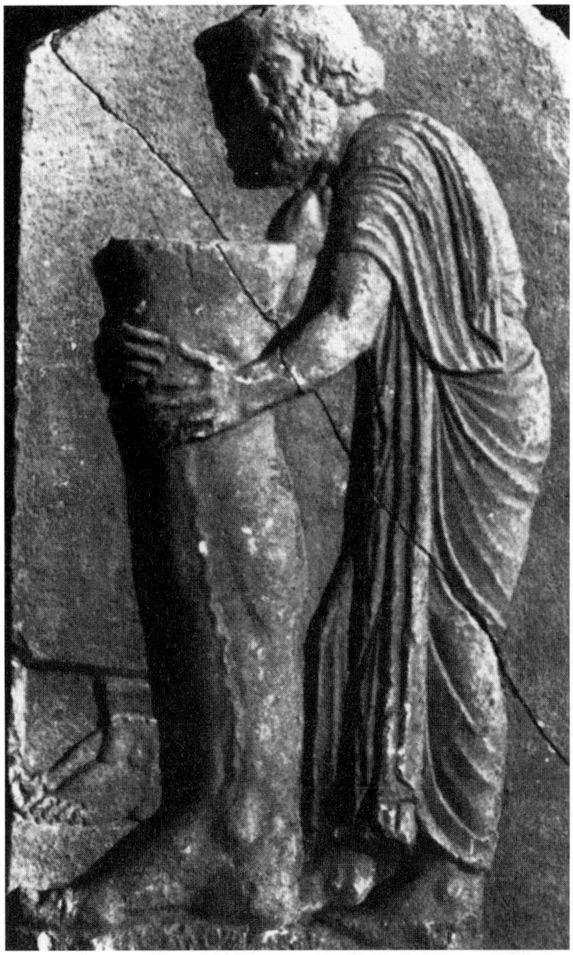

Figure 1.2 *Votive offering from a grateful Greek patient to his doctor, apparently commemorating successful treatment of a varicose vein. (Reproduced with permission from Bergan JJ. Historical highlights. In Bergan JJ, Yao JST.* Venous Disorders. *Philadelphia: WB Saunders, 1991: 4)*

VARICOSE VEINS

Varicose veins have been recognized since recorded history began. There is a stone votive offering in the National Museum in Athens, Greece, dedicated to a physician by a grateful patient, which clearly shows a long varicose vein (apparently with an incompetent perforator distal to the area that is being compressed)[2] (Fig. 1.2). Although multiple methods for their treatment have been investigated, the Arab statement, 'cut skin, expose varix, insert probe under it . . . pull out varix and cut'[3] has perhaps not been improved upon as we enter the twenty-first century – although it was made in c. 400 AD! Homans eloquently described the pathophysiology, etiology and treatment of varicose veins in 1916, using ideas and descriptions that remain startlingly modern today.[29]

CHRONIC VENOUS DISEASE

As discussed above, the observation that venous ulceration and edema are made worse with standing seems to have been made well before the birth of Christ. Compression therapy is mentioned in the Old Testament (Isaiah I:6), and Roman foot soldiers knew that tightly wrapping their legs alleviated discomfort induced by prolonged standing. Both Celsus (before Christ) and Chauliac (1363) used linen and plaster wraps for chronic venous disease, obviously antedating Unna by many centuries. Apart from its spelling, Paré's observation in the sixteenth century that '[in bandaging, wrap] the leg beginning at the foote and finishing at the knee, not forgetting a little bolster upon the varicose veins' remains an absolutely perfect statement today.[2]

Brodie, in 1846, was the first to succinctly describe the signs and symptoms of chronic venous insufficiency in a scientific manner and described visible superficial venous reflux, and was followed by Trendelenburg's classic clinical test to distinguish superficial from deep reflux in 1891.[2,30] Once again, Homans was among the first to accurately describe the relationship between varicose veins, deep venous thrombosis, and venous ulceration, and pointed out that valvular incompetence does not necessarily have to follow deep venous thrombosis.[29] Interestingly, he also seems to have been the first to point out (anticipating the results of the North American Subfascial Endoscopic Perforator Surgery registry by many decades) that venous ulcers behave quite differently whether they are associated with superficial reflux only or follow deep vein thrombosis and recanalization.[31] Although many others contributed, it was Linton in 1953 who most eloquently described what has become the best-accepted modern pathophysiologic theory of chronic venous ulceration and dermatitis, apparently coining the term 'ambulatory venous hypertension' in the process.[32]

As discussed above, even the Romans empirically knew the value of compression therapy for venous insufficiency. Richard Wiseman, surgeon to Charles II of England, introduced a lace-up boot for venous compression for 'varicose ulcers' in 1676,[2] whilst Gay coined the term 'venous ulcer' in 1867 and pointed out that such ulcers can occur in the absence of varicose veins.[33] Unna's boot, a combination of a moist, occlusive dressing and leg compression, has been used since the turn of the century.[34]

Elastic stockings first arose in the twentieth century when such fibers became available, but original stockings were crude, 'one-size-fits-all' and did not significantly improve outcome. Conrad Jobst, a successful engineer, developed refractory varicose veins and ulcerations in the 1930s, apparently suffering recurrences and nonhealing despite superficial venous ablation for at least a decade. He noticed that his symptoms were alleviated while standing in his pool, and came to the conclusion that the graduated pressure naturally created by the water was the beneficial factor involved. After experimentation and invention, he made his own graduated compression stockings, which promptly alleviated his symptoms.[35] Despite other advances, graduated compression stockings remain the essential and most widely accepted therapeutic measure for chronic venous insufficiency today.

Operative therapy for hemodynamic venous disease also dates from the early part of the twentieth century. Gay described the perforators in 1867,[33] and though perforator interruption had apparently been practiced before, Robert Linton first widely publicized the procedure in 1938.[36] Originally involving three separate incisions as well as ligation of the superficial femoral vein, the 'modern' Linton procedure eventually included division of the medial perforators only.[32] Of course, wound complications proved the major problem, which prompted Linton to note carefully that all ulcers must be healed and the skin in as good a condition as possible before proceeding. Modifications were designed to reduce wound complications, including DePalma's parallel transverse incisions and Rob and Felder's posterior, 'stocking-seam' approach,[5] but operative perforator ligation remained morbid and cumbersome, and hence little-used by the majority of surgeons.

Edwards seems to have first thought of dividing the perforators through a remote incision.[37] His technique, described in 1976, was to blindly shear the perforators with a 'phlebotome' inserted proximally into the superficial posterior compartment, and results were acceptable. With the advent of improved technology and familiarization with endoscopic techniques in general, however, attention shifted to this method as a way of gaining visual access to the perforators without a long incision (Fig. 1.3). Extensive clinical work has been carried out by Hauer, Gloviczki,[38] O'Donnell and Iafrati, Bergan, and Padberg, among others, in the USA, and by groups in Germany, England and the Netherlands. Although proponents of subfascial endoscopic perforator surgery (SEPS) believe it offers significant clinical benefit over nonoperative therapy and superficial venous ablation alone, this has not been proven.

Efforts have also been directed toward correction of incompetence in the deep system, by means of direct valvular reconstruction (Kistner) or transposition of a venous segment bearing functional valves (Raju and others), techniques that date from the 1970s and 1980s, respectively.[39,40] Bypass for occluded infrainguinal veins (most commonly the superficial femoral vein) was first discussed as early as 1954,[41] and popularized in the 1970s as the May–Husni operation.[42] Crossover femoral grafts (the contralateral saphenous; Palma operation, ipsilateral saphenous, or even prosthetic) with or without arteriovenous fistulae for iliac occlusion were similarly popularized in the 1960s[43] and continue to be performed today in appropriate settings.

EFFORT THROMBOSIS

Venous thrombosis of the upper extremity was first described by Paget and von Schroetter in 1875 and 1884, respectively,[44] but seems not to have been widely recognized as an important clinical entity until 1949.[45,46] By the late 1930s, the observation that intermittent axillo-subclavian venous obstruction can be caused by careful positioning of the arm in a substantial number of persons had been made.[47] Because exercise is often associated with its acute clinical presentation or exacerbates chronic symptoms, this entity is today most commonly referred to as 'effort thrombosis'.[45]

Treatment was originally conservative, but after it became apparent that these patients have a substantial risk of both pulmonary embolus and functional morbidity, anticoagulation was added.[46] What differentiates these patients from those with lower extremity clot, however, is that there is a correctable causative factor, compression at the thoracic outlet, in many or most such patients. In the 1980s and 1990s, various

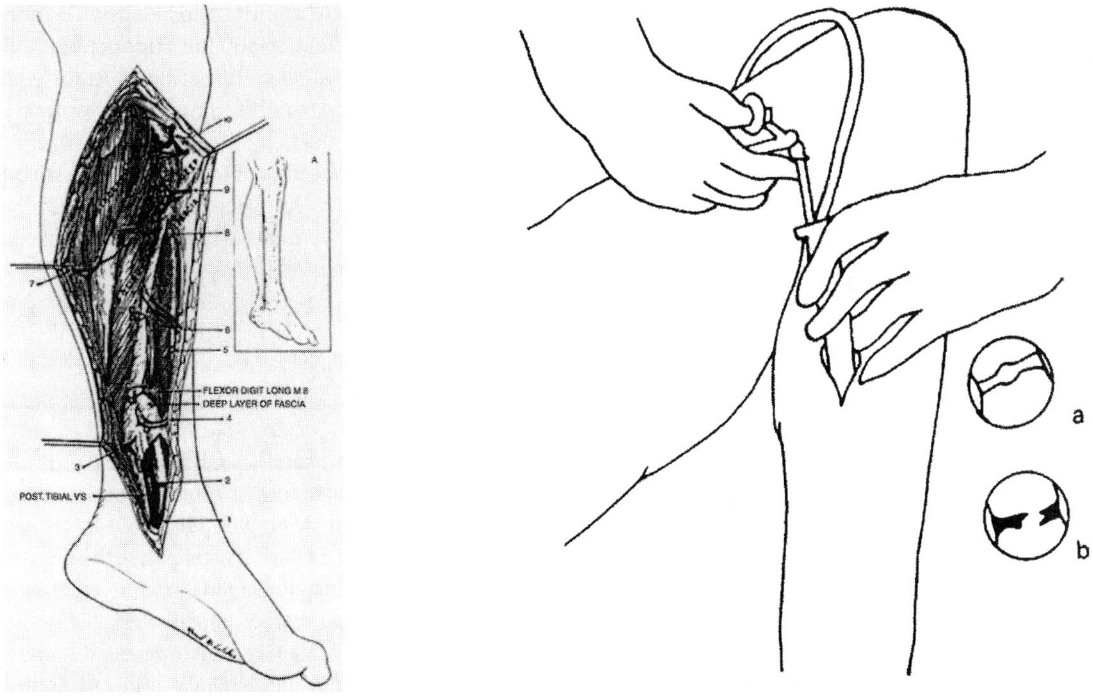

Figure 1.3 *(a) Linton's technique of ligation of the communicating veins. (From Linton RR. The communicating veins of the lower leg and the operative technic for their ligation.* Ann Surg *1938;* ***107****: 582–93). (b) The first illustration of endoscopic subfascial perforator vein surgery by Hauer in 1985. (From Hauer G. The endoscopic subfascial division of the perforating veins – preliminary report [in German].* Vasa *1985;* ***14****: 59–61.)*

methods for alleviating this compression, usually by resection of the first rib or medial clavicle, sometimes combined with venous thrombectomy, were used. With the advent of thrombolysis and its success in this situation, however, many have become more aggressive in attempts to clear the axillary vein of clot, and subsequently relieve the compression and reconstruct the vein, if necessary, although timing remains somewhat controversial.[48]

LYMPHATIC DISEASE

Once again, it was Hippocrates who first seemed to have left an historical record of the lymphatics, describing 'glands, that everybody has in the armpit' and 'white blood'.[49] Although several others described lymphatics before the birth of Christ, the discovery of the lymphatic system in a scientifically accurate sense is attributed to Asellius, who observed and described the mesenteric lymphatic in a well-fed dog. Pecquet subsequently described the cysterna chyli and thoracic duct (1651), while Bartholin (1653) and Rudbeck (1942) clarified the anatomy of the major lymphatic structures (Fig. 1.4). Finally, Hunter in the eighteenth century, Starling in the nineteenth, and Rusznyák, Földi, and Szabó in the twentieth all elucidated modern concepts of lymphatic physiology.[6]

Diagnosis and treatment of lymphatic disorders have only been relatively recently developed. Direct contrast lymphangiography was the first diagnostic method to be investigated, being first described in 1944,[50] but it is now felt to contribute to further lymphatic damage. For this reason, lymphoscintigraphy, first described by Taylor in 1957,[51] has become the diagnostic test of choice. Although his original report described injection of ^{131}I-labeled protein, imaging today is usually performed using technetium-99.

Treatment of lymphedema in antiquity is not widely described (perhaps because the entity was confused with or lumped together with venous insufficiency), although undoubtedly elevation and compression therapy were used. Modern treatment strategies designed to directly treat the swelling itself date from the 1960s and 1970s, when various algorithms, including manual lymphatic drainage and general limb massage, pneumatic compression devices, simple and adjustable compression stockings, and elevation were all used in various protocols.[50,52] Operative attempts to improve lymphatic drainage, either by direct lymphatic reconstruction[53] or transposition of lymphatic-rich tissues[54,55] to drainage basins, have been described since the 1970s, but only a few centers have had much experience with them.

'Reduction' or debulking operations have been attempted since the early 1900s. Early attempts involved complete excision of all tissue, including skin, to the level of the fascia, with reconstruction by grafting. Originally described by Charles in 1912 and still bearing his name, this procedure is still sometimes used today for selected

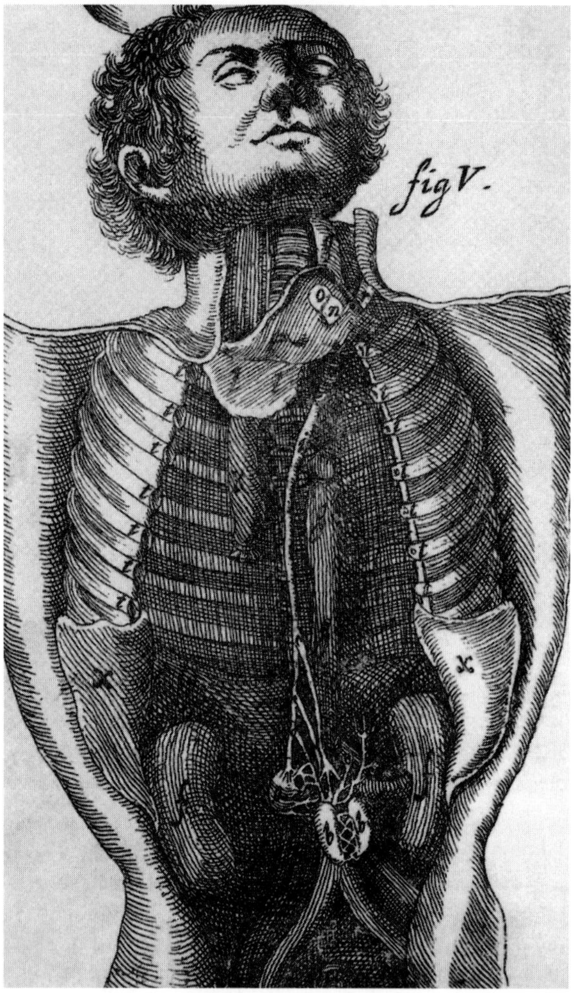

Figure 1.4 *One of Bartholin's illustrations (1653) depicting the cysterna chyli and thoracic duct. (Reproduced with permission from Gloviczki P. Lymphedema: introduction and historical highlights. In Rutherford RB, ed.* Vascular Surgery, *4th edn. Philadelphia: WB Saunders, 1995: 1884)*

patients.[56] Thompson described (in 1962) and later popularized his 'buried dermal flap' procedure, designed to both debulk the limb and provide improved drainage,[57] whilst Sistrunk (1918) described a straight debulking procedure for excision of the involved tissue alone.[58] Homans modified and popularized this procedure in 1936,[59] and it now bears his name and has become the most commonly used debulking operation in this situation.

SUMMARY

Venous (and probably lymphatic) disease certainly deserves a prominent position as one of the earliest known and understood medical conditions. Although names such as Hunter, Virchow, Homans, Linton, Jobst and others are rightly associated with modern knowledge in this field, so too are Hippocrates, Celsus and the anonymous Greeks, Romans and Arabs whose writings have survived to this day. Whilst progress continues, sparked, in part, by the increasing operative options available for both problems, it is impressive to note how well developed knowledge of the pathophysiology and treatment of venous and lymphatic problems was before the scientific age.

REFERENCES

1. Callam MJ, Ruckley CV, Harper DR, Dale JJ. Chronic ulceration of the leg: extent of the problem and provision of care. *Br Med J* 1985; **290**: 1855–6.
2. Bergan JJ. Historical highlights in treating venous insufficiency. In Bergan JJ, Yao JST, eds. *Venous Disorders.* Philadelphia: WB Saunders, 1991: 3–15.
3. Johnson G. Management of venous disorders: introduction and general considerations. In Rutherford RB, ed. *Vascular Surgery*, 4th edn. Philadelphia: WB Saunders, 1995: 1671–3.
4. DeWeese JA. Treatment of venous disease: the innovators. *J Vasc Surg* 1994; **20**(5): 675–83.
5. Bergan JJ, Ballard JL. Historical perspectives. In Gloviczki P, Bergan JJ, eds. *Atlas of Endoscopic Perforator Vein Surgery.* London: Springer-Verlag, 1998: 1–13.
6. Gloviczki P. Lymphedema: introduction and general considerations. In Rutherford RB, ed. *Vascular Surgery*, 4th edn. Philadelphia: WB Saunders, 1995: 1883–8.
7. Adams F. *The Genuine Works of Hippocrates.* Baltimore: Williams & Wilkins, 1939: 333.
8. Dodd H, Cockett FB. *The Pathology and Surgery of the Veins of the Lower Limb.* Edinburgh: E&S Livingstone, 1956: 8.
9. Virchow R. Neuer fall von todlicher Emboli der Lungenarterie. *Arch Pathol Anat* 1856; **10**: 225–8.
10. Homans J. Thrombosis of the deep veins of the lower leg, causing pulmonary embolism. *N Engl J Med* 1934; **211**(22): 993–7.
11. Homans J. Thrombophlebitis of the leg. *N Engl J Med* 1938; **218**(14): 594–9.
12. Homans J. Exploration and division of the femoral and iliac veins in the treatment of thrombophlebitis of the leg. *N Engl J Med* 1941; **224**(5): 179–86.
13. Barner HB, DeWeese JA. An evaluation of the sphygmomanometer pain test in venous thrombosis. *Surgery* 1960; **48**(5): 915–24.
14. Neiman HL. Phlebography in the diagnosis of venous thrombosis. In Bergan JJ, Yao JST, eds. *Venous Problems.* Chicago: Year Book Medical Publishers, 1978: 111–22.
15. Brodie TG, Russell AE. On the determination of the rate of blood flow through an organ. *J Physiol* 1905; **32**: 47P.
16. Eriksson E. Plethysmographic studies of venous diseases of the legs. *Acta Chir Scand Suppl* 1968; **398**: 7–18.

17. Mullick SC, Wheeler HB, Songster GP. Diagnosis of deep venous thrombosis by measurement of electrical impedance. *Am J Surg* 1970; **119**(4): 417–22.
18. Gomez RL, Wheeler HB, Belko JS, Warren R. Observations on the uptake of a radioactive fibrinolytic enzyme by intravascular clots. *Ann Surg* 1963; **158**(5): 905–11.
19. Satomura S. Study of the flow patterns in peripheral arteries by ultrasonics. *J Acoust Soc Jpn* 1959; **15**: 151.
20. Sigel B, Popky GL, Boland JP, Wagner DK, Mapp EM. Diagnosis of venous disease by ultrasonic flow detection. *Surg Forum* 1967; **18**: 185–7.
21. Strandness DE, Sumner DS. Ultrasonic velocity detector in the diagnosis of thrombophlebitis. *Arch Surg* 1972; **104**(2): 180–3.
22. Homans J. Diseases of the veins. *N Engl J Med* 1944; **231**(2): 51–60.
23. DeWeese JA, Jones TI, Lyon J, Dale WA. Evaluation of thrombectomy in the management of iliofemoral venous thrombosis. *Surgery* 1960; **47**(1): 140–59.
24. Johnsson H, Schulman S. Anticoagulation treatment in deep vein thrombosis. In Eklof B, Gjores JE, Thulesius O, Bergqvist D, eds. *Controversies in the Management of Venous Disorders.* London: Butterworth and Co., 1989: 105–14.
25. Illig KA, DeWeese JA. Operative inferior vena caval interruption. In Ernst CB, Stanley JC, eds. *Current Therapy in Vascular Surgery*, 4th edn. St Louis: Mosby, 2001: 892–4.
26. Mobin-Uddin H, McLean R, Bolooki H, Jude JR. Caval interruption for prevention of pulmonary embolism. *Arch Surg* 1969; **99**(6): 711–15.
27. Whitehill TA. Caval interruption methods: comparison of options. *Semin Vasc Surg* 1996; **9**(1): 59–69.
28. Semba CP, Dake MD. Venous thrombolysis. In Ouriel K, ed. *Lower Extremity Vascular Disease.* Philadelphia: WB Saunders, 1995: 321–30.
29. Homans J. The operative treatment of varicose veins and ulcers, based upon a classification of these lesions. *Surg Gynecol Obstet* 1916; **22**: 143–58.
30. Greenfield LJ. Venous and lymphatic disease. In Schwartz SI, Shires GT, Spencer FC, eds. *Principles of Surgery*, 6th edn. New York: McGraw-Hill, 1994: 989–1014.
31. Homans J. The etiology of treatment of varicose ulcer of the leg. *Surg Gynecol Obstet* 1917; **24**: 300–11.
32. Linton RR. The post-thrombotic ulceration of the lower extremity: its etiology and surgical treatment. *Ann Surg* 1953; **138**(3): 415–32.
33. Wittens CHS, Pierik RGJM, van Urk H. The surgical treatment of incompetent perforating veins. *Eur J Vasc Endovasc Surg* 1995; **9**: 19–23.
34. Kitka MJ, Schuler JJ, Meyer JP, *et al.* A prospective, randomized trial of Unna's boots versus hydroactive dressing in the treatment of venous stasis ulcers. *J Vasc Surg* 1988; **7**(3): 478–86.
35. Bergan JJ. Conrad Jobst and the development of pressure gradient therapy for venous disease. In Bergan JJ, Yao JST, eds. *Surgery of the Veins.* Orlando, FL: Grune and Stratton, 1985: 529–40.
36. Linton RR. The communicating veins of the lower leg and the operative technic for their ligation. *Ann Surg* 1938; **107**(4): 582–93.
37. Edwards JM. Shearing operation for incompetent perforating veins. *Br J Surg* 1976; **63**: 885–6.
38. Gloviczki P, Bergan JJ, Rhodes JM, Canton LG, Harmsen S, Ilstrup DM. Mid-term results of endoscopic perforator vein interruption for chronic venous insufficiency: lessons learned from the North American Subfascial Endoscopic Perforator Surgery registry. *J Vasc Surg* 1999; **29**: 489–502.
39. Kistner RL. Surgical repair of the incompetent femoral valve. *Arch Surg* 1975; **110**: 1336–42.
40. Raju S. Valvuloplasty and valve transfer. *Int Angiol* 1985; **4**: 419–24.
41. Warren R, Thayer T. Transplantation of the saphenous vein for postphlebitic stasis. *Surgery* 1954; **35**(6): 867–76.
42. Husni EA. In situ saphenopopliteal bypass graft for incompetence of the femoral and popliteal veins. *Surg Gynecol Obstet* 1970; **130**(2): 279–84.
43. Palma EC, Esperon R. Vein transplants and grafts in surgical treatment of the postphlebitic syndrome. *J Cardiovasc Surg* 1960; **1**: 94–107.
44. Adams JT, DeWeese JA. 'Effort' thrombosis of the axillary and subclavian veins. *J Trauma* 1971; **11**(11): 923–30.
45. Kleinsasser L. 'Effort' thrombosis of axillary and subclavian veins: analysis of 16 personal cases and 56 cases collected from the literature. *Arch Surg* 1949; **59**: 258–74.
46. Adams JT, McEvoy RK, DeWeese JA. Primary deep venous thrombosis of the upper extremity. *Arch Surg* 1965; **91**: 29–42.
47. McLaughlin CW, Popma AM. Intermittent obstruction of the subclavian vein. *JAMA* 1939; **113**: 1960–3.
48. Green RM. Acute axillosubclavian venous thrombosis: twenty years of progress. In Yao JST, Pearce WH, eds. *Progress in Vascular Surgery.* Stamford, CT: Appleton and Lange, 1997: 505–14.
49. Kanter MA. The lymphatic system: an historical perspective. *Plast Reconstr Surg* 1987; **79**: 131.
50. Rooke TW, Gloviczki P. Nonoperative management of chronic lymphedema. In Rutherford RB, ed. *Vascular Surgery*, 4th edn. Philadelphia: WB Saunders, 1995: 1920–7.
51. Taylor GW, Kinmonth JB, Rollinson E. Lymphatic circulation studied with radioactive plasma protein. *Br Med J* 1957; **1**: 133–7.
52. Felty CL, Rooke TW. Modern treatment of lymphedema. In Yao JST, Pearce WH, eds. *Progress in Vascular Surgery.* Stamford, CT: Appleton and Lange, 1997: 535–47.
53. Gloviczki P, Fisher J, Hollier LH, Pairolero DC, Schirger A, Wahner HW. Microsurgical lymphovenous anastomosis for treatment of lymphedema: a critical review. *J Vasc Surg* 1988; **7**: 647–52.
54. Goldsmith HS. Long-term evaluation of omental transposition for chronic lymphedema. *Ann Surg* 1974; **180**(6): 847–9.
55. Hurst PAE, Stuart G, Kinmonth JB, Browse NL. Long term

results of the enteromesenteric bridge operation in the treatment of primary lymphoedema. *Br J Surg* 1985; **72**: 272–4.
56. Abdou MS, Ashby ER, Miller TA. Excisional operations for chronic lymphedema. In Rutherford RB, ed. *Vascular Surgery*, 4th edn. Philadelphia: WB Saunders, 1995: 1928–36.
57. Thompson N. Surgical treatment of chronic lymphedema of the lower limb. With preliminary report of a new operation. *Br Med J* 1962; **2**: 1566–73.
58. Sistrunk WE. Further experiences with the Kondoleon operation for elephantiasis. *JAMA* 1918; **71**: 800–6.
59. Homans J. The treatment of elephantiasis of the legs. *N Engl J Med* 1936; **215**: 1099–104.

2

Development and anatomy of the venous system

GÉZA MÓZES, STEPHEN W CARMICHAEL AND PETER GLOVICZKI

Description of the venous anatomy and embryology is frequently underrepresented in anatomy textbooks. However, surgical practice requires a more sophisticated knowledge of certain veins of the lower limb. This chapter, therefore, includes a detailed description of the lower limb veins, with less emphasis on the veins of the trunk and upper limb. [The current *Terminologia Anatomica*[1] suggests terms that are somewhat different than those used in the surgical practice. In this text we follow the surgical terminology and anatomic terms are listed here in parenthesis: peroneal vein (fibular vein), lesser and greater saphenous veins (small and great saphenous veins), common and superficial femoral vein (femoral vein).] A description of the visceral veins and the veins of the head and neck are beyond the scope of this text.

EMBRYOLOGY AND COMMON DEVELOPMENTAL VARIATIONS

The development of veins is generally preceded by the appearance of complex capillary plexuses, with certain channels being preferred as development progresses, these channels becoming veins.[2] Also, the venous system first appears in the trunk as bilaterally symmetrical vessels, with the left vessels regressing and the right vessels dominating as the superior and inferior vena cavae. These patterns of development lend themselves to differences among individuals. The prevalent patterns of venous development in the trunk and in the limbs are discussed with explanations of how the relatively common variations can occur.

Veins of the trunk

Blood is initially returned to the heart tube via the paired sinus venosus.[2] The portion of the body cranial to the developing heart drains through the *bilateral anterior cardinal veins*, and the caudal portion of the body drains through the *bilateral posterior cardinal veins* (Fig. 2.1). The anterior and posterior cardinal veins flow together as the *common cardinal veins*, with the right and left common cardinal veins draining centrally into the sinus venosus. The common cardinal veins also receive *vitelline* and *umbilical veins*, which initially drain the yolk sac and allantois, but later drain the intestines and the placenta, respectively. The anastomosing vitelline veins become the *hepatic portal system*. The *right umbilical vein* regresses, leaving the *left umbilical vein* (called simply the *umbilical vein*) to carry blood from the placenta.

The anterior cardinal veins form an anastomosis through which blood normally drains from the *left anterior cardinal vein* into the *right anterior cardinal vein*. This left to right channel becomes the *left brachiocephalic vein*. The portion of the left anterior cardinal vein cranial to the anastomosis becomes the *left internal jugular vein*, receiving the *left subclavian vein* from the developing upper limb. The portion of the left anterior cardinal vein caudal to the anastomosis regresses but does not disappear; it remains as the *oblique vein of the left atrium (vein of Marshall)* and the *coronary sinus*. Occasional persistence of the left caudal anterior cardinal vein with small or absent left brachiocephalic vein results in *double superior vena cava* (Fig. 2.2a).[3] In the rare case of the absence of the right proximal superior vena cava, the blood from

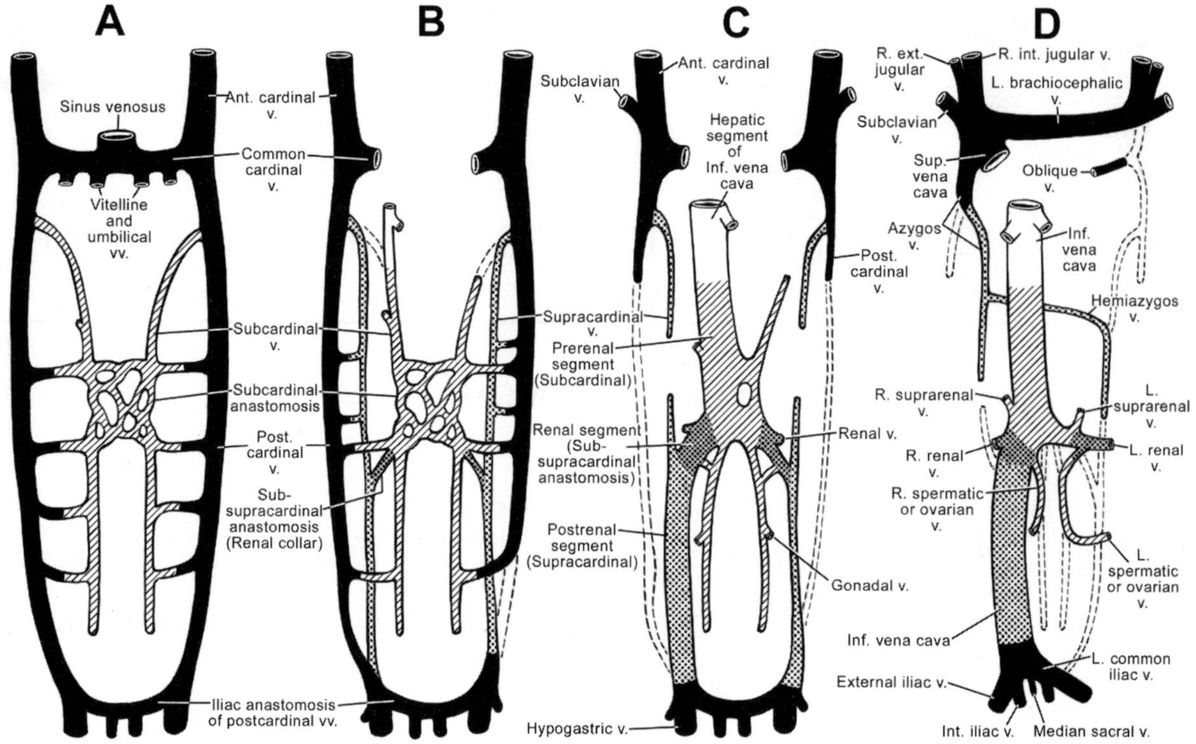

Figure 2.1 *Development of the major veins. (Redrawn from Avery LB.* Developmental Anatomy, *revised 7th edn. Philadelphia: WB Saunders, 1974)*

the right upper body flows via the right brachiocephalic vein into a *left superior vena cava* (Fig. 2.2b).

The developmental pattern of the veins caudal to the heart is more complicated. The paired *posterior cardinal veins* originally extend into the region that will become the pelvis, and are joined together at the *iliac anastomosis* (Fig. 2.1). Most of the posterior cardinal veins disappear, the most cranial portion on the right persists as the *arch of the azygos.* The very caudal portion of the posterior cardinal veins and iliac anastomosis form the *common, external and internal iliac veins*, and the *median sacral vein.* The posterior cardinal veins are mostly replaced by the ventral *subcardinal*, and the dorsal *supracardinal veins.* Drainage of the more cranial region of the abdomen goes mostly into the subcardinal and that of the more caudal portion into the supracardinal veins. Most of the *azygos system* develops from the supracardinal veins. Lastly, veins of the left side regress, resulting in a right-sided *inferior vena cava.*

The sub- and supracardinal veins anastomose on both sides to form the *sub-supracardinal anastomoses.* The anastomosing veins form a venous ring around the aorta; therefore it is also called the *renal collar.* Later, the posterior portion of the renal collar regresses and the anterior portion forms the *left renal vein.*

The complex development of the inferior vena cava can be summarized as follows: the most inferior portion (*postrenal segment*) develops from the right supracardinal vein; therefore it is relatively posterior in position (this is demonstrated by the confluence of the common iliac veins forming behind the common iliac arteries). At the level of the kidneys, the inferior vena cava is formed from the right sub-supracardinal anastomosis (*renal segment*), thereby becoming more anterior in position. Above the kidneys, the inferior vena cava is formed from the right subcardinal *vein (prerenal segment)*, which is still more anterior as is demonstrated by the inferior vena cava diverging anterior to the aorta. The *hepatic segment* of the inferior vena cava is formed directly by hepatic sinusoids.

Since the inferior vena cava develops from bilateral veins, with the right veins usually persisting, variations are to be expected, although they are unusual. If the right subcardinal vein fails to make connection with the liver, *absence of the suprarenal inferior vena cava* results, so that the inferior vena cava drains into the arch of the azygos and the hepatic veins drain independently through the diaphragm to the right atrium.[3] *Double inferior vena cavae* (2–3%) occur usually in the infra-renal portion due to bilateral persistence of the supracardinal veins (Fig. 2.2c). *Left inferior vena cava* (<0.5%) results from caudal regression of the right supracardinal vein with persistence of the left supracardinal vein (Fig. 2.2d). Renal vein anomalies include the *persistent (circumaortic) renal collar* (1–9%) and the *posterior (retroaortic) left renal vein* (1–2%) (Fig. 2.3).

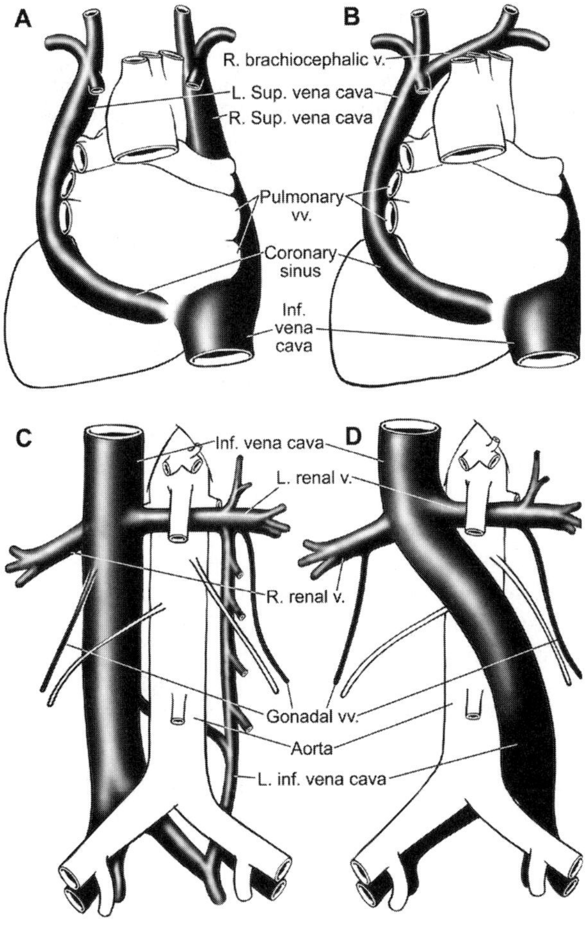

Figure 2.2 *Anomalies of the vena cava. (a) Double superior vena cava. (b) Left superior vena cava. (c) Double inferior vena cava. (d) Left inferior vena cava. (a, b) Posterior view; (c, d) anterior view.*

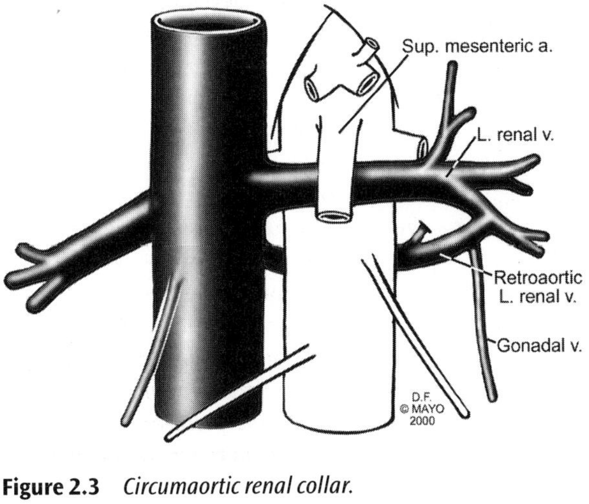

Figure 2.3 *Circumaortic renal collar.*

Veins of the limbs

The general pattern for the development of the vasculature of the limbs begins as a fine capillary network arising from several segmental branches of the aorta. As the limb begins to extend from the body, a channel from within this network predominates as the *axial* or *central artery*. The blood returning to the body from capillary networks is first collected in a *marginal sinus* that extends around the apex of the limb bud, just deep to the apical ectodermal ridge. The capillary networks and the marginal sinus itself send out new vascular sprouts in response to growth of the limbs. Early on, blood drains from the marginal sinuses of the limbs into superficial venous plexuses of the body, but the blood is progressively shunted into deeper channels as development progresses. Valves form in the veins relatively early. It is thought that the definitive number of valves is reached by the sixth month of fetal life.

The role of the vasculature directing the development of the limb is not clear. Some embryologists claim that the vessels play an important role in organizing the muscles, bones and other structures during development, whereas others claim that the vessels develop after the onset of cartilage and muscle differentiation, indicating a secondary role for vessels in directing limb formation.

The original *axial artery of the lower limb* develops into the *internal iliac artery*, the *inferior gluteal artery*, the *artery to the sciatic nerve*, the *popliteal artery* and the *peroneal (fibular) artery*. Later, the *femoral artery* develops from the *external iliac artery* and grows distally to join the popliteal artery. Blood returning to the body is first collected into the marginal sinus, then into superficial plexuses, then into deeper channels that become the *deep veins*. The deep veins form the *femoral vein* and flow into the external iliac vein that developed from the iliac anastomosis of the posterior cardinal veins.

The axial artery of the upper limb forms the *brachial artery* in the arm and the interosseous artery in the forearm, with the *ulnar* and *radial arteries* forming later. As the digits are forming, the apical marginal sinus regresses, but the proximal marginal channels persist as the *cephalic and basilic veins.*

ANATOMY

Veins of the lower extremity

'The (leg) veins may be divided into three sets, the saphenous, the deep and the intercommunicating (veins) ... perforating the intervening aponeurosis ...' stated John Gay (1812–85) first in a Lettsomian Lecture in 1868.[4] Indeed, the venous network of the lower extremity is composed of the superficial veins draining the cutaneous microcirculation, and the deep, axial veins draining muscles and muscular venous sinuses (Fig. 2.4). Perforating veins (in the European literature perforating veins are frequently called 'communicating veins') connect the superficial to the deep veins perforating the deep fascia which separates these two venous systems. Communicating veins connect veins within the same system.[5]

CUTANEOUS MICROCIRCULATION

Cutaneous branches of arteries reach the skin either directly or following the penetration of skeletal muscles.[6] In the skin the arteries form a reticular and a more superficial subpapillary dermal plexus.[7] Capillary loops of the dermal papillae emerge from the latter plexus and drain through venules into the subpapillary venous plexus, which again drained into the deeper reticular venous plexus at the dermal-subcutaneous junction (Fig. 2.4). Vertically oriented, small-valved veins connect the reticular venous plexus to the superficial veins.

SUPERFICIAL VEINS OF THE LEG

Few veins of the human body have more variability in their gross anatomy than the superficial veins of the leg. Superficial veins, the lesser and the greater saphenous veins and their tributaries, course in the subcutaneous fat outside the deep fascia and drain blood from the skin and subcutaneous tissues (Fig. 2.1).

Venous drainage of the foot is somewhat different from that of the calf and the thigh in response to the special requirements of weight bearing. In the foot there are two superficial systems, the *plantar* and the *dorsal venous plexuses*, which anastomose extensively with each other and the intervening *deep plantar venous plexus.* The superficial plantar plexus is particularly rich in communicating branches in the weight-bearing areas (on the heel and over the metatarsophalangeal joints).[8] On the dorsum of the foot small superficial veins are collected into the *dorsal venous arch* at the level of the proximal end of the metatarsals. The medial end of this arch continues in the greater, the lateral end in the lesser saphenous veins (Fig. 2.5).

The *greater saphenous vein* begins just anterior to the medial malleolus, crosses the tibia and ascends medial to the knee (Fig. 2.6). At the knee it courses about 8 cm dorsal to the medial edge of the patella, just behind the medial condyle of the tibia. In the upper calf and in the lower third of the thigh it has a fibrous sheet attached to the outer surface of the deep fascia. The greater saphenous vein is doubled in the calf in 25% and in the thigh in 8%.[9,10] In the calf it usually has two main tributaries: an anterior and a more constant posterior, the *posterior*

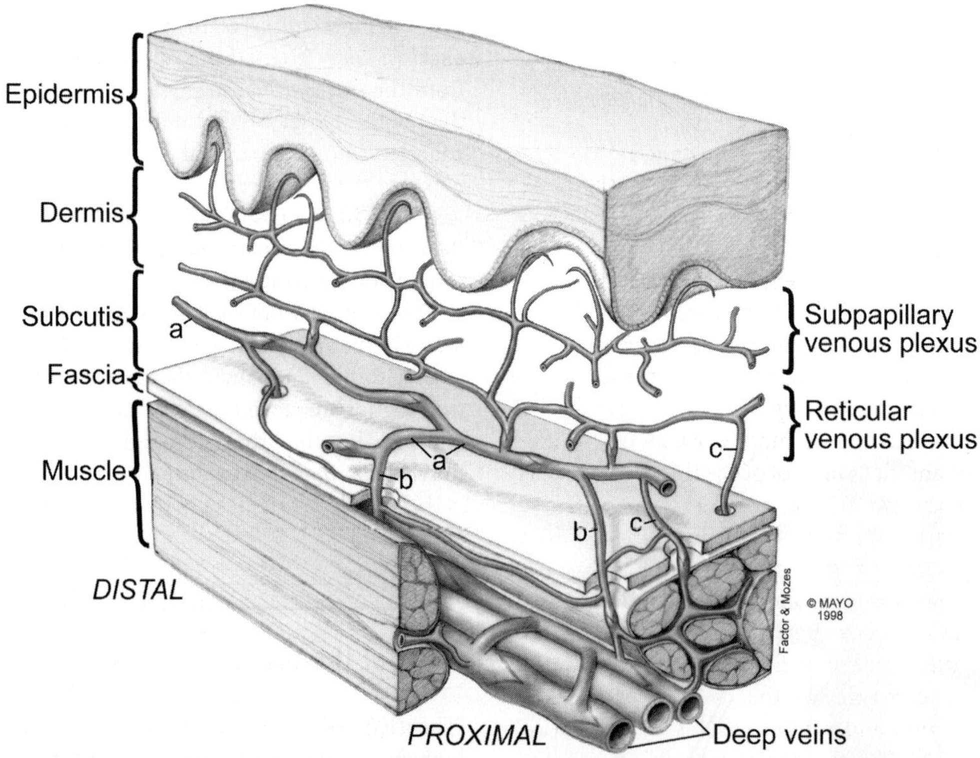

Figure 2.4 *Venous networks in the lower extremity. Capillaries of dermal papillae are drained by the subpapillary venous plexus, which in turn joins to the reticular venous plexus. Superficial veins (a) drain dermal veins and empty into the deep axial veins through direct perforating veins (b). Perforating veins communicate with each other through small branches. Muscular venous sinuses fill from the superficial veins or from the reticular venous plexus through indirect perforating veins (c) and they are drained into the deep axial veins.*

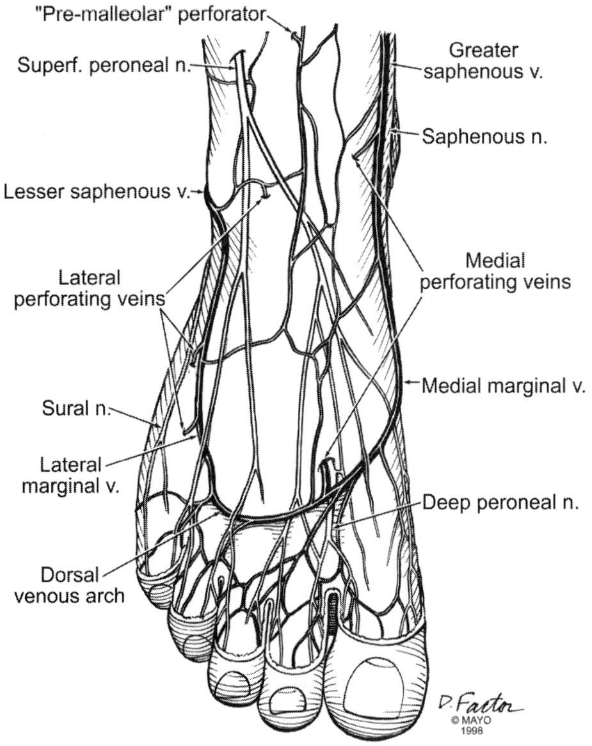

Figure 2.5 *Superficial and perforating veins of the foot.*

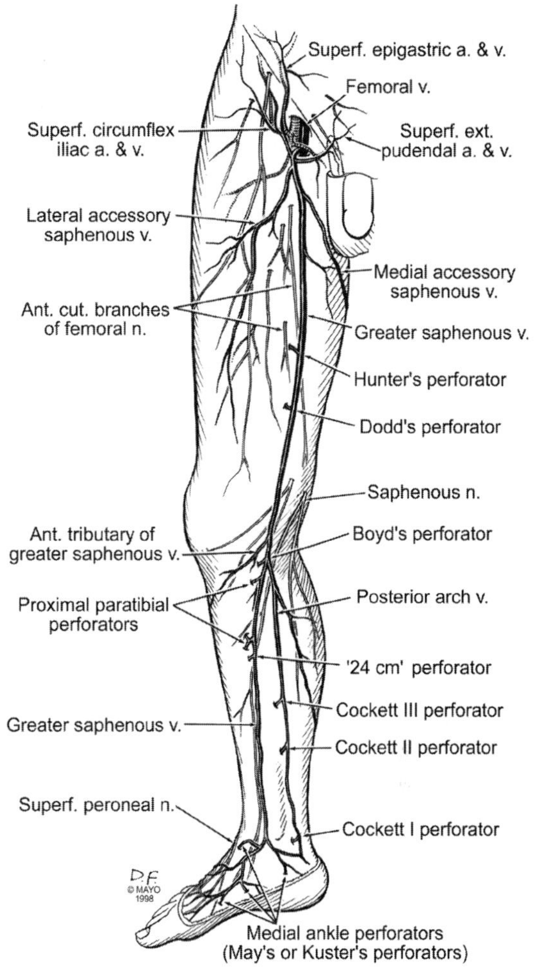

Figure 2.6 *Medial superficial and perforating veins of the leg.*

arch vein or Leonardo's vein (presumably first depicted on Leonardo da Vinci's drawings).[11] The posterior arch vein begins posterior to the medial ankle, ascends on the posteromedial aspect of the calf and joins the greater saphenous vein distal to the knee (Fig. 2.6). Major medial perforating veins (Cockett perforators) connect the posterior arch vein with the posterior tibial veins. Proximal to the knee the greater saphenous vein ascends anteriorly, enters the fossa ovalis below the inguinal ligament and empties into the femoral vein at two fingerbreadths (3–4 cm) inferior and lateral to the pubic tubercle.[12] Just before the greater saphenous vein ends, it receives one or two large tributaries from the thigh, the *lateral* and *medial accessory saphenous veins.* The lateral accessory saphenous vein is more constant and drains the lateral and anterior surfaces of the thigh. The medial accessory saphenous vein is present in 8–20% and receives tributaries from the posterior surface.[8] Both accessory saphenous veins may be large enough to be mistaken for the greater saphenous vein during surgical dissection. The *superficial circumflex iliac* and *superficial (inferior) epigastric veins* as well as the *superficial external pudendal vein* converge to the area of the saphenofemoral junction and confluence in several different ways (Fig. 2.7).[8,13] The superficial circumflex iliac and superficial (inferior) epigastric veins drain the lower lateral abdominal wall and through the thoracoepigastric vein they communicate with the lateral thoracic and axillary veins. Rarely, the greater saphenous vein joins the femoral vein low and some of the aforementioned tributaries empty individually into the femoral vein or the greater saphenous vein terminates high in one of the veins of the lower abdomen.[14]

The *lesser saphenous vein* begins on the lateral side of the foot and ascends lateral to the Achilles tendon in the calf.[15] It runs in the subcutaneous fat until the upper third of the calf, where it usually pierces the deep fascia and courses between the two heads of the gastrocnemius. Duplication of the lesser saphenous vein is very rare (<1%). The lesser saphenous vein joins the popliteal vein in the proximal popliteal fossa in 57% (Fig. 2.8). In 33% it ends high and empties into the femoral vein or it courses superficially on the posteromedial aspect of the thigh to join the greater saphenous vein.[8] Uncommonly, the lesser saphenous vein ends below the knee and empties into the posterior tibial veins. In about 15% of legs a vein in the posterior thigh, named after Giacomini, connects the most proximal part of the lesser saphenous to the greater saphenous vein.[16] There are several other, smaller connections between the two saphenous veins which are usually located around the knee.

In the superficial veins bicuspid valves secure unidirectional venous blood flow towards the heart. There are

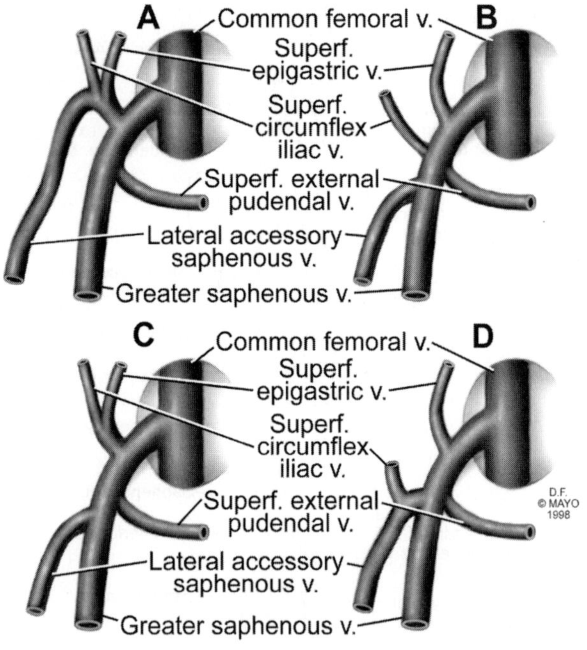

Figure 2.7 *Most common anatomic variations (a, 33%; b, 15%; c, 15%; d, 13%) of the venous tributaries at the saphenofemoral junction based on Daseler's observations.*

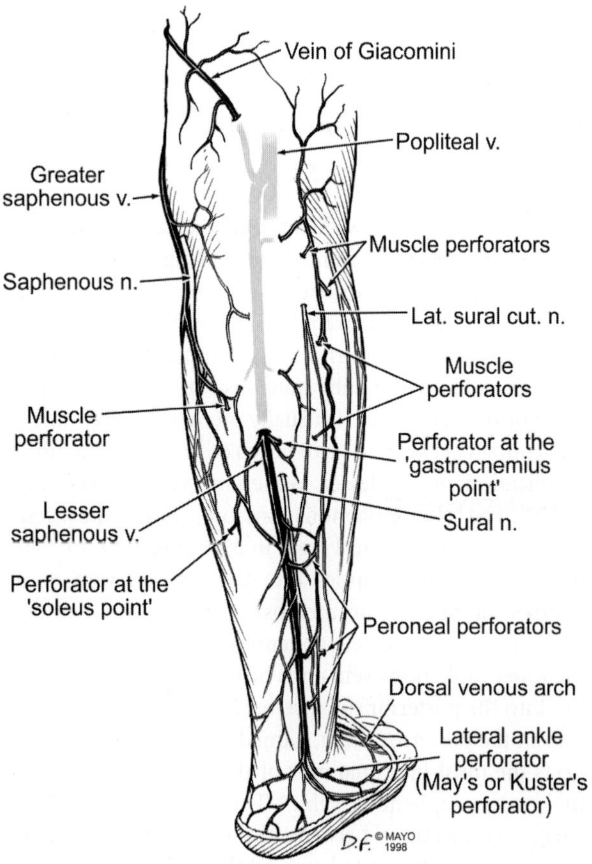

Figure 2.8 *Posterior superficial and perforating veins of the leg.*

more constant valves, which are usually placed at the termination of the major venous trunks. These valves have strong, white cusps and marked sinusoid dilatation of the venous wall at the origin of the valves. Other valves are delicate, almost transparent structures.[17] In the greater saphenous vein there are usually at least six valves (maximum 14–25).[8] In about 85% of veins a constant valve is present in the greater saphenous vein within 2–3 cm to the saphenofemoral junction.[18] The frequency of valves is greater below than above the knee. In the lesser saphenous vein valves are numerous (median 7–10; range 4–13) and more closely spaced.[15] The highest valve is usually situated close to the termination of the lesser saphenous vein. Valves in communicating tributaries between the two saphenous veins are always oriented to direct blood from the lesser to the greater saphenous vein.

Superficial veins are accompanied by major cutaneous nerves which accidentally avulsed may result in significant postoperative morbidity. The *saphenous nerve*, a cutaneous branch of the femoral nerve, emerges from the deep through the hiatus in the tendon of the adductor magnus muscle and approaches the greater saphenous vein at the knee.[19] In the middle and lower third of the calf the anatomic relation between the vein and the nerve is very intimate and frequently the perineum and the adventitia are histologically indistinguishable (Fig. 2.6).[20] The *sural nerve* courses close to the lesser saphenous vein in the foot and the lower calf (Fig. 2.8). The most intimate relation occurs in the lateral retromalleolar space, although these structures are rarely attached so tightly as the greater saphenous vein and saphenous nerve.

PERFORATING VEINS OF THE LEG

Perforating veins origin from the superficial veins, perforate the deep fascia underlying the subcutaneous fat and join either deep veins (*direct perforators*) or venous sinuses of the calf muscles (*indirect perforators*).[21] Direct perforating veins show a relatively constant anatomic distribution, while the more frequent indirect ones are irregularly distributed. Small communicating branches on both sides of the fascia connect the perforating veins to each other, and direct perforating veins often have small side branches communicating with muscle veins as well; therefore distinction between direct and indirect perforators may seem somewhat arbitrary (Fig. 2.4). In the thigh and the calf, cutaneous arteries and occasionally small subcutaneous nerves accompany some of the perforating veins. In the foot, perforators pierce the fascia always alone.[22] In the thigh and the calf, major perforators usually have one to three bicuspid valves, all of which are subfascially located and oriented to direct flow from the superficial to the deep veins.[23] Perforating veins smaller than 1 mm are valveless. In the foot, perforating veins are either valveless or valves are oriented to allow an outward flow into the superficial veins, which refers to a normally bidirectional flow.[24] Besides valves the oblique run-off of the perforators between the deep fascia and the muscles and their location often in dense intermuscular septa can all contribute to maintain perforator sufficiency. The number of perforating veins in the leg varies considerably in different studies. Sophisticated anatomic dissection may demonstrate as much as 150 perforating veins in the lower extremity; however, most of these are very small without any clinical significance. Gross dissection or radiological imaging discloses four groups of clinically significant perforators: those of the foot, the medial and lateral calf, and the thigh.

In the foot there is an average of nine direct perforator veins.[25] A constant, large perforator in the first metatarsal interosseous space connects the superficial dorsal venous arch to the deep dorsalis pedis veins (Fig. 2.5).[26] On the medial aspect of the foot, perforating veins emerge from the greater saphenous vein and end in the dorsalis pedis and medial plantar deep veins (Fig. 2.6). On the lateral aspect, the lesser saphenous vein usually has one proximal connection to the dorsalis pedis veins and several others to the lateral plantar deep vein (Fig. 2.8). The medial and lateral ankle perforators sometimes are named after Kuster or May.[5]

The medial calf perforators are clinically the most significant. In our anatomic study on cadaver legs, an average of seven to eight direct and five to six indirect perforators were found in this region.[27] Indirect muscle perforators are randomly distributed, mostly located in the proximal half of the calf. Direct perforating veins clustered in four groups (Table 2.1). The lowest, the retromalleolar *Cockett I* is situated just behind the medial ankle (Fig. 2.6).[28–31] *Cockett II and III perforators* are usually at 7–9 and 10–12 cm proximal from the tip of the medial malleolus, in a distance within 2–4 cm from the medial edge of the tibia. These perforating veins connect the posterior arch vein or other tributaries of the greater saphenous vein with the deep posterior tibial veins. In the proximal half of the medial calf, direct perforating veins are more closely (<1 cm) located to the tibia (paratibial). *Paratibial direct perforators* at 18–22 cm from the medial malleolus were earlier described as *24 cm perforators* because of their usual distance from the sole.[5] Two other groups of paratibial perforators are located at 23–27 and 28–32 cm from the medial malleolus (Fig. 2.6). Less than half of these perforators make immediate connections between the greater saphenous and the posterior tibial deep veins; the majority drain the tributaries of the greater saphenous vein (Fig. 2.9). Perforators located just distal to the knee at about 1–2 cm medial to the tibia are called *Boyd's perforators.*[32] Boyd's perforators connect the main trunk or tributaries of the greater saphenous vein to either the posterior tibial or the tibioperonal or the popliteal deep veins (Figs 2.6 and 2.9). The exact anatomic relation of the medial calf perforators to the fascial compartments gained attention with the advent of subfascial endoscopic perforator surgery. Most of the medial calf perforators cross the superficial posterior compartment because they join the deep veins in the deep posterior compartment (Table 2.2) (Fig. 2.10).[33,34] However, some of the more distal perforators enter the deep posterior compartment without crossing the superficial one. The primary working space for the endoscopic perforator surgery is the superficial posterior compartment; therefore an additional incision on the fascia between the two posterior compartments is needed to access some of the important distal perforators.[35]

On the distal part of the posterolateral side of the calf, the *peroneal perforators* directly connect tributaries of the lesser saphenous to the peroneal veins (*Bassi's perforator* at 5–7 cm and *12 cm perforator* at 12–14 cm from the lateral ankle) (Fig. 2.5).[5] More proximal on the posterolateral region, numerous indirect perforating veins connect the tributaries of the lesser saphenous vein to either muscular venous sinuses or to veins draining the

Table 2.1 *Studies on the location of direct medial perforating veins in the leg*

First author (year)	Number of legs		Location of medial perforating veins*		
	Anatomic dissections	Surgical findings	Cockett II	Cockett III	Proximal paratibial PVs
Linton (1938)	10	50	Distal third of the leg	Middle third of the leg	Proximal third of the leg
Sherman (1948)	92	901	13.5 cm	18.5 cm	24 cm, 30 cm, 35 cm, 40 cm
Cockett (1953)	21	201	13–14 cm	16–17 cm	At the knee
O'Donnell (1977)	–	39	Half of the incompetent PVs is between 10 and 15 cm† (15–20 cm*)		Few incompetent PVs
Fischer (1992)	–	194	Random distribution of incompetent PVs		
Mózes (1996)	40	–	7–9 cm† (12–14 cm*)	10–12 cm† (15–17 cm*)	18–22 cm†, 23–27 cm†, 28–32 cm† (23–27 cm*), (28–32 cm*), (33–37 cm*)

* Distances measured from the sole.
† Distances measured from the lower tip of the medial malleolus.

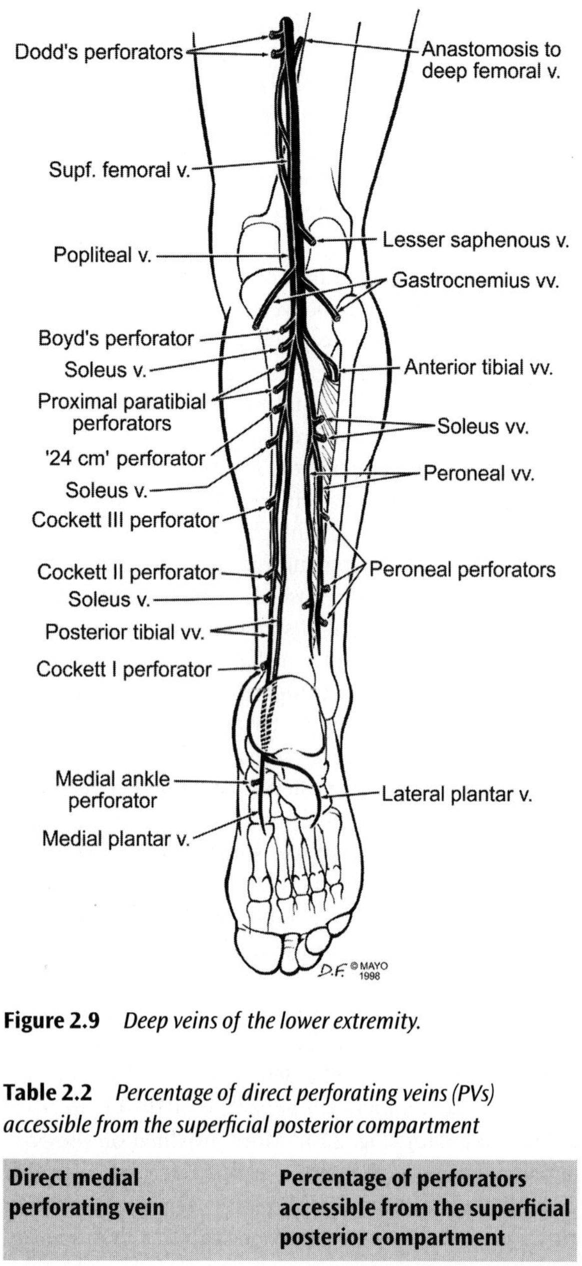

Figure 2.9 *Deep veins of the lower extremity.*

Table 2.2 *Percentage of direct perforating veins (PVs) accessible from the superficial posterior compartment*

Direct medial perforating vein	Percentage of perforators accessible from the superficial posterior compartment
Cockett I	c. 0
Cockett II	32
Cockett III	84
Proximal paratibial PVs including '24 cm' PV	25

gastrocnemius and soleal muscles into the deep veins.[36,37] The locations of the greatest muscle perforators in this area are referred as the *gastrocnemius and soleus points* (Fig. 2.8).[5]

On the anterior side of the calf, direct perforators connect the anterior tributary of the greater saphenous vein to the deep anterior tibial veins. Anterior perforators are irregularly distributed in a line 2–5 cm lateral from the crest of the tibia.[38,39] The *pre-malleolar* and the *mid-crural* are the relatively constant perforating veins in this area (Fig. 2.5).

In the thigh, direct perforating veins are less numerous, but clinically they can be equally important (Figs 2.6 and 2.9). Two major groups at the medial aspect of the thigh are the *Dodd's perforators* and the *Hunterian perforators*, connecting directly the greater saphenous vein with the proximal popliteal or distal superficial femoral vein.[5,36] Unnamed perforators connect the lateral and medial accessory saphenous veins or the vein of Giacomini to the profunda femoris (deep femoral) vein. There are several indirect perforators in the thigh connecting tributaries of the saphenous system to the muscular veins.

DEEP VEINS OF THE LEG

In the foot, similarly to the rest of the lower extremity, deep veins accompany the corresponding arteries. On the sole the richly anastomosing *deep plantar venous arch* collects blood from the toes and the metatarsum. The deep plantar venous arch continues into the *medial* and *lateral plantar veins*, which become the posterior tibial veins behind the medial ankle (Fig. 2.9).[40] On the dorsum of the foot, the major deep veins, the *dorsalis pedis veins*, continue into the anterior tibial veins.

In the calf, the deep veins run in richly anastomosing pairs. The *posterior tibial veins* run between the edges of the flexor digitorum longus and tibialis posterior muscles, under the fascia of the deep posterior compartment (Fig. 2.10). They drain the muscles of the deep and superficial posterior compartments and they are connected to the greater saphenous and posterior arch veins by perforators (Fig. 2.9). The posterior tibial veins pierce the soleus muscle close to its bony adherence and continue into the popliteal vein. The *anterior tibial veins* ascend in the anterior compartment. They drain the muscles of this compartment and receive perforators from the anterior calf. Distally there is a constant connection between the anterior tibial and the peroneal veins.[39] The *peroneal veins* originate in the distal third of the calf and ascend deep to the flexor hallucis longus muscle. They receive the peroneal perforators and several large veins from the soleus muscle. The anterior tibial and peroneal veins form the short tibioperoneal trunk which joins the posterior tibial veins to form the *popliteal vein.*

The popliteal and femoral veins are usually duplicated in segments of various length and form a plexus around the corresponding arteries similarly to the deep veins of the calf (Fig. 2.9).[17] In the popliteal fossa, the popliteal vein is deep to the artery; however, as the vein ascends, it crosses the artery from medial to lateral in a superficial position. The gastrocnemius and the lesser saphenous veins are the main tributaries of the popliteal vein. In the adductor canal the popliteal vein becomes the *(superficial) femoral vein* and runs initially lateral and then medial to the femoral artery. (It is important to remember, that the segment of the femoral vein between the

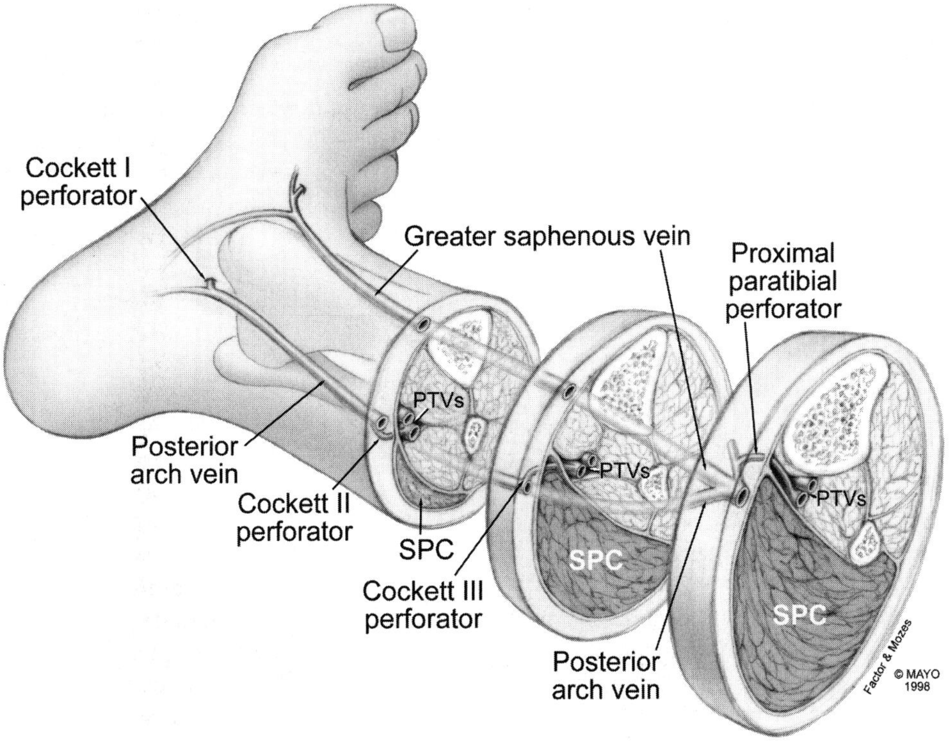

Figure 2.10 *Relation of the medial direct perforating veins to the deep and superficial posterior fascial compartments (SPC). PTVs, posterior tibial veins.*

adductor canal and the profunda femoris vein is frequently called superficial femoral vein, although this segment is part of the deep venous system.) It drains the muscles of the medial side of the thigh and it is connected to the greater saphenous vein through the Dodd's and Hunterian perforators. The (superficial) femoral vein unites with the *profunda femoris (deep femoral) vein* at about 9 cm below the inguinal ligament.[17] The profunda femoris vein drains muscles of the lateral aspect of the thigh and receives perforators from the lateral accessory saphenous vein. In the adductor canal or more distal from it there is a constant (c. 84%) anastomosis between the profunda femoris and the superficial femoral or popliteal veins which provides an important collateral avenue in case of deep venous thrombosis. The *common femoral vein* is the continuation of the superficial femoral vein after joining by the deep femoral vein. The greater saphenous vein empties into the common femoral vein at the saphenofemoral junction. Further tributaries of the common femoral vein are the *lateral and medial circumflex femoral veins*, which can anastomose with the internal iliac vein. The common femoral vein is medial to the corresponding artery and ends at the inguinal ligament as it continues in the external iliac vein.

The frequency of *valves* in deep veins increases from proximal to distal. Deep veins of the foot, the posterior and anterior tibial and the peroneal veins are profusely valved containing valves at about 2 cm intervals. The popliteal vein and the most distal part of the (superficial) femoral vein have usually one or two valves.[17] There are an additional three or more valves in the (superficial) femoral vein up to the junction with the profunda femoris vein. One of these valves is constantly (c. 90%) found just distal to this junction.[41] In the common femoral vein usually there is only one valve. It is important to emphasize that in the external iliac and common femoral veins proximal to the saphenofemoral junction there is only one or in 37% of cases there is no valve at all. The common iliac and cava veins are completely valveless.[17]

VENOUS SINUSES OF CALF MUSCLES

Venous sinuses are thin-walled, large veins in the calf muscles, which have a capacity to hold great volumes of venous blood. They are embedded in skeletal muscles which contract rhythmically during ambulation; therefore, they serve as 'chambers' of the 'peripheral heart', the calf muscle pump.[17] The soleus muscle is particularly rich in venous sinuses, it may contain 1–18 of them.[42] They are less developed in the gastrocnemius muscle. Venus sinuses are filled from the superficial veins and from the reticular venous plexus through indirect, muscular perforators and from the muscles through postcapillary venules and small muscular veins (Fig. 2.4). Venous sinuses of the soleus muscle are drained into the posterior tibial and peroneal veins by the soleus veins (Fig.

2.6). Soleus veins are large, short and tortuous to accommodate the considerable range of muscular movements.[17] In the lower third of the leg, soleus veins frequently join direct perforating veins before entering the deep veins. Bilateral *gastrocnemius veins* draining the two heads of the gastrocnemius muscle usually empty into the popliteal vein, distal to the confluence of the lesser saphenous vein with the popliteal trunk (Fig. 2.6). The venous sinuses themselves are valveless; however, the small intramuscular veins linking them and the muscular veins draining venous sinuses into the deep veins contain numerous valves.[17,42] Indirect perforating veins feeding venous sinuses are also valved. Sufficiency of these valves plays a critical role in the efficient work of the calf muscle pump.

Veins of the abdomen and pelvis

The *external iliac vein* begins at the inguinal ligament, courses along the pelvic brim and ends anterior to the sacroiliac joint by joining the internal iliac to form the common iliac vein.[43] Its tributaries are the *(deep) inferior epigastric*, the *deep circumflex iliac* and the *pubic veins*, which freely anastomose with the corresponding superficial veins and with the obturator vein. The *internal iliac vein* is a short trunk, formed by the union of its extra- and intrapelvic tributaries. The extrapelvic tributaries are the gluteal (superior and inferior), the internal pudendal and the obturator veins. The *gluteal veins* anastomose with the medial circumflex femoral vein and receive numerous perforating veins from the corresponding superficial veins (Fig. 2.11). Intrapelvic tributaries of the internal iliac vein, such as the *lateral sacral* and several visceral (middle rectal, vesical, uterine and vaginal) veins, drain the *presacral venous plexus* and the pelvic *visceral plexuses* (rectal, vesical, prostatic, uterine and vaginal).[17] These plexuses and the additional *superficial (pudendal)* plexus provide free communication for venous flow between the two sides of the pelvis.[44]

The *common iliac veins* begin at the sacroiliac joints and confluence at the right side of the fifth lumbar vertebra to form the inferior vena cava. The only tributary of the right common iliac vein is the right ascending lumbar vein, whereas the left drains the *median sacral vein* too.[14] The *ascending lumbar vein* runs vertically along the column, collects blood from lumbar veins and proximally anastomoses with the azygos system.

The *inferior vena cava* ascends on the right side of the vertebral column and terminates in the right atrium very shortly after passing through the diaphragm (Fig. 2.11). Its tributaries are the lumbar veins, the right gonadal vein, the renal veins, the right suprarenal, the right inferior phrenic and the hepatic veins. The left gonadal and suprarenal veins join the left renal vein and the left inferior phrenic opens into the left suprarenal vein. In case of inferior vena cava obstruction, the anastomoses between

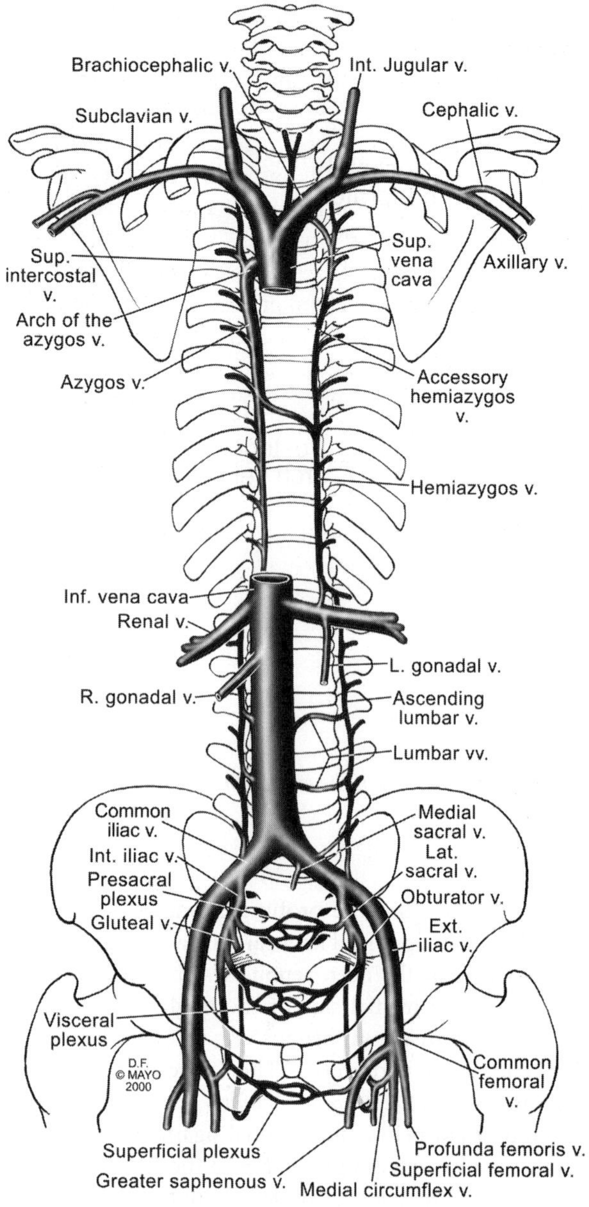

Figure 2.11 *Major veins of the pelvis, abdomen and thorax.*

the veins of the chest and abdominal wall (thoracoepigastric, internal thoracic and epigastric veins), the lumbar–azygos connections and the vertebral plexuses can provide important collateral avenues.[43]

Veins of the upper extremity and the thorax

UPPER EXTREMITY VEINS

Venous return from the arm is mostly maintained by the work of the heart.[14] Valves do not play an important role in the venous circulation. Deep veins of the arm are paired and follow their corresponding arteries.

Perforators between the deep and superficial veins are less numerous in the arm than in the leg.

Superficial veins of the upper limb are the cephalic and basilic veins and their tributaries (Fig. 2.12).[43] The *dorsal venous plexus* of the hand continues into the cephalic vein on the radial and into the basilic on the ulnar side. The *cephalic vein* begins at the 'anatomical snuff box', courses over the distal radius to the ventral aspect of the forearm, ascends on the lateral side of the arm and in the deltopectoral groove. It enters the infraclavicular fossa, pierces the clavipectoral fascia and empties into the axillary vein. The *basilic vein* ascends on the ulnar side of the forearm, perforates the deep fascia about midway in the arm and, after receiving the deep brachial vein, it continues in the axillary vein. The *median cubital vein* connects the cephalic and basilic veins in front of the elbow. Variations are common, including the presence of additional major venous trunks, such as the *accessory cephalic* or *antebrachial veins.*

The *axillary vein* begins at the lower border of the teres major, which corresponds with the lateral border of the scapula on anteroposterior chest roentgenogram. At the outer border of the first rib it becomes the *subclavian*, which ends at the medial border of the scalenus anterior muscle where it joins the *internal jugular vein* to form the brachiocephalic vein. The *brachiocephalic (innominate) vein* begins behind the sternoclavicular joint. The left brachiocephalic vein descends obliquely to join the right one. Constant tributaries of the brachiocephalic vein are the *vertebral, internal thoracic* and *inferior thyroid veins.* The *superior intercostal vein* drains the upper intercostal veins and opens into the brachiocephalic vein on the left, whereas on the opposite side it joins the azygos vein.

The *superior vena cava* is formed behind the first right costal cartilage by the union of the brachiocephalic veins. It descends right to the ascending aorta and opens into the right atrium at the level of the third right costal cartilage. Halfway along its length, before it enters the pericardium, it receives the azygos vein from behind.[45]

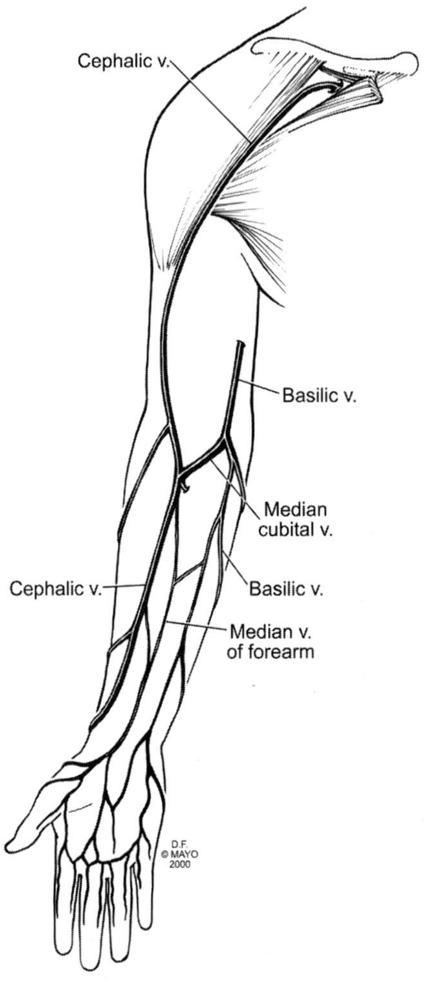

Figure 2.12 *Superficial veins of the upper extremity.*

AZYGOS VEINS

The origin of the azygos vein is not constant. It may arise from the back of the inferior vena cava at the level of the renal veins or it may be the continuation of the right ascending lumbar vein (Fig. 2.11).[43] The azygos vein ascends on the right until the fourth thoracic vertebra, then passes anteriorly to join the superior vena cava. Major tributaries of the azygos vein are the right superior intercostal, the hemiazygos and the accessory hemiazygos veins. The *hemiazygos vein* courses on the left side of the vertebral column; its origin is similar to that of the azygos vein. At the level of the eighth thoracic vertebra, it crosses the column and joins the azygos vein. Often the left renal vein communicates with the hemiazygos vein. The *accessory hemiazygos vein* descends left to the vertebral column, parallel with the azygos vein. Proximally it anastomoses with the left brachiocephalic vein; it ends distally when it joins to the azygos or the hemiazygos veins at the level of the seventh thoracic vertebra. The azygos veins drain the intercostal veins on both sides, they receive several visceral tributaries and freely anastomose with the vertebral venous plexuses. The azygos veins and their tributaries provide important collateral circulation in superior or inferior vena cava obstruction.

HISTOLOGY

The venous wall is three layered: intima, media and adventitia.[46,47] The *intima* uniformly consists of a single layer of endothelial cells resting on scant connective tissue. The *internal elastic lamina*, a layer of thick elastic fibers at the base of the intima, is frequently incomplete in medium sized veins and absent in the smaller ones. Venous valves are bicuspid infoldings of the intima covered by endothelium on both sides with an intervening connective tissue skeleton (Figs 2.13, 2.14). At the origin

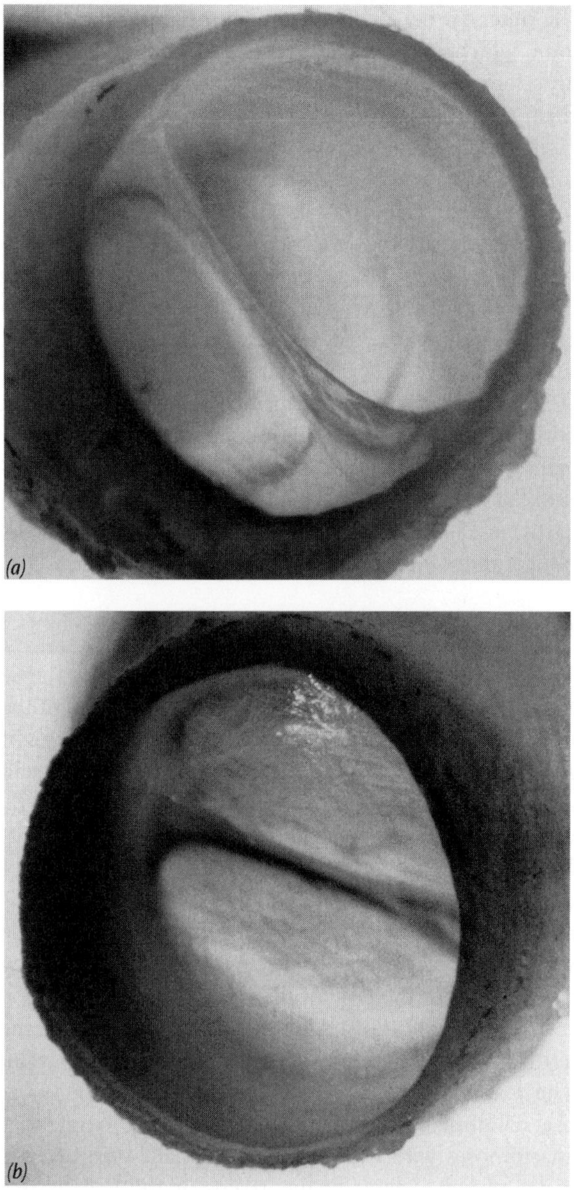

Figure 2.13 *Proximal (a) and distal (b) aspect of a venous valve (stereo microscopy, magnification × 11.2).*

of valves, veins may be focally distended, forming small sinusoid dilation, probably in response to the hemodynamic consequences of focally reversed flow.

The *media* is composed of layers of smooth muscle cells and connective tissue. The relative thickness of media, as well as the proportion of the two major components, smooth muscle and collagen, varies considerably with different size and function. Major superficial veins, such as the greater and lesser saphenous, have thick, muscular media providing ability to contract and a resistance to varicosity. Tributaries of the saphenous veins have thinner media and they can become varicose more easily. Media of the deep veins of the calf contain as much smooth muscle as do saphenous veins; however, their collagen content is more abundant, resulting in a

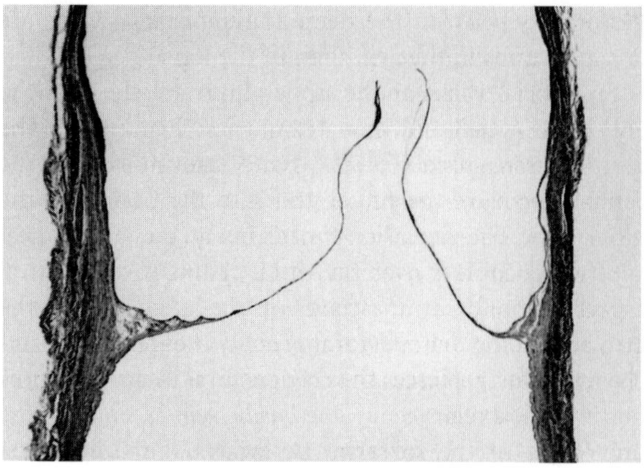

Figure 2.14 *Histology of a venous valve (orcein, magnification × 1.25).*

more rigid wall. Larger deep veins (femoral, iliac, axillary, subclavian, innominate) contain less and less smooth muscle cell; the almost complete lack of these cells in the media of the caval veins is remarkable.[14]

The *adventitia* is poorly demarcated and contains loose connective tissue with lymphatics, vessels (vasa vasorum) and adrenergic nerve fibers. The greater saphenous vein is ensheathed in further layers of fibrous tissue associated with the deep fascia, which makes this vein even more resistant to varicosity.[48]

REFERENCES

1. *Terminologia Anatomica.* International Anatomical Terminology, Federative Committee on Anatomical Terminology. Stuttgart, New York: Thieme, 1998.
2. Carlson BM. The development of the circulatory system. In Carlson BE, ed. *Patten's Foundations of Embryology*, 5th edn. New York: McGraw-Hill, 1988: 586–627.
3. Nicholson CP, Gloviczki P. Embryology and development of the vascular system. In White RA, Hollier LH, eds. *Vascular Surgery. Basic Science and Clinical Correlations.* Philadelphia: JB Lippincott, 1994: 3–20.
4. Gay J. *On Varicose Disease of the Lower Extremities.* London: John Churchill and Sons, 1868.
5. May R. Nomenclature of the surgically most important connecting veins. In May R, Partsch H, Staubesand J, eds. *Perforating Veins.* Baltimore: Urban & Schwarzenberg, 1981: 13–18.
6. Zbrodowski A, Gumener R, Gajisin S, Montandon D, Bednarkiewicz M. Blood supply of subcutaneous tissue in the leg and its clinical application. *Clin Anat* 1995; **8**: 202–7.
7. Braverman IM. The cutaneous microcirculation: ultrastructure and microanatomical organization. *Microcirculation* 1997; **4**: 329–40.

8. Hollinshead WH. The back and limbs. In Hollinshead WH, ed. *Anatomy for Surgeons*. New York: Harper & Row, 1969: 617–31, 754–8, 803–7.
9. Kaiser A, Duff C, Scherrer C, Enzler M, Hauser M, Brunner U. Proximo-distal course of the diameter of the greater saphenous vein and the distribution of the number of side branched as an inherent difficulty in infra-inguinal arterial in-situ bypass. [In German] *Helv Chir Acta* 1993; **59**: 893–6.
10. Thomson H. The surgical anatomy of the superficial and perforating veins of the lower limb. *Ann R Coll Surg Engl* 1979; **61**: 198–205.
11. Negus D. The blood vessels of lower limb: applied anatomy. In Negus D, ed. *Leg Ulcers: a Practical Approach to Management*, 2nd edn. London: Butterworth-Heinemann, 1995: 14–29.
12. Gardner E, Gray DJ, O'Rahilly R, eds. Vessels and lymphatic drainage of the lower limb. In *Anatomy, a Regional Study of Human Structure*, 5th edn. Philadelphia: WB Saunders, 1986: 190–6.
13. Daseler EH, Anson BJ, Reimann AF, Beaton LE. The saphenous venous tributaries and related structures in relation to the technique of high ligation: based chiefly upon a study of 550 anatomical dissection. *Surg Gynecol Obstet* 1946; **82**: 53–63.
14. Browse NL, Burnand KG, Irvine AT, Wilson NM, eds. Embryology and radiographic anatomy. In *Diseases of the Veins*, 2nd edn. London: Arnold, 1999: 23–48.
15. Kosinski C. Observations on the superficial venous system of the lower extremity. *J Anat* 1926; **60**: 131–42.
16. Bergan JJ. Surgical management of primary and recurrent varicose veins. In Gloviczki P, Yao JST, eds. *Handbook of Venous Disorders. Guidelines of the American Venous Forum*. London: Chapman & Hall Medical, 1996: 394–415.
17. Dodd H, Cockett FB. Surgical anatomy of the veins of the lower limb. In Dodd H, Cockett FB, eds. *The Pathology and Surgery of the Veins of the Lower Limb*. London: E&S Livingstone, 1956: 28–64.
18. Pang AS. Location of valves and competence of the great saphenous vein above the knee. *Ann Acad Med Singapore* 1991; **20**: 248–50.
19. Garnjobst W. Injuries to the saphenous nerve following operation for varicose veins. *Surg Gynecol Obstet* 1964; **119**: 359–61.
20. Murakami G, Negishi N, Tanaka K, Hoshi H, Sezai Y. Anatomical relationship between saphenous vein and cutaneous nerves. *Okajimas Folia Anat Jpn* 1994; **71**: 21–33.
21. Le Dentu A. *Anatomic research and physiologic considerations of the venous circulation of the foot and leg*. [In French] Thèse Agrégat, Paris, 1867.
22. Schäfer K. The course, structure and passage through the fascia of the perforating veins. In May R, Partsch H, Staubesand J, eds. *Perforating Veins*. Baltimore: Urban & Schwarzenberg, 1981: 37–45.
23. Pirner F. On the valves of the perforating veins. In May R, Partsch H, Staubesand J, eds. *Perforating Veins*. Baltimore: Urban & Schwarzenberg, 1981: 46–8.
24. Tibbs DJ. The role of the perforator. In: Tibbs DJ, ed. *Varicose Veins and Related Disorders*. Oxford: Butterworth-Heinemann, 1992: 204–32.
25. Kuster G, Lofgren EP, Hollinshead WH. Anatomy of the veins of the foot. *Surg Gynecol Obstet* 1968; **127**: 817–23.
26. Stolic E. Terminology, division and systematic anatomy of the communicating veins of the lower limb. In May R, Partsch H, Staubesand J, eds. *Perforating Veins*. Baltimore: Urban & Schwarzenberg, 1981: 19–34.
27. Mozes G, Gloviczki P, Menawat SS, Fisher DR, Carmichael SW, Kadar A. Surgical anatomy for endoscopic subfascial division of perforating veins. *J Vasc Surg* 1996; **24**: 800–8.
28. Cockett FB, Jones DEE. The ankle blow-out syndrome: a new approach to the varicose ulcer problem. *Lancet* 1953; **1**: 17–23.
29. Cockett FB. The pathology and treatment of venous ulcers of the leg. *Br J Surg* 1956; **44**: 260–78.
30. O'Donnell TF, Burnand KG, Clemenson G, Thomas ML, Browse NL. Doppler examination vs. clinical and phlebographic detection of the location of incompetent perforating veins. *Arch Surg* 1977; **112**: 31–5.
31. Fischer R, Fullemann HJ, Alder W. About a phlebological dogma of the localization of the Cockett perforators. [In French] *Phlébologie* 1992; **45**: 207–12.
32. Boyd AM. Discussion on primary treatment of varicose veins. *Proc R Soc Med* 1948; **61**: 633–9.
33. Linton RR. The communicating veins of the lower leg and the operative technic for their ligation. *Ann Surg* 1938; **107**: 582–93.
34. Gloviczki P, Canton LG, Cambria RA, Rhee RY. Subfascial endoscopic perforator vein surgery with gas insufflation. In Gloviczki P, Bergan JJ, eds. *Atlas of Endoscopic Perforator Vein Surgery*. London: Springer-Verlag, 1998: 125–38.
35. Mozes G, Gloviczki P, Kadar A, Carmichael SW. Surgical anatomy of perforating veins. In Gloviczki P, Bergan JJ, eds. *Atlas of Endoscopic Perforator Vein Surgery*. London: Springer-Verlag, 1998: 17–28.
36. Sherman RS. Varicose veins: anatomic findings and an operative procedure based upon them. *Ann Surg* 1944; **120**: 222–232.
37. Sherman RS. Varicose veins: further findings based on anatomic and surgical dissections. *Ann Surg* 1949; **130**: 218–32.
38. Fischer R. Insufficient perforating vein on the antero-medial surface of the tibia. [In German] *Vasa* 1985; **14**: 168–9.
39. Green NA, Griffiths JD, Lavy GAD. Venous drainage of the anterior tibio-fibular compartment of the leg, with reference to varicose veins. *Br Med J* 1958: 1209–10.
40. White JW, Katz ML, Cisek P, Kreithen J. Venous outflow of the leg: anatomy and physiologic mechanism of the plantar venous plexus. *J Vasc Surg* 1996; **24**: 819–24.

41. Basmajian JV. Distribution of valves in femoral, external iliac and common iliac veins and their relationship to varicose veins. *Surg Gynecol Obstet* 1952; **95**: 537–42.
42. Moneta GL, Nehler MR. The lower extremity venous system: anatomy and physiology of normal venous function and chronic venous insufficiency. In Gloviczki P, Yao JST, eds. *Handbook of Venous Disorders. Guidelines of the American Venous Forum.* London: Chapman & Hall Medical, 1996: 3–26.
43. Gabella G. Venous system. In Williams PL, Bannister LH, *et al. Gray's Anatomy*, 38th edn. New York: Churchill Livingstone, 1995: 1574–605.
44. Mavor GE, Galloway JM. Collaterals of the deep venous circulation of the lower limb. *Surg Gynecol Obstet* 1967; **125**: 561–71.
45. Walls EW. Veins. In Romanes GJ, ed. *Cunningham's Textbook of Anatomy*, 12th edn. Oxford: Oxford University Press, 1981: 942–79.
46. Patrick JG. Blood vessels. In Sternberg SS, ed. *Histology for Pathologists.* New York: Raven Press, 1992: 195–213.
47. Parum DV. Histochemistry and immunochemistry of vascular disease. In Stehbens WE, Lie JT, eds. *Vascular Pathology.* London: Chapman & Hall, 1995: 313–27.
48. Thomson H. The surgical anatomy of varicose veins. *Phlébologie* 1982; **35**: 11–18.

3

The physiology and hemodynamics of the normal venous circulation

FRANK PADBERG, JR

Although venous disease has been recognized since antiquity, it is only in the last 150 years that substantial progress in therapy and understanding has been realized. Anatomy and function are better appreciated now from the perspective of twentieth century testing modalities. Ambulatory pressure manometry, dynamic phlebography, plethysmographic evaluations and, most recently, color-flow duplex, have contributed substantially to the advancement of current knowledge. Although the interactions can be confusing, consideration of both volume and pressure relationships are essential for understanding normal and abnormal venous function. Many studies from the middle of the twentieth century assess useful and unique physiologic concepts. Although somewhat limited by the available diagnostic modalities of the time, small sample size and minimal descriptive statistics, these studies continue to offer valuable physiologic and hemodynamic data on normal individuals. Detailed discussions of the major pathologic conditions affecting the venous circulation – obstruction and reflux – can be found in later chapters.

The primary purpose of the venous circulation is to return blood to the heart for reoxygenation and recirculation; however, the enormous capacity of the venous reservoir plays a major role in the maintenance of cardiovascular homeostasis by accommodating volume shifts. Regulation of venous tone is an important aspect of volume accommodation and works in concert with arterial control mechanisms which effect changes in the distribution of cardiac output. Sympathetic mediated adjustments of smooth muscle tone are most pronounced in the splanchnic and cutaneous distributions, which are also the most densely innervated. In the upright posture, the physiologic effects of gravity and hydrostatic pressure would appear to oppose return flow; but these effects are largely offset by valves and an efficient peripheral pump mechanism.

VENOUS RETURN

Venous return is defined as the rate of blood flow toward the heart, which in homeostatic circumstances must equal cardiac output. It is expressed as volume per unit time, and varies with age, gender and physical conditioning. The normal resting cardiac output (5.040 l/min) is the product of stroke volume (70 ml) and heart rate (72 b.p.m.).[1] Increasing fiber length (volume) or heart rate will increase cardiac output.

Active venoconstriction of capacitance vessels was once thought to have been a major contributor to changes in cardiac output. The accumulated evidence has now demonstrated that reflex-mediated control of the resistance (precapillary) vessels is the major determinant of the distribution of the circulation.[2–4] However, depending on activity and posture, 60–80% of human resting blood volume (70 ml/kg in men, and 65 ml/kg in women) resides in the splanchnic network.[1–3]

The interaction of multiple components are required for effective venous return: a central pump, a pressure gradient, a peripheral venous pump, and venous valves.

Central circulation

Blood moves through both arteries and veins because of the pumping action of the heart. Fluid flow follows a pressure gradient toward the entry port of the central pump – the right atrium. In the normal individual, atrial pressures of 4–7 mmHg are relatively constant regardless of position. When supine, pressures at the venular end of the capillary bed are estimated to be 12–18 mmHg, which is consistent with venous pressure measured in ankle veins.[5] Thus, flow moves toward the lower pressures of the right atrium. Pressures in the upper extremity in the upright posture are increased by approximately 6 mmHg, at the level of the first rib.[1] In an upright posture, or in the raised arm, gravitational or hydrostatic forces propel upper extremity and cerebral blood toward the heart. The pliable venous wall collapses above the height of the central venous pressure, a fact utilized clinically during bedside estimation of this pressure in the jugular vein. Whether standing or sitting, gravity is additive to both arterial and venous pressures in the lower extremity. However, since the force of gravity is equilibrated between the arterial and venous circulation, it is not a significant factor when considering the pressure gradients influencing venous return in the normal lower extremity.

Venous return is enhanced by negative and neutral (usually 0 mmHg) intra-abdominal and intrathoracic pressures. However, during inspiration, the increase in intra-abdominal pressure causes a transient reduction in flow from the lower extremities to the right atrium by acting as an external compressive force on flow through a collapsible tube (the inferior vena cava, IVC). When the intraperitoneal pressures are chronically elevated (i.e. ascites, morbid obesity may be 15–20 mmHg), venous pressure in the lower extremities must rise above this level to effect flow through the collapsible IVC.

In normal circumstances, a pressure gradient begins with the 12–18 mmHg at the venous end of the capillary, and falls steadily to 5.5 mmHg at the extrathoracic great veins.[6] When blood reaches the right atrium, it is actively pulled into the pump, oxygenated in the pulmonary circuit, and recirculated. Since there are no valves in the large venous conduits, the pathophysiologic consequences are generally those of obstruction to venous flow. The consequences of elevated central venous pressures are well characterized by congestive heart failure, ascites, Budd–Chiari syndrome, and superior vena cava syndrome.

Peripheral venous circulation

Venous return from the dependent lower extremity is achieved by active pumping of the calf muscle assisted by competent venous valves. Normal valve closure effectively prevents retrograde flow of blood. In the normal extremity, competent saphenofemoral and saphenopopliteal valves make consideration of lower extremity venous return primarily a function of the deep veins. Valves are distributed throughout upper and lower extremity veins and seem to be more numerous in the more distal segments. The minimal extent and anatomic distribution of valvular incompetence necessary to produce clinical symptoms remains incompletely understood. As might be anticipated, the greater the valvular dysfunction or reflux, the greater the likelihood of symptoms from peripheral venous insufficiency.[7–11]

The plantar venous plexus probably serves to fill or prime the calf pump. Since most investigators have focused on the calf pump, the role of the foot and thigh components are less well defined. The calf pump is very efficient in the normal limb; however, it is unknown whether or how it might compensate for deficiencies such as outflow obstruction, proximal valvular failure, distal valvular failure, muscle weakness, or loss of joint motion.

PHYSIOLOGIC COMPONENTS OF THE VENOUS CIRCULATION

The prominent role of hydrostatic pressure and capacitance are unique to the venous circulation. Both interact with other physiologic and hemodynamic factors to exert a variable influence relative to circumstances such as posture, volume depletion, physical exercise and ambient temperature. The splanchnic circulation is largely controlled by adrenergic-mediated reflexes; blood flow to skin and skeletal muscle fluctuates over a wide range of volume in response to local, hormonal, and reflex stimuli.[2–4,12,13]

Hydrostatic and dynamic pressure relationships

Although local venous pressure varies with the recumbent, sitting, and standing positions, venous flow still follows a pressure gradient. The peripheral calf muscle pump/valvular mechanism is quite effective at returning venous blood, but it only functions when there are active muscle contractions. Transient inactivity of this mechanism may lead to edema in otherwise normal individuals when the extremity is immobilized for an extended period of time, such as an intercontinental flight in the 'economy' or coach section. When active movement is artificially constrained, the capacitance increases, and the pressure slowly rises to that produced by gravity – the hydrostatic pressure. Exposure to elevated hydrostatic pressures is transmitted to the capillary bed where the balance of filtration favors transudation into the extracellular fluid. Clinically, the result is transient edema.

This pressure, the static or hydrostatic pressure, represents the weight of the column of blood from the point where active recirculation begins – usually the right atrium. Topographically this is assigned to the level of the 4th costosternal junction. The hydrostatic pressure at a given anatomic point is determined by measuring the vertical distance below this landmark.[5,14] The effect of gravity increases 0.77 mmHg/cm of height below the atria; the constant being derived from the product of the density of blood (1.056 g/ml) times the acceleration of gravity (960 cm/s^2) divided by 1333 dynes/cm^2.[1,6] As demonstrated in Table 3.1, the hydrostatic pressure at the distal calf in the average 174 cm tall American male is 94 mmHg when standing.

Chronic, sustained venous pressure elevation, or venous hypertension, is closely associated with pathologic consequences. In the peripheral venous circulation, the major outcomes are reflected in the skin and subcutaneous tissues and include the typical changes described in the CEAP clinical classifications three through six: edema, pigmentation, fibrosis and ulceration. The frequency of cutaneous ulceration increases with increasing end-exercise venous pressures above 30 mmHg.[10] This condition, termed venous hypertension, is not the only abnormality producing these symptoms, but remains a major focus for surgical correction.[7,11] Reflux, the most common pathophysiology associated with venous hypertension, may result from primary valvular insufficiency of either deep or superficial system, or from secondary deep valvular insufficiency.

Capacitance and pressure relationships

The total body venous reservoir has an enormous capacity for fluid volume, which permits accommodation of as much as 20–30% additional volume in the normal individual.[1,2] The normal blood volume is approximately 65 ml/kg in women and 70 ml/kg in men, of which 60–80% resides in the venous circulation. The change to upright posture alone is responsible for a 10% volume shift (7 ml/kg or 250–500 ml) into the lower extremity.[2,3]

The shape of the venous wall varies greatly depending upon pressure, volume and flow as demonstrated in Fig. 3.1.[15] When empty or flaccid, the walls are coapted and the pressure low. As the cross-sectional profile changes to that of a dumbbell or ellipse, large shifts in flow (or volume) are accommodated with minimal change in pressure. Until the vein becomes circular in shape, the pressures remain low. The enormous flow carried by an incompletely distended vein can be deceiving; the experienced surgeon learns to avoid even a small nick in a flaccid iliac vein or the vena cava!

Once a circular geometry is achieved, further distension is accompanied by a rather sharp increase in pressure per unit volume (Fig. 3.1). Over the normal pressure range of 5–25 mmHg, capacitance volume may change in large amounts without effecting flow or pressure.[2,15] As a result, within the range of normal pressures, the venous hydrostatic pressure becomes an inactive factor in the mechanics of venous return. The circular distension pressure is very close to that defined as 'abnormal' by ambulatory venous pressure studies (30 mmHg).[10] Likewise, this threshold is similar to the pressures associated with pulmonary dysfunction from obstructive or regurgitant valvular disease, and the threshold for neuromuscular dysfunction in compartmental syndromes.

The venous wall is considerably thinner than the arterial wall, but consists of the same elements – intima, media and adventitia. The walls of the subfascial deep veins have a relatively uniform thickness; in comparison, the walls of the major superficial venous trunks, the saphenous and cephalic veins, are relatively thick. Pliability and the capacity to constrict or dilate over a

Table 3.1 *Venous pressures when standing*

Pressure (mmHg)	Dynamic	Hydrostatic	Height in reference to RA or HIP (cm), for an average male	Supine (mmHg)
Arm – above head	15	0	75	
Head (ear lobe)		0	34	
Neck (clavicle)		0	19	
Arm – at side		49	45	
IVC at RA	0	0	–	4.6
Iliac bifurcation		15	20	7.5
Femoral bifurcation		31	40	
Popliteal at knee		59	76	
Ankle at malleolus	15	94	122	10
Ankle at end-exercise		22	122	

Pressures at various venous sites are calculated for standing and supine positions for an individual with a height of 174 cm. Gravitational effects: 0.77 mmHg/cm height represents the product of (the density of blood)(acceleration of gravity)/(constant for mercury) × (cm from the right atrium). Acceleration of gravity is 980 cm/s^2; density of blood is 1.056 g/ml; Hg constant is 1333 dynes/cm^2.

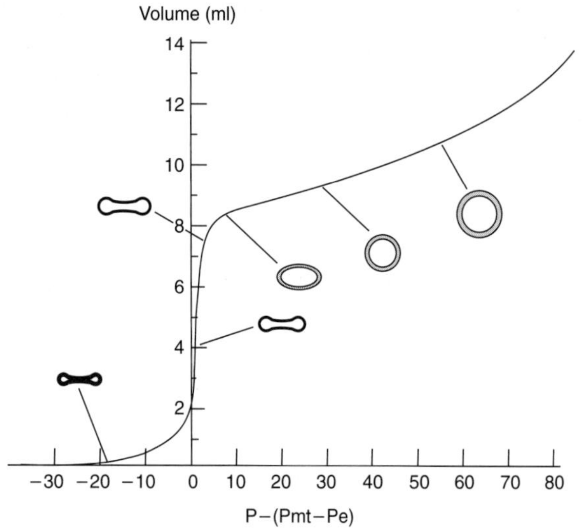

Figure 3.1 *Volume in a collapsible tube as a function of transmural pressure. Typical transverse cross-sections are shown at various points on the curve. (Reproduced with permission from Katz AI, Chen Y, Moreno AH. Flow through a collapsible tube; experimental analysis and mathematical model.* Biophys J *1969;* ***9****: 1262)*

wide range of diameters is a key feature of the venous or capacitance vessels. In the operating room this quality is most readily appreciated by observing the rapid venoconstriction of a vein exposed for harvest and the venodilation after application of warm towels! However, when fully distended with high pressures, a vein loses this pliability and becomes as stiff as an artery.[6]

Physiologic control: reflex, hormonal and local mechanisms

In response to various stimuli, flow through splanchnic, muscle, and cutaneous veins can vary by an enormous volume. Reflex impulses are transmitted through sympathetic nerves, which predominantly exert their effects as arterial constriction. Baroreceptor- and chemoreceptor-mediated effects are the most effective acute adjustments to distribution of blood flows.[1] Fluid shifts and hormonal mechanisms become more important with later adjustments to volume status. Whilst flow is largely controlled by the small resistance arterial beds, capacity is largely adjusted by dilation or constriction of the venous network.

Adrenergic innervation is distributed to both arteries and veins. Furness *et al.*, in an elegant physiologic/anatomic study demonstrated that the relative density of these adrenergic endings in the microcirculatory bed is far greater in the arterial (resistance) circulation[16] (Fig. 3.2). The splanchnic and cutaneous distributions receive the greatest venous concentration of adrenergic fibers. These distributions also have the largest complement of smooth muscle.[1] Marked arteriolar smooth muscle hypertrophy is one of many adaptations in extremity skin, which facilitate adaptation of the giraffe to extreme physiologic stress.[17]

The splanchnic circulation normally contains approximately 18 ml/kg or about 25% of the total blood volume and accounts for approximately 27% of the total blood flow. While normal splanchnic demand is determined from local regulatory mechanisms, acute adjustments of splanchnic volume may be mediated by baroreceptors via adrenergic fibers.[2,4] In severe hypotension, circulating vasopressin and catecholamines may exert a substantial additive effect to the splanchnic adjustments. These redistributions account for approximately 50% of the acute volume compensation following an acute hemorrhage. Whilst a small proportion of this volume shift may result from active venoconstriction, the majority results from passive elastic recoil and redistribution of arterial flow.

Blood flow to inactive skeletal muscle is only 3–4 ml/min/100 g tissue, but because of its large tissue mass, this accounts for approximately 15% of the total blood volume. Adrenergic stimulation has little influence on skeletal muscle flow, which is primarily controlled by locally mediated stimuli.[1,2] Skeletal muscle flow may increase as much as 20-fold to 80 ml/min/100 g tissue with sustained exercise. Venoconstriction occurs in response to exercise although this is abolished by local heating.[3] The increased volume of flow with exercise, along with the heat generated secondarily, recruits dilation of the cutaneous venous network.

The core temperature is maintained at a constant 36–37.5°C, while the skin temperature varies markedly with the ambient temperature. Cutaneous circulation responds to both reflex innervation and direct local stimuli, but overall temperature control is maintained by the hypothalamus. Cutaneous blood flow may vary by as much as 30-fold. Cutaneous blood flow is approximately 3 ml/min/100 g tissue in cool weather, which accounts for approximately 6% of the total blood flow.[12] Conservation of body heat is achieved by constriction of the cutaneous network which lowers flow even further. The deep veins are unaffected by cold.[13] Thus, extreme cold also concentrates venous flow in the deep veins, where a countercurrent heat exchange efficiently preserves thermal energy. Reduction of body temperature markedly enhances venoconstriction in response to local cooling through potentiation of the threshold of the adrenergic receptors of cutaneous veins.[13] In a warm environment, heat loss is facilitated to maintain homeostatic body temperature. Skin blood flow increases with reduced adrenergic impulses, leading to both arterial and venous dilation.[12] In severe heat stress, the skin blood flow may reach 2–3 l/min.

Local injury leads to release of histamine and bradykinin, which produce localized vasodilation. There is mounting evidence to suggest that the vasodilatory actions of progesterone seem to increase venodilation

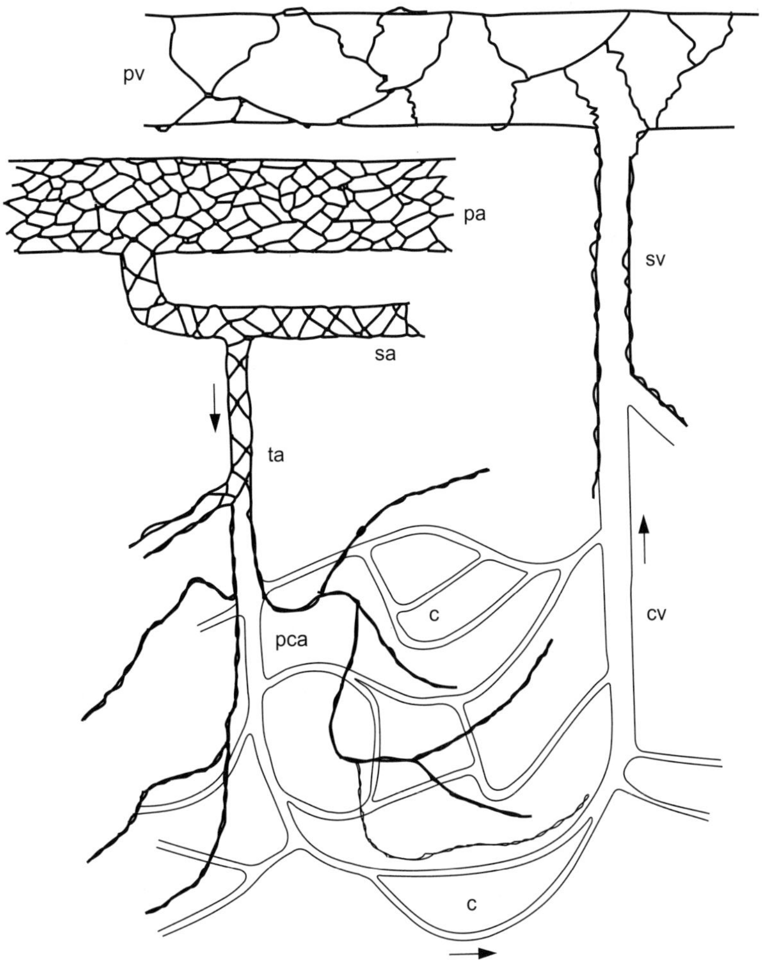

Figure 3.2 *Innervation diagram. Diagrammatic representation of the relationship between adrenergic nerves and the mesenteric blood vessels: pa, principal artery; pv, principal vein; sa, small artery of the microvasculature; ta, terminal arteriole; pca, precapillary arteriole; c, capillary; cv, collecting venule; sv, small vein. The adrenergic nerves are represented by the heavy lines. Arrows indicate the direction of blood flow. Note that the precapillary arterioles and the collecting venules are not innervated. (Reproduced with permission from Furness JB, Marshall JM. Correlation of the directly observed responses of mesenteric vessels of the rat to nerve stimulation and noradrenaline with the distribution of adrenergic nerves.* J Physiol *1974;* ***239****: 79)*

and even the incidence of varicose veins.[4] Although evaluated by a number of investigators, only a limited role has been identified for nitric oxide in venous regulation.[18,19]

THE PERIPHERAL MUSCLE PUMP MECHANISM

Flow against gravity is maintained using a system of muscle pumps to eject the blood, and internal valves to prevent retrograde flow (Fig. 3.3). In normal individuals, this mechanism is remarkably efficient. The complex relationship between pressure and volume is integral to comprehension of venous function, and may be difficult to sort out even though the patterns are similar.

Valvular function

Duplex surveys have defined normal valvular function as a duration of retrograde flow which is <0.5 seconds for all deep and superficial veins of the lower extremities, except the common femoral vein (<1.5 seconds).[20,21] Soleal sinuses have no valves, and a relatively fixed volume.[22] The paired gastrocnemius muscles also have sinuses, but apparently of less volume and number. Although the role of valves in prevention of reflux flow is obvious, the importance of dysfunction (incompetence) of a single or even several valves is not clear. Incompetence of a single valve produces no known physiologic consequence.[20]

The importance of various anatomic sites of valvular dysfunction is incompletely resolved. While some have

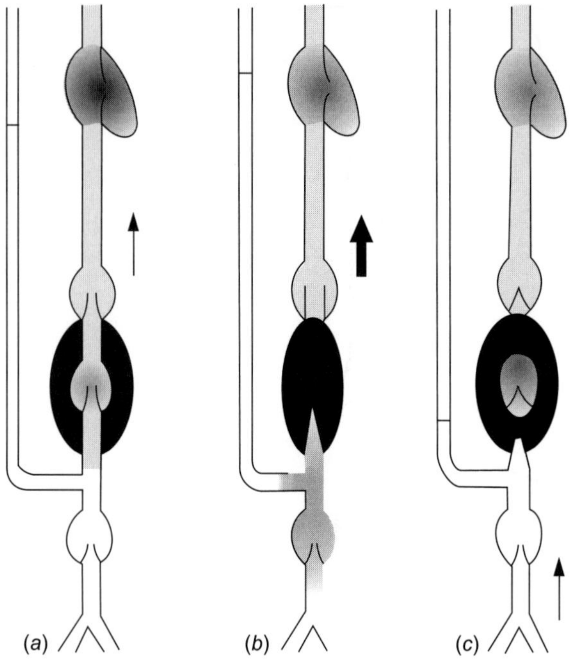

Figure 3.3 *Drawing illustrating 'operation of the muscle pump': (a) resting; (b) muscle contraction; (c) muscle relaxation. Venous pressure in the distal leg is indicated by the length of the hydrostatic column. (Reproduced with permission from Sumner DS. Hemodynamics and pathophysiology of venous disease. In Rutherford RB, ed.* Vascular Surgery, *4th edn. Philadelphia: WB Saunders, 1995: 1679)*

ascribed great pathophysiologic significance to the femoral and popliteal valves, others have emphasized abnormalities of the distal valves.[20,23–25] In an analysis of 155 patients from a series of randomized trials, incompetence of the popliteal vein valve was the only significant risk factor for delayed healing.[23] Rosfors determined that distal valvular dysfunction was of greater significance than popliteal valvular dysfunction; but combined disease categories were most likely to be associated with severe CVI.[9,25] The increased number of valves in the infrapopliteal segments suggests that their functional importance is greater in that location.

Perforating vein valves prevent outward flow when functioning properly.[22,26] This concept is consistent with the pressure/flow relationships of the calf pump. However, even with modern Doppler interrogation, valvular function and flow patterns of perforator veins in the calf continue to remain unclear in a substantial proportion of patients.[27] Cockett colorfully captured the image of perforating vein malfunction with his description of the 'ankle blow-out' syndrome.

The calf pump

Contracting gastrocnemius and soleus muscles expel blood into the large capacity popliteal vein. The normal limb has a calf volume range of 1500–3000 ml, a venous volume of 100–150 ml, and ejects over 60% of the venous volume with a single contraction.[8,28,29] Christopoulos normalized the reporting of air plethysmographic volumes to facilitate comparison of clinical groups and eliminate such effects as edema and variance in calf size.[28] An ejection volume of 2.5–3.7 ml/100 ml calf tissue volume was described for normal limbs. Expression of ejection fraction as a ratio serves the same comparative function.

Measurements of changes in venous pressure and volume during repetitive contractions of the normal calf transcribe similar curves (Fig. 3.4).[5,28,29] Beginning at the resting hydrostatic pressure, the venous pressure is substantially reduced after the initial contractions. This end-exercise pressure, referred to as the ambulatory venous pressure (AVP), is maintained at a lower value by repetitive contractions. When active contraction ceases, 31 seconds are required to restore hydrostatic pressure in the normal limb.[5] Restoration of >90% of volume requires over 70 seconds to refill the calf.[28]

In the normal resting state, the veins of the calf are filled at a rate of 1–2 ml/s by both active and passive mechanisms. The calf pump is actively primed by compression of the plantar venous plexus. Passive filling occurs during muscle relaxation when blood flows into the just emptied deep veins from the muscle itself, the distal deep veins, and the superficial veins. Venous blood flows through perforating veins to follow the pressure gradient from elevated hydrostatic pressures in the superficial veins to the rhythmically decreased mean pressure in the deep veins of the calf. Not all perforating veins have valves, but those which do are oriented to prevent flow from the deep to the superficial system.[22,27] Abnormal function of either the deep or superficial venous system will commonly result in an increased venous pressure, an increased venous volume, and a shortened refill time.[5,10,28] Notably, external compression would benefit this flow pattern by actively encouraging flow into the deep system and reducing calf volume, thus effectively priming the peripheral pump.

Radiographic visualization of contrast movement during active calf contraction was described by Almén.[26] The intramuscular soleal and gastrocnemial sinuses fill from the deep muscle compartment and empty completely with a single calf contraction. The intermuscular, paired, deep tibial veins, which lie between the muscle bundles, are substantially compressed, but are never completely empty. The proximal valves open during active calf contraction. The distal deep vein valves close during active calf contraction, along with those in the perforating veins, thus preventing retrograde or outward flow during the contraction cycle.[26] In addition, video phlebography of the foot suggests a major role for the plantar venous plexus in filling the deep tibial veins.[30]

Use of direct pressure measurements in the tibial, popliteal, and saphenous veins have provided invaluable

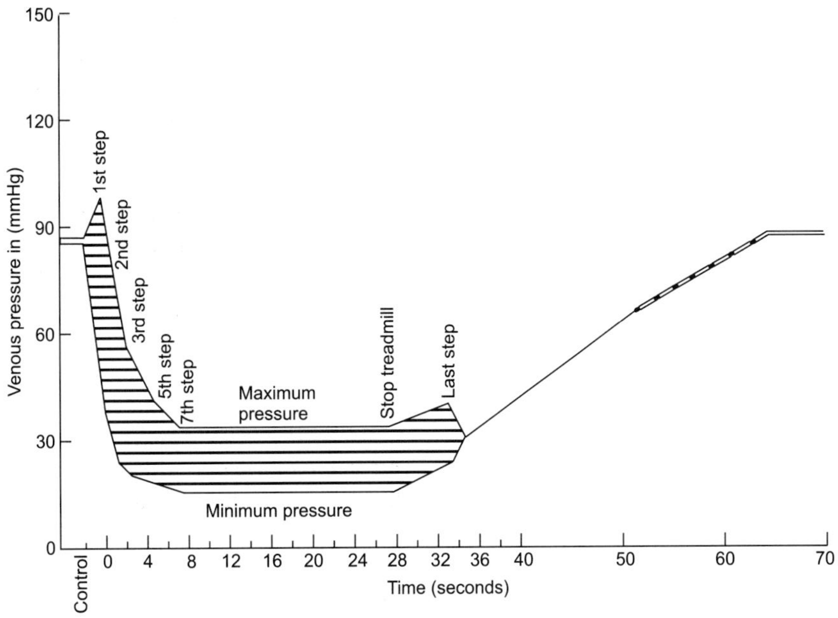

Figure 3.4 *The drawing illustrates mean pressure changes in the dorsal foot vein during standing, calf exercise, and the subsequent resting state. Limb ambulatory pressure curve. (Reproduced with permission from Pollack AA, Wood EH. Venous pressure in the saphenous vein at the ankle in man during exercise and changes in posture.* J Appl Physiol *1949;* ***1****: 656)*

measures of hydrostatic pressure, pressure reduction with single and multiple calf contractions, and time for recovery of resting pressure. However, despite innovative and extensive experimental observations, the invasive aspects of these investigations have precluded repetitive examination. Plethysmography, whether by foot volume, air, or strain gauge is noninvasive and well accepted such that this type of longitudinal data is now appearing. Various authors have described the volume changes associated with elastic compression, surgical intervention, CEAP clinical class, late-day deterioration of venous function, and diminished joint function.[7,8,11,28,31,32]

Thigh and foot contributions to the peripheral venous pump

Although the thigh veins are surrounded by muscle, the contribution of active contraction of thigh muscle to venous return is thought to be minimal. Ludbrook was surprised by his data demonstrating that it required less than 10 seconds for normal venous filling in the thigh as compared with over a minute for the calf.[29] The virtually instantaneous refill of the segment is consistent with end-exercise pressure measurements in the popliteal vein.[14,33] A thigh segment ejection fraction of 20% was measured with a 15 cm air plethysmographic cuff.[29] Considerably less efficient venous return from the thigh segment was attributed to the observed rapid refill and less compressible intermuscular location of the deep veins in the thigh.

Compression of the plantar venous plexus actively pumps blood proximally.[30] Although the medial and lateral plantar veins are also intermuscular in location, intrinsic muscle contraction coincides with the timing of maximal weight-bearing on the full foot; compression then forces blood out of the foot. Blood flow from the plantar venous plexus is primarily directed into the paired, deep tibial veins; however, there is disagreement about whether it is all retained in the deep system. Several investigators describe findings that suggest that flow passes from these and other deep foot veins into both the deep and superficial venous networks.[34,35] Kuster studied the veins communicating between the deep and suprafascial systems of the foot in 10 unembalmed limbs and identified 6–12 veins per foot. Approximately 50% of these veins had valves which, unlike the perforating veins of the calf and thigh, only allowed flow from the deep veins toward the superficial veins.[35] Even with intraosseus tarsal phlebography, an ankle tourniquet was still needed to direct flow into the deep veins.[34] Notably, this flow pattern would also be improved by the addition of external compression.

Although the interaction between the various leg pumps is not fully understood, all work with competent valve function to return the venous blood from one segment of the extremity to another.

STROKE VOLUME AND CALF PUMP OUTPUT

Like many biologic systems, the provision for normal venous return from the peripheral muscle pump greatly exceeds the minimum required for normal function. If we postulate a conservative normal walking cadence of 100 steps/min, and a median ejection volume of 3.0 ml/100 ml in a 2.0 liter calf, the calf pump output (CPO) would be 6.0 l/min. The CPO per limb would be half this figure, or 3.0 l/min. Even by employing conservative assumptions, these estimates for CPO exceed the resting cardiac output. Logically, if venous volume is increased, the proportion ejected would be reduced, resulting in a less efficient pump and a decreased CPO. For example, in deep venous insufficiency, with a median ejection volume of 1.7 ml/100 ml, the CPO would be 3.4 l/min.

PRESSURE RELATIONSHIPS IN THE LOWER EXTREMITY

In the normal limb, the pressure is reduced from the resting hydrostatic pressure to a mean of 22 mmHg with ambulatory calf contractions, a value which is reached within 7–12 steps.[5] Two contraction–relaxation cycles occur with each step corresponding to lift off, swing and restrike. Similar pressure changes were observed with standing ankle plantar flexion or heel-raising which transfers weight to the forefoot (the tip-toe maneuver).[5,10] When resuming a static standing position, the hydrostatic pressure is restored in a mean of 31 seconds (Fig. 3.4). As a practical matter, venous pressure studies have generally been obtained from the dorsal foot veins, since the pressures accurately reflect the pressures determined from direct cannulation of the deep veins of the calf (posterior tibial). Several authors have compared simultaneous pressures from deep and superficial vein catheters placed at the same anatomic height.[14,33,35] The incidence of ulceration has a linear relationship to increases in ambulatory venous pressures above 30 mmHg; ulceration and an increased AVP was also associated with a 90% refill time of <20 seconds.[10] In addition, rapid reflux (i.e. venous filling of greater than 7 ml/s) is also associated with a high incidence of ulceration.[28]

Contracting muscle and an intact limb fascia are integral components of the peripheral musculovenous pump. During maximal contraction, intramuscular pressures of 250 mmHg are generated in the soleus muscle; and 215 mmHg in the gastrocnemius.[29] Pressures within the fascial envelope of the leg were estimated to reach 100–150 mmHg. Intravenous pressures taken from the proximal posterior tibial vein rise to greater than 200 mmHg during initial calf contraction, with subsequent peak pressures of >150 mmHg on repetitive contractions; pressures were 30 mmHg on relaxation.[14] Saphenous vein measurements at the same anatomic height had a lesser initial peak pressure and demonstrated declining peak pressures with each contraction. The pressure gradient thus favors superficial to deep flow only during the post-contraction, relaxation phase of the calf muscle cycle. Pressures in the popliteal vein demonstrate a short rise during the initial calf contraction, which corresponds to expulsion of blood from the calf, but popliteal pressures do not sustain a decrease following relaxation; thus, the baseline, resting popliteal vein pressure remains close to the hydrostatic pressure for the greater proportion of the walking cycle.[14,33] The fixed, non-elastic investing fascia of the lower leg provides an unyielding envelope which permits generation of these high pressures, but also prevents dilation of the capacitance chamber, thus eliminating an increase in stroke volume as a potential compensatory mechanism for calf pump failure.

Unlike the fascia, normal skin is elastic and can stretch in response to a sustained increase in subcutaneous pressure. The combination of stretched skin, edema, venous hypertension, and minor injury may predispose to ulceration. Study of the giraffe, with its exaggerated physiologic demands, identified several physical adaptations including an elevated interstitial fluid pressure (mean 40–50 mmHg) supported by a skin structure with characteristics of a tight and unyielding fascia.[17] Clinically, these considerations are incorporated into therapeutic devices such as the adjustable Velcro wrap, and Unna's boot which also provide an unyielding external envelope. The gradient compression stocking utilizes elastic to provide similar external support.

PHYSIOLOGIC COMPENSATIONS

Compensation for upright posture

In man, the primary peripheral circulatory adaptation to assumption of upright posture is made by changes in arterial resistance and not by adjustments in venous tone or capacitance.[3,36] Circulatory homeostasis with this change in position is largely achieved by immediate changes in heart rate and then adjustment in arterial resistance.[2,5,36] When the dependent capacitance vessels (veins) are allowed to continue to fill passively without emptying, the resulting redistribution of blood volume may result in syncope, a common problem in fresh military recruits learning to stand in formation. Normal individuals, standing in a static position, fidget and shift weight from one leg to another at least once per minute; this frequency was not diminished by extremes of heat or cold.[33,37]

Volume depletion: hemorrhage (acute), dehydration (chronic)

Compensation for acute reduction in blood volume and the resulting decrease in venous return is mediated by baroreceptor stimulation and increased sympathetic output. Loss of approximately 10% of circulating volume may be accommodated without change in cardiac output or systemic pressure by sympathetic-mediated arteriolar constriction and venoconstriction and increases in heart rate. Acute loss of approximately 30–40% of volume can be tolerated without death, but requires maximal utilization of compensatory mechanisms. Reflex vasoconstriction, which is most prominent in the splanchnic and cutaneous distributions, is accompanied by circulating catecholamines in severe acute blood loss. Canine studies suggest that acute volume depletion of approximately 29% (20 ml/kg), can be compensated by the combination of vasoconstriction and transcapillary fluid resorption (6 ml/kg). Thus, 10–15 ml/kg is able to be compensated by active venoconstriction and passive elastic recoil resulting from both reduced arterial pressure and vasoconstriction.[1,2]

Over a prolonged time interval, an individual can compensate for loss of almost 50% of blood volume (35 ml/kg). Accommodation for chronic volume loss is achieved by transfer of extracellular fluid volume to circulating volume and the hormonal effects of aldosterone and the renin–angiotensin system.[1,2] Both acute and chronic adjustments to volume depletion are primarily achieved through control of arterial resistance, with veins playing a passive, but essential role.

Musculoskeletal activity

To supply the enormous blood flow to required by exercising muscle, three major circulatory accommodations take place.[1] Cardiac output may increase five to seven times normal resting values. Mean arterial pressure rises 20–80 mmHg. Third, mass sympathetic discharge produces diffuse arteriolar constriction and venoconstriction. Local effects produce vasodilation of the muscle arterioles because local metabolic effects override the sympathetic signals to vasoconstriction.

Deterioration of calf pump function at the end of the day was reported using both photo- and air-plethysmography.[31,32] Although the variance was relatively limited, these findings did suggest that venous return from the limb does deteriorate with prolonged upright activity. The explanation for these findings may be related to stress relaxation of venous smooth muscle. It is unclear whether, or how, the calf pump can compensate for valvular insufficiency, whether it can adjust the components of outflow, or if it reaches a finite level of failure. While the role of the calf pump in venous insufficiency is well recognized, little has been done in a direct attempt to effect a therapeutic intervention. Data has demonstrated a progressive reduction in calf pump function and ankle range of motion with increasing severity of CVI.[7,8] Physical conditioning, directed to improve calf pump function, may be of therapeutic value. A current program at our institution includes interventions directed at both calf muscle strengthening and joint mobility.

Temperature adjustment

Regulation of heat loss from the body is a major determinant of skin blood flow. A decrease in temperature produces cutaneous arterial vasoconstriction as well as subcutaneous venoconstriction. The combined effects of local and central effects can reduce skin blood flow to less than 3 ml/100 g/min.[12] Additional physiologic compensations for cold include shivering, hunger, and catecholamine secretion.

Compensatory mechanisms for increased temperature include increased cutaneous arterial flow and increased subcutaneous venous capacitance. Maximal skin blood flow may increase by over 10-fold to 30 ml/100 g/min with flows of 2–3 l/min.[12] Additional physiologic compensations for heat include sweating, increased respiration, and decreased activity.

At the extremes of ambient temperature (0–55°C) venous pressure measurements in normal individuals exhibit pathologic findings.[37] By gradually adjusting ambient temperatures between 0 and 55°C, toe temperatures of 22 and 40°C respectively were recorded, while subjects were stressed to clinical endpoints of shivering or sweating[37] (Fig. 3.5). A cold extremity never achieved a full hydrostatic pressure head and required prolonged filling to reach even a reduced hydrostatic pressure. A warm extremity achieved a full hydrostatic pressure almost immediately, making assessment of post-exercise pressures difficult.[37] Although specifically determined in relatively extreme temperatures, these findings for ambulatory venous pressure determinations have implications for other methods of venous testing as well. Because of this, rooms for these examinations must be maintained within a reasonable range of comfortable ambient temperatures.

Other

Active venoconstriction occurs with hyperventilation, cold showers, strong emotion, and muscular exercise and is mediated by the adrenergic (sympathetic) nervous system.[3] Ongoing research continues to seek effective pharmacologic solutions for venotonic therapy.[4]

Although a specific neural pathway for venodilation has not been identified in humans, the paracrine mechanism of endothelial-derived relaxing factor has been an important focus of recent research. Now recognized as

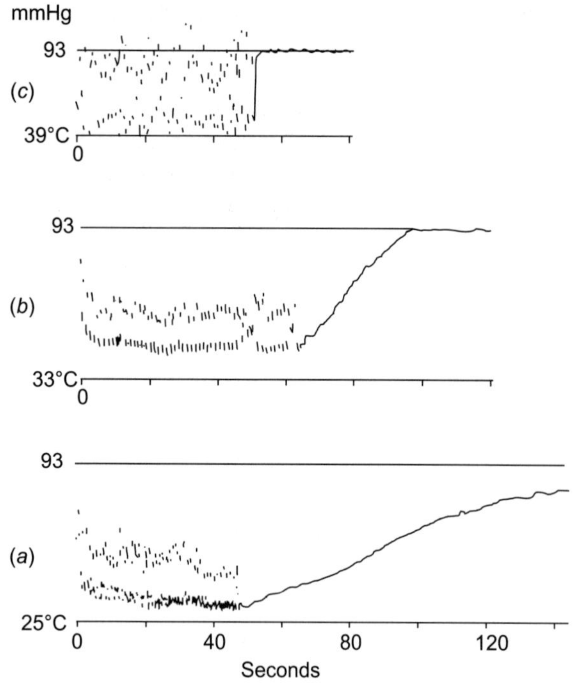

Figure 3.5 *The three panels illustrate the changes in an ambulatory venous pressure tracing at extremes of ambient temperature (the temperature markings indicate toe temperatures). Note the absence of a return to the baseline hydrostatic pressure (93 mmHg) in (a) cold; and the immediate return to baseline hydrostatic pressure in (c) hot. (Reproduced with permission from Henry JP, Gauer OH. Influence of temperature on venous pressure in the foot.* J Clin Invest *1950;* ***29****: 857)*

nitric oxide, the vasodilator effect in the venous circulation is minimal in comparison to its effects in the arterial circulation. A clinical correlate was described by Lüscher who studied internal mammary arteries, internal mammary veins, and saphenous veins harvested for coronary arterial bypass grafts. The relaxation response of the veins was markedly reduced in comparison to the artery (Fig. 3.6). They postulated that these physiologic characteristics influenced patency of the bypass grafts.[19]

SUMMARY

Understanding the normal venous circulation requires mastery of complex hemodynamic and physiologic concepts. Gravity-induced hydrostatic pressure encourages flow into the dependent capacitance network. The distensibility of the venous wall permits the system to accept (or contribute) large volume adjustments with a minimal rise (or fall) in pressure.

Venous return flows along a pressure gradient, just as the arterial and microcirculations do. Return of venous blood against gravity is accomplished by breaking the system into multiple pumped segments with internal valves preventing the return of ejected blood. The muscle pumping mechanism is very efficient, and empties into a capacious valved popliteal vein. Acute circulatory adjustments associated with standing, volume deficiencies, or changes in temperature are largely compensated by reflex alterations in resistance vessels, in conjunction with adjustments of venous tone. The complex physiologic interactions of the return circulation provide a homeostatic milieu that supports reasonable human function in a wide variety of circumstances.

REFERENCES

1. Guyton AC, Hall J. *Medical Physiology*, 9th edn. Philadelphia: Saunders, 1996.
2. Rothe CF. Venous System: Physiology of the capacitance vessels. In Shepherd JT, Abboud FM, eds. *Handbook of Physiology, Volume III, Peripheral Circulation and Organ*

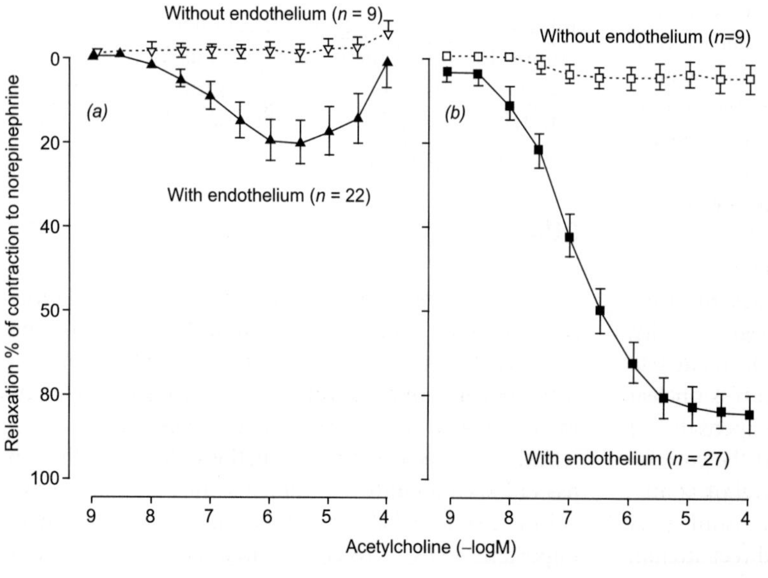

Figure 3.6 *Endothelium-dependent relaxation responses to ACH in human internal mammary arteries (■, □ and saphenous veins (▲, ▽). (Reproduced with permission from Lüscher TF, Diederich D, Siebenmann R,* et al. *Difference between endothelium-dependent relaxation in arterial and in venous coronary bypass grafts.* N Engl J Med *1988;* ***319****: 464)*

Blood Flow, Section 2 The Cardiovascular System. Bethesda, MD: American Physiological Society, 1983: 397–452.

3. Shepherd JT. Role of the veins in the circulation. *Circulation* 1966; **33**: 484–91.
4. Vanhoutte PM. Venous wall and venous disease. In Vanhoute PM, ed. *Return Circulation and Norepinephrine: an Update*. Paris: John Libby, 1991: 1–14.
5. Pollack AA, Wood EH. Venous Pressure in the saphenous vein at the ankle in man during exercise and changes in posture. *J Appl Physiol* 1949; **1**: 649–62.
6. Sumner DS. Hemodynamics and pathophysiology of venous disease. In Rutherford RB, ed. *Vascular Surgery*, 4th edn. Philadelphia: WB Saunders, 1995: 1673–95.
7. Araki C, Back TL, Padberg FT, *et al*. Significance of calf muscle pump function in venous ulceration. *J Vasc Surg* 1994; **20**: 872–9.
8. Back T, Padberg F, Araki C, Thompson PN, Hobson RW. Ankle range of motion and reduced venous function is associated with progression of chronic venous insufficiency. *J Vasc Surg* 1995; **22**: 519–23.
9. Lees TA, Lambert D. Patterns of venous reflux in limbs with skin changes associated with chronic venous insufficiency. *Br J Surg* 1993; **80**: 725–8.
10. Nicolaides AN, Hussein MK, Szendro G, Christopoulos D, Vasdekis S, Clarke H. The relation of venous ulceration with ambulatory venous pressure measurements. *J Vasc Surg* 1993; **17**: 414–19.
11. Padberg R. Surgical intervention in venous ulceration. *Cardiovasc Surg* 1999; **7**: 83–90.
12. Roddie IC. Circulation to skin and adipose tissue. In Shepherd JT, Abboud FM, eds. *Handbook of Physiology, Volume III, Peripheral Circulation and Organ Blood Flow, Section 2 The Cardiovascular System*. Bethesda, MD: American Physiological Society, 1983: 285–317.
13. Vanhoutte PM, Shepherd JT. Thermosensitivity and veins. *J Physiol (Paris)* 1971; **63**: 449–51.
14. Arnoldi CG. Venous pressure in the leg of healthy human subjects at rest and during muscular exercise in the nearly erect position. *Acta Chir Scand* 1965; **130**: 570–83.
15. Katz AI, Chen Y, Moreno AH. Flow through a collapsible tube; experimental analysis and mathematical model. *Biophys J* 1969; **9**: 1261–79.
16. Furness JB, Marshall JM. Correlation of the directly observed responses of mesenteric vessels of the rat to nerve stimulation and noradrenaline with the distribution of adrenergic nerves. *J Physiol* 1974; **239**: 75–88.
17. Hargens AR, Millard RW, Petterssen K, Johansen K. Gravitational hemodynamics and edema prevention in the giraffe. *Nature* 1987; **329**: 59–60.
18. DeMey JG, Vanhoutte PM. Heterogenous behavior of the canine arterial and venous wall; importance of the endothelium. *Circ Res* 1982; **51**: 439–47.
19. Lüscher TF, Diederich D, Siebenmann R, *et al*. Difference between endothelium-dependent relaxation in arterial and in venous coronary bypass grafts. *N Engl J Med* 1988; **319**: 462–7.
20. Araki C, Back TL, Padberg FT, Refinements in detection of popliteal vein reflux. *J Vasc Surg* 1993; **18**: 742–8.
21. Van Bemellen PJ, Bedford G, Beach K, Strandness DE. Quantitative segmental evaluation of venous valvular reflux with the duplex ultrasound scanner. *J Vasc Surg* 1989; **10**: 425–31.
22. Cockett FG. The pathology and treatment of venous ulcers of the leg. *Br J Surg* 1955; **43**: 260–78.
23. Brittenden J, Bradbury AW, Allan PL, Prescott RJ, Halper DR, Ruckley CV. Popliteal vein reflux reduces healing of chronic venous ulcer. *Br J Surg* 1998; **85**: 60–2.
24. Dalsing MC, Raju S, Wakefield TW, Taheri S. A multicenter, phase 1 evaluation of cryopreserved venous valvular allografts for treatment of chronic deep venous insufficiency. *J Vasc Surg* 1999; **30**: 854–66.
25. Rosfors S, Lamke L-O, Nordstrom E, Bygdman S. Severity and location of venous valvular insufficiency: the importance of distal valve function. *Acta Chir Scand* 1990; **156**: 689–94.
26. Almén T, Nylander G. Serial phlebography of the normal lower leg during muscle contraction and relaxation. *Acta Radiol* 1963; **57**: 264–72.
27. Sarin S, Scurr JH, Coleridge Smith PD. Medial calf perforators in venous disease: the significance of outward flow. *J Vasc Surg* 1992; **16**: 40–6.
28. Christopoulos DG, Nicolaides AN, Szendro G, Irvine AT, Bull M-I, Eastcott HHG. Air-plethysmography and the effect of elastic compression on venous hemodynamics of the leg. *J Vasc Surg* 1987; **5**: 148–59.
29. Ludbrook J. Musculovenous pumps of the human lower limb. *Am Heart J* 1966; **71**: 635–41.
30. Gardner AMN, Fox RH. The venous pump of the human foot – preliminary report. *Bristol Med Chir J* 1983; **98**: 109–12.
31. Bishara RA, Sigel B, Rocco K, Socha E, Schuler JJ, Flanigan DP. Deterioration of venous function in normal lower extremities during daily activity. *J Vasc Surg* 1986; **3**: 700–6.
32. Katz ML, Comerota AJ, Kerr RP, Caputo GC. Variability of venous hemodynamics with daily activity. *J Vasc Surg* 1994; **19**: 361–5.
33. Hojensgard IC, Sturup H. Static and dynamic pressures in superficial and deep veins of the lower extremity in man. *Acta Physiol Scand* 1953; **27**: 49–67.
34. Jacobsen BH. Venous drainage of the foot. *Surg Gynecol Obstet* 1970; **131**: 22–4.
35. Kuster G, Lofgren EP, Hollinshead WH. Anatomy of the veins of the foot. *Surg Gynecol Obstet* 1968; **127**: 817–23.
36. Samuelhoff SI, Browse NL, Shepherd JT. Response of capacity vessels in human limbs to head up tilt and suction on the lower body. *J Appl Physiol* 1966; **21**: 47–54.
37. Henry JP, Gauer OH. The influence of temperature upon venous pressure in the foot. *J Clin Invest* 1950; **29**: 855–61.

4

The epidemiology and natural history of acute deep venous thrombosis

MARK H MEISSNER AND D EUGENE STRANDNESS, JR

Clinically recognized acute deep venous thrombosis (DVT) has been estimated to occur with an incidence of 116 000 to over 250 000 new cases per year in the USA.[1,2] However, thrombotic risk is not uniformly distributed in the population and an appreciation of the associated risk factors provides insight into the underlying pathophysiology. As initially postulated by Virchow, three factors are of primary importance in the development of venous thrombosis – abnormalities of blood flow, abnormalities of blood, and vessel wall injury. However, recent advances in our understanding of coagulation and vascular biology, accompanied by improvements in noninvasive venous studies, have further defined Virchow's model.

It is increasingly apparent that Virchow's 'abnormalities of blood', which include aberrations of both the coagulation and fibrinolytic systems, are of primary importance in the origin of venous thrombi. The formation of thrombi in the venous system depends in large measure on imbalances within the coagulation and fibrinolytic systems and similar interactions continue to be important throughout the subsequent evolution of these thrombi. Over time, the processes of recanalization and organization compete with thrombus extension and rethrombosis.

Although animal models have contributed an understanding of the mechanisms of thrombogenesis, organization and recanalization, duplex ultrasonography has been the most important development in characterizing the natural history of venous thrombi in humans. Noninvasive natural history studies have provided critical information about the frequency and rate at which changes in the venous system occur after an episode of acute DVT. Although our understanding remains incomplete, the most important chronic manifestations of acute DVT, valvular incompetence and persistent venous obstruction, can now be related to its natural history. More importantly, identification of the determinants of valvular incompetence and persistent obstruction may provide opportunities to correct or modify the changes contributing to a poor outcome.

VENOUS THROMBOGENESIS

Despite the accuracy of Virchow's initial postulates, all three components are not equally important in individual patients. The role of structural injury to the venous wall is disputable; even in the presence of stasis, overt endothelial injury appears to be neither a necessary or sufficient condition for thrombosis.[3] With the notable exceptions of direct venous trauma, hip arthroplasty and central venous catheters, there is little evidence that either gross or microscopic endothelial injury plays a significant role in venous thrombogenesis. By contrast, data are accumulating that biologic injury to the endothelium may have a very important role in the origin of DVT. The venous endothelium is normally antithrombotic, producing prostaglandin I_2, thrombomodulin, tissue-type plasminogen activator (t-PA), and glycosaminoglycan cofactors of antithrombin. Under conditions favoring thrombosis, the endothelium may become prothrombotic, producing tissue factor, von Willebrand factor, and fibronectin. Leukocytes may be a key mediator of both endothelial injury and hypercoagulability, with the early phases of thrombosis marked by increases in permeability followed by leukocyte adhesion, migration and endothelial disruption.[4,5] Associated cytokines may also be of importance, factors such as interleukin 1 (IL-1) increasing tissue factor expression while diminishing protein C activation.[6]

Although most venous thrombi originate in areas of low blood flow, stasis alone is also an inadequate stimulus in the absence of low levels of activated coagulation factors.[7,8] Stasis may facilitate endothelial leukocyte adhesion[4] and cause endothelial hypoxia leading to a procoagulant state,[9] but its most important role may be in permitting the accumulation of activated coagulation factors in areas prone to thrombosis. Stasis may thus be a permissive factor for the other events required for thrombosis.

Imbalanced activation of the coagulation system appears to be the most important factor underlying many episodes of acute DVT. Although the hemostatic system is continuously active, thrombus formation is ordinarily confined to sites of local injury by a precise balance between activators and inhibitors of coagulation and fibrinolysis. A prethrombotic state may result either from imbalances in the regulatory and inhibitory systems or from activation exceeding antithrombotic capacity.[10] An appreciation of the importance of activated coagulation has been facilitated by the development of assays for stable byproducts of thrombin activation, including prothrombin fragment 1+2, fibrinopeptide A, and thrombin–antithrombin complex. Some component of imbalanced coagulation appears to be associated with many thrombotic risk factors including age, malignancy, surgery, trauma, primary hypercoagulable states, pregnancy, and oral contraceptive use.

PREVALENCE AND RISK FACTORS

The incidence of deep venous thrombosis is highly dependent on the population studied and their underlying risk factors for thromboembolism as well as the means by which DVT is documented. True estimates of the incidence of DVT are limited by the few population-based studies, the clinically silent nature of most thromboses, and the need for objective documentation of the diagnosis. It is generally believed that incidence rates from epidemiologic studies are underestimates. Community-based studies of hospitalized patients have suggested an annual incidence of 56 per 100 000, whereas population-based studies of healthy volunteers have produced estimates of 122 per 100 000.[2] Studies of venographically confirmed DVT in Sweden have suggested a somewhat higher incidence of 160 cases of new or recurrent DVT per 100 000 population per year.[11] Extrapolated to the population of the USA, this represents 116 000 to over 250 000 new cases of clinically recognized DVT per year.[1,2]

Despite the imprecision in estimating the incidence of DVT in the general population, multiple risk factors for deep venous thrombosis have been identified and the degree of risk associated with these factors established to a variable extent. Most of these risk factors can be associated with the components of Virchow's triad. Well-established risk factors for thrombosis are shown in Table 4.1, although the development of clinically manifest thrombosis most often occurs with the convergence of several genetic and acquired risk factors.[12] Multiple risk factors often act synergistically to increase risk dramatically above the sum of individual risk factors.

Not surprisingly, the risk of venous thromboembolism appears to increase with the number of risk factors. In symptomatic outpatients, the odds ratio for an objectively documented DVT increases from 1.26 for one risk factor to 3.88 for three or more risk factors.[13] The general population of hospitalized patients has an average of 1.5 risk factors per patient, with 26% having three or more risk factors.[14] Three or more risk factors are present in 80% of inpatients with venous thromboembolism[2] and 30% of outpatients with confirmed DVT.[13]

Demographic risk factors

Age, gender and race may potentially influence the incidence of deep venous thrombosis. Among these, age has been most consistently associated with an increased incidence of DVT. Population-based studies have shown the incidence of DVT to increase exponentially by a factor of 200 between 20 and 80 years of age with a relative risk of 1.9 for each 10-year increase in age.[2] This increased risk is related to multiple age-associated factors including an increased number of major thrombotic risk factors, an acquired prothrombotic state as suggested by increased levels of thrombin activation markers, and changes in the venous system associated with increased stasis.[15] Three or more risk factors are present in 30% of hospitalized patients over age 40 in comparison with only 3% of those less than age 40.[14]

Gender differences in the incidence of DVT have been variable, and may be related to other thrombotic risk factors. Although Coon and associates[1] found a higher frequency of DVT in young women, one-half of thromboembolic events in women less than 40 years old were associated with pregnancy. Some have noted no significant differences in incidence between men and women,[11,13] whilst others have noted a slightly increased risk (relative risk 1.4) in males.[2]

Geographic differences in the incidence of DVT do exist. In the USA, the incidence of venous thromboembolism is higher in the interior than on either coast.[16] However, regional variations in medical and surgical diseases, prophylactic measures, and methods of diagnosis

Table 4.1 *Thromboembolic risk factors*

Risk factor	Risk	Reference
Age	Relative risk 1.9 per 10-year increase	2
Surgery	General surgery – 19%	23
	Neurosurgery – 24%	
	Hip/knee – 48–61%	
Trauma	58% of patients	82
Malignancy	15% of patients	83
History of VTE	2–9% of VTE patients	1
	(40% of patients with factor V Leiden – 2.4×)	74
Primary hypercoagulable states		
Antithrombin, protein C/S deficiency	10×	
Factor V Leiden		
Heterozygous	8×	12
Homozygous	80×	
Prothrombin 20210A	4×	
Increased factor VIII	6×	
Hyperhomocysteinemia	2.5–4×	
Family history	2.9×	84
Oral contraceptives	2.9×	28
	(30–50× with factor V Leiden)	
Estrogen replacement	2–4×	30
Immobilization	2× (preoperative)	85
Pregnancy & puerperium	Pregnancy – 0.075% of pregnancies	31
	Postpartum – 2.3–6.1 per 1000 deliveries	
Femoral catheters	12% of trauma patients	86
Antiphospholipid antibodies	Lupus anticoagulant – 6×	87
	Anticardiolipin antibody – 2×	
Inflammatory bowel disease	1.2–7.1% of patients	88
Obesity	Variable	
Varicose veins	Variable	
Myocardial infarction/CHF	Variable	

CHF, congestive heart failure.

make conclusions regarding ethnic differences difficult. Among elderly Medicare patients, the incidence of pulmonary embolism is higher among blacks, while the incidence of DVT is lower.[16] Autopsy series suggest an identical prevalence of thromboembolism among American black and white patients.[17] Neither have racial differences been found in the rate of hospital diagnosis of DVT based on coded discharge data.[18] Although there is suggestive evidence that the incidence of postoperative DVT may be lower in Asian, Arab and African populations than among Europeans,[19] the incidence of postoperative DVT is similar among South African European and non-European patients.[20] Nevertheless, racial and ethnic differences in genetic risk factors, including blood group and the factor V Leiden mutation, do exist and corresponding differences in rates of thromboembolism can not be excluded.[21,22]

Surgery

Like age, the risk associated with surgery also appears to be multifactorially related to perioperative immobilization, activated coagulation, and transient depression of fibrinolysis. Increases in thrombin activation as well as elevated levels of plasminogen activator inhibitor-1 (PAI-1) have been well documented perioperatively. The degree of risk is variable with the age of the patient, length and type of procedure, and the presence of other thrombotic risk factors.[23]

Trauma

The trauma patient perhaps best represents the convergence of all components of Virchow's triad. Direct venous injury, multiple coagulation and fibrinolytic derangements, and immobilization by skeletal injuries, paralysis and critical illness may all contribute to the high incidence of DVT in the injured patient. Factors identified as important determinants of DVT in this population have included advanced age; blood transfusion; surgery; fractures of the pelvis, femur or tibia; spinal cord injury; Injury Severity Score (ISS); Trauma Injury Severity Score (TRISS); major venous injury; and femoral venous catheters.[24]

Malignancy

Although classically associated with mucinous gastrointestinal tumors, DVT may complicate a spectrum of malignancies, with carcinoma of the lung now most frequently associated with thrombosis. Deep venous thrombosis may complicate 19–30% of malignancies, may be present at the time of diagnosis in 3–23% of patients with idiopathic thrombosis, and may develop 1–2 years after presentation in another 5–11% of patients. Abnormalities of the coagulation system are present in up to 90% of patients with cancer, with activation of coagulation mediated by tissue factor, cancer procoagulant, and macrophage-associated cytokines.

Immobilization

A relationship between bed rest and DVT has long been recognized. Prior to the use of DVT prophylaxis, the autopsy incidence of lower extremity thrombosis was noted to increase within 3 days of bed rest and to rapidly rise to 15%, 77% and 94% after 1, 2 and 4 weeks of confinement, respectively.[25] The importance of immobilization is further emphasized by the observations that thrombosis following bed rest is frequently bilateral whereas that associated with stroke is often confined to the paralyzed limb. The relationship between DVT and prolonged travel has been controversial. However, suggestive evidence tends to be supported by one case–control study demonstrating an association between DVT and travel of greater than 4 hours' duration.[26]

History of venous thromboembolism

As many as 26% of cases will have a previous history of DVT, whereas, depending on sex and age, recurrent thromboembolism will affect one in every 11–50 persons per year.[1] The incidence of recurrent DVT is higher among those having irreversible thrombotic risk factors and those with idiopathic DVT. Some[27] have also noted a significantly higher incidence in patients less than 65 years of age.

Primary hypercoagulable states

The primary hypercoagulable states constitute those thrombophilic conditions that have a genetic basis. Among these, deficiencies of the naturally occurring anticoagulants antithrombin, protein C, and protein S are present in only 5–10% of DVT patients. Several recently described abnormalities are substantially more common.[12] The factor V Leiden mutation, present in approximately 20% of DVT patients, results from a point mutation in the factor V gene rendering it less sensitive to degradation by activated protein C. A mutation in the 3′ region of the prothrombin gene, prothrombin 20210, is associated with increased plasma levels of prothrombin and is present in approximately 6% of those with venous thrombosis. An increased risk associated with hyperhomocysteinemia and increased plasma concentrations of factor VIII has recently been described and may be present in 10% and 25% of those with DVT, respectively. The phenotypic expression of these abnormalities varies both within and between families, although the risk is higher and the age at first thrombosis earlier among those with a family history of thrombosis. Thrombophilic families appear to have a significant incidence of combined, multigenic defects.

Oral contraceptives and hormonal therapy

Epidemiologic studies have clearly established an association between oral contraceptives and venous thromboembolism. Pharmacologic doses of estrogen are associated with increased factor VIIa levels as well as depressed antithrombin and protein S activity. The overall summary relative risk from eight case–control, six follow-up, and one randomized study in the literature is 2.9, corresponding to a calculated absolute risk of approximately 3.3 per 10 000 users.[28] However, some populations, particularly those with congenital thrombophilias, are at substantially higher risk. Thrombotic risk is correlated with estrogen dose, preparations containing more than 50 μg of estrogen being associated with the highest risk. Although cautious interpretation has been advised and there is substantial potential for bias,[29] the progestin components in third-generation oral contraceptives have also been associated with a slightly increased thrombotic risk in comparison to other formulations. Pharmacologic doses of estrogen, such as those used for suppression of lactation have similarly been associated with an increased risk of thromboembolism. Although estrogen doses used for postmenopausal replacement therapy are approximately one-sixth those in oral contraceptives, recent data supports an increased thromboembolic risk at these doses as well. However, the risk of replacement therapy must be kept in perspective, as it contributes only approximately two new cases of venous thromboembolism per 10 000 women per year.[30]

Pregnancy

Venous thromboembolism is second only to abortion as leading causes of death associated with pregnancy. The increased thrombotic risk associated with pregnancy has been attributed to an acquired prethrombotic state in combination with impaired venous outflow due to uterine compression. Population-based studies performed since the introduction of venous ultrasound suggest an incidence of 0.75 per 1000 deliveries.[31] The risk of postpartum DVT is thought to be two- to threefold higher than that during pregnancy. Other concurrent risk factors, notably documented hypercoagulable states including the factor V Leiden mutation, suppression of lactation, increased maternal age, and assisted delivery, are associated with an increase thrombotic risk.

Other risk factors

Although lacking the strong epidemiologic support of the above factors, a number of other circumstances have been consistently associated with an increased incidence of deep venous thrombosis. These include central venous instrumentation, antiphospholipid antibodies, and inflammatory bowel disease. Other risk factors such as obesity, varicose veins, myocardial infarction, and congestive heart failure have been inconsistently identified as independent risk factors for acute DVT.[15] Many studies examining these conditions have been performed in high-risk inpatients with other risk factors for DVT, making an independent association difficult to establish.

THE NATURAL HISTORY OF ACUTE DVT

Lower extremity thrombi originate in areas where imbalanced coagulation is localized by stasis – in the soleal sinuses, behind venous valve pockets and at venous confluences. The calf veins are the most common site of origin, although 40% of proximal thrombi arise primarily in the femoral or iliac veins, presumably in the regions behind the valves.[32] In flow models, vortices produced beyond the valve cusps tend to trap red cells in a low shear field near the apex of the cusp.[33] Red cell aggregates forming within these eddies are likely the early niduses for thrombus formation.[34] However, such aggregates are probably transient until stabilized by fibrin in the setting of locally activated coagulation. After their formation, these early thrombi may become anchored to the endothelium near the apex of the valve cusp,[35,36] a process postulated to be mediated by adherent leukocytes.[5]

Propagation of thrombi beyond areas of stasis probably depends largely on the relative balance between activated coagulation and thrombolysis. If local conditions favor propagation, laminated appositional growth occurs outward from the apex as platelets are surrounded by a red cell, fibrin, and leukocyte network. In contrast to arterial thrombi, venous thrombi are composed largely of red cells and fibrin with relatively few platelets and leukocytes. Once luminal flow is disturbed, prograde and retrograde propagation may also be promoted by hemodynamic factors. Conversely, such early thrombi may fail to propagate, aborted thrombi appearing as endothelialized fibrin fragments within the valve pockets.

The competing processes of recanalization and recurrent thrombosis determine the further natural history of acute DVT. The venous lumen is most often re-established after both experimental and clinical thrombosis,[37] although the primary process responsible for this and nomenclature to be employed remains the subject of debate. Often referred to interchangeably as recanalization or spontaneous lysis, this is actually a complex series of both cellular and humoral processes. The ultimate outcome, with respect to both luminal patency and chronic sequelae, is determined by the balance between organization, thrombolysis, propagation, and re-thrombosis.

The mechanisms of organization and recanalization have been extensively investigated in animal models of DVT. Both the vein wall and thrombus play important roles in these processes. The endothelium has traditionally been considered the primary source of tissue plasminogen activator (t-PA) and there is a global increase in the fibrinolytic activity of distant veins after DVT.[37,38] Furthermore, although evidence suggests that the endothelium underlying a thrombus initially disappears, rapid regeneration of a fibrinolytically active neoendothelium soon occurs.[38,39] However, the activation of plasminogen intrinsic to the thrombus appears to be quantitatively more important than systemically activated extrinsic fibrinolysis.[39] An early neutrophilic infiltrate appears within the thrombus followed by a predominantly monocyte infiltrate by day 8.[40] A similar tumor necrosis factor (TNF)-mediated inflammatory response occurs in the vein wall, an early neutrophil infiltrate being replaced by monocytes.[41] Monocytes may play a particularly important role in thrombus organization and recanalization, functioning as a source of both fibrinolytic and cytokine mediators. Thrombus-associated monocytes appear to be the primary source of t-PA as well as urokinase-type plasminogen activator (u-PA) and may also direct cytokine-mediated neovascularization of the thrombus.[39,40] Although the mechanism is not entirely clear, monocyte chemotactic protein-1 (MCP-1) has been shown to significantly accelerate thrombus resolution.[42] Experimental thrombi show complete recanalization by 3 weeks, with the thrombus reduced to an endothelialized subintimal streak.

Although less extensively investigated, histologic studies suggest that human thrombi follow a similar course. As in the animal models, recanalization appears to be a complex process involving a combination of both intrinsic and extrinsic fibrinolysis, peripheral fragmentation, neovascularization and retraction. Thrombus organization begins in the attachment zone with the migration of surfacing cells, presumably arising from the endothelium, over the thrombus.[35] Pockets formed between the thrombus and the vein walls then progressively enlarge through peripheral fragmentation and fibrinolysis. Some[43] have found thrombus resolution in humans to be associated with early and sustained increases in plasma t-

PA activity, whilst others[44] have found PAI-1 levels at presentation to be significantly higher in patients with poor thrombus resolution at 6 months. The thrombus simultaneously undergoes central softening as well as contraction. In the absence of propagation, the ultimate result is a restored venous lumen with a slightly raised fibroelastic plaque at the site of initial thrombus adherence to the vein wall.

The development of noninvasive diagnostic tests, permitting venous thrombi to be serially followed, has confirmed the clinical importance of these processes. Impedance plethysmography was the first widely available test for the serial evaluation of venous outflow obstruction due to an acute DVT. Although unable to distinguish between recanalization and development of collateral venous outflow, such studies were found to normalize in 67% of patients by 3 months and 92% of patients by 9 months.[45] Duplex ultrasonography, with its ability to localize flow to specific venous segments, has advanced these observations and confirmed the importance of recanalization. Among 21 patients prospectively followed with ultrasound, Killewich[43] noted that some recanalization was present by 7 days in 44% of patients and by 90 days in 100% of patients (Fig. 4.1). The percentage of initially involved segments that remained occluded decreased to a mean of 44% by 30 days and 14% by 90 days (Fig. 4.2). Van Ramshorst *et al.*[46] similarly noted an exponential decrease in thrombus load over the first 6 months after femoropopliteal thrombosis. Most recanalization occurred within the first 6 weeks, with flow re-established in 87% of 23 completely occluded segments during this interval. Using a somewhat different approach, measuring thrombus thickness when maximally compressed, Prandoni and colleagues[47] noted the most significant reduction in thrombus mass over the first 3 months after thrombosis – 62% in the common femoral vein and 50% in the popliteal vein.

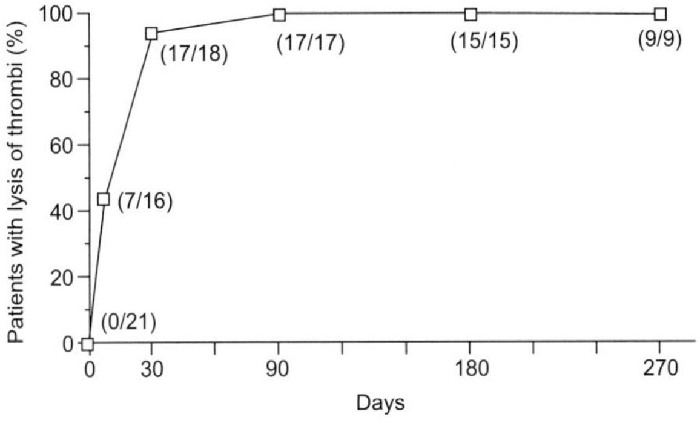

Figure 4.1 *Rate of recanalization among 21 patients followed with serial ultrasonography. Percent of patients with lysis in any originally occluded segment. Numbers in parentheses represent the proportion of patients with lysis at each interval. (Reproduced with permission from Killewich LA, Bedford GR, Beach KW, Strandness DE. Spontaneous lysis of deep venous thrombi: rate and outcome.* J Vasc Surg *1989;* ***9****: 89–97)*

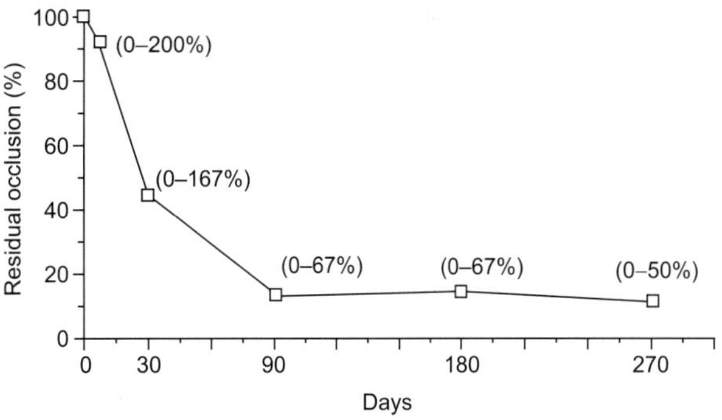

Figure 4.2 *Mean percentage of initially occluded segments remaining occluded at follow-up among 21 patients with acute DVT (percentage residual occlusion = number of segments occluded at follow-up/number of segments occluded at presentation). Numbers in parentheses are the ranges for individual cases, with numbers greater than 100% indicating extension of the initial thrombus. (Reproduced with permission from Killewich LA, Bedford GR, Beach KW, Strandness DE. Spontaneous lysis of deep venous thrombi: rate and outcome.* J Vasc Surg *1989;* ***9****: 89–97)*

Although thrombus resolution appears to proceed at a similar rate in the proximal venous segments,[46] some[48] have found more rapid clearance from the tibial segments, perhaps reflecting the increased efficiency of thrombolysis in small veins. As in animal studies, these clinical observations suggest that recanalization begins early after an episode of acute DVT, with the majority of thrombus regression occurring within the first 3 months after the event. Approximately 55% of subjects will show complete recanalization within 6–9 months of thrombosis.[43,44] However, some reduction in thrombus load may continue, albeit at a slower rate, for months to years after the acute event.

Recurrent thrombotic events compete with recanalization early after an acute DVT. Most clinical studies have included both symptomatic recurrent DVT and pulmonary embolism, with rates depending on treatment, proximal or distal location of thrombus, and duration of follow-up. Among patients with proximal DVT, recurrent thromboembolic events have been reported in 5.2% of patients treated with standard anticoagulation measures for 3 months[49] in comparison with 47% of patients inadequately treated with a 3-month course of low-dose subcutaneous heparin.[50] Sarasin and Bounameaux[51] calculated a theoretical recurrence rate of 0.9% per month after discontinuing anticoagulant therapy for proximal DVT, whilst others[27] have noted a 13% cumulative incidence of symptomatic recurrent thromboembolism 5 years after diagnosis. In patients with isolated calf vein thrombosis, proximal propagation occurred in 23% of untreated patients and 10% of patients treated with only intravenous heparin.[52]

However, since most episodes are asymptomatic, noninvasive natural history studies have also been important in defining the true incidence of recurrent thrombotic events. Serial duplex studies have shown propagation of thrombus in 26–38% of treated patients within the first few weeks after presentation (Fig. 4.3).[53,54] In a larger series of 177 patients followed for a median of 9.3 months, recurrent thrombotic events were observed in 52% of patients.[55] Among initially involved extremities, propagation to new segments occurred in 30% and rethrombosis of a partially occluded or recanalized segment in 31%. New thrombi were also observed in 6% of initially uninvolved contralateral extremities. Although these events have not been associated with identifiable clinical risk factors, they are related to the adequacy of anticoagulation. Several clinical trials have demonstrated failure to achieve an activated partial thromboplastin time (aPTT) 1.5 times the control value within 24 hours to be associated with a significantly higher risk of recurrent thrombosis. Others[54] have shown a 1.4-fold increase in the risk of new thrombotic events for each 20% reduction in the time that anticoagulation is adequate according to standard laboratory measures.

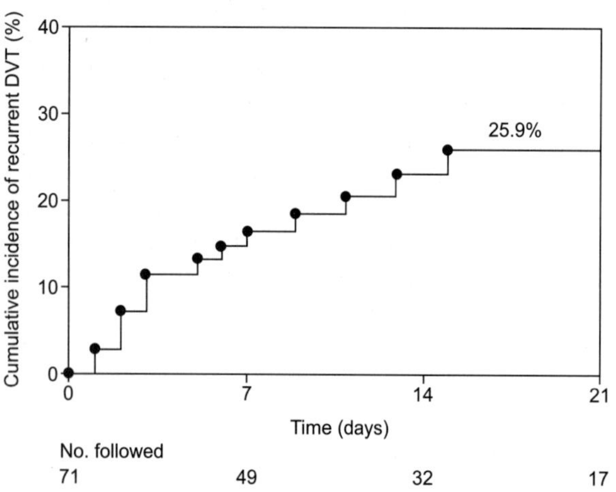

Figure 4.3 *Cumulative incidence of ultrasound documented recurrent thrombotic events during the first 3 weeks of therapy. (Reproduced with permission from Caps MT, Meissner MH, Tullis MJ,* et al. *Venous thrombus stability during acute phase of therapy.* Vasc Med *1999; 4: 9–14)*

COMPLICATIONS OF ACUTE DVT

Pulmonary embolism

The potentially life-threatening consequences of pulmonary embolism make it the most important short-term complication of acute DVT. Diagnosed pulmonary embolism accompanies approximately 10% of deep venous thromboses[27] and an incidence of 23 per 100 000 population has been reported based on hospital discharge data.[2] Extrapolated to the population of the USA, this would correspond to an incidence of 55 000 initial diagnoses of pulmonary embolism per year. Mathematical estimates, based on a number of assumptions, have yielded a substantially higher incidence of 630 000 cases per year in the USA.[56]

However, respiratory symptoms correlate poorly with the presence or absence of objectively documented pulmonary embolism and as many as 75% of pulmonary emboli may be asymptomatic.[57,58] Routine diagnostic testing suggests that pulmonary embolism accompanies acute DVT much more frequently than appreciated. As many as 25–52% patients with documented DVT but no symptoms of pulmonary embolism will have high-probability lung scans at presentation.[57–60] Although regarded as an unusual source of symptomatic pulmonary embolism, high-probability scans have also been noted in 18–29% of patients with isolated calf vein thrombosis. The high incidence of asymptomatic pulmonary embolism suggests that DVT and pulmonary embolism are, indeed, a 'pathophysiologic continuum'.[59]

The post-thrombotic syndrome

The post-thrombotic syndrome is the most common late complication of acute DVT, with as many as two-thirds of patients developing symptoms of pain, edema, hyperpigmentation, or ulceration. Although some post-thrombotic symptoms may be present in 29–79% of patients, severe manifestations and ulceration occur in only 7–23% and 4–6% of patients respectively.[61–65] Population-based studies have suggested that skin changes and ulceration are present in 6–7 million and 400 000–500 000 people in the USA, respectively.[1] In addition to the substantial economic costs, the physical limitations of patients with post-thrombotic symptoms are comparable to those of patients with other serious chronic medical conditions.[27]

REFLUX, OBSTRUCTION AND THE POST-THROMBOTIC SYNDROME

Ambulatory venous hypertension, resulting from a combination of venous reflux and persistent venous obstruction, is the hemodynamic mechanism underlying the more severe post-thrombotic sequelae. Valvular incompetence appears to be clinically more important, symptoms correlating more closely with a reduction in venous refilling time than with residual abnormalities of venous outflow.[66] However, limbs developing edema, hyperpigmentation, or ulceration are more likely to have a combination of reflux and residual obstruction than either abnormality alone (Fig. 4.4).[67] In addition to its direct effects on ambulatory venous pressure, obstruction may indirectly contribute to the development of reflux. Although the majority of incompetent venous segments have been rendered so by the presence of thrombus, as

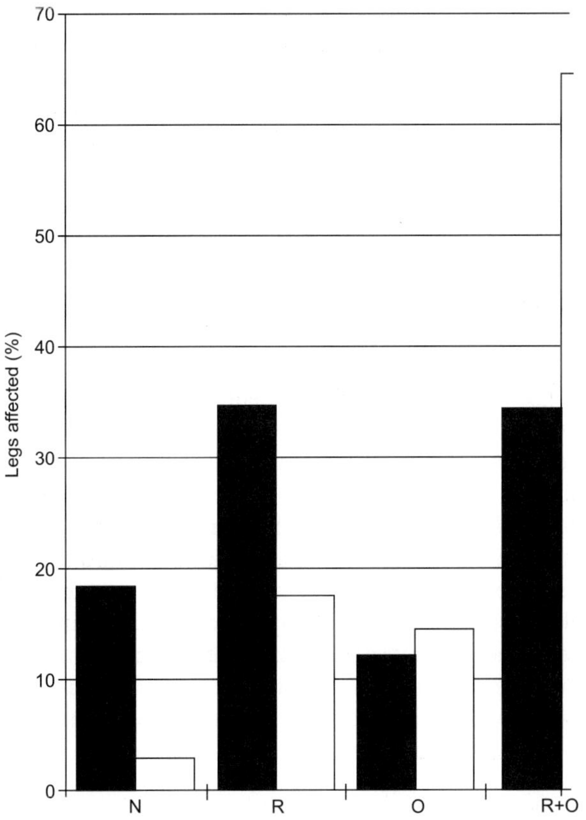

Figure 4.4 *Proportion of limbs demonstrating no abnormality (N), reflux alone (R), obstruction alone (O), and reflux with obstruction (R+O) after DVT with respect to symptoms. Dark bars indicate asymptomatic legs; white bars indicate legs with post-thrombotic symptoms. (Reproduced with permission from Johnson BF, Manzo RA, Bergelin RO, Strandness DE. Relationship between changes in the deep venous system and the development of postthrombotic syndrome after an acute episode of lower limb deep vein thrombosis: a one- to six-year follow-up.* J Vasc Surg *1995;* ***21****: 307–313)*

many as 30% of segments developing reflux during follow-up have not been previously thrombosed.[68] Although the precise mechanism remains unclear, reflux in these initially uninvolved segments may be related to persistent proximal obstruction. There may therefore be at least two different mechanisms by which reflux develops – a more common mechanism related to recanalization of a thrombosed segment and a less common mechanism related to proximal obstruction of uninvolved segments. The risk of developing reflux in segments involved by thrombus is almost three times that in uninvolved segments.[68]

Although experimentally produced thrombi frequently recanalize to produce a patent but valveless lumen, valvular destruction is not a universal consequence of clinical DVT. As many as one-third of patients may remain free of chronic symptoms after an episode of acute DVT and only 69% of extremities show evidence of reflux by duplex ultrasonography one year after the event.[69] The incidence of reflux in individual venous segments is even lower, with only 33–59% of involved segments becoming incompetent.

Histologic examination of the consequences of thrombosis provides some explanation for the differential development of reflux after DVT. In extremities with established post-thrombotic syndrome, approximately 50% of popliteal valves will demonstrate thrombus formation on the valve leaflets, whilst others show endothelial erosion with basement membrane thickening and atypical subintimal collagen fibers.[70] However, most episodes of acute DVT are not associated with such extensive histologic changes. In contrast to the observations in patients with established post-thrombotic syndrome, early fibrocellular organization after an acute DVT rarely involves the valve cusps.[35,71] Thrombus adherence to the valve cusp was noted in only 4 of 44 specimens examined by Sevitt.[71] In the majority of cases, the thrombus was separated from the valve cusp by a cleft postulated to arise from the local fibrinolytic activity of the valvular endothelium. These observations are consistent with the intense plasminogen activator activity associated with the venous valve cusps and may act to preserve some valves during recanalization.

These histologic observations are consistent with the natural history of valvular reflux. Serial duplex studies have shown the development of reflux to coincide with or slightly precede complete recanalization of a segment.[48] As with recanalization, the rate at which reflux develops is highest during the first 6–12 months after DVT.[68] Reflux may be transient in up to 23% of involved segments, resolving during the course of follow-up.[68] This phenomenon conceivably occurs when valves protected by the lytic clefts described above remain partially encumbered by residual thrombus. Normal valvular function then presumably returns with complete recanalization.

DETERMINANTS OF THE POST-THROMBOTIC SYNDROME

As the treatment options for the prevention of post-thrombotic syndrome expand to include adjuncts such as thrombolytic therapy, compression stockings and various surgical procedures, an appreciation of the factors involved in the development of these sequelae becomes important. Most investigators have not found a clear relationship between the initial extent of thrombus and ultimate outcome. However, other potential determinants of post-thrombotic manifestations include the rate of recanalization, recurrent thrombotic events, the global extent of reflux and the anatomic distribution of reflux and obstruction.

The application of thrombolytic therapy to acute DVT would appear an ideal model for examining the relationship between the rate of recanalization and ultimate valve function. Unfortunately, although thrombolytic therapy clearly has the ability to restore a patent lumen, implications for preservation of valve function are limited by the absence of well-controlled follow-up studies. Other evidence does, however, suggest a relationship between early recanalization and valve function. In the long-term ultrasound follow-up of 113 patients with an acute DVT, the majority of whom were treated with standard anticoagulation measures, the time to complete recanalization was related to the ultimate development of reflux.[48] Depending upon the venous segment involved, complete recanalization required 2.3–7.3 times longer in segments developing reflux than in segments in which valve function was preserved (Fig. 4.5).

Although routine use of venous thrombolytic therapy awaits further clinical trials, there is evidence that the adequacy of anticoagulation may influence the rate of recanalization. Among patients treated with a 6-month course of warfarin, complete resolution of thrombus was significantly associated with an INR (international normalized ratio) in the therapeutic range during follow-up.[72] There is also early, suggestive evidence that thrombus resolution may proceed at a more rapid rate during treatment with low molecular weight heparin in comparison with warfarin. Although the mechanism underlying the association between the level of anticoagulation and recanalization has not been established, it may relate to the prevention of recurrent thrombotic events.

Recurrent thrombotic events also have a detrimental effect on valvular competence and development of the post-thrombotic syndrome. Extension of thrombus to initially uninvolved segments obviously places these segments at risk for valvular destruction. Re-thrombosis of a partially occluded or recanalized segment further increases the risk of reflux.[55] Reflux has been noted to develop in 36–73% of such segments, considerably higher than the incidence in segments without re-thrombosis (Fig. 4.6). Consistent with these observations, recurrent thrombotic events have been noted in 45% of patients with post-thrombotic symptoms in comparison with only 17% of asymptomatic subjects.[27] Others have reported the risk of post-thrombotic syndrome to be six times greater among patients with recurrent thrombosis.[63]

Factors important in the development of recurrent venous thrombosis may include the adequacy of anticoagulation as well as abnormalities of the fibrinolytic and coagulation systems. A relationship between impaired fibrinolysis and recurrent DVT has been suggested by several investigators, although the methodological validity of these findings has been questioned.[73] It is also conceivable that fibrinolytic deficiencies could contribute to the development of reflux by prolonging lysis times or failing to prevent early thrombus adherence to the valve cusp. Recognized thrombophilic states, particularly the factor V Leiden mutation,[74] lupus anticoagulant[75] and homocysteinemia,[76] may also be associated with recurrent thromboembolic events.

The development of clinical signs and symptoms is also related to the global extent of reflux[77] and the anatomic distribution of reflux and obstruction. Reflux in the distal deep venous segments, particularly the popliteal and posterior tibial veins, is most significantly associated with post-thrombotic skin changes.[78–80]

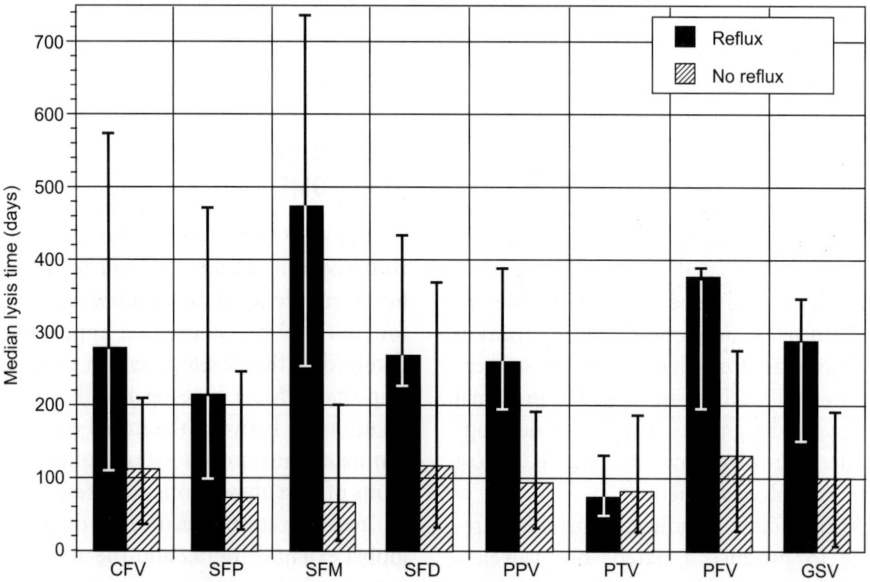

Figure 4.5 *Median time from thrombosis to complete recanalization, grouped according to ultimate reflux status. Error bars denote interquartile range. Segments: common femoral vein (CFV), proximal superficial femoral vein (SFP), mid-superficial femoral vein (SFM), distal superficial femoral vein (SFD), popliteal vein (PPV), posterior tibial vein (PTV), profunda femoris vein (PFV), and greater saphenous vein (GSV). (Reproduced with permission from Meissner MH, Manzo RA, Bergelin, RO, Markel A, Strandness DE. Deep venous insufficiency: the relationship between lysis and subsequent reflux.* J Vasc Surg *1993;* ***18****: 596–608)*

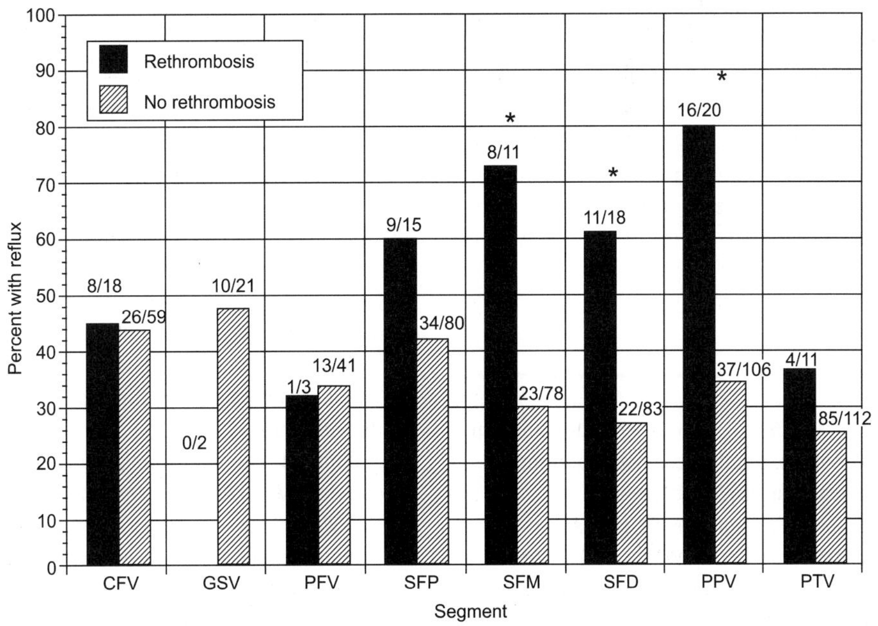

Figure 4.6 *The development of reflux in initially involved venous segments with and without subsequent re-thrombosis. Numbers above bars indicate the number of segments in which reflux was observed over the number of segments in which reflux could be definitively assessed. Differences between segments with and without re-thrombosis are statistically significant (**P <0.005*) for the SFM, SFD, and PPV segments. (Reproduced with permission from Meissner MH, Caps MT, Bergelin RO, Manzo RA, Strandness DE. Propagation, rethrombosis, and new thrombus formation after acute deep venous thrombosis.* J Vasc Surg *1995;* ***22****: 558–67)*

However, associated superficial reflux has been reported in 84–94% of patients with chronic skin changes and 60–100% of patients with venous ulceration. Although pressure transmission through incompetent perforating veins may play a role, direct thrombotic involvement of the superficial veins and thrombus-independent degenerative processes also appear important in the development of superficial venous incompetence.[81] With respect to venous obstruction, the severity of post-thrombotic manifestations is most significantly related to persistent popliteal thrombosis.[77]

Mortality after acute DVT

Many investigators have noted that mortality after an episode of acute DVT exceeds that expected in an age-matched population. Excess mortality is likely due to the frequency of co-morbid medical conditions. Although the in-hospital case-fatality rate for DVT is only 5%, 3- and 5-year mortality rates of 30% and 39%, respectively have been noted.[2,27] Most deaths are related to malignancy or cardiovascular disease.

CLINICAL APPLICATIONS OF NATURAL HISTORY STUDIES

Although many questions remain, these natural history studies have some application to the clinical management of acute DVT. It is perhaps valuable to view an episode of acute DVT as a dynamic balance between recanalization and recurrent venous thrombosis, with the most dramatic changes occurring over the first 3–6 months after presentation. Both these processes effect ultimate valve function and long-term outcome. This is important since some measures are available to alter their outcomes. With respect to recanalization, the rate at which this proceeds is a determinant of ultimate valve function and thrombolytic therapy potentially has a role in promoting rapid and complete recanalization in at least some patients. These considerations must, however, be qualified, since no well designed randomized study exists to prove that thrombolytic therapy preserves valve function and reduces the incidence of the post-thrombotic syndrome. Ensuring an adequate duration and intensity of anticoagulation is critical in preventing recurrent thrombosis. The incidence of recurrent thromboembolic events is 15 times higher among patients with inadequate early anticoagulation.[49] Determining the optimal duration of anticoagulation is more difficult, since most theoretical models are necessarily based on balancing the life-threatening risks of pulmonary embolism and hemorrhage rather than the long-term morbidity of the post-thrombotic syndrome. Although a shorter course may be acceptable in patients with reversible risk factors, the incidence of recurrent thromboembolism may be as high as 27.4% per patient-year in patients with idiopathic thrombosis and such patients warrant more protracted anticoagulation.[75] Finally, it appears the risk of post-thrombotic sequelae may be predicted in at least some patients. Certain anatomic patterns of reflux, particularly those involving the popliteal and posterior tibial veins as well as the superficial veins, appear to be associated with a higher incidence of the post-thrombotic syndrome. These patients may warrant particular attention to the use of adjunctive measures such as compression stockings.

REFERENCES

1. Coon WW, Willis PW, Keller JB. Venous thromboembolism and other venous disease in the Tecumseh Community Health Study. *Circulation* 1973; **48**: 839–46.
2. Anderson FA, Wheeler HB, Goldberg RJ, *et al.* A population-based perspective of the hospital incidence and case-fatality rates of deep vein thrombosis and pulmonary embolism. *Arch Intern Med* 1991; **151**: 933–8.
3. Thomas DP, Merton RE, Wood RD, Hockley DJ. The relationship between vessel wall injury and venous thrombosis: an experimental study. *Br J Haematol* 1985; **59**: 449–57.
4. Schaub RG, Simmons CA, Koets MH, *et al.* Early events in the formation of a venous thrombus following local trauma and stasis. *Lab Invest* **51**: 218–24.
5. Stewart GJ. Neutrophils and deep venous thrombosis. *Haemostasis* 1993; **23**(Suppl 1): 127–40.
6. Nawroth PP, Handley DA, Esmon CT, Stern DM. Interleukin 1 induces endothelial cell procoagulant while suppressing cell-surface anticoagulant activity. *Proc Natl Acad Sci U S A* 1986; **83**: 3460–4.
7. Aronson DL, Thomas DP. Experimental studies on venous thrombosis: effect of coagulants, procoagulants and vessel contusion. *Thromb Haemost* 1985; **54**: 866–70.
8. Thomas DP, Merton RE, Hockley DJ. The effect of stasis on the venous endothelium: an ultrastructural study. *Br J Haematol* 1983; **55**: 113–22.
9. Lawson CA, Yan SD, Yan SF, *et al.* Monocytes and tissue factor promote thrombosis in a murine model of oxygen deprivation. *J Clin Invest* 1997; **99**: 1729–38.
10. Amiral J, Fareed J. Thromboembolic diseases: biochemical mechanisms and new possibilities of biological diagnosis. *Semin Thromb Hemost* 1996; **22**: 41–8.
11. Nordstrom M, Lindblad B, Bergqvist D, Kjelstrom T. A prospective study of the incidence of deep-vein thrombosis within a defined urban population. *J Intern Med* 1992; **232**: 155–60.
12. Rosendaal FR. Venous thrombosis: a multicausal disease. *Lancet* 1999; **353**: 1167–73.
13. Oger E, Leroyer C, Le Moigne E, *et al.* The value of risk factor analysis in clinically suspected deep venous thrombosis. *Respiration* 1997; **64**: 326–30.
14. Anderson FA, Wheeler HB, Goldberg RJ, *et al.* The prevalence of risk factors for venous thromboembolism among hospital patients. *Arch Intern Med* 1992; **152**: 1660–4.
15. Meissner MH, Strandness DE. Pathophysiology and natural history of deep venous thrombosis. In Rutherford RB, ed. *Vascular Surgery*, 5th edn. Philadelphia: WB Saunders, 2000: 1920–37.
16. Kniffen WD, Baron JA, Barrett J, *et al.* The epidemiology of diagnosed pulmonary embolism and deep venous thrombosis in the elderly. *Arch Intern Med* 1994; **154**: 861–6.
17. Thomas WA, Davies JNP, O'Neal RM, Dimakaulangan AA. Incidence of myocardial infarction correlated with venous and pulmonary thrombosis and embolism. *Am J Cardiol* 1960; **5**: 41–7.
18. Gillum RF. Pulmonary embolism and thrombophlebitis in the USA, 1970–1985. *Am Heart J* 1987; **114**: 1262–4.
19. Chumnijarakij T, Poshyachinda V. Postoperative thrombosis in Thai women. *Lancet* 1975; **1**: 1357–8.
20. Joffe SN. Racial incidence of postoperative deep vein thrombosis in South Africa. *Br J Surg* 1974; **61**: 982–3.
21. Hooper WC, Dilley A, Ribeiro MJ, *et al.* A racial difference in the prevalence of the Arg506→Gln mutation. *Thromb Res* 1996; **81**: 577–81.
22. Rees DC, Cox M, Clegg JB. World distribution of factor V Leiden. *Lancet* 1995; **346**: 1133–4.
23. Hull RD, Raskob GE, Hirsh J. Prophylaxis of venous thromboembolism. An overview. *Chest* 1986; **89**: 374S–83S.
24. Meissner MH. Deep venous thrombosis in the trauma patient. *Semin Vasc Surg* 1998; **11**: 274–82.
25. Gibbs NM. Venous thrombosis of the lower limbs with particular reference to bed rest. *Br J Surg* 1957; **45**: 209–36.
26. Ferrari E, Chevallier T, Chapelier A, Baudouy M. Travel as a risk factor for venous thromboembolic disease: a case–control study. *Chest* 1999; **115**: 440–4.
27. Beyth RJ, Cohen AM, Landefeld CS. Long-term outcome of deep-vein thrombosis. *Arch Intern Med* 1995; **155**: 1031–7.
28. Koster T, Small R-A, Rosendaal FR, Helmerhorst FM. Oral contraceptives and venous thromboembolism: a quantitative discussion of the uncertainties. *J Intern Med* 1995; **238**: 31–7.
29. Lewis MA. The epidemiology of oral contraceptive use: a critical review of the studies on oral contraceptives and the health of young women. *Am J Obstet Gynecol* 1998; **179**: 1086–97.
30. Perez Gutthann S, Garcia Rodriguez LA, Castellsague J, Duque Oliart A. Hormone replacement therapy and risk of venous thromboembolism: population based case-control study. *Br Med J* 1997; **314**: 796–800.
31. Andersen BS, Steffensen FH, Sorensen HT, *et al.* The cumulative incidence of venous thromboembolism during pregnancy and puerperium – an 11 year Danish population-based study of 63,300 pregnancies. *Acta Obstet Gynecol* 1998; **77**: 170–3.

32. Browse NL, Thomas ML. Source of non-lethal pulmonary emboli. *Lancet* 1974; **1**: 258–9.
33. Karino T, Motomiya M. Flow through a venous valve and its implications for thrombus formation. *Thromb Res* 1984; **36**: 245–57.
34. Quarmby J, Smith A, Collins M, *et al.* A model of in vivo human venous thrombosis that confirms changes in the release of specific soluble adhesion molecules in experimental venous thrombogenesis. *J Vasc Surg* 1999; **30**: 139–47.
35. Sevitt S. Organization of valve pocket thrombi and the anomalies of double thrombi and valve cusp involvement. *Br J Surg* 1974; **61**: 641–9.
36. Sevitt S. The structure and growth of valve-pocket thrombi in femoral veins. *J Clin Pathol* 1974; **27**: 517–28.
37. Northeast AD, Soo KS, Bobrow LG, *et al.* The tissue plasminogen activator and urokinase response in vivo during natural resolution of venous thrombus. *J Vasc Surg* 1995; **22**: 573–9.
38. Northeast AD, Burnand KG. The response of the vessel wall to thrombosis: the in vivo study of venous thrombolysis. *Ann N Y Acad Sci* 1992; **667**: 127–40.
39. Soo KS, Northeast AD, Happerfield LC, *et al.* Tissue plasminogen activator production by monocytes in venous thrombolysis. *J Pathol* 1996; **178**: 190–4.
40. Wakefield TW, Linn MJ, Henke PK, *et al.* Neo-vascularization during venous thrombus organization: a preliminary study. *J Vasc Surg* 1999; **30**: 885–93.
41. Wakefield TW, Strieter RM, Wilke CA, *et al.* Venous thrombosis-associated inflammation and attenuation with neutralizing antibodies to cytokines and adhesion molecules. *Arterioscler Thromb Vasc Biol* 1995; **15**: 258–68.
42. Humphries J, McGuiness CL, Smith A, *et al.* Monocyte chemotactic protein-1 (MCP-1) accelerates the organization and resolution of venous thrombi. *J Vasc Surg* 1999; **30**: 894–900.
43. Killewich LA, Macko RF, Cox K, *et al.* Regression of proximal deep venous thrombosis is associated with fibrinolytic enhancement. *J Vasc Surg* 1997; **26**: 861–8.
44. Arcelus JI, Caprini JA, Hoffman KN, *et al.* Laboratory assays and duplex scanning outcomes after symptomatic deep vein thrombosis: preliminary results. *J Vasc Surg* 1996; **23**: 616–21.
45. Huisman MV, Buller HR, ten Cate JW. Utility of impedence plethymography in the diagnosis of recurrent deep-vein thrombosis. *Arch Intern Med* 1988; **148**: 681–3.
46. van Ramshorst B, van Bemmelen PS, Honeveld H, *et al.* Thrombus regression in deep venous thrombosis. Quantification of spontaneous thrombolysis with duplex scanning. *Circulation* 1992; **86**: 414–19.
47. Prandoni P, Cogo A, Bernardi E, *et al.* A simple ultrasound approach for detection of recurrent proximal vein thrombosis. *Circulation* 1993; **88**: 1730–5.
48. Meissner MH, Manzo RA, Bergelin RO, *et al.* Deep venous insufficiency: the relationship between lysis and subsequent reflux. *J Vasc Surg* 1993; **18**: 596–608.
49. Hull RD, Raskob GE, Hirsch J, *et al.* Continuous intravenous heparin compared with intermittent subcutaneous heparin in the initial treatment of proximal-vein thrombosis. *N Engl J Med* 1986; **315**: 1109–14.
50. Hull R, Delmore T, Genton E, *et al.* Warfarin sodium versus low-dose heparin in the treatment of venous thrombosis. *N Engl J Med* 1979; **301**: 855–8.
51. Sarasin FP, Bounameaux H. Duration of oral anticoagulant therapy after proximal deep vein thrombosis: a decision analysis. *Thromb Haemost* 1994; **71**: 286–91.
52. Philbrick JT, Becker DM. Calf deep venous thrombosis. A wolf in sheep's clothing? *Arch Intern Med* 1988; **148**: 2131–8.
53. Krupski WC, Bass A, Dilley RB, *et al.* Propagation of deep venous thrombosis by duplex ultrasonography. *J Vasc Surg* 1990; **12**: 467–75.
54. Caps MT, Meissner MH, Tullis MJ, *et al.* Venous thrombus stability during the acute phase of therapy. *Vasc Med* 1999; **4**: 9–14.
55. Meissner MH, Caps MT, Bergelin RO, *et al.* Propagation, rethrombosis, and new thrombus formation after acute deep venous thrombosis. *J Vasc Surg* 1995; **22**: 558–67.
56. Dalen JE, Alpert JS. Natural history of pulmonary embolism. *Prog Cardiovasc Dis* 1975; **17**: 259–70.
57. Kistner R, Ball J, Nordyke R, Freeman G. Incidence of pulmonary embolism in the course of thrombophlebitis of the lower extremities. *Am J Surg* 1972; **124**: 169–76.
58. Plate G, Ohlin P, Eklof B. Pulmonary embolism in acute ileofemoral venous thrombosis. *Br J Surg* 1985; **72**: 912–15.
59. Huisman MV, Buller HR, ten Cate JW, *et al.* Unexpected high prevalence of silent pulmonary embolism in patients with deep venous thrombosis. *Chest* 1989; **95**: 498–502.
60. Monreal M, Barroso R-J, Ruiz Manzano J, *et al.* Asymptomatic pulmonary embolism in patients with deep vein thrombosis. Is it useful to take a lung scan to rule out this condition? *J Cardiovasc Surg* 1989; **30**: 104–7.
61. Monreal M, Martorell A, Callejas J, *et al.* Venographic assessment of deep vein thrombosis and risk of developing post-thrombotic syndrome: a prospective trial. *J Intern Med* 1993; **233**: 233–8.
62. Strandness DE, Langlois Y, Cramer M, *et al.* Long-term sequelae of acute venous thrombosis. *J Am Med Assoc* 1983; **250**: 1289–92.
63. Prandoni P, Lensing A, Cogo A, *et al.* The long term clinical course of acute deep venous thrombosis. *Ann Intern Med* 1996 **125**: 1–7.
64. Prandoni P, Villalta S, Polistena P, *et al.* Symptomatic deep-vein thrombosis and the post-thrombotic syndrome. *Haematologica* 1995; **80**: 42–8.
65. Lindner DJ, Edwards JM, Phinney ES, *et al.* Long-term hemodynamic and clinical sequelae of lower extremity deep vein thrombosis. *J Vasc Surg* 1986; **4**: 436–42.

66. Killewich LA, Martin R, Cramer M, *et al.* An objective assessment of the physiological changes in the postthrombotic syndrome. *Arch Surg* 1985; **120**: 424–6.
67. Johnson BF, Manzo RA, Bergelin RO, Strandness DE. Relationship between changes in the deep venous system and the development of the postthrombotic syndrome after an acute episode of lower limb deep vein thrombosis: a one- to six- year follow-up. *J Vasc Surg* 1995; **21**: 307–13.
68. Caps MT, Manzo RA, Bergelin RO, *et al.* Venous valvular reflux in veins not involved at the time of acute deep vein thrombosis. *J Vasc Surg* 1995; **22**: 524–31.
69. Markel A, Manzo RA, Bergelin RO, Strandness DE. Valvular reflux after deep vein thrombosis: incidence and time of occurrence. *J Vasc Surg* 1992; **15**: 377–84.
70. Budd TW, Meenaghan MA, Wirth J, Taheri SA. Histopathology of veins and venous valves of patients with venous insufficiency syndrome: ultrastructure. *J Med* 1990; **21**: 181–99.
71. Sevitt S. The mechanisms of canalisation in deep vein thrombosis. *J Pathol* 1973; **110**: 153–65.
72. Caprini JA, Arcelus JI, Reyna JJ, *et al.* Deep vein thrombosis outcome and the level of oral anticoagulation therapy. *J Vasc Surg* 1999; **30**: 805–12.
73. Prins MH, Hirsch J. A critical review of the evidence supporting a relationship between impaired fibrinolytic activity and venous thromboembolism. *Arch Intern Med* 1991; **151**: 1721–31.
74. Simioni P, Prandoni P, Lensing AW, *et al.* The risk of recurrent venous thromboembolism in patients with an Arg506→Gln mutation in the gene for factor V (factor V Leiden). *N Engl J Med* 1997; **336**: 399–403.
75. Kearon C, Gent M, Hirsh J, *et al.* A comparison of three months of anticoagulation with extended anticoagulation for a first episode of idiopathic venous thromboembolism. *N Engl J Med* 1999; **340**: 901–7.
76. den Heijer M, Blom HJ, Gerrits WB, *et al.* Is hyperhomocysteinaemia a risk factor for recurrent venous thrombosis? *Lancet* 1995; **345**: 882–5.
77. Meissner MH, Caps MT, Zierler BK, *et al.* Determinants of chronic venous disease after acute deep venous thrombosis. *J Vasc Surg* 1998; **28**: 826–33.
78. Gooley NA, Sumner DS. Relationship of venous reflux to the site of venous valvular incompetence: implications for venous reconstructive surgery. *J Vasc Surg* 1988; **7**: 50–9.
79. Rosfors S, Lamke LO, Nordstroem E, Bygdeman S. Severity and location of venous valvular insufficiency: the importance of distal valve function. *Acta Chir Scand* 1990; **156**: 689–94.
80. van Bemmelen PS, Bedford G, Beach K, Strandness Jr DE. Status of the valves in the superficial and deep venous system in chronic venous disease. *Surgery* 1991; **109**: 730–4.
81. Meissner MH, Caps MT, Zierler BK, *et al.* Deep venous thrombosis and superficial venous reflux. *J Vasc Surg* 2000; **32**: 48–56.
82. Geerts WH, Code KI, Jay RM, *et al.* A prospective study of venous thromboembolism after major trauma. *N Engl J Med* 1994; **331**: 1601–6.
83. Falanga A, Ofosu FA, Oldani E, *et al.* The hypercoagulable state in cancer patients: evidence for impaired thrombin inhibitions. *Blood Coag Fibrinol* 1994; **5**(Suppl 1): S19–23.
84. Bloemenkamp KWM, Rosendaal FR, Helmerhorst FM, *et al.* Enhancement by factor V Leiden mutation of risk of deep-vein thrombosis associated with oral contraceptives containing a third generation progestagen. *Lancet* 1995; **346**: 1593–6.
85. Sigel B, Ipsen J, Felix WR. The epidemiology of lower extremity deep venous thrombosis in surgical patients. *Ann Surg* 1974; **179**: 278–90.
86. Meredith JW, Young JS, O'Neil EA, *et al.* Femoral catheters and deep venous thrombosis: a prospective evaluation with venous duplex sonography. *J Trauma* 1993; **35**: 187–91.
87. Wahl DG, Guillemin F, de Maistre E, *et al.* Risk for venous thrombosis related to antiphospholipid antibodies in systemic lupus erythematosus – a meta-analysis. *Lupus* 1997; **6**: 467–73.
88. Koenigs KP, McPhedran P, Spiro HM. Thrombosis in inflammatory bowel disease. *J Clin Gastroenterol* 1987; **9**: 627–31.

5

The physiology and hemodynamics of chronic venous insufficiency of the lower limb

KEVIN G BURNAND

Chronic venous insufficiency of the lower limb is a poorly defined term and means a different set of symptoms and signs to different clinicians. To some it means all venous disorders that are not acute venous thromboses, occlusions or injuries.[1–5] To others it implies venous disease causing symptoms in the leg, including swelling (venous edema) and the skin changes of lipodermatosclerosis and ulceration.[6] The latter definition excludes uncomplicated varicose veins and has certain advantages, because many patients with varicose veins only seek medical advice for the cosmetic problem and do not progress to develop skin problems or limb swelling.[7] Therefore, the definition that will be utilized in this chapter is chronic venous disease producing chronic lipodermatosclerosis or ulceration within the limb (clinical classes 4, 5 and 6).

VENOUS (CALF) PUMP FUNCTION

The calf muscle pump and to a lesser extent the thigh and foot pumps have a vital role in returning venous blood against gravity from the lower limbs in the erect individual. Abnormalities in the valves or lumen of the superficial, deep and communicating veins can impede or negate the function of these pumps. This causes persistent ambulatory venous hypertension or more correctly an inability to reduce the superficial venous pressure that is achieved by normal calf pump function. The calf pump is the most important of the three venous pumps because it contains the largest venous capacitance (the soleal sinusoids), and it generates the highest pressures (200 mmHg) during muscular contraction.[8] Muscle action drives blood up the stem veins of the limb, where competent valves prevent reflux and retrograde flow during relaxation.

When muscular relaxation occurs, the veins open up and suck in blood from the superficial system through the competent valves of the communicating veins. This in turn reduces the pressure in the superficial veins. This effect is incremental, until the arterial inflow equals the venous outflow capacity of the venous pumps. The efficiency of the calf pump in normal subjects is in the region of 70%. The resting venous pressure is approximately 100 mmHg, depending on the patient's height, reducing to about 30 mmHg after 10 or more repetitive calf contractions. Additional calf contractions fail to reduce the venous pressure further once a steady state has been reached. The normal foot venous pressure during exercise is shown in Fig. 5.1.

The thigh pump is not as efficient as the calf pump, but the foot pump may well be more important than was originally thought, especially as the perforating veins of the foot have a reversed direction of flow (in to out) under normal circumstances.[9] Once exercise ceases, capillary inflow from the vis a tergo slowly fills the superficial veins, which empty during exercise, as the blood is sucked through the communicating veins into the empty deep veins. This causes a slow rise in venous pressure over the next 20–35 seconds as the veins refill back to their original resting pressure (see Fig. 5.1). The recovery time is rapid if there is incompetence of the valves in the superficial or communicating veins (Figs 5.2, 5.3 and

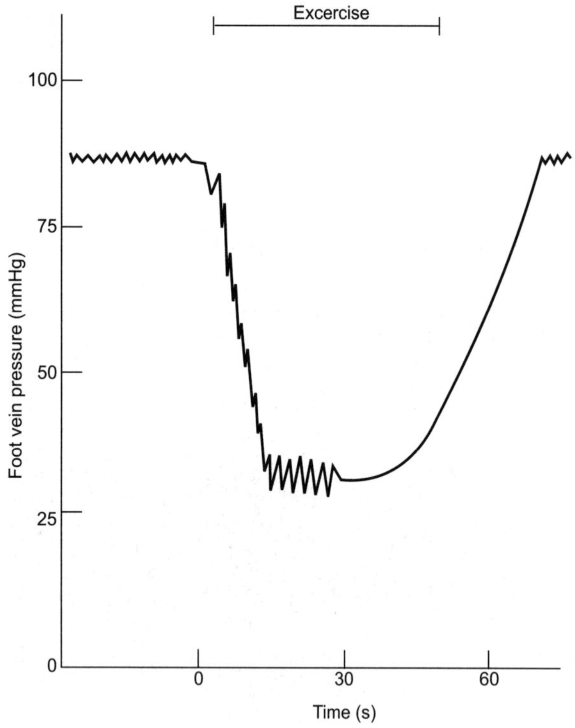

Figure 5.1 *The changes in foot vein pressure during heel-raising exercise. In a normal limb the pressure drops by 80–90% and after exercise, takes 13–25 seconds to return to resting levels. (Reproduced with permission from Browse NL, Burnand KG, Irvine A, Wilson N, eds.* Diseases of the Veins. *London: Arnold, 1999)*

5.4). When there is deep venous occlusion obstruction or agenesis (Figs 5.2 and 5.5), there is little reduction in superficial venous pressure, and this may actually rise above the resting pressure during calf contraction, although persistent venous hypertension is rare. Deep valvular incompetence, with or without associated incompetence of the calf communicating veins, is responsible for blood 'yo-yoing' up and down the deep veins (Fig. 5.6), with accompanying flux through any associated incompetent perforating veins. This produces little in the way of venous pressure fall on calf contraction and a rapid return to a high resting pressure (Fig. 5.2).

All these mechanisms, described above, can cause persistently elevated ambulatory pressure, which in turn leads to raised pressure at the venous end of the capillary (the venule). This causes increased capillary hydrostatic pressure which encourages both transudation and exudation.[10] In 1953, Pappenheimer and Soto-Rivera[11,12] described the stretched pore phenomenon to explain the high protein content of interstitial fluid which occurs when the pressure in the venular capillaries is elevated. These authors suggested that raised pressure distended the lumen enlarging the intra-endothelial pores, which in turn allowed and encouraged large molecules, especially protein, to enter the interstitial space. These observations confirmed the studies by Landis *et al.*,[13] who had demonstrated that the interstitial protein content increases as the capillary pressure rises. A persistently elevated venous pressure is associated with increased tissue fluid production, which has the composition of an exudate, having a high protein content.

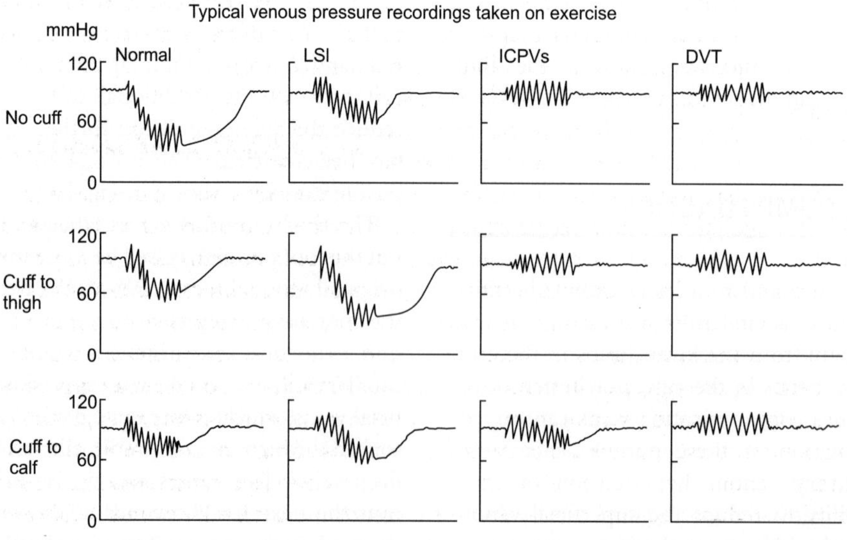

Figure 5.2 *Foot vein pressure measurements. LSI, long saphenous incompetence; ICPVs, incompetent perforating veins; DVT, post-thrombotic legs.*

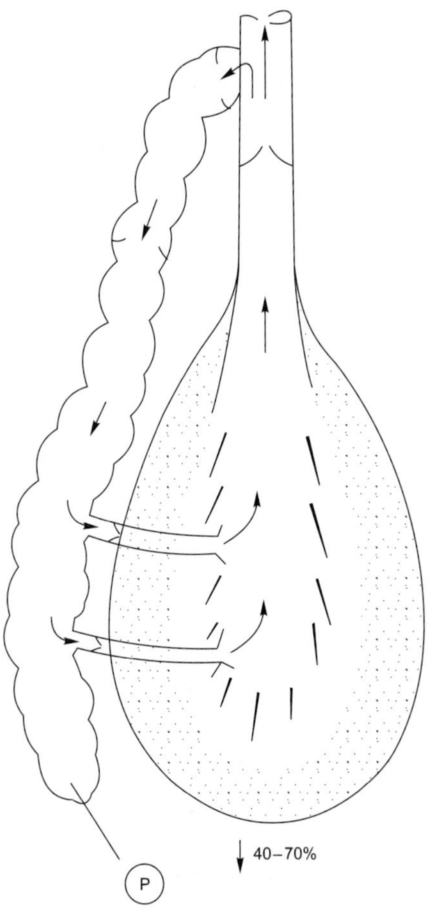

Figure 5.3 *Superficial vein incompetence allows blood to reflux down the superficial veins but, providing the communicating veins are competent, the calf pump can usually cope with the additional load and reduce the foot vein pressure during exercise by 40–70%. This is why simple superficial varicose veins are an uncommon cause of venous ulceration. (Reproduced with permission from Browse NL, Burnand KG, Irvine A, Wilson N, eds.* Diseases of the Veins. *London: Arnold, 1999)*

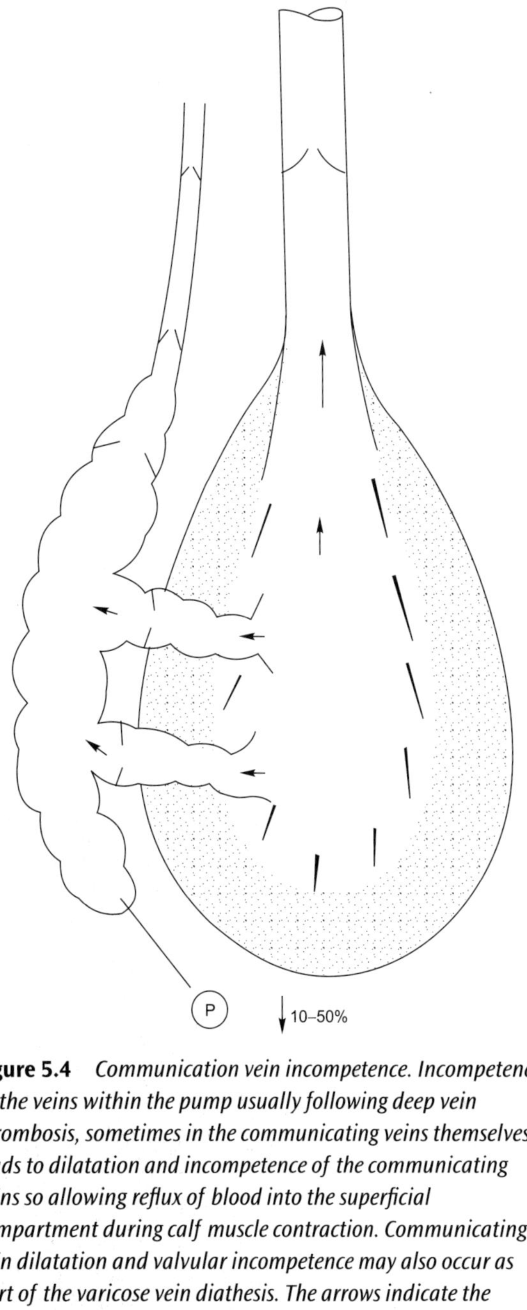

Figure 5.4 *Communication vein incompetence. Incompetence of the veins within the pump usually following deep vein thrombosis, sometimes in the communicating veins themselves, leads to dilatation and incompetence of the communicating veins so allowing reflux of blood into the superficial compartment during calf muscle contraction. Communicating vein dilatation and valvular incompetence may also occur as part of the varicose vein diathesis. The arrows indicate the direction of blood flow. During exercise the foot vein pressure falls by 10–40%. (Reproduced with permission from Browse NL, Burnand KG, Irvine A, Wilson N, eds.* Diseases of the Veins. *London: Arnold, 1999)*

SUPERFICIAL VENOUS INCOMPETENCE

The mechanism of valvular incompetence in the saphenous systems is still disputed, although the bulk of evidence seems to favor a weakness of the vein wall producing venous dilatation, which causes secondary valvular incompetence, as the valve ring enlarges and the valve leaflets are unable to coapt. Numerous biochemical abnormalities have been reported, including elevated levels of collagenases, elastases, acid phosphatase, and lactic dehydrogenase, as well as collagen defects and lysosomal abnormalities.[14,15] Urokinase type plasminogen activator,[16] free radicals[17] and mast cells have also been shown to be elevated within the vein walls.

An important study by Akroyd *et al.*[18] showed that the valve ring and its leaflets had far greater tensile strength than the vein wall itself. It has also been pointed out that saphenous veins that have been deliberately denuded of valves for in situ vein bypass hardly ever become varicose.[19] These studies and observations all support the theory that valvular incompetence is secondary to a defect in the vein wall. This concept was originally proposed by Cotton[20] after he demonstrated, using anatomical casts, that venous dilatation developed below rather than above the valves in patients with varicose veins. This effectively destroyed the descending valvular incompetence theory[21] that had been popular since

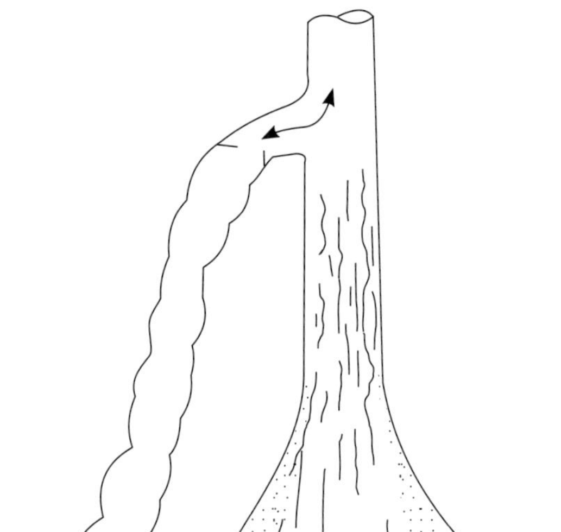

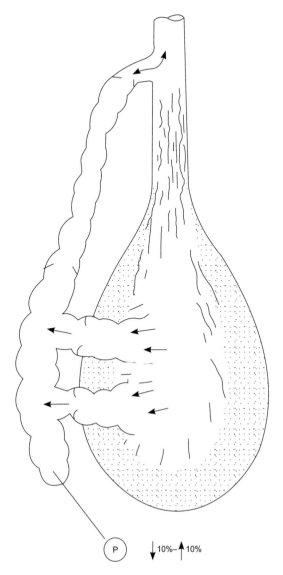

Figure 5.5 *Outflow tract obstruction. Deep vein obstruction causes upstream dilatation of the veins in the pump chamber and secondary incompetence of the communicating veins because these veins become part of the collateral outflow tract. During exercise the foot vein pressure will fall slightly. (Reproduced with permission from Browse NL, Burnand KG, Irvine A, Wilson N, eds.* Diseases of the Veins. *London: Arnold, 1999)*

Trendelenburg had first ligated the saphenofemoral junction.[22]

THE CALF COMMUNICATING VEINS (PERFORATING VEINS)

The dilating process that affects the saphenous system can also affect the communicating veins including the important perforating veins of the medial calf (Cockett's veins).[23] This may explain the observation of Campbell[24] (subsequently confirmed by the Edinburgh Group[25]) that in many patients where saphenous and perforator incompetence coexist, postoperative duplex re-examination shows that perforator valve competence is restored after the saphenous system has been ablated. This has led to the theory that in many patients the perforating veins simply act as 're-entry' veins, allowing blood refluxing down the saphenous system to flow back into the deep system.

Incompetent calf perforating veins are also often associated with deep vein obstruction or incompetence, where the primary abnormality is in the deep veins, and under these circumstances the perforating veins act as 'safety valves' or 'collaterals', allowing blood under high pressure in the calf pump to escape as it either yo-yos up and down, or is unable to pass up the axial limb veins. Under these circumstances the high pressures developed as the calf muscles attempt to drive blood up the deep veins are directly transmitted via the overlying perforating veins to the superficial venous system of the calf.[8] This in turn leads to enlargement of the dermal capillary bed[26] and exudation of proteins including fibrinogen into the interstitial space.[27,28]

THE DEEP VEINS

Post-thrombotic damage within the deep veins is the most important cause of chronic venous insufficiency. Venous thrombi rarely lyse completely unless they are subjected to pharmacological lysis. The residual thrombus organizes, becoming replaced by fibrous tissue and covered by a neoepithelium, which prevents further lysis from occurring. Thrombus filling the lumen and adhering to the vein wall can cause complete venous obstruction which becomes permanent after it has been organized (Fig. 5.7), whilst thrombus arising in a valve pocket, or in direct contact with valve cusps, can irreparably damage their function.[29] Synechiae, which are permanent endothelialized strands of residual organized thrombus, often develop across the vein wall, producing a cribriform meshwork within the venous lumen, which obstructs outflow and impedes valve function, often binding valve leaflets to the vein wall. When the axial veins remain obstructed, collaterals develop, and the extent of the obstruction and the collateral pathways determine the severity of the hemodynamic changes and the extent of the post-thrombotic symptoms (Fig. 5.8). When the popliteal vein has been obliterated, the calf perforating veins become important collaterals and popliteal obstruction, either in isolation or in combination with calf vein and iliofemoral damage, is usually indicative of severe symptoms and subsequent ulceration.[30]

Deep venous valvular incompetence without coexisting obstruction can be compensated for by the presence of a powerful calf pump, provided the perforating veins remain competent. When these also become incom-

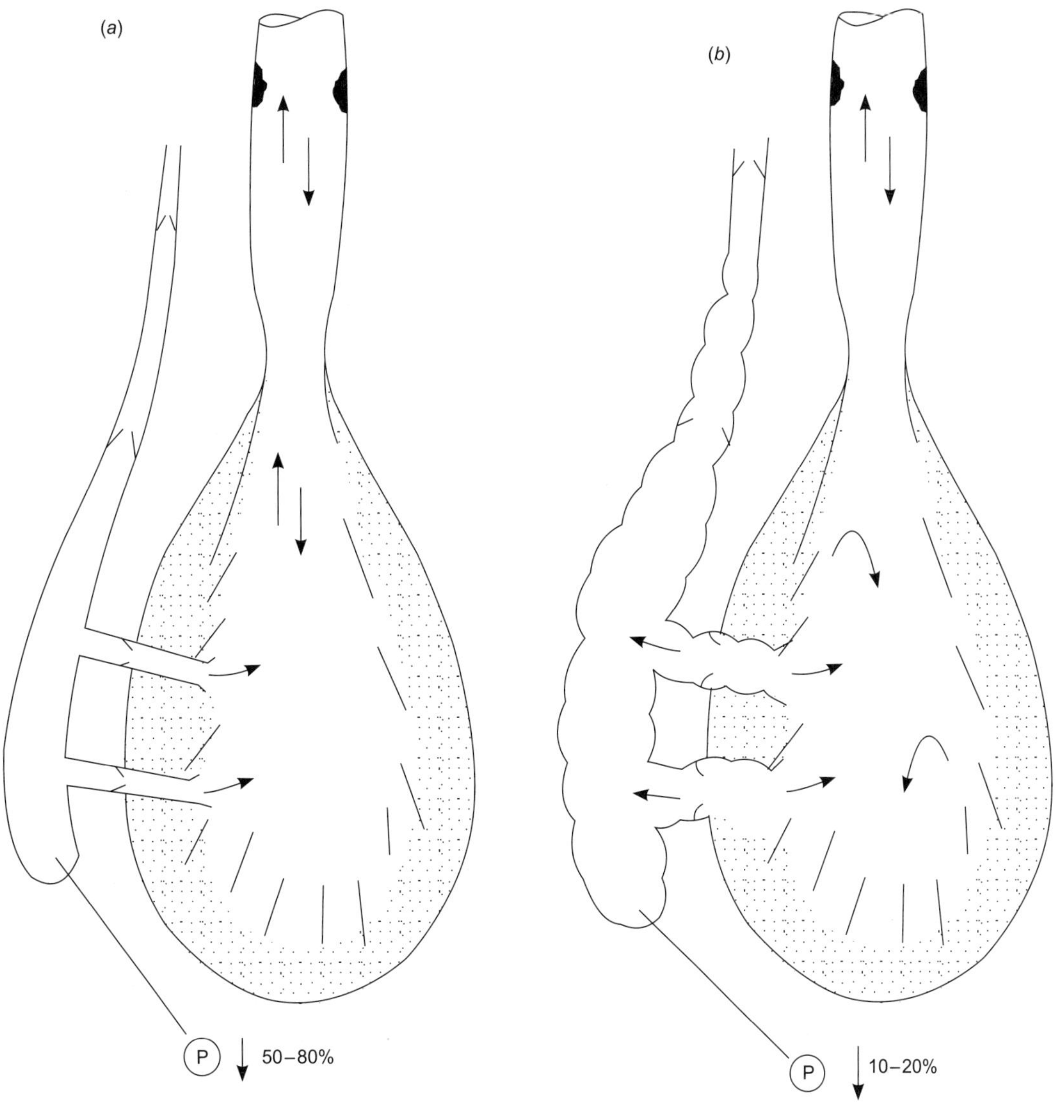

Figure 5.6 *Outflow tract incompetence. (a) The calf pump can compensate for pure deep vein (outflow tract) incompetence by increasing its output. (b) If the dilatation of the veins within the pump affects the communicating veins, the pump begins to fail and foot vein pressure is only reduced by 10–20% during exercise. (Reproduced with permission from Browse NL, Burnand KG, Irvine A, Wilson N, eds.* Diseases of the Veins. *London: Arnold, 1999)*

petent, the calf pump can no longer compensate and the superficial venous pressure rises, leading to the changes already described above. In many patients the perivenous fibrosis which follows thrombosis prevents venous distension and may also act as a functional obstruction.

A small group of patients have primary deep valvular incompetence, with no evidence of a thrombotic etiology. Whether this is a consequence of abnormal valves (the floppy valves of Kistner),[31] or true congenital valvular agenesis, remains a matter of conjecture. Both may coexist. It is also possible that valvular incompetence is secondary to dilatation of the wall of the deep veins. In some patients, particularly with Klippel–Trenaunay syndrome, the deep veins are completely absent, being replaced by a primitive axial vein.[32] This may be the result of true venous agenesis.

Deep vein damage and obstruction may also be a consequence of direct or indirect injury, surgical mishap, leiomyomas and leiomyosarcomas. These and a few other unusual causes of deep venous obstruction are, however, very rare causes of chronic venous insufficiency.

MECHANISM OF SKIN CHANGES

Homans[33] was the first to suggest that venous stasis was the cause of skin changes and ulceration that accompany the development of the post-thrombotic limb, although John Gay,[34] 100 years earlier had described the presence of 'matter' in the deep veins of ulcerated limbs dissected at postmortem examination. Gay was also the first person to describe perforating vein incompetence in the cadaver limbs.

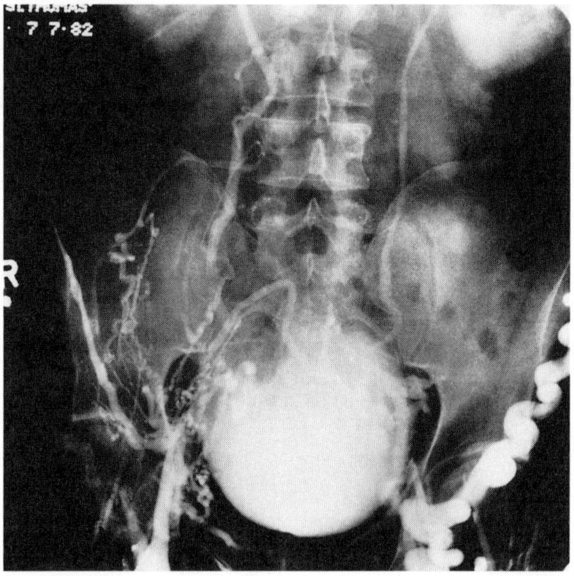

Figure 5.7 *A venogram showing obstructed iliac veins with collateral flow going up the anterior abdominal wall.*

The concept of stasis was later challenged when Blalock[35] and subsequently a number of others[36–38] demonstrated that the oxygen content of the venous blood was high rather than low in the venous effluent of limbs with venous ulceration. This finding, taken in conjunction with the observation that angiography in these limbs demonstrated rapid passage of contrast material into the veins,[39] led to the suggestion that arteriovenous fistulae opened up in response to chronic venous hypertension. There were even claims that arteriovenous fistulae could be demonstrated on histologic examination,[40] although these claims were subsequently qualified when the paper's author accepted that he could not differentiate an arteriovenous fistula from a thick-walled capillary or venule. Nevertheless, the consistent finding of a raised venous oxygen content in ulcerated limbs led Fontaine[41] to propose again that arteriovenous shunts situated in the dermis below the ulcer-bearing area were responsible for ulcer development. Schalin[42] has continued to champion the theory that arteriovenous fistulae are the major cause of both varicose veins and venous ulceration. Much of his evidence is, however, speculative and open to interpretation. Ryan and Copeman[43] suggested that the arteriovenous shunts in the dermis, which control temperature regulation, might open up in response to raised venous pressure and shunt blood away from the skin. The whole theory of arteriovenous shunts being responsible for venous ulceration was challenged by the work of Hugo Partsch,[44] who as a young researcher in the department of dermatology at Vienna showed that radiolabelled macroaggregates injected into the femoral veins of ulcerated limbs failed to enter the lungs in greater quantities than those injected into the control 'normal' limbs. Instead the macroaggregates were trapped in the capillary bed beneath the ulcer, causing a hot area in the leg. This work was unable to show evidence of excessive shunting in ulcerated limbs, but merely confirmed that the capillary bed had increased in size. Hopkins and Jamieson,[45] using positron emission tomography in patients with leg ulcers and lipodermatosclerosis, found that the metabolic and flow measurements suggested excessive blood flow through the local capillary bed with

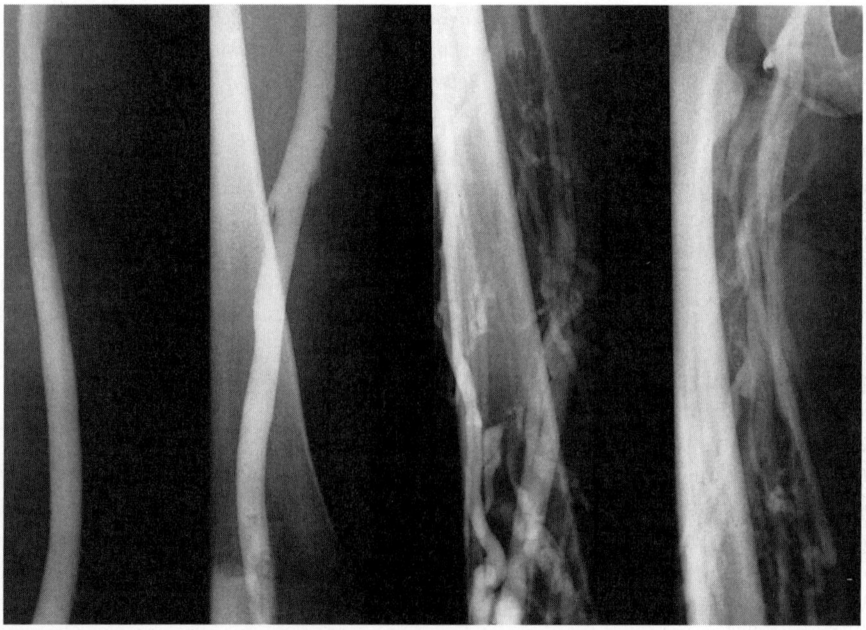

Figure 5.8 *On the left two panels, a normal set of deep veins. On the right two panels, post-thrombotic femoral veins with synechiae and collateral pathways.*

reduced metabolic uptake of oxygen, consistent with a diffusion block. Taken together, these two pieces of work provide fairly convincing evidence that physiological arteriovenous shunting is not present in the ulcer bed.

Bollinger reported that 'halos' were present around the dermal calf capillaries in the ulcer-bearing skin,[46] and Browse and Burnand went on to expand these observations by showing pericapillary fibrin cuffs in the same dermal capillary bed (Fig. 5.9).[26,27] These were associated with an expanded capillary bed, venous hypertension and defective local and systemic fibrinolytic capacity. The presence of pericapillary fibrin cuffs led us to speculate[47] that these, in combination with other molecules and interstitial fibrin, might interfere with the passage of oxygen and other nutrients to the overlying skin. Although evidence was provided that a thick film of fibrin did interfere with oxygen diffusion, subsequent theoretical estimations have cast doubt that pure fibrin would be an effective diffusion block.[48]

More recently, the finding of white cell depletion in the venous effluent of dependent limbs led initially to the concept of white cells plugging or trapping with the white cells theoretically blocking the dermal capillaries.[49,50] Subsequently, refinements of this theory have suggested that white cell margination, activation and even escape into the tissues may cause local damage and eventually lead to ulceration.[51] At present there is no evidence that white cells are activated before skin changes become apparent, and therefore no proof that these changes are the cause rather than the effect of venous hypertension and lipodermatosclerosis, and of course ulceration.

A number of studies have shown that changes in white cells are produced by short-term (tourniquet-induced) venous hypertension,[52] but its relationship to chronic venous hypertension is less well understood.

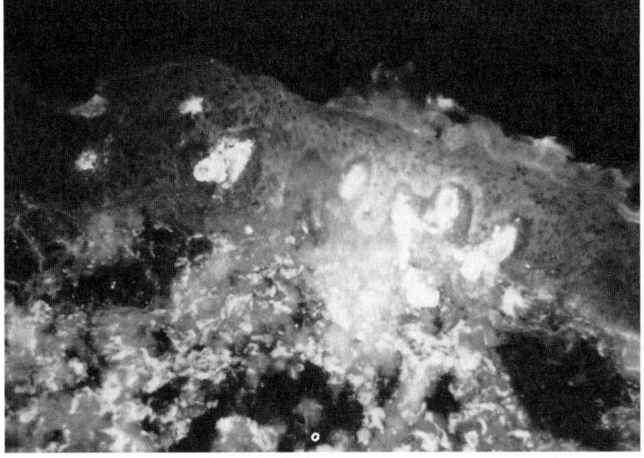

Figure 5.9 *The skin of the ulcer bearing area in a patient with lipodermatosclerosis. Immunofluorescent staining with an antifibrin antibody showing bright halos of fibrin around the dermal capillaries. (Courtesy of Professor H Partsch)*

Other theories that have recently been put forward for the development of venous ulcers include release of free radicals,[53] mast cell activation[54] and mechanical damage based upon the venous hypertension.[55] Falanga and Eaglestein[56] have suggested that the fibrin cuff acts as a trap to block or slow down growth factors reaching the skin and Herrick *et al.*[57] have carried out a nice histologic study that has demonstrated that the pericapillary halos not only contain fibrinogen but also lamisin and other proteins. The presence of crosslinked fibrin within the cuff has been confirmed by Brakman *et al.*[58]

CONCLUSIONS

The importance of persistent ambulatory venous hypertension in the development of lipodermatosclerosis and ulceration is not disputed. The relative frequency of deep and superficial venous obstruction and reflux seems to vary in different studies and the true role of perforator incompetence in the development of venous ulcers remains to be established. The precise mechanisms that cause skin breakdown are not known. A number of theories have been put forward but these need to be confirmed or refuted by further studies. A better understanding of the mechanisms that cause ulceration should lead to better methods of preventing ulcers developing and treating them once they have developed.

REFERENCES

1. Kurz X, Kahn SR, Benhaim EA, *et al.* Chronic venous disorders of the leg: epidemiology, outcomes, diagnosis and management. *Int Angiol* 1999; **18**: 83–101.
2. Porter JM, Rutherford RB, Clagett GP, Raju S. Reporting standards in venous disease. *J Vasc Surg* 1988; **8**: 172–9.
3. Porter D, Rosen M, Skillman J, *et al.* Clinical-anamnestic and instrumental data in out patients suffering from venous disease. *Int Angiol* 1995; **14**: 400–3.
4. Da Silva A, Widmer LK, Martin H, *et al.* Varicose veins and chronic venous insufficiency – prevalence and risk factors in 4376 subjects in the Basle study. *Vasa* 1974; **3**: 118–25.
5. Perrin M. *Chronic Venous Insufficiency in the Lower Limbs.* Paris: McGraw-Hill, 1990.
6. Browse NL, Burnand KG, Irvine A, Wilson N, eds. *Diseases of the Veins.* London: Arnold, 1999.
7. Bradbury A, Evans C, Allan P, Lee A, Ruckley CV, Fowkes FGR. What are the symptoms of varicose veins? Edinburgh vein study cross-sectional population survey. *Br Med J* 1999; **318**: 353–6.
8. Bjordal RI. Circulation patterns in the saphenous system and the perforating veins of the calf in patients with previous deep vein thrombosis. *Vasa Suppl* 1974; **3**: 1–41.
9. Pegum JM, Fegan WG. Physiology of venous return from the foot. *Cardiovasc Res* 1967; **1**: 249–51.

10. Landis EM. Capillary pressure and capillary permeability. *Physiol Rev* 1934; **14**: 404–81.
11. Pappenheimer JR, Soto-Rivera A. An effective osmotic pressure of plasma proteins and other quantities associated with the capillary circulation in the hind limbs of cats and dogs. *Am J Physiol* 1948; **52**: 471–91.
12. Pappenheimer JR. Passage of molecules through capillary walls. *Physiol Rev* 1953; **33**: 387.
13. Landis EM, Jonas L, Angevine M, Erb W. The passage of fluid and protein through the human capillary wall during venous congestion. *J Clin Invest* 1932; **11**: 717.
14. Urbanova D, Prerovsky I. Enzymes in the wall of normal and varicose veins. Histochemical study. *Angiologica* 1972; **9**: 53–61.
15. Wegmann R, Elsammannoudy FA, Oliver C, Rettori R. Histochemical studies on the walls of human varicose veins: the saphenous varicose vein. *Ann Histochem* 1974; **19**: 285–92.
16. Shireman PR, McCarthy WJ, Pearce WH, *et al.* Plasminogen activator levels are influenced by location and varicosity in great saphenous vein. *J Vasc Surg* 1996; **24**: 719–24.
17. Farbiszewski R, Glowinski PJ, Makarewicz-Plonska M, *et al.* Oxygen-derived free radicals as mediators of varicose vein wall damage. *Vasc Surg* 1996; **30**: 47–52.
18. Ackroyd JS, Pattison M, Browse NL. A study on the mechanical properties of fresh and preserved human femoral vein wall and valve cusps. *Br J Surg* 1985; **72**: 117–19.
19. Rose S, Ahmed A. Some thoughts on the aetiology of varicose veins. *J Cardiovasc Surg* 1986; **27**: 534–43.
20. Cotton L. Varicose veins. Gross anatomy and development. *Br J Surg* 1961; **48**: 589–98.
21. Ludbrook J. Valvular defect in primary varicose veins. Cause or effect? *Lancet* 1963; **2**: 1289–92.
22. Trendelenburg F. Uber die unterbildung der vena saphena magna bei unterschenkel varicen. *Beitr Klin Chir* 1891; **7**: 195–210.
23. Cockett FB, Jones DE. The ankle blowout syndrome. A new approach to the varicose ulcer problem. *Lancet* 1953; **1**: 17–23.
24. Campbell WA, West A. Duplex ultrasound of operative treatment of varicose veins. In Negus D, Jantet G, Coleridge Smith P, eds. *Phlebology* Berlin: Springer, 1995.
25. Stuart WP, Adam DJ, Allan PL, Ruckley CV, Bradbury AW. Saphenous surgery does not correct perforator incompetence in the presence of deep venous reflux. *J Vasc Surg* 1998; **28**: 834–8.
26. Burnand KG, Whimster I, Clemenson G, Lea Thomas M, Browse NL. The relationship between the number of capillaries in the skin of the venous ulcer bearing area of the lower leg and the fall in foot vein pressure during exercise. *Br J Surg* 1981; **68**: 297–300.
27. Burnand KG, Whimster I, Naidoo A, Browse NL. Pericapillary fibrin in the ulcer bearing skin of the leg. *Br Med J* 1982; **285**: 1071–2.
28. Burnand KG, Clemenson G, Whimster I, Gaunt J, Browse NL. The effect of sustained venous hypertension on the skin capillaries of the canine hind limb. *Br J Surg* 1982; **69**: 41–4.
29. Edwards EA, Edwards JE. The effect of thrombophlebitis on the venous valves. *Surg Gynecol Obstet* 1937; **65**: 310–20.
30. Brittenden J, Bradbury AW, Allan PL, Ruckley CV. Popliteal vein reflux reduces the healing of chronic venous ulcer. *Br J Surg* 1998; **85**: 60–2.
31. Kistner RL. Primary venous valve incompetence of the leg. *Am J Surg* 1980; **140**: 218–24.
32. Gloviczki P, Stanson AW, Stickler AW, *et al.* Klippel–Trenaunay syndrome: the risks and benefits of vascular interventions. *Surgery* 1991; **110**: 469–79.
33. Homans J. The etiology and treatment of varicose ulcer of the leg. *Surg Gynecol Obstet* 1917; **24**: 300–11.
34. Gay J. *Vascular Disease of the Lower Extremities and its Allied Disorders: Skin Discoloration, Induration and Ulcer.* London: Churchill, 1868.
35. Blalock A. Oxygen content of blood in patients with varicose veins. *Arch Surg* 1929; **19**: 898–905.
36. Blumoff RL, Johnson G. Saphenous vein Po_2 in patients with varicose veins. *J Surg Res* 1977; **23**: 35–6.
37. Clyne CAC, Ramsden WH, Chant ADR, Webster JH. Oxygen tension in the skin of the gaiter area of limbs with venous disease. *Br J Surg* 1985; **72**: 644–7.
38. Holling HE, Beecher HK, Linton RR. Study of the tendency to edema formation associated with incompetence of the valves of the communicating veins of the leg. *J Clin Invest* 1938; **17**: 555–61.
39. Haimovici H. Abnormal arterio-venous shunts associated with chronic venous insufficiency. *J Cardiovasc Surg* 1976; **17**: 473–82.
40. Guis JA. Arteriovenous anastomoses and varicose veins. *Arch Surg* 1960; **81**: 299–308.
41. Fontaine R. Remarks concerning venous thrombosis and its sequelae. *Surgery* 1957; **41**: 6–25.
42. Schalin S. Arteriovenous communications localised by thermography and identified by operative microscopy. *Acta Chir Scand* 1981; **147**: 409–20.
43. Ryan TJ, Copeman PMW. Microvascular patterns and blood stasis in skin diseases. *Br J Dermatol* 1970; **8**: 563–70.
44. Lindemayr W, Loefferer O, Mostbeck A, Partsch H. Arteriovenous shunts in primary varicoses? A critical essay. *Vasc Surg* 1972; **6**: 9–14.
45. Hopkins NFG, Spinks TJ, Rhodes CG, Ranicar ASO, Jamieson CW. Positron emission tomography in venous ulceration and liposclerosis: study of regional tissue function. *Br Med J (Clin Res Ed)* 1983; **286**: 333–6.
46. Bollinger A, Jager K, Geser A, Sgier F, Seglias J. Transcapillary and interstitial diffusion of Na fluorescein in chronic venous insufficiency with white atrophy. *Int J Microcirc Clin Exp* 1982; **1** 5–17.
47. Browse NL, Burnand KG. The cause of venous ulceration. *Lancet* 1982; **2**: 243–5.
48. Michel CC. Aetiology of venous ulceration. *Br J Surg* 1990; **77**: 1071.

49. Thomas PRS, Nash GB, Dormandy JA. White cell accumulation in the dependent legs of patients with venous hypertension. *Br Med J* 1988; **296**: 1693–5.
50. Coleridge-Smith PD, Thomas P, Scurr JH, Dormandy JA. Causes of venous ulceration: a new hypothesis. *Br Med J* 1988; **296**: 1726–7.
51. Scott HJ, McMullin GM, Coleridge-Smith PD, Scurr JH. Venous ulceration the role of the white blood cell. *Phlebology* 1989; **4**: 153–9.
52. Shields DA, Andaz S, Abeysinghe RD, Porter JB, Scurr JH, Coleridge-Smith PD. Soluble markers of leucocyte adhesion in patients with venous disease. *Phlebol Suppl* 1994; **9**: 55–8.
53. Edwards AT, Herrick SE, Suarez-Mendez VJ, McCollum CN. Oxidants, antioxidants and venous ulceration. *Br J Surg* 1992; **79**(5): 443–4.
54. Pappas PJ, Defouw DO, Venezio LM, *et al.* Morphometric assessment of dermal microcirculation in patients with venous insufficiency. *J Vasc Surg* 1997; **26**: 784–95.
55. Chant A. The biomechanics of leg ulceration. *Ann R Coll Surg Engl* 1999; **81**: 80–5.
56. Falanga V, Eaglestein WH. The 'trap' hypothesis of venous ulceration. *Lancet* 1993; **341**: 1006–8.
57. Herrick SE, Sloan P, McGurie M, Freak L, McCollum CN, Ferguson MW. Sequential changes in histologic patterns and extracellular matrix deposition during the healing of chronic venous ulcers. *Am J Pathol* 1992; **141**: 1085–95.
58. Brakman M, Faber WR, Kerckhaert JA, *et al.* Immunofluorescence studies of atrophie blanche with antibodies against fibrinogen, fibrin, plasminogen activator inhibitor, factor VIII related antigen and collagen type IV. *Vasa* 1992; **21**(2): 143–8.

6

Pathology and cellular physiology of chronic venous insufficiency

PETER J PAPPAS, WALTER N DURÁN AND ROBERT W HOBSON II

Failure of venous valve apposition causes valvular reflux. Over time, patients with persistent valvular reflux will develop venous hypertension and an increase in ambulatory venous pressure. This scenario, sometimes associated with venous outflow obstruction, initiates a cascade of pathologic events that clinically manifests itself as lower extremity edema, pain, itching, skin discoloration, varicose veins, venous ulceration and, in its severest form, limb loss. These clinical symptoms collectively refer to the disorder known as chronic venous insufficiency (CVI).[1] The purpose of this chapter is to review the pathologic alterations that occur at the tissue level as a result of chronic venous hypertension. Chapter 5 provides an overview of the pathology and hemodynamics of CVI.

HISTORICAL THEORIES

In the twentieth century, numerous theories have been postulated regarding the etiology of venous ulceration and CVI. No one theory completely explains the entire process and the majority of these postulates have been disproved. However, for historical interest, several of these theories are presented below.

Venous stasis theory

In 1917, a manuscript entitled 'The etiology and treatment of varicose ulcer of the leg' was published by John Homans.[2] In this manuscript, Dr Homans coined the term 'postphlebitic' syndrome and speculated on the cause of venous ulceration. He stated that:

> Overstretching of the vein walls and destruction of the valves upon which the mechanism principally depends, brings about a degree of surface stasis which obviously interferes with the nutrition of the skin and subcutaneous tissues.... It is to be expected, therefore, that skin which is bathed under pressure in stagnant venous blood will readily form permanent, open sores or ulcers.[2]

It is now known that hypoxia is not the cause of venous ulceration. However, this hypothesis stimulated numerous investigators to try and identify a causal relationship between hypoxia, stagnant blood flow and the development of CVI. It was not until the early 1980s that this theory came into disfavor.

Arteriovenous fistula theory

Increased venous flow in the dermal venous plexus was suggested as a possible etiology for venous ulceration by Pratt.[3] He reported that increased venous flow in patients with CVI could be clinically observed and attributed the development of venous ulceration to the presence of arteriovenous connections. In a series of 272 patients with varicose veins who underwent vein ligation, 24% had observable arteriovenous connections. Of the 61 patients who developed recurrences, 50% occurred in patients with arteriovenous communications identified clinically by the presence of arterial pulsations in venous conduits. Pratt hypothesized that increased venous flow shunted nutrient and oxygen-rich blood away from the dermal plexus, leading to areas of ischemia and hypoxia and resulting in venous ulceration. Pratt's clinical observations, however, have never been confirmed with objective scientific evidence. Experiments with radioactively labeled microspheres have never demonstrated shunting, casting serious doubts on the validity of this theory.[4]

Diffusion block theory

Hypoxia and alterations in nutrient blood flow were again proposed as the underlying etiology of CVI in 1982 by Burnand *et al.*[5] These authors studied skin biopsies obtained from 109 CVI limbs and 30 normal limbs. Foot vein pressures were measured in CVI patients at rest and after 5, 10, 15 and 20 heel raises. Vein pressure measurements were then correlated with the number of capillaries observed on histologic section. The authors reported that venous hypertension was associated with increased capillary number in the dermis of patients with CVI . Whether the histologic sections represented true increases in capillary quantity or an elongation and distension of existing capillaries is not known. However, in a canine hind limb model, experimentally induced venous hypertension caused an enlargement in dermal capillaries.[6] This important investigation was one of the first studies to demonstrate a direct effect of venous hypertension on the venous microcirculation. In a later study, Browse and Burnand noted that the enlarged capillaries observed on histologic examination exhibited pericapillary fibrin deposition and coined the term 'fibrin cuff'.[5] They speculated that venous hypertension caused a widening of inter-endothelial gap junctions with subsequent extravasation of fibrinogen and pericapillary fibrin deposition. The cuffs would therefore act as a barrier to oxygen diffusion and nutrient blood flow, resulting in epidermal cell death. Although pericapillary cuffs do exist, deficiencies in nutrient flow or oxygen diffusion have never been demonstrated.

Leukocyte activation

Dissatisfaction with the fibrin cuff theory and subsequent observations of decreased circulating leukocytes in blood samples obtained from the greater saphenous veins in CVI patients stimulated Coleridge Smith *et al.* to propose the leukocyte trapping theory.[7] This theory proposes that circulating neutrophils are trapped in the venous microcirculation secondary to venous hypertension, resulting in sluggish capillary blood flow. Circulating leukocytes come into contact with the dermal microcirculation, migrate into the dermal interstitium and become activated. Release of toxic metabolites leads to tissue damage and eventual ulcer formation. Unfortunately, leukocyte trapping of neutrophils has never been directly observed, suggesting alternative mechanisms for leukocyte activation.

Role of leukocyte activation and function

Leukocyte involvement in CVI dermal pathology was first suggested by Thomas *et al.* in 1988.[8] They reported that 24% fewer white cells left the venous circulation after a period of recumbency in patients with CVI as compared with normal patients. They suggested that their results were secondary to some element of leukocyte trapping in the dermal circulation of CVI patients. Scott *et al.* provided further evidence for leukocyte involvement by demonstrating alterations in the number of white cells observed in CVI dermal biopsies.[9] Punch biopsies from patients with primary varicose veins, lipodermatosclerosis, and patients with lipodermatosclerosis and healed ulcers were obtained and the number of white blood cells (WBCs) per high power field (40× magnification) quantified. No patients with active ulcers were included and no attempt to identify the type of leukocytes was made. The authors reported that in patients with primary varicose veins, lipodermatosclerosis and healed ulceration, there was a median of 6, 45 and 217 WBCs per mm^2, respectively. This study demonstrated that with clinical progression and increasing severity of CVI, there was a progressive increase in the number of leukocytes in the dermis of CVI patients. Although WBC infiltration into the dermis of CVI patients was now confirmed, the types and distribution of cells was unknown. In a study performed by Wilkinson *et al.*, skin biopsies were obtained from 23 patients who required surgical ligation, stripping and/or avulsion for their varicose veins.[10] The condition of the skin was recorded as liposclerotic, eczematous or normal. Lipodermatosclerosis was defined clinically as palpable induration of the skin and subcutaneous tissues and eczema as visible erythema with scaling of the skin. Using immunohistochemical techniques, the authors stained for leukocyte specific cell surface markers and reported that macrophages and lymphocytes were the predominant leukocytes observed in this patient population. Neutrophils and B-lymphocytes were rarely observed. T-lymphocytes and macrophages were predominantly observed perivascularly and in the epidermis. However, Pappas *et al.* performed a quantitative morphometric assessment of the dermal microcirculation using electron microscopy and reported that macrophages and mast cells were the predominant cells observed in patients with CVI dermal skin changes.[11] Furthermore, lymphocytes were never observed. This discrepancy may reflect the types of patients that were studied. Wilkinson *et al.* biopsied patients with erythematous and eczematous skin changes whereas Pappas predominantly evaluated older patients with dermal fibrosis. Patients with eczematous skin changes may have an autoimmune component to their CVI whereas patients with dermal fibrosis may reflect changes consistent with chronic inflammation and altered tissue remodeling.

Given the predominant role of leukocytes in CVI pathology, there has been great interest in the activation state and functional status of leukocytes in CVI patients. Pappas *et al.* explored the hypothesis that circulating leukocytes in CVI patients were in an altered state of activation and therefore may be involved in leukocyte-mediated injury. They measured the expression of cell surface activation markers of circulating leukocytes using fluorescence flow cytometry.[12] Relative to normal individuals, patients with chronic venous stasis ulcers had a decreased expression of the CD3+/DR+ and CD3+/CD38+ markers on T-lymphocytes and an increased expression of CD14+/CD38+ markers on monocytes. Circulating neutrophils demonstrated no evidence of activation.

Although Pappas *et al.* identified a population of circulating cells demonstrating altered activation markers, their results did not test the functional status of these cells. In a follow-up study, Pappas *et al.* tested the hypothesis that circulating mononuclear cells in CVI patients were dysfunctional by challenging monocytes with test mitogens.[13] Lymphocyte and monocyte cell function was measured as the degree of proliferation in response to a mitogenic challenge. Fifty patients were separated into four groups:

- group 1, 14 patients with normal limbs;
- group 2, 10 patients with class II CVI (stasis dermatitis only);
- group 3, 15 patients with active venous ulcers;
- group 4, 11 patients with healed venous ulcers and current evidence of lipodermatosclerosis.

Systemically circulating lymphocytes and monocytes were obtained by antecubital venipuncture from groups 1–4. Cells were cultured in the presence of staphylococcal enterotoxins (SEs) A, B, C1, D and E (mitogens) and PHA (phytohemagglutinin), a control mitogen. Proliferative responses to PHA indicated that lymphocytes and monocytes from CVI patients were not globally depressed. However, patients in group 2 did not exhibit the same degree of proliferation to PHA as did groups 1, 3 and 4. Differences in proliferative responses between group 2 and 1 (44.38 ± 43.9 versus 118.87 ± 27.1, $P \leq 0.05$) and groups 2 and 3 (44.38 ± 43.9 versus 105.95 ± 60.99, $P \leq 0.05$), were significant. Challenges with staphylococcal enterotoxin A and B revealed significant diminution of proliferative responses in groups 2 (42.73 ± 11.55, $P \leq 0.05$) and 3 (45.57 ± 9.1, $P \leq 0.05$) and groups 3 (36.81 ± 6.9, $P \leq 0.05$) and 4 (35.04 ± 7.5, $P \leq 0.05$), compared to SEA controls (68.68 ± 9.9) and SEB controls (66.25 ± 13.56), respectively. A trend towards diminished cellular function with progression of CVI was observed with staphylococcal enterotoxins B, C1, D and E, strongly suggesting biologic significance. Furthermore, patients with LDS and a history of healed ulcers, uniformly exhibited the poorest proliferative responses (Fig. 6.1). This study indicated that deterioration of mononuclear cell function was associated with CVI and suggested that lymphocyte and monocyte function diminished with

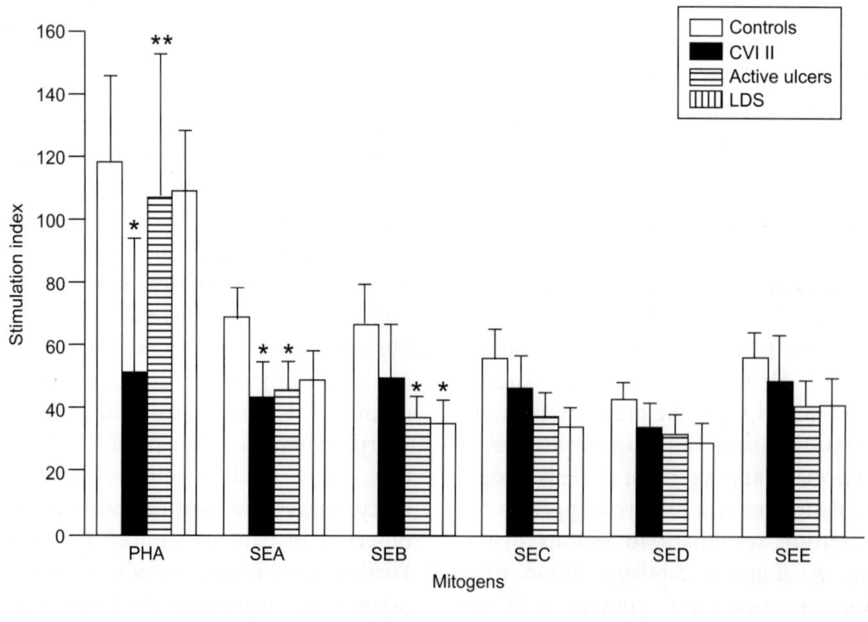

Figure 6.1 *Histogram of leukocyte proliferative responses upon exposure to phytohemagglutinin (PHA) and staphylococcal enterotoxins A, B, C1, D and E (*P ≤0.05 compared with controls. **P ≤0.05 PHA group 2 compared with PHA group 3).*

clinical disease progression. The authors speculated that the decreased capacity for mononuclear cell proliferation in response to various challenges may manifest itself clinically as poor and prolonged wound healing.

THE VENOUS MICROCIRCULATION

Numerous investigations have attempted to evaluate the microcirculation of patients with CVI.[11,14–17] The majority of these investigations were qualitative descriptions of vascular abnormalities that lacked uniformity of biopsy sites and patient stratification. Prior to 1997, it was widely accepted that endothelial cells from the dermal microcirculation appeared abnormal, contained Weibel–Palade bodies, were edematous and demonstrated widened inter-endothelial gap junctions.[16] Based on these descriptive observations, it has been assumed that the dermal microcirculation of CVI patients has functional derangements related to permeability and ulcer formation. It was not until 1997 that a quantitative morphometric analysis of the dermal microcirculation was reported.[11] The objectives of this investigation were to quantify differences in endothelial cell structure and local cell type with emphasis on leukocyte cell type and their relationship to arterioles, capillaries and post-capillary venules (PCVs). Variables assessed were number and types of leukocytes, endothelial cell thickness, endothelial vesicle density, inter-endothelial junctional width, cuff thickness and ribosome density. Thirty-five patients had two 4-mm punch biopsies obtained from the lower calf (gaiter region) and lower thigh. Patients were separated into one of four groups according to the 1995 ISCVS/SVS (International Society for Cardiovascular Surgery/Society for Vascular Surgery) CEAP classification 1. Group 1 consisted of five patients with no evidence of venous disease. Skin biopsies from these patients served as normal controls. Groups 2–4 consisted of patients with CEAP class 4 (n = 11), class 5 (n = 9) and class 6 (n = 10) CVI.

Endothelial cell characteristics

No significant differences were observed in endothelial cell thickness of arterioles, capillaries and PCVs from either gaiter or thigh biopsies. Qualitatively, endothelial cells appeared metabolically active. Many nuclei exhibited an euchromatic appearance, implying active mRNA transcription. In most instances, ribosome numbers were so abundant that they exceeded the resolution capacity of the image analysis system and were unable to be quantified. The prominence in ribosome content and the euchromatic appearance of the endothelial cell nucleus strongly suggested active protein production. No significant differences in vesicle density were observed in gaiter biopsies between groups. Class 6 patients exhibited an increased number of vesicles in arterioles and PCV endothelia from thigh biopsies but did not differ compared with gaiter biopsies. Mean inter-endothelial junctional width varied within a normal range of 20–50 nm. Significantly widened inter-endothelial gap junctions were not observed and thus conflicted with the reports of Wenner *et al.*[16] Mean basal lamina thickness differed significantly at the capillary level in both gaiter and thigh biopsies. Differences were most pronounced in patients with class 4 disease. These data indicated that endothelial cells from the dermal microcirculation of CVI patients were far from abnormal. They demonstrated increased metabolic activity suggestive of active cellular transcription and protein production. Most surprising was the observation of uniformly tight gap junctions. Previously these gap junctions were reported to be as wide as 180 nm and it was assumed that these widened junctions were responsible for macromolecule extravasation and edema formation.[5,6,16,18] Pappas *et al.* suggested that alternative methods for tissue edema, such as increased transendothelial vesicle transport, formation of transendothelial channels, and alterations in the glycocalyx lining the junctional cleft, may be involved in CVI edema and macromolecule transport.[11]

Types and distribution of leukocytes

The most striking differences in cell type and distribution were observed with mast cells and macrophages (Figs 6.2–6.4). In both gaiter and thigh biopsies, mast cell numbers were two to four times greater than control in class 4 and 5 patients around arterioles and PCVs (P <0.05). Class 6 patients demonstrated no difference in mast cell number compared to controls. Mast cell numbers around capillaries did not differ across groups in either gaiter or thigh biopsies. Macrophages demonstrated increased numbers in class 5 and 6 patients around arterioles and PCVs, respectively (P <0.05). Differences in macrophage numbers around capillaries were observed primarily in class 4 patients in both gaiter and thigh biopsies. Surprisingly, lymphocytes, plasma cells and neutrophils were not present in the immediate perivascular space. Fibroblasts were the most common cells observed in both gaiter and thigh biopsies. Pappas *et al.* speculated that mast cells and macrophages may function to regulate tissue remodeling resulting in dermal fibrosis.[11] The mast cell enzyme chymase is a potent activator of matrix metalloproteinases 1 and 3 (collagenase and stromelysin).[19–21] In an *in vitro* model using the human mast cell line HMC-1, these cells were reported to spontaneously adhere to fibronectin, laminin and collagen types I and III, all components of the perivascular cuff (see below).[21] Chymase also causes release of latent TGF-β_1 secreted by activated endothelial cells, fibroblasts and platelets from extracellular

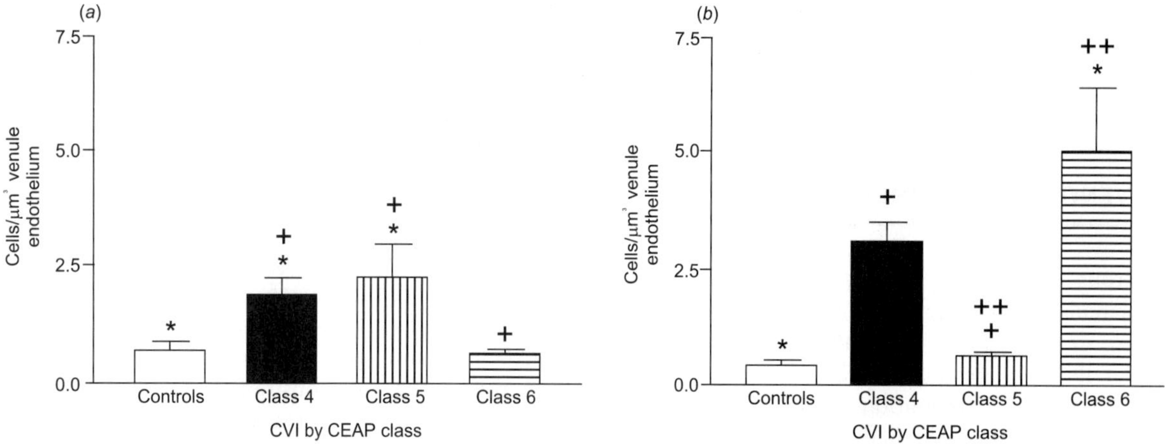

Figure 6.2 *Histogram demonstrating (a) mast cell and (b) macrophage density surrounding postcapillary venules according to disease classification. Increased mast cell content was observed in class 4 and 5 patients compared with controls and class 6 patients (P ≤0.05). Increased macrophage content was observed in class 6 patients compared with control and class 4 and 5 patients (P ≤0.05).*

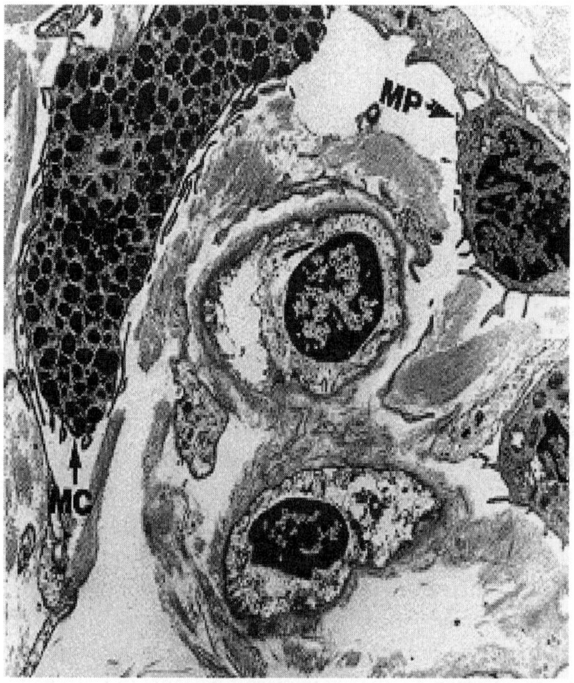

Figure 6.3 *Photomicrograph of a mast cell (MC), fibroblast, and macrophage (MP) surrounding a capillary (×3440).*

matrices.[22] Release and activation of TGF-β_1 initiates a cascade of events in which macrophages and fibroblasts are recruited to wound healing sites and stimulated to produce fibroblast mitogens and connective tissue proteins, respectively.[23] Mast cell degranulation leading to TGF-β_1 activation and macrophage recruitment may explain why decreased mast cell and increased macrophage numbers were observed in class 6 patients. Macrophage migration, as evidenced by the frequent appearance of cytoplasmic tails in perivascular macrophages, further substantiates the concept of inflammatory cytokine recruitment (Fig. 6.4).

Extracellular matrix (ECM) alterations

Once leukocytes have migrated to the extracellular space, they localize around capillaries and postcapillary venules. The perivascular space is surrounded by extracellular matrix (ECM) proteins and forms a perivascular cuff. Adjacent to these perivascular cuffs, and throughout the dermal interstitium, is an intense and disorganized collagen deposition.[5,11] Perivascular cuffs and the accompanying collagen deposition are the *sine qua non* of the dermal microcirculation in CVI patients (Fig. 6.4). The perivascular cuff was originally thought to be the result of fibrinogen extravasation and erroneously referred to as a 'fibrin cuff'.[5] It is now known that the cuff is a ring of ECM proteins consisting of collagens type I and III, fibronectin, vitronectin, laminin, tenascin and fibrin.[24] The role of the cuff and its cell of origin is not completely understood. The investigation by Pappas *et al.* suggested that the endothelial cells of the dermal microcirculation were responsible for cuff formation. The cuff was once thought to be a barrier to oxygen and nutrient diffusion; however, recent evidence suggests that cuff formation is an attempt to maintain vascular architecture in response to increased mechanical load.[25] Although perivascular cuffs may function to preserve microcirculatory architecture, several pathologic processes may be related to cuff formation. Immunohistochemical analyses have demonstrated transforming growth factor-β_1 (TGF-β_1) and α_2-macroglobulin in the interstices of perivascular cuffs.[26] It has been suggested that these 'trapped' molecules are abnormally distributed in the dermis leading to altered tissue remodeling and fibrosis. Cuffs may also serve as a lattice for capillary

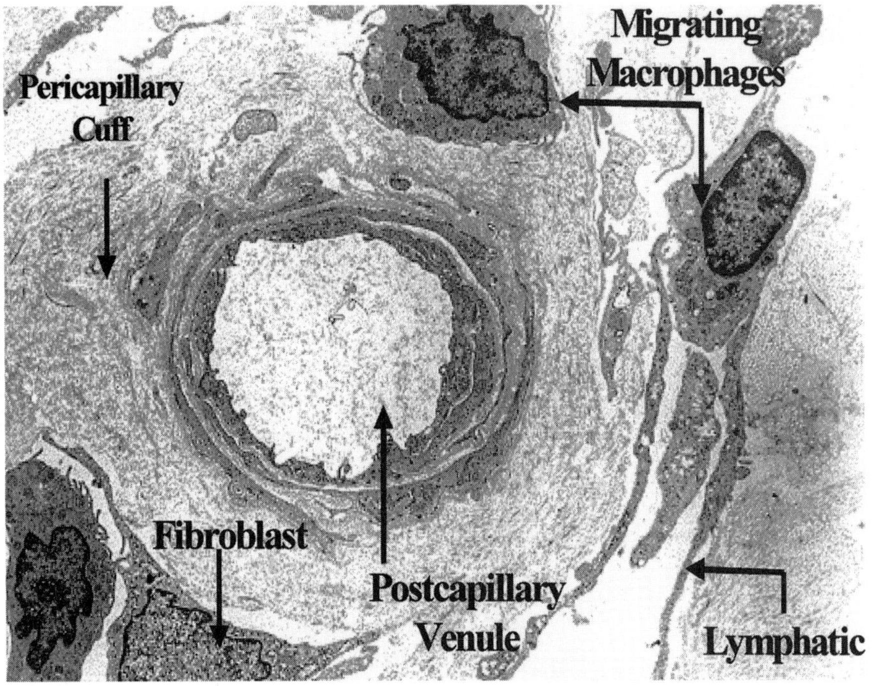

Figure 6.4 *Photomicrograph demonstrating a well developed perivascular cuff, a cytoplasmic tail from a migrating macrophage, a macrophage entering a lymphatic, a fibroblast and interstitial collagen deposition (×2450).*

angiogenesis explaining the capillary tortuosity and increased capillary density observed in the dermis of CVI patients.

PATHOPHYSIOLOGY OF STASIS DERMATITIS AND DERMAL FIBROSIS

The mechanisms modulating leukocyte activation, fibroblast function and dermal extracellular matrix alterations have been the focus of investigation in the 1990s. CVI is a disease of chronic inflammation due to a persistent and sustained injury secondary to venous hypertension. It is hypothesized that the primary injury is extravasation of macromolecules (i.e. fibrinogen and α_2-macroglobulin) and red blood cells (RBCs) into the dermal interstitium.[16] RBC degradation products and interstitial protein extravasation are potent chemoattractants and presumably represent the initial underlying chronic inflammatory signal responsible for leukocyte recruitment. It has been assumed that these cytochemical events are responsible for the increased expression of ICAM-1 (intercellular adhesion molecule-1) on endothelial cells of microcirculatory exchange vessels observed in CVI dermal biopsies.[10] ICAM-1 is the activation-dependent adhesion molecule utilized by macrophages, lymphocytes and mast cells for diapedesis. As stated above, all these cells have been observed by immunohistochemistry and electron microscopy in the interstitium of dermal biopsies.[10,11]

Cytokine regulation and tissue fibrosis

Our laboratory has been interested in the mechanisms regulating dermal tissue remodeling in CVI patients. Leukocyte recruitment, ECM alterations and tissue fibrosis are characteristic of chronic inflammatory diseases caused by alterations in TGF-β_1 gene expression and protein production. To determine the role of TGF-β_1 in CVI, dermal biopsies from normal patients and CEAP classes 4, 5 and 6 CVI patients were analyzed for TGF-β_1 gene expression, protein production and cellular location.[27] Quantitative RT-PCR for TGF-β_1 gene expression was performed on 24 skin biopsies obtained from 24 patients. Patients were separated into four groups according to the ISCVS/SVS classification for CVI: normal skin ($n = 6$), CEAP class 4 ($n = 6$), CEAP class 5 ($n = 5$) and CEAP class 6 ($n = 7$). TGF-β_1 gene transcripts for controls, classes 4, 5 and 6 patients were 7.02 ± 7.33, 43.33 ± 9.0, 16.13 ± 7.67 and 7.22 ± 0.56 × 10^{-14} mol/μg total RNA, respectively. The differences in TGF-β_1 gene expression in class 4 patients was significantly elevated compared with control and class 5 and 6 patients (Fig. 6.5, $P < 0.05$).[27] An additional 38 patients had 54 biopsies from the lower calf (LC) and lower thigh (LT) analyzed for TGF-β_1 protein concentration. The amount of active TGF-β_1 in picograms/gram (pg/g) of tissue from LC and LT biopsies compared with normal skin biopsies were as follows: normal skin (<1.0 pc/g), class 4 (LC, 5061 ± 1827; LT 317.3 ± 277), class 5 (LC, 8327 ± 3690; LT 193 ± 164) and class 6 (LC, 5392 ± 1800; LT, 117 ± 61) (Fig. 6.6). Differences between normal skin

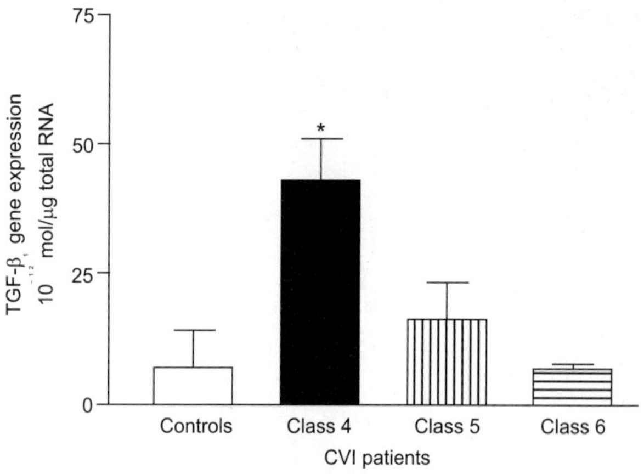

Figure 6.5 *Quantitative RT-PCR results demonstrating increased TGF-β_1 gene transcript levels from skin biopsies in class 4 patients compared with controls and class 5 and 6 patients (*P ≤0.05).*

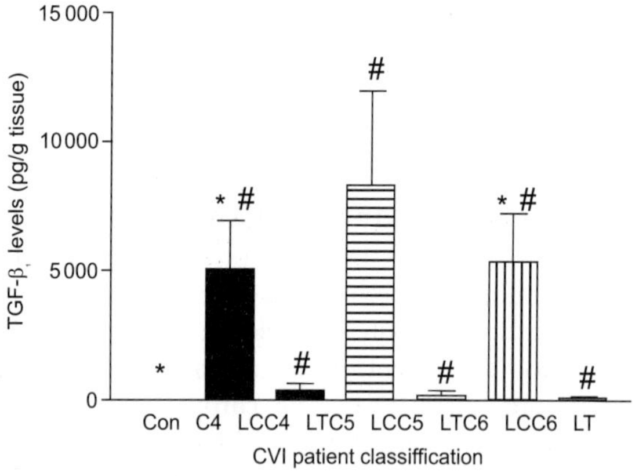

Figure 6.6 *Bioactive TGF-β_1 protein levels from dermal skin patients in CVI patients. Differences in active TGF-β_1 protein concentration between and within CVI groups compared with controls. Increased active TGF-β_1 protein was observed in class 4 and 6 patients compared to control (Con) and class 5 patients (P ≤0.05). Differences between calf and thigh biopsies were significant within CVI groups (P ≤0.05).*

and class 4 and 6 patients were significant ($P \leq 0.05$ and $P \leq 0.01$, respectively). No differences between class 4, 5 and 6 patients were observed. Differences between LC and LT within each CVI group were significant (class 4, $P \leq 0.003$; class 5, $P \leq 0.008$; class 6, $P \leq 0.02$). These data demonstrate that in areas of clinically active CVI, increased amounts of active TGF-β_1 are present compared with normal skin. Furthermore, active TGF-β_1 protein concentrations of biopsies from the LT did not differ from normal skin, demonstrating a regionalized response to injury.[27]

Immunohistochemistry and immunogold labeling experiments were performed to identify the sources of active TGF-β_1 protein production. Immunohistochemistry of normal skin and ipsilateral thigh biopsies of CVI patients demonstrated mild TGF-β_1 in the basal layer of the epidermis. The dermis demonstrated few capillaries, ordered collagen architecture and no interstitial leukocytes. CVI dermal biopsies from areas of clinically active disease demonstrated staining of the basal layer of the epidermis, interstitial leukocytes and fibroblasts. Many perivascular leukocytes demonstrated positive staining of intracellular granules and appeared morphologically similar to previously reported mast cells (Fig. 6.7).[27] Numerous capillaries with perivascular cuffs were observed; however, cuffs did not stain positively for TGF-β_1.[27] This study conflicts with the observations reported by Higley *et al.* in which they reported positive TGF-β_1 staining in perivascular cuffs and an absence of TGF-β_1 in the provisional matrix of the venous ulcer compared to healing donor skin graft sites.[26] They concluded that TGF-β_1 was therefore abnormally 'trapped' in the perivascular cuff and therefore unavailable for normal granulation tissue development. Differences between the two studies may relate to biopsy site selection. Higley *et al.* biopsied chronic, non-healing venous ulcer edges and ulcer bases, whereas patients with active ulcers in the study by Pappas *et al.* were biopsied 5–10 cm away from an active ulcer. Therefore, the former study reflects the biology of chronic wound healing whereas our data suggests active tissue remodeling in response to a chronic injury stimulus.

Immunogold labeling confirmed the presence of TGF-β_1 in dermal leukocytes. Positive labeling of gold particles were similarly observed in collagen fibrils of the ECM. This observation may explain why the molecular regulation of TGF-β_1 in CVI patients demonstrates differential gene and protein production according to disease classification. As stated above, the gene expression of TGF-β_1 was increased in class 4 patients only while the protein production was essentially increased in class 4, 5 and 6 patients. These differences may be related to disease severity and the pluripotential responses of TGF-β_1. TGF-β_1 can have inhibitory and stimulatory effects that are primarily dependent on local concentration, cell source and surrounding ECM. In the study by Pappas *et al.*, class 4 patients were younger than the other study groups, never experienced an episode of venous stasis ulceration and clinically demonstrated less dermal tissue fibrosis. TGF-β_1 in these patients may therefore be involved in limiting the response to injury. Indeed, one could speculate that early on in the disease process, a low-grade production of TGF-β_1 is a normal wound healing response and may serve to prevent the onset and development of tissue fibrosis. With continued and prolonged exposure, an imbalance in tissue remodeling in patients with class 5 and 6 disease clinically manifests itself as dermatofibrosis. A pathologic effect of increased ECM deposition is an alteration in the storage and release of growth factors.[22] The latent form of

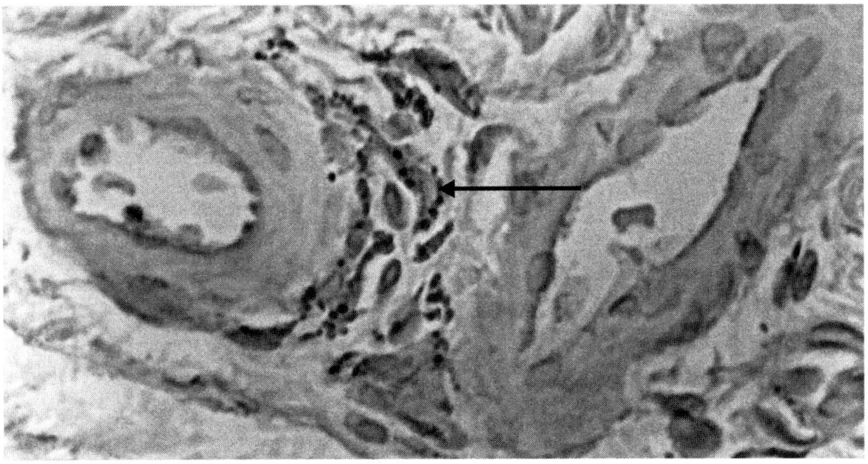

Figure 6.7 *Immunohistochemistry for TGF-β_1 demonstrating positive in granules of perivascular leukocytes (arrow) which appear morphologically to mast cells (×495).*

TGF-β_1 is secreted from cells bound to one of three latent TGF-β_1 binding proteins (LTBP). Once secreted, LTBPs mediate binding of latent TGF-β_1 to matrix proteins. Matrix release of TGF-β_1 is mediated by multiple serine proteinases including plasmin, mast cell chymase and leukocyte elastase.[23,28–30] An increase in the number of mast cells and circulating leukocyte elastase have been previously reported in CVI patients.[11,31] The increase in active TGF-β_1 observed in class 5 and 6 patients may therefore result from ECM release of latent TGF-β_1, resulting in tissue fibrosis. This hypothesis is consistent with the demonstration of immunogold labeling to collagen fibrils in the ECM of CVI patients. The modulation of TGF-β_1 release from the ECM may therefore provide a faster means of signal transduction than simple control of gene expression and therefore explain the sustained increase of TGF-β_1 in class 5 and 6 patients in the absence of increased gene expression. This study did not demonstrate increased TGF-β_1 staining in the ECM by ICC because the primary antibody used was specific only for active TGF-β_1 and therefore may have missed LAP- and LTBP-associated TGF-β_1.

In summary, the study by Pappas *et al.* demonstrated increased gene expression of TGF-β_1 in patients with class 4 CVI and increased protein production in patients with class 4, 5 and 6 CVI. Active TGF-β_1 protein appeared to originate from leukocytes, many of which morphologically were similar to mast cells. Similarly, fibroblasts stained positively for TGF-β_1, suggesting that they are the target cells for activated leukocytes. The authors hypothesized that increased active TGF-β_1 protein observed in class 5 and 6 patients, in the absence of a corresponding increase of gene expression, is the result of ECM storage of TGF-β_1. Immunogold labeling of collagen fibrils containing active TGF-β_1 gold-labeled particles supports this position. These data therefore suggest that activated leukocytes traverse perivascular cuffs and release TGF-β_1, which binds to interstitial dermal fibroblasts. Once bound, collagen production is stimulated and if the process proceeds unabated, tissue fibrosis and end-organ dysfunction ensue.

Dermal fibroblast function

Several studies have reported aberrant phenotypic behavior of fibroblasts isolated from venous ulcer edges when compared with fibroblasts obtained from ipsilateral thigh biopsies of normal skin in the same patients. Hasan *et al.* compared the ability of venous ulcer fibroblasts to produce αI procollagen mRNA and collagen after stimulation with TGF-β_1.[32] These authors were not able to demonstrate differences in αI procollagen mRNA levels after stimulation with TGF-β_1 between venous ulcer fibroblasts and normal fibroblasts (control) from ipsilateral thigh biopsies. However, collagen production was increased by 60% in a dose-dependent manner in controls whereas venous ulcer fibroblasts were unresponsive. This unresponsiveness was associated with a fourfold decrease in TGF-β_1 type II receptors. A similar investigation reported a decrease in collagen production from venous ulcer fibroblasts and similar amounts of fibronectin production when compared with normal controls.[33]

Fibroblast responsiveness to growth factors was further delineated by Stanley *et al.*[34] These investigators characterized the proliferative responses of venous ulcer fibroblasts when stimulated with basic fibroblastic growth factor (bFGF), epidermal growth factor (EGF) and interleukin 1β (IL-1β). In their initial study, they reported that venous ulcer fibroblast growth rates were markedly suppressed when stimulated with bFGF, EGF and IL-1β. They noted that normal fibroblasts appeared compact and tapered with well defined nuclear morphologic features, whereas venous ulcer fibroblasts appeared larger, polygonal and with varied nuclear morphologic features. Venous ulcer fibroblasts appeared morphologically similar to fibroblasts undergoing cellular senescence. The authors therefore concluded that the blunted growth response of their cells was associated with cellular senescence.[34]

Other characteristics of senescent cells are an overexpression of matrix proteins such as fibronectin (cFN) and enhanced activity of β-galactosidase (SA-β-Gal). In an evaluation of seven patients with venous stasis ulcers, the same group of investigators noted a higher percentage of SA-β-Gal positive cells in venous ulcers compared with normal controls (6.3% versus 0.21%, $P \leq 0.0.6$).[35] They also reported that venous ulcer fibroblasts produced one to four times more cFN by Western blot analysis compared with controls. In a follow-up investigation they noted an increase in fibronectin mRNA and protein production but reported that the previously observed growth inhibition could be reversed with bFGF.[36] These data support the hypothesis that venous ulcer fibroblasts phenotypically behave like senescent cells. However, these responses may not be reflective of events occurring in the lower extremity dermis of CVI patients. The biology of a stasis ulcer is similar to that of chronic nonhealing wounds and may not be reflective of active ongoing tissue remodeling observed in CVI patients without venous ulcers. Furthermore, what role senescence has on disease progression has yet to be determined.

Role of matrix metalloproteinases (MMPs) and their inhibitors in venous ulcer healing

The signaling event responsible for the development of a venous ulcer and the mechanisms responsible for prolonged wound healing are poorly understood. Wound healing is an orderly process that involves inflammation, re-epithelialization, matrix deposition and tissue remodeling. Tissue remodeling and matrix deposition are processes controlled by matrix metalloproteinases (MMPs) and tissue inhibitors of matrix metalloproteinases (TIMPs). In general, MMPs and TIMPs are not constitutively expressed. They are induced temporarily in response to exogenous signals such as various cytokines, or growth factors, cell–matrix interactions and altered cell–cell contacts. TGF-β_1 is a potent inducer of TIMP-1 and inhibitor of MMP-1. Several studies have demonstrated that prolonged and continuous TGF-β_1 production causes tissue fibrosis by stimulating ECM production and inhibiting degradation by affecting MMP and TIMP production. Alterations in MMP and TIMP production may similarly modulate the tissue fibrosis of the lower extremity in CVI patients. In patients with active ulcers, increases in MMP activity from ulcer exudates and decreased expression of TIMP-1 in keratinocytes from venous ulcers have been reported.[37,38] These observations suggest that excessive proteolysis may be responsible for the decreased healing rates seen with venous stasis ulcers.

CONCLUSION

Venous hypertension causes extravasation of RBCs and macromolecules that results in leukocyte migration into the dermis. Once in the dermis, a cascade of pathologic events occurs which results in dermal fibrosis. One of these events is an increase in TGF-β_1. TGF-β_1 is either released by macrophages and mast cells or autoinduced by dermal fibroblasts. This increase presumably causes an imbalance in tissue remodeling, resulting in increased collagen synthesis. The role of other growth factors and matrix metalloproteinases in CVI dermal pathology is currently being investigated. Very little is understood regarding the mechanisms of CVI dermal angiogenesis and keratinocyte physiology. The answers to these questions will help in the development of future tissue-engineered products and techniques for the prevention of venous ulceration. It is our hope that these chapters will stimulate future and current investigators to include CVI in their research endeavors in order to better serve patients with chronic venous insufficiency.

REFERENCES

1. Porter JM. International Consensus Committee on Chronic Venous Disease. Reporting standards in venous disease: an update. *J Vasc Surg* 1995; **21**: 635–45.
2. Homans J. The etiology and treatment of varicose ulcer of the leg. *Surg Gynecol Obstet* 1917; **24**: 300–11.
3. Pratt GH. Arterial varices: a syndrome. *Am J Surg* 1949; **77**: 456–60.
4. Lyndemayr WLOMAPH. Arteriovenous shunts in primary varicosis: a critical essay. *Vasc Surg* 1972; **6**: 9–14.
5. Burnand KG, Whimster I, Naidoo A, Browse NL. Pericapillary fibrin deposition in the ulcer bearing skin of the lower limb: the cause of lipodermatosclerosis and venous ulceration. *Br Med J* 1982; **285**: 1071–2.
6. Burnand KG, Clemenson.G., Gaunt J, Browse NL. The effect of sustained venous hypertension in the skin and capillaries of the canine hind limb. *Br J Surg* 1981; **69**: 41–4.
7. Smith PDC, Thomas P, Scurr JH, Dormandy JA. Causes of venous ulceration: a new hypothesis. *Br Med J* 1988; **296**: 1726–7.
8. Thomas P, Nash GB, Dormandy JA. White cell accumulation in dependent legs of patients with venous hypertension: a possible mechanism for trophic changes in the skin. *Br Med J* 1988; **296**: 1693–5.
9. Scott HJ, Smith PDC, Scurr JH. Histological study of white blood cells and their association with lipodermatosclerosis and venous ulceration. *Br J Surg* 1991; **78**: 210–11.

10. Wilkinson LS, Bunker C, Edward JCW, Scurr JH, Smith PDC. Leukocytes: their role in the etiopathogenesis of skin damage in venous disease. *J Vasc Surg* 1993; **17**: 669–75.
11. Pappas PJ, DeFouw DO, Venezio LM, *et al.* Morphometric assessment of the dermal microcirculation in patients with chronic venous insufficiency. *J Vasc Surg* 1997; **26**: 784–95.
12. Pappas PJ, Fallek SR, Garcia A, *et al.* Role of leukocyte activation in patients with venous stasis ulcers. *J Surg Res* 1995; **59**: 553–9.
13. Pappas PJ, Teehan EP, Fallek SR, *et al.* Diminished mononuclear cell function is associated with chronic venous insufficiency. *J Vasc Surg* 1995; **22**: 580–6.
14. Leu AJ, Leu HJ, Franzeck UK, Bollinger A. Microvascular changes in chronic venous insufficiency: a review. *Cardiovasc Surg* 1995; **3**: 237–45.
15. Leu HJ. Morphology of chronic venous insufficiency-light and electron microscopic examinations. *Vasa* 1991; **20**: 330–42.
16. Wenner A, Leu HJ, Spycher M, Brunner U. Ultrastructural changes of capillaries in chronic venous insufficiency. *Exp Cell Biol* 1980; **48**: 1–14.
17. Scelsi R, Scelsi L, Cortinovis R, Poggi P. Morphological changes of dermal blood and lymphatic vessels in chronic venous insufficiency of the leg. *Int Angiol* 1994; **13**: 308–11.
18. Browse NL, Burnand KG. The cause of venous ulceration. *Lancet* 1982; **2**: 243–5.
19. Saarien J, Lalkkinen N, Welgus HG, Kovannen PT. Activation of human interstitial procollagenase through direct cleavage of the Leu83-Thr84 bond by mast cell chymase. *J Biol Chem* 1994; **269**: 18134–40.
20. Lees M, Taylor DJ, Woolley DE. Mast cell proteinases activate precursor forms of collagenase and stromelysin, but not of gelatinases A and B. *Eur J Biochem* 1994; **223**: 171–7.
21. Kruger-Drasagakes S, Grutzkau A, Baghramian R, Henz BM. Interactions of immature human mast cells with extracellular matrix: expression of specific adhesion receptors and their role in cell binding to matrix proteins. *J Invest Dermatol* 1996; **106**: 538–43.
22. Taipale J, Keski-oja J. Growth factors in the extracellular matrix. *FASEB J* 1997; **11**: 51–9.
23. Roberts AB, Flanders KC, Kondaiah P, *et al.* Transforming growth factor β: biochemistry and roles in embryogenesis, tissue repair and remodeling, and carcinogenesis. *Recent Prog Horm Res* 1988; **44**: 157–97.
24. Herrick S, Sloan P, McGurk M, Freak L, McCollum CN, Ferguson WJ. Sequential changes in histologic pattern and extracellular matrix deposition during the healing of chronic venous ulcers. *Am J Pathol* 1992; **141**: 1085–95.
25. Bishop JE. Regulation of cardiovascular collagen deposition by mechanical forces. *Mol Med Today* 1998; **4**: 69–75.
26. Higley HR, Kasander GA, Gerhardt CO, Falanga V. Extravasation of macromolecules and possible trapping of transforming growth factor-β_1 in venous ulceration. *Br J Dermatol* 1995; **132**: 79–85.
27. Pappas PJ, You R, Rameshwar P, *et al.* Dermal tissue fibrosis in patients with chronic venous insufficiency is associated with increased transforming growth factor-$\beta_1$gene expression and protein production. *J Vasc Surg* 1999; **30**: 1129–45.
28. O'Kane S, Ferguson WJ. Transforming growth factor βs and wound healing. *Int J Biochem Cell Biol* 1997; **29**: 63–78.
29. Border WA, Noble NA. Transforming growth factor β in tissue fibrosis. *N Engl J Med* 1994; **331**: 1286–92.
30. Grande JP. Role of transforming growth factor-β in tissue injury and repair. *Proc Soc Exp Biol Med* 1997; **214**: 27–40.
31. Shields DA, Sarin AS, Scurr JH, Smith PDC. Plasma elastase in venous disease. *Br J Surg* 1994; **81**: 1496–9.
32. Hasan A, Murata H, Falabella A, *et al.* Dermal fibroblasts from venous ulcers are unresponsive to the action of transforming growth factor-β_1. *J Dermatol Sci* 1997; **16**: 59–66.
33. Herrick SE, Ireland GW, Simon D, McCollum CN, Ferguson MW. Venous ulcer fibroblasts compared with normal fibroblasts show differences in collagen but not in fibronectin production under both normal and hypoxic conditions. *J Invest Dermatol* 1996; **106**: 187–93.
34. Stanley AC, Park H, Phillips TJ, Russakovsky V, Menzoian JO. Reduced growth of dermal fibroblasts from chronic venous ulcers can be stimulated with growth factors. *J Vasc Surg* 1997; **26**: 994–1001.
35. Mendez MV, Stanley A, Park H, Shon K, Phillips TJ, Menzoian JO. Fibroblasts cultured from venous ulcers display cellular characteristics of senescence. *J Vasc Surg* 1998; **28**: 876–83.
36. Mendez MV, Stanley A, Phillips TJ, Murphy M, Menzoian JO, Park H. Fibroblasts cultured from distal lower extremities in patients with venous reflux display cellular characteristics of senescence. *J Vasc Surg* 1998; **28**: 1040–50.
37. Vaalamo M, Weckroth M, Puolakkainen P, *et al.* Patterns of matrix metalloproteinase and TIMP-1 expression in chronic and normally healing human cutaneous wounds. *Br J Dermatol* 1996; **135**: 52–9.
38. Saarialho-Kere UK, Kovacs SO, Pentland AP, Olerud JE, Welgus HG, Parks WC. Cell-matrix interactions modulate interstitial collagenase expression by human keratinocytes actively involved in wound healing. *J Clin Invest* 1993; **92**: 2858–66.

PART 2

Evaluation and diagnosis

7

Clinical assessment of patients with venous disease

ANDREW BRADBURY AND C VAUGHAN RUCKLEY

Most patients referred to vascular surgeons because of venous symptoms and signs undergo some form of further investigation, usually duplex ultrasound, in addition to clinical assessment. One interpretation of this observation would be that most practitioners believe history and examination alone to be unreliable, even misleading, in the assessment of venous pathology. Although there are circumstances where this is undoubtedly true, much useful information can be gleaned from a thorough clinical assessment based upon a sound understanding of the underlying anatomy and pathophysiological mechanisms. It may be the case that the modern vascular surgeon has become rather spoilt by the availability, in most health care settings, of duplex and other investigative modalities. However, we must not become lazy and dispense with clinical assessment as:

- further investigations are not always obtainable, for example, in the emergency situation or in less well developed health care settings;
- it may guide the choice of investigation(s) and enable questions posed to the technologist to be framed in a more clinically (and cost) effective manner;
- it may allow a more meaningful interpretation of the results of investigations.

THE UPPER LIMB

The upper limb is less frequently involved with venous disease than the leg. However, such disease can have serious consequences for the patients because:

- morbidity of symptoms may be considerable, especially in the dominant arm, because the patients affected are often young and otherwise active;
- for an increasing number of patients, ready access to and normal function of the veins of the upper limb offer the only prospect of long-term survival, for example, hemodialysis, parenteral nutrition, long-term antibiotic administration, chemotherapy;
- there is an increased realization that the long-term patency of femorodistal bypass with prosthetic material may be unacceptably poor. That observation, together with an increase in graft infection [particularly methicillin-resistant *Staphylococcus aureus* (MRSA)], has led many surgeons to more frequent use of arm vein for limb salvage.

Anatomic considerations

SUPERFICIAL VEINS

The superficial veins of the hand are highly variable and drain into the cephalic vein laterally and the basilic vein medially (Fig. 7.1). The cephalic vein:

- begins on the radial side of the wrist in the anatomic snuff box;
- ascends to the lateral margin of the antecubital fossa;
- continues lateral to the biceps muscle;
- passes through the deltopectoral groove;
- finally pieces the coracoclavicular fascia to join the axillary vein just below the clavicle.

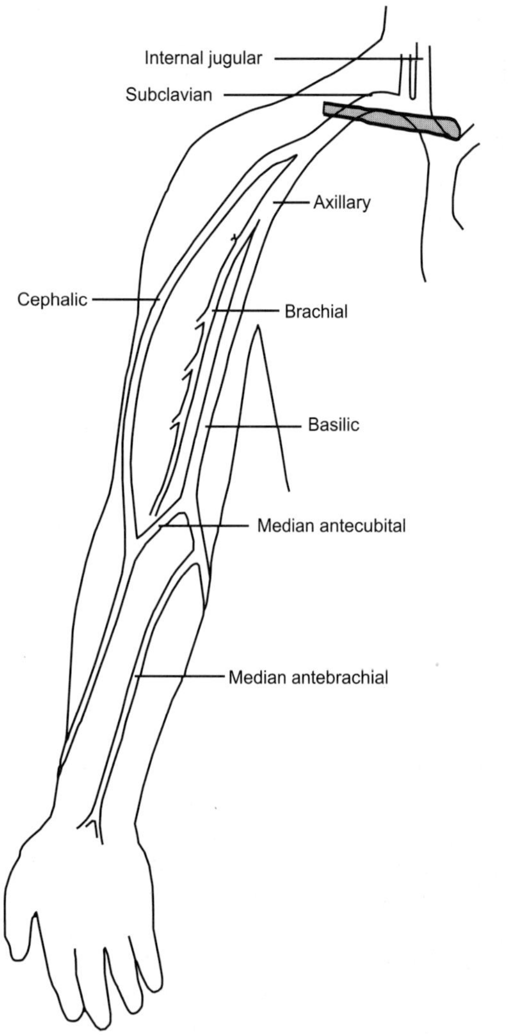

Figure 7.1 *Major veins of the arm: on the radial side of the arm the cephalic vein begins at the anatomic snuff box, ascends to the antecubital space and then remains lateral to the biceps in the upper arm and in the deltopectoral groove pierces the coracoclavicular fascia to join the axillary vein. The veins on the ulnar side of the forearm and the medial antecubital vein drain into the basilic vein, which is joined in the upper arm by the brachial vein to become the axillary vein. The axillary vein becomes the subclavian vein at the outer border of the first rib and the internal jugular vein joins it in the base of the neck to become the innominate vein. (Reproduced with permission from DeWeese JA. Management of subclavian venous obstruction. In Bergan JJ, Yao JST, eds.* Surgery of the Veins. *New York: Grune & Stratton, 1985;* ***26****: 365–72)*

The basilic vein:

- ascends the forearm on its medial side, curling to the ventral from its dorsal aspect;
- is joined by the median antecubital veins;
- passes medial to biceps; and
- joins the brachial vein in the upper arm.

DEEP VEINS

These follow the respective arteries and may be paired. The basilic vein joins the brachial vein in the upper arm to form the axillary vein, which is joined by the cephalic vein just below the clavicle. The axillary vein becomes the subclavian vein as it enters the costoclavicular space, which is bounded by:

- the first rib below;
- the clavicle, subclavius muscle and the costocoracoid ligament above (Fig. 7.2).

The subclavian vein is separated from the subclavian artery by the scalenus anterior muscle and joins with the internal jugular vein to become the innominate vein.

Intermittent subclavian vein obstruction

In the authors' practice this is a rare presentation as most patients seem to seek medical attention only once the vein has thrombosed (see below). However, identification of patients at the pre-occlusive stage may allow pre-emptive treatment to be considered.[1] Patients typically complain of:

- intermittent swelling;
- discomfort and tightness (not usually true pain) in the arm, which is relieved by rest;
- abnormally prominent superficial veins.

These symptoms are aggravated in the erect position or when the arm is raised above the head; for example, typing, playing the piano, driving the car, standing to attention, playing the flute or painting a ceiling.

Patients with these symptoms should be evaluated with their shoulders braced in the military position (Fig. 7.3) or with their arms hyperabducted and externally rotated at the shoulder (Fig. 7.4), as this will result in the subclavian vein being compressed by the scissor-like closure of the costoclavicular space. Arm discomfort, swelling and venous distension in this position suggests intermittent venous outflow obstruction. However, as with arterial thoracic outlet obstruction, these findings can be reproduced in certain otherwise normal individuals at the extremes of movement.

Superficial thrombophlebitis

This is characterized by localized pain, redness and swelling over a segment of a superficial vein. The great majority of cases are iatrogenic due to cannulation site infection. Palpation will reveal tenderness over an underlying thrombus in the vein with surrounding induration. If the thrombus in the vein is localized and not infected, there will not be significant distal swelling. Thrombus that propagates to involve the deep vein may, at least

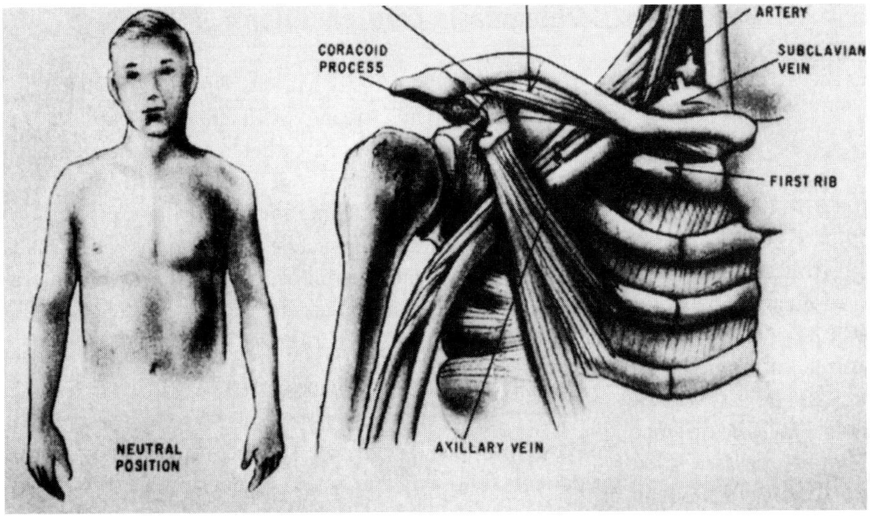

Figure 7.2 *Course of the subclavian vein: the subclavian vein begins at the lateral border of the first rib and enters the costoclavicular space which is bordered by the first rib posteriorly and the clavicle with its underlying subclavius muscle and costocoracoid ligament anteriorly. The subclavian vein remains anterior to the anterior scalene muscle as opposed to the subclavian artery which lies posterior to that muscle. (Adapted from Adams JT, DeWeese JA, Mahoney EB,* et al. *Intermittent subclavian vein obstruction without thrombosis.* Surgery *1968;* ***63****: 147–65)*

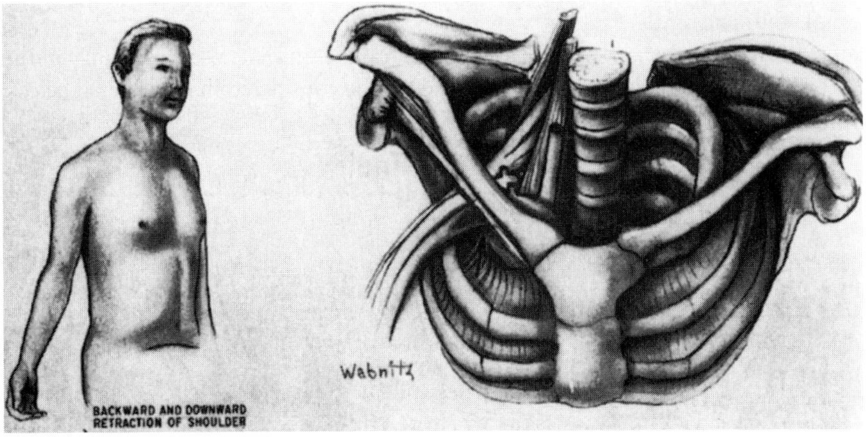

Figure 7.3 *Compression of the subclavian vein in the military position: when the shoulder is retracted backward and downward the subclavian vein is narrowed by the scissoring action of the clavicle and first rib. (Adapted from Adams JT, DeWeese JA, Mahoney EB,* et al. *Intermittent subclavian vein obstruction without thrombosis.* Surgery *1968;* ***63****: 147–65)*

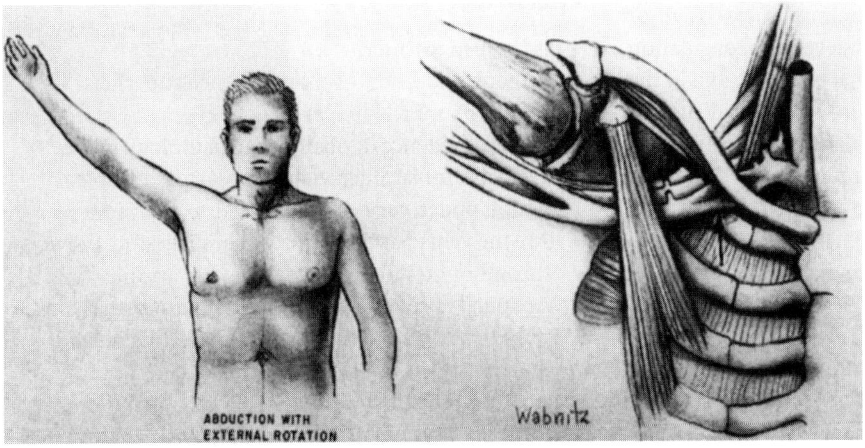

Figure 7.4 *Compression of the subclavian vein with hyperabduction of the arm: with hyperabduction and external rotation of the arm the clavicle rotates backward and downward and causes compression of the subclavian vein secondary to narrowing of the costoclavicular space. (Adapted from Adams JT, DeWeese JA, Mahoney EB,* et al. *Intermittent subclavian vein obstruction without thrombosis.* Surgery *1968;* ***63****: 147–65)*

theoretically, lead to pulmonary embolus, but is rare. A history of thrombophlebitis is important as it may have important consequences for venous access and the utility of arm vein for arterial bypass.

Primary axillary-subclavian vein thrombosis

Once considered rare, patients with this condition are now increasingly presented to the vascular surgeon for consideration of active intervention. Thrombosis originates in a chronically traumatized subclavian vein that has been repeatedly compressed by the costo-clavicular scissors, and propagates for a variable distance both proximally and distally. It is said to be associated with pulmonary embolus in up to 10% of cases but in the authors' experience this has not been observed. Patients present with arm swelling and discomfort, often following a particularly strenuous activity (hence the alternative term 'effort thrombosis'),[2] associated with either backward or downward traction on the shoulders, or hyperabduction of the arm. The pain, swelling, rubor and venous distension may be quite severe. Associated arterial and neurological features of thoracic outlet compression are unusual. On examination the arm is obviously swollen, has a bluish discoloration with distended collateral veins over the shoulder. Treatment remains controversial but comprises various combinations of anticoagulation, thrombolysis and surgical decompression.

Secondary axillary-subclavian thrombosis

As the numbers of patients requiring central venous cannulation increases so does the incidence of this complication. Because the onset of venous stenosis and thrombosis is more gradual leading to the development of collaterals, and because other outflow veins are less likely to be affected than in primary disease, the patient is often only mildly symptomatic or asymptomatic. The first presentation may be non-function of the line and duplex or a 'linogram' shows thrombosis. Treatment involves thrombolysis if the thrombus is extensive or simply removal of the line and whatever anticoagulation may be feasible. Lines should be placed if possible in the internal jugular vein, cephalic vein or external jugular vein as this complication is particularly common following direct subclavicular vein cannulation. A history of central venous cannulation is important in patients being considered for:

- hemodialysis access and
- arterial reconstruction using arm vein

as subclinical subclavian vein thrombosis or stenosis is common and may lead to unacceptable limb swelling postoperatively.

Phlegmasia cerulea dolens

This typically occurs in patients with advanced malignancy, often being treated with chemotherapy via an indwelling central venous catheter. It is associated with intense swelling, pain and discoloration and may progress to venous gangrene requiring amputation. Pulmonary embolus is relatively common. Phlegmasia is due to widespread thrombosis in main stem, collateral veins and venous microcirculation.

Post-thrombotic syndromes

Post-thrombotic symptoms are reported in 30–70% of patients following a primary subclavian vein thrombosis and comprise discomfort and swelling, particularly in positions that compress collaterals in the costoclavicular space (see above). However, the skin changes commonly found in the lower limb are extremely rare in the upper limb.

Arteriovenous malformations

These are rare but can be misdiagnosed, especially in the lower limb, and will be considered in more detail below.

Examination findings

INSPECTION

Most of the available clinical information can be gained by simply inspecting the arm and comparing it with the contralateral limb.

- Is the arm swollen?
- Is the arm hypertrophied?
- Is the arm discolored?
- Are venous collaterals apparent?
- Are there scars and/or puncture sites?
- Is there evidence of previous trauma?
- Are there any indwelling lines or cannulae?

PALPATION

- Is the arm warmer?
- Is there tenderness over an inflamed superficial vein or in the supraclavicular fossa?
- Is there evidence of obstructing pathology in the axilla and/or supraclavicular fossa, for example, lymph nodes, cervical rib?
- Are the veins hard and 'cord-like', suggesting previous thrombophlebitis?
- Are pulses present and are there any abnormal pulsations, either venous or arterial (AV fistula, malformation)?
- Are there any thrills?
- Is there any edema and is it pitting?

- Allen's test should be performed to confirm the arterial inflow to the hand and completeness of the palmar arch.

PERCUSSION

As in the leg, the course of superficial veins can be outlined using the 'tap' test (see below).

AUSCULTATION

The blood pressure should be measured in each arm. Are there any murmurs?

ADDITIONAL STEPS

If the arm is swollen, examination should include the axilla for adenopathy and the breast to exclude malignancy. If there is concern about the adequacy of the deep venous outflow (for example, if an AV fistula or particularly a brachial vein transposition is being considered), then the arm can be observed for swelling after application of a light superficial tourniquet around the upper arm. Obviously, symptoms of pulmonary embolism should prompt a full cardiorespiratory examination.

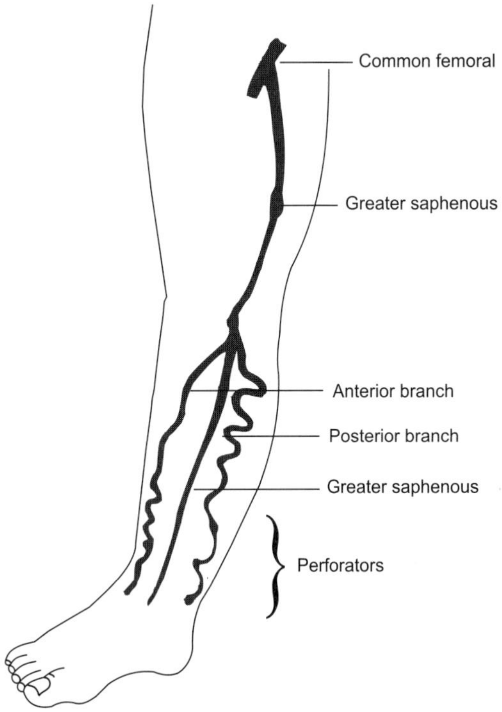

Figure 7.5 *Usual course of the greater saphenous vein and its major branches: the saphenous vein begins just anterior to the medial malleolus and passes behind the knee and to the groin where it inserts into the common femoral vein. Varicosities that are seen in the lower leg are usually the anterior and posterior branches of the greater saphenous vein. Perforating veins originate from the posterior branch. (Adapted from DeWeese JA. Chapter 22. In Schwartz SI, ed.* Venous and Lymphatic Disease, Principles of Surgery, *4th edn. New York: McGraw-Hill, 1984)*

THE LOWER LIMB

Venous disease of the lower limb is perhaps the commonest human affliction. Indeed, it is so common that it may be considered an almost normal part of the ageing process.

Anatomic considerations

SUPERFICIAL VEINS

The long (greater, internal) saphenous vein (LSV) and the short (lesser, external) saphenous veins (SSV) begin at the medial and lateral ends of the dorsal venous arch respectively. It is important to appreciate that there are numerous connections at many different levels between the long and short systems both in health and disease. The LSV passes anterior to the medial malleolus, then two fingerbreadths posterior to the medial condyle of the tibia (Fig. 7.5) and joins the common femoral vein 2.5 cm below and lateral to the pubic tubercle at the saphenofemoral junction (SFJ). The LSV tributaries are highly variable but the four most constant are:

- anterolateral thigh branch, which often gives rise to varices on the lateral thigh and front of the knee;
- posteromedial thigh branch, which may join the short saphenous system and a major medial branch in the thigh;
- anterior arch vein, which gives rise to varices over the tibia;
- posterior arch vein, which gives rise to most of the medial calf perforating veins (Fig. 7.6).

The main LSV runs in a fascial tunnel bound to the deep fascia and, because of this support, the main trunk itself rarely becomes varicose; it is the tributaries that form varicose veins. The saphenous nerve joins the LSV at the level of the knee.

The SSV passes posterior to the lateral malleolus, ascends the posterior calf, pierces the deep fascia at a variable point and usually enters the popliteal vein about 2 cm above the knee crease (Fig. 7.6). However, the level of saphenopopliteal junction (SPJ) is highly variable and may be absent. The sural nerve runs closely applied to the SSV.

DEEP VEINS

The deep veins of the lower leg accompany the three major arteries, the anterior tibial, posterior tibial, and peroneal (Fig. 7.7). The veins are usually paired until they reach the popliteal vein, which is also often paired. The popliteal vein becomes the superficial femoral vein at the level of the adductor magnus tendon and continues to the groin where it joins the deep femoral vein

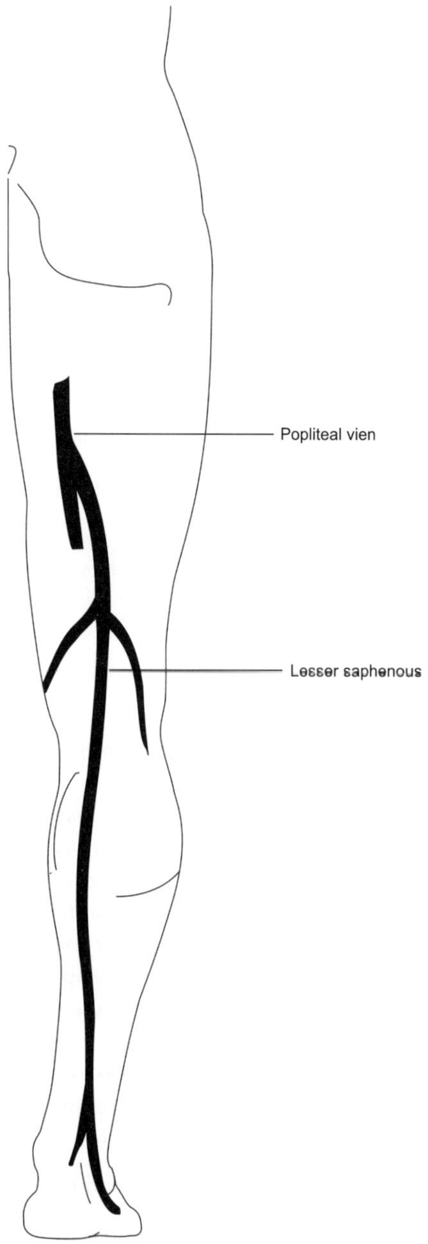

Figure 7.6 *The deep veins of the lower extremity: the deep veins of the calf are paired veins that accompany the anterior tibial, peroneal and posterior tibial arteries. These veins may remain double until they enter the popliteal vein but may also enter the popliteal vein individually. The popliteal vein becomes the superficial femoral vein in Hunter's canal and ascends to the groin where it joins the deep femoral vein to become the common femoral vein.*

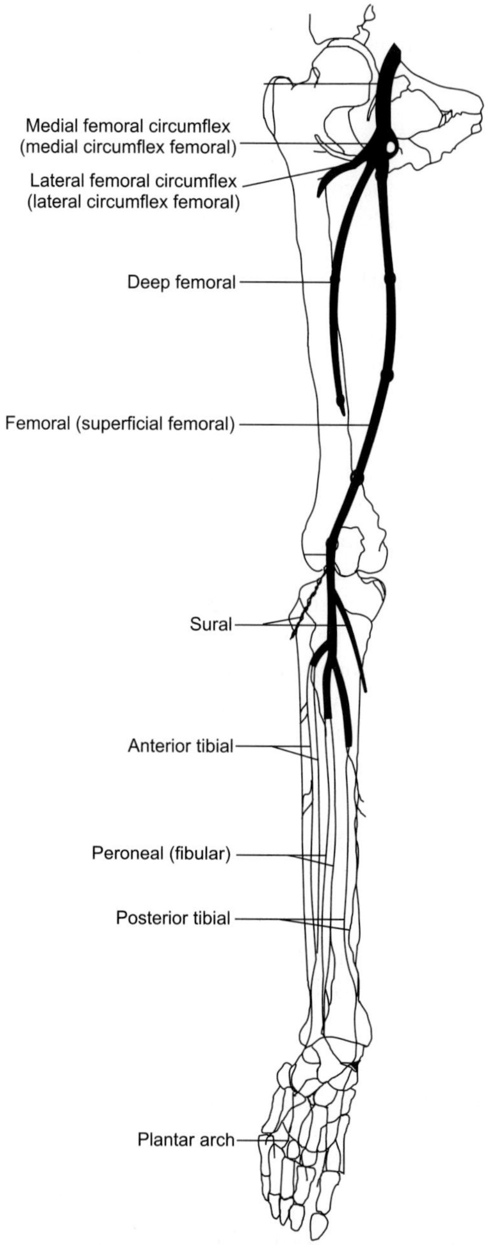

Figure 7.7 *Venous drainage of the lower leg: the superficial veins drain into the deep veins of the lower leg through perforating veins. The major perforators are posterior and superior to the medial malleolus and drain from the posterior branch of the greater saphenous vein into the posterior tibial vein. Normal valves prevent retrograde flow in the perforating, superficial and deep veins. (Adapted from DeWeese JA. Chapter 22. In Schwartz SI, ed.* Venous and Lymphatic Disease, Principles of Surgery, *4th edn. New York: McGraw-Hill, 1984)*

to become the common femoral vein. The common femoral vein becomes the external iliac vein at the inguinal ligament and ascends to join the internal iliac veins to become the common iliac veins, which join to become the inferior vena cava. The deep and superficial venous systems are joined by non-junctional perforators (Fig. 7.8).

Superficial thrombophlebitis

Two types of superficial thrombophlebitis are recognized, that arising in:

- a normal vein;
- a diseased, usually varicose, vein.

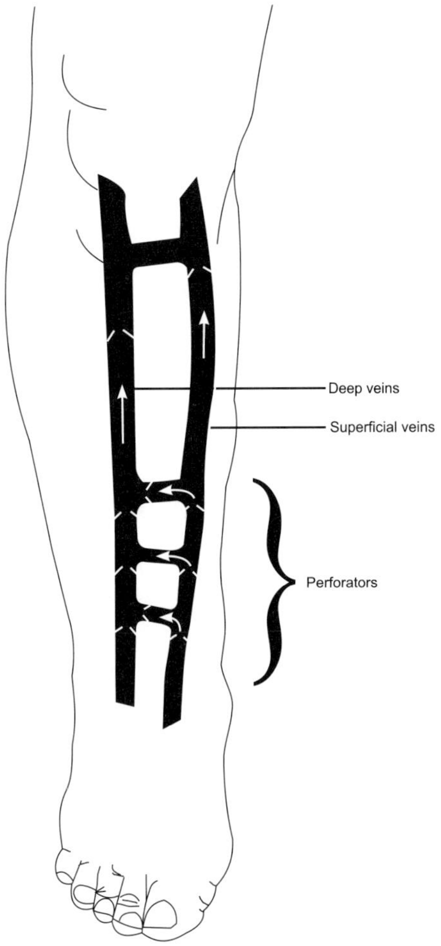

Figure 7.8 *Lesser saphenous vein: the lesser saphenous vein begins posterior to the lateral malleolus and ascends the leg to pierce the deep fascia in the superior portion of the lower leg to join the popliteal vein. (Adapted from DeWeese JA. Chapter 22. In Schwartz SI, ed.* Venous and Lymphatic Disease, Principles of Surgery, *4th edn. New York: McGraw-Hill, 1984)*

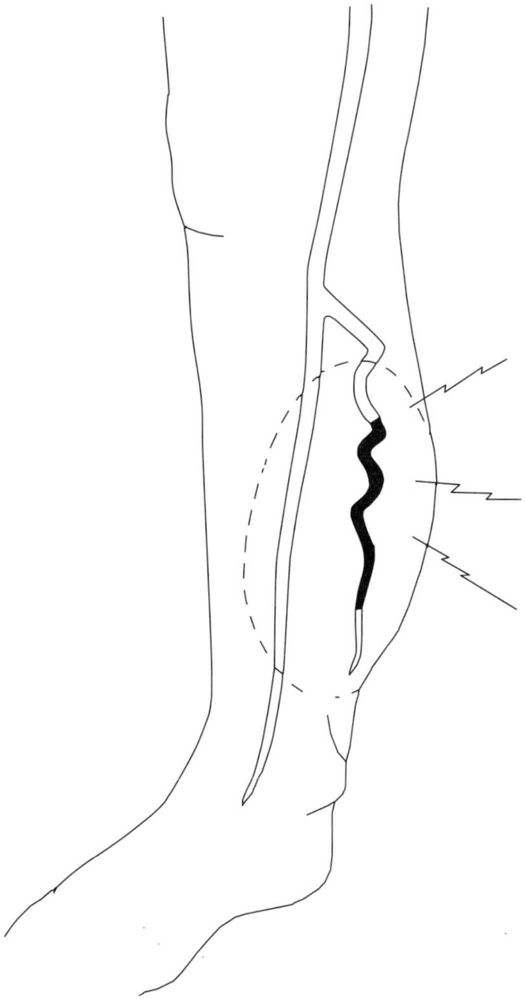

Figure 7.9 *Superficial venous thrombosis: localized redness, tenderness, and swelling surround a palpably thrombosed superficial vein. (Adapted from DeWeese JA. Chapter 22. In Schwartz SI, ed.* Venous and Lymphatic Disease, Principles of Surgery, *4th edn. New York: McGraw-Hill, 1984)*

The former is usually iatrogenic, bacterial and is treated by removal of the line or cannula, with or without antibiotics. Occasionally, it can arise in association with known or occult malignancy and, in this circumstance, is often migratory.

The latter usually complicates varicose veins (VV) and is particularly common in pregnancy. It is usually due to sterile thrombosis. There is intense pain and redness over the affected segment and, if clot propagates through junctional and non-junctional perforators, there is a risk of pulmonary embolism. Systemic upset (pyrexia, tachycardia) and abscess formation are uncommon. Treatment is usually conservative with analgesia and anti-inflammatory agents, although some surgeons believe that ligation with or without stripping of the LSV may be indicated in some circumstances to prevent embolism. On examination, there is rubor, calor and dolor around the affected segment. Upon resolution, there is often a residual mass or cord (Fig. 7.9).

Deep venous thrombosis

Deep venous thrombosis, leading to pulmonary embolism, is the commonest cause of potentially preventable death in adult patients. It is important to remember that most patients dying of pulmonary embolism in hospital have no symptoms or signs in their legs. Management therefore depends crucially upon prophylaxis, a high index of suspicion in 'at-risk' patients regardless of symptoms, and early recourse to definitive investigation.

It is helpful to consider the development of DVT in two phases. In the early phase the thrombus is:

- non-occlusive and may be free floating in a fast moving column of blood;
- not yet adherent to the vein wall.

As a result there is no:

- swelling
- inflammation (pain, heat and tenderness)
- distension of superficial collateral veins.

In other words, the leg may appear quite normal although the risk of embolism is high. In the late phase, when the thrombus becomes occlusive and incites a phlebitis anchoring it to the vein wall, the patient develops all the 'typical' symptoms and signs of DVT. At this stage, however, the risk of pulmonary embolism is low. Even when 'typical' symptoms and signs are present, studies show that less than half are due to DVT, the remainder being due to a range of other pathologies. So, the symptoms and signs of DVT are highly insensitive and nonspecific. Homans' sign is also unreliable, painful and in patients with DVT may precipitate embolism; in the authors' view it should not be performed.

Anatomically, it is useful to consider three patterns of disease (calf, femoral, and iliofemoral) although thrombosis is a dynamic process and proximal propagation is common (Fig. 7.10).

CALF VEIN THROMBOSIS

Calf vein thrombosis is usually localized to one or two of the three major veins of the lower leg. The thrombi are usually not completely obstructive and, since tibial and peroneal veins are paired, there is usually adequate venous drainage. Calf tenderness may be present but significant swelling is nearly always absent and in fact, most patients have no symptoms or signs whatsoever. About 20% if untreated may propagate above the knee.

FEMORAL VEIN THROMBOSIS

Femoral vein thrombosis may propagate to the common femoral vein. As the great majority of lower limb DVTs

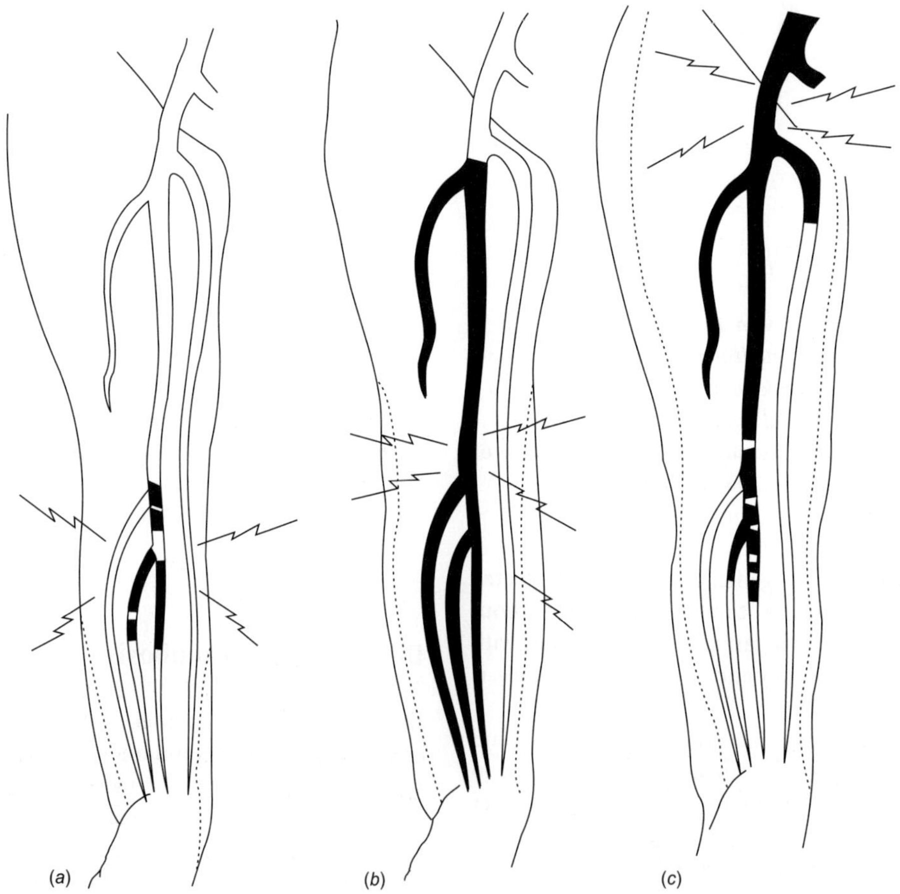

Figure 7.10 *(a) Calf vein thrombosis: the thrombosis is limited to the veins of the calf and the popliteal vein. There is minimal, if any, swelling at the level of the ankle. Tender deep cords may be palpable. Homans' sign may be present. (b) Femoral vein thrombosis: there is thrombosis of the femoral vein, which is usually associated with thrombosis in the calf veins. Swelling is usually present and extends to just above the level of the knee. Popliteal tenderness and calf tenderness may be present. Homans' sign may or may not be present. (c) Iliofemoral venous thrombosis: there is thrombosis of iliac and proximal femoral vein and frequently calf veins are also involved. Edema is present from the foot to the level of the inguinal ligament. Tenderness is usually present in the groin and sometimes at the popliteal level and in the calf. Homans' sign may or may not be present. (Adapted from DeWeese JA. Chapter 22. In Schwartz SI, ed.* Venous and Lymphatic Disease, Principles of Surgery, *4th edn. New York: McGraw-Hill, 1984)*

arise in the calf veins, it is not surprising that thrombus is also present at that level in most patients. Tenderness is often present over the femoral vein. There is swelling at the ankle and calf of greater than 1 cm in most patients but it rarely extends above the patella unless outflow via the deep femoral vein is also compromised.

ILIOFEMORAL THROMBOSIS

Iliofemoral venous thrombosis, since it commonly originates in the pelvic veins, does not involve the distal femoral or calf veins in over one-third of patients. There is swelling of thigh as well as the leg. If the cava is involved then the symptoms and signs are usually bilateral.

PHLEGMASIA CERULEA DOLENS

As described above with respect to the arm, extensive thrombosis may lead to phlegmasia, which in turn may precipitate venous gangrene.

Varicose veins

EPIDEMIOLOGY

Varicose veins (VV) are so common that they could be considered a variant of normal. The prevalence of VV increases markedly with age and they are an almost universal finding in individuals over the age of 60 years.

TRUNK VARICES

These involve the main stem and/or major tributaries of the LSV (80%) and/or SSV (20%), are usually >4 mm in diameter (and may be much larger), lie subcutaneously, are palpable, do not usually discolor the overlying skin and are present in about a third of the adult population. Although five times more women than men present for treatment, the prevalence is roughly equal between the sexes. There appears to be a familial tendency and obesity, pregnancy, constipation and prolonged standing may be aggravating factors.

RETICULAR VARICES

These lie deep in the dermis, are <4 mm in diameter, are impalpable and may render the overlying skin dark blue. They may or may not be associated with trunk varices and are present in about 80% of the adult population.

TELANGECTASIA

These are also termed spider or hyphen web veins. They lie superficially in the dermis, are usually 1 mm or less in diameter, are impalpable and render the overlying skin purple or bright red. Again, they may be associated with trunk and reticular varices and are present in 90% of adults. Like reticular veins, they are slightly commoner in women.

SYMPTOMS

The great majority of individuals with VV are asymptomatic, or at least they do not seek treatment. Those that do attend the surgical clinic do so because they are unhappy about the appearance of their leg(s), and/or they associate lower limb symptoms with their VV, and/or they are concerned about developing complications.

Many patients, especially young women, seek treatment because they consider their veins to be unsightly and want them removed. In general, the UK National Health Service does not fund minor cosmetic surgery. Patients are aware of this, and because they may also be embarrassed to admit that cosmesis is the main issue, they frequently complain of various lower limb symptoms as well.

A wide variety of lower limb symptoms have been attributed to VV. These include:

- aching
- heaviness and tension
- a feeling of swelling
- tiredness
- restless legs
- nocturnal cramps
- itching.

Epidemiological studies[3–5] show that:

- such symptoms are present in about half the adult population;
- there is little or no relationship between these symptoms and the presence and severity of VV on clinical examination;
- nor is there a good correlation between symptoms and the pattern and severity of reflux on duplex ultrasonography disease.

Experience in the vascular clinic confirms this to be the case and it can be difficult to determine to what extent a patient's symptoms are due to VV and whether they will benefit from (surgical) treatment.

Only a small proportion of patients with VV go on to develop the complications of chronic venous insufficiency, for example, lipodermatosclerosis, leg ulcers, hemorrhage and thrombophlebitis. It is difficult to predict which patients will progress and there is no evidence that early VV surgery will prevent these complications from developing.

Chronic venous insufficiency

DEFINITION

Chronic venous insufficiency (CVI) may be defined as the presence of (irreversible) skin damage in the lower leg as a result of sustained venous hypertension.

PATHOPHYSIOLOGY

Venous hypertension is due to failure of the mechanisms which normally lower venous pressure upon ambulation; namely:

- venous reflux due to valvular incompetence (90%), which may affect the superficial veins, the deep veins or both; and may be due to primary valvular insufficiency (as in VV) or post-thrombotic damage (see below);
- venous obstruction (10%), which is usually post-thrombotic in nature.

EPIDEMIOLOGY

CVI affects 5–10% of the adult population. Chronic venous ulceration, the end result of CVI, affects 2–3% of people over the age of 65 years and its treatment accounts for 1–2% of health care spending in developed countries. The female: male ratio is 3:1. Approximately 70% of all leg ulcers are venous in etiology. Another 20% are due to mixed arterial and venous disease. In many cases the situation is aggravated by old age, poor social circumstances, obesity, trauma, immobility, osteoarthritis, rheumatoid arthritis, diabetes and neurological problems (e.g. stroke). All these many and varied factors must be included in a 'holistic' clinical assessment of the patient. It is usually possible to differentiate venous from arterial ulceration on clinical examination alone (see below).

SYMPTOMS

All the symptoms described above for VV may be associated with CVI and there is a stronger relationship between such symptoms and the features of disease in this group. However, such patients are significantly older and, as such, other co-morbidity is much more common. In particular, arterial disease and musculoskeletal problems should not be overlooked and falsely attributed to venous pathology. Unlike patients with simple VV where actual swelling is unusual, the majority of patients with CVI have a degree of edema. This is usually of mixed etiology; venous hypertension, right heart failure and a degree of lymphedema, for example. Severe pain is unusual and suggests coexisting arterial disease and/or infection.

HISTORY

This should include the history of the present and previous episodes of ulceration; previous thrombotic episodes; previous venous and non-venous surgery to the leg, pelvis and abdomen; arterial symptoms; diabetes; autoimmune disease; other medical conditions; locomotor problems; current medications, and allergies.

Examination findings

POSITION

The patient should be examined standing in a warm room and, in these circumstances, significant VV soon become apparent. Patients often feel faint and some form of support should be available. The examiner can sit on the floor. Better still, the patient can be provided with a platform and the examiner can sit on a low chair.

INSPECTION

The cardinal features of varicose veins are that they are dilated, elongated, tortuous and sacculated. These features only arise when there is reverse flow (reflux) and are commonly seen below an incompetent valve. The main trunks themselves may be dilated and may exhibit sacculation but they are rarely, if ever, tortuous or elongated because they are supported by the deep fascia (see above). The distribution of varices will usually indicate whether they are tributaries of the long or short saphenous system or both. However, in an obese patient, or one that has undergone previous surgery, the anatomic connections may be obscure.[6,7] In thin, particularly athletic, patients there may be highly visible and enlarged veins and these may be erroneously considered to be pathological when they are physiological. Such veins are dilated uniformly and do not exhibit elongation, tortuosity or sacculation.

PALPATION

Percussion over a varix while palpating with the other hand at a higher or lower level will help trace out the pattern (the 'tap' test of Chevrier). This is particularly helpful in the obese. There may be a cough impulse, even a thrill over a large varix, particularly a saphena varix in the groin.

TRENDELENBURG TEST

This test (Fig. 7.11) comprises two parts.

- Part 1: with the patient lying down the leg is elevated to 45° and a tourniquet or the examiner's hand compresses the greater saphenous vein in the high thigh. With compression in place, the patient stands in a well-lit room. Previously noted superficial veins are then carefully observed for filling with blood.
- Part 2: the compression is then released. The superficial veins are then carefully observed for increased filling with blood.

There are four possible results of the findings:

- negative-negative (Fig. 7.11a). Part 1 is negative when there is only gradual filling of normal veins from arterial inflow in the distal one-third of the lower leg, indicating the valves in the perforating veins are normal. Part 2 is negative when the following release of the compression there is only continued gradual filling of the veins indicating the valves in the greater saphenous veins are normal.

- negative-positive (Fig. 7.11b). Part 1 is negative because the perforating veins have competent valves. Part 2 is positive when the release of compression results in sudden filling of all the superficial veins, indicating the valves in the greater saphenous veins are incompetent.
- positive-negative (Fig. 7.11c). Part 1 is positive when there is rapid filling of the veins in the lower leg, indicating these are incompetent valves in the deep and perforating veins. Part 2 is negative if there is only continued slow filling of the greater saphenous vein, indicating there are competent valves in the greater saphenous vein.
- positive-positive (Fig. 7.11d). Part 1 is positive, indicating there are incompetent valves in the deep and perforating veins. Part 2 is positive when the greater saphenous vein shows rapidly increased filling following release of its compression indicating the valves in the greater saphenous vein are incompetent.

A more effective way to demonstrate reflux is to insonate over the site of incompetence and reflux with a portable continuous wave Doppler ultrasound probe. This is particularly valuable in obese patients or those with recurrent VV, where the anatomy may be obscure.

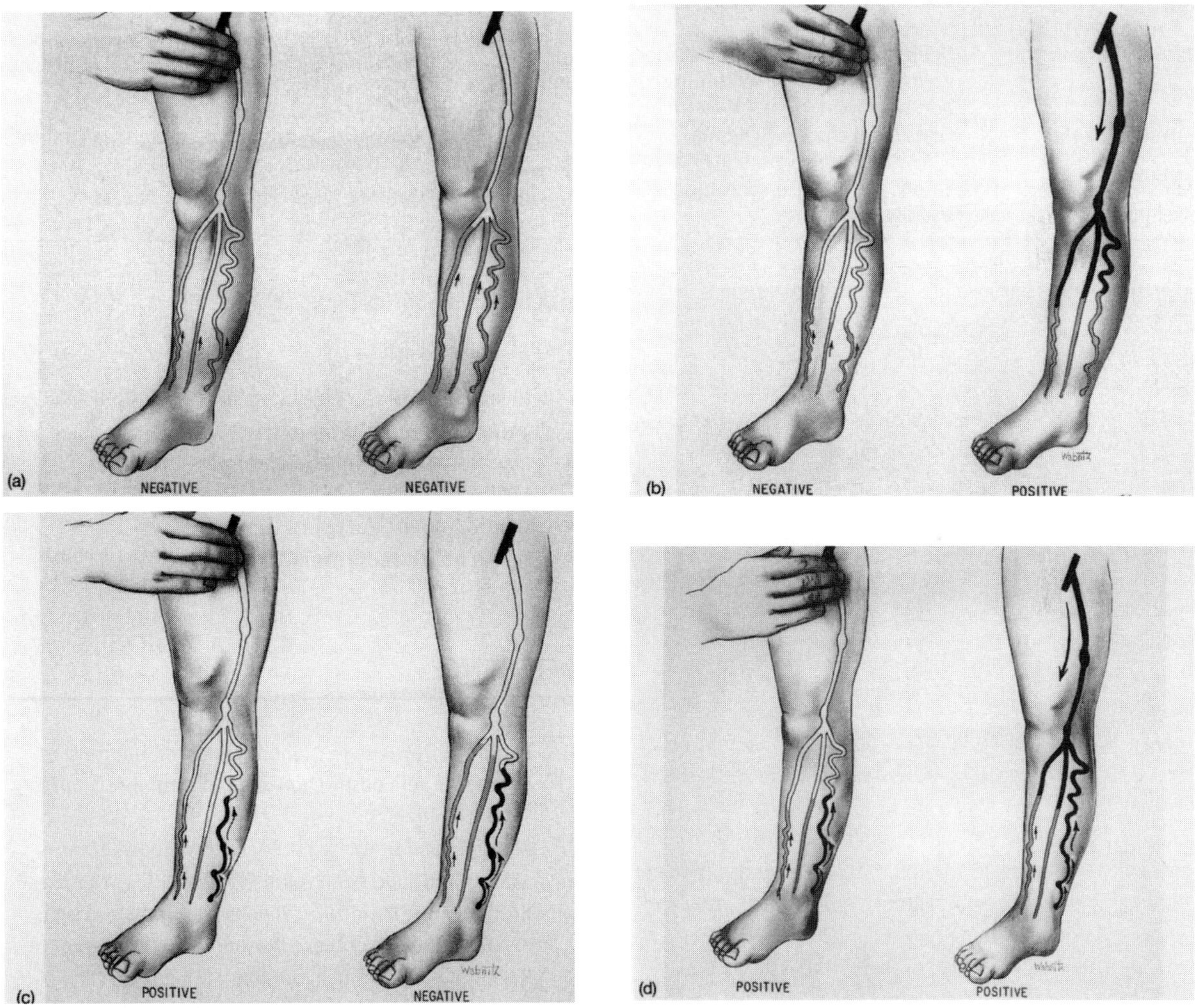

Figure 7.11 *Trendelenburg test: initially the patient is lying down with his leg elevated and then stands up with compression over the saphenofemoral junction with the hand or tourniquet. (a) Negative-negative response: there is gradual filling of the veins at the ankle over a 30-second period and there is continued slow filling after release of the hand. (b) Negative-positive response: on standing there is again only gradual filling of the distal vein but on release of compression there is a rapid retrograde filling of the saphenous vein. (c) Positive-negative response: with saphenous vein compressed there is rapid filling of the superficial veins through incompetent perforators. With release of compression there is further slow filling of all of the veins. (d) Positive-positive response: on standing with the saphenous vein compressed there is again rapid filling of varices through incompetent perforators. On release of compression there is additional rapid filling of the saphenous vein through incompetent valves. (Adapted from DeWeese JA. Chapter 22. In Schwartz SI, ed.* Venous and Lymphatic Disease, Principles of Surgery, *4th edn. New York: McGraw-Hill, 1984)*

Table 7.1 *Differential diagnosis of leg ulceration*

Clinical features	Arterial ulcer	Venous ulcer
Gender	Men > women	Women < men
Age	Usually presents > 60 years	Typically develops 40–60 years but patient may not present for medical attention until much older, multiple recurrences are the norm
Risk factors	Smoking, diabetes, hyperlipidemia and hypertension	Previous DVT, thrombophilia, varicose veins
Past medical history	Most have a clear history of peripheral, coronary and cerebrovascular disease	More than 20% have clear history of DVT, many more have a history suggestive of occult DVT i.e. leg swelling after childbirth, hip/knee replacement or long bone fracture
Symptoms	Severe pain is present unless there is (diabetic) neuropathy, pain maybe relieved by dependency	About a third have pain but it is not usually severe and may be relieved on elevation
Site	Normal and abnormal (diabetics) pressure areas (malleoli, heel, metatarsal heads, 5th metatarsal base)	Medial (70%), lateral (20%) or both malleoli and gaiter area
Edge	Regular, 'punched-out', indolent	Irregular, with neoepithelium (whiter than mature skin)
Base	Deep, green (sloughy) or black (necrotic) with no granulation tissue, may comprise major tendon, bone and joint	Pink and granulating but may be covered in yellow-green slough
Surrounding skin	Features of chronic ischemia	Lipodermatosclerosis (pigmentation, induration, varicose dermatitis, atrophe blanche)
Veins	Empty, 'guttering' on elevation	Full, usually varicose
Swelling	Usually absent	Usually present

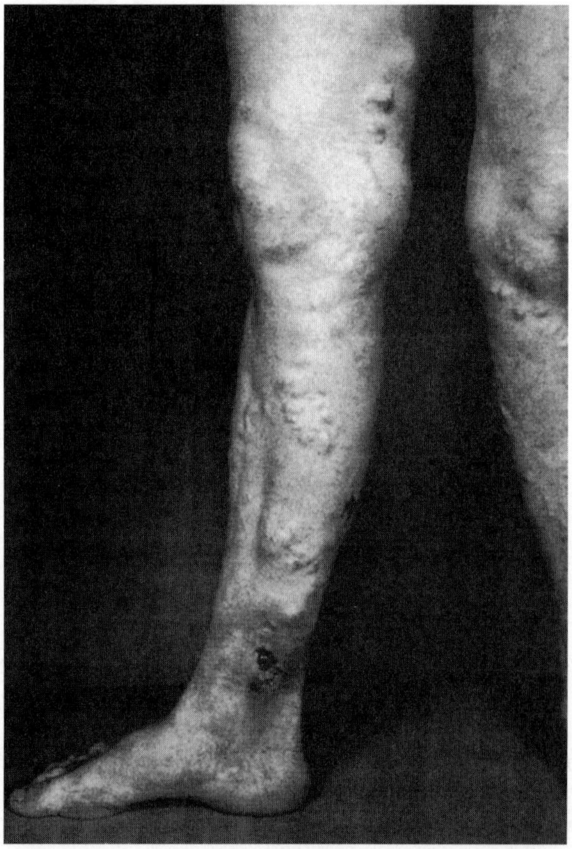

Figure 7.12 *Post-thrombotic leg: there is visible swelling and secondary varicosities. There is brownish discoloration and brawny induration at the ankle level and ulceration is present over the site of an incompetent perforator just posterior and superior to the medial malleolus.*

ULCER ASSESSMENT

This should include

- a description of the ulcer, concentrating on the features outlined in Table 7.1 (Fig. 7.12);
- pulse status and ankle brachial pressure index (ABPI);
- gait and, in particular, ankle mobility;
- general physical examination.

REFERENCES

1. Adams JT, DeWeese JA, Mahoney EB, *et al.* Intermittent subclavian vein obstruction without thrombosis. *Surgery* 1968; **63**: 147–65.
2. Adams JT and DeWeese JS. 'Effort' thrombosis of the axillary and subclavian veins. *J Trauma* 1971; **11** 923–30.
3. Bradbury AW, Ruckley CV. Venous symptoms and signs and the results of duplex ultrasound: do they agree? In Ruckley CV, Fowkes FGR, Bradbury AW, eds. *The Epidemiology and Management of Venous Disease.* London: Springer-Verlag, 1998.
4. Bradbury AW, Ruckley CV. Venous reflux and chronic venous insufficiency. In Yao JST, Pearce WH, eds. *Practical Vascular Surgery.* Stamford, CT: Appleton & Lange, 1998: 475–89.
5. Bradbury AW, Evans CJ, Allan PL, Lee AJ, Ruckley CV, Fowkes FGR. What are the symptoms of varicose veins? Edinburgh vein study cross-sectional population survey. *Br Med J* 1999; **318**: 353–6.

6. Bradbury AW, Stonebridge PA, Ruckley CV, Beggs I. Recurrent varicose veins: correlation between preoperative clinical and hand-held Doppler ultrasonographic examination, and anatomical findings at surgery. *Br J Surg* 1993; **80**: 849–51.

7. Bradbury AW, Stonebridge PA, Callam M, *et al.* Recurrent varicose veins: assessment of the saphenofemoral junction. *Br J Surg* 1994; **81**: 373–5.

8

Hypercoagulable states in venous disease

KELLIE R BROWN AND JONATHAN B TOWNE

Hereditary thrombotic disease is more common than is generally appreciated. Venous thrombosis occurs in approximately 1 in 1000 people per year.[1] A variety of inherited and acquired conditions have been described which can lead to abnormal thrombosis. The formation of a hemostatic clot requires the coordinated action of the vessel wall, endothelium, platelets and plasma coagulation factors. There exists a balance between thrombus formation and dissolution in the normal physiologic response. On occasion, congenital or acquired defects destroy this balance, resulting in clinical scenarios of abnormal bleeding or exaggerated thrombosis. Approximately 50% of all patients who die from thrombotic events have a definable coagulation or platelet defect.[2] The clinical manifestations of most hypercoagulable states present as spontaneous onset of deep venous thrombosis at an early age. Virchow proposed that thrombus formation was the result of an interaction between an injured surface, stasis and the hypercoagulability of blood. One or more components of Virchow's triad can be invoked when determining the cause of thrombosis. This chapter reviews the normal hemostatic mechanisms, and describes the pathophysiology and treatment of hypercoagulable states that result in venous thrombosis.

NORMAL HEMOSTATIC MECHANISMS

The normal hemostatic response requires interaction between the vessel wall, endothelium, platelets, and the coagulation cascade responsible for thrombin generation. Control of hemostasis occurs by balancing thrombosis with fibrinolysis through multiple anticoagulant pathways.

Vasoconstriction

When vessel injury occurs, the endothelium and the forming thrombus generate several factors, which lead to smooth muscle contraction in the vessel wall. The injured endothelium and activated platelets produce thromboxane, a potent vasoconstrictor. Endothelin, a small peptide, is released from injured endothelium and also leads to vasoconstriction. Thrombin and the fibrinopeptide B released by thrombin's action on fibrinogen also stimulate smooth muscle contraction.

Endothelial response

The normal endothelium is a non-thrombogenic barrier between the blood and the thrombogenic subendothelial constituents. The metabolic activity of the endothelium is complex, generating a number of molecules involved in both preventing thrombosis in the normal state and forming platelet plugs when endothelial continuity is disrupted. Prostacyclin (PGI_2) is a potent vasodilator and antiplatelet compound produced by endothelial cell metabolism of arachidonic acid. Thromboxane A_2 (TxA_2), a potent vasoconstrictor and platelet activator usually associated with platelet granules, is also released by the endothelium. The relative excess of PGI_2 to TxA_2 production (100:1) in the endothelial cell may be an important determinant of the endothelium's antithrombotic state.[3] PGI_2 release is stimulated by endothelial cell contact with thrombin, platelets and adenosine diphosphate.[4]

Nitric oxide, the endothelium-derived relaxing factor, is important in the maintenance of normal vasorelaxation and is also an inhibitor of platelet activation and adhesion.[5] Endothelial cell injury can therefore result in increased vasospasm and platelet adherence.

Thrombomodulin is another membrane receptor on the endothelium, which contributes to a non-thrombogenic surface. The receptor combines with thrombin and decreases its ability to generate fibrin, and increases its ability to activate the protein C anticoagulant pathway.[6] The endothelium also modulates the fibrinolytic system by producing tissue plasminogen activator (t-PA) and plasminogen activator inhibitor-1 (PAI-1). The net balance of t-PA and PAI-1 activities determines the fibrinolytic activity of the vessel wall.[7]

Platelets

Platelets are involved in the initial phase of hemostasis by forming a hemostatic plug at the site of vessel injury. The binding of the platelet membrane glycoprotein (GPI-b) to von Willebrand's factor (vWF) on the subendothelial collagen leads to platelet adherence and subsequent platelet activation. Activated platelets release dense granules and alpha granules. Dense granules release both ADP, a potent stimulus of aggregation, and serotonin, a vasoconstrictor. Platelet activation also results in the synthesis of TxA_2, a potent vasoconstrictor and platelet aggregator, and in a conformational change in the platelet which is instrumental in thrombin generation. These events all lead to platelet aggregation which requires fibrinogen to link platelets by binding the GP IIa–IIIa receptor expressed on the surface membrane after activation. Stabilization of the platelet plug occurs when fibrin is formed and crosslinked in the platelet mass.[8]

Coagulation cascades

Fibrin formation is dependent on thrombin, the central enzyme in the hemostatic mechanism. The cascades involved in thrombin generation have been divided into extrinsic and intrinsic pathways (Fig. 8.1). The two pathways interact at two points (XIIa can activate VII, and VIIa–tissue factor complex can activate IX) and they converge at the step of factor X activation. It is unlikely that the two pathways ever function individually *in vivo*. The extrinsic pathway seems relatively more important than the intrinsic since individuals with a deficiency in the factors of the early steps of the intrinsic pathway have no significant bleeding problems.

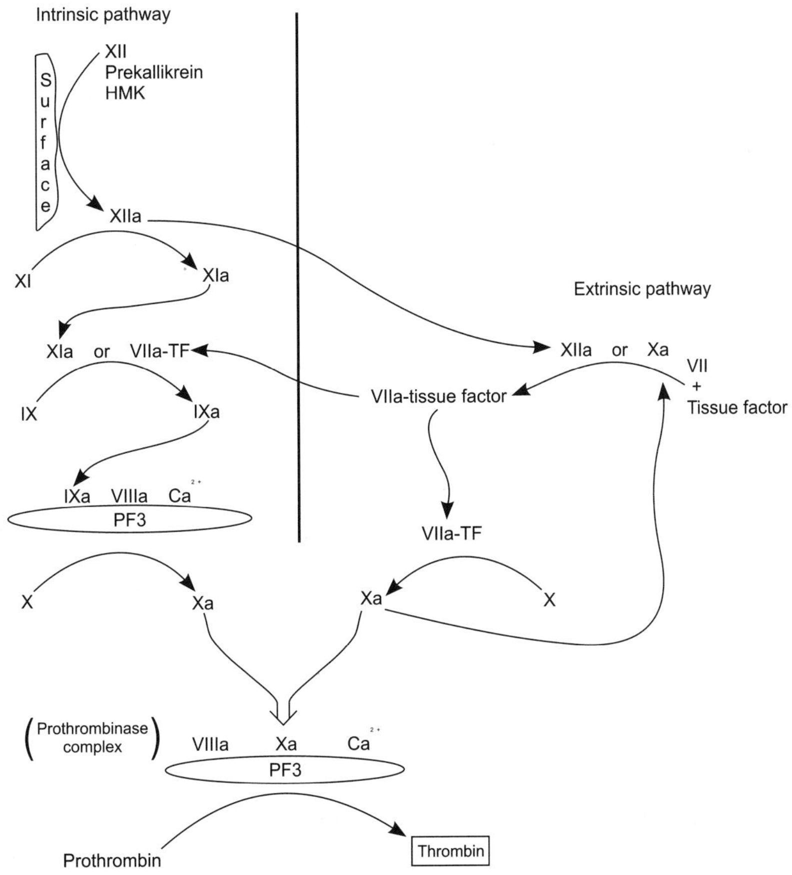

Figure 8.1 *Thrombin generation. HMK, high molecular weight kininogen; TF, tissue factor; PF3, platelet factor-3; Ca^{2+}, calcium ion.*

The extrinsic pathway is initiated by the expression of tissue factor (tissue thromboplastin) on the cells of injured tissue or from activated endothelial cells and monocytes. Tissue factor is a transmembrane protein, which is not fully expressed until tissue injury occurs. The exposure of blood to the injured tissue stimulates complex formation between factor VII and tissue factor. This complex (factor VII–tissue factor) can activate factor X. Factor Xa is a primary junction point of the extrinsic and intrinsic pathways. Factor Xa cleaves prothrombin to thrombin by the prothrombinase complex.

The intrinsic pathway is activated by contact with a negatively charged surface such as glass, or a biological activator such as collagen or endotoxin. The initial phase of the pathway, also known as the contact phase, involves the precursors factor XII, factor XI, and prekallikrein, which are converted to their active serine protease forms by surface contact and high molecular weight (HMW) kininogen as a cofactor. In contrast to most other complex formations in the coagulation cascade, the contact phase requires no calcium and is not vitamin K dependent. The second phase of the intrinsic pathway is the activation of factor IX by Xa, which combines with cofactors to convert factor X to Xa. Factor IX, a vitamin K-dependent protein also known as Christmas factor, is deficient in hemophilia B. Factor IX is converted to the serine protease IXa by XIa in the presence of calcium ion or by the tissue factor–VIIa complex of the extrinsic pathway. Factor VIII, also known as antihemophilic factor, is deficient in hemophilia A and is present in plasma as a stable complex with vWF. Factor VII in the presence of calcium ion acts as a cofactor for the factor IXa conversion of X to Xa. Factor Xa is the point of final convergence of the intrinsic and extrinsic pathways and goes on to participate in the prothrombinase complex (Fig. 8.1). The final step in thrombin generation is the cleavage of prothrombin to thrombin by Xa in the presence of factor Va, calcium, and platelet factor 3. Thrombin cleaves fibrinogen to fibrin, which is involved in clot stabilization. Thrombin also activates factors XIII, V and VIII, prothrombin, and protein C. Thrombin can also aggregate platelets and stimulate endothelial cell release of PGI_2, vWF, and PAI-1.[9,10]

Fibrin is the cohesive substance of the mature clot whose formation is central to secondary hemostasis. Fibrin formation occurs in three steps (Fig. 8.2):

- splitting of fibrinogen by thrombin into fibrin monomer and fibrinopeptides A and B;
- polymerization of monomers to fibrin strands;
- action of factor XIII (activated by thrombin) and calcium ion to crosslink the fibrin strands.

Fibrinopeptide A release is essential for the polymerization of fibrin monomers to occur. Fibrinopeptide B release appears to be important before crosslinking can occur.[11]

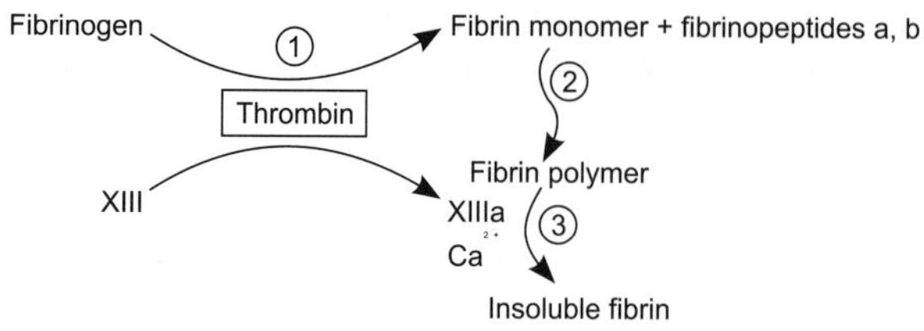

Figure 8.2 *Three steps of fibrin formation: 1, cleavage of fibrinogen by thrombin; 2, spontaneous polymerization of fibrin monomers; 3, crosslinking of fibrin strands.*

FIBRINOLYSIS AND ANTICOAGULANT PATHWAYS

Plasmin is active in the degradation of fibrin and facilitates the lysis of thrombus. Plasmin also limits thrombus formation by digestion of coagulation factors V, VIII, XII and prekallikrein. Plasmin is derived from plasminogen by the proteolytic action of multiple activators. Intrinsic activators include the contact plasmoproteins factor XII, prekallikrein, and HMW kininogen.[12] Extrinsic activators include t-PA, urokinase and streptokinase.

Plasmin is inhibited by PAI-1, which is released by endothelial cells. A second mechanism to inhibit plasmin is α_2-antiplasmin, produced by endothelial cells. Control of the fibrinolytic system is dependent on the relative activities of the plasminogen activators and inhibitors.

Control of hemostasis occurs by balancing thrombosis and the dissolution of thrombus. Besides the fibrinolytic system, there are natural anticoagulants which inhibit the coagulation pathways and activate the fibrinolytic system. Antithrombin III is the major inhibitor of thrombin and is the most important natural anticoagulant.[13] Heparin functions as an anticoagulant by binding to antithrombin III and increasing its activity. Antithrombin III is also an inhibitor of the activated clotting factors XIIIa, XIa, Xa, IXa, and kallikrein.

The protein C anticoagulant pathway consists of two vitamin K-dependent proteins, protein C and protein S, and the thrombin receptor thrombomodulin. Thrombin combines with thrombomodulin and becomes less active at catalyzing fibrin formation and more active at converting protein C to the activated form. Active protein C forms a complex with protein S, which acts to decrease thrombus formation by selectively degrading factors Va and VIIIa. The protein C and S complex also increases the rate of fibrinolysis by neutralizing PAI-1. Protein C and S deficiencies both result in thrombotic tendencies. These deficiencies are discussed in the following section on hypercoagulable states.

HYPERCOAGULABLE STATES

Hypercoagulable states as a cause of acute arterial or venous thrombosis pose a difficult problem. The ability of blood to remain fluid within the intravascular system and to form a thrombus when there is disruption or injury to the endothelial lining depends on complex interactions between the various components of the vascular system. These components previously discussed in this chapter include the endothelium, platelets, plasma, the coagulation cascade, and fibrinolytic factors. In 80–90% of patients with thrombosis a definable cause can be determined, and 50–80% have an underlying hereditary or acquired defect causing thrombosis.[2] Abnormal thrombosis may be secondary to deficiencies in protein C and protein S, activated protein C resistance, abnormalities in the antithrombin system, abnormalities of the fibrinolytic system, t-PA or factor XII deficiency, prothrombin mutations, heparin-induced platelet aggregation, the antiphospholipid antibody syndrome, lupus anticoagulant, or hyperhomocysteinemia. The remainder of the chapter is dedicated to the discussion of these abnormalities, their clinical significance and known treatment strategies.

Protein C deficiency

Protein C is a vitamin K-dependent proenzyme, synthesized in the liver, which is involved in clotting and thrombolysis. Protein C is activated by thrombin and this activation is greatly enhanced when thrombin forms a complex with thrombomodulin and endothelial cell membrane protein. Protein S acts as a cofactor for protein C which inactivates factors V and VIII:C, the two cofactors necessary for thrombin and factor Xa activation. In addition, thrombomodulin-bound thrombin cannot convert fibrinogen to fibrin or activate XIII or platelets.[2] Factors Va and VIIIa are cofactors in the rate-limiting steps of thrombin generation via both the intrinsic and extrinsic pathways.[14]

Heterozygous protein C deficiency is inherited in the autosomal dominant fashion. There are two types of deficiency. Type 1 involves a decrease in both the immunologic and biologic function of the protein. Type 2, which is uncommon, consists of a dysfunctional protein, which has normal antigen levels. The prevalence of protein C deficiency is 1 in 500 individuals, who have an 8- to 10-fold increase in the risk of thrombosis.[1] Heterozygous individuals have protein C levels in the range of 30–60%. As not all individuals with a low level of protein C develop thrombosis, asymptomatic patients who have low levels of protein C should not be given prophylactic anticoagulation. They should be given prophylactic anticoagulants or fresh frozen plasma if major surgery or prolonged immobilization is required.[14] The vast majority of thrombotic events are venous. Sixty-three percent of these events consist of DVT, and 40% are pulmonary embolus. Superficial thrombophlebitis is common, but arterial events are rare.[2] The typical age of onset is between 15 and 30 years of age, and this delay in the onset of the first thrombotic event is not fully understood. When protein C deficiency is homozygous it is associated with a severe deficiency and a condition termed 'neonatal purpura fulminans', which is usually fatal.

In patients with protein C-related thrombosis, heparin therapy, either regular or low molecular weight, is the preferred medical treatment. In the preoperative period when heparin therapy may be relatively contraindicated, fresh frozen plasma (one unit every 6 hours) may be given to supply the necessary protein C. Because of the risk of recurrent thrombotic events, long-term therapy with warfarin or low molecular weight heparin is indicated. Many patients with protein C or S deficiency develop skin and fat necrosis with warfarin; therefore no loading dose should be administered.[15,16] When skin necrosis associated with warfarin therapy is encountered, protein C or S deficiency should be ruled out.

Protein S deficiency

Protein S is also a vitamin K-dependent protein; it functions as a cofactor in the anticoagulant activity of activated protein C. The liver is the major source of synthesis, but endothelial cells and megakaryocytes have been identified as other sites of synthesis. Protein S is bound to protein in serum. Three types of protein S deficiency have been described. Type 1 is a decrease in the total and free portions of protein S. Type 2 consists of a functional defect in the protein S. Type 3 is a decrease only in the free portion of protein S. Protein S functions by expediting the binding of activated protein C to lipid and platelet surfaces. Symptomatic patients often have protein S levels 50% of normal and, as in protein C deficiency, protein S likewise causes primarily venous thrombosis.[17] Homozygotes are severely affected and may have a form of purpura fulminans shortly after birth.[18] Protein S has been estimated by some to be the cause of approximately 10% of spontaneous venous thrombosis. In a review of 71 patients, 71% had a DVT, 72% had superficial thrombophlebitis, and 38% had pulmonary embolus.[19] The mechanism by which protein S deficiency leads to a hypercoagulable state is similar to that of protein C deficiency. As with patients with protein C problems, the clotting abnormalities tend to be recurrent; therefore it is essential that symptomatic patients remain on long-term warfarin or low molecular weight heparin therapy.

It is important to note that protein C and S levels decrease 40–60% within the first 48 hours of starting warfarin therapy; therefore these deficiencies cannot be tested for during this time period. The levels return to

70% of normal after 2 weeks of therapy, thus the protein C and S assay should be done after the patient has been on warfarin for several weeks if not completed prior to the initiation of therapy.[2]

Antithrombin III deficiency

Antithrombin III, produced in the liver and in endothelial cells, is a potent plasma inactivator of thrombin and other serine proteases, most significantly factor X, but also activated factors VII, IX, XI and XII. Antithrombin III deficiency is inherited as an autosomal dominant trait. Most patients with hereditary antithrombin deficiency are heterozygous, although kindreds with homozygous deficiency have been reported.[20] There are two types of antithrombin deficiency. In most patients with classic hereditary type I deficiency of antithrombin, there is reduced synthesis of the antithrombin molecule. Type II antithrombin deficiency is characterized by normal antigen levels but decreased functional activity. Type II deficiency typically results from point mutations.

There is a wide variety of defects that clinically are manifested as antithrombin deficiency; therefore functional antithrombin assays are the preferred method to be used in the screening for antithrombin deficiency. The best single test for screening purposes is the antithrombin-heparin cofactor assay.[2,21] Patients with hereditary deficiency of antithrombin have a marked increased risk for venous thrombotic events, which usually occur in the second or third decades of life. Two-thirds of these patients have an event by the age of 35.[2] The most common sites of thrombosis are of the deep veins of the lower extremities, followed by the iliofemoral veins. The usual presentation is that of recurrent deep vein thrombosis with or without pulmonary embolism. The deficiency need not be severe for thrombotic events to happen. Some patients with DVT and pulmonary embolism have levels between 50 and 70% biologic activity, whereas others with lower levels experience no thrombotic event. Although antithrombin deficiency usually results in venous thrombosis, acute arterial thrombosis and thrombosis from arterial reconstructions can occur and antithrombin deficiency should be suspected in any patient with unsuspected thrombosis.[22] A common presentation of antithrombin III deficiency is that of a patient who has a thrombotic event and manifests an inability to anticoagulate adequately in response to heparin therapy. The prevalence of this defect in a population with thrombotic or thromboembolic events is 3–8%.[1]

Antithrombin deficiency can also be acquired. Causes of acquired antithrombin deficiency include acute thrombosis, disseminated intravascular coagulation, liver disease, nephrotic syndrome, oral contraceptive use and, rarely, following heparin administration. Postoperative measurements have demonstrated that antithrombin levels can drop 63% after major vascular procedures with a nadir around the third postoperative day. Also, the administration of heparin can decrease antithrombin III levels presumably due to increased clearance of antithrombin III after complexing with heparin.[23,24] Conversely, oral anticoagulants have been reported to increase the level of antithrombin III into the normal range in individuals with known inherited antithrombin III deficiency.[25] Estrogens may decrease antithrombin III levels by 15% in normal patients, and greater decreases are associated with higher doses of estrogens.[2]

Treatment of individuals with symptomatic antithrombin deficiency requires the use of lifelong warfarin anticoagulation. Warfarin not only achieves anticoagulation by decreasing vitamin K-dependent factors, but also increases antithrombin III levels, as noted above. Asymptomatic conditions of antithrombin deficiency are not prophylactically treated unless the individuals are thought to be at an increased risk for thrombosis, including pregnancy or the preoperative period. Treatment of an acute thrombosis in a patient with antithrombin III deficiency requires replacement of antithrombin III using antithrombin III concentrates or fresh frozen plasma and heparin anticoagulation until adequate anticoagulation is achieved. Data that are currently available suggest that antithrombin concentrates used with or without concomitant heparin administration are safe and effective in the prevention of thrombosis in high-risk patients and for the treatment of acute thrombotic episodes in deficient patients.[21]

Prothrombin defects

A point mutation in the 3′ untranslated region of the prothrombin gene has been identified.[26] This is a G to A transition at nucleotide position 20210 that appears to be associated with increased prothrombin levels. The prevalence of this mutation is approximately 6% in patients with thrombosis, and 2% in healthy controls.[1] Carriers of this mutation have two times the risk for thrombotic events as compared to noncarriers, and the majority of these events are venous. There has been no noted association with arterial thrombosis.[27]

Fibrinolytic system defects

Decreased fibrinolytic activity and predisposition to thrombus formation can be secondary to either decreased plasminogen levels or abnormal plasminogen, decreased plasminogen activator activity, or increased plasminogen inhibitor activity. Decreased fibrinolytic activity has been noted in patients with myocardial infarction, generalized atherosclerosis, diabetes, scleroderma, thrombotic thrombocytopenic purpura, recurrent deep venous thrombosis, oral contraception and in most postoperative patients.[28–30]

Congenital plasminogen deficiency is regulated by autosomal dominant inheritance. Patients with this disorder begin to experience thrombotic events in their late teenage years. The most common manifestations are deep venous thrombosis and pulmonary embolism. Venous thrombotic and thromboembolic events occur when the plasminogen level is less than 40% of normal biologic activity.[31] It is estimated that congenital plasminogen deficiency may account for as many as 2–3% of unexplained deep venous thrombosis in young patients. There are two types of plasminogen deficiency, quantitative hypoplasminogenemia and a dysfunctional plasminogen disorder. The presence of a genetically determined plasminogen variant has been reported, resulting in a functional deficiency of the plasminogen system, causing a reduction of fibrinolytic activity and a latent thrombotic tendency.[32] Deficiency can be identified by a synthetic substrate assay for biological activity of plasminogen, and a comparison of biological activity with immunologic levels will distinguish those patients who have dysfunctional plasminogen from those with quantitative hypoplasminogenemia.[21] Successful therapy for this disorder has included the use of heparin, and long-term warfarin or low molecular weight heparin therapy.

Congenital deficiency of plasminogen activator is extremely uncommon and only a few cases have been reported. Congenital increased plasminogen activator inhibitor has also been reported, but is very rare.[33] Acquired deficiency of plasminogen activator has been associated with multiple conditions, including myocardial infarction, post-coronary angioplasty, diabetes, ulcerative colitis, Crohn's disease, oral contraceptives and heavy smoking. The actual risk of thrombosis with this deficiency is not known.

Congenital dysfibrinogenemia represents the presence of a functionally abnormal fibrinogen, which results from a multitude of different molecular defects.[2] The majority of these patients are asymptomatic; however, about 10% of the dysfibrinogenemias are associated with thrombosis.[34] Most of these events consist of venous thrombosis, and are a result of abnormal fibrin monomer polymerization, impaired activation, or resistance to fibrinolysis.[2]

Heparin-induced thrombocytopenia

Up to 30% of patients may manifest a decrease in their platelet count after starting heparin therapy, but the incidence of significant thrombocytopenia and resulting thrombotic or hemorrhagic complications is approximately 5%.[34] Two types of heparin-induced thrombocytopenia are described. Type I, or the acute form, occurs relatively early and results in a benign course with improvement in the platelet count during continued heparin therapy. Type II, or the delayed form, occurs 5–14 days after the institution of heparin therapy in a patient not previously exposed to heparin and after 3–9 days in patients with a history of previous heparin therapy. Type II heparin-induced thrombocytopenia is reported to have a 23–60% thrombotic or hemorrhagic complication rate and a 12–18% mortality rate. Early recognition and treatment results in a significant improvement in the associated morbidity and mortality.[35]

In type I heparin-induced thrombocytopenia, the mechanism of action is thought to be a non-immune-mediated direct effect of heparin on platelets that causes aggregation. Type II heparin-induced thrombocytopenia is due to an immune mediated (IgG and IgM) platelet aggregation. Heparin is not the antigen against which the antibody is directed. Instead, heparin is thought to bind to the platelet, causing the expression of a neoantigen against which the immune response is directed.[36]

The clinical features of this syndrome are often dramatic. Heparin-induced aggregation of platelets should be considered in any patient who has thrombotic complications while receiving heparin therapy. This is especially important in patients with arterial occlusions who do not have any other evidence of atherosclerotic vascular disease. At operation in these patients, the finding of white clot at thrombectomy should alert the surgeon to the possibility of a heparin-induced thrombosis. Also, platelet aggregating tests should be performed on any patient in whom recurrent deep venous thrombosis or pulmonary embolism develops while receiving adequate heparin therapy.[37] A prompt increase in platelet count seen after discontinuing heparin therapy confirms the diagnosis of heparin-induced thrombocytopenia. Additionally, confirmation of the diagnosis of the immune-mediated thrombocytopenia requires the measurement of platelet aggregation using donor platelets in the presence of the patient's plasma and heparin.

All sources of heparin exposure, including heparin flushes of intravascular catheters and heparin-coated catheters, must be eliminated. Continued exposure to heparin at these very low doses can still evoke a heparin-induced thrombocytopenia. Therefore, patients on heparin therapy should have daily platelet counts. If the platelet count drops below 100 000/mm$_3$, or if there is a significant drop (>100 000), the heparin should be stopped and platelet aggregation tests performed. When the diagnosis is made, heparin treatment should be reversed with protamine. Aspirin may be used as an antiplatelet medication in the acute setting and is continued until adequate anticoagulation has been achieved by alternative agents such as dextran or warfarin if long-term anticoagulant therapy is needed.

Patients who require re-exposure to heparin for other vascular or cardiac procedures require special management. Patients who develop heparin-induced platelet aggregation usually have their aggregation tests revert to normal within 6 weeks to 3 months. It is preferable to delay the vascular or cardiac procedure until these tests revert to normal. The patient is tested at 6 weeks, then every 2 weeks thereafter to determine when their platelet-aggregation tests are negative. When they are negative, the patient is then brought into the hospital. Cardiac catheterization or angiography is done as required without the use of heparin flush solutions. This is extremely important since even small amounts of heparin in the flush solutions can stimulate the development of the heparin-induced antiplatelet antibodies. The patient then has the vascular or cardiac procedure done with the usual administration of heparin. At the conclusion of the procedure, all heparin is reversed with protamine and care is taken during the postoperative period to ensure the patient does not receive heparin inadvertently either through flushing central venous catheters or arterial lines. Using this protocol, one can effectively avoid heparin-induced thrombocytopenia.[17]

However, for those patients who require an additional vascular or cardiac procedure and cannot wait until the heparin-induced platelet aggregation tests are negative, a different strategy is necessary. In patients requiring procedures that can be done without the use of heparin, such as resection of abdominal aortic aneurysms, heparin is not used. However, in patients who require complex lower extremity revascularization or cardiopulmonary bypass, some sort of anticoagulation is necessary. There are basically two approaches to this. One approach consists of giving the patients aspirin and Persantine (dipyrimadole) for several days preoperatively, and using heparin for the operative procedure as is customary. In addition to the aspirin and Persantine, low molecular weight dextran can be used, which, in addition to its rheologic properties, coats the platelets and interferes with platelet adhesion. In some patients, however, as noted by Kappa and his group, the administration of aspirin had no effect on the heparin-induced platelet aggregation tests.[38] Makhoul *et al.* noted that aspirin abolished the aggregation in 9 of 16 patients with heparin-induced platelet aggregation, and only decreased the aggregation in the remaining 7, suggesting that aspirin is not able to reverse the abnormal aggregation in all patients.[39] Therefore, on the day of the procedure, the platelet-aggregation tests should be performed with the addition of heparin. If the addition of heparin causes abnormal platelet aggregation, the platelet-aggregation test should be repeated with the addition of danaparoid rather than heparin.[39] Danaparoid sodium, a mixture of anticoagulant glycosaminoglycans (predominantly low-sulfated heparin sulfate and dermatan sulfate) can be used if it does not cause platelet aggregation. There is an approximately 10% cross-reactivity of danaparoid with heparin. Prior to its use however, *in vitro* testing must be done to assure that danaparoid will not aggregate the patient's platelets. Newer agents such as recombinant hirudin can be used. The advantage of hirudin is the lack of cross-reactivity with heparin-induced thrombosis antibodies.

Sobel *et al.* reported an alternative technique of having patients on coumadin (warfarin) anticoagulation combined with dextran as a means of preventing intraoperative thrombosis during reconstruction.[40] This is a reasonable alternative for peripheral vascular reconstructions, but is not possible for cardiopulmonary bypass. In the future, different substances may be available to allow for adequate anticoagulation. Makhoul noted that *in vitro* heparinoids did not cause platelet aggregation in patients with heparin-induced platelet aggregation. It is essential to perform *in vitro* aggregation tests prior to use, since the reactivity to these new heparins and heparin substitutes ranges from 19.6 to 60.8%.[41,42]

Cole and Bormanis have reported the use of ancrod, which is made from the venom of the Malaysian pit viper, as an anticoagulant in patients who have heparin-induced platelet aggregation.[43] Ancrod acts enzymatically on the fibrinogen molecule to form a product that cannot be clotted by physiologic thrombin. At the present time this medication is in the investigational phase, and may be cleared by the FDA in the not too distant future.

Antiphospholipid antibodies

Antiphospholipid (APL) antibodies are acquired antibodies to phospholipid-bound protein and prothrombin. These antibodies can react with the phospholipid components of the phospholipid-dependent coagulation tests and prolong the coagulation times *in vitro*. APL antibodies occur in approximately 5% of the general population, and are more common in patients with systemic lupus erythematosus (SLE). Ten to thirty percent of patients with SLE may exhibit such plasma inhibitors of *in vitro* coagulation, hence their designation as lupus anticoagulant.[44] However, these antibodies are associated clinically with a hypercoagulable state. There are really two distinct antiphospholipid antibody syndromes that are known. The first involves the lupus anticoagulant, and the second involves the anticardiolipin antibody. Anticardiolipin antibody is more common than the lupus anticoagulant; however, both may be associated with arterial or venous thrombosis, thrombocytopenia and recurrent pregnancy loss. Although sometimes associated with SLE, APL antibodies can also be associated with other connective tissue disorders, malignancy, HIV, drug ingestion and possibly estrogens.[45] They can also be found in healthy patients without other underlying conditions.

Approximately 30% of patients with these antibodies have a history of a thrombotic event. Both venous and arterial thromboses can occur with a 50% incidence of thrombosis after vascular procedures reported in a series of patients positive for antiphospholipid antibody.[46] Both the lupus anticoagulant and anticardiolipin antibodies are more commonly associated with venous thrombosis. APL antibodies are found in 10–25% of patients presenting with DVT.[45] They can also be associated with pulmonary embolus, intravenous catheter (IVC) thrombosis, hepatic, portal, renal or retinal vein thromboses.

The mechanism by which these antibodies produce thrombosis is not clear. There are several proposed theories, including:

- interference with endothelial release of prostacyclin;
- interference with activation, via thrombomodulin, of protein C or S activity;
- interference with antithrombin activity;
- interaction with platelet phospholipids, causing activation and release;
- interference with prekallikrein activation;
- interference with endothelial t-PA release.[2]

As yet, there is not a single prevailing theory for the mechanism of thrombosis caused by the antiphospholipid antibodies.

Diagnosis of the presence of antiphospholipid antibodies can be made by demonstration of a prolongation of the coagulation times, which do not correct with the addition of normal plasma. The platelet neutralization assay utilizes the APL antibodies' ability to inhibit platelet binding to collagen as evidence of their presence in a patient's plasma. Reactivity of a patient's plasma with cardiolipin by an enzyme-linked immunoadsorbent assay (ELISA) is also a useful screening test; however, it is not a specific test and may be confirmed by one of the above-mentioned assays.

Prophylactic therapy in asymptomatic patients with a known lupus anticoagulant who are undergoing vascular reconstruction is recommended. This consists of preoperative antiplatelet therapy, intraoperative dextran 40, heparin and postoperative warfarin.[46] Therapy for a symptomatic patient with antiphospholipid antibody consists of heparin for the acute event and chronic oral anticoagulation subsequently. Steroids have also been used to decrease the level of anticoagulant antibodies. Monitoring of the partial thromboplastin time can be problematic due to the anticoagulant effect of the antibody on the test. Measurement of the thrombin time or measurements of the heparin levels are an alternative method of monitoring heparin therapy.

Activated protein C resistance

A recurring theme throughout this chapter has been the fact that procoagulant and anticoagulant properties of blood are delicately balanced by a complex system of cofactors and inhibitors. The thrombomodulin/protein C anticoagulant pathway is an essential anticoagulant system. As thrombin is generated at sites of vascular injury it activates and aggregates platelets and clots fibrinogen. It also binds to the endothelial membrane protein thrombomodulin. Upon binding to thrombomodulin, thrombin takes on anticoagulant properties by activating protein C. The activated protein C (APC) cleaves and inactivates factor Va and VIIIa in the presence of protein S. This endothelial-based anticoagulant system allows blood to clot while maintaining intravascular fluidity. Defects in this anticoagulant pathway can provoke thrombosis and, indeed, protein C and protein S deficiencies, which were discussed previously, are associated with an increased risk of thrombosis in heterozygotes.

A family history of thrombotic events is frequently obtained in young adults with venous thrombosis; however, the inherited deficiencies in anticoagulant proteins, such as protein C and protein S, are found in only approximately 5% of patients.[47] APC resistance is another risk factor for venous thrombosis which is frequently found in these patients. It is, in fact, the most common genetic risk factor for venous thrombosis described to date.[2] It is caused by a point mutation in the factor V gene which causes increased resistance to the anticoagulant effect of APC. This defect was discovered in 1993 by Dahlbäck *et al.*, and has been named factor V Leiden.[47]

Dahlbäck originally postulated that a defect in the protein C pathway interfered with the anticoagulant action of APC. He devised assays to test this possibility in which the clotting time of blood was measured in the presence and absence of exogenous APC. In the normal response, the clotting time was prolonged in the presence of APC because of the inactivation of factors Va and VIIIa. A defect was detected as a failure of prolongation of the clotting time resulting from resistance to added APC. Dahlbäck showed that this test detects an autosomal dominant trait associated with thrombosis. Further work done by Bertina and his group demonstrated that the phenotype of APC resistance is associated with a heterozygous or homozygous single point mutation in the factor V gene which predicts the synthesis of a factor V molecule that is not properly inactivated by APC (factor V Leiden).[48] Other data confirming these results were published by Zoller and Dahlbäck who studied 50 Swedish families with inherited APC resistance.[49] They found that the specific point mutation in the factor V gene was present in 47 out of 50 families. In their study, by age 33 years 20% of the heterozygous and 40% of the homozygous patients had had manifestations of venous thrombosis.

Factor V Leiden is present in 3–7% of all Caucasians, but is more rare in other ethnic populations.[1] It is present in up to 20% of unselected patients with DVT, and confers a 5- to 10-fold increased risk of thrombosis in heterozygotes; homozygotes have a 50- to 100-fold increased risk.[1]

The laboratory diagnosis is made by measuring the responsiveness of plasma to APC as the ratio of two activated partial thromboplastin times (aPTTs), one in the presence of APC and one in its absence. The APC sensitivity ration is normalized to the ratio obtained with reference plasma. Resistance to APC is defined by an APC sensitivity ratio of <0.84.[48] A more recent way of identifying this factor V resistance to APC is by a direct assay for the factor V molecule which is resistant to inactivation by APC (factor V Leiden). The question arises what can be done about these point mutations which cause factor V to be resistant to APC. It is clear that this is a major risk factor for thromboembolic disease; however, the majority of patients with these mutant proteins will not suffer thrombosis. The risks of lifelong anticoagulation therapy in an asymptomatic patient must be weighed against the benefit of preventing infrequent although devastating thrombotic attacks. At this point, it would be a logical course of action to treat those patients who have already suffered thrombotic attacks with long-term warfarin therapy.

Hyperhomocysteinemia

Homocysteine is a thiol-containing amino acid derived from the metabolism of methionine. Re-methylation of homocysteine with a methyl group from methyltetrahydrofolate (MTHF) reproduces methionine. This reaction is B_{12} dependent and is catalyzed by methyltetrahydrofolate reductase (MTHFR). Homocysteine can also be metabolized via transulferation to cysteine, a reaction that requires cystathionine synthase and B_6 cofactor. Homozygous deficiency of cystathionine synthase produces classical homocystinuria, in which levels of homocysteine in the blood and urine are quite elevated. This defect is associated with early onset of vascular disease and venous thrombosis; however, it is quite rare.

Recent attention has been turned to evaluating other factors that might contribute to elevated levels of homocysteine in the plasma, and determining their association with thrombosis. A defect in either MTHFR or cystathionine synthase can be associated with increased homocysteine levels in the blood. Elevated levels of homocysteine have been found to be present in 10–25% of patients with venous thrombosis, which is approximately 2.5 times the number of control patients with increased homocysteine levels.[50,51] In one multicenter trial, homocysteine levels were followed in 264 patients with documented DVT after their 3-month course of oral anticoagulants was stopped. Twenty-five percent of these patients had increased homocysteine levels, and these patients had a 19% recurrence of DVT after 2 years, in comparison with a 6.3% recurrence rate in those patients without increased homocysteine levels.[51] It appears that elevated homocysteine levels increase the risk of venous thrombosis by up to fourfold.[51]

Normalization of homocysteine levels can be accomplished by giving folic acid with or without B_{12}. It remains to be proved, however, that normalizing homocysteine levels confers any benefit. Treatment therefore, is unclear. In asymptomatic patients, vitamin supplementation is probably reasonable. In patients who have had DVT, anticoagulation with warfarin or low molecular weight heparin should be undertaken, but the time course of this therapy is uncertain. There is evidence that these patients are at high risk for recurrent DVT, and lifetime anticoagulation should be considered.

REFERENCES

1. Rosendaal F. Risk factors for venous thrombosis: prevalence, risk and interactum. *Semin Hematol* 1997; **34**: 171–87.
2. Bick R, Kaplan H. Syndromes of thrombosis and hypercoagulability. *Med Clin North Am* 1998; **82**: 409–58.
3. Goldsmith J, Neddleman SW. A comparative study of thromboxane and prostacyclin release from ex vivo and cultured bovine vascular endothelium. *Prostaglandin* 1982; **24**: 173.
4. Mehta J, Roberts A. Human vascular tissue produce thromboxane as well as prostacyclin. *Am J Physiol* 1983; **244**: R839.
5. Radomski MW, Palmer, RM, Moncada S. The antiaggregating properties of vascular endothelium: interactions between prostacyclin and nitric oxide. *Br J Pharmacol* 1987; **92**: 639–46.
6. Esmon CT. The regulation of natural anticoagulant pathways. *Science* 1987; **235**: 1348.
7. Loskutoff DJ, Curriden SA. The fibrinolytic system of the vessel wall and its role in the control of thrombosis. *Ann N Y Acad Sci* 1990; **598**: 238.
8. Crawford N, Scutton MC. Biochemistry of the blood platelets. In Bloom AL, Thomas DP, eds. *Haemostasis and Thrombosis*, 2nd edn. Edinburgh: Churchill Livingtone, 1987: 47.
9. DeGroot PG, Gonsalves MD, Loesburg C, *et al.* Thrombin induced release of von Willebrand factor from endothelial cells is mediated by phospholipid methylation. *J Biol Chem* 1984; **259**: 13329.
10. Gelehrter TD, Synycer-Laszuk R. Thrombin induction of plasminogen activator inhibitor in cultured human endothelial cells. *J Clin Invest* 1986; **77**: 165.
11. Olexa SA, Budzynski AZ. Localization of a fibrin polymerization site. *J Biol Chem* 1981; **256**: 3544.
12. Coleman RW. Surface mediated defense reactions: the plasma contact activation system. *J Clin Invest* 1984; **73**: 1249.

13. Rosenburg RD. Biochemistry of heparin antithrombin interactions, and the physiologic role of this natural anticoagulant mechanism. *Am J Med* 1989; **87**(Suppl 3B): 2S.
14. Tollefson DFJ, Bandyk DF, Towne JB, *et al.* Protein C deficiency – a cause of unusual or unexplained thrombosis. *Arch Surg* 1988; **123**: 881.
15. Kazmier FJ. Thromboembolism, coumarin necrosis and protein C. *Mayo Clin Proc* 1985; **60**: 673.
16. Peterson CE, Kwann HC. Current concepts of warfarin therapy. *Arch Intern Med* 1986; **146**: 581.
17. Towne JB. Hypercoagulable states and unexplained vascular thrombosis. In Bernhard VM, Towne JB, eds. *Complications in Vascular Surgery*, 3rd edn. St Louis, MO: Quality Medical Publishing, 1991: 101.
18. Griffin J, Heeb M, Schwarz H. Plasma protein S deficiency and thromboembolic disease. *Prog Hematol* 1987; **15**: 39.
19. Engesser L, Broekmans A, Briet E, *et al.* Hereditary protein S deficiency: clinical manifestations. *Ann Intern Med* 1987; **106**: 677–82.
20. Fischer AM, Cornu P, Sternberg C, *et al.* Antithrombin III Alger: a new homozygous ATIII variant. *Thromb Haemost* 1986; **55**: 218–21.
21. Bick RL, Pegram M. Syndromes of hypercoagulability and thrombosis. *Semin Thromb Hemost* 1994; **20**(1): 109.
22. Towne JB, Bernhard VM, Hussey C, *et al.* Antithrombin deficiency a cause of unexplained thrombosis in vascular surgery. *Surgery* 1981; **89**: 735.
23. Buller HR, TenCate JW. Acquired antithrombin III deficiency: laboratory diagnosis, incidence, clinical implications and treatment with antithrombin III concentrate. *Am J Med* 1989; **87**(Suppl 3B): 44S.
24. Marciniak E, Gockeman JP. Heparin induced clearance of circulating antithrombin III. *Lancet* 1978; **2**: 581.
25. Kitchens CS. Amelioration of antithrombin III deficiency by coumarin administration. *Am J Med Sci* 1987; **293**: 403.
26. Poort S, Rosendaal F, Reitsma P, *et al.* A common genetic variation in the 3′- untranslated region of the prothrombin gene is associated with elevated plasma prothrombin levels and an increase in venous thrombosis. *Blood* 1996; **88**: 3698–703.
27. Ridker P, Hennekens C, Miletich J. G20210A mutation in prothrombin gene and risk of myocardial infarction, stroke, and venous thrombosis in a large cohort of US men. *Circulation* 1999; **99**: 999–1004.
28. Colleen D, Juhan-Vague I. Fibrinolysis and atherosclerosis. *Semin Thromb Hemost* 1988; **14**: 180.
29. Almer LD, Pandolfi M, Osterlin S. The fibrinolytic system in patients with diabetes mellitus with special reference to diabetic retinopathy. *Ophthalmologica* 1975; **170**: 353.
30. Nalbandian RM, Henry RL, Bick RL. Thrombotic thrombocytopenic purpura: an extended editorial. *Semin Thromb Hemost* 1979; **5**: 216.
31. Hasegawa DH, Tyler BJ, Edson JR. Thrombotic disease in three families with inherited plasminogen deficiency. *Blood* 1982; **60**: 213.
32. Towne JB, Bandyk DF, Hussey CV, *et al.* Abnormal plasminogen: a genetically determined cause of hypercoagulability. *J Vasc Surg* 1984; **1**(6): 896.
33. Nilsson IM, Tengborn LA. A family with thrombosis associated with high level of tissue plasminogen activator inhibitor. *Haemostasis* 1984; **14**: 24.
34. Silver D. Heparin-induced thrombocytopenia. *Semin Vasc Surg* 1988; **1**: 228.
35. Laster J. Cikrit D, Walker N, *et al.* The heparin-induced thrombocytopenia syndrome: an update. *Surgery* 1987; **102**: 763.
36. Anderson GP. Insights into heparin-induced thrombocytopenia. *Br J Haematol* 1992; **80**: 504.
37. Towne JB, Bernhard VM, Hussey C, *et al.* White clot syndrome-peripheral vascular complications of heparin therapy. *Arch Surg* 1979; **114**: 372.
38. Kappa JR, Fisher CA, Berkowitz HD, *et al.* Heparin-induced platelet activation in sixteen surgical patients: diagnosis and management. *J Vasc Surg* 1987; **5**: 101.
39. Makhoul RG, Greenberg CS, McCann RL. Heparin-associated thrombocytopenia and thrombosis: a serious clinical problem and potential solution. *J Vasc Surg* 1986; **4**: 522.
40. Sobel M, Adelman B, Szaboles S, *et al.* Surgical management of heparin-associated thrombocytopenia. *J Vasc Surg* 1988; **8**: 395.
41. Rhodes GR, Dixon RH, Silver D. Heparin-induced thrombocytopenia. *Ann Surg* 1977; **186**: 752.
42. Spadeon D, Clark F, James E, Laseter J, Silver D. Heparin-induced thrombocytopenia. *J Vasc Surg* 1992; **15**: 306.
43. Cole CW, Fournier LM, Bormanis J. Heparin-associated thrombocytopenia and thrombosis: optimal therapy with ancrod. *Can J Surg* 1990; **33**: 207.
44. Espinoza LR, Hartman RC. Significance of the lupus anticoagulant. *Am J Haematol* 1986; **22**: 331.
45. Petri M. 1998 update on antiphospholipid antibodies. *Curr Opin Rheumatol* 1998; **10**: 426–30.
46. Ahn SS, Kalunian L, Rosove M, *et al.* Postoperative thrombotic complications in patients with the lupus anticoagulant: increased risk after vascular procedures. *J Vasc Surg* 1988; **7**: 749.
47. Svensson PJ, Dahlbäck B. Resistance to activated protein C as a basis for venous thrombosis. *N Engl J Med* 1994; **330**: 517–21.
48. Bertina RM, Koeleman BP, Koster T, *et al.* Mutation in blood coagulation factor V associated with resistance to activated protein C. *Nature* 1994; **369**: 64–7.
49. Zoller B, Svensson PJ, Xuhua H, Dahlbäck B. Identification of the same factor V gene mutation in 47 out of 50 thrombosis-prone families with inherited resistance to activated protein C. *J Clin Invest* 1994; **94**: 2521.
50. Bos G, Den Heijer M. Hyperhomocysteinemia and venous thrombosis. *Semin Thromb Hemost* 1998; **24**: 387–91.
51. Eichinger S, Stumpflen A, Hirschl M, *et al.* Hyperhomocysteinemia is a risk factor of recurrent venous thromboembolism. *Thromb Haemost* 1998; **80**: 566–9.

9

Classification and diagnostic evaluation of chronic venous disease

ROBERT L KISTNER AND BO EKLOF

The truism that good treatment begins with a good diagnosis applies to venous disease as well as to other problems. Chronic venous disease (CVD) includes a variety of problems that affect the lower limbs of the erect human, ranging from the most minor cosmetic blemishes to disabling conditions that may impair the individual's ability to work and dominate his/her way of life. With the development in recent years of accurate noninvasive testing of the veins and new surgical abilities to correct reflux and obstruction throughout the venous tree, the expectations of an adequate diagnosis have changed. This chapter describes the elements of a complete diagnosis that fulfill the criteria for the new CEAP classification, and will present an orderly method of reaching the diagnosis that is appropriate to the clinical condition under consideration.

The clinical diagnosis of chronic venous problems has been dominated in the past by clinical appearance and external patterns of varicose veins, skin discoloration and thickening, and ulceration. This was adequate when treatment was limited to external support and medications for the ulcers, but the newer developments that allow definitive surgical repair of both reflux and obstruction demand much more precise information. The new attitude in CVD is to establish the etiology of the venous condition by determining if the problem is due to primary, secondary (post-thrombotic), or congenital causes, to discover the process by which it acts whether this is reflux or obstruction, or both, and to establish which segments of the venous tree are affected by the pathologic changes. The sophistication of the work-up in each case is dictated by the seriousness of the clinical problem in that patient's way of life. Simple conditions merit simple diagnostics, but complex problems require a thorough diagnostic work-up which delineates the abnormalities throughout the venous tree and provides a template to outline the treatment alternatives appropriate to a given clinical setting. These alternatives result from an understanding of the etiology, pathophysiology, and anatomic distribution of pathologic changes in the extremity.

DIAGNOSTIC PROCESS

The diagnostic process in CVD should be a logical one in which the sophistication of the diagnostic testing is tuned to the magnitude of the problem and its effect upon the patient's lifestyle. The nature of the problem and its severity should be defined in the initial interview, and used to guide the rest of the work-up. The main steps in diagnosing chronic venous patients are listed in Fig. 9.1.

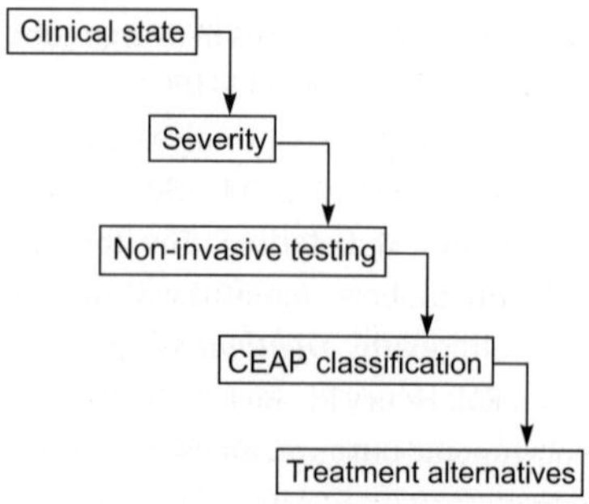

Figure 9.1 *Five steps in the definitive diagnosis of the CVD patient outlined in their logical sequence when evaluating a new CVD patient.*

The clinical state can readily be defined in terms of objective and subjective manifestations. The objective signs of varicose veins, swelling, and skin changes of pigmentation, thickening, and ulceration need to be detailed. The more subjective effects of pain and interference with work or other aspects of lifestyle determine the severity of the venous problem for the individual, and define whether there is a need for definitive surgery to supplement conservative management. The patient with more significant problems will go to the vascular laboratory for noninvasive testing, which begins with duplex scanning and may progress through plethysmographic and pressure testing to define the physiologic derangement. These tests provide sufficient data to create the CEAP classification[1] that includes the etiologic, anatomic and pathophysiologic aspects of the problem, and from this the treatment alternatives can be outlined. For those who may go on to definitive deep venous reconstruction, further work-up by venography will be needed.

Most of the problems in CVD are due to reflux rather than obstruction. All of the saphenous and perforator problems are ones of reflux rather than obstruction, and these constitute about 80% of CVD problems.[2,3] In the deep veins, acute DVT is an obstructive condition which matures in the chronic phase through the process of recanalization (which includes clot retraction, fibrinolysis and neovascularization) into varying degrees of reflux, and it is this combination of partial obstruction and progressive reflux that leads to post-thrombotic ulcers. With the use of objective imaging by duplex scan and descending venography, primary valve incompetence (PVI) has been more frequently recognized. In an increasing number of reports, PVI represents the cause of proximal reflux in one half or more of the cases that have severe sequelae.[3–5] In our series of 100 venous ulcers being prepared for publication, the etiology of the ulceration was PVI in 72% of the cases (unpublished data).

The separation of primary from secondary disease is very important because reflux is the only physiologic problem in primary disease while both reflux and obstruction, alone or in combination, may be found in secondary and in congenital disease. These are important differences for the surgeon who would do different operations for these different problems. Duplex scan and plethysmography are the most frequent ways of differentiating primary from secondary disease since they are the most frequently performed noninvasive tests and scanning is a definitive method for showing reflux. The more subtle changes of secondary disease, such as synechiae and luminal strands, are better shown by venography in some cases, and the pattern of venous flow is better determined by venography, factors that make venography a complementary method for differentiating secondary from primary disease.

In cases where deep vein obstruction is present, the most common cause is post-thrombotic disease affecting the femoropopliteal and/or iliocaval veins, although other causes such as tumor, retroperitoneal fibrosis, or compression by anatomical anomalies such as the iliac compression syndrome (May–Thurner syndrome) or the femoral vein compression syndrome (Gullmo syndrome) may also occur. Even the recanalized, apparently patent post-thrombotic vein may act as a physiologic obstruction due to its retained luminal strands and synechiae. The symptoms depend upon which segments of veins are involved and the degree of collateral circulation, and may range from asymptomatic to severe venous claudication and ulceration.

Work-up of patients with chronic venous disease

A practical approach to the venous work-up is to divide the evaluation into the initial office visit, a subsequent noninvasive vascular laboratory visit, and selective use of invasive venography, as detailed in the algorithm in Fig. 9.2. By using this approach, those with mild-to-moderate disease are clearly identified with a minimum of testing and those with advanced disease are objectively studied until the alternatives for treatment are thoroughly defined.

The diagnostic process is organized into three phases beginning in the office, progressing to the vascular laboratory, and culminating in the radiology suite for selected problems.

PHASE I: OFFICE PHASE

The initial evaluation is one in which the clinical diagnosis is defined and the effect the chronic venous state has upon the patient is estimated. An apparently minor cosmetic blemish may be very important in the life of an actor or a dancer whilst it is of no import to a truck driver. Similarly, a venous ulcer may disable the truck driver from work whereas it is of little import to the sedentary elderly person with many other ailments.

During this visit all of the appropriate history and general physical findings are detailed. The list includes, but is not limited to, prior history of venous problems such as varicose veins and thrombophlebitis, coagulation problems, family history of venous disease, severity of swelling and pain, and arterial insufficiency. A question sheet that can be used in the office for the patient to initiate and the office nurse to elaborate is shown in Fig. 9.3.

The office examination should include a venous Doppler examination in addition to the clinical evaluation of telangiectases, varicose veins, and skin changes of discoloration, thickening and ulceration typical of CVD. The Doppler examination by the physician will detect reflux in the saphenous and deep veins of the thigh, popliteal and calf, and provide an estimate of probable perforator disease.

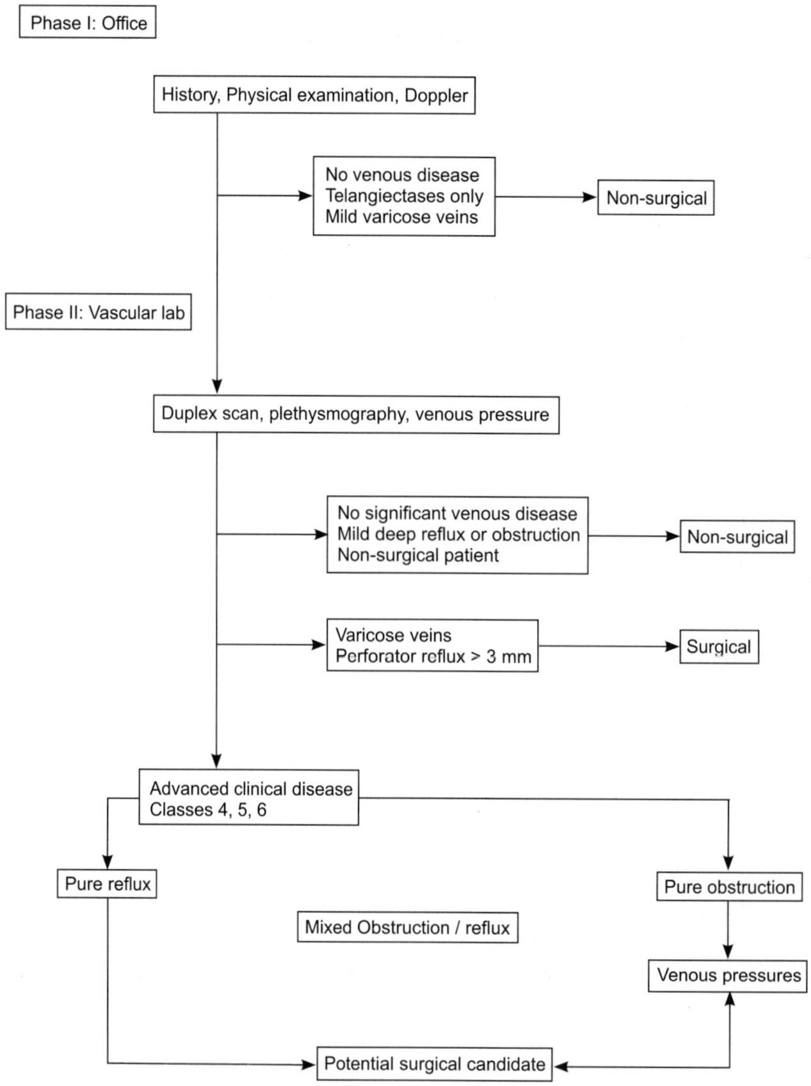

Figure 9.2 *(a) Algorithm for CVD work-up (1). Diagnostic examinations and definitive results obtained in phase 1: office and phase II: vascular lab. The results of these two phases are definitive for the majority of CVD patients who are in classes 1, 2 and 3. For those in classes 4, 5 and 6 who are potential candidates for deep venous reconstruction, further work-up by radiologic testing is needed.*

At the completion of the office phase the clinical state, its severity, and its effect upon the patient's life will have been detailed. This is the data set needed to decide the appropriate next step. For those with absence of detectable venous disease, or with minor problems of telangiectasia or peripheral varices without saphenous reflux, the office visit is adequate for the full work-up because further evaluation will not change the management. Those with more complicated problems should be sent for vascular laboratory testing.

PHASE II: THE VASCULAR LABORATORY

Vascular laboratory work-up is necessary for the patient who would be a candidate for correction of a specific abnormality, or whose management would change depending upon the exact diagnosis. The purpose is to reach a sufficiently precise knowledge of the condition to classify its etiology, whether due to primary valvular incompetence (PVI) or secondary (post-thrombotic syndrome) (PTS), its mechanism of development by reflux or obstruction, or both, and its distribution in the anatomic segments of the extremity. This information will lead to the alternative treatment choices available for the individual.

The duplex scan, especially with color flow, is today's mainstay of noninvasive evaluation. It provides real-time observation of venous flow in the leg and permits one to watch and record the effects of muscle contraction, of proximal and distal compression, and of the Valsalva maneuver, on each segment of the veins. It can be done in any position, supine, sitting or erect. The veins throughout the extremity can be observed for patency and for reflux. Incompetent saphenous and perforator

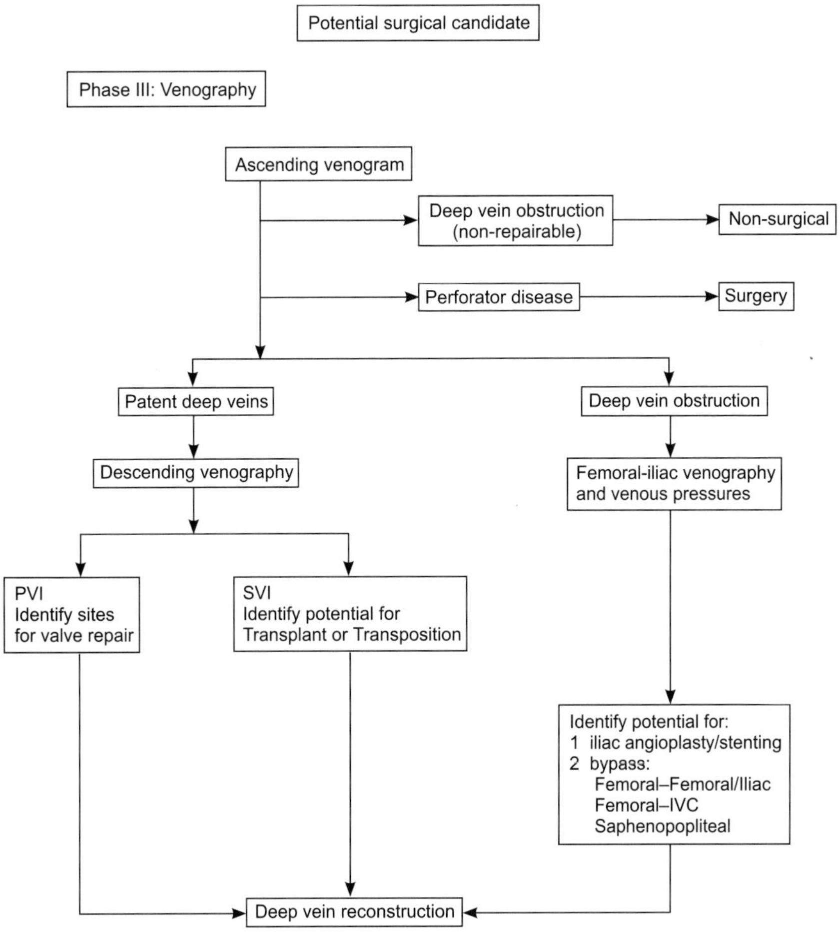

Figure 9.2 *(b) Algorithm for CVD work-up (2). Potential candidates for deep venous reconstruction are separated into those who are appropriate for various surgical operations through a series of logical steps.*

veins are clearly identified. All segments of the deep veins, including common femoral vein (CFV), superficial femoral vein (SFV), profunda femoris vein (PFV), and popliteal and tibial veins should be individually studied both for patency and competence. As the technology improves, even the moving venous valves can be observed in many instances, and reflux through these valves can be observed and measured.

Plethysmographic and pressure studies may be used to substantiate and partially quantify the pathologic findings noted by scan. Plethysmography has many forms of which the most thorough may be the air plethysmograph (APG),[6] and the simplest is the photoplethysmograph (PPG). The APG provides data on both obstruction and reflux in the extremity and estimates calf muscle function in the leg. It is a convenient way to confirm whether there is an obstructive element in the extremity, and may be used to provide a physiologic correlation when anatomic obstruction had been seen on duplex scan.

Venous pressure studies are particularly helpful in assessing the physiologic importance of anatomic obstruction, because collaterals may or may not provide adequate physiologic compensation for an obstructed major pathway. Since just seeing that collaterals are present does not give accurate assessment of their functional adequacy, further study with plethysmographic and pressure data is important when trying to determine the need for surgical bypass or valve replacement. Venous pressure does not discriminate between obstruction and reflux, although it does have value in identifying severe abnormal function compared with mild dysfunction. Arm–foot differential pressure[7] for calf and thigh obstruction and femoral venous pressure for iliac vein obstruction are useful in quantifying the degree of physiologic occlusion present in a given individual. Valsalva foot pressure is useful in reflux disease.

As noted in Fig. 9.2, the vascular laboratory tests provide definitive testing for varicose veins and most of the perforator problems, and are decisive in eliminating those without significant venous disease. They are also adequate for knowledge of the superficial and deep circulation in those who are non-candidates for surgical reconstruction. Furthermore, patients with more severe disease can be categorized into those few with pure obstruction, a larger group with obstruction and reflux,

VENOUS PATIENT QUESTIONNAIRE

Please mark yes or no to those which apply and circle where appropriate.

YES	NO	
☐	☐	VARICOSE VEINS (visibly enlarged, bulging veins beneath the skin).
☐	☐	SPIDER VEINS (small, visible blood vessels in the skin which take on a blue or red color).
☐	☐	SLOW HEALING SORES (ULCERS) ON YOUR LEGS OR FEET.
☐	☐	SKIN CHANGES IN LOWER LEGS (discoloration/thickening).
☐	☐	DISCOMFORT/HEAVINESS/PAIN IN YOUR LEGS.
☐	☐	SWELLING (right/left) (legs/ankles/feet).
☐	☐	DO YOU WEAR SUPPORT STOCKINGS? (never/sometimes/always).
☐	☐	OTHER VEIN PROBLEM (please explain or describe).

YES	NO	Medical history	MEDICATIONS:
☐	☐	Did you experience injury or trauma to affected area?	
☐	☐	Are you diabetic?	
☐	☐	Do you smoke cigarettes?	
☐	☐	Did you smoke cigarettes in the past?	
☐	☐	Have you had a previous blood clot or phlebitis?	
☐	☐	Is it possible that you may be pregnant?	

YES	NO	Past surgeries
☐	☐	Previous varicose vein surgery?
☐	☐	Previous injections (sclerotherapy) of varicose veins or spider veins?
☐	☐	Leg bypass surgery?
☐	☐	Heart bypass surgery?
☐	☐	Knee/hip surgery (replacement)?

YES	NO	Family history. Please mark those which apply to any of your family members.
☐	☐	History of blood clots or phlebitis?
☐	☐	Varicose veins or spider veins?
☐	☐	History of vascular or bypass surgery?
☐	☐	Bleeding problems?
☐	☐	Diabetes?

SIGNATURE: ____________________

CEAP: ____________________

Figure 9.3 *Sample of a patient questionnaire that can be initiated by the patient and refined by the nursing staff to facilitate definitive office consultation in CVD.*

and the largest group with pure reflux. From these findings, a group will emerge who are potential surgical candidates, and they will need to go on for venography to develop a reliable surgical plan.

PHASE III: RADIOLOGIC IMAGING

This third phase of diagnosis is not warranted for the patient whose diagnosis is clear, and whose treatment is defined, by less invasive and less expensive testing. Venography is complementary to duplex scanning in several ways and should be looked upon as an additional way to learn about the veins that will aid in deciding upon a specific surgical approach.

Ascending venography

Ascending venography is important in all candidates for deep vein reconstruction and some who require additional information prior to perforator surgery. It is useful in the CVI patient to map the patent veins in the extremity and to identify the incompetent perforator veins in the calf. It is done through a needle in a dorsal foot vein with the patient semi-erect at 45–60°. With an occluding tourniquet at the ankle to prevent filling of the superficial veins, contrast is injected while flow is followed by fluoroscopy as it fills the tibial veins and ascends above the knee. In this way, flow from deep veins to the surface veins identifies that the perforating veins are incompetent. The addition of a second tourniquet near the knee may help to identify incompetent perforator veins. The conventional ascending venogram of the popliteal, femoral and iliac veins is then obtained to visualize the entire patent venous tree from the ankle into the pelvis, and ideally up to the inferior vena cava (IVC). When the ascending venogram is performed in this manner, it will identify incompetent perforator veins, obstructed vein segments in the calf and thigh and pelvis, and most of the recanalized post-thrombotic segments; it will also provide a map of patent veins in the extremity. Careful search of the veins, especially the tibial veins, for an irregular pattern will identify the recanalized post-thrombotic vein and distinguish it from the normal. Interpretation of valve function by ascending venography is not reliable.

Descending venography

Descending venograms are necessary to plan deep vein valve reconstruction or valve substitution procedures and are the most reliable means to differentiate PVI from secondary valve incompetence (SVI) as a cause of deep vein reflux in the proximal thigh (Fig. 9.2b). The study is best performed by selective technique with a catheter introduced from the opposite groin.[8] The patient is placed in the 60° erect position, and the separate vein segments (GSV, PFV, SFV) are examined under conditions of both quiet breathing and forced Valsalva after teaching the patient how to perform a forced Valsalva maneuver. Individual study of the GSV, SFV and PFV is done to identify the presence of valves and their state of competence with and without Valsalva. When reflux occurs through a proximal valve, the contrast is followed distally in that segment until it dissipates.

When a valve shows reflux with quiet breathing but becomes competent with Valsalva, it is deemed a competent valve. Conversely, when a valve is competent with quiet breathing but develops reflux with Valsalva, it is termed incompetent. The Valsalva is important and must be taught to the patient who can be instructed to inflate a balloon or blow a mercury manometer to 40 mmHg pressure to standardize the force of the Valsalva.

The descending venogram is interpreted in light of the distal extent of reflux.[9] When reflux is limited to the thigh in the deep veins, the patient is not considered to be a candidate for deep valve surgery. When reflux passes through the popliteal vein and into the calf, surgical correction is deemed appropriate.

Because the descending venogram is a dynamic study, it must be performed under fluoroscopy. For post-procedural study, the entire venogram should be recorded on videotape, and the video should include sound to clarify when the patient is straining or moving in order to accurately interpret valvular function. Still films alone can be very misleading when reviewing the results of descending venography.

THE CEAP CLASSIFICATION

In 1994 an ad hoc committee of the American Venous Forum with international representation gathered to develop a new classification system for CVD to address the considerations imposed by modern diagnostic and treatment capabilities. It met in a consensus format under the chairmanship of Professor Andrew Nicolaides and produced a document entitled the CEAP classification.[1] This classification was adopted by the board of the American Venous Forum and by the joint council of the SVS and ISCS surgical societies who approved its publication in the updated reporting standards for venous disease.[10] The CEAP system has been widely adopted around the world, having been published in at least six languages on five continents and in over 20 journals. The importance of the worldwide dissemination is that it is necessary for a single classification to be used universally in order to facilitate accurate communication between institutions and countries about the details of CVD and the results of new forms of treatment.

Since the classification is presented in its entirety in Chapter 52, the individual tables will not be repeated here. The design of the classification is to provide a framework around which the key elements of CVD can be organized. These elements are the clinical condition 'C' denoted in six categories, the etiological (E) basis of the venous dysfunction as primary, secondary, or congenital in nature, the anatomic distribution of the disease 'A' in superficial, perforator and deep divisions, and the pathophysiologic 'P' mechanisms of development as reflux, or obstruction, or both, denoted as occurring in 18 defined segments of the lower extremity veins.

This classification forces consideration of the cause of the venous problem, its pathogenetic mechanism of development through reflux or obstruction or both, and the distribution of pathologic changes in universally agreed-upon anatomic segments of the veins (Fig. 9.4), and by doing so it provides a description of the venous problem that is reproducible from one institution to another. In this way, the natural history of similar venous problems can be traced and the results of treatment in specific categories can be analyzed. This provides the basis for future inter-institutional studies in chronic venous disease and is the basis from which a more scientific analysis of chronic venous disease can be developed.

Use of the classification is facilitated by employing a form such as the one in Fig. 9.5. This format guides the recording of details during the work-up, and results in an orderly presentation of the CEAP classification at the end of the work-up. In addition, this form records the elements that are included in the clinical severity scoring system that was published along with the CEAP

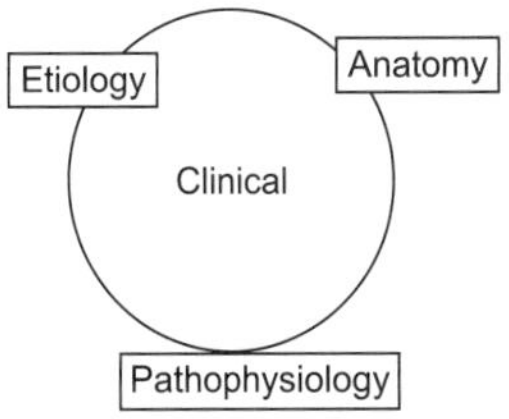

Figure 9.4 *Diagram of the four important elem... diagnosis of the chronic venous condition. The etic... anatomy and pathophysiology of the chronic veno... interact with one another and each brings a special influence to the clinical state and to its treatment. The diagram is meant to connote that any of the four elements could be in the center of the ring, and would be influenced by the other three.*

CEAP: Clinical Score			RIGHT	LEFT
PAIN	None	0		
	Occasional-no analgesics	1		
	Daily-some analgesics	2		
	Daily-regular analgesics	3		
VARICOSE VEINS	None	0		
	Scattered-branch varices	1		
	Multiple-thigh or calf only	2		
	Extensive-thigh and calf	3		
VENOUS EDEMA	None	0		
	Evening, ankle edema	1		
	Afternoon edema, above ankle	2		
	Morning edema, above ankle	3		
SKIN PIGMENTATION	None	0		
	Limited area, old (brown)	1		
	Gaiter distribution, recent	2		
	Above lower 1/3, recent	3		
INFLAMMATION	None	0		
	Mild cellulitis, limited area	1		
	Gaiter area distribution	2		
	Severe, above gaiter distribution	3		
INDURATION	None	0		
	Focal, <5 cm	1		
	Up to lower third of leg	2		
	> lower third of leg	3		
NUMBER OF ACTIVE ULCERS	None	0		
	One	1		
	Two	2		
	> Two	3		
ACTIVE ULCERATION, DURATION	None	0		
	<3 months	1		
	>3 months, <1 year	2		
	Unhealed >1 year	3		
ACTIVE ULCER, SIZE	None	0		
	<2 cm diameter	1		
	2–6 cm diameter	2		
	>6 cm diameter	3		
COMPRESSIVE THERAPY	Not used or non-compliant	0		
	Intermittent stockings	1		
	Uses stockings most of time	2		
	Full compliance with stockings, elevation	3		
TOTAL CLIN SCORE (C)				
ANATOMIC SCORE (A)	(Segmental score of reflux and obstruction)			

			RIGHT	LEFT
DISABILITY SCORE (D)	Asymptomatic	0		
	Symptomatic, normal activity without support	1		
	Requires support for normal activity	2		
	Limited activity even with support	3		

Severity (CAD) Score: (C+A+D=Total Score)	RIGHT	LEFT

				RIGHT	LEFT
CLINICAL		No visible sign of venous disease	0		
		Telangiectases or reticular	1		
		Varicose veins	2		
		Edema	3		
		Skin changes	4		
		Skin changes + healed ulcer	5		
		Skin changes + active ulcer	6		
		ASYMPTOMATIC	A		
		SYMPTOMATIC	S		
ETIOLOGIC		Congenital (at birth or later)	C		
		Primary (undetermined cause)	P		
		Secondary (PTS, Other)	S		
ANATOMIC	Reflux:	Lesser Saphenous	(0.5)		
		Greater Saphenous	(1.0)		
		Perforators, Thigh	(0.5)		
		Perforators, Calf	(1.0)		
		Calf Veins, Multiple	(2.0)		
		Calf Veins, PT Alone	(1.0)		
		Popliteal Vein	(2.0)		
		Superficial Femoral V	(1.0)		
		Profunda Femoral V	(1.0)		
		Common Femoral V	(1.0)		
	Obstruction:	Greater Saphenous	(1.0)		
		Calf Veins, Multiple	(1.0)		
		Popliteal Vein	(2.0)		
		Superficial Femoral V	(1.0)		
		Profunda Femoral V	(1.0)		
		Common Femoral V	(2.0)		
		Iliac Vein	(1.0)		
		IVC	(1.0)		
PATHOPHYSIOLOGY		Reflux	R		
		Obstruction	O		
		Both	RO		

CEAP Classification:	RIGHT	LEFT

Figure 9.5 *A sample format of a method to record the cogent data in a venous work-up that will be useful in recording the CEAP classification, and will result in analysis of the severity score for that extremity. (Adapted from J Jerome Guex, MD and Michel Perrin, MD, by personal communication). Adapted from Rutherford RB, Padberg FT, Comerota AJ, Kistner RL, Meissner MH, Moneta GL* Venous Severity Scoring: adjunct to venous outcome assessment. J Vasc Surg *2000,* ***21:*** *1307–12, Tables 1, 2 and 3.*

classification.[1,11] This scoring system provides a numerical score to estimate the severity of the venous condition by combining a numerical score for the clinical state (C), another score for the anatomic distribution (A) of the involved segments, and a third score for the disability (D) rating at the time the examination was done. This 'C-A-D' score can be used for longitudinal follow-up of the patient's progress over time because it permits quantification of improvement after treatment or of worsening due to complications from new disease over time.

An important step toward standardization in chronic venous diagnosis was taken in 1997 when Professor Nicolaides organized a consensus conference on the indications and limitations of testing procedures in chronic venous disease. This is published in the journal *Circulation* in late 1999.[12] The last step in standardizing venous diagnosis will be taken when standards for performing each test are established to ensure that the diagnoses made from these tests are similar around the world.

A shorthand method of writing the classification provides an acronym for the patient's condition, and with practice it can be readily used to denote the entire CEAP classification for any chronic venous problem very quickly. For instance, uncomplicated telangiectases may be identified by the acronym

$$C_1 \text{ (s or a)}$$

where C_1 represents the condition, and s or a denotes symptomatic or asymptomatic for those with and without pain. Varicose veins may be:

$$C_2 \text{ (s or a), Ep, As, Pr}_{2,3}$$

to denote varicose veins with or without pain (a or s), due to primary disease (Ep), affecting the superficial veins only (As), and with reflux found in the segments 2 and 3 ($r_{2,3}$). Very complicated disease would be a more detailed acronym, such as

$$C_{2,3,4,6}\text{-Es-As,p,d-Pr}_{2,3,13,14,15,17,18}///o_{13,14}$$

to represent a case with varicose veins, swelling, skin changes, and active ulceration ($C_{2,3,4,6}$), due to post-thrombotic disease (Es), found in the superficial, perforator and deep veins (As,p,d), with the pathogenetic mechanisms of reflux in the entire greater saphenous, the superficial femoral, popliteal, and crural veins and in both thigh and calf perforators ($r_{2,3,13,14,15,17,18}$), and obstructive post-thrombotic changes in the superficial femoral and popliteal veins ($o_{13,14}$).

By employing all these features of the CEAP approach, the chronic venous condition can be thoroughly classified, its severity can be graded, and its findings can be noted and communicated very quickly.

CONCLUSION

A new way of thinking about chronic venous disease is needed to permit scientific analysis of its manifestations and to support new advances in its treatment. It is no longer enough to settle for the simple diagnosis of 'venous ulcer' or of the 'post-phlebitic syndrome' without defining the cause and pathogenetic mechanisms involved in development of the problem, and the anatomic segments involved in the process. With advances in noninvasive diagnosis, especially by duplex scanning, every case of CVD can be objectively studied in a safe, painless, and affordable manner. The need for complete diagnosis results from the advances in treatment, which now allow surgical correction of both reflux and obstructive states throughout the lower extremity. This provides the opportunity for the patient to have the CVD state improved to fit his/her way of life rather than requiring the patient to adapt his/her way of life to the CVD limitations.

REFERENCES

1. Classification and grading of chronic venous disease. A consensus statement. *J Vasc Surg* 1995; **21**: 635–45.
2. Labropoulos N. CEAP in clinical practice. *Vasc Surg* 1997; **31**: 224–5.
3. Kistner RL, Eklof B, Masuda EM. Diagnosis of chronic venous disease of the lower extremities: the CEAP classification. *Mayo Clin Proc* 1996; **71**(4): 338–45.
4. Bauer G. The etiology of leg ulcers and their treatment by resection of the popliteal vein. *J Int Chir* 1948; **8**: 937–61.
5. Raju S, Fredericks R. Valve reconstruction procedures for nonobstructive venous insufficiency: rationale, technique, and results in 107 procedures with two- to eight-year follow-up. *J Vasc Surg* 1988; **7**: 301–10.
6. Nicolaides AN, Christopoulos DC. Methods of quantification of chronic venous insufficiency. In Bergan JJ, Yao JST, eds. *Venous Disorders.* Philadelphia: WB Saunders, 1991: 77–90.
7. Raju S. New approaches to the diagnosis and treatment of venous obstruction. *J Vasc Surg* 1986; **4**: 42–54.
8. Kamida CB, Kistner RL. Descending phlebolography: the Straub technique. In Bergan JJ, Kistner RL, eds. *Atlas of Venous Surgery.* Philadelphia: WB Saunders, 1992: 105–9.
9. Kistner RL, Ferris EB, Randhawa G, Kamida CB. A method of performing descending venography. *J Vasc Surg* 1986; **4**: 464–8.
10. Porter JM, Moneta GL. Reporting standards in venous disease: an update. International Consensus Committee on Chronic Venous Disease. *J Vasc Surg* 1995; **21**(4): 635–45.

11. Nicolaides AN (Chairman), Bergan JJ, Eklof B, Kistner RL, Moneta GL (exec comm.), *et al.* Classification and grading of chronic venous disease in the lower limbs: a consensus statement. *Phlebology* 1995; **10**: 42–5.

12. Nicolaides AN (Chairman), *et al.* The investigation of chronic venous disorders of the lower limb: a consensus statement. *Circulation* Accepted for publication 1999.

10

Indirect noninvasive tests (plethysmography)

CLIFFORD T ARAKI AND ROBERT W HOBSON II

Optimal testing for chronic venous disease should quantify the severity of venous incompetence and venous obstruction and be able to map the distribution of disease. Two forms of testing, duplex ultrasonography and plethysmography, are commonly employed. Although they appear to be competing modalities, neither is capable of providing all information adequately. Active centers use both modalities, with the complementary data providing a more complete picture of the insufficient limb.

This chapter discusses the plethysmographic instruments currently employed to evaluate patients for chronic venous insufficiency (CVI). Whilst a previous review on plethysmography included a discussion of testing for acute DVT,[1] it has been omitted from this presentation because current practices using duplex ultrasonography have supplanted these techniques.

INSTRUMENTATION

Plethysmography ('to record an increase') is a term applied to the measurement of volume and volume displacement. A number of different electronic instruments are included which do not measure volume directly but measure a volume-related parameter. Some provide global information on limb hemodynamics whilst others target local tissue hemodynamics. The measurement of 'volume' change is loosely common to all methods.

While ultrasound provides its best hemodynamic data directly on specific vein segments, plethysmography provides information that is indirectly related to venous volume changes. The data obtained is not specific to venous function because limb volume changes may be caused by several factors. Still, rapid changes are typically associated with changes in blood volume or movement artifact and if movement is controlled, information specific to blood volume can be obtained. Further separation of arterial and venous flow effects can be obtained through electronic filtration. Venous flow changes typically involve long, transient time constants, lasting several seconds or minutes. Venous displacement measurements are typically associated with shifts in body position and limb compressions, which allow the quantitative measurement of magnitude and duration.

Plethysmographic techniques maintain their popularity because of their ability to quantify CVI information that can be compared serially for assessing operative efficacy and disease progression. The major forms of plethysmography used clinically include strain-gauge, impedance, air, and photoelectric plethysmography. Air plethysmography is currently the most popular.

Air plethysmography (APG)

The air plethysmograph measures volume displacement in a limb segment. The measurement device is an air-filled plastic sleeve, placed around an extremity segment, usually the calf. The sleeve is inflated to 6 mmHg to hold it in place. Air pressure in the sleeve is calibrated to reflect calf volume changes by injecting then withdrawing a known volume of air into the sleeve. When the patient is asked to then perform a standardized series of maneuvers, pressure in the pneumatic sleeve is used to monitor the changes in limb volume in milliliters. Some of the volume change may be associated with shifts in tissue mass but the bulk of the measured volume change is ascribed to shifts in venous volume in the monitored segment.

Photoelectric plethysmography (PPG)

Photoplethysmography provides a qualitative assessment of changes in cutaneous blood volume. The PPG electrode is composed of an infrared light emitting diode and a photo-sensor. Light transmitted into the skin is scattered and absorbed by tissues in the illuminated field. Blood, being more opaque than surrounding tissue, attenuates the reflected light in greater proportion. The intensity of reflected light changes with tissue blood density. The measurement is localized to the microvasculature of the cutaneous layer underlying the electrode. The instrument may be used to measure arterial pulsations or transient venous volume. To measure changes in venous volume, the voltage signal generated in the photosensor is amplified through a DC coupled circuit, which dampens higher frequency arterial pulsations, leaving a low frequency response with a longer time constant. This produces a relatively stable tracing, which corresponds to blood density in the underlying tissue. The PPG is able to monitor alterations in tissue venous filling as the patient is asked to perform certain maneuvers.

LIGHT REFLECTION RHEOGRAPHY (LRR)

Light reflection rheography is a modification of the PPG. It is composed of three light-emitting diodes concentrically arranged around a single, centrally placed photosensor. The LRR electrode also incorporates a thermistor to measure skin temperature. The three diodes, instead of the one used for the PPG, are thought to provide a more uniform illumination of the tissue underlying the sensor and better information on blood density.[2]

PPG and LRR testing should be performed in temperature controlled environments and skin temperature should be maintained near thermoneutral 28–32°C. Thermoregulatory adjustments in cutaneous blood flow may otherwise affect test results. The results of PPG and LRR testing are most often used to evaluate venous hemodynamics of the entire limb. However, both provide localized superficial assessment. Extrapolating the results of testing to the whole limb is of questionable value.[3] The potential use of either instrument for evaluating local derangements in venous hemodynamics has not been adequately explored.

Strain-gauge plethysmography (SPG)

A strain-gauge is a mechanical transducer that expresses deformation as a change in electrical resistance. For clinical plethysmographic studies, the transducer is an elastic tube filled with mercury or an indium–gallium metal alloy conductor. Stretching the strain-gauge decreases the diameter of the conductor and increases its electrical resistance. The transducer is calibrated by incrementally stretching the conductor, then measuring the change in voltage that is produced. When wrapped around a limb segment, e.g. the calf, the strain-gauge provides a circumferential measurement that is used to calculate an area. The 'slice volume' of the limb segment changes as the calf volume expands and contracts. The strain-gauge can be used for both arterial and venous applications. Strain-gauge measurements are typically determined from voltage tracings. Measurement error may be caused by temperature changes in the conductor, which affects electrical resistance, shifting of the transducer with limb repositioning, and selecting a limb area less sensitive to volume expansion.

Impedance plethysmography (IPG)

Impedance plethysmography is used to measure electrolyte fluid volume through changes in electrical conductivity. The instrument passes a weak (1 mA) alternating current through a limb and measures the electrical resistance to current flow. To perform the measurement, four conductive bands are taped around the limb as outer and inner pairs of electrodes. The outer pair applies the alternating current. The inner pair is used to measure electrical resistance. The technique is termed impedance plethysmography to coincide with the use of an alternating current, which has an impediment composed of resistive, capacitive and inductive elements. The latter two are reactive to the cyclical current. The major portion of the impedance remains resistive. The current is imperceptible to the patient because of its low amperage and the 22–100 kHz alternating current reduces its interference with neuromuscular processes.

The results are quantitative in resistive units but not easily translated into volume. Electrolyte concentration, red blood cell velocity, hematocrit, and other factors make the conversion inexact.[4] Still, short duration volume changes in the order of seconds to minutes are principally associated with shifts in venous blood volume. Once extensively used for acute DVT detection, it has not fared well in the transition to CVI testing.

APPLICATIONS

All forms of plethysmography applied to CVI testing are able to provide quantitative information that is complementary to duplex ultrasonography. Plethysmographic testing has been used for the following forms of CVI testing.

Venous outflow obstruction

Venous obstruction is of first concern, particularly if surgical intervention is contemplated. The success of any reconstructive or ablative procedure depends upon adequate venous outflow. Only plethysmography provides quantitative physiologic information that is able to gauge the severity of outflow obstruction.

Plethysmographic techniques grade outflow by measuring the rate of volume change in an elevated limb. For the lower extremities, the volume-measuring device, whether APG, IPG, SPG, or PPG, is positioned on the calf and a pneumatic cuff is placed around the thigh. With the extremity elevated above heart level, the thigh cuff is inflated to 60–80 mmHg, to occlude venous outflow while maintaining arterial inflow. Blood volume accumulates in the calf until it reaches a stable plateau. The timed period takes 1–2 minutes. Once calf volume has stabilized, the thigh cuff is rapidly vented.

The entire period of calf filling and drainage is monitored and recorded. The output tracing is used to measure the venous blood volume capacity during thigh cuff inflation and the rate of venous outflow rate after thigh cuff is vented. The outflow rate is typically determined as the reduction in calf volume at 1 or 3 seconds after the start of venting (Fig. 10.1). In normal limbs, the rate of outflow is determined in part by total venous volume (venous capacitance). Outflow is normalized by indexing it against capacitance. Abnormal outflow is discriminated from normal by applying an empirically derived range of normal outflow or a regression line.[5,6] Using APG, capacitance and outflow are expressed as an outflow fraction (OF), which is calculated as the outflow volume at 1 second divided by the total calf volume.[7] Normal venous flow is determined if 40% or more of the venous volume drains from the calf within 1 second of the release of thigh cuff pressure.

It is generally felt that plethysmographic testing has a low false-negative rate for iliofemoral obstruction. There is a higher false-positive rate caused by venous compression through patient positioning, or extrinsic masses. Congestive heart failure may also impede outflow in an otherwise normal venous system. To reduce the possibility of a falsely positive examination, repetitive testing is performed to maximally normalize the results. Longer calf filling and patient repositioning with knee flexed, the hip rotated externally may improve outflow.[8]

Whilst the negative predictive value for an iliofemoral obstruction is good, the test is much less diagnostic for obstruction in the popliteal and calf veins because of increased venous collateralization at these levels. Plethysmography may not be as sensitive as ultrasound in determining the presence of occlusive disease in specific vein segments but it is much better than ultrasound in grading the severity of residual obstruction. Serial testing through plethysmography offers particular advantage in following recanalization or the effect of reconstructive surgery. To date, no other method, invasive or noninvasive, is able to quantitatively follow venous outflow obstruction to its ultimate degree of resolution in the postphlebitic limb.

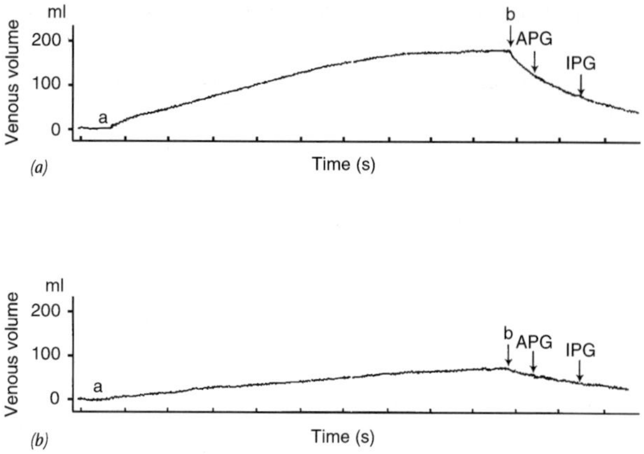

Figure 10.1 *Lower extremity venous obstruction is determined plethysmographically through calf venous capacitance and maximal venous outflow (MVO). Patient is supine with limb elevated and externally rotated. A thigh cuff is inflated at (a) to prevent venous outflow. Venous filling in the calf occurs until volume plateaus at full or near full capacitance. The thigh cuff is then vented at (b), which provokes venous outflow from the calf. Capacitance is determined as the difference in volume between (b) and baseline (a). MVO is determined as the difference between (b) and outflow volume at 1 second (for APG) or at 3 seconds (for IPG). Fig. 10.1(a) represents normal outflow pattern. Fig. 10.1(b) represents the effect of chronic obstruction, which can cause a reduction in both capacitance and outflow.*

Valvular incompetence

With ambulatory venous pressure (AVP) long considered the gold standard test for CVI, numerous attempts have been made to duplicate the invasive AVP techniques noninvasively. Post-exercise venous refill time was the most readily adapted, using plethysmographic testing. Through AVP measurement, venous pressure in the foot was found to normally remain low after exercise. The return to baseline hydrostatic pressure takes longer than 20 seconds,[9] as blood refills vein valve segments through the microvasculature. When valves are incompetent, the slow refill component is overwhelmed by large volume reflux through the incompetent valves. Refill times of 15 seconds or less can be encountered with significant reflux.

To duplicate the AVP measurement, the patient is usually tested while sitting or standing and is asked to perform a repetitive, stationary calf exercise using knee bends or ankle flexions. The common protocol described for the PPG[10] is performed with the patient sitting, legs dependent and non-weight bearing. The PPG electrode is taped to the ankle, 10 cm above the medial malleolus. The patient is then asked to perform plantar/dorsiflexion maneuvers at 1-second intervals for five repetitions. The patient then relaxes to allow passive calf vein refilling.

The transducer should be placed distally in the leg. Published reports have demonstrated that distal valvular incompetence is important with shorter refill times demonstrated in normal limbs at mid-calf than at ankle. Ankle refill times also appeared more strongly affected by incompetence and may be more clinically relevant measures of incompetence.[11,12] It is not uncommon for the venous filling curve to drift gently upward, blurring the endpoint for refill time.

Using the APG, venous filling time is expressed as a venous filling index (VFI). Instead of performing a stationary exercise, the patient is guided in a maneuver from supine with the leg elevated to standing with the leg unweighted.[7] This maximally empties the calf veins then rapidly refills them. Pressure in the APG pneumatic sleeve, calibrated to volume, is recorded throughout the maneuver to yield a pattern of venous filling (Fig. 10.2) that is similar to the PPG. The rate of filling through 90% of total venous volume is used to determine VFI. The use of a 90% end point serves as a refinement to the PPG technique by removing much of the drift error encountered when timing refill in the PPG tracing. At 90%, the end point is tightened by positioning it at a steeper portion of the filling curve.

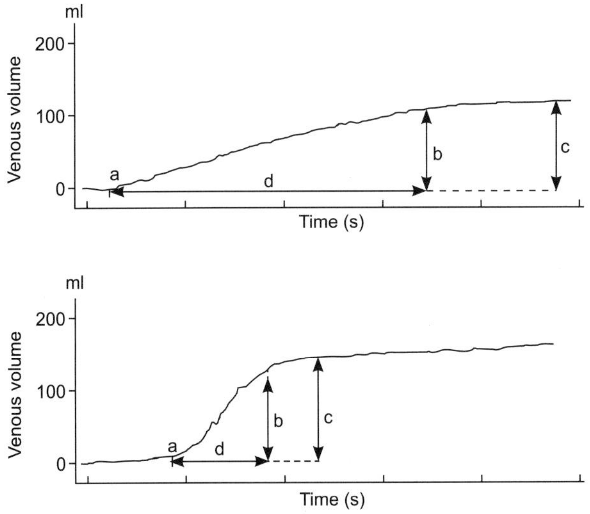

Figure 10.2 *Venous refill time. Venous filling can be monitored using strain-gauge or PPG following stationary calf exercise and using the APG through supine-standing maneuver. The SPG and PPG protocols estimate maximal capacitance (c) then measure a venous refill time (a–c), with refill durations greater than 23 seconds considered normal valvular competence. The APG protocol calculates a venous filling index (VFI) to determine competency. For the latter, the total venous volume (c) is estimated and used to calculate the 90% total venous volume (b). The time (d) to reach (b) is then determined. VFI is then calculated as: VFI = b/d in ml/s. A VFI of less than 2 ml/s is considered normal.*

Tourniquets are used routinely to exclude superficial reflux and to evaluate the deep system separately. Results have been found to be unpredictable.[13,14] The lack of an empirically derived standard for the use of a tourniquet has made this a major problem in separating deep and superficial effects through plethysmographic testing. Pneumatic cuffs, latex ligatures and wedged Velcro straps have been applied above knee, below knee and segmentally to exclude the effects of superficial incompetence. In most applications, the tourniquet was applied but the impact of the tourniquet on the underlying deep and superficial vasculature was not evaluated at the time of testing.

Calf muscle pump function

Noninvasive testing of calf muscle pump function did not receive much attention until APG testing was introduced in 1987.[7] Calf pump function is described in terms of ejection fraction (EF) and residual volume fraction (RVF), which compares the percentage of venous volume ejected by the calf (EF) against the percent venous volume which cannot be expelled (RVF). Ejection volume is measured as the volume of blood ejected when the patient performs a single tiptoe maneuver in a maximal calf muscle contraction. Residual volume is measured as the minimum venous volume retained in the calf during a series of 10 standing tiptoe maneuvers (Figs. 10.3 and 10.4). To remove interlimb variability, EF and RVF are calculated by indexing ejection and residual volumes against total calf venous volume. This greatly improves the comparability of data among limbs.

Residual volume has been proposed as an estimate of AVP, the second invasive measurement that can be estimated through plethysmography. Presumably, the lowest residual venous volume retained in the calf during 10 tiptoe exercises corresponds to the decrease in venous pressure attained when walking. A linear correlation between AVP and RVF of $r = 0.83$ has been reported. Other forms of plethysmography have shown similar correlation with AVP and AVP-venous refill time.[1]

CURRENT STATUS

Protocols and instrumentation for venous plethysmography were principally developed in the 1970s and 1980s. Much of this work addressed the quantitation of venous obstruction and refill time. Noninvasive testing of the calf muscle pump did not receive much attention until 1987, when the APG testing protocol was introduced.[7]

The 1990s has shown little new development in equipment or applications. The APG and SPG have been the

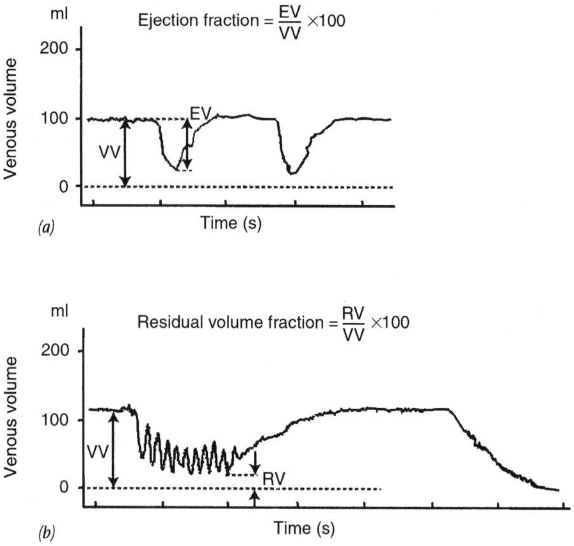

Figure 10.3 *A good calf muscle pump ejects most (>60%) of the venous blood in the calf during maximal exercise. The ejection fraction (EF) and residual volume fraction (RVF) can be determined through plethysmography. In (a), ejection fraction is determined from a single maximal tiptoe maneuver. The ejection volume (EV) is obtained by measuring the volume displaced during tiptoe. EF is calculated by dividing it by the venous volume (VV) measured during the VFI determination. In (b), a separate maneuver is used to determine the RVF. A series of 10 standing tiptoe maneuvers is used to maximally extract venous blood from the calf. The residual volume (RV), is measured relative to baseline volume and divided by VV.*

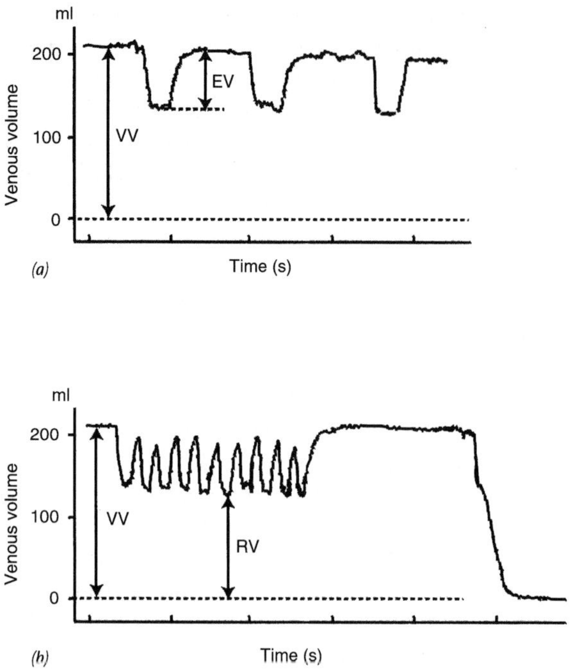

Figure 10.4 *Poor calf muscle pump function is often demonstrated (a) by an increase in VV. Only a small proportion of the total volume may be expressed from the calf (EV and EF) and (b) RV and RVF are increased. Superficial varicosities may make a sizeable contribution to increased venous volume (VV) and residual volume (RV) and decrease ejection volume (EV). Calf pump efficiency may also be limited by inadequate ankle flexion and perforator incompetence.*

most enduring among plethysmographic instrumentation. Strain-gauge testing protocols have been devised for calf pump function,[15] with protocols that differ from that of the APG. Most studies which reference plethysmography note successes and limitations in application. Studies have shown a clinically relevant relationship between venous ulceration, calf muscle pump dysfunction, and restricted ankle range of motion.[16–18] Others have found little utility in RVF and EF calculations.[19] Tourniquets continue to be problematic in isolating deep venous hemodynamics.[19] Technique refinements are few and far between.

CONCLUSION

With direct testing offered by ultrasound, the role of plethysmography for the diagnosis of acute DVT has diminished dramatically. However, it continues to have an important role in the assessment of chronic venous insufficiency. Whilst ultrasound provides direct information on the distribution of valvular reflux, plethysmography provides global data on venous outflow, calf muscle pump function, and overall venous incompetence. Through PPG testing it also has the capacity of providing information on tissue level venous function. These capabilities make it a valuable complement to ultrasound in providing a more complete understanding of limb venous function.

However, a literature review will demonstrate a dilemma in the need for clinical refinements that is not being addressed in research and development. Criticisms leveled against plethysmography may be caused by inadequate instrumentation, by uncertainties associated with CVI pathophysiology, and by the lack of protocol refinements. It may be argued that plethysmographic testing is relying upon equipment and protocols that are not developing at a pace that keeps up with the needs of testing.

REFERENCES

1. Araki CT, Back TL, Meyers MG, Hobson RW. Indirect noninvasive tests (plethysmography). In Gloviczki P, Yao SJT, eds. *The Handbook of Venous Disorders, Guidelines of The American Venous Forum.* London: Chapman & Hall, 1996: 97–111.

2. Shepard AD, Mackey WC, O'Donnell TF, *et al.* Light reflection rheography (LRR): a new non-invasive test of venous function. *Bruit* 1984; **8**: 266–70.
3. Illig KA, Shortell CK, Ouriel K, Greenberg RK, Waldman D, Green RM. Photoplethysmography and calf muscle pump function after subfascial endoscopic perforator ligation. *J Vasc Surg* 1999; **30**: 1067–76.
4. Wheeler HB, Penny BC, Anderson FA. Impedance plethysmography: theoretic, experimental, and clinical considerations. In Bernstein EF, ed. *Vascular Diagnosis*, 4th edn. St Louis: Mosby-Year Book, 1993: 194–204.
5. Wheeler HB, O'Donnell JA, Anderson FA, Benedict K. Occlusive impedance phlebography: a diagnostic procedure for venous thrombosis and pulmonary embolism. *Prog Cardiovasc Dis* 1974; **17**: 199–205.
6. Hull R, van Aken WG, Hirsh J, *et al.* Impedance plethysmography using the occlusive cuff technique in the diagnosis of venous thrombosis. *Circulation* 1976; **53**: 696–700.
7. Christopoulos DG, Nicolaides AN, Szendro G, Irvine AT, Bull M, Eastcott HHG. Air-plethysmography and the effect of elastic compression on venous hemodynamics of the leg. *J Vasc Surg* 1987; **5**: 148–59.
8. Hull R, Taylor DW, Hirsh J, *et al.* Impedance plethysmography: the relationship between venous filling and sensitivity and specificity for proximal vein thrombosis. *Circulation* 1978; **58**: 898–902.
9. Schanzer H, Peirce EC. A rational approach to the chronic venous stasis syndrome. *Ann Surg* 1982; **195**: 25–9.
10. Abramowitz HB, Queral LA, Flinn WR, *et al.* The use of photoplethysmography in the assessment of venous insufficiency: a comparison to venous pressure measurements. *Surgery* 1979; **86**: 434–41.
11. Struckman JR, Mathiesen FR. A noninvasive plethysmographic method for evaluation of the musculovenous pump in the lower extremities. *Acta Chir Scand* 1985; **151**: 235–40.
12. Rosfors S, Lamke LO, Nordstrom E , Bygdeman S. Severity and location of venous valvular insufficiency: the importance of distal valve function. *Acta Chir Scand* 1990; **156**: 689–94.
13. Neglen P, Raju S. A rational approach to detection of significant reflux with duplex Doppler scanning and air plethysmography. *J Vasc Surg* 1993; **17**: 590–5.
14. van Bemmelen PS, Mattos MA, Hodgson KJ, *et al.* Does air plethysmography correlate with duplex scanning patients with chronic venous insufficiency? *J Vasc Surg* 1993; **18**: 796–807.
15. Struckmann JR. Assessment of the venous muscle pump function by ambulatory strain gauge plethysmography. *Dan Med Bull* 1993; **40**: 460–77.
16. Araki CT, Back TL, Padberg FT, *et al.* The significance of calf muscle pump function in venous ulceration. *J Vasc Surg* 1994; **20**: 872–9.
17. Back TL, Padberg FT, Araki CT, Thompson PN, Hobson RW. Limited range of motion is a significant factor in venous ulceration. *J Vasc Surg* 1995; **22**: 519–23.
18. Padberg FT, Pappas PJ, Araki CT, Back TL, Hobson RW. Hemodynamic and clinical improvement after superficial vein ablation in primary combined venous insufficiency with ulceration. *J Vasc Surg* 1996; **24**: 711–18.
19. Criado E, Farber MA, Marston WA, Daniel PF, Burnham CB, Keagy BA. The role of air plethysmography in the diagnosis of chronic venous insufficiency. *J Vasc Surg* 1998; **27**: 660–70.

11

Direct noninvasive tests (duplex scan) for the evaluation of acute venous disease

SERGIO X SALLES-CUNHA AND HUGH G BEEBE

The specter of pulmonary embolism and its link to venous thromboembolism of the extremities[1] has led to the common practice of investigating extremity veins by laboratory testing in patients with relevant symptoms or above-average risk of developing deep venous thrombosis. Virchow's classical triad remains important today and identifies patients at risk of venous thrombosis as having increased blood coagulability, decreased blood flow, and venous wall abnormality. Signs and symptoms of deep venous thrombosis are the consequence of venous obstruction causing swelling from edema, and pain from muscle compartment pressure, or perivenous inflammation. However, the reliability of clinical diagnosis is so poor that objective confirmation is required, especially in the hospitalized patient.[2]

This chapter addresses diagnosis of deep venous thrombosis of the lower and upper extremities by use of direct ultrasound testing. In a limited but growing number of patients, when indicated, examination of the lower extremity is also extended to the iliac veins and inferior vena cava. Upper extremity evaluation also includes the subclavian and innominate veins. Thrombosis in these veins is increasing due to increasing invasion of the subclavian vein with catheters and other devices.[3,4]

The advantages of noninvasive ultrasonography over phlebography have increased its use to rule in or out deep venous thrombosis.[5–8] As a consequence of an increasing number of vascular examinations, the percentage of positive tests has dropped below 10 or 20% in many centers. Often, the cause of calf pain and swelling is not acute venous disease, particularly in the outpatient, ambulatory population. Gender differences may dictate type of testing with interpretation focusing on valvular insufficiency besides deep venous thrombosis.[9] A complete vascular laboratory evaluation should focus not only on deep venous thrombosis but should identify other potential causes of signs or symptoms such as venous valvular incompetence, extravascular masses or even arteriovenous fistulas and popliteal or femoral artery aneurysms.[10–12] A high frequency of negative tests has resulted in suggestions of limited protocols.[13] On the other side of the spectrum, several investigators have emphasized the importance of complete examination with inclusion of calf vein scanning.[14–16]

In recent years, during attempts to make vascular laboratories more cost-effective, the question has arisen whether both lower extremities must always be examined. It has been argued that, when evaluating a patient with unilateral leg symptoms only, the yield in studying the contralateral leg for occult deep venous thrombosis is so low that is not worthwhile incurring the cost of a longer examination.[17] If leg venous duplex scanning is being done to support the diagnosis of pulmonary embolism made by other means, a positive scan in the first leg might obviate the need for studying the other. However, since defining the extent of deep venous thrombosis at the time of its development is so useful in subsequent evaluation for recurrent acute thrombosis, it seems prudent to study both legs nearly always.

Alternative treatment such as low molecular weight heparin[18] and alternative diagnostic methods such as D-dimer tests[19] may alter protocols for diagnostic and follow-up ultrasound testing. New protocols for stat and emergency-room late-hour testing may evolve. Appropriate indications with integration of risk factors, symptoms and signs are analyzed in detail.[20–22] A word of caution is warranted: when using statistics to analyze databases containing a majority of negative cases, results will be distorted in favor of limited testing at the expense of complete evaluation of patients at high risk of developing deep venous thrombosis. The effectiveness of limited protocols should be fully investigated.[23]

INDICATIONS FOR TESTING

Patients examined for acute venous disease in the vascular laboratory can be grouped into three categories:

- those with signs or symptoms of pulmonary embolism who may have both lower extremities examined seeking the most probable embolic source;
- patients with extremity pain and/or swelling as common indications for performing a bilateral or unilateral examination of upper or lower extremities;
- patients at increased risk of developing deep venous thrombosis because of known factors such as trauma, joint replacement surgery, other major surgery, prolonged mobility limitation, or hypercoagulability, often associated with cancer;
- patients with superficial thrombophlebitis, who should be tested for progression of disease and deep venous thrombosis.[24,25]

EXAMINATION TECHNIQUE

In a comfortable warm room, the patient is positioned supine in a slightly reversed Trendelenburg position with the legs or arms dependent to take advantage of the venous dilation caused by temperature and gravity. A warm blanket wrapped around the limb aids venodilation. During lower extremity examination slight external rotation of the hip together with slight knee flexion avoids venous compression by normal anatomic structures.

There are three essential phases to the venous examination, applied successively in each venous segment: thrombus visualization, venous coaptability or compressibility, and detection of venous flow.[26–28] We prefer to start the examination proximally in the thigh, following the veins distally as needed. Calf examination does not need to be performed if venous thrombi are detected within the femoropopliteal segments. Similarly, upper extremity evaluation may be interrupted if thrombus is found in the innominate or subclavian veins.

Thrombus visualization is sought with B-mode imaging but may be impossible to detect by direct B-mode methods, especially when the thrombus is acute. Color flow imaging is supplemental but can greatly facilitate detection of non-occluding thrombi. Cross-sectional scanning is preferred for complete visualization of the vein. The coaptation or compressibility maneuver is performed by application of topical pressure using the ultrasound transducer while observing the vein with B-mode. This should be performed in cross-section because a longitudinal scan intersects the vein in only one plane and usually misses most of the lumen. Longitudinally, the plane of insonation may be displaced away from the vein, giving the misleading impression that the vein is compressed or coapted when in reality the vein is in another plane not being insonated. Coaptation of the vena cava, iliac, innominate and subclavian veins is difficult or virtually impossible because of limited access to apply pressure with the ultrasound probe. Full coaptation testing is also impaired by the inguinal ligament, structures of the adductor canal, tendons in the popliteal fossa, and bones of the lower leg.

Because velocity quantification is not important in this venous examination, venous flow assessment can be performed with either cross-sectional or longitudinal insonation. The latter aids optimization of the ultrasonic beam angulation, increasing the sensibility to slow-flow velocity or low-flow volume. Doppler spectrum analysis and/or color flow can be used. A large sampling volume facilitates detection of the Doppler waveform. Color sensitivity should be set for low flow.

Flow study comprises observation of respiratory fluctuation inflow or phasicity and response to external extremity compression proximal and distal to the segment being observed by ultrasound. During leg studies, manual abdominal compression is often faster and more effective than instructing the patient in a Valsalva maneuver.

Scanning for thrombus visualization and venous coaptability should encompass as much vein length as possible, while flow study may be restricted to a few anatomic locations. In the lower extremity, flow signals are detected at the common femoral, mid-thigh (superficial) femoral, popliteal, and posterior and anterior tibial and peroneal veins. Because anterior tibial veins can be small or absent, their study is often overlooked. The superficial veins are examined by direct observation and palpation or by ultrasound in a similar manner as the deep veins. Flow waveforms are detected in the greater saphenous vein in the thigh and calf and at the lesser saphenous vein. In the upper extremity, flow signals are detected at selected locations, often in midsegment of the veins being examined: subclavian, axillary, brachial, ulnar and radial. The cephalic and basilic veins are important contributors to the venous drainage and are evaluated at the upper arm and forearm.

With pressure applied distally to the foot, lower calf, hand or distal forearm, venous flow is increased, facilitating identification of a patent vein by Doppler spectrum or color flow. Because we have yet to find a person with 'three hands', one to press the buttons of the instrument, a second to hold the transducer, and a third to compress the extremities, we have in the past used a rhythmic pulsatile pump to compress the limb. This automatic technique, however, has limitations: it quickly depletes the blood reservoir in the extremity and eventually may produce the false impression that venous flow is decreased. We prefer to compress the limb upon demand. A simple way to accomplish this objective is to interconnect two pneumatic cuffs, place one loosely around the distal limb and the other on the floor. After inflating them to a light comfortable pressure, the one on the floor is stepped on when a flow augmentation testing is performed.

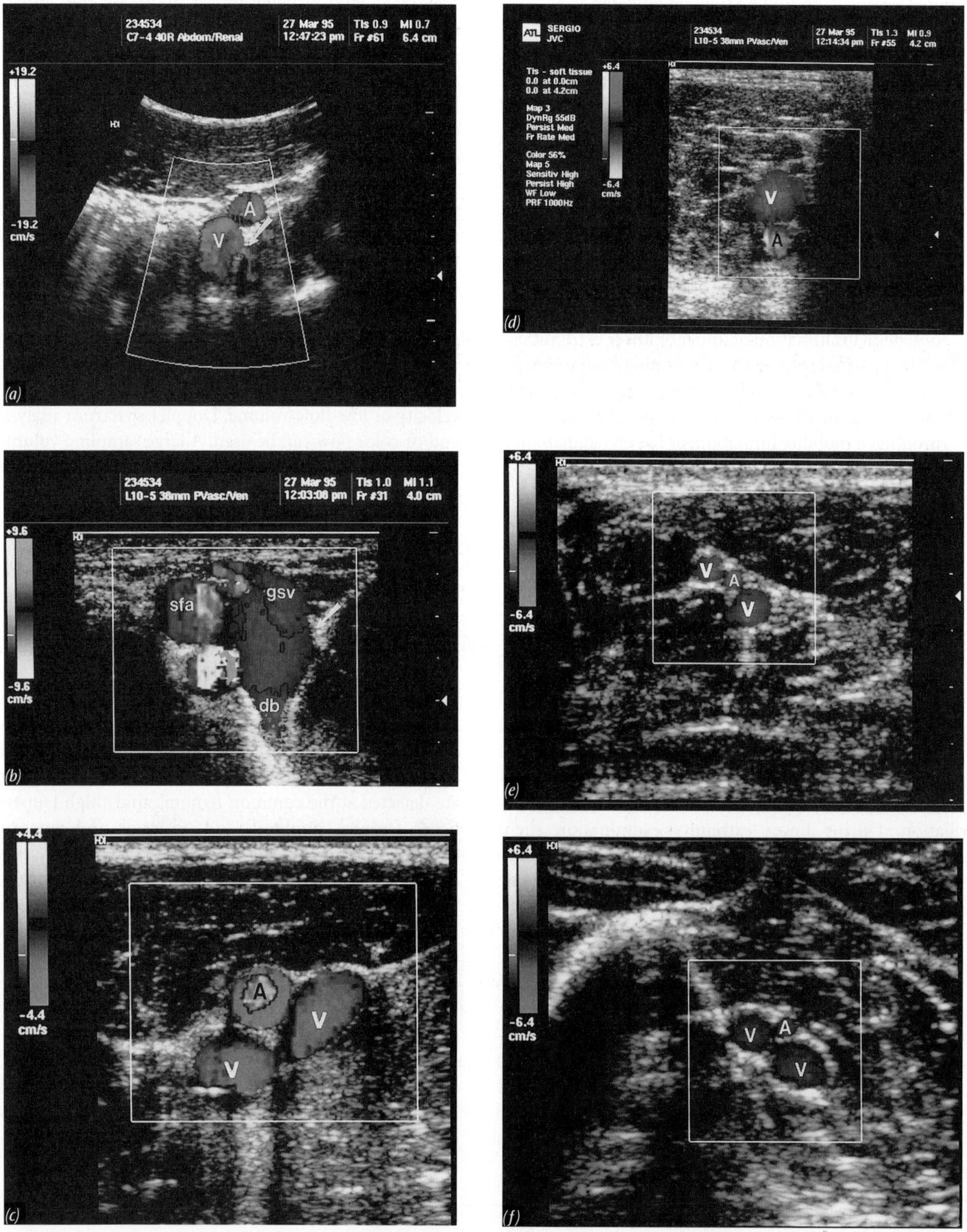

INTERPRETATION

Normal findings

Figure 11.1 shows a series of images of patent lower extremity veins, the most commonly studied. Figure 11.2 shows how the appearance of normal veins changes as

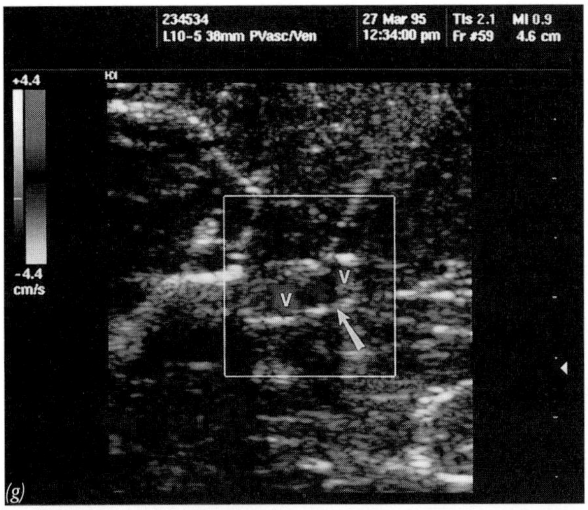

Figure 11.1 (left and above) *Cross-sections of blood vessels. (a) Iliac vessels: the common iliac artery (A) is the smaller vessel on top; the common iliac vein (V) is the larger vessel at the bottom. A branch can be seen entering the vein (arrow). (b) Vessels at the saphenofemoral junction: the larger vessel on the right is the common femoral vein (arrow) receiving blood from the greater saphenous vein on top (gsv) and a deep branch from the bottom (db); the two vessels on the left are the superficial femoral artery (sfa) on top and the deep femoral artery below. (c) Femoral vessels at mid-thigh: in the middle, the superficial femoral artery (A) has low flow near the wall and high flow in the center, as shown in this picture taken during late systole. The other two vessels are femoral veins (V); this duplicate variant occurs in about one-third of patients. Use of the phrase/term 'superficial' femoral vein should be discouraged because it has been misinterpreted as superficial rather than deep venous thrombosis. (d) Vessels in the popliteal fossa: the larger vein (V) is on the top (superficial) with the smaller artery (A) below. The shadow on the right is caused by probe placement over tendon, which may impair the probe compressibility maneuver. (Picture taken using a posterior approach). (e) Posterior tibial vessels underneath muscular fascia: the smaller vessel in the center is the artery (A), surrounded by the larger veins (V). (Picture taken using a medial approach, the tibia being on the left). (f) Peroneal vessels by the fibula: the smaller vessel in the center is the artery (A), surrounded by the larger veins (V). (Picture taken using a lateral approach). (g) Anterior tibial vessels: the vessel in the center is the artery (arrow) surrounded by two veins (V). The anterior tibial veins are often small or undetectable. (Picture taken using an anterior-lateral approach with the tibia on the left).*

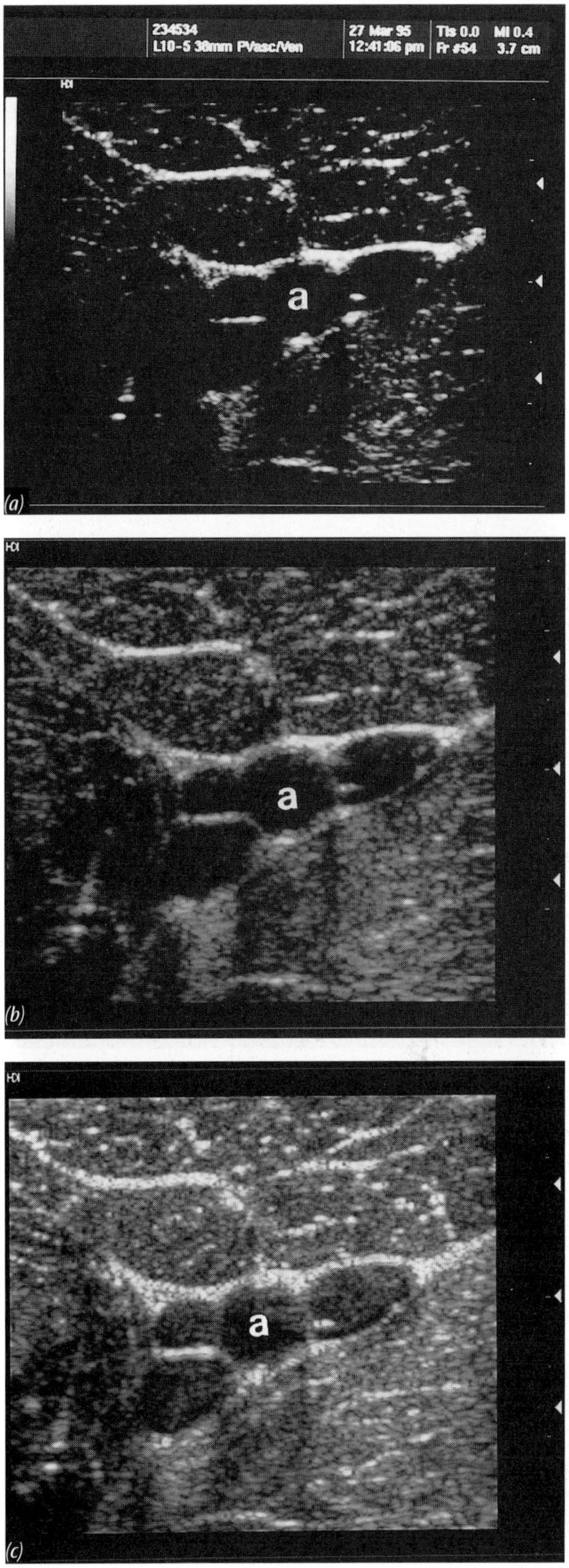

Figure 11.2 *Appearance of the intraluminal image changes as the gain of the instrument is increased progressively from (a) to (c). Fresh thrombus may be missed at low gains. If excessive gain is used, even the lumen of a normal vein may become hyperechoic, giving the false impression of thrombosis. (Uncommon configuration at mid-thigh with the superficial femoral artery (a) surrounded by three veins).*

the gain setting of the instrument is increased. Figure 11.3 is a sequence of changes during compression of a normal coaptable vein. Figure 11.4 shows normal Doppler spectral flow findings: phasicity with respiration, interruption of flow with proximal leg compression and flow augmentation with release of proximal compression followed by flow augmentation with distal leg compression. Phasicity with respiration in the upper extremities is reversed from that of the lower extremities. Inspiration lowers intrathoracic pressure and increases abdominal pressure, resulting in opposite forces on venous return.

Abnormal findings and differential diagnosis

All characteristics of veins, as observed by ultrasound, should be taken into account. Contradictions or inconsistencies should alert the observer to the possibility of a false impression. Thus, the process of performing a venous duplex is not separable from continuous interpretation as the examination proceeds. Knowledge of conditions associated with similar signs or symptoms as deep venous thrombosis along with certain specific ultrasound findings greatly aids this examination.

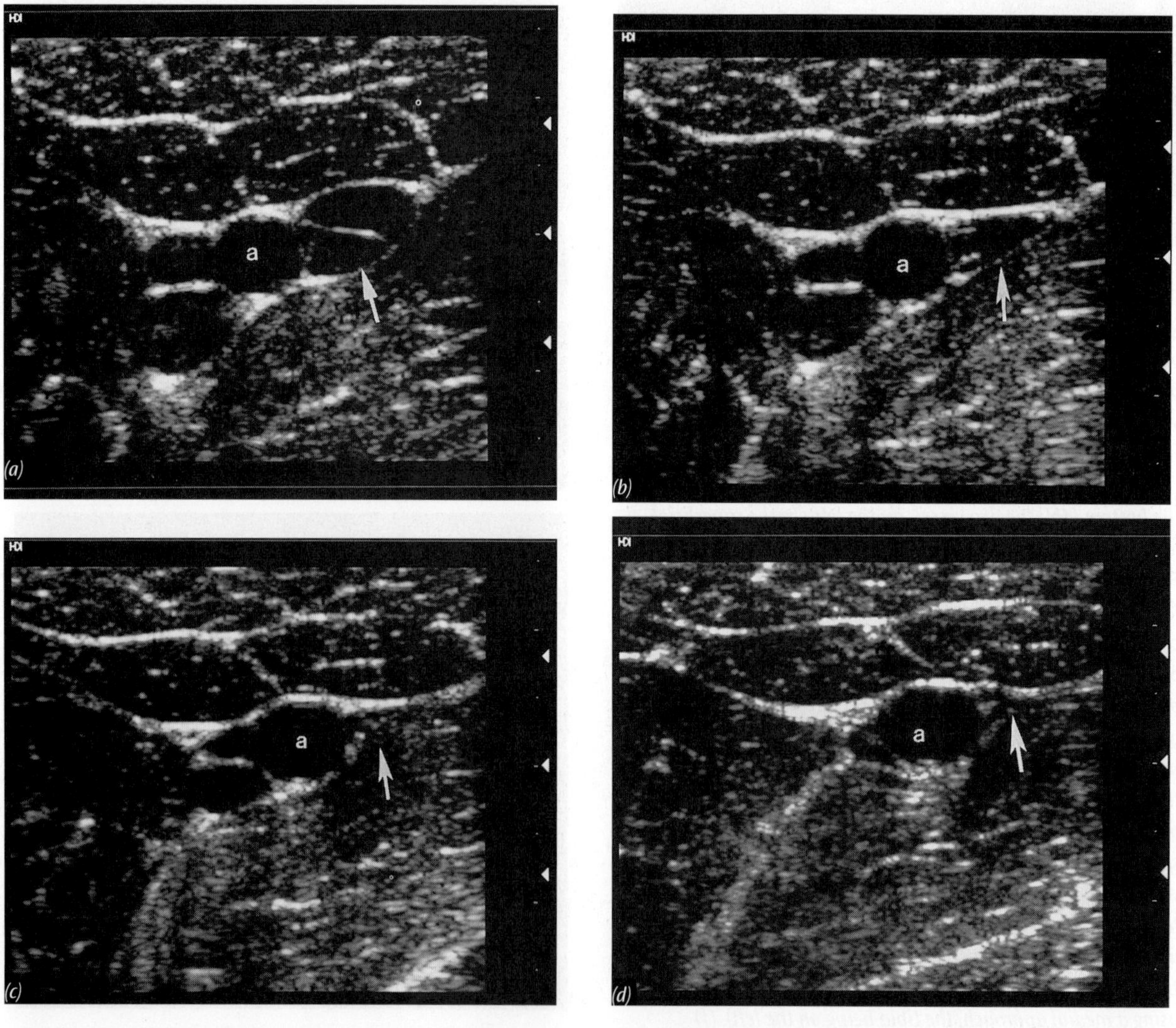

Figure 11.3 *Coaptability or compressibility of four femoral vessels at mid-thigh. (a) Minimal pressure applied to the transducer: the two vessels on the left are veins; on the right, a valve leaflet can be seen within a large vein (arrow); the superficial femoral artery (a), is the most circular of these vessels. (b) As pressure applied to the transducer increases, the cross-section of veins diminishes. The most significant change occurred first in the vein on the right (arrow); only the origin of the valve leaflet is now noted. (c) With additional pressure applied to the transducer, the vein on the right coapts (arrow), while the other veins change in shape and diminish in size. (d) As applied pressure increases, the veins coapt while the smallest vein is almost closed. Note that the artery (a) is only minimally compressed. (Uncommon configuration at mid-thigh with the superficial femoral artery surrounded by three veins).*

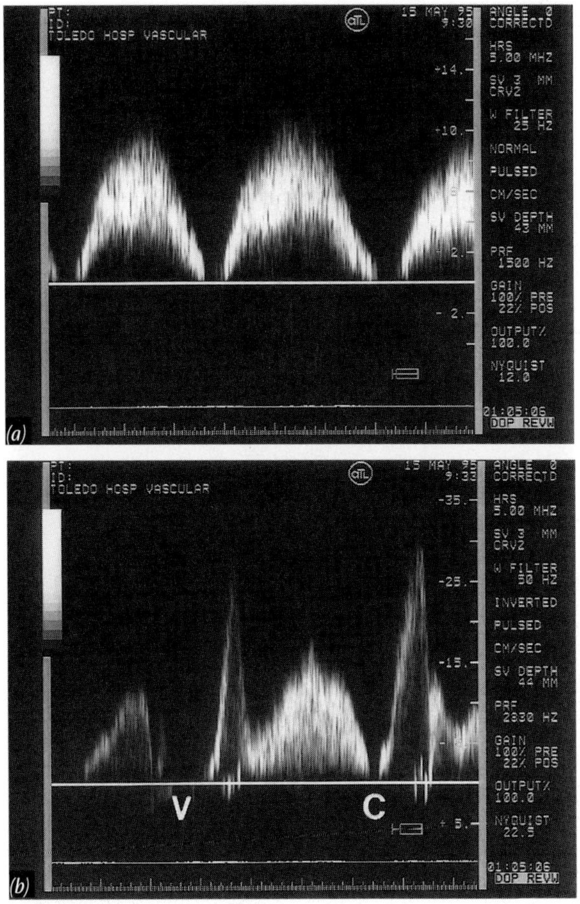

Figure 11.4 *Normal venous flow in the superficial femoral vein at mid-thigh. (a) At rest, venous flow is phasic with respiration; the respiratory cycle lasts about 3 seconds. (b) Valsalva maneuver (V) interrupts venous flow during the respiratory wave. When this is relieved, venous flow increases suddenly. The following respiratory wave also has increased flow. At the end of this respiratory wave, compression of calf muscles (C) causes another increase in venous flow.*

Lower extremity pain and edema may be caused by a variety of pathology including:

- incompetent superficial system
- incompetent perforator veins
- incompetent deep system
- arteriovenous fistulas
- arteriovenous malformations
- popliteal or femoral aneurysms
- enlarged lymph nodes compressing veins
- lymphatic obstruction
- obstruction by tumors
- synovial cyst (Baker's cyst)
- hematoma
- bony abnormalities and exostoses.

VENOUS COAPTABILITY OR COMPRESSIBILITY

The primary criterion of a positive duplex scan for deep vein thrombosis is an incompressible vein, clearly visualized in cross-section and subjected to adequate pressure forces from the ultrasound probe.[29] Even fresh thrombi, barely detected during B-mode imaging, impede complete collapse of a vein under compression. The innominate and subclavian veins, segments of the iliac veins, and inferior vena cava usually cannot be compressed because of their anatomic location. Therefore, diagnosis in these segments is based on thrombus visualization and study of flow patterns.

If the only abnormal finding is incompressibility of a very localized segment of the common femoral vein near the inguinal ligament, femoral vein at the adductor canal, popliteal vein, or tibial and peroneal veins near the calf bones, false-positive venous incompressibility should be suspected. The compression maneuver should be repeated with the patient in a different position or the angle of compression should be changed.

VENOUS ECHOGENICITY

Thrombus echogenicity increases with age.[30,31] The appearance of the ultrasonic image progresses from 'black' blood to lack of ultrasound reflection to densely speckled hyperechoic old thrombi (Fig. 11.5). At an intermediary level, a new thrombus has a spongy appearance with noticeable echo reflection at the blood–thrombus interface. Such fresh thrombi may appear to 'float' inside the vein (Fig. 11.6). When relatively acute and not attached to the venous wall, such thrombi may occasionally be seen to change position within the vein in response to compression. As thrombus ages, the ratio of black-to-gray echoes decreases. If a catheter is present inside a vein, it acts as a catalyst for thrombus formation, and a layer of mildly echogenic thrombus observed layered against the catheter (Fig. 11.7).

Once fresh thrombus fills the vein, venous diameter enlargement occurs and the diameter difference between the thrombosed vein and the corresponding contralateral vein may be observed. If recanalization occurs, the open lumen is usually surrounded by a thickened venous wall with an irregularly contoured flow lumen (Fig. 11.8). Venous thrombosis stimulates development of collateral veins, and superficial venous enlargement can occur as soon as the deep system becomes occluded. Small deep veins dilate and are noted by their tortuosity and irregular pathway through muscles.

Venous flow

Most Doppler spectrum and color flow findings are similar. Persistent lack of flow signal indicates total obstruction. Decreased flow augmentation either after release of proximal compression or during distal compression suggests venous obstruction proximal to the site of observation.[32] Lack of phasicity with respiration is

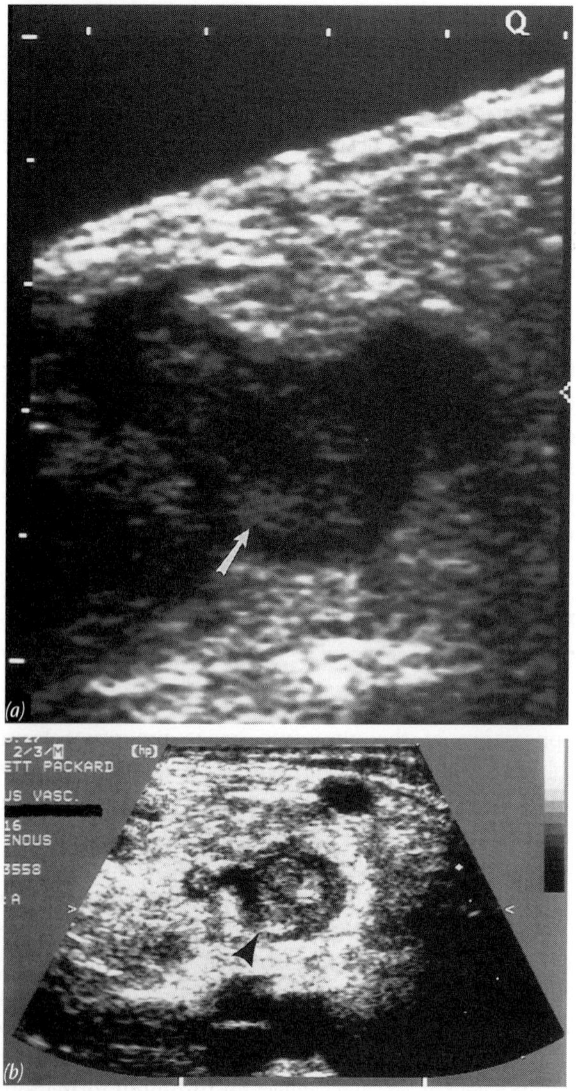

Figure 11.5 *(a) Fresh, barely detected hypoechoic and apparently unattached thrombus (arrow head) at the saphenofemoral junction. This classical 'Mickey Mouse' appearance is formed by the common femoral vein (face), common femoral artery (right ear) and greater saphenous vein (left ear). (b) Old, hyperechoic and apparently attached thrombus in an enlarged saphenous vein (arrow head).*

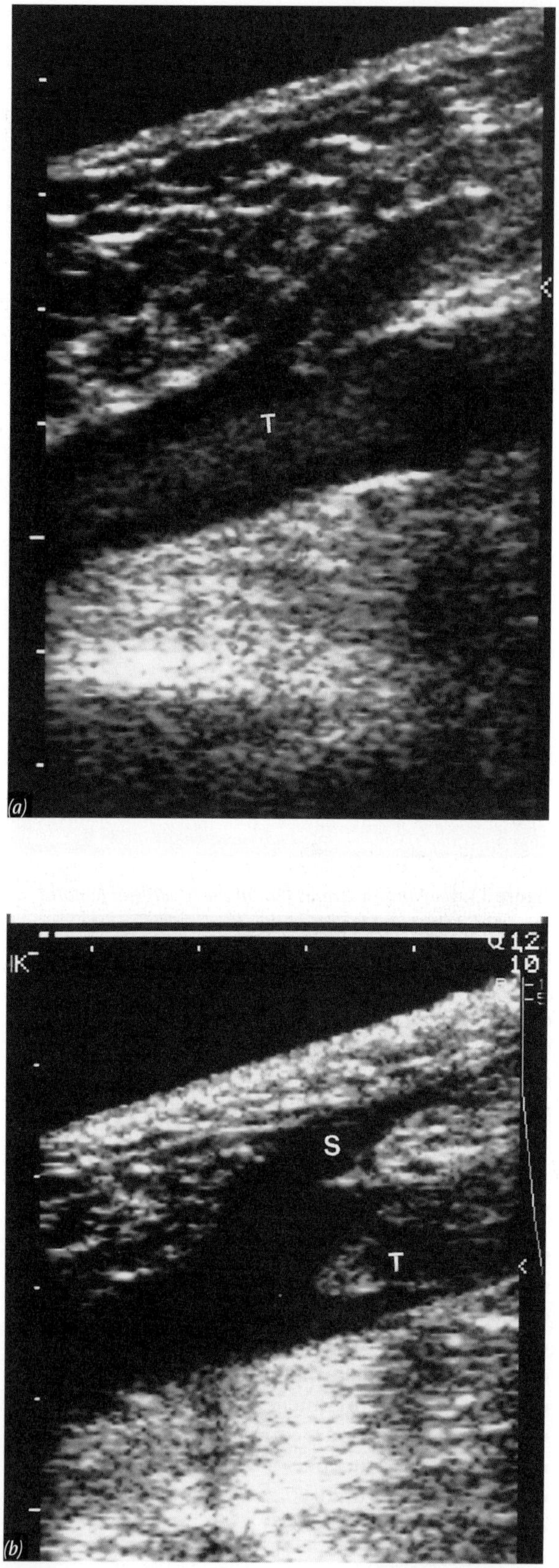

Figure 11.6 *Unattached thrombi. (a) An apparently unattached thrombus (T) is seen at the saphenofemoral junction. Note that it is surrounded on both sides by non-echoic channels. (b) Floating tip of a thrombus (T) in the common femoral vein distal to the saphenous vein orifice (S).*

indicative of venous flow obstruction. Before an abnormal finding leads to a positive interpretation, the flow test should be confirmed by repeating with the knee and hip slightly flexed at a different angle.

Of the various signs observable by duplex scan for diagnosis of acute venous disease, flow changes are the least reliable. Any presumed abnormal Doppler finding, either spontaneous or induced, should be confirmed by additional observations before being heavily weighted. This is especially true when ruling out thrombosis. The reason for this is that even though the vein under observation may be 90% occluded by acute thrombus, even this small remaining patent portion of the lumen

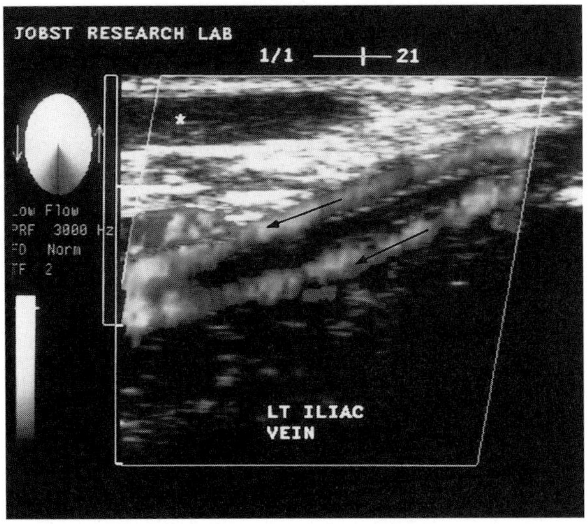

Figure 11.7 *Experimental laboratory study showing catheter coated with thrombus. The catheter is in the center of the vein, pictured in longitudinal section. Flow is present between the catheter and the venous wall (arrows).*

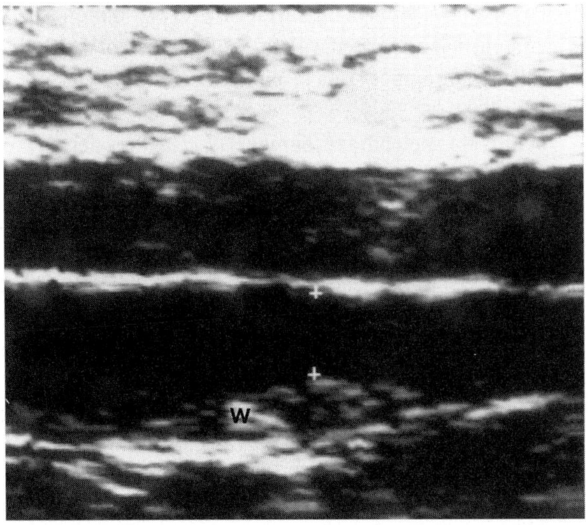

Figure 11.8 *Recanalization with wall thickening (W) and irregularities in a post-thrombotic deep vein. The diameter measured between markers is only 3.5 mm in a femoral vein that originally was 7 mm in diameter.*

may allow sufficient flow to produce readily observable Doppler signals.

Laboratory quality

Duplex ultrasonography with B-mode imaging and Doppler, aided or not by color flow, has become the standard of practice to evaluate the extremity veins. If the hospital or clinic has a vascular laboratory performing at the level required for Intersocietal Commission for Accreditation of Vascular Laboratories certification, phlebography is probably being performed in less than 10% of patients.

Thus quality control issues are important for continuing validation of a test which is so necessarily dependent upon operator skills. There should also be formal comparison with phlebography whenever it may be obtained, realizing, however, that the patient set having contrast phlebograms represents a highly selected 'problem' group. Blinded duplicate scanning programs by different technologists for a percentage of routine examinations also offers a method of documenting quality control of this important diagnostic test.

Systematic review by interpreting physicians is only a part of maintaining excellent results of scanning for deep venous thrombosis. Although complete physician review of negative examinations is probably not of practical value, all positive findings should be submitted for formal confirmation by physician interpretation. Physicians who are responsible for interpretation of findings and vascular laboratory oversight must be personally skilled in techniques of venous duplex scanning and the equipment used.

Accuracy

In the past, the results of venous ultrasonography for detection of deep venous thrombosis have been extensively compared with phlebography. Accuracy greater than 90% has been consistently reported for detection of femoropopliteal thrombosis.[7,8,27,33,34] Lower accuracies, in a widespread range from 50 to 90%, have been reported for calf vein thrombosis, and in particular, in asymptomatic patients in the immediate postoperative period.[35–38] These results are affected by several factors:

- technologists are not as well trained in calf vein scanning, often lacking experience;
- scanners without enough resolution have been employed;
- venous scanning below the knee is time consuming and uneconomical, and, consequently, often avoided;
- a mental attitude exists, minimizing the importance of calf thrombosis, created by the myth that thrombus below the knee is not relevant;
- there are physical hindrances to the performance of the test, for example, in orthopedic patients with casts or awkwardly positioned in bed;
- serial tests are not performed regularly in patients at risk, with thrombus developing after a negative study.

CONTINUOUS-WAVE DOPPLER

Venous flow signals may be detected by use of simple, hand-held, continuous-wave Doppler ultrasound instruments readily available in many settings throughout most hospitals. In the authors' opinion, the use of such instruments for diagnosis of deep venous thrombosis has extremely limited value, if any.

The unreliability of flow signal information in ruling out deep venous thrombosis and difficulty of proving that flow signals are being obtained from named, deep venous structures, make the possibility of error in establishing the most important diagnosis of deep venous thrombosis unacceptable. Furthermore, the ready availability of duplex scanning equipment capable of removing these variables makes the use of continuous-wave Doppler generally unwise.

An exception might be simple confirmation of common femoral vein occlusion in a patient with a clinical syndrome suggesting the diagnosis of iliofemoral deep venous thrombosis or vena cava thrombosis in a setting or time when vascular laboratory examination was not available. This might be a useful test if applied either by a physician or technologist completely familiar with groin vascular anatomy, since the likelihood of anatomic variance producing false information in that specific anatomic locus is exceedingly small. Even so, subsequent examination and documentation by more reliable duplex scanning, also yielding formal recording of images, should be obtained.

REFERENCES

1. Nicholls SC, O'Brian JK, Sutton MG. Venous thromboembolism: detection by duplex scanning. *J Vasc Surg* 1996; **23**: 511–16.
2. Cranley JJ, Canos AJ, Sull WJ. The diagnosis of deep venous thrombosis. Fallibility of clinical symptoms and signs. *Arch Surg* 1976; **111**: 34–6.
3. Hingorani A, Ascher E, Lorenson E, *et al.* Upper extremity deep venous thrombosis and its impact on morbidity and mortality rates in a hospital-based population. *J Vasc Surg* 1997; **26**: 853–60.
4. Hingorani A, Ascher E, Hanson J, *et al.* Upper extremity versus lower extremity deep venous thrombosis. *Am J Surg* 1997; **174**: 214–17.
5. Talbot SR. Use of real-time imaging in identifying deep venous obstruction. *Bruit* 1982; **6**: 41–2.
6. Barnes RW, Nix ML, Barnes CL, *et al.* Perioperative asymptomatic venous thrombosis: role of duplex scanning versus venography. *J Vasc Surg* 1989; **9**: 251–60.
7. Persson AV, Jones C, Zide R, *et al.* Use of triplex scanner in diagnosis of deep venous thrombosis. *Arch Surg* 1989; **124**: 593–6.
8. Killewich LA, Bedford GR, Beach KW, *et al.* Diagnosis of deep venous thrombosis. A prospective study comparing duplex scanning to contrast venography. *Circulation* 1989; **79**: 810–14.
9. Beebe HG, Scissons RP, Salles-Cunha SX, *et al.* Gender bias in use of venous ultrasonography for diagnosis of deep venous thrombosis. *J Vasc Surg* 1995; **22**: 538–42.
10. Muller C, Muller R, Andros G, *et al.* Pitfalls in the comparison of phlebographic and ultrasonic-based diagnosis in the evaluation of the lower extremity. *J Vasc Tech* 1992; **16**: 136–9.
11. Lohr JM, James KV, Hasselfeld KA, *et al.* Vascular laboratory personnel on-call: effect on patient management. *J Vasc Surg* 1995; **22**: 548–52.
12. Langsfeld M, Matteson B, Johnson W, *et al.* Baker's cysts mimicking the symptoms of deep vein thrombosis: diagnosis with venous duplex scanning. *J Vasc Surg* 1997; **25**: 658–62.
13. Gottlieb RH, Widjaja J. Clinical outcomes of untreated symptomatic patients with negative findings on sonography of the thigh for deep vein thrombosis: our experience and a review of the literature. *AJR Am J Roentgenol* 1999; **172**: 1601–4.
14. Cornuz J, Pearson SD, Polak JF. Deep venous thrombosis: complete lower extremity venous US evaluation in patients without known risk factors – outcome study. *Radiology* 1999; **211**: 637–41.
15. Passman MA, Moneta GL, Taylor LM Jr, *et al.* Pulmonary embolism is associated with the combination of isolated calf vein thrombosis and respiratory symptoms. *J Vasc Surg* 1997; **25**: 39–45.
16. Mattos MA, Melendres G, Sumner DS, *et al.* Prevalence and distribution of calf vein thrombosis in patients with symptomatic deep venous thrombosis: a color-flow duplex study. *J Vasc Surg* 1996; **24**: 738–44.
17. Blebea J, Kihara TK, Neumyer MM, *et al.* A national survey of practice patterns in the noninvasive diagnosis of deep venous thrombosis. *J Vasc Surg* 1999; **29**: 799–804, 806.
18. Rodger M, Bredeson C, Wells PS, *et al.* Cost-effectiveness of low-molecular-weight heparin and unfractionated heparin in treatment of deep vein thrombosis. *Can Med Assoc J* 1998; **159**: 931–8.
19. Wahlander K, Tengborn L, Hellstrom M, *et al.* Comparison of various D-dimer tests for the diagnosis of deep venous thrombosis. *Blood Coag Fibrinol* 1999; **10**: 121–6.
20. Glover JL, Bendick PJ. Appropriate indications for venous duplex ultrasonographic examinations. *Surgery* 1996; **120**: 725–30.
21. Criado E, Burnham CB. Predictive value of clinical criteria for the diagnosis of deep vein thrombosis. *Surgery* 1997; **122**: 578–83.
22. Kahn SR. The clinical diagnosis of deep venous thrombosis: integrating incidence, risk factors, and symptoms and signs. *Arch Intern Med* 1998; **158**: 2315–23.
23. Hirsch AT, Zierler RE, Bendick PJ. Commentary re: 'A national survey of practice patterns in the noninvasive diagnosis of deep venous thrombosis.' Intersocietal Commission for the Accreditation of Vascular Laboratories. *J Vasc Surg* 1999; **29**: 939–40.

24. Blumenberg RM, Barton E, Gelfand ML, *et al.* Occult deep venous thrombosis complicating superficial thrombophlebitis. *J Vasc Surg* 1998; **27**: 338–43.
25. Hanson JN, Ascher E, DePippo P, *et al.* Saphenous vein thrombophlebitis (SVT): a deceptively benign disease. *J Vasc Surg* 1998; **27**: 677–80.
26. Salles-Cunha S, Andros G. *Atlas of Duplex Ultrasonography: Essential Images of the Vascular System.* Pasadena, CA: Appleton Davies, 1988.
27. Talbot SR, Oliver MA. *Techniques of Venous Imaging.* Pasadena, CA: Appleton Davies, 1991.
28. Baxter BT, Blackburn D, Payne K, *et al.* Noninvasive evaluation of the upper extremity. *Surg Clin North Am* 1990; **70**: 87–97.
29. Lensing AW, Prandoni P, Brandjes D, *et al.* Detection of deep-vein thrombosis by real-time B-mode ultrasonography. *N Engl J Med* 1989; **320**: 342–5.
30. Salles-Cunha SX, Fowlkes JB, Wakefield TW. B-mode ultrasonographic quantification of deep vein thrombi. *J Vasc Tech* 1994; **18**: 207–9.
31. Fowlkes JB, Strieter RM, Downing LJ, *et al.* Ultrasound echogenicity in experimental venous thrombosis. *Ultrasound Med Biol* 1998; **24**: 1175–82.
32. Sumner DS, Baker DW, Strandness DE Jr. The ultrasonic velocity detector in a clinical study of venous disease. *Arch Surg* 1968; **97**: 75–80.
33. Elias A, Le Corff G, Bouvier JL, *et al.* Value of real time B mode ultrasound imaging in the diagnosis of deep vein thrombosis of the lower limbs. *Int Angiol* 1987; **6**: 175–82.
34. Nix ML, Nelson CL, Harmon BH, *et al.* Duplex venous scanning: image versus Doppler accuracy. *J Vasc Tech* 1989; **13**: 121–6.
35. Monreal M, Montserrat E, Salvador R, *et al.* Real-time ultrasound for diagnosis of symptomatic venous thrombosis and for screening of patients at risk: correlation with ascending conventional venography. *Angiology* 1989; **40**: 527–33.
36. Mussurakis S, Papaioannou S, Voros D, *et al.* Compression ultrasonography as a reliable imaging monitor in deep venous thrombosis. *Surg Gynecol Obstet* 1990; **171**: 233–9.
37. Habscheid W, Hohmann M, Wilhelm T, *et al.* Real-time ultrasound in the diagnosis of acute deep venous thrombosis of the lower extremity. *Angiology* 1990; **41**: 599–608.
38. Fletcher JP, Kershaw LZ, Barker DS, *et al.* Ultrasound diagnosis of lower limb deep venous thrombosis. *Med J Aust* 1990; **153**: 453–5.

12

Direct noninvasive tests (duplex scan) for the evaluation of chronic venous obstruction and valvular incompetence

MARK A MATTOS AND DAVID S SUMNER

Despite the frequency with which chronic venous disease is encountered in clinical practice and the extraordinary amount of research that has been done, its etiology remains poorly understood. What is known is that venous valvular incompetence, venous obstruction, or both are present in the limbs of most patients suffering from this malady and that these physiologic aberrations are in some way ultimately responsible for the clinical manifestations. In most cases, the diagnosis is easily made by inspecting the leg. Physical findings are characteristic and are among the most specific of any disease. Yet, physical findings (other than the identification of varicose veins) provide little clue to the presence, location, or extent of venous valvular incompetence or residual obstruction. This information is valuable, not only for establishing an accurate diagnosis, but also for planning an effective therapeutic approach and for understanding the natural history of the disease.

Indirect noninvasive tests (described in Chapter 10) play an important role in detecting and evaluating the severity of the hemodynamic changes caused by venous obstruction or valvular incompetence, but do not contribute anatomic information. Before the advent of ultrasonic technology, phlebography was the only method capable of defining the underlying pathologic morphology. Aside from being invasive, relatively expensive, and associated with some risk, phlebography is significantly limited in its ability to detect incompetence of the calf veins and in its ability to identify obstruction of non-axial veins. Although continuous-wave (CW) Doppler examinations furnish only segmental information and although the anatomic detail provided by ultrasonic imaging is generally inferior to that of phlebography, these methods are noninvasive, repeatable, widely applicable, and (at least theoretically) do not suffer from the same limitations that plague phlebography. At present, duplex scanning is widely accepted as the most clinically useful test for detecting, locating, and evaluating venous valvular incompetence and chronic venous obstruction. When duplex scanning is not available, a simple CW Doppler examination may provide sufficient, albeit less precise, information.

CONTINUOUS-WAVE DOPPLER

Any of a variety of CW Doppler devices is suitable for venous examinations. Because the depth of sonic penetration is inversely related to frequency of the transmitted ultrasound, lower frequencies (5 MHz) are usually best for studying deep veins. On the other hand, the relatively low velocity of blood flow in superficial veins is often more clearly detected when higher frequencies (10 MHz) are used. Although panel meters indicating the direction of flow are useful for the assessment of venous valvular incompetence, for most purposes the audible signal is all that is required.

Examinations are conducted in a warm room with the patient supine, preferably in a slightly reversed

Trendelenburg position (10–15°) to ensure adequate venous filling. The patient should be comfortable and the legs must be relaxed. This is best achieved when the legs are slightly externally rotated at the hip and flexed a few degrees at the knee.

The initial step at all levels of the leg is to locate the corresponding artery. Arteries are easily identified by their characteristic signal and by the direction of flow. In most cases, when the vein is patent, the venous signal will be heard in the background. By shifting the probe slightly in the proper direction, the venous signal can be optimized. Using the corresponding artery as a guide, the examiner studies the common femoral, superficial femoral, popliteal and posterior tibial veins in descending or ascending order. After the deep veins have been surveyed, the saphenous veins, both above and below the knee, are examined. Because even deep veins are easily collapsed, care must be taken to apply the probe with the least external pressure necessary to obtain a good signal. When the posterior tibial veins at the ankle and superficial veins are examined, sonic coupling should be achieved with the acoustic gel. The probe should not actually touch the skin.

At each location, particular attention should be given to the 'spontaneous' (unaugmented) Doppler signal. The normal spontaneous venous signal sounds much like a windstorm and typically varies with respiration, increasing with expiration and decreasing with inspiration. Venous signals can be augmented by compressing the leg above or below the site of probe application. Compressing the leg below the probe displaces blood up the leg, producing an increase in the volume of the audible signal detected by the Doppler probe. Compressing the leg cephalad to the probe temporarily restricts venous outflow and allows blood to back up in the veins below the site of compression. Upon release of compression, the accumulated blood rushes up the leg to fill the void left in veins collapsed by manual compression. Augmentation maneuvers are most useful when small veins with low flow velocities are examined. In these veins spontaneous signals may be absent. In the authors' experience, spontaneous signals are almost always present in normal veins at the popliteal and more proximal level and provided the patient is warm and the legs are relaxed, they are present in most posterior tibial veins.

Venous obstruction

Methods similar to those used to detect acute venous thrombosis are employed to identify chronic venous obstruction (see Chapter 11). Because collateral development and partial recanalization of previously thrombosed veins often complicate the picture, a few additional points need to be made. It is important to emphasize that the major veins lie immediately adjacent to the corresponding artery. If one has to search for a signal in the leg at a distance more than a centimeter from the artery, the vessel located is more likely to be a collateral of the vein whose patency is in question. This is potentially a major source of error, since a signal arising from well developed collaterals in the vicinity of a chronic venous occlusion might lead to a false-negative interpretation.

Normal Doppler signals imply patency but can be obtained when a vein has recanalized or when only one of a pair of duplicated veins is occluded. Although total absence of a signal suggests that the insonated vein is occluded, a weak signal can be hard to interpret. Such signals may arise from small collaterals that are closely applied to an occluded vein, may represent flow in an incompletely recanalized segment, or may be due to physiologic or technical factors. Augmentation maneuvers are best applied after spontaneous signals have been assessed. If no signal is obtained when the leg is compressed distal to the probe, one can assume that the vein is occluded at the point of interrogation. The examiner must be aware that confusing signals may be obtained when small collateral channels are present or when the vein is only partially occluded. These signals may be erroneously interpreted as indicating venous patency.

Despite these problems, the hand-held Doppler technique has proved useful for identifying chronic venous obstruction in the clinic or at the bedside.

Venous valvular incompetence

Venous valvular incompetence can be detected by demonstrating flow reversal in a venous segment. Having the patient perform a Valsalva maneuver increases intra-abdominal pressure, which forces blood out of the inferior vena cava and iliac veins. In limbs with at least one functionally competent iliac or common femoral venous valve, retrograde flow is prohibited by valve closure. Under these circumstances, the 'spontaneous' phasic common femoral flow signal ceases abruptly. In the absence of a functioning valve, a Valsalva maneuver will generate retrograde flow in the common femoral vein, which is easily detected by a properly positioned CW Doppler probe. The meters on a direction-sensing instrument will confirm reversal of flow. If the instrument lacks direction-sensing capabilities, the occurrence of a signal during the Valsalva maneuver is sufficient to diagnose valvular incompetence.

Although the Valsalva maneuver may produce retrograde flow as far distally as the posterior tibial or ankle saphenous vein when all intervening valves are incompetent, the presence of a single competent valve at any level proximal to the site of the probe will prevent reflux and may lead to a false-negative result. The test, therefore, is most useful for examining the common femoral vein or the superficial femoral vein when reflux is detected at the common femoral level. At other sites, limb compression is better adapted to the demonstration of segmental reflux.

If the intervening valves are incompetent, manual compression of the leg above the site of the probe will produce a retrograde surge of blood.[1] Upon release of compression, blood rushes back up the leg, producing an easily recognized to-and-fro sound (Fig. 12.1). Although a directional Doppler is helpful for distinguishing retrograde from antegrade flow, a non-directional instrument usually suffices.

Although these studies can be conducted with the patient supine, the upright position more closely approximates the physiologic conditions in which reflux is important. The patient stands, holding onto a rail, a walker, or other support, with his or her weight shifted to the limb opposite that being examined. When the limb is manually compressed below the site of the probe, a surge of antegrade flow will be detected (provided the intervening segment is patent). Upon release of compression, competent valves close rapidly and there will be little or no reflux flow.[1] If, however, valves in the intervening segment are absent or incompetent, blood displaced upward during compression will fall back down the leg once the compression is released, refilling the evacuated veins (Fig. 12.1).

Reflux detected in the common femoral vein in response to a Valsalva maneuver or release of leg compression implies not only incompetence of the iliac and common femoral valves but also incompetence of the saphenofemoral junction, the upper superficial femoral vein, or both.[2] If reflux is abolished by manual pressure over the greater saphenous vein or by the application of a tourniquet to the thigh 10 cm below the groin, reflux can be attributed to an incompetent saphenofemoral junction. Persistence of reflux despite compression of the saphenous vein suggests incompetence of the superficial femoral vein. If the popliteal valves are competent, significant reflux in the upper superficial femoral vein may indicate incompetence of thigh-perforating veins.

The popliteal vein and the lesser saphenous junction are studied with the knee slightly bent and the patient facing away from the examiner. Absence of retrograde flow upon release of calf compression implies competence of the popliteal valves. Reflux indicates incompetence of either the popliteal or lesser saphenous veins, or both.[2] Persistence of reflux while the lesser saphenous vein is digitally compressed below the probe is indicative of popliteal valvular incompetence.

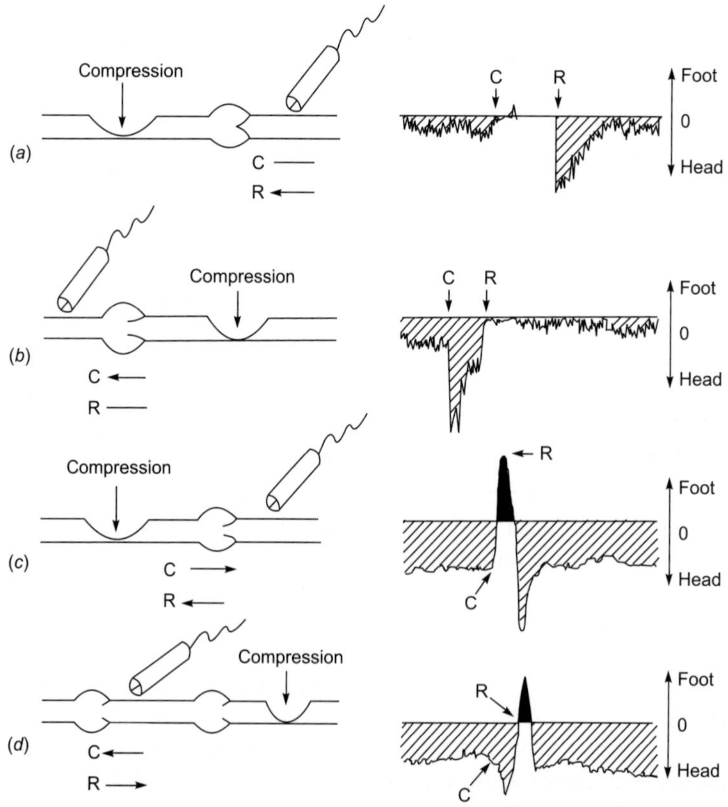

Figure 12.1 *Continuous-wave directional Doppler recordings of venous blood flow responses to augmentation maneuvers. (a, b) Normal response. (c, d) Abnormal responses typical of venous valvular incompetence. Flow in the normal (antegrade) direction is indicated by downward deflection of the tracing, and retrograde flow is indicated by an upward deflection. C, application of manual limb compression; R, release of compression. (Reproduced with permission from Sumner DS. Diagnosis of deep venous thrombosis. In Rutherford RB, ed.* Vascular Surgery, *4th edn. Philadelphia: WB Saunders, 1995: 1698–743)*

CW Doppler examination of superficial veins should include the greater saphenous vein both above and below the knee and the lesser saphenous vein. Any superficial varicosities can be examined, but they always demonstrate incompetence. Reflux is easily demonstrated by the methods mentioned above or by having the patient slowly shift his or her weight from one leg to the other. Bidirectional flow detected along the medial calf when the calf is manually compressed above the site of the Doppler probe can be used to identify incompetent perforating veins.[3] A tourniquet is applied to the leg between the site of compression and the probe to avoid confusing signals produced by reflux flow in the superficial veins. This technique, unfortunately, is not very sensitive or specific.[4]

Limitations

A major drawback of CW Doppler examinations is the inability to be absolutely sure which veins in the ultrasound beam are being interrogated. Errors may occur when veins are duplicated or when collateral veins are in close proximity to the vein being studied. At the groin, it can be difficult to differentiate reflux in a tributary of the saphenous vein from reflux in the saphenous vein itself or in the common femoral vein. (Tourniquets may not compress superficial veins adequately, leading to an erroneous diagnosis of deep venous insufficiency.) Similarly, confusion may occur in the popliteal area between reflux in the popliteal, lesser saphenous, gastrocnemius or Giacomini vein. Moreover, the extent of obstruction and the precise location of incompetent valves cannot be determined with certainty. Lastly, reflux severity is not easily estimated with the CW Doppler.

Little has been written regarding the accuracy of CW Doppler for identifying incompetence. One study found that incompetence of the greater saphenous vein was diagnosed with a sensitivity of 73% and a specificity of 85% compared with duplex scanning.[5] The sensitivity for identifying lesser saphenous and deep vein incompetence was only 33% and 48%, respectively, but the specificity for both exceeded 90%.

DUPLEX SCANNING

Most of the limitations of CW Doppler examinations have been overcome by Duplex scanning. The B-mode image allows veins to be visualized and ensures accurate placement of the pulsed-Doppler sample volume. These features avoid confusing a major vein with a collateral, permit individual interrogation of paired veins, and allow non-axial veins (such as the profunda femoris, gastrocnemius, and soleal veins) to be examined. Because the greater and lesser saphenous veins and their junctions with the common femoral and popliteal veins are easily identified, tourniquets are not required to differentiate between reflux in the two systems.

Although obstruction of major veins can be detected with real-time B-mode scanning alone, recognition of valvular incompetence is difficult. Duplex instruments, which incorporate a pulsed-Doppler flow-velocity detector, provide additional information necessary to make studies of chronic venous insufficiency clinically feasible. Spectral analysis of the Doppler signal is used to confirm the presence or absence of flow, to indicate the direction of flow, and to record flow patterns. The addition of a color-coded flow map confers advantages that simplify the examination and make it more expeditious.[6,7] Color immediately identifies vascular structures and distinguishes arteries from veins. Flow is visible over a relatively long region and simultaneously in multiple vessels, making it less necessary to interrogate the leg every centimeter or so with the Doppler. Absence of flow in an occluded segment is immediately apparent and encroachment by clot on the flow image is easily detected. The direction of flow is clearly depicted. By convention, color assignments are blue for flow toward the heart and red for flow toward the periphery. Color immediately identifies the presence of reflux by the change from blue to red (Fig. 12.2).

Venous obstruction

Chronic venous obstruction is detected by the same methods used to identify acute deep venous thrombosis (see Chapter 11). Patients are positioned as described for the CW Doppler examination. After a vein is identified, its patency is ascertained by evaluating its compressibility and by assessing the Doppler signal. A totally thrombosed vein will be incompressible and will be devoid of Doppler signals. A partially thrombosed vein will be incompletely compressible and Doppler signals will be obtained from part of the lumen area. With color, total thrombosis is immediately evident since no color will be detected in the vein identified by the B-mode scan. With partial occlusion there will be encroachment on the flow image, which will no longer fill the entire lumen. Flow in collateral channels is easily located. Collateral channels are less likely to be confused with the major vein when duplex or color-flow scanning is used since the location of the vein from which the signals are detected is apparent. Chronic venous obstruction may be differentiated from acute DVT in various ways. Whereas an acutely thrombosed vein tends to be distended beyond the usually normal diameter, chronically occluded veins are often shrunken and have thick walls that may be more echogenic owing to fibrosis. Occasionally calcification is present. The residual clot may also be more echogenic.

When the vein in question cannot be visualized because of its deep location or overlying bowel gas (iliac

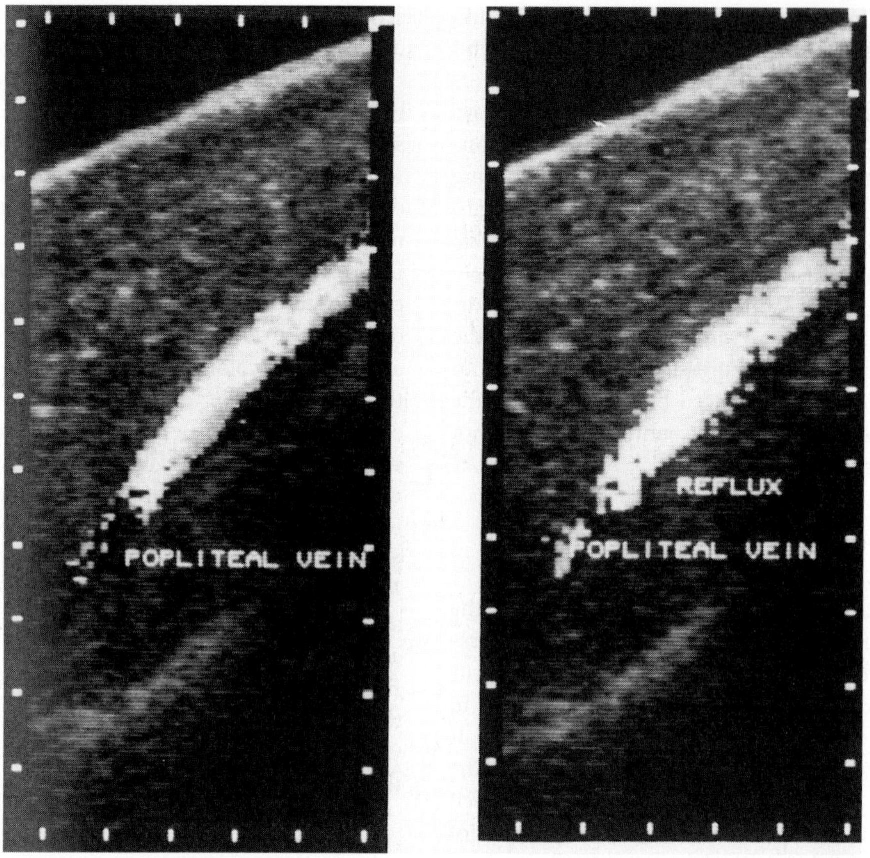

Figure 12.2 *Color-flow duplex scan of incompetent lesser saphenous vein. (a) Antegrade flow during calf compression. (b) Reflux flow during release of calf compression.*

veins, for example, or the superficial femoral vein at the adductor canal level), Doppler signals can be assessed in a manner analogous to that used when the CW Doppler is employed.

As in surveys for acute DVT, the entire venous system from the common femoral to the ankle are studied. Duplex scanning has the advantage of allowing each of the three axial vein pairs below the knee to be identified and studied, including the posterior tibial, anterior tibial and peroneal. In addition, the gastrocnemius and soleal veins can be examined, as well as the profunda femoris vein, at least in its distal segment near the junction with the common femoral. Although the IVC and the iliac veins are deeply located, they can be examined in an appreciable number of patients.

Venous valvular incompetence

Techniques for detecting and evaluating venous valvular incompetence with duplex and color-flow scanning are essentially refinements of those employed with the CW Doppler. After the vein to be studied has been located on the B-mode image and its identity confirmed by the characteristic audible Doppler signal, velocity spectrum, or color-flow map, the position of the probe is adjusted to provide a long-axis view that encompasses the segment of interest. The pulsed-Doppler sample volume is then placed in the center of the flow stream at an angle approximating 60°. While the velocity spectrum is being displayed on the monitor, maneuvers designed to reverse the normal peripheral to central venous pressure gradient are performed. Retrograde flow is indicated by an inverted spectrum or by a change in the flow-map color from blue to red. In some cases, the color image alone may be sufficient, thus obviating the need for time-consuming spectrum analyses (Fig. 12.2).[6,7] Pertinent portions of study may be preserved on video tape, and a hard copy of the velocity spectrum can be made.

Venous valves are often seen on the gray-scale image (Fig. 12.3).[8] Normal valve sinuses have an elliptical configuration and the leaflets are thin and mobile. Diseased valve sinuses are distorted, may contain echogenic material, and the leaflets, when visible, are short and thick. When the leaflets are adequately visualized in real time and their motion clearly discerned, valvular competence may be assessed directly. Precise location of an incompetent valve is of clinical importance but is not always possible. Owing to the echogenicity of slowly moving blood (a phenomenon attributed to erythrocyte aggregation), the motion of blood may be perceptible on the B-mode image. Prior to

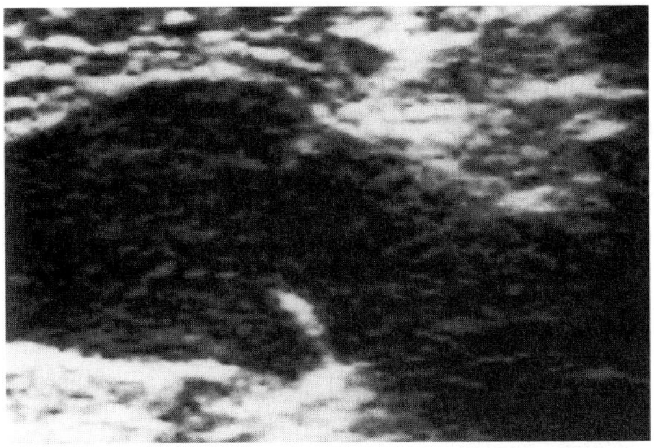

Figure 12.3 *B-mode image of normal venous valve, showing elliptical configuration of the sinus and the presence of delicate valve cusps.*

the introduction of duplex scanning, this feature was used to indicate the direction of blood flow. Doppler assessment, however, provides much more information and is less subjective.

A variety of positions have been advocated for conducting the examination. These include the 10–15° and 30–40° reversed Trendelenburg,[7,9] the 45° semi-Fowler,[10] and the standing position.[11,12] Popliteal and calf veins can be studied with the patient sitting, the foot resting on a stool or on the examiner's lap.[9,7,13] As mentioned previously, the leg being studied should be relaxed. In the supine patient, this is best achieved when the legs are externally rotated at the hip and slightly flexed at the knee. In the standing position, the patient holds on to a support and is instructed to shift his or her weight to the opposite leg.

At the groin, reflux may be assessed by having the patient perform a Valsalva maneuver. Pressures generated by the Valsalva maneuver depend on the patient's ability to cooperate and on the rapidity and force with which the maneuver is performed. Having the patient blow into a mercury manometer to achieve a pressure of 40 mmHg is one way of standardizing the test.[14] A period of reversed flow lasting longer than 1.5 seconds is considered abnormal at the common femoral area.[14] Because Valsalva maneuvers produce reflux only down to the first competent valve, this technique is usually of value only for examining veins in the groin or proximal leg and may overlook valvular incompetence located more distally.[15]

Further down the leg, manual compression either above or below the probe may be used to evaluate valvular competence. The techniques are identical to those used with the CW Doppler. When the patient is supine, compression of the limb above a competent valve results in valve closure, provided that compression is sufficiently rapid and forceful; but when the valve is incompetent reversed flow occurs. Reflux flow persisting for more than 1.0 second is considered abnormal. If the velocity of retrograde blood flow generated by compression is less than a critical value (30 cm/s, according to one study), a normal valve may not close, leading to a false-positive interpretation.[16] Manual compression of the limb below the probe is best performed with the patient standing or sitting. Retrograde flow appearing after release of compression and persisting for 1.0 second or more is indicative of valvular incompetence (Fig. 12.4). Calf contraction and relaxation has also been used to demonstrate reflux flow in the standing position.[12]

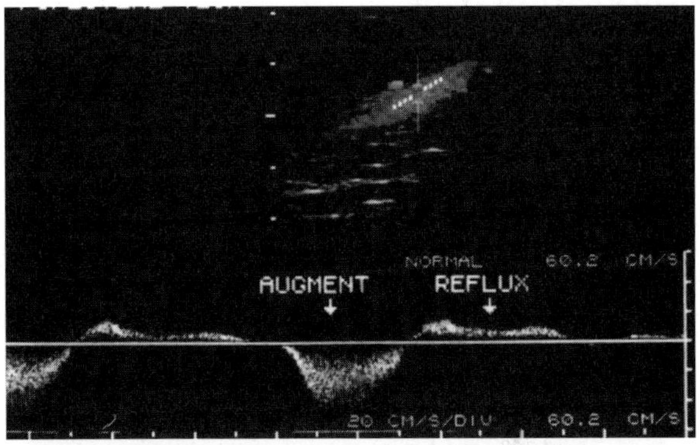

Figure 12.4 *Doppler frequency spectrum of flow in an incompetent popliteal vein of a patient lying supine in the reversed Trendelenburg position. Antegrade flow occurs during manual calf compression (augmentation). Reflux flow occurs with the release of compression.*

The method proposed by van Bemmelen and associates is preferred by many investigators, who argue that it provides a more reliable and consistent way of identifying and quantifying valvular incompetence.[11] Studies are performed with the patient standing, as described above. At a minimum, the common femoral, superficial femoral, popliteal, and posterior tibial veins (at mid-calf and at the ankle) are examined with the probe positioned over the appropriate vein after it has been identified on the B-mode scan. Other veins such as the profunda femoris vein and the greater and lesser saphenous veins can be examined to complete the study. In each position, a pneumatic cuff is positioned around the leg about 5 cm below the transducer site. To provide adequate compression, the cuff width should be approximately 24 cm at the thigh, 12 cm at the calf, and 7 cm at the foot. Cuffs are connected to an automatic cuff inflator. Inflation is maintained for about 3 seconds, after which the cuff is deflated rapidly within 0.3 seconds or less. At the thigh, cuffs are inflated to 80 mmHg. To overcome hydrostatic pressure and ensure complete venous evacuation, higher pressures are required at the calf (100 mmHg) and foot (120 mmHg).

The velocity spectrum is recorded continuously during cuff inflation and for at least 4 seconds after deflation. Normal valves close rapidly when the cuff is deflated in response to temporary flow reversal

(Fig. 12.5a). As van Bemmelen *et al.*[11] have shown, the duration of reflux flow is less than 0.5 seconds in 95% of normal veins and rarely exceeds 1.0 seconds. Therefore, retrograde flow persisting longer than 0.5 seconds is considered to be indicative of valvular incompetence (Fig. 12.5b). In most cases, when the valve is incompetent, the median duration of reflux flow is about 3–4 seconds with a range of 2–8 seconds. Discrimination is therefore quite good between competent and incompetent valves.

PERFORATING VEINS

Perforating veins may be studied with the patient in an exaggerated 45° reversed Trendelenburg position, sitting with the legs dependent, or standing without weight-bearing.[4,17,18] The medial calf is surveyed systematically. Perforators are identified as veins arising from the superficial system which penetrate the deep fascia to enter the muscle compartment, where they join the deep veins (Fig. 12.6). Outward flow detected with manual calf compression (either above or below the sampling site) or active calf contraction is used to identify those perforators that are incompetent.[12,17,18] Outward flow, however, may be observed in 21% of normal limbs and therefore may not always represent a pathologic finding.[18]

Color duplex is very helpful in confirming bi-directional flow, which is indicated by the color change that occurs when compression is applied and released. Prior to subfascial endoscopic surgery, the location of incompetent perforators may be marked on the skin with an indelible pen. Although incompetent perforators identified by duplex scanning are usually verified at surgery, additional incompetent perforators not identified by duplex scanning may be found during surgical exploration.

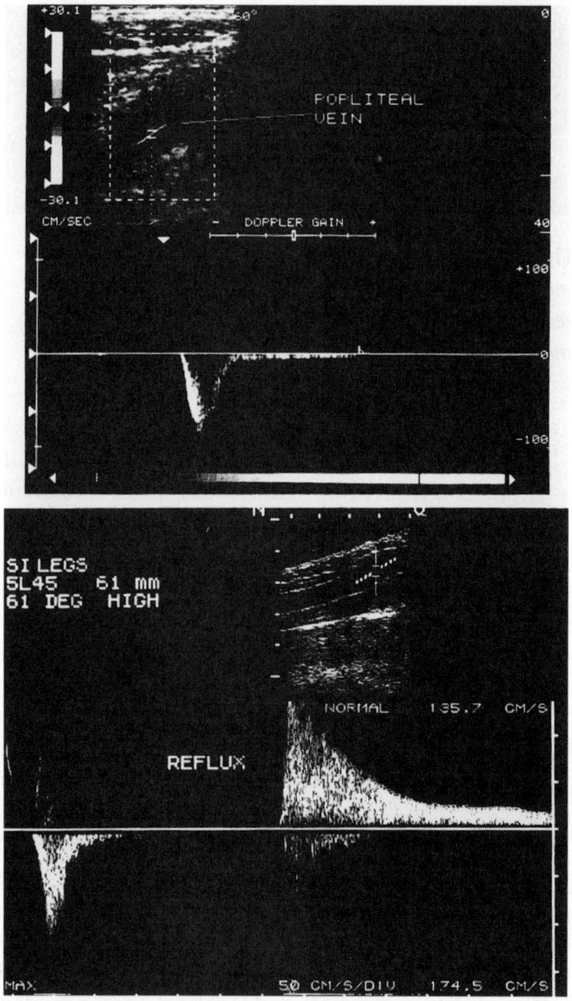

Figure 12.5 *(a) Doppler frequency spectrum of flow in a normal popliteal vein (standing cuff technique) showing antegrade flow (downward deflection) during cuff inflation and only a minute amount of reversed flow with cuff deflation. (b) Doppler frequency spectrum of flow in an incompetent greater saphenous vein. Antegrade flow (downward deflection) occurs during cuff inflation. Release of compression 3 seconds later is followed by reflux flow (upward deflection) that persists for several seconds. (Fig. 12.5b courtesy Dr Paul S. van Bemmelen)*

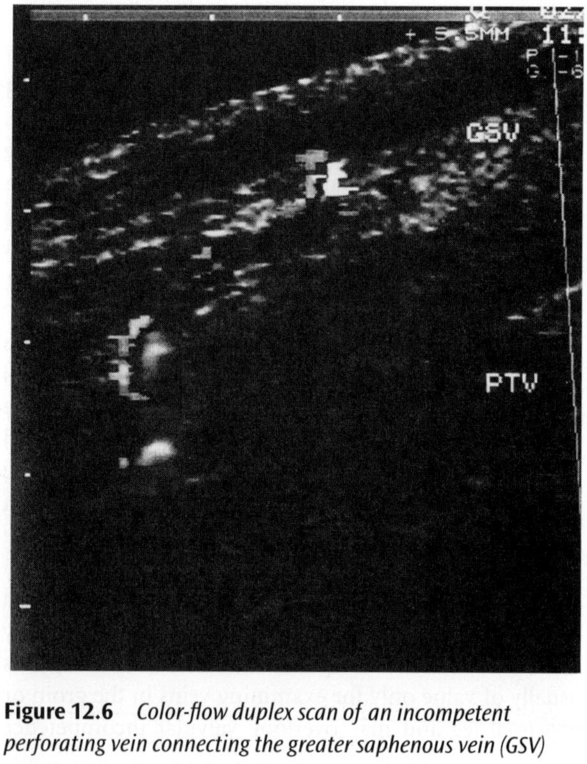

Figure 12.6 *Color-flow duplex scan of an incompetent perforating vein connecting the greater saphenous vein (GSV) and the posterior tibial vein (PTV).*

QUANTIFICATION OF REFLUX

There have been efforts to quantify the magnitude of the reflux flow and to correlate this with clinical manifestations of chronic venous insufficiency. Peak reversed flow velocities may be recorded directly from the Doppler spectrum. Features incorporated on many duplex instruments permit the diameter of the vein to be estimated. With the sample volume expanded to insonate the entire venous lumen, the machine can then determine the mean reflux flow velocity and multiply this by the cross-sectional area (considered to be circular) to determine the mean rate of flow. Using this method, Vasdekis and associates found that 66% of limbs with peak reflux flows in excess of 10 ml/s had ulcers, while none of those with lower velocities did.[19] This method of quantifying reflux, however, has not been widely adopted.

Other investigators have proposed scoring systems based on the number of incompetent valve sites[20–22] or on the total or mean duration of reflux flow (obtained by adding the duration of reflux flow from each of the venous segments that were studied).[6,23–25] Average scores and mean reflux times correlate with disease severity, but individual results may have little predictive value. In some studies, reflux times have correlated with the venous filling index obtained with the air plethysmograph,[25] but, in others, no relationship has been found.[24]

ACCURACY

Although phlebography may fail to disclose thrombi in non-axial and tributary veins (such as the profunda femoris, internal iliac, gastrocnemius, and soleal veins), it serves as an acceptable, albeit flawed, gold standard for the detection of venous obstruction. Nothing, however, really qualifies as a gold standard for identifying and quantifying reflux in individual veins. Because descending phlebography cannot evaluate the competency of valves in peripheral veins when there is a competent valve in the upper part of the leg, results with this test may be falsely negative. False-positive interpretations are also possible owing to the relatively high density of the contrast medium, which may trickle down the relaxed leg through normal but partially open valves. It is not surprising, therefore, that the reported correlation between duplex findings and descending phlebography ranges from about 60% to 90%.[22,26,27] Most of the errors relate to disease below the knee. Until something better comes along, duplex scanning must act as its own gold standard.

Results obtained with the different methods of duplex scanning may also differ significantly.[14] It appears, however, that the standing-cuff technique may be substantially more sensitive than the supine-manual compression or Valsalva methods.[15]

INTERPRETATION

Unlike the assessment of arterial disease, in which angiography, duplex scanning, and ankle pressure indices are highly predictive of disease severity, the assessment of chronic venous disease is frustrated by relatively poor and inconsistent correlations between objective findings and the clinical manifestations of chronic venous insufficiency (see Chapter 52). There are a number of possible explanations for this.

First, although venous congestion and elevated venous pressure appear to be responsible for instigating the events leading to the cutaneous and subcutaneous changes typical of chronic venous insufficiency, the events themselves occur at the microvascular level and remain poorly understood. Second, although the physiologic aberrations associated with venous valvular incompetence probably appear immediately, their clinical effect is gradual, and overt signs and symptoms may not become evident for several years. It is possible that patients may move from clinical class 0 through classes 1, 2 and 3 to reach classes 4, 5, or 6 without ever having any further deterioration in venous function. In fact, classes 4, 5 and 6 may be hemodynamically indistinguishable.[28] Thus, studies that attempt to correlate valve function with clinical staging are obtaining a 'snapshot' of what is almost certainly a dynamic process. For example, some patients with class 3 or 4 disease may have physiologic changes sufficient only to reach class 3 or 4, whereas others with more severe changes are destined to progress to higher stages. Third, it is likely that the physiologic consequences of venous incompetence depend on the location of the incompetent valve or valves. In some areas, incompetence may have little effect on overall venous function. Although the effect of separate arterial lesions is roughly additive, the same may not be true of venous disease. In other words, clinical severity may relate poorly to the number of incompetent valves. A single incompetent valve in a crucial location may be more detrimental to venous function than several incompetent valves in a less important location. Furthermore, valvular incompetence in the superficial or perforating venous systems may develop as a result of incompetence (or obstruction) in other areas and may not be directly or even indirectly responsible for clinical signs.

Venous obstruction

Chronic thrombotic obstruction of a major axial vein may have major physiologic implications. For example, iliac vein obstruction may limit venous outflow during exercise-induced hyperemia. This in turn leads to venous congestion and an elevation of venous pressure. Patients experience a painful, tight sensation in their calves after walking, a condition known as 'venous claudication'. The combination of increased venous outflow resistance and venous valvular incompetence is particularly detrimental to the proper function of the calf muscle pump mechanism.[20,21,28,29] Consequently, limbs with the most severe cutaneous manifestations of chronic venous insufficiency often have an element of venous obstruction. On the other hand, when an obstruction does not involve significant inflow or outflow collaterals, physiologic impairment is usually minimal.

Doppler studies and duplex examinations cannot measure venous resistance. This is best done with plethysmography (venous outflow plethysmography) or with pressure measurements. However, the location and extent of the occlusion may provide clues to the severity of the obstruction and allow one to make some clinical predictions.

Venous valvular incompetence

Venous valves may become incompetent following an episode of DVT, the delicate valve leaflets having been damaged during resolution of the thrombotic process. Through mechanisms that are not entirely clear, valves in venous segments not directly involved with clot may also become incompetent. Approximately two-thirds of patients with venous insufficiency give no history of DVT.[13,30,31] In these patients, valvular incompetence or the predisposition to venous incompetence may have been present since birth.

The reported distribution of venous valvular incompetence in limbs with class 4, 5 or 6 disease (lipodermatosclerosis, healed or active ulcers) varies widely (Table 12.1).[32–34] Superficial venous incompetence has been the only abnormality detected by some authors in an appreciable fraction of patients with chronic venous insufficiency.[9,12,34] Other investigators have found relatively few patients with chronic venous insufficiency in whom incompetence was confined to the superficial veins.[6,10,20,30,32] In their studies, most limbs with venous ulcers have deep venous insufficiency alone or in combination with superficial venous incompetence. That superficial venous incompetence is found in a majority of limbs with stasis changes is not disputed, but its role as a primary causative factor is. Many patients with large, ropey varicose veins that have been present for many years have no symptoms and no cutaneous manifestations of chronic venous insufficiency. Only 5% of the limbs of patients referred to a tertiary clinic with reflux confined to the greater saphenous system had stasis ulcers,[35] and it is probable that the incidence in the general population is much less.

There is little difference between clinical class 4 and class 5–6 disease in the distribution of venous incompetence. In patients with class 1 and 2 disease, however, the relative frequency of isolated superficial incompetence tends to be somewhat higher and the incidence of deep venous incompetence (either alone or in combination with superficial incompetence) somewhat lower than they are in the more severe categories.[12,20,30,33] It is worthy of emphasis that patients in any of the three groups may exhibit similar patterns.

About 15% of 'normal' limbs have reflux in the common femoral vein. Reversal of flow in this area may, however, predispose to the development of primary varicose veins (if one accepts the descending valvular incompetence theory). Incompetence limited to the superficial femoral valves may also be a normal variant, since reflux of contrast to the knee level on descending phlebography is often observed in patients with none of the typical signs of chronic venous insufficiency. On the other hand, many studies suggest that incompetence of the popliteal vein and deep veins of the calf (alone or in combination with proximal venous incompetence) may be a factor of great importance in the production of signs and symptoms associated with chronic venous insufficiency.[13,29,36] In several reports, the frequency of posterior tibial vein or popliteal vein incompetence in limbs with class 2 or 3 disease (42–68%) was appreciably higher than that in limbs less severely affected (3–35%).[20,30,32,33]

Table 12.1 *Distribution of venous valve incompetence in class 4–6 disease (lipodermatosclerosis, healed or active ulcers)*

Authors	Number of limbs	SVI only (%)	SVI + DVI (%)	DVI only (%)	Perf only (%)	None (%)
Araki *et al.* (1994)[10]	25 a	0	71	20	C	4 b
Moore *et al.* (1986)[30]	35	3	69	23	C	6
van Bemmelen *et al.* (1991)[32]	25	4	84	8	4	0
Neglén, Raju (1993)[20]	31	6	65	29	0	0
Araki *et al.* (1994)[10]	18 c	6	88	6	C	0
Weingarten *et al.* (1993)[6]	192	16	42	19	C	23
Hanrahan *et al.* (1991)[31]	95	36	43 d	6 d	8	6
Myers *et al.* (1995)[33]	96	38	48	8	2	4
Labropoulos *et al.* (1995)[13]	112	44	39	11	3	4
Lees, Lambert (1993)[12]	25	52	44	4	0	0
Shami *et al.* (1993)[34]	79	53	32	15	0	0
van Rij *et al.* (1994)[9]	120	70	20	8	2	<1

SVI, superficial venous insufficiency; DVI, deep venous insufficiency; Perf, incompetent perforating veins.
a, Active ulcers (class 6); b, authors' figures do not equal 100%; c, healed ulcers (class 5); d, deep calf veins not studied.

Likewise, incompetence of the distal superficial veins (below-knee greater saphenous and lesser saphenous veins), either alone or in combination with above-knee greater saphenous incompetence, appears to be more strongly associated with ulcer development than incompetence limited to the proximal superficial veins.[13,31,33,37] In one study, only 4% of limbs with reflux confined to the above-knee saphenous vein exhibited skin changes and none had ulcers.[35] These observations are consistent with the pivotal role that calf veins play in the function of the muscle pump mechanism.[29,36,38]

Incompetent perforating veins are detected by duplex examination in approximately two-thirds of limbs with lipodermatosclerosis or stasis ulcers (classes 4, 5 and 6).[12,13,20,33] They are somewhat less common (23–57%) in class 0–3 disease. Most are located in the medial calf and are associated with concomitant insufficiency of the deep and superficial venous systems. Isolated perforator incompetence is rare, occurring in only 0–8% of legs with class 5–6 disease (Table 12.1). Although many investigators now believe that incompetent perforating veins are of major importance in the genesis of stasis ulceration, the issue is still debated. In one study, 46% of ulcer beds were devoid of incompetent perforators. Other perforators, such as those in the thigh, may serve as the source of reflux flow to the greater saphenous vein when the saphenofemoral junction is competent.

APPLICATIONS

The symptoms and signs of chronic venous insufficiency are usually sufficient to make the diagnosis. Indeed, one might argue that objective confirmation is required only when clinical findings are in some respect atypical. Only a few patients with class 4, 5, or 6 disease have no evidence of venous reflux (Table 12.1), and in some of these cases incompetence may have been overlooked because of an incomplete examination. The role of objective anatomic studies, therefore, is to identify the location of incompetent valves (or obstructed veins). As pointed out above, duplex or Doppler studies do not discriminate well between clinical classes of disease and are only marginally useful in a prognostic sense.

The extent of the examination may be varied depending on the approach that is to be adopted in treating the patient with suspected chronic venous insufficiency. If the choice is to use elastic support, inelastic compression, or other nonoperative measures such as Unna paste boots to treat edema, ulceration, or lipodermatosclerosis, it is only necessary to rule out concomitant arterial disease (by ankle indices or other noninvasive methods). If there is any doubt concerning the diagnosis, a hand-held Doppler examination may be sufficient to establish the presence of venous reflux; otherwise, a duplex scan is indicated.

When the patient's condition proves recalcitrant to conventional treatment, operative therapy may be considered. In such cases, it is critical to know the location and extent of disease. This requires careful duplex examination. For example, if the treatment options include venous valvuloplasty or valve transplantation, the incompetent segments must be identified and extensive venous occlusion or severe damage to veins in the area to be reconstructed must be excluded. Usually, the valves to be surgically addressed are those in the upper superficial femoral vein or popliteal vein. Once the decision has been made to intervene surgically, the anatomic detail provided by phlebography is necessary. Postoperative follow-up examinations should be performed to demonstrate that the procedure has successfully re-established venous competency.

In some cases, open subfascial or extrafascial ligation of incompetent perforating veins may be the chosen form of therapy. In this event, not only must the presence of perforator incompetence be established but the incompetent perforators should be located accurately to ensure the proper placement of surgical incisions. When the procedure to be performed is subfascial endoscopic perforator ligation, duplex scanning is the only diagnostic examination required. Phlebography is necessary only when lateral perforators are suspected.

Optimum treatment of varicose veins requires identification of incompetent venous segments and the location of communications with the deep system that feed the varicosities. It is necessary to ligate, strip, or sclerose only those segments that are incompetent, preserving normal segments. Superficial venous incompetence may involve the entire greater saphenous vein or it can be confined to the greater saphenous vein above the knee, the saphenous vein below the Hunterian perforator, the saphenous vein below the knee, the lesser saphenous vein, or any combination of the above. When ulcers are the indication for treating superficial venous insufficiency, it is particularly important to identify which veins are incompetent since stripping of the greater saphenous vein alone would correct only about 6% of the hemodynamic abnormalities in patients with ulcers.[13] Superficial venous ligation and stripping is indicated only when the below-knee greater saphenous or lesser saphenous veins are incompetent.[13,35]

Because of the variable anatomy of veins in the popliteal fossa, duplex scanning is recommended prior to operations for lesser saphenous varicosities. According to one study,[39] the saphenopopliteal junction was located within 2 cm of the popliteal skin crease in 51% of the limbs surveyed and within 2–4 cm in 36%. In 14%, however, the junction was 4 to more than 10 cm above the skin crease. Incompetent gastrocnemius veins or Giacomini veins, which represent a continuation of the lesser saphenous vein above the knee and drain into the greater saphenous, femoral, or gluteal systems, were found in 18% of the limbs. Without preoperative mapping, surgical therapy is apt to be unsuccessful, leading to recurrence of varicose veins.

Duplex scanning is especially helpful for determining the cause of recurrent varicose veins. Among the problems identified are incompetent saphenofemoral junctions with or without residual greater saphenous veins, incompetent mid-thigh perforators, incompetent saphenopopliteal junction with or without residual lesser saphenous veins, and incompetent calf perforators.[40] Multiple sites are the rule. Associated deep venous incompetence is common, especially in patients with ulcers.

In patients with symptoms suggesting venous claudication, in whom arterial obstructive disease has been ruled out, the leg should be surveyed for chronic venous obstruction. This is most likely to involve a major axial vein, such as the iliac and common femoral. If obstruction is the major culprit, the obstruction must be localized so that it can be effectively bypassed. It is of little avail to perform a cross-pubic venous graft if in addition there is extensive distal obstruction.

Finally, duplex scanning applied prospectively to the study of patients recovering from an episode of DVT has contributed important information concerning the natural history of the disease. This information may aid in establishing better methods for the initial treatment of DVT and disclose which patients are most at risk for developing the signs and symptoms of chronic venous insufficiency. In addition, we need to know what proportion of patients with a particular pattern of venous incompetence have or go on to develop class 4–6 clinical signs. These data are sadly lacking.

REFERENCES

1. Sumner DS. Diagnosis of deep venous thrombosis. In Rutherford RB, ed. *Vascular Surgery*, 4th edn. Philadelphia: WB Saunders, 1995: 1698–743.
2. Nicolaides AN, Sumner DS. *Investigation of Patients with Deep Venous Thrombosis and Chronic Venous Insufficiency*. London: Med-Orion, 1991.
3. Folse R, Alexander RH. Directional flow detection for localizing venous valvular incompetency. *Surgery* 1970; **67**: 114–21.
4. Schultheiss R, Billeter M, Bollinger A, Franzeck UK. Comparison between clinical examination, cw-Doppler ultrasound and colour-duplex sonography in the diagnosis of incompetent perforating veins. *Eur J Vasc Endovasc Surg* 1997; **13**: 122–6.
5. McMullin GM, Coleridge Smith PD. An evaluation of Doppler ultrasound and photoplethysmography in the investigation of venous insufficiency. *Aust N Z J Surg* 1992; **62**: 270–5.
6. Weingarten MS, Branas CC, Czeredarczuk M, *et al.* Distribution and quantification of venous reflux in lower extremity chronic venous stasis disease with duplex scanning. *J Vasc Surg* 1993; **18**: 753–9.
7. Magnusson M, Kälebo P, Lukes P, *et al.* Colour Doppler ultrasound in diagnosing venous insufficiency, a comparison to descending phlebography. *Eur J Vasc Endovasc Surg* 1995; **9**: 437–43.
8. Rollins DL, Semrow CM, Friedell ML, Buchbinder D. Use of ultrasonic venography in the evaluation of venous valve function. *Am J Surg* 1987; **154**: 189–91.
9. van Rij AM, Solomon C, Christie R. Anatomic and physiologic characteristics of venous ulceration. *J Vasc Surg* 1994; **20**: 759–64.
10. Araki CT, Back TL, Padberg FT, *et al.* The significance of calf muscle pump function in venous ulceration. *J Vasc Surg* 1994; **20**: 872–9.
11. van Bemmelen PS, Bedford G, Beach K, Strandness DE. Quantitative segmental evaluation of venous valvular reflux with duplex ultrasound scanning. *J Vasc Surg* 1989; **10**: 425–31.
12. Lees TA, Lambert D. Patterns of venous reflux in limbs with skin changes associated with chronic venous insufficiency. *Br J Surg* 1993; **80**: 725–8.
13. Labropoulos N, Leon M, Geroulakos G, *et al.* Venous hemodynamic abnormalities in patients with leg ulceration. *Am J Surg* 1995; **169**: 572–4.
14. Masuda EM, Kistner RL, Eklof B. Prospective study of duplex scanning for venous reflux: comparison of Valsalva and pneumatic cuff techniques in the reverse Trendelenburg and standing positions. *J Vasc Surg* 1994; **20**: 711–20.
15. Markel A, Meissner MH, Manzo RA, *et al.* A comparison of the cuff deflation method with Valsalva's maneuver and limb compression in detecting venous valvular reflux. *Arch Surg* 1994; **129**: 701–5.
16. van Bemmelen PS, Beach K, Bedford G, Strandness DE. The mechanism of venous valve closure. Its relationship to the velocity of reverse flow. *Arch Surg* 1990; **125**: 617–19.
17. Hanrahan LM, Araki CT, Fisher JB, *et al.* Evaluation of the perforating veins of the lower extremity using high resolution duplex imaging. *J Cardiovasc Surg* 1991; **32**: 87–97.
18. Sarin S, Scurr JH, Coleridge Smith PD. Medial calf perforators in venous disease: the significance of outward flow. *J Vasc Surg* 1992; **16**: 40–6.
19. Vasdekis SN, Clarke GH, Nicolaides AN. Quantification of venous reflux by means of duplex scanning. *J Vasc Surg* 1989; **10**: 670–7.
20. Neglén P, Raju S. A rational approach to detection of significant reflux with duplex Doppler scanning and air plethysmography. *J Vasc Surg* 1993; **17**: 590–5.
21. van Bemmelen PS, Mattos MA, Hodgson KJ, *et al.* Does air plethysmography correlate with duplex scanning in patients with chronic venous insufficiency. *J Vasc Surg* 1993; **18**: 796–807.

22. Neglén P, Raju S. A comparison between descending phlebography and duplex Doppler investigation in the evaluation of reflux in chronic venous insufficiency: a challenge to phlebography as the 'gold standard'. *J Vasc Surg* 1992; **16**: 687–93.
23. Welch HJ, Faliakou EC, McLauglin RL, *et al.* Comparison of descending phlebography with quantitative photoplethysmography, air plethysmography, and duplex quantitative valve closure time in assessing deep venous reflux. *J Vasc Surg* 1992; **16**: 913–20.
24. Rodriguez AA, Whitehead CM, McLaughlin RL, *et al.* Duplex derived valve closure times fail to correlate with reflux flow volumes in patients with chronic venous insufficiency. *J Vasc Surg* 1996; **23**: 606–10.
25. Weingarten MS, Czeredarczuk M, Scovell S, *et al.* A correlation of air plethysmography and color flow-assisted duplex scanning in the quantification of chronic venous insufficiency. *J Vasc Surg* 1996; **24**: 750–4.
26. Baker SR, Burnand KG, Sommerville KM, *et al.* Comparison of venous reflux assessed by duplex scanning and descending phlebography in chronic venous disease. *Lancet* 1993; **341**: 400–3.
27. Masuda EM, Kistner RL. Prospective comparison of duplex scanning and descending venography in the assessment of venous insufficiency. *Am J Surg* 1992; **164**: 254–9.
28. Welkie JF, Comerota AJ, Katz ML, *et al.* Hemodynamic deterioration in chronic venous disease. *J Vasc Surg* 1992; **16**: 733–40.
29. Shull KC, Nicolaides AN, Fernandes é Fernandes J, *et al.* Significance of popliteal reflux in relation to ambulatory venous pressure and ulceration. *Arch Surg* 1979; **114**: 1304–6.
30. Moore DJ, Himmel PD, Sumner DS. Distribution of venous valvular incompetence in patients with the postphlebitic syndrome. *J Vasc Surg* 1986; **3**: 49–57.
31. Hanrahan LM, Araki CT, Rodriguez AA, *et al.* Distribution of valvular incompetence in patients with venous stasis ulceration. *J Vasc Surg* 1991; **13**: 805–12.
32. van Bemmelen PS, Bedford G, Beach K, Strandness DE. Status of the valves in the superficial and deep venous system in chronic venous disease. *Surgery* 1991; **109**: 730–4.
33. Myers KA, Ziegenbein RW, Zeng GH, Mathews PG. Duplex ultrasonography scanning for chronic venous disease: patterns of venous reflux. *J Vasc Surg* 1995; **21**: 605–12.
34. Shami SK, Sarin S, Cheatle TR, *et al.* Venous ulcers and the superficial venous system. *J Vasc Surg* 1993; **17**: 487–90.
35. Labropoulos N, Leon M, Nicolaides AN, *et al.* Superficial venous insufficiency: correlation of anatomic extent of reflux with clinical symptoms and signs. *J Vasc Surg* 1994; **20**: 953–8.
36. Gooley NA, Sumner DS. Relationship of venous reflux to the site of venous incompetence: implications for venous reconstructive surgery. *J Vasc Surg* 1988; **7**: 50–9.
37. Labropoulos N, Leon M, Nicolaides AN, *et al.* Venous reflux in patients with previous deep venous thrombosis: correlation with ulceration and other symptoms. *J Vasc Surg* 1994; **20**: 20–6.
38. Rosfors S, Lamke L-O, Nordström E, Bygdeman S. Severity and location of venous valvular insufficiency: the importance of distal valve function. *Acta Chir Scand* 1990; **156**: 689–94.
39. Farrah J, Saharay M, Georgiannos SN, Scurr JH, Smith PD. Variable venous anatomy of the popliteal fossa demonstrated by duplex scanning. *Dermatol Surg* 1998; **24**: 901–3.
40. Jiang P, van Rij AM, Christie R, *et al.* Recurrent varicose veins: patterns of reflux and clinical severity. *Cardiovasc Surg* 1999; **7**: 332–9.

13

Lower extremity ascending and descending phlebography

CURTIS B KAMIDA, ROBERT L KISTNER, BO ELKOF AND ELNA M MASUDA

Proper management of the patient with venous disease requires an accurate and objective diagnosis. Contrast phlebography has historically been considered the 'gold standard' against which all modalities are measured.[1] Recently, the widespread availability of duplex Doppler, color Doppler and compression ultrasound has reduced the role of contrast phlebography in the diagnosis of venous disease.[2] These noninvasive imaging methods have been shown to be accurate, relatively inexpensive, and safer than phlebography.[3] However, there are still instances where the use of more invasive phlebographic procedures is necessary. This chapter discusses the current role of these procedures in the clinical evaluation of the patient with venous disease.

Phlebography in the lower extremity can be done by several techniques depending upon the need of the individual case. Classical ascending phlebography is performed through a needle placed into the dorsum of the foot. Contrast is injected in order to outline the veins of the foot, calf, thigh and pelvis. Direct puncture of the popliteal vein or common femoral vein and subsequent passage of a catheter for selective injection of contrast will often show vein detail not easily seen with a foot injection. Similarly, puncture of the greater saphenous vein or the posterior tibial veins at the ankle can be performed as a prelude to catheter-directed thrombolysis. Varicography is a method that can be used to locate the sites of origin and termination of individual varices and to identify perforators. This is performed by injecting contrast directly into the varix itself.

Descending phlebography, first performed by Bauer,[4] is a method of identifying the site of valves in the veins and studying their degree of competence.[5–7] It is done by placing the contrast into the common femoral or external iliac vein with the patient in a semi-erect position.

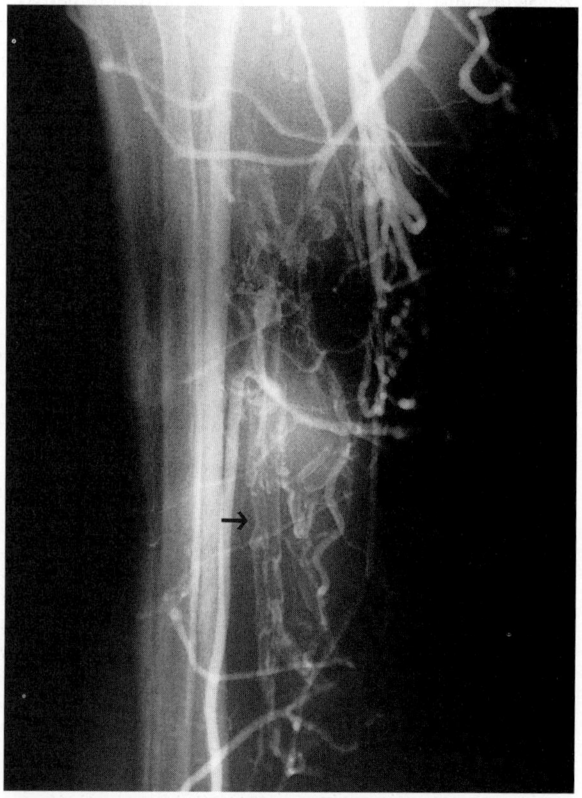

Figure 13.1 *Arrow points to clot in tibial veins, which were not adequately seen with ultrasound.*

INDICATIONS FOR PHLEBOGRAPHY

Acute deep venous thrombosis

In the diagnosis of acute deep venous thrombosis, the ultrasound examination has largely replaced phlebography for routine diagnosis, and the indications for phlebography are now selective.[8] These include cases:

- when the duplex scan is not definitive. Infrapopliteal veins are often difficult to evaluate (Fig. 13.1). Three studies that evaluated conventional duplex for diagnosis of calf vein deep thrombosis had a cumulative positive predictive value of 81%, with a range of 69–85%.[9–11]
- where iliofemoral venous thrombosis exists and thrombectomy is planned (Fig. 13.2). In this instance, the precise location of the top of the thrombus is needed. Due to overlying bowel gas and the depth of the vessels, iliac veins can often be difficult to visualize on an ultrasound examination.[3]
- when catheter-directed thrombosis is being considered (Fig. 13.3).
- where the duplex scan does not satisfy the suspicions of the clinician. In particular, patients with a duplicated superficial femoral vein may be a significant source of error in the diagnosis of deep vein thrombosis.[12,13] In one study, 46% of phlebograms demonstrated duplicated or even more complex superficial femoral veins.[12]

In all these instances, phlebography can clarify intraluminal details that are suggested by the ultrasound scan. A detailed and comprehensive duplex scan may be the only test required, but adoption of abbreviated ultrasound examination protocols may lead to a decrease in

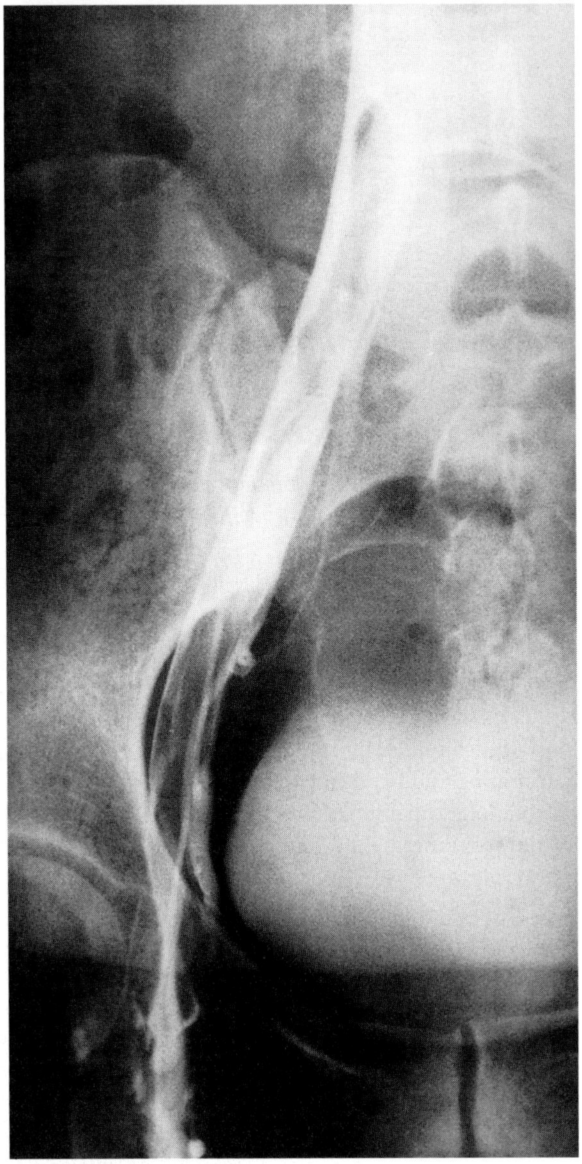

Figure 13.2 *Large thrombus in common iliac vein. The top of the thrombus is well visualized. A contralateral catheter can be pulled back into the opposite common iliac vein to determine the precise location of iliac vein confluence.*

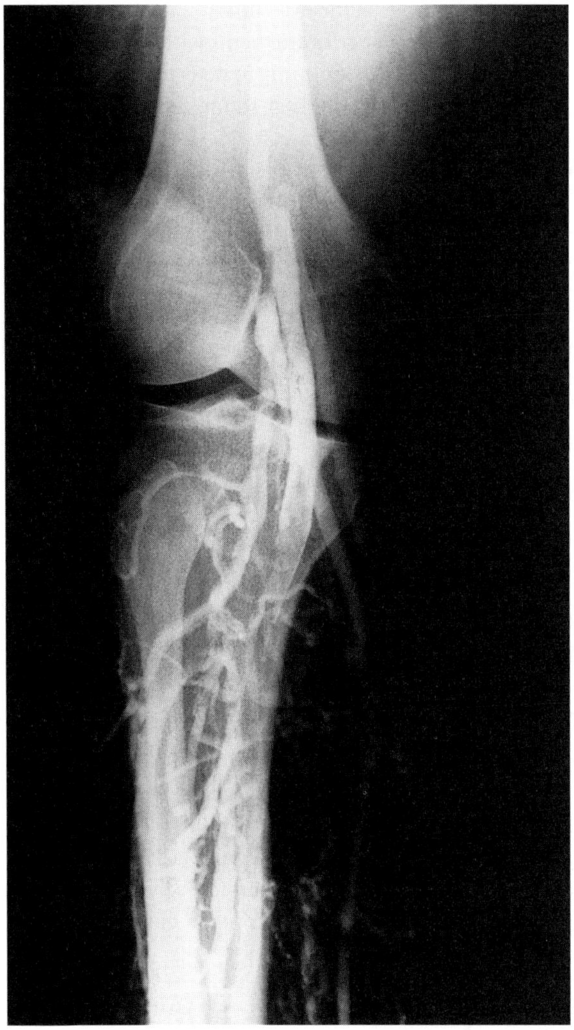

Figure 13.3 *Clot in popliteal vein. In planning catheter-directed thrombolysis, the catheter should be directed into the vein containing clot.*

sensitivity and the need for a more definitive imaging procedure such as phlebography.[14]

Chronic venous disease

The indications for phlebography in chronic venous disease depend upon the type of treatment that will be considered for the patient. Where the diagnosis is only a prelude for use of elastic support, there is little practical need to know the details of reflux and obstruction in a given extremity since the treatment will always be the same and phlebography will rarely be needed. Quite the converse is the case for those who are candidates for surgical therapy, since the treatment will depend upon the precise details of obstruction and reflux, segment by segment, throughout the extremity. The contributions made by ascending phlebography in chronic venous disease are the following:

- a map of the entire venous system in the extremity that is useful for study of the relationship between the various findings in the extremity;
- detailed study of perforator veins with the use of tourniquets and positioning to determine the site and size of perforators and their connections to the deep and superficial veins (Fig. 13.4);
- differentiation of primary venous disease from secondary (post-thrombotic) disease (Fig. 13.5);
- identification of collateral patterns, especially in the thigh, around the knee, and at the iliofemoral level.

In cases where these advantages are useful in planning surgery or deciding whether the patient is a surgical candidate, ascending phlebography is indicated.

The points gained from descending phlebography are as follows:[15]

- identification of the site of proximal valves down to the first component valve in each axial vein of the extremity, including greater saphenous vein, superficial femoral vein and profunda femoris vein;
- definition of the degree of competence of each valve;
- an accurate differential diagnosis between primary and secondary valve incompetence;
- determination of the distal extent of incompetence in the femoral and popliteal segments down to the tibial and perforator veins.

Descending phlebography is an absolute necessity for the patient who is considered for valvuloplasty operations in primary venous insufficiency or for valve substitution procedures in secondary venous insufficiency.

TECHNIQUES OF PHLEBOGRAPHY

Patient preparation for phlebography involves the usual precautions taken before administration of any intra-vascular x-ray contrast material. Anticoagulation is not a contraindication. A tilting table capable of fluoroscopy, spot filming and overhead 14 × 17 inch films is desired. Videotaping capabilities are often useful but not an absolute requirement. The contrast material most commonly used is of moderate concentration. This is generally 200–400 mg iodine per ml. Higher concentrations of contrast are associated with an increase in patient discomfort and an increased risk of contrast-associated thrombosis.[16] The use of non-ionic or low-osmolality contract media reduces patient discomfort, 'allergic' reactions, nephrotoxicity and post-phlebographic thrombosis, but with a considerable increase in the cost of the examination. The American College of Radiology has not taken a position on whether non-ionic contrast media should be used universally or selectively, but it does publish guidelines for identifying high-risk patients who would benefit from non-ionic contrast media.[17]

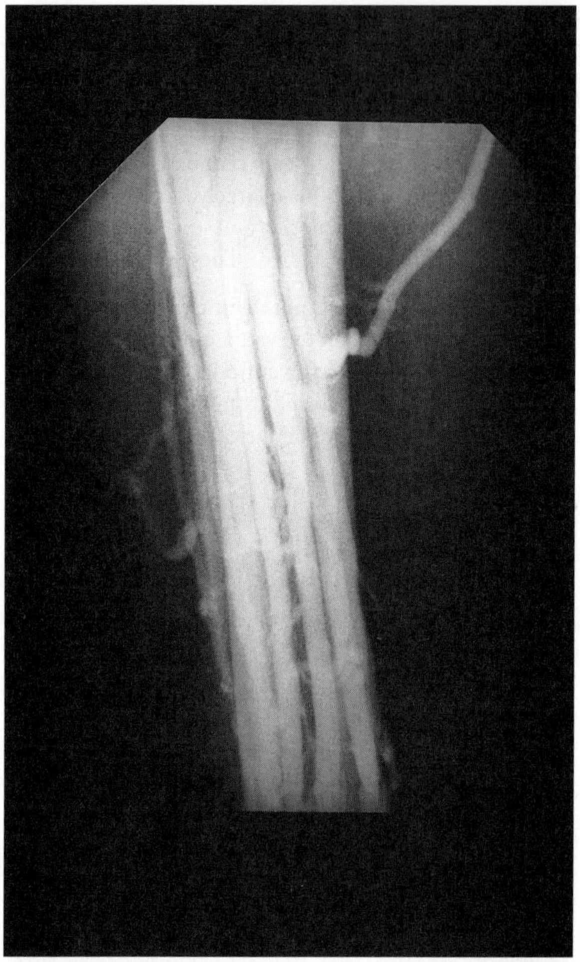

Figure 13.4 *Incompetent perforating vein observed during phlebogram performed with ankle tourniquet which forces contrast into deep system.*

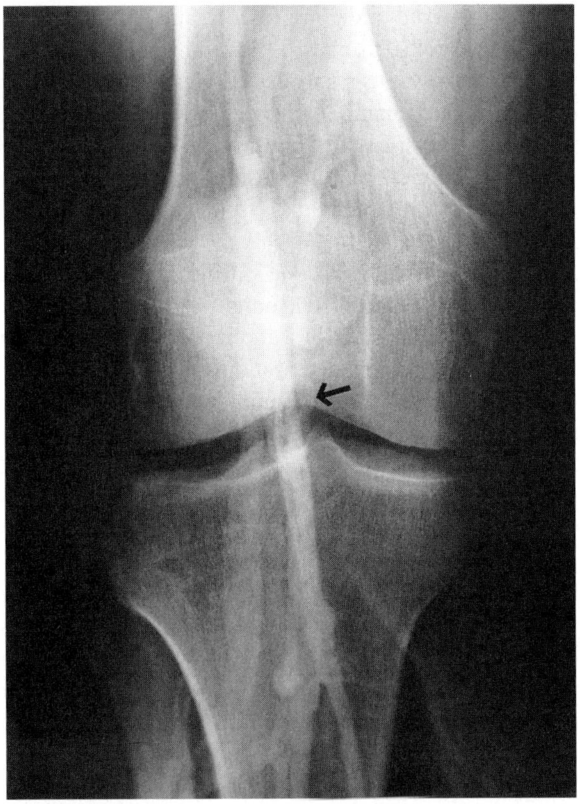

Figure 13.5 *Webs and synechiae in the popliteal vein are evidence of a previous thrombosis and recanalization.*

Ascending phlebography

An adaptation of the method of Rabinov and Paulin[18] is used in our institution. Approximately 100 ml contrast is injected per leg. Venipuncture is performed with a small needle (usually a 22 or 21 gauge butterfly) inserted into a vein on the dorsum of the foot. Ideally, the examination is done with the patient upright. The leg to be examined is made non-weight-bearing by placing a box under the other foot. Since muscle contractions decrease deep venous filling, the patient is instructed to relax the non-weight-bearing leg. The upright position (60° is usually sufficient) produces an increase in hydrostatic pressure, which results in better opacification of the veins and delays venous emptying, giving the examiner more time for positioning and filming. Directing the needle toward the toes may give better filling of the foot veins.[19]

The use of an ankle tourniquet increases the risk of contrast extravasation at the venipuncture site. It can also cause non-filling of the anterior tibial veins and poor opacification of the gastrocnemius muscular veins.[20] We do not initially use an ankle tourniquet unless there is so much superficial vein filling that the deep veins are inadequately visualized. However, the use of a tourniquet above the knee can aid in calf filling if the patient cannot be examined in the upright position, and can be used if the only available venipuncture site is a superficial vein in an area other than the dorsum of the foot.[21] When ascending phlebography is performed to evaluate perforating veins, ankle tourniquets are used initially. Contrast selectively enters the deep veins and incompetent perforating veins can be identified when the contrast flows from the deep to the superficial system.

Overhead 14 × 17 inch films are taken of the entire extremity. In the upright position, orthogonal views of the calf and then the knee and lower thigh are obtained after 50–70 ml contrast has been injected. The table is lowered to 15–30° and a film of the upper thigh and groin is obtained. The last film is an overhead supine view of the iliac veins and lower inferior vena cava. This is obtained by rapidly lowering the table, elevating the leg, or having the patient dorsiflex the foot against resistance and immediately taking a radiograph. Better opacification of the pelvic veins and lower inferior vena cava can also be obtained by manual compression over the femoral vein at the groin prior to lowering the table. This decrease in vein emptying can be augmented by having the patient perform a Valsalva maneuver. When the table is brought to the horizontal position, the compression is released and a deep inspiration is performed.[22]

Direct puncture of varices can be done with a small needle and contrast injected with fluoroscopic observation. The table tilt may be adjusted to guide filling in the proximal or distal direction. This test is used to find the communications of varices with the deep system, and to identify sites of perforator veins. It is particularly useful in the thigh, whereas ascending phlebography with foot injection and ankle tourniquets usually adequately identifies perforators in the calf.[24]

Ascending popliteal, femoral, posterior tibial and saphenous phlebography

In angiographic evaluation of the arterial system, it is a well-known fact that selective or super-selective catheterization with contract injection close to the area to be evaluated usually gives better visualization. In a similar fashion, contrast injection close to areas of concern in the venous system allows for better delineation of normal and abnormal anatomy. In fact, although aortic injection is often used for opacification of pedal arteries, injection of contrast in foot veins does not usually result in adequate opacification of the inferior vena cava. This is predominantly due to the inflow of unopacified blood and venous return, which dilutes contrast injected at a site distant from the area to be examined. Several techniques have been developed to aid in the evaluation of the larger axial veins. These all involve either a venipuncture site close to the area of interest, or the passage of angiographic catheters from a distant site to the area of interest.

Ascending popliteal phlebography is done by puncturing the popliteal vein in the popliteal fossa and introducing a catheter into the popliteal vein by the Seldinger technique.[25] Puncture is aided by ultrasound guidance or by fluoroscopic identification of the popliteal vein after foot injection. In the prone position, contrast injection through a catheter can locate perforators, duplications, valves and post-thrombotic changes. In a similar fashion, optimal visualization of the pelvic veins and inferior vena cava is easily obtained with direct puncture of the common femoral vein and passage of a multi-sidehole angiographic catheter with power injection.

Although primarily used as a prelude to catheter-directed thrombolysis, access to the venous system via the posterior tibial veins or great saphenous vein at the ankle allows for catheter passage into many of the veins for more selective contrast injections.[26]

INTERPRETATION OF THE ASCENDING PHLEBOGRAPHY

The definitive finding on ascending phlebography in acute deep venous thrombosis is the presence of an intraluminal filling defect. A non-filling segment of vein or the abrupt termination of a contrast column is not a reliable sign of deep venous thrombosis. Both extrinsic and intrinsic pressure phenomena can change the flow pattern within the veins and can lead to interpretive errors. The presence of 'well-developed' collaterals implies venous occlusion, but the age is often difficult to determine and the cause may not be intraluminal thrombus.[18] Linear webs and synechiae within the veins usually implies chronic changes, but acute clot can be superimposed and present as more rounded and larger filling defects. Difficulty in interpretation can often be reduced by a more careful and detailed examination using appropriate amounts of contrast, positioning the patient to facilitate deep vein filling, and the judicious use of tourniquets. Fluoroscopic observation of the pattern of vein filling is mandatory when the site of incompetent perforators is being determined.

Descending phlebography

This is performed on a fluoroscopic table of at least 60° of tilt. We strongly believe in videotaping the procedure and obtaining spot films during the course of the examination. An audio tract is usually necessary for independent review of the tape after the procedure. The catheter generally needs to be positioned above the valve to be examined so that contrast can be injected retrograde to venous return. The contralateral common femoral vein is the usual site of the venipuncture, although a brachial or antecubital approach can also be used. Contrast is hand injected in boluses of 10–20 ml with the patient in an upright position. The examined leg is non-weight-bearing, similar to ascending phlebography. The level of reflux is observed under fluoroscopy and graded according to the classification of Kistner and associates.[6]

Controversy exists regarding the ideal patient position during the performance of descending phlebography. We feel that the semi-erect position is ideal, and have found that the horizontal (supine) position underestimates the extent and degree of reflux, as published by Raju and Fredericks.[7]

Contrast injection is done during a forced Valsalva maneuver, and heparin (5000 units) is given intravenously prior to selective catheterization of any of the vein segments. Selective catheterization of the axial veins is usually easy to perform. All manipulations across the valve are done while the patient is supine. Slight ankle plantar flexion against resistance increases venous return flow and prevents valve leaflet closure when maneuvering across the valve. Selective catheterization is used to define venous incompetence in any segment independent of the dynamics in an adjacent segment. For example, if the greater saphenous vein shows massive reflux when contrast is injected in the common femoral vein, it is possible to mask important reflux in the superficial femoral or profunda femoral vein. Catheter manipulation with injection below the greater saphenous vein orifice allows for separate evaluation of the other axial veins (Figs 13.6,

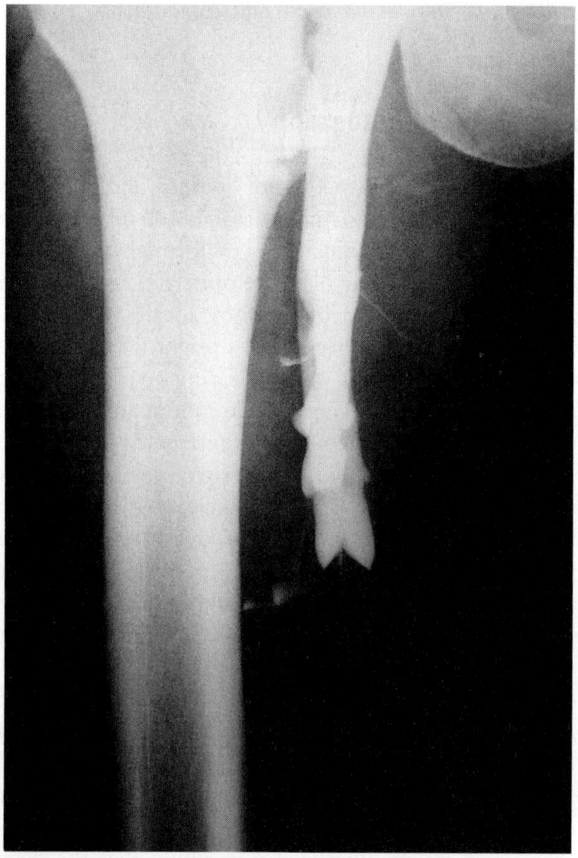

Figure 13.6 *Descending venogram spot film showing competent valves. The proximal axial veins are often superimposed on the AP view.*

13.7). With a catheter of sufficient length, selective catheterization can be done down the superficial femoral vein to search for perforators and to study the popliteal vein valves more directly.

INTERPRETATION OF DESCENDING PHLEBOGRAPHY

Accurate interpretation requires demonstration of the valves in each major axial segment, including the greater saphenous vein, superficial femoral vein, profunda femoris vein, and any collateral pathways. Normally, blood flow is toward the heart with quiet breathing. A Valsalva maneuver initially causes cessation of prograde flow, and then actual flow reversal. It is this retrograde blood flow that causes the valve cusps to close. Contrast will outline the cusps in sharp relief, with the vein at the valve station visibly dilating in its sinus portion. No contrast leaks through the competent valve except for a small wisp, which may be accepted as normal physiologic reflux occurring as the valve cusps close. If the proximal valves are fully competent, descending phlebography will not visualize the more distal vein unless selective catheterization through the valve is performed (Fig. 13.8).

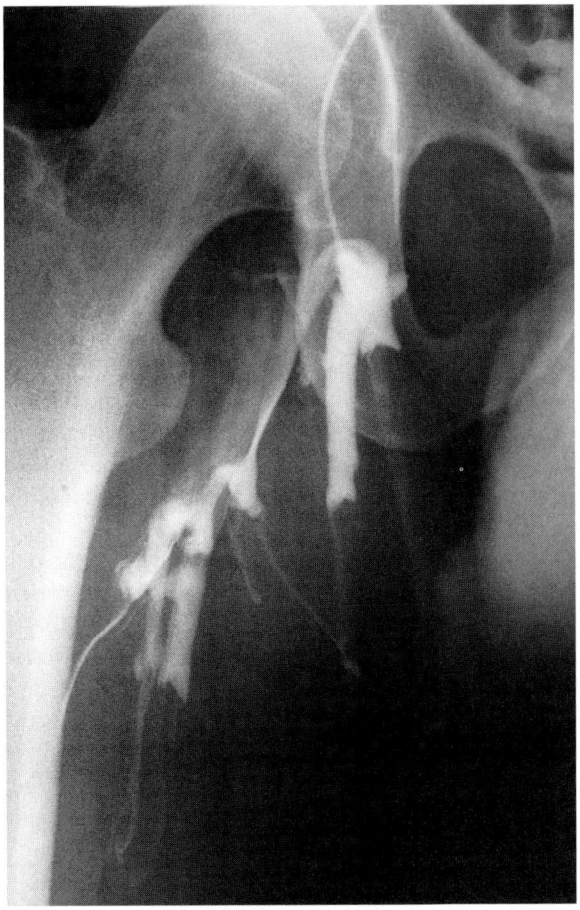

Figure 13.7 *Same patient as in Fig. 13.6. In the ipsilateral anterior oblique view and with selective catheterization, the origins of the axial veins are no longer superimposed.*

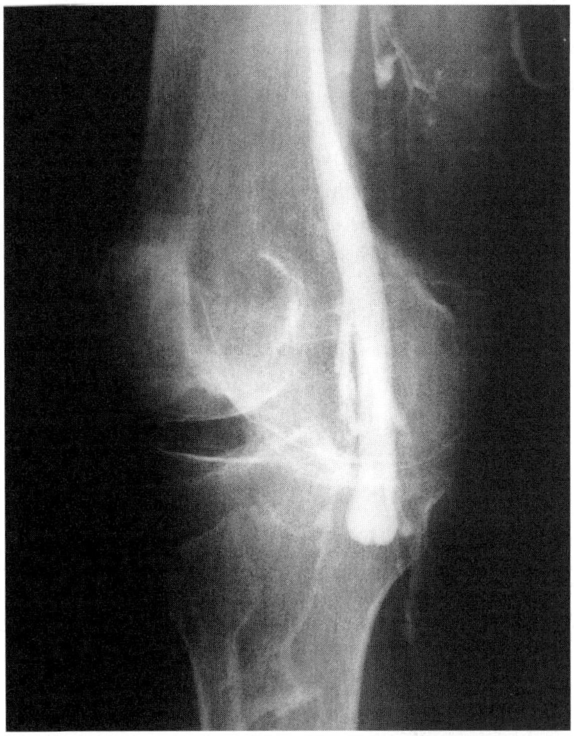

Figure 13.8 *Competent popliteal vein valve. Selective injection into superficial femoral vein beyond a competent common femoral vein valve.*

The Valsalva maneuver is essential to the performance of accurate descending phlebography. It can be standardized by having the patient practice the maneuver prior to the venogram by blowing against a blood pressure manometer up to 40 mmHg resistance. The inability to perform an adequate and effective Valsalva maneuver limits the phlebographic accuracy in an uncooperative patient.

We strongly feel that videotaping the examination is important as real-time visualization of the flow dynamics and a narrated description of the position of the patient and the performance of the Valsalva maneuver are essential for the clinician. Since the valves remain open to allow blood flow to return in the erect position, normal reflux of small amounts of contrast with quiet breathing can be erroneously reported as reflux. Slight retrograde flow of contrast will also occur in the beginning stages of the forced Valsalva maneuver, as the initial retrograde blood flow is insufficient to cause the proximal resistance which forces the competent valve to close. A spot film obtained during these stages can give the erroneous appearance of reflux and a false-positive result. A false-negative result can also be obtained if the injection of contrast and the Valsalva maneuver are too weak. In this instance, poorly opacified blood will flow toward the heart along with normal venous return, and no information regarding the valve's competency will be elicited.

The grading of reflux is according to the system previously reported:[6]

- grade 0: competent valve with no reflux. There is a clear outline of the valve cusps during the Valsalva maneuver (Fig. 13.9).
- grade 1: wisps of reflux limited to upper thigh.
- grade 2: definite reflux, but limited to the upper thigh by competent valves in the distal thigh or popliteal vein.
- grade 3: reflux through the popliteal vein and into the calf.
- grade 4: massive cascading reflux through the popliteal vein, into the calf, and frequently through incompetent perforating veins.

COMPLICATIONS OF PHLEBOGRAPHY

Phlebography introduces expense, discomfort and risks to the patient, which need to be taken into account in the work-up of the patient with a venous disorder.[27] These risks include the usual reactions to iodinated contrast. This does not differ from other procedures such as intravenous pyelography. An important risk is the potential for post-procedural vein thrombosis. Contrast agents are an irritant to the intima, and can result in thrombosis. Prospective clinical trial data suggest that this occurs in 1–2% of cases.[28] This can be reduced by frequent flushing of the veins with saline to minimize prolonged contact of the contrast with the venous intima, using dilute contrast for certain examinations such as varicography, the use of non-ionic contrast material, and the concurrent use of 3000–5000 units of heparin during selective catheterization. Extravasation of contrast can result in skin necrosis and can be avoided by careful monitoring of the injection site with fluoroscopy. Treatment of extravasation is controversial and can include cold compresses to reduce pain as well as hot compresses to increase local blood flow and absorption of the extravasated dye.[17]

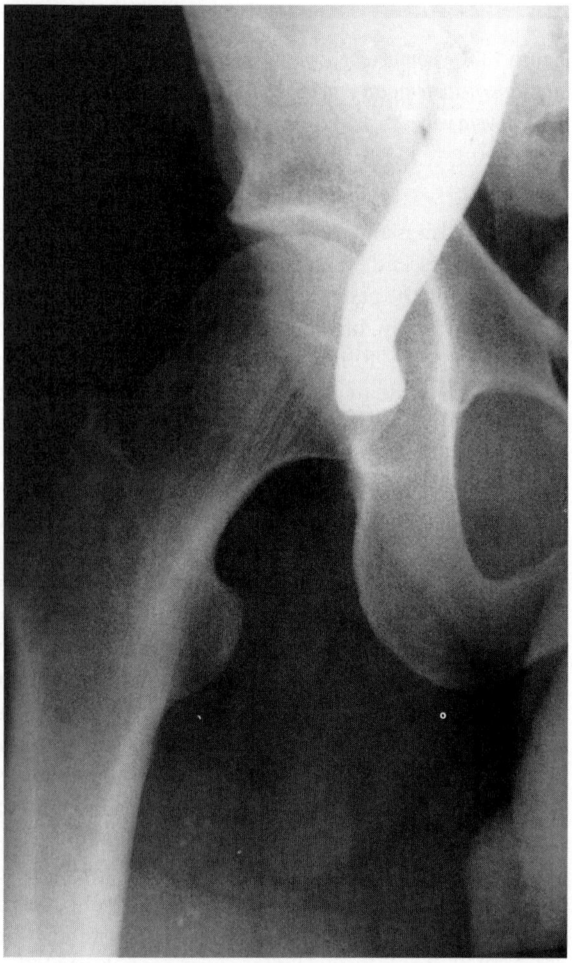

Figure 13.9 *Descending phlebogram demonstrates a competent valve in the common femoral vein, which precludes filling of the superficial femoral, greater saphenous, and profunda femoral veins.*

CONCLUSION

The diagnosis of acute and chronic venous disease requires accurate delineation of the venous system, including the deep veins, superficial veins, and perforators. With the development of sophisticated duplex scan techniques, the need for contrast phlebography has been drastically reduced, but it remains a valuable tool in selected circumstances.

Ascending phlebography is often more accurate than ultrasound in detecting thrombi in the calf and pelvis. In the instance of a difficult duplex exam, phlebography can be used to resolve unanswered questions. Phlebography is still the most accurate method to differentiate primary from secondary causes of chronic venous disease. We believe that descending phlebography is necessary in the candidate for deep venous reconstructive surgery, and gives better anatomic detail of the valves and valve stations.

Although ultrasound is the initial and often the only imaging modality used in the work-up of the patient with venous disease, contrast phlebography continues to be a necessary part of the definitive evaluation of venous disease in the difficult diagnostic case and in the preoperative evaluation for deep vein reconstructive surgery. A recent letter by Reid and Hardwick in the *British Medical Journal* makes an interesting point. When communicating on an abbreviated duplex ultrasonography scanning protocol, they state that 'venography is as invasive as taking a blood sample, and reactions to modern contrast material are as rare as hen's teeth. Slavish pursuit of non-invasive alternatives to an accurate test which can never be considered a serious intervention may not be worth the trade-off'.[29]

Phlebography is a necessity in acute deep vein thrombosis to:

- identify the top of the thrombus before surgery for iliofemoral DVT. 'Fracture' of a thrombus popping up into the IVC can kill the patient;
- identify the extent of the thrombus before catheter-directed thrombolysis, and to evaluate morphology and function of treated valves.

Phlebography is important in chronic venous disease to:

- differentiate between primary and secondary disease;
- identify the extent and nature of any obstruction, particularly of the common femoral and iliac veins;
- evaluate the degree of reflux and the morphology of the valves.

REFERENCES

1. Cranley JJ, Canos AJ, Sull WF. The diagnosis of deep venous thrombosis: fallability of clinical symptoms and signs. *Arch Surg* 1976; **111**: 34–6.
2. Montefusco-van Kliest CM, Bakal C, Spraygen S, *et al.* Comparison of duplex ultrasonography and ascending venography in the diagnosis of venous thrombosis. *Angiology* 1993; **44**: 169–75.
3. Douglas MG, Sumner DS. Duplex scanning for deep vein thrombosis: has it replaced both phlebography and non-invasive testing? *Semin Vasc Surg* 1996; **9**: 3–12.
4. Bauer G. The etiology of leg ulcers and their treatment by resection of the popliteal vein. *J Int Chir* 1948; **8**: 937–67.
5. Herman RJ, Neiman HL, Yao JST, *et al.* Descending venography: a method of evaluating lower extremity venous valvular function. *Radiology* 1980; **137**: 63–9.
6. Kistner, RL, Ferris RG, Randhawa G, Kamida CB. A method of performing descending venography. *J Vasc Surg* 1986; **4**: 464–8.
7. Raju S, Fredericks R. Evaluation of methods for detecting venous reflux. *Arch Surg* 1990; **125**: 1463–7.
8. Quintavalla R, Larini P, Miselli A, *et al.* Duplex ultrasound diagnosis of symptomatic proximal deep vein thrombosis of lower limbs. *Eur J Radiol* 1992; **15**: 32–6.
9. Elias A, LeCorff G, Bouvier JL. Value of real-time ultrasound imaging in the diagnosis of deep vein thrombosis of the lower limbs. *Int Angiol* 1987; **6**: 175–82.
10. Fletcher JP, Kershaw LZ, Barker DS, *et al.* Ultrasound diagnosis of lower limb deep venous thrombosis. *Med J Aust* 1990; **153**: 453–5.
11. Mitchell DC, Grasty MS, Stebbings WSL, *et al.* Comparison of duplex ultrasonography and venography in the diagnosis of deep venous thrombosis. *Br J Surg* 1991; **78**: 611–13.
12. Screaton NJ, Gillard JH, Berman LH Kemp PM. Duplicated superficial femoral veins: a source of error in the sonographic investigation of deep vein thrombosis. *Radiology* 1998; **206**: 397–401.
13. Pasquariello F, Kurol M, Wilberg S, *et al.* Diagnosis of deep venous thrombosis of the lower limbs: is it premature to introduce ultrasound as a routine method. *Angiology* 1999; **50**: 31–6.
14. Cogo A, Lensing AWA, Koopman MMW, *et al.* Compression ultrasonography for diagnostic management of patients with clinically suspected deep vein thrombosis: prospective cohort study. *Br Med J* 1998; **316**: 17–20.
15. Kistner RL, Kamida CB. 1994 Update on phlebology and varicography. *Dermatol Surg* 1995; **21**: 71–6.
16. Albrightson U, Olsson CG. Thrombotic side effects of lower limb phlebography. *Lancet* 1976; **1**: 723–4.
17. American College of Radiology. *Manual on Contrast Media*, 4th edn. Reston, VA: American College of Radiology, 1998.
18. Rabinov K, Paulin S. Roentgen diagnosis of venous thrombosis in the leg. *Arch Surg* 1972; **104**: 134–44.
19. Kadir S. *Diagnostic Angiography.* Philadelphia: WB Saunders, 1986: 536–83.
20. Kalebo P, Anthmyr BA, Erikkson BI, Zachrisson BE. Optimization of ascending phlebography of the leg for screening of deep vein thrombosis in thromboprophylactic trials. *Acta Radiol* 1997; **38**: 320–6.
21. Gordon DH, Glanz S, Stillman R, Sawyer PN. Descending varicose venography of the lower extremities: an alternate method to evaluate the deep venous system. *Radiology* 1982; **145**: 832–4.
22. Kim D, Orron DE, Porter DH. Venographic anatomy, technique and interpretation. In Kim D, Orron DE, eds. *Peripheral Vascular Imaging and Intervention.* St Louis, MO: Mosby Year Book, 1992: 269–350.
23. Thomas ML, Bowles JN. Incompetent perforating veins: comparison of varicography and ascending phlebography. *Radiology* 1985; **154**: 619–23.
24. Savolainen H, Toivio I, Mokka R. Recurrent varicose veins: is there a role for varicography? *Ann Chir Gynecol* 1998; **77**: 70.
25. Perrin J, Bolot JE, Genevois A, Hiltbrand B. Dynamic popliteal phlebography. *Phlebology* 1998; **3**: 227–35.
26. Cragg AH. Lower extremity deep venous thrombolysis: a new approach to obtaining access. *J Vasc Interv Radiol* 1996; **7**: 283–8.
27. Bettmann MA, Paulin S. Leg phlebography: the incidence, nature and modification of undesirable side effects. *Radiology* 1977; **122**: 101–4.
28. Hull R, Hirsch J, Sackett DL, *et al.* Clinical validity of a negative venogram in patients with clinically suspected venous thrombosis. *Circulation* 1981: **64**: 622–5.
29. Reid JH, Hardwich DJ. Compression ultrasonography for diagnosing deep vein thrombosis: venography is more accurate. *Br Med J* 1998; **316**: 1532.

14

Direct venous pressure: role in the assessment of venous disease

ELNA M MASUDA, BERNDT ARFVIDSSON, BO EKLOF AND ROBERT L KISTNER

Elevated venous pressure in the leg is acknowledged as the fundamental pathology which leads to symptoms and signs of venous insufficiency. There are generally two sites in the leg where venous pressures are measured: the dorsal foot vein and/or the femoral vein. Abnormal venous pressures at these sites are the result of either venous obstruction, valvular dysfunction and/or calf muscle pump dysfunction that may lead to symptoms of swelling, pain, lipodermatosclerosis, hyperpigmentation and ulceration.

Historically, the ambulatory venous pressure (AVP) was considered the 'gold standard' test for the physiologic derangement observed in chronic venous insufficiency. AVP represents the global measurement of venous insufficiency in the limb and is the product of venous obstruction, valvular reflux and calf muscle pump failure. It cannot be used to separate the effects of each of these three contributing factors. Since pressure measurements are obtained by placing a needle into the foot, it is not an ideal test for screening or repeat examinations. Currently, AVP testing is used primarily as a research tool and has been replaced in the clinical setting by noninvasive tests such as color-flow duplex scanning, air plethysmography and photoplethysmography.

In contrast to AVP testing, direct femoral vein pressures has been applied more often in the clinical setting. Femoral venous pressures provide information of the venous outflow tract in the iliac and inferior vena cava, and may be useful in determining whether femoral crossover bypass or iliac balloon angioplasty and stenting may be physiologically beneficial.

The goal of this chapter is to describe the techniques of venous pressure measurements for the researcher and clinician, and discuss the interpretation of these values.

HISTORY

At rest, venous pressures are no different between limbs normal and those with varicose veins.[1,2] In 1895, Perthes observed that in normal limbs, pressures in veins decreased with ambulation.[3] By contrast, those with varicose veins showed pressures that failed to fall with exercise unless the superficial veins were occluded above the area examined. Perthes' conclusion was made by placing a rubber band around the calf and venous pressure fall was estimated by contraction of the band. This was one of the first descriptions of ambulatory venous pressures.

With more direct methods of testing, Pollack and Wood showed that ambulation produced a normal drop in the venous pressure at the foot as a result of the emptying of veins by the calf muscle pump.[4] When walking stopped, there was a gradual rise in foot pressures back to baseline.

Others studied the effects of straining on venous pressures in normals and varicose limbs. Delbet found a tremendous increase in pressure on straining when saphenous vein pressure was measured in the thigh with a mercury manometer.[5] In 1939, Adams showed that straining in patients with varicose veins caused venous pressures to increase as high as 224 mmHg, over twice the pressures induced by straining in normal limbs.[1]

METHOD

The examination is performed by inserting a small butterfly needle such as a 20 or 21 gauge into a superficial dorsal foot or ankle vein. Alternatively, a small catheter with 0.5 mm internal diameter may be used. Preferably, the largest vein in the foot or ankle such as the greater saphenous vein should be selected to allow the needle to lie comfortably inside the vein, without impinging on the vein wall which may cause damping of the tracing. Measurements are taken in the standing position with or without tourniquet followed by exercise in the form of toe lifts. In order to localize the level of disease and distinguish between superficial and deep venous disease, tourniquets are applied at the ankle, below the knee, and above the knee. The ideal tourniquet pressure would be that which occludes the superficial veins but not the deep veins. The recommended tourniquet pressures are based on the study by Nicolaides and Yao who showed that a pressure of 120 mmHg at the ankle and 180 mmHg at the thigh was adequate for occlusion of the superficial veins without obstructing the deep system.[6] This was observed when a narrow 2.5 cm cuff was used in subjects with average soft tissue thickness. Since several variables can affect the efficacy of the cuff, such as the width of the tourniquet, thickness of the limb, anatomy of the veins and presence of arterial occlusive disease, the inflation pressure may need to be adjusted based on these factors.

EXERCISE

To test the efficacy of the calf muscle pump in emptying the veins, the subject must be studied in the standing position. The most common form of exercise is to have the patient raise the heel off the ground repeatedly at the rate of once per second. A metronome can be used to regulate the rate. Exercise is continued until the maximal pressure fall is reached and stabilizes. The subject stops exercising and the time for the pressure to return to baseline is recorded as the refill time. Some centers have advocated measuring the time at 90% of the total time required to reach baseline, which may be more accurately defined than the end point of full recovery.[7]

INTERPRETATION OF STUDY

Ambulatory venous pressure measurements are assessed by examining two parameters: the maximum drop in foot pressure or percentage fall during ambulation, and refill rate. Normal values for ambulatory venous pressure may vary from laboratory to laboratory and therefore it is essential that each laboratory establish its own normal values. Resting foot venous pressure when the subject is quietly standing is usually 80–90 mmHg, and represents the hydrostatic pressure created by a column of blood between the atrium and the foot. With exercise, most groups report a fall in pressure from 80–90 mmHg to 20–30 mmHg, or a pressure drop greater than 50%.[4,8] Normal refill time is defined as greater than 20 seconds.[9] An example of a normal ambulatory venous pressure tracing is shown in Fig. 14.1.

Abnormal values of ambulatory venous pressure are defined by lack of sufficient drop in pressure with ambulation and/or short refill time. In both reflux disease (Fig. 14.2) and obstructive disease (Fig. 14.3),

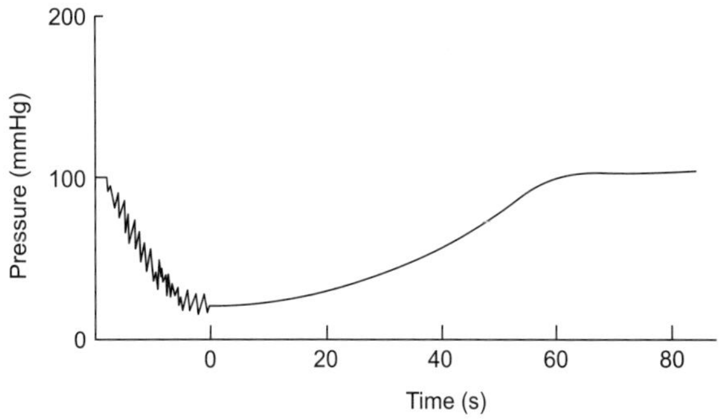

Figure 14.1 *Ambulatory venous pressure tracing in normal limb. (Adapted from Schanzer H, Peirce EC II. Pathophysiologic evaluation of chronic venous stasis with ambulatory venous pressure studies.* Angiology *1982;* ***33****: 183–91).*

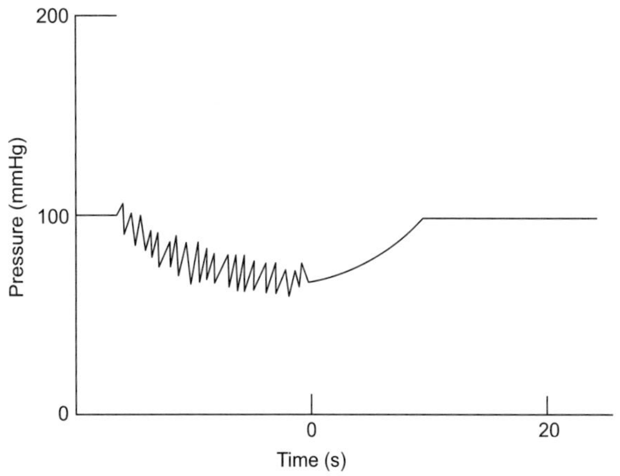

Figure 14.2 *Ambulatory venous pressure tracing deep vein incompetence. Note the lack of fall in pressure during exercise (less than 50% drop) and the short refill time (less than 20 seconds). (Adapted from Schanzer H, Peirce EC II. Pathophysiologic evaluation of chronic venous stasis with ambulatory venous pressure studies.* Angiology *1982;* ***33****: 183–91).*

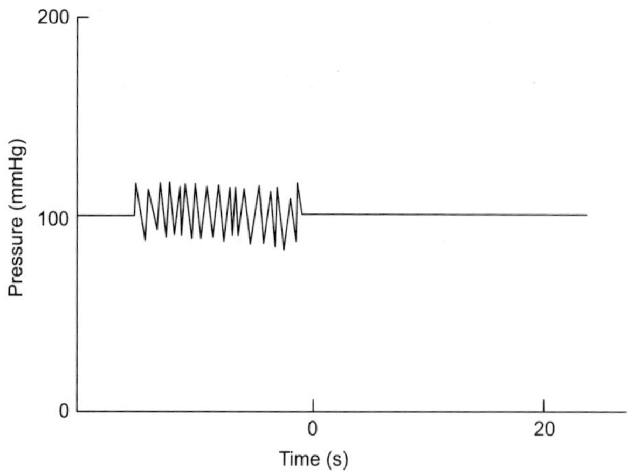

Figure 14.3 *Ambulatory venous pressure tracing deep vein obstruction. Note that the venous pressure does not decrease with exercise, and in fact may increase. (Adapted from Schanzer H, Peirce EC II. Pathophysiologic evaluation of chronic venous stasis with ambulatory venous pressure studies.* Angiology *1982;* **33***: 183–91).*

lack of fall in pressure and short refill times may be present. In severe venous obstruction, a rise in venous pressure may occur with ambulation. If an abnormal ambulatory venous pressure normalizes with tourniquet, this suggests that the disease is in the superficial system or perforators above the tourniquet. If pressures do not normalize with tourniquet, this suggests deep venous disease and/or perforator disease may exist below the tourniquet.

ACUTE OBSTRUCTION

Measurements of ambulatory venous pressure probably serve no useful application in the assessment of acute venous obstruction because, as a rule, physiologic obstruction produced by deep venous thrombosis improves with time as a result of thrombus lysis and recanalization. Therefore, hemodynamically significant obstruction following deep venous thrombosis is not frequently observed. Hemodynamic compromise is observed with phlegmasia cerulea dolens where venous obstruction is so extensive that circulatory compromise ensues. In the most extreme cases of phlegmasia cerulea dolens, venous pressures may reach values 16–17 times normal within 6 hours.[10] Trivial elevations in foot pressures are found in cases of 'silent' deep venous thrombosis[11] and, in the supine position, Husni[12] found mean pressures of 17 mmHg, or 2.5 times that in normal limbs. This difference is not detected when subjects are asked to stand quietly and is probably masked by the hydrostatic pressure produced by the erect position. With exercise, limbs with acute deep venous thrombosis produce sustained high venous pressures that fail to drop with ambulation.

CHRONIC OBSTRUCTION

The most important practical application of direct venous pressure measurements is to determine the hemodynamic significance of chronic venous obstruction in order to select cases that may benefit from venous bypass or endovascular procedures. The presence of an anatomic blockage of the venous system does not always produce abnormal venous hemodynamics and symptoms of venous insufficiency. It has been well demonstrated by Raju that phlebographic occlusion does not directly relate to severity of symptoms, and that limb compensation is strongly dependent on the presence of venous collaterals.[13] In order to determine significance of obstruction, several provocative tests have been described to determine severity of outflow obstruction.

Foot venous pressures

Ordinarily, in chronic venous obstruction, foot pressures are normal while standing quietly. However, with exercise, lack of drop in pressure, or in some cases an actual rise in foot pressure will signal the presence of significant outflow obstruction.[14] A method of determining outflow obstruction by arm and foot venous pressures was described by Raju[15] and is summarized in Table 14.1.[16] Needles were placed in the arm and foot and

Table 14.1 *Grading of obstruction*

		Arm/foot venous pressure differential (normal < 4 mmHg)	Reactive hyperemia foot venous pressure elevation (normal < 6 mmHg)
Grade I*	Fully compensated	<4 mmHg	<6 mmHg
Grade II	Partially compensated	<4 mmHg	>6 mmHg
Grade III	Partially decompensated	>4 mmHg	>6 mmHg
Grade IV	Fully decompensated	>4 mmHg	<6 mmHg†

*Paradoxical response.
†Since pressure parameters for both tests are normal, accurate diagnosis depends on Doppler and/or venography.

pressures were measured with and without a tourniquet around the thigh to induce reactive hyperemia. In normal limbs, the pressure difference between the arm and the foot was found to be less than 4 mmHg. Patients with obstruction but with partial compensation showed a resting differential of less than 4 mmHg but under induced reactive hyperemia (ischemic cuff occlusion for 2 minutes), showed an elevation in foot pressure greater than 6 mmHg. Paradoxically, in the highly decompensated obstruction, pressure under reactive hyperemia was found to be less than 6 mmHg due to fixed venous outflow, that restricted the expected increased inflow with hyperemia.

Venous pressures at the foot can be applied in four ways to assess severity of outflow obstruction:

- venous pressure with exercise or ambulatory venous pressure;
- venous pressure differential between foot and arm;[13]
- venous pressure changes after reactive hyperemia induced by thigh tourniquet;[13]
- simultaneous pressure and volume changes to calculate venous outflow resistance.[17]

Femoral vein pressures

Direct venous pressures can be measured at the femoral level for iliofemoral or iliocaval thrombosis. Femoral vein pressures serve as an important tool in determining the adequacy of pelvic collaterals in subjects with iliofemoral or caval obstruction. When combined with ascending femoral phlebography and cavography, Albrechtsson *et al.* showed that data from bilateral femoral pressures at rest and after exercise correlated with severity of post-thrombotic symptoms.[18] From their study of 50 patients with post-thrombotic disease, they concluded that noncompensated limbs were characterized by pressure elevation after exercise, pressure difference between limbs after exercise, and prolonged normalization time after exercise. In normal limbs, femoral venous pressures remain unchanged with exercise. The examination was performed on an x-ray tilt table, tilted 30–45° from the horizontal plane, and exercise was induced by repeated toe lifts.

Physiologic obstruction of the iliac system is suggested by a resting femoral pressure difference of ≥5 mmHg between affected and normal limb, or an increase in femoral pressure ≥5 mmHg with exercise. Gloviczki advocates using a pressure gradient of at least 5 mmHg between central circulation and femoral vein not only with exercise but also at rest.[19] Negus and Cockett propose that a pathological block is present when the resting pressure difference is greater than 2 mmHg and the rise in pressure with exercise greater than 3 mmHg.[20] Finally, Gottlob and May state that the noncompensated limb will have a pressure increase of greater than three times that of the normal limb with exercise.[21] These parameters provide guidelines for choosing the patient who may benefit from cross-femoral bypass, iliocaval or femorocaval bypass, or iliac balloon angioplasty and stenting.

AMBULATORY VENOUS PRESSURE IN VALVULAR REFLUX

Whilst venous obstruction tends to subside with time, venous valvular incompetence increases and is accompanied by gradual hemodynamic deterioration as the veins recanalize and valves are destroyed.[22] The utility of ambulatory venous pressure measurements for reflux disease has had a diminishing role since color-flow duplex scanning and plethysmographic techniques have become more widespread. Ambulatory venous pressure is limited because it provides an overall assessment of disease, and the exact site of reflux is not apparent. Duplex provides information of valve function and furthermore has the advantage of showing the location of disease. For screening of reflux disease, duplex is a superior test because it is noninvasive and provides details of the anatomy and function of specific venous segments. Furthermore, duplex enables the clinician to distinguish between reflux and obstruction.

AVP may have prognostic significance. The frequency of ulceration and stasis changes appear to directly increase with values of ambulatory venous pressures. In a study of 220 patients with primarily venous reflux disease, Nicolaides *et al.* showed that when the AVP exceeded 90 mmHg the prevalence of ulcers was 100%, whereas if pressures were less than 30 mmHg, no ulceration occurred.[23] Aside from this potential use, ambulatory venous pressure measurements do not have a major role in evaluating venous reflux.

CURRENT AND NEW APPLICATIONS

The best application for venous pressures today is for preoperative and postoperative evaluation for venous reconstruction of chronic obstruction, for diagnostic testing in cases of equivocal findings by noninvasive testing, and for venous research. Direct femoral vein pressures have a more practical application than AVP in the intervention of iliac vein obstruction for balloon angioplasty and stenting.

Alternative noninvasive tests such as duplex scanning and air plethysmography are more practical for screening and follow-up. Duplex scanning provides both anatomic and functional information, whereas air plethysmography separates superficial and deep reflux, obstruction and calf muscle pump dysfunction.

Table 14.2 *Femoral vein and intra-abdominal pressures (taken from urinary bladder pressures) in morbidly obese patients versus normal weight controls*

BMI (kg/m^2)	SAD (cm)	Femoral vein pressure (cmH_2O)	Bladder pressure (cmH_2O)
Morbidly obese patients ($n = 15$)			
50.2 ± 1.2	32.7 ± 0.8	19.7 ± 3.7	19.1 ± 4.1
Normal weight controls ($n = 4$)			
24.8 ± 2.1	19.7 ± 1.2	7.5 ± 0.6	8.5 ± 1.7

BMI, body mass index; SAD, sagittal abdominal diameter.

Direct femoral vein pressures in severe obesity

A stimulating research project is currently under way by members of the Straub Clinic and Hospital in Honolulu to study the relationship between femoral vein pressures, intra-abdominal pressures (IAP), and lower extremity manifestations of venous disease in severely obese patients. This project is based on the observation that obese patients often have leg problems such as swelling, skin changes and ulceration. The landmark paper by Sugerman showed that IAP was significantly higher in obese patients compared to normal controls.[24] The Honolulu group's hypothesis is that obese patients develop leg ulcers and swelling as a result of high intra-abdominal pressure, and the pressure is transmitted to the iliac veins. This leads to elevated femoral pressures and subsequent impairment of normal venous physiology.

Preliminary results of a pilot study of 19 patients confirm that obese patients have higher intra-abdominal pressures than normal controls. The latest finding is that femoral vein pressures appear to be higher in obese compared with normal controls, and correlate well with elevated IAP. Table 14.2 shows the relationship between femoral vein pressures and IAP measured by obtaining bladder pressures. Whether these elevated femoral and intra-abdominal pressures eventually lead to the development of limb symptoms of swelling, pain and ulceration over time is being actively studied.

SUMMARY

At rest, hydrostatic foot vein pressure is equal to the pressure created by a column of blood from the heart to the foot and is not affected by the presence of incompetent valves, and is only minimally affected by venous obstruction. With exercise, lack of appropriate fall in pressure and rapid refill with cessation of exercise is observed with venous incompetence, obstruction, calf muscle pump dysfunction, or combinations of these factors.

Ambulatory venous pressure can be used to provide an overall estimate of calf pump efficiency in expelling venous blood. Direct femoral venous pressures, with provocative measures, can be used to identify physiologically important iliac or caval obstruction and may be helpful in selecting patients for venous bypass or endovascular procedures. By contrast, other modalities such as venography, duplex scanning and air plethysmography may be more useful in selecting patients for venous reconstruction for valvular incompetence.

REFERENCES

1. Adams JC. Etiological factors in varicose veins of the lower extremities. *Surg Gynecol Obstet* 1939; **69**: 717–25.
2. Beecher HK. Adjustment of the flow of tissue fluid in the presence of localized sustained high venous pressures as found with varices of the great saphenous system during walking. *J Clin Invest* 1937; **16**: 733–9.
3. Perthes G. Ueber die operation der unterschenkel-varicen nach Trendelenburg. *Dtsch Med Wochenschr* 1895; **21**: 253–7.
4. Pollack AA, Wood EH. Venous pressure in the saphenous vein at the ankle in man during exercise and changes in position. *J Appl Physiol* 1949; **1**: 649–62.
5. Delbet P. Du role de l'insufficence de la saphene interne dans les varices du membre inferieur. *Semaine Med* 1897; **17**: 372.
6. Nicolaides A, Yao JST. *The Investigation of Vascular Disorders.* Edinburgh: Churchill Livingstone, 1980.
7. Zukowski AJ, Nicolaides AN, Szendro A, *et al.* Haemodynamic significance of incompetent calf perforating veins. *Br J Surg* 1991; **78**: 625–9.
8. Browse NL. Venous pressure measurements. In Bernstein EF, ed. *Vascular Diagnosis*, 4th edn. St Louis, MO: Mosby Year Book, 1993: 893–6.
9. Schanzer H, Peirce EC II. Pathophysiologic evaluation of chronic venous stasis with ambulatory venous pressure studies. *Angiology* 1982; **33**: 183–91.
10. Snyder MA, Adams JT, Schwartz SI. Hemodynamics of phlegmasia cerulea dolens. *Surg Gynecol Obstet* 1967; **125**: 342–6.

11. Ellwood RA, Lee WB. Pedal venous pressure: correlation with presence and site of deep-venous abnormalities. *Radiology* 1979; **131**: 73–4.
12. Husni EA, Ximenes JO, Goyett EM. Elastic support of the lower limbs in hospital patients – a critical study. *J Am Med Assoc* 1970; **214**: 1456–62.
13. Raju S, Fredericks R. Venous obstruction: an analysis of 137 cases with hemodynamic, venographic and clinical correlations. *J Vasc Surg* 1991; **13**: 91–100.
14. DeCamp PT, Schramel RJ, Roy CJ, *et al.* Ambulatory venous pressure determinations in postphlebitic and related syndromes. *Surgery* 1951; **29**: 44–52.
15. Raju S. A pressure-based technique for the detection of acute and chronic venous obstruction. *Phlebology* 1988; **3**: 207–16.
16. Raju S, Fredericks R. Venous obstruction: an analysis of one hundred thirty-seven cases with hemodynamic, venographic, and clinical correlations. *J Vasc Surg* 1991; **14**: 305–13.
17. Neglén P, Raju S. Detection of outflow obstruction in chronic venous insufficiency. *J Vasc Surg* 1993; **17**: 583–9.
18. Albrechtsson U, Einarsson E, Eklof B. Femoral vein pressure measurements for evaluation of venous function in patients with postthrombotic iliac veins. *Cardiovasc Interv Radiol* 1981; **4**: 43–50.
19. Gloviczki P, Pairolero PC. Prosthetic replacement of large veins. In Bergan JJ, Kistner RL, eds. *Atlas of Venous Surgery.* Philadelphia: WB Saunders, 1992: 191–214.
20. Negus D, Cockett FB. Femoral vein pressures in postphlebitic iliac vein obstruction. *Br J Surg* 1967; **54**: 522–5.
21. Gottlob R, May R. Der Fruhverschluss der Palma-operation. *Vasa* 1977; **6**: 263–9.
22. Killewich LA, Bedfor GR, Beach KW, Strandness DEJ. Spontaneous lysis of deep venous thrombi: rate and outcome. *J Vasc Surg* 1989; **9**: 89–97.
23. Nicolaides AN, Hussein MK, Szendro G, *et al.* The relation of venous ulceration with ambulatory venous pressure measurements. *J Vasc Surg* 1993; **17**: 414–19.
24. Sugerman H, Windsor A, Bessos M, Wolfe L. Intra-abdominal pressure, sagittal abdominal diameter and obesity comorbidity. *J Intern Med* 1997; **241**: 71–9.

15

Upper extremity venography (phlebography)

JAMES S T YAO

Venography of the upper extremity was first introduced by Sgalitzer and his colleagues in 1931.[1] Unlike the ascending venography of the lower extremity, this technique has received relatively little attention. With increasing use of indwelling catheters for chemotherapy, hyperalimentation, and transvenous placement of cardiac pacemakers, the incidence of venous thrombosis has increased significantly.[2–4] In addition, the introduction of various interventional techniques and the use of thrombolytic therapy have placed venography as an essential diagnostic and therapeutic technique in patients with thrombosis of major veins of the upper part of the body. This chapter reviews the current technique of upper extremity venography in the evaluation of upper extremity venous problems.

NORMAL ANATOMY OF THE UPPER EXTREMITY VENOUS SYSTEM

Venous return of the upper extremity is by two sets of veins: superficial and deep. The deep veins are usually paired, have cross-connections between them, and accompany the ulnar, radial and brachial arteries with similar names. The deep veins drain into the axillary vein. The superficial veins lie in the subcutaneous tissue for most of the course and drain most of the blood from the upper extremity. The most prominent superficial veins are the basilic and cephalic veins. The cephalic vein begins in the radial part of the dorsal venous network of the hand. It communicates with the basilic vein at the antecubital fossa, through the medial cubital vein. The cephalic vein ascends laterally, empties into the axillary vein and is an important collateral pathway in the presence of occlusion of the lower segment of the axillary vein. The cephalic vein may be double, for it may communicate with the internal jugular or subclavian vein.

The basilic vein runs from the ulnar part of the dorsal venous network of the hand and ascends on the medial side of the arm. It pierces the fascia at the middle part of the arm, where it joins the brachial veins of the deep venous system and becomes the axillary vein. The veins of the forearm contain 8–15 valves.

The axillary vein begins at the lower border of the teres major, at the outer border of the first rib, and continues as the subclavian vein. The subclavian vein unites with the internal jugular vein behind the corresponding sternoclavicular joint to form the innominate (brachiocephalic) vein. The right and left innominate veins join to form the superior vena cava. The latter descends on the right side of the ascending thoracic aorta, receives the azygos vein, and ends in the right atrium.

The venous system of the upper thorax is of interest because significant differences exist between the right and left sides. The right and left innominate (brachiocephalic) veins are asymmetric, the left being 6 cm in length as compared with 2.5 cm on the right. A second important anatomic landmark is the anterior scalenus muscle, which lies posterior to both right and left subclavian vein. Consequently, the subclavian vein is unaffected by the scalene muscles, and compression of the vein is often due to an abnormal costoclavicular space between the clavicle and first rib.

INDICATIONS FOR VENOGRAPHY

Indications for venography are, first, to establish the diagnosis of acute venous thrombosis of the subclavian-axillary vein or superior vena cava. Etiologies for venous thrombosis of the upper extremity are multiple (Table 15.1). Venographic finding is essential for treatment strategy.[5] A second indication is to examine venous malformation or varicose veins, and a third is to determine operability for venous bypass in patients with an intractable chronic venous obstruction. Venous bypass graft is an uncommon surgical procedure and, in selected cases, bypass graft yields gratifying results.[6] In patients with subclavian vein thrombosis in the presence of a hemodialysis fistula, bypass graft helps to reduce the selling and to preserve the fistula.[7] Similarly, a spiral vein graft from the jugular vein to the atrium provides immediate symptomatic relief of intractable swelling of the face in patients with superior vena cava syndrome.[8]

Table 15.1 *Etiologies of deep venous thrombosis of the upper extremity*

- Nonocclusive thrombosis
  - Intermittent compression of the subclavian vein due to thoracic outlet bony anomaly or pectoris minor tendon
- Occlusive thrombosis
  - Traumatic
    - External
      - Clavicular fracture or shoulder dislocation
      - Thoracic-outlet syndrome
    - Internal (intimal injury)
      - Indwelling catheters: hyperalimentation, dialysis and chemotherapy
      - Transvenous cardiac pacemakers
- Non-traumatic
  - Associated with underlying malignancy
  - Radiation therapy
  - Blood dyscrasias
  - Infections
  - Deficiency of antithrombin III, protein C, protein S
  - Antiphospholipid syndrome
- Superior vena cava syndrome
  - Malignancy
  - Aneurysm
  - Mediastinal fibrosis
  - Radiation injury

TECHNIQUE OF VENOGRAPHY (PHLEBOGRAPHY)

Upper extremity venography is a readily performed procedure. The examination is done with the patient in a supine position. For visualization of the entire upper extremity, a vein on the dorsum of the patient's hand or distal forearm is cannulated with a 20 or 22 gauge intravenous catheter. Smaller veins may be more readily entered with a 19 or 21 gauge butterfly needle. A small amount of saline solution is forcefully injected through the needle to be certain of its intraluminal position. If the site appears to swell, or if the patient complains of a burning sensation, the procedure should be terminated immediately. A different site should then be selected for continuation of the examination. Once the site is secured, the deep venous system is opacified by injecting 40–60 ml of 43–60% contrast medium while visually monitoring the injection site. Either digital subtraction or plain film techniques can be used to acquire images.

To visualize the central venous anatomy, it is better to place an 18–20 gauge intravenous catheter into a vein within the antecubital fossa. A manual injection of 30–50 ml of 60% contrast medium is performed. Digital subtraction angiographic techniques are preferable but require patients to hold their breath for a prolonged period of time. This may not be feasible in all patients. The superior vena cava system is best delineated by bilateral upper extremity venography; 30–50 ml of contrast is simultaneously injected into each upper extremity via intravenous catheters in the antecubital veins. Optimal visualization of the central venous system may require selective catheterization of the subclavian vein from a femoral or antecubital approach. Larger volumes of contrast can be injected to better define the venous anatomy.

When placing a catheter in the antecubital vein, it is important to avoid the pitfall of selectively catheterizing the cephalic vein. Subsequent contrast administration will opacify the cephalic and axillary veins and not the basilic vein. This may lead to an erroneous diagnosis of basilic vein thrombosis (Fig. 15.1).

In patients suspected of having compression of the axillary-subclavian vein by the thoracic outlet, a positional venogram must be performed. This is done by placing the arm in hyperabduction and external rotation to simulate the stress position (Fig. 15.2).

ADJUNCTIVE VENOUS PRESSURE MEASUREMENT

Venous pressure measurement at the time of venography provides physiological information that may help to supplement venographic findings.[9] A simple water manometer, readily available in all institutions, can be utilized. Initially, pressures are obtained in a resting position. The patient is then asked to open and close the fist repetitively as fast as possible for 2 minutes, or until the exercise becomes fatiguing. Pressure measurements are then repeated. This physiologic evaluation complements the venous contrast study and is particularly helpful in equivocal cases, such as patients with nonocclusive, intermittent compression of the subclavian vein. In this situation, measurement can be easily done in neutral and

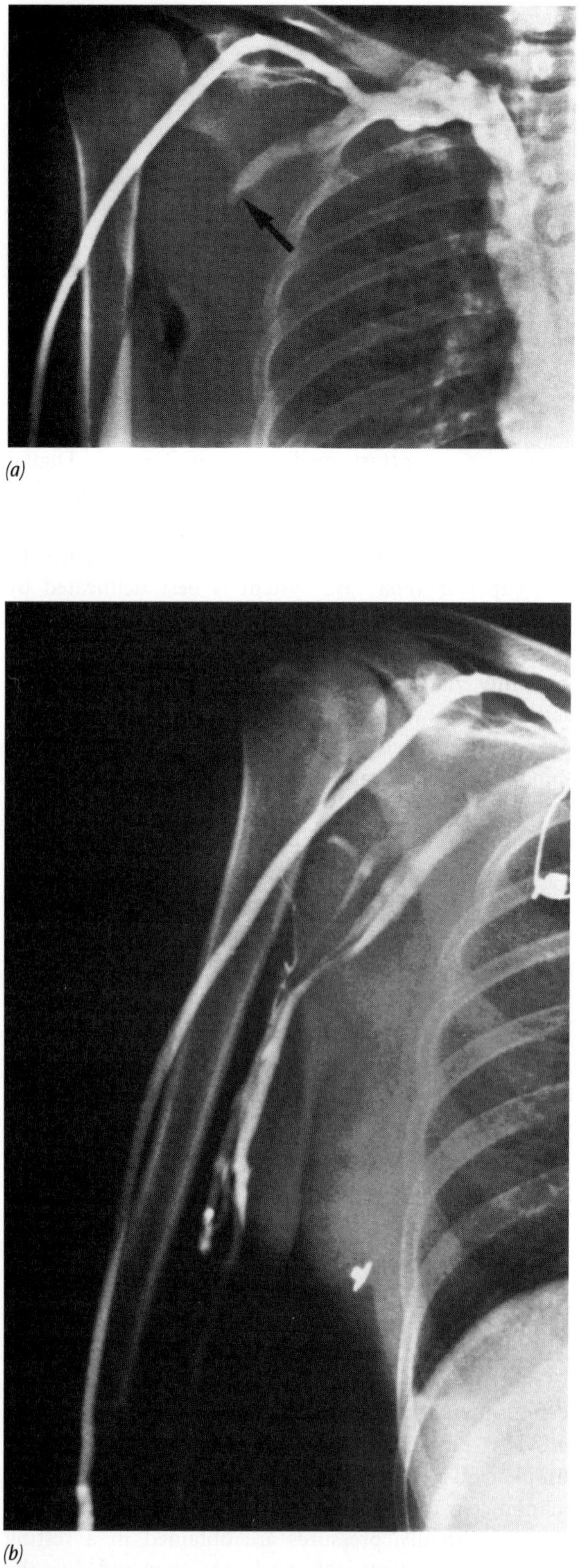

(a)

(b)

Figure 15.1 *(a) Injection of contrast media into the cephalic vein may give pseudo-occlusion of the axillary vein (arrow). (b) In the same patient, replacement of the needle in the basilic vein shows patent axillary vein. (Reproduced with permission from Yao JST, Neiman HL. Upper-extremity venography. In Neiman HL, Yao JST, eds.* Angiography of Vascular Disease. *Edinburgh, Churchill Livingstone, 1985: 484).*

adduction-external rotation positions to determine whether there is significant compression by the thoracic outlet. In the normal individual, venous pressures will remain unchanged after exercise or, more commonly, will fall below the baseline level. By contrast, the patient with significant obstruction to flow will show pressure elevation after exercise (Fig. 15.2).

ADJUNCTIVE THROMBOLYTIC THERAPY

Urokinase is no longer available for infusion thrombolytic therapy. Currently, tissue plasminogen activator (t-PA) is used at the completion of venography to offer complete thrombolysis of the occluded segment and restoration of venous return (Fig. 15.3). After complete thrombolysis, the underlying pathology causing the thrombosis may be better defined (Fig. 15.4). Although interventional procedures such as balloon dilation or stent placement have been attempted in patients with focal stenosis after thrombolytic therapy, the high recurrent rates of thrombosis have made many interventional radiologists abandon these procedures. Stent placement in patients with superior vena cava syndrome, however, offers immediate relief in patients with terminal malignancy.

Thrombolysis of axillary-subclavian occlusions is approached from the periphery of the affected arm. Venography or ultrasound is used to gain access into a vein that can accept up to a 6-French catheter. The basilic vein is the preferred peripheral venous access site. A steerable guidewire is used to traverse the thrombosed venous segment. Successful crossing of the thrombosed segment with a guidewire is a good prognostic sign. An infusion catheter is embedded within the thrombus. The side holes of the infusion catheter are distributed throughout the clot to saturate the largest surface area possible.

During thrombolysis, the patient's affected extremity is elevated to mobilize the edema. The patient's fibrinogen level is monitored to assess conversion from a local anticoagulation state into a systemic anticoagulation state. If the fibrinogen level drops below 100 units, the thrombolysis is temporarily discontinued. Following an interval of 1-2 hours, the thrombolysis can be restarted if the fibrinogen level has risen.

Venography is used to assess the efficacy of the thrombolysis. Venography is performed at approximately 24-hour intervals during the thrombolysis. Venography can be performed when either logistically feasible or clinically indicated. Venography is used to reposition the catheter within the thrombus. Adjunctive angioplasty of underlying stenoses or difficult-to-dissolve thrombus is performed.

When an antegrade approach cannot traverse an occluded vein, a retrograde femoral approach may be

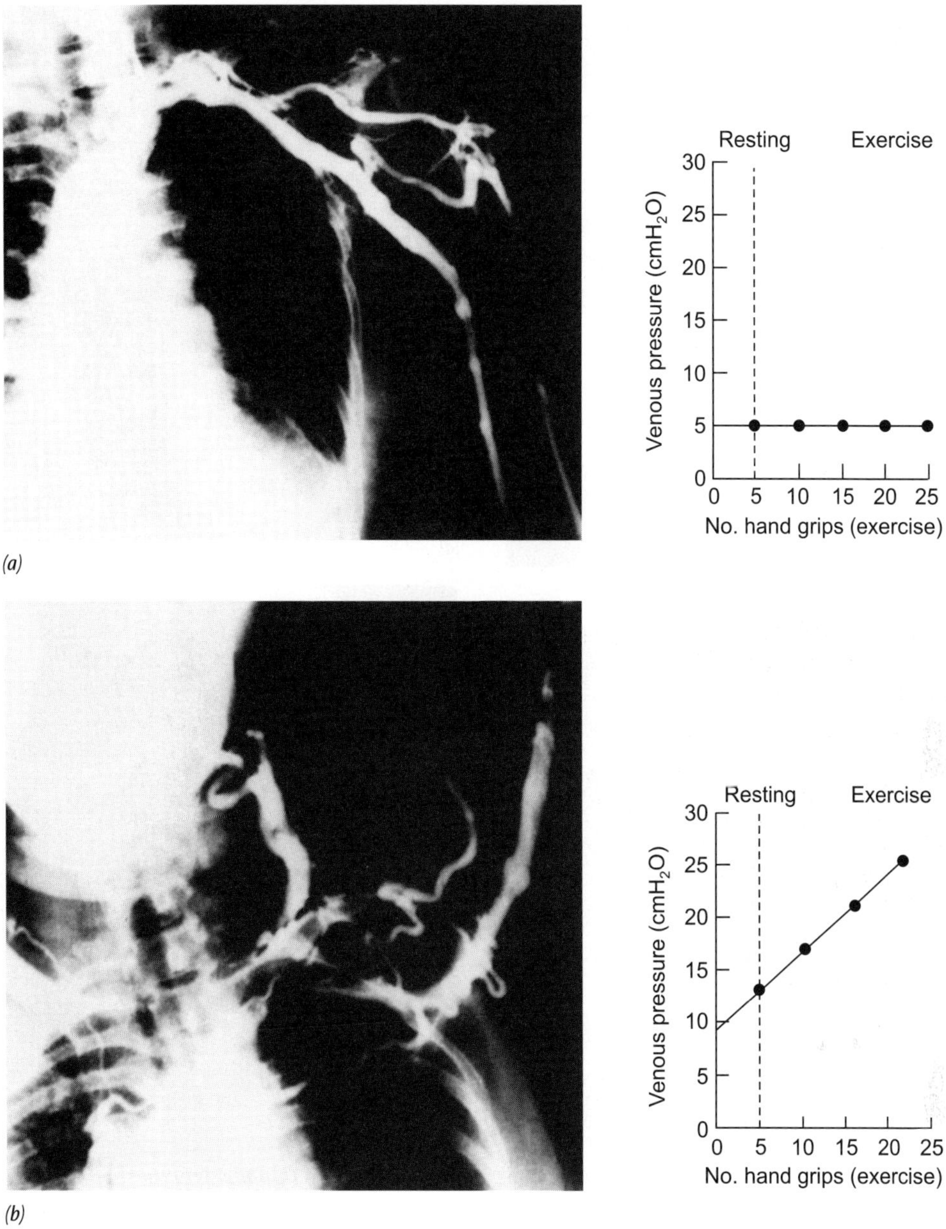

Figure 15.2 *(a) Venous pressure response in a patient with arm in the neutral position. The subclavian vein is normal. There is no change in venous pressure after repetitive hand grips (right panel). (b) In the same patient with intermittent compression of the subclavian vein when the arm is hyperabducted. Note the steady increase of venous pressure following repetitive hand grips. (Reproduced with permission from Yao JST, Neiman HL. Upper-extremity venography. In Neiman HL, Yao JST, eds.* Angiography of Vascular Disease. *Edinburgh, Churchill Livingstone, 1985: 484).*

successful. It is often necessary to remove or reposition venous access catheters or ports to optimize venous thrombolysis results.

COLLATERAL PATHWAYS

In the presence of axillary-subclavian vein or superior vena cava thrombosis, extensive collateral networks may be seen in the shoulder region and veins between the superior and inferior caval systems via the iliac veins.[10] Figure 15.5 shows the diagrammatic sketch of various collateral pathways. The major collateral pathways are as follows:

- azygos system via the ascending lumbar veins or intercostal veins;
- thoracoepigastric–external iliac vein;
- internal thoracic vein–inferior epigastric vein–external iliac vein or iliolumbar vein to the internal iliac vein;

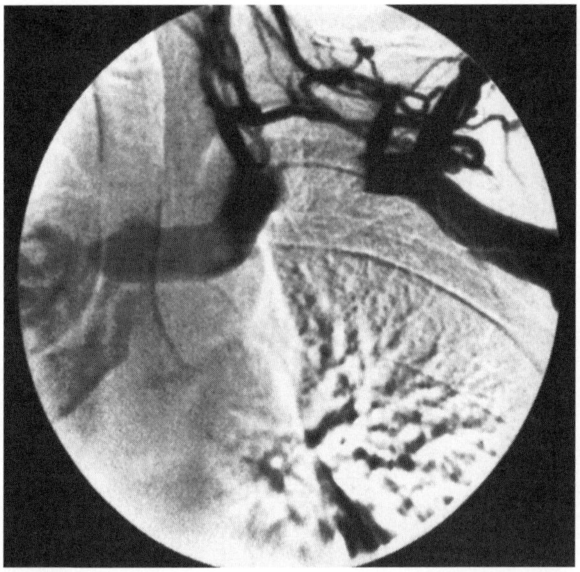

(a)

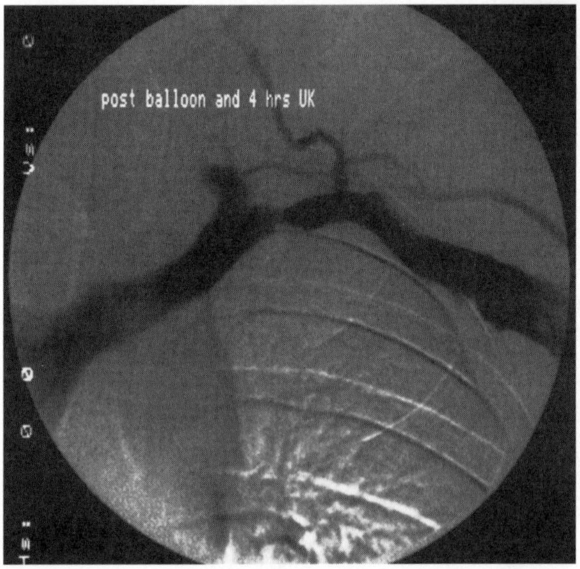

(b)

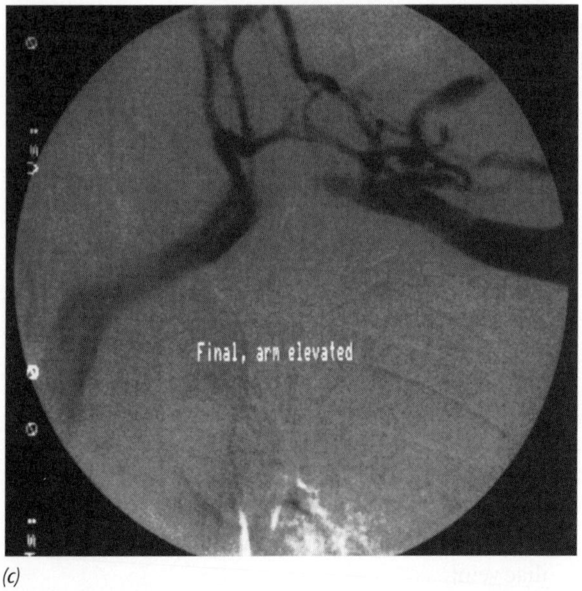

(c)

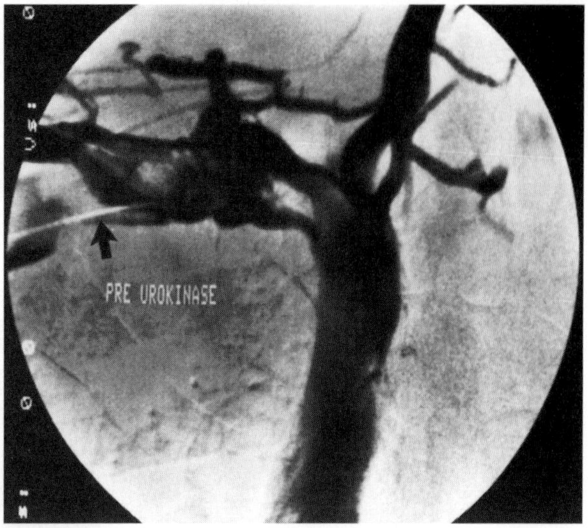

(a)

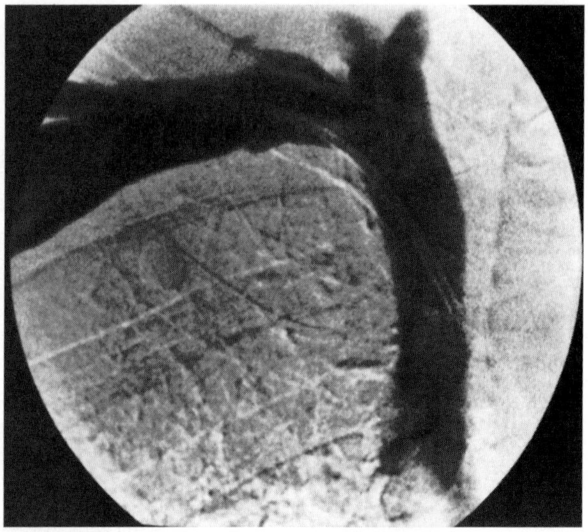

(b)

Figure 15.4 *(a) Thrombosis of the subclavian vein in a patient receiving chemotherapy. Note the thrombi surrounding the catheter (arrow). (b) Complete lysis of the thrombi after 6 hours of urokinase infusion. (Reproduced with permission from McCarthy WJ, Vogelzang RL, Bergan JJ. Changing concepts and present-day etiology of upper extremity venous thrombosis. In Bergan JJ, Yao JST, eds.* Venous Disorders. *Philadelphia: WB Saunders, 1991: 418).*

Figure 15.3 (left) *(a) Acute effort thrombosis of the left subclavian vein treated with urokinase infusion. (b) Urokinase was followed by balloon dilation of the subclavian vein. (c) Despite restoration of patency by balloon angioplasty, a high-grade stenosis is detected with the arm placed in hyperabduction. (Reproduced with permission from McCarthy WJ, Vogelzang RL, Bergan JJ. Changing concepts and present-day etiology of upper extremity venous thrombosis. In Bergan JJ, Yao JST, eds.* Venous Disorders. *Philadelphia: WB Saunders, 1991: 417).*

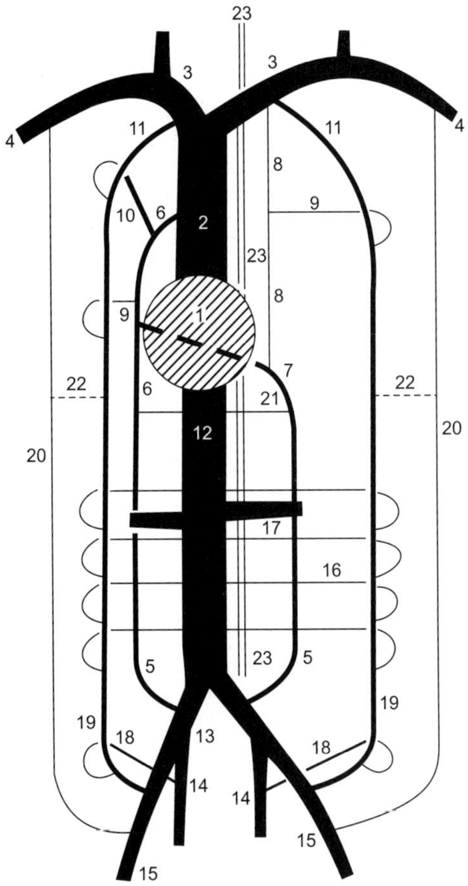

Figure 15.5 *Diagrammatic sketch of various collateral pathways between the inferior and the superior vena cava: 1, right atrium; 2, superior vena cava; 3, brachiocephalic veins; 4, axillary vein; 5, ascending lumbar vein; 6, azygos vein; 7, hemiazygos veins; 8, accessory hemiazygos vein; 9, posterior intercostal veins; 10, right superior intercostal vein; 11, internal thoracic vein; 12, inferior vena cava; 13, common iliac vein; 14, internal iliac vein; 15, external iliac vein; 16, lumbar veins; 17, renal vein; 18, iliolumbar vein; 19, inferior epigastric vein; 20, thoracoepigastric vein; 21, inferior and superior phrenic veins; 22, anastomosis between thoracoepigastric and internal thoracic veins; 23, vertebral venous plexus. (Reproduced with permission from Luzsa G.* X-Ray Anatomy of the Vascular System. *Published jointly by JB Lippincott Co., Butterworth & Co. and Akadémiai Kiadoó, 1974: 49. © Akadémiai Kiadoó, 1974).*

- vertebral veins with communication between the superior and inferior vena cava via the intercostal, lumbar and sacral veins;
- internal jugular–endocranial traverse sinuses.

COMPLICATIONS

The complications of venography are allergic reactions, contrast nephrotoxicity, extravasation of contrast medium, and venous thrombosis. Patients with allergies to contrast media are best studied using alternative techniques. Both duplex scan and magnetic resonance imaging may offer valuable diagnostic information. When a venogram is necessary, the use of non-ionic contrast medium is treated by elevation of the extremity and application of a hot pack. Venous thrombosis and contrast nephrotoxicity are infrequent complications of upper extremity venography because of the small volume of contrast utilized.

REFERENCES

1. Sgalitzer M, Kollert V, Demel R. Kootrast dar Stellung der Venen im Rotgenbilde. *Klin Wochenschr* 1931; **10**: 1659.
2. McCarthy WJ, Vogelzang RL, Bergan JJ. Changing concepts and present-day etiology of upper extremity venous thrombosis. In Bergan JJ, Yao JST, eds. *Venous Disorders.* Philadelphia: WB Saunders, 1991: 407–20.
3. Lindblad B, Tengborn L, Berqvist D. Deep vein thrombosis of the axillary-subclavian veins: epidemiologic data, effect of different types of treatment and late sequelae. *Eur J Vasc Surg* 1988; **2**: 161–5.
4. Becker DM, Philbrick JT, Walder FB IV. Axillary and subclavian venous thrombosis: prognosis and treatment. *Arch Intern Med* 1991; **151**: 1934–43.
5. Machleder HI. Evaluation of a new treatment strategy for Paget–Schroetter syndrome: spontaneous thrombosis of the axillary-subclavian vein. *J Vasc Surg* 1993; **17**: 306–17.
6. DeWeese JA. Results of surgical treatment of axillary-subclavian venous thrombosis. In Bergan JJ, Yao JS, eds. *Venous Disorders.* Philadelphia: WB Saunders, 1991: 421–33.
7. Currior CB Jr, Widder S, Ali A, *et al.* Surgical management of subclavian and axillary vein thrombosis in patients with a functioning arteriovenous fistula. *Surgery* 1986; **100**: 25–8.
8. Doty DB, Doty JR, Jones KW. Bypass of superior vena cava: fifteen years' experience with spiral vein graft for obstruction of superior vena cava caused by benign disease. *J Thorac Cardiovasc Surg* 1990; **99**: 889–95.
9. Yao JST, Neiman JL. Upper-extremity venography. In Nieman HL, Yao JST, eds. *Angiography of Vascular Disease.* Edinburgh: Churchill Livingstone, 1985: 481–94.
10. Okay NH, Bryk D. Collateral pathways in occlusion of the superior vena cava and its tributaries. *Radiology* 1969; **92**: 1493–8.

16

Computed tomography and magnetic resonance imaging in venous disorders

ANTHONY W STANSON AND JEROME F BREEN

Computed tomography and magnetic resonance imaging are each complex imaging modalities that provide global views of the body. Whilst the anatomic display of the images produced are somewhat similar in appearance, the technologies are very different in their respective harnessing of the energy spectrum to display anatomic and pathologic information.

COMPUTED TOMOGRAPHY AND MAGNETIC RESONANCE IMAGING MODALITIES

Computed tomography scan

A computed tomography scanner is an x-ray machine that produces cross-sectional images displayed in shades of black, white, and gray representing tissue densities that are similar to what we are accustomed to seeing on plain x-ray films, that is, bone is white, air is black, and all other tissues are various shades of gray, indicating the degree of attenuation of the x-ray beam. A computed tomography image is much more sensitive to display differences in soft tissue density than is a plain film; that is, the range of the gray scale is much larger for computed tomography. For instance, an acute hematoma will have a higher computed tomography density than flowing blood or a fluid collection. Such distinctions cannot be made from a plain film. Also, soft tissue calcifications, such as in atheromatous disease of arteries, are identified at a much earlier stage by computed tomography than by plain film. Intravenous contrast material is often used to enhance the lumen of vessels and to identify vascular perfusion of soft tissue structures, thus making the computed tomography images even more revealing in most instances.

Magnetic resonance imaging

On the other hand, magnetic resonance imaging is a completely different technology. It is a process of stimulated pulses of radiofrequency energy perturbing proton spins of the hydrogen nucleus (primarily in water molecules) within complex and controlled magnetic fields. This results in the production of resonant radiofrequency signals as echoes of the original, stimulating radiofrequency signal. The body's tissues are identified in shades of gray depending upon the intensity of the echo signal; high signal is white. By contrast, the images show no signal from cortical bone or air as they are devoid of sufficient hydrogen protons and are thus displayed as black on the images. However, another structure that may be black on a magnetic resonance image is a blood vessel with flowing blood. It is also possible to set up a sequence that displays flowing blood as a white image (high signal intensity). There are many protocols for manipulating the radiofrequency signals and the timing of collecting the echo data, such that the images produced have great variations in the appearance of gray scale for any given organ or vascular structure. Also, magnetic resonance imaging sequences can be set up to display information about flow velocity of blood. This type of flexibility makes magnetic resonance imaging unique as an imaging modality. Intravenous contrast material is also available to use with magnetic resonance scanning, although it is a different compound than that used for computed tomography scanning.

Computed tomography versus magnetic resonance imaging: image planes

Another major difference between computed tomography and magnetic resonance imaging is the orientation of the imaging plane. Computed tomography is performed in a single plane, transaxial to the orientation of the table. The images are cross-sections of the body. With magnetic resonance the plane of imaging is chosen by the examiner. There is, however, the possibility of multiplanar reformatting of the computed tomography images. This is a computer manipulation of the cross-sectional image data, to create views in other planes and even in three dimensions. However, when computed tomography images are reformatted, the spatial resolution of such derived images is much less than that of the original transaxial images (Fig. 16.1a, b). This is because the thickness of the computed tomography slice is much

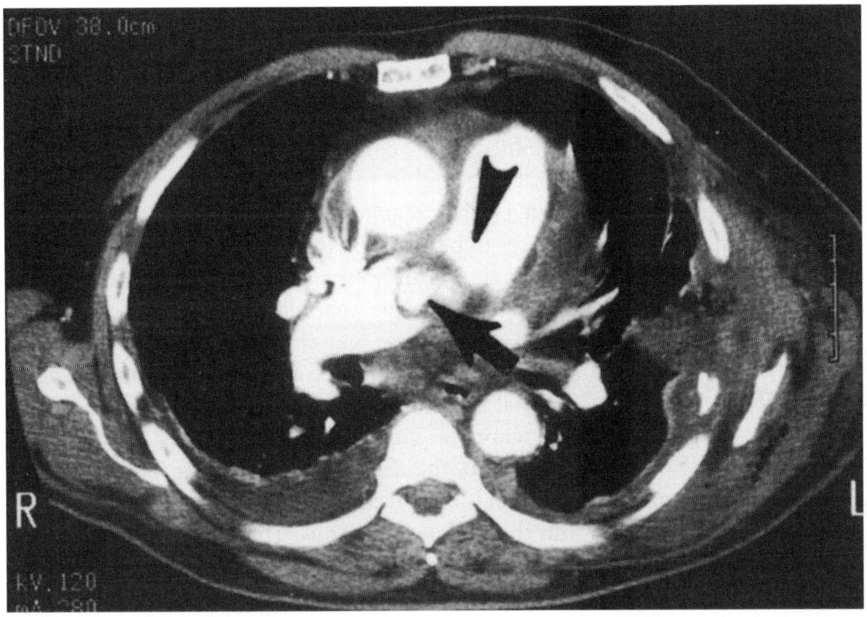

(a)

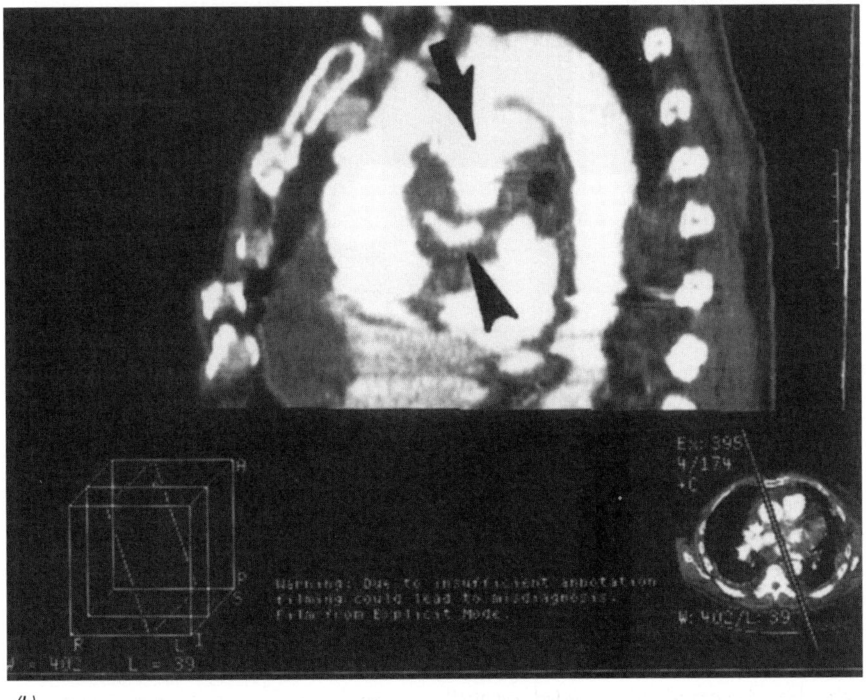

(b)

Figure 16.1 *Spiral computed tomography scan through the chest in a patient with a false aneurysm at the bottom of the aortic arch. (a) Axial scan, with contrast opacification, taken a few centimeters below the level of the aortic arch shows an arch aneurysm (arrow) compressing the superior margin of the right pulmonary artery (arrowhead). (b) The reformatted image in oblique sagittal plane shows a view somewhat like an angiogram. The size of the aneurysm (arrow and its position relative to the right pulmonary artery (arrowhead) is more fully appreciated. Note that the spatial resolution of this reconstructed image is much less than that of the cross-section image in (a).*

greater (5–10 mm) than the pixel size (0.2 mm) on the acquired axial image. The thickness of the slice becomes profiled on the reconstructed sagittal or coronal image and a staircase-like, irregular border is seen on the margin of an axially oriented structure such as the aorta or vena cava. The reason for the imperfect margins is patient motion in conjunction with the thick slice of data. The sources of motion include patient movement, differences in respiratory level from one scan to the next, and cardiac pulsation transmitted through the aorta and other large arteries which is subsequently transmitted to adjacent structures.

The choice of the imaging plane for a magnetic resonance imaging study is selected by the examiner for each sequence performed. The data are always collected in each of three planes, and the precise orientation of these planes can be changed. This means that a particular anatomic structure can be displayed in sagittal, coronal, or axial view, or indeed in any off-axis plane selected and the spatial quality of the images is always maintained because the original acquisition data are used to create them. There is no secondary manipulation of images that inherently creates low-resolution images as there is with computed tomography scan reformatting.

Conventional computed tomography scanners

The type of scanner used for a computed tomography examination will largely determine the quality of the study, which may in turn have an impact on the accuracy of the diagnosis. Conventional computed tomography scanners take several seconds to acquire a single section and usually only one or two pictures can be obtained in one breath hold. Because it would be rare to find a person who can duplicate respiratory level from one breath to the next, it is not likely that the major organs are accurately recorded, in sequence from one scan level to the next. Scans taken at end-expiratory level will be the most accurately reproducible. This technical point is important to consider when evaluating a series of images to determine accurately the site of a vascular occlusion or a small lesion.

Fast-computed tomography scanners

There are two types of newer scanners that by their design produce higher-quality images because they minimize motion artifacts: electron beam and spiral computed tomography. These are the so-called fast-computed tomography scanners. The electron beam scanner (Imatron, South San Francisco) uses incremental exposures of 0.1 s and can be gated to the heartbeat for certain types of cardiovascular studies. This eliminates motion artifact from the heart, aorta and major arteries, thus ensuring that the position of the walls of these structures are exactly in the same place on all images. For most body scanning applications, it is not necessary to use cardiac gating, thereby allowing longer exposure times to produce better image quality. Furthermore, many scans can be obtained in a single breath hold, thus eliminating respiratory differences as a source of inter-scan variation of anatomic position.[1] This scan technology has been available for about a decade and has greatly contributed to the ability to diagnose cardiovascular diseases such as cardiac masses (Fig. 16.2), pericardial constriction, aortic dissection and pulmonary embolism.[2] The latest improvement of this scanner is a feature of constant table movement which further allows more rapid image acquisition.

The other newer scan technology is *spiral computed tomography*. This uses a conventional type scanner modified to have a constantly spinning x-ray tube combined with a constantly moving table, resulting in a 'spiral' acquisition of data from which the images are created. This scanner is also fast and allows many pictures to be acquired in a short period of time so that in a single breath hold a large zone of the body can be scanned. All major manufacturers produce a 'spiral' model. With these newer scan technologies, motion artifacts are much reduced and the utilization of contrast material infusion is maximized. Furthermore, patient throughput is greatly increased because of their high speed. Also, the capacity for multiplanar image reconstruction is improved because dedicated software is built into the keyboard controls. The image quality will also be much better because thinner slices can be analyzed and motion artifact is reduced.

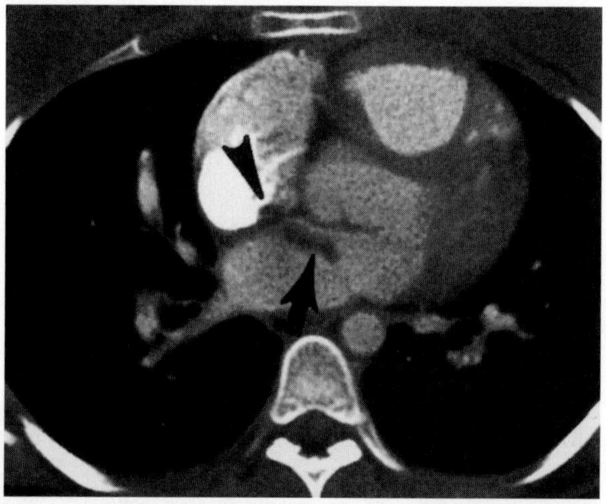

Figure 16.2 *Electron beam computed tomography scan shows an embolus crossing a patent foramen ovale. Intraluminal filling defect within the left atrium (arrow) is a tail of thrombus extending across a patent foramen ovale from the right atrium. Small filling defect in the right atrium (arrowhead) is the right-sided end of this embolus.*

COMPUTED TOMOGRAPHY SCANNING TECHNIQUE

Contrast material

Because of the diverse anatomic relationships of the major veins and the time variation in venous return at the different sites, performing the computed tomography scan requires close monitoring by the radiologist to maximize the degree of contrast opacification of the venous system.

A preliminary set of scans before the injection of contrast material is not often performed in the study of venous disease. However, sometimes it is helpful to have these images to identify the high computed tomography density of acute hematoma or thrombus, and to look for calcified deposits that may otherwise become obscured by the presence of contrast material. The use of intravenous contrast material is almost always necessary for computed tomography scanning of venous disorders. Intravenous, iodinated contrast material opacifies the lumens of all patent venous structures. It outlines their pathways, anomalous routes, identifies occlusions, collateral venous drainage, distinguishes between adjacent lymph nodes and venous structures as well as aids in the detection of thrombosed veins.

In most patients, an arm vein is chosen for the administration of contrast material. An indwelling catheter is acceptable to use as long as the injection rate does not exceed the structural integrity of the catheter. The inflow of contrast material from an arm vein offers direct opacification of the drainage through the ipsilateral subclavian and innominate vein segments and subsequently the superior vena cava. Scans of the upper thorax display these opacified venous segments as having a very high computed tomography density, similar to that of the bone.

Contrast flow artifacts

Contrast material has different physical properties from blood, and at major venous junctions the wash-in of unopacified blood does not mix homogeneously with the opacified venous blood. This produces filling defects downstream that may be large and give the false appearance of a thrombus or a mass (Fig. 16.3). In the thorax, this occurs at the junctions of the ipsilateral jugular vein, the opposite innominate vein, and in the right atrium. When studying the superior vena cava, it is best to have bilateral infusions of contrast material from the arms. This will produce homogeneous opacification of the innominate veins and the superior vena cava. It can be difficult at times to identify tumor or thrombus within the right atrium as a result of incomplete mixing of contrast material with inflow from the inferior vena cava. When the contrast reaches the right ventricle, the opacification will become homogeneous in density and will remain homogeneous throughout the pulmonary vessels, the left heart, the aorta and its branches. However, within the inferior vena cava at the levels of the renal and hepatic veins, prominent wash-in artifacts are often seen, especially with fast scanners (Figs 16.4 and 16.5). These flow artifacts can be misinterpreted as thrombus. They occur because of the rapid, high flow through the tributary veins while the cava, caudal to this, receives only a small amount of blood flow from the lower extremities.

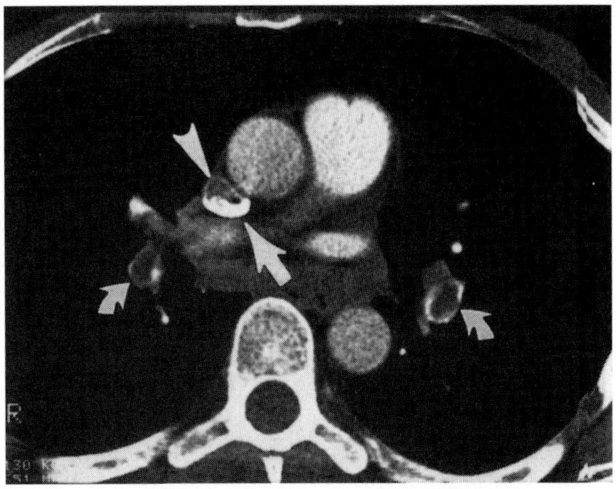

Figure 16.3 *Electron beam computed tomography scan through the chest at the pulmonary valve level. Contrast material within the superior vena cava is present in the posterior portion only (arrow), indicating that only one arm was injected and the wash-in from the contralateral innominate vein results in incomplete mixing of contrast. This gives a false appearance of thrombus in the superior vena cava (arrowhead). Also note the bilateral pulmonary embolism (curved arrows) in the lower lobe pulmonary arteries with a thin rim of contrast opacification peripherally. This is a typical appearance by computed tomography scanning of acute pulmonary embolism.*

Venous opacification

Understanding the timing of venous opacification is important in performing a diagnostic computed tomography examination. Once the contrast material leaves the aorta, the timing of venous opacification is dependent upon the proximity of the organ and the volume of blood flow to it as well as its distance from the central veins. For example, the jugular veins opacify quickly but opacification of the inferior vena cava, renal, portal, and iliofemoral venous segments occurs later and at different times from each other. The mesenteric and portal venous segments fill almost as fast as the renal veins, and contrast opacification of their tributaries will be seen at approximately the same scanning time. However, the hepatic veins take a little longer – perhaps another 15 seconds – to opacify fully. The low inferior vena cava and

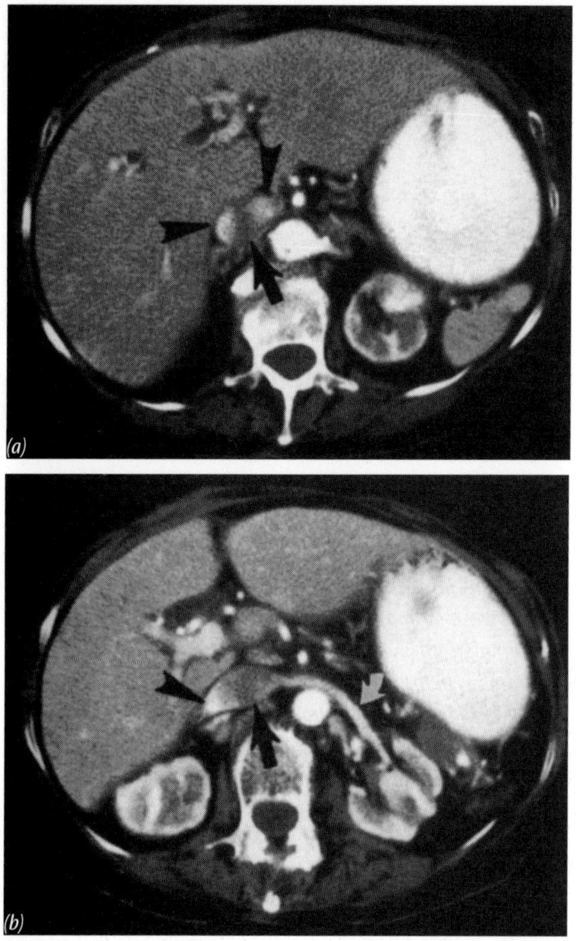

Figure 16.4 *Computed tomography scan at the renal vein level shows incomplete opacification of the upper inferior vena cava. (a) Shows lateral zones of opacification (arrowheads) in the inferior vena cava while the central portion is unopacified (arrow). (b) Computed tomography scan taken 2 cm caudal to (a) shows right lateral opacification within the cava from the right renal vein (arrowhead). Note the opacification of the left renal vein (curved arrow). The majority of the inferior vena cava is devoid of opacification (arrow).*

the iliofemoral vein segments will opacify relatively late because of the long return transit time through the legs (Fig. 16.6).

Capturing adequate opacification levels of all venous structures by computed tomography scanning is challenging. It is somewhat difficult to opacify all major venous segments adequately on one scan sequence because of the complex relationships of the venous system in certain parts of the body. The timing of the scanning must be coordinated with the delivery of the contrast material.

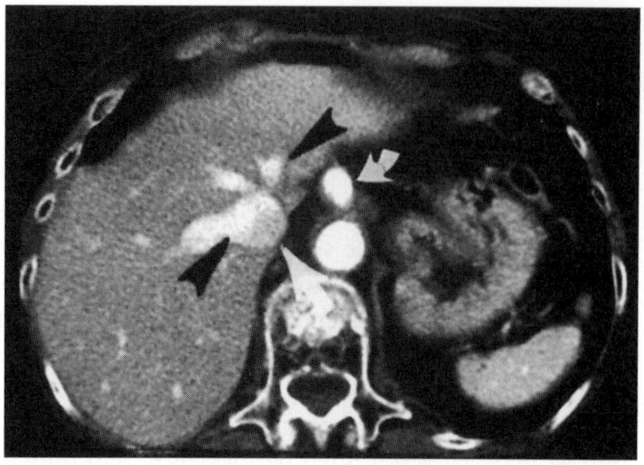

Figure 16.5 *Computed tomography scan through the mid-liver shows hepatic vein opacification (arrowheads) with mixed density in the inferior vena cava from wash-in of blood from the lower inferior vena cava (arrow). The scan was performed for evaluation of the celiac artery aneurysm (curved arrow).*

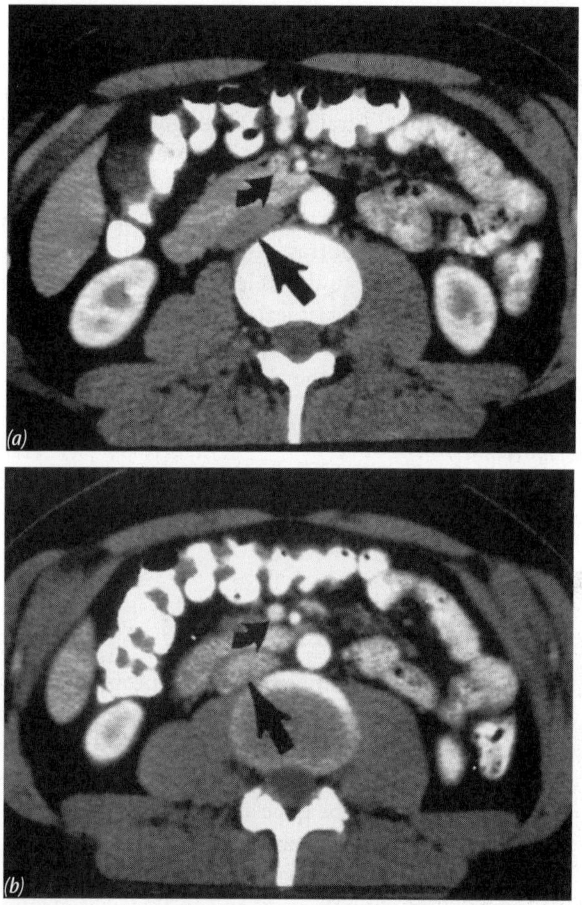

Fig. 16.6 *Computed tomography scan through the mid-abdomen. (a) At this level and time, the inferior vena cava (arrow) is not yet opacified with contrast material. Also note the opacification of the superior mesenteric artery (arrowhead) and the lack of opacification of the mesenteric vein (curved arrow). (b) This scan is taken 1 cm caudal to (a) and 2 seconds later. Note that now the inferior vena cava (arrow) and the mesenteric vein (curved arrow) have become opacified.*

COMPUTED TOMOGRAPHY IMAGING

Peripheral veins

Examination of peripheral veins in not often performed with computed tomography scanning in view of the cost-effectiveness of ultrasound. However, when examining the pelvis, the lower sections include the common femoral vessels. Thrombus within the iliofemoral veins is sometimes discovered by coincidence either in a patient with a protracted hospital course or in someone who is having an abdominal computed tomography scan for other indications (Fig. 16.7). Computed tomography scanning of the neck sometimes reveals occlusion of a jugular vein (Fig. 16.8), which is readily identified because of the high volume and rapid flow in the carotid arteries. However, ultrasound provides a more cost-effective imaging modality.

Vena cava

The superior and inferior vena caval segments are anatomically oriented in the long axis of the body which is ideal for cross-section views as provided by computed tomography scans. A routine series of scans will capture the entire length of the cava. The fat-tissue planes surrounding the caval segments allow most of their course to be well seen without contrast material. However, contrast enhancement usually will be necessary to completely evaluate for most disorders.[3] In most clinical situations, magnetic resonance imaging duplicates this imaging capacity. Thrombosis, extrinsic compression, tumors and postoperative states are the most frequent caval disorders encountered and an aneurysm (Fig. 16.9) would be one of the rarest.[4] The consequence of obstruction of the superior vena cava is the superior vena cava syndrome: the result of venous hypertension to the head and arms[5] (see Chapter 41).

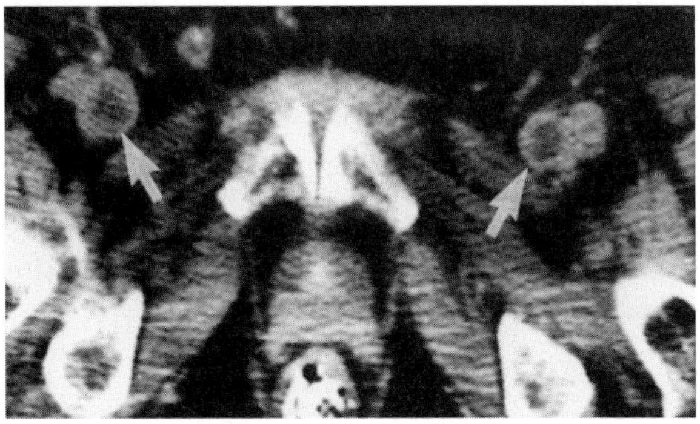

Figure 16.7 *Thrombosis of the femoral veins. Computed tomography scan taken through the femoral vein level shows bilateral intraluminal filling defects (arrows) of acute thrombosis.*

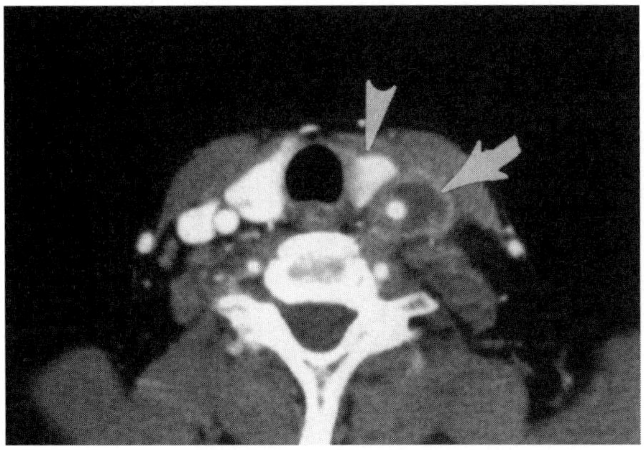

Figure 16.8 *Computed tomography scan taken through the low neck shows a low-density zone (arrow) around the left common carotid artery. This is an infection in the carotid sheath. Note that the internal jugular vein does not opacify because of occlusion. The high-density zone anterior to the left carotid artery is the thyroid gland (arrowhead).*

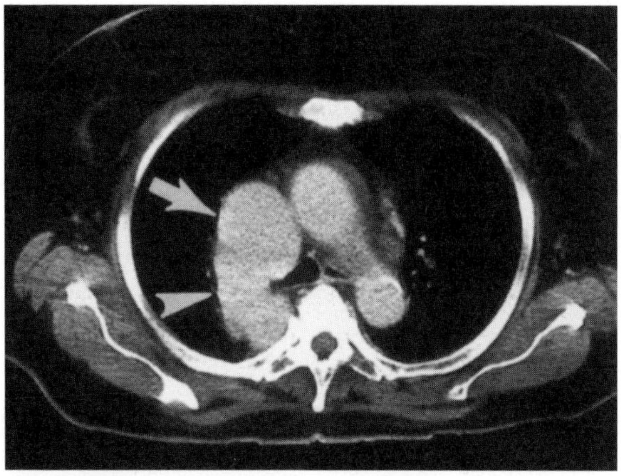

(a)

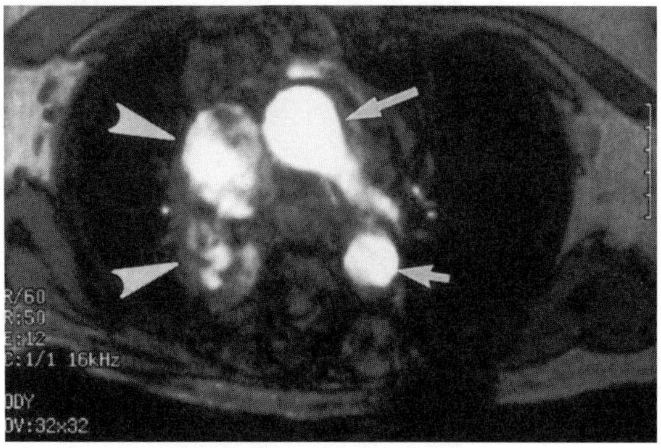

(b)

Figure 16.9 *Aneurysm of the superior vena cava with extension into the azygos vein. (a) Computed tomography scan of the thorax taken through the azygos arch shows an aneurysm of the superior vena cava (arrow) and of the azygos arch (arrowhead). (b) Magnetic resonance image taken through the same thoracic level with a sequence of gradient echo shows high signal of flowing blood in the aorta (arrows) and mixed signal intensity in the venous aneurysm (arrowheads).*

ANOMALIES

Anomalies of the cava reflect remnant embryological pathways and subsequent development.[6] Therefore, the expected possibilities are large left-sided venous structures and absence of some of the right-sided cava. Usually, the persistent left-sided caval segment is only partially represented. For instance, in the low abdomen, a persistent left-sided cava usually crosses to the right by entering the left renal vein. It may be the only cava at this site. But, if it is a duplication, its diameter may not be equal to its mate on the right. At times it is found to have the diameter of a large gonadal vein. When its caliber is intermediate in size it may be confused for a lymph node when viewed on a single computed tomography slice.

Interruption of the inferior vena cava at or just above the renal vein level is sometimes encountered (Fig. 16.10). This can be related to either a right- or left-sided inferior vena cava. The cephalic continuation is via the azygos vein on the right or the hemiazygos on the left. In this condition, the hepatic veins drain into the cephalic remnant of the inferior vena cava. These variants can appear as confusing images when first encountered, but remembering the double-sided embryological development and mentally considering variations in regression and persistence of various segments during growth usually allows accurate interpretation.

In the chest, the most common variant of the superior vena cava is duplication manifested by a left-sided superior vena cava which empties to either the coronary sinus or the hemiazygos vein. The size of the left-sided superior vena cava is variable and rarely is it equal to the right. Its origin may be directly and solely from the left innominate vein or just a remnant branch from it.[5] Its appearance on computed tomography scan is that of a round or oval mass of variable size along the left lateral side of the aortic arch (Fig. 16.11). During contrast injection of the right arm the left-sided superior vena cava will not opacify and therefore may be misinterpreted as a lymph node adjacent to the aortic arch. Obviously, if the contrast is given via the left arm, then only the left superior vena cava will be opacified. Enlargement of the azygos arch and the caudal portion of this vein and its companion the hemiazygos vein may be an indication of anomalous drainage from a left superior vena cava or from azygos continuation of an interrupted inferior vena cava.[6] However, it is important to consider that there may be an acquired occlusion resulting in large venous collaterals. A search must be made to distinguish between a congenital variation and collateral drainage secondary to obstruction of a major venous structure or portal hypertension (Fig. 16.12).

A major venous anomaly within the thorax that produces unusual computed tomography findings is partial or complete anomalous pulmonary venous connections. Magnetic resonance imaging is the best noninvasive imaging modality for this entity because of its multiplanar imaging capacity.[7]

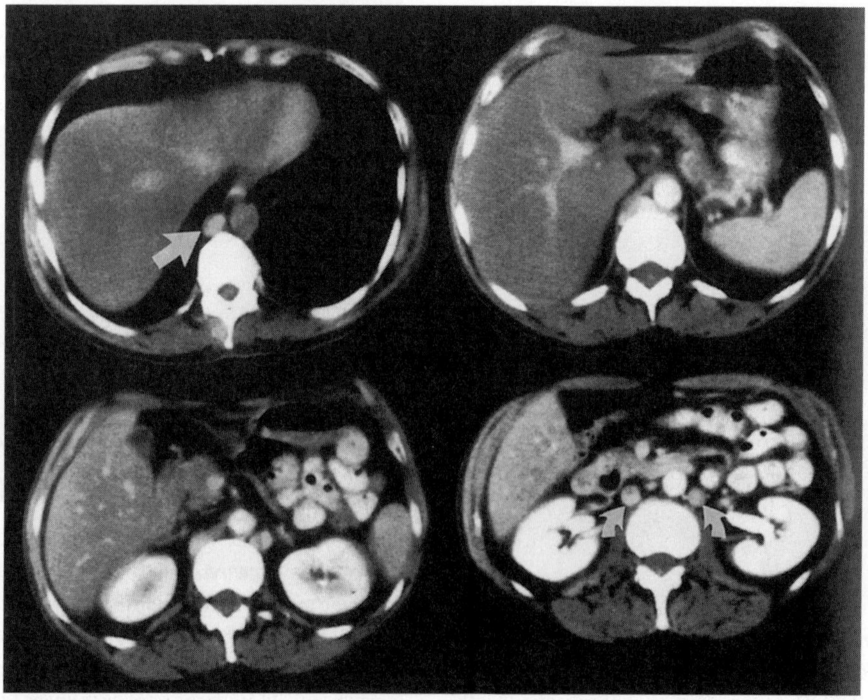

Figure 16.10 *Duplication of the low inferior vena cava with azygos continuation into the thorax. The left upper computed tomography image shows a large azygos vein (arrow). The right lower image through the abdomen shows bilateral inferior venae cavae (curved arrows).*

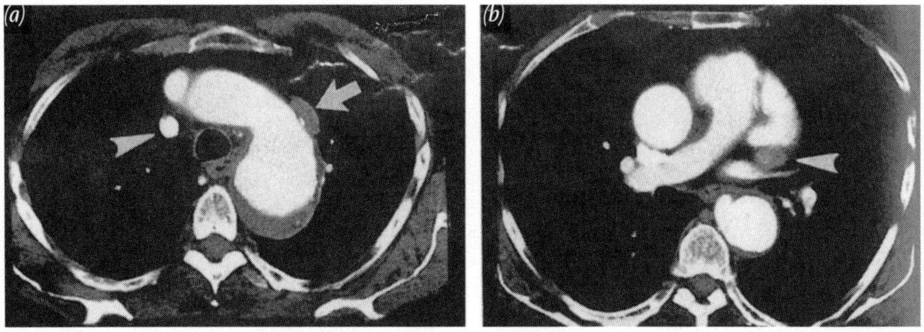

Figure 16.11 *Left-sided superior vena cava. (a) Electron beam computed tomography scan taken across the aortic arch shows a non-opacified vascular structure (arrow) representing the left superior vena cava. This drains from the left innominate vein; however, the contrast material was injected from the right arm which opacifies the right superior vena cava (arrowhead). (b) Computed tomography scan taken a few centimeters caudal to (a) shows the course of the left superior vena cava (arrowhead) between the atrial appendage anteriorly and the pulmonary vein posteriorly.*

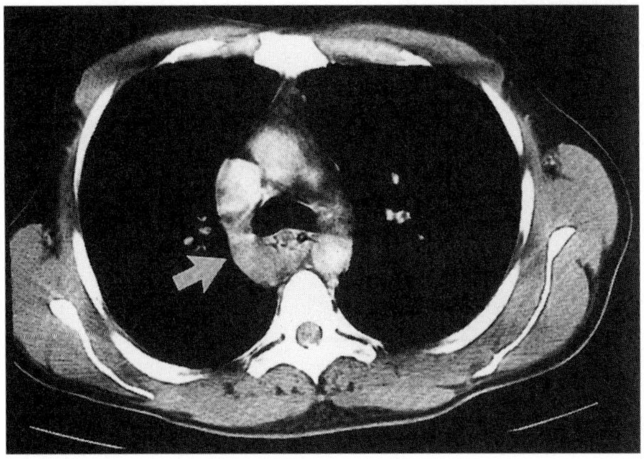

Figure 16.12 *Computed tomography scan through the azygos arch (arrow) shows enlargement secondary to high flow through the azygos system decompressing gastroesophageal varices from portal hypertension.*

THROMBUS

Thrombus within the cava is readily detected (Fig. 16.13), provided the contrast material is correctly delivered and accurately captured on the scans at the various venous segments as previously mentioned. Acute thrombus presents as a filling defect within the lumen of the cava, often expanding the lumen to a moderate degree, in the acute phase, and making it appear round and large in cross-section. Often, the normal cava is not round, but instead it has an irregular oval configuration reflecting normal compression by adjacent structures such as the ascending thoracic aorta, the intrahepatic portion of the liver, and infrarenal abdominal aortic aneurysms. The normal cross-sectional shape of the cava reflects its compliance and wide range of distensibility (Fig. 16.14). Its shape readily changes with forced respiratory efforts – inspiration, expiration and Valsalva maneuver – made during the scanning sequence. A sustained Valsalva maneuver causes distension of the inferior vena cava and the major tributaries as well as reduction of the flow.

Rarely, a fresh thrombus within any major vein will be found to have a high density by computed tomography.[8] This is true also for hematomas within the first 2–3 weeks of duration. It may be difficult to discover such a high-density thrombus because almost always the computed tomography scan sequence would initially be performed with intravenous contrast material. Old thrombus that does not dissolve or recanalize may convert to a fibrotic scar and obliterate the vessel to a thin cord. Rarely, old thrombus may calcify and present as a calcified mass within the occluded lumen.

INFERIOR VENA CAVA FILTERS

The status of an inferior vena cava filter sometimes needs to be evaluated by computed tomography scanning to determine if there has been migration of the legs outside the cava and into adjacent bowel or the aorta or to determine if there is thrombus above the filter. Computed tomography scanning is the best method to rule out these problems (Fig. 16.15).

TUMORS

Tumors of the cava are either primary, such as leiomyosarcoma (Fig. 16.16), or secondary due to invasion by tumors of adjacent organs (see Chapter 43). Indeed, a retroperitoneal source of leiomyosarcoma may also spread into the inferior vena cava through draining veins or from the veins of organs such as the uterus. Renal tumors (hypernephromas) are the most common source of tumor thrombus extending into the inferior vena cava.[9] This phenomenon is also found to occur rarely with some adrenal tumors. Intraluminal tumor from any source causes expansion of the venous lumen (Fig. 16.17) and, therefore, often can be recognized even without contrast enhancement. In the superior vena cava, tumor within the lumen is a rare finding and usually arises from primary or secondary thyroid cancers extending from the inferior thyroidal veins. When obstruction of the superior vena cava is suspected, it is important to deliver

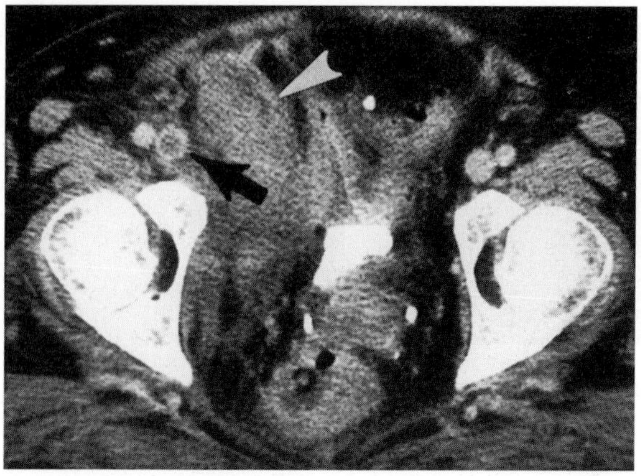

(a)

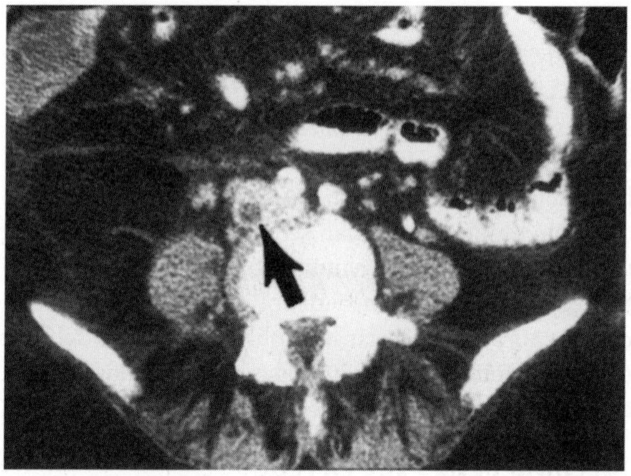

(b)

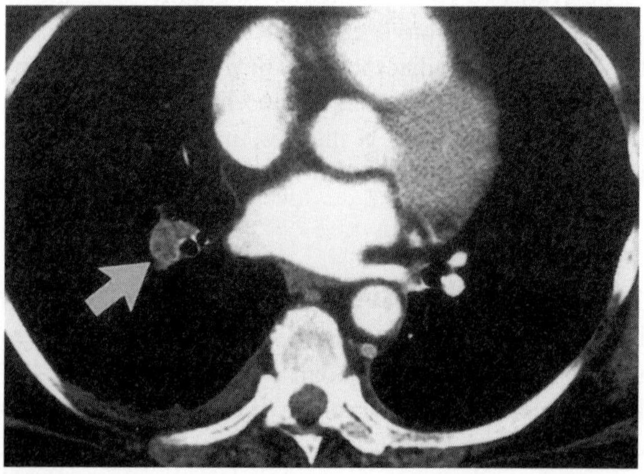

(c)

Figure 16.13 *Thromboembolism. (a) Computed tomography scan taken through the femoral vein level shows acute thrombus within the right common femoral vein (arrow) with adjacent hematoma medially (arrowhead) secondary to complication of cardiac catheterization. (b) Computed tomography scan taken through the junction of the left and right common iliac veins shows thrombus (arrow) extending from the right common iliac vein up to the inferior vena cava. (c) Electron beam computed tomography scan through the mid-chest shows a large embolus in the right lower pulmonary artery (arrow).*

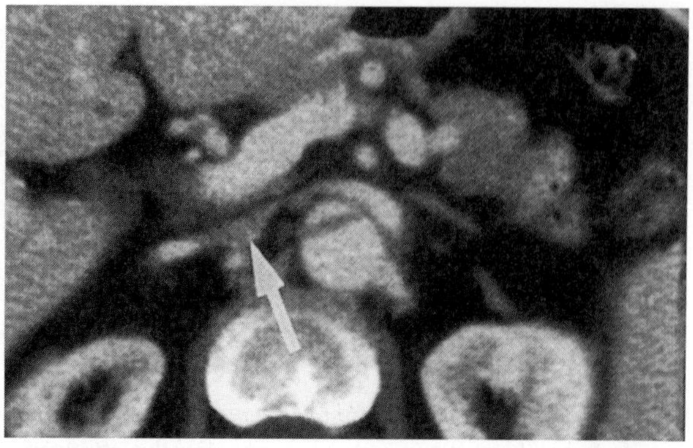

(a)

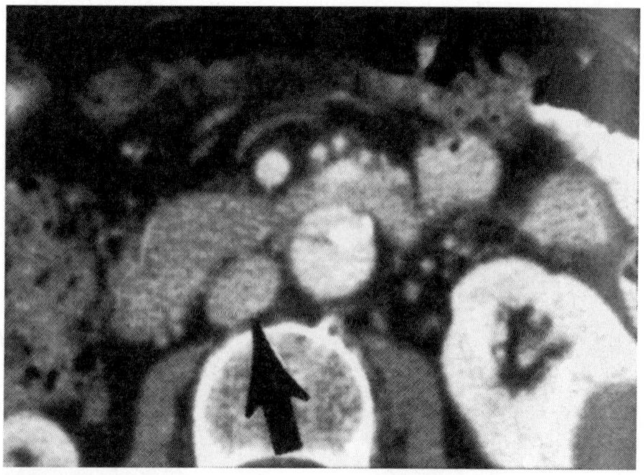

(b)

Figure 16.14 *There is a large change in diameter of the inferior vena cava secondary to voluntary respiratory control. (a) Computed tomography scan shows the cava to be a narrow slit (arrow). (b) The cava has a much more rounded configuration (arrow) on this computed tomography scan taken 3 cm caudal to (a).*

intravenous contrast material from both arms simultaneously to fully opacify both innominate veins.

Extrinsic compression of the cava can occur from aortic aneurysms, adjacent tumors (Figs 16.18 and 16.19) and from surrounding inflammatory conditions.[3,10] Aneurysms of the ascending thoracic aorta cause compression deformity of the superior vena cava (Fig. 16.20). However, it is unusual for this to result in obstruction of the venous drainage of the superior vena cava. In very rare cases, a large, chronic abdominal aortic aneurysm can erode into the adjacent inferior vena cava or the iliac vein, causing a fistula to develop. This can be recognized on the computed tomography scan by rapid and dense opacification of the infrarenal inferior vena cava. Fistula formation can also occur as a complication of performing laminectomy for protruded lumbar disc disease (Fig. 16.21).

Neoplasm in the mediastinum causing occlusion of the superior vena cava or innominate veins is a late

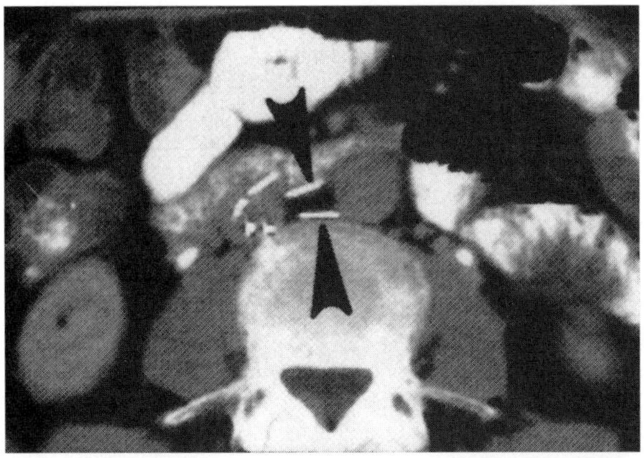

(a)

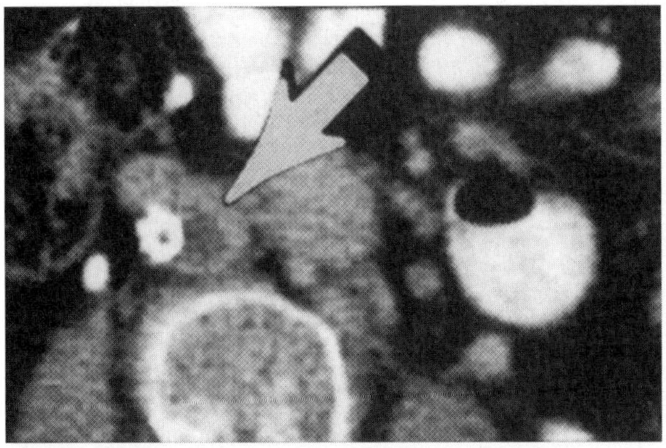

(b)

Figure 16.15 *Inferior vena cava filter. (a) Computed tomography scan taken through the low inferior vena cava shows the legs of the caval filter (arrowheads) have penetrated through the wall of the cava. (b) Computed tomography scan at the level of the low inferior vena cava. The cava contains thrombus (arrow) alongside the cephalad tip of a caval filter, indicating extension of thrombus beyond the filter.*

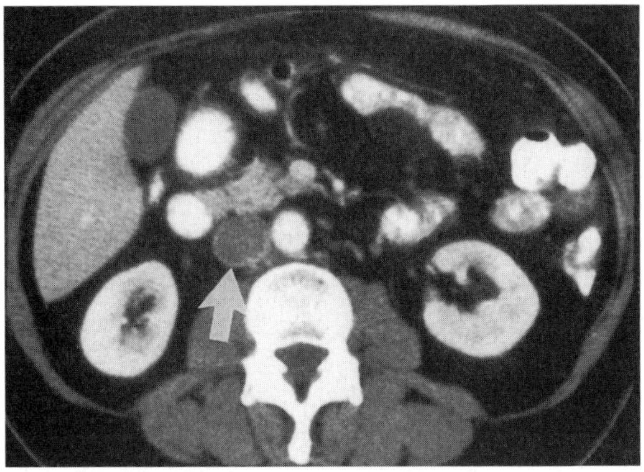

Figure 16.16 *Computed tomography scan through the low inferior vena cava shows a low-density filling defect (arrow) within it, indicating leiomyosarcoma within the cava.*

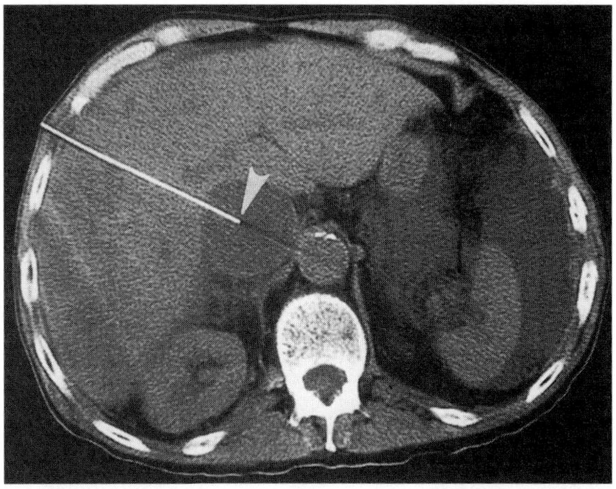

Figure 16.17 *Large tumor thrombus within the inferior vena cava from a hypernephroma. Computed tomography scan taken through the upper inferior vena cava with a biopsy needle (arrowhead) positioned in the center of the tumor thrombus. Note the marked dilation of the inferior vena cava.*

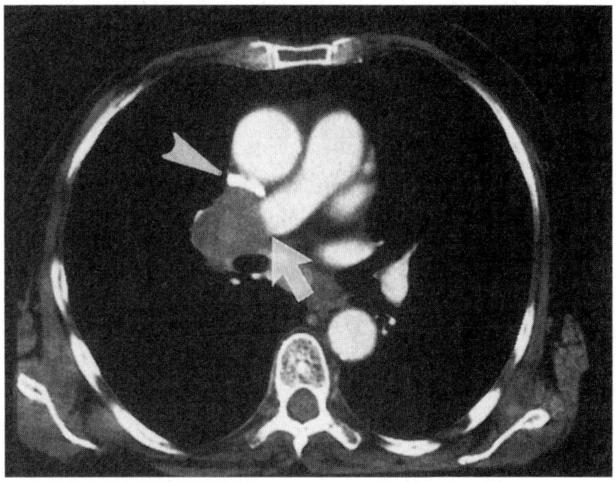

Figure 16.18 *Carcinoma of the lung obstructing the right main pulmonary artery (arrow) and causing stenosis of the superior vena cava (arrowhead).*

manifestation of the disease process (see Chapter 41). The computed tomography findings are those of compressive occlusion of the superior vena cava with poorly developed venous collaterals draining the blood around the obstruction through the intercostal veins or through mediastinal collaterals into the azygos and hemiazygos systems. From there, venous drainage is either antegrade into the lower aspect of the superior vena cava or retrograde into abdominal veins with subsequent drainage into the inferior vena cava. These collateral veins are not well developed in cases of malignant obstruction of the superior vena cava, unlike the situation of benign, chronic obstruction.

In the abdomen, primary malignancies of the retroperitoneum may cause extensive displacement, effacement, or occlusion of the inferior vena cava. Injecting the

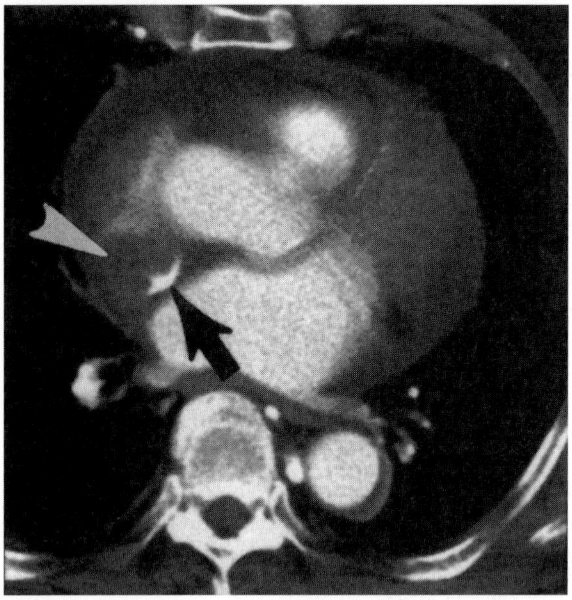

Figure 16.19 *Lymphoma at the junction of the superior vena cava and right atrium. Computed tomography scan taken through the low superior vena cava shows marked stenosis (arrow) secondary to the tumor mass (arrowhead) within the superior vena cava.*

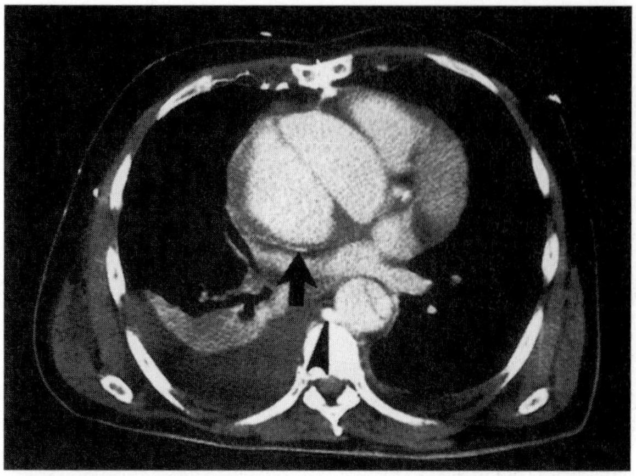

(a)

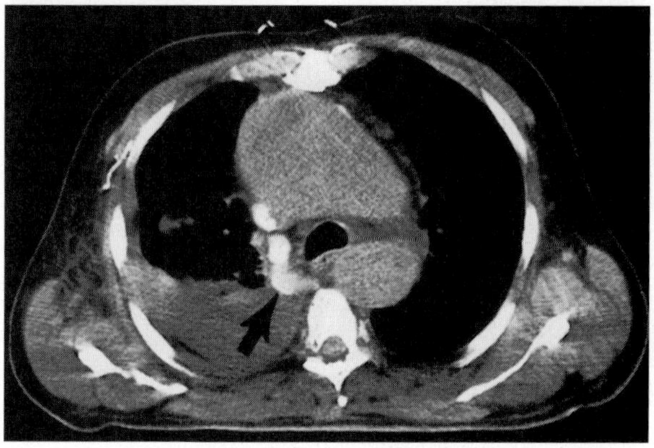

(b)

Figure 16.20 *Dissection of the thoracic aorta with aneurysm of the ascending segment and marked effacement of the superior vena cava. (a) Computed tomography scan shows the superior vena cava to be a thin slit (arrow) compressed by the dissecting aneurysm of the ascending aorta. The azygos vein is densely opacified (arrowhead). (b) Computed tomography scan taken at the level of the azygos arch shows dense opacification of the azygos vein (arrow) which is draining the superior vena cava to a subdiaphragmatic site.*

intravenous contrast material through one or both saphenous veins will also allow identification of the collateral venous drainage. The network of collaterals is usually found to be over the abdominal wall and in the paraspinal region with subsequent drainage into the upper lumbar and lower intercostal veins. There can also be collateral drainage into the portal system and through the capsule of the liver into the hepatic veins. A benign cause of inferior vena cava compression by a mass is found in severe cases of polycystic liver disease. This may cause severe symptoms for the patient because in such a situation the obstruction is high in the abdomen and potential drainage through the liver is blocked by the presence of massive hepatic cysts.

INFLAMMATION

Inflammatory conditions that can stenose or occlude the cava include mediastinitis and retroperitoneal fibrosis. In the central part of the USA, histoplasmosis is the most common etiology of mediastinitis (Fig. 16.22).

Retroperitoneal fibrosis has several etiologies and several different appearances on computed tomography scan. The most common type encountered is periaortitis (or inflammatory aneurysm if the aorta actually has a diameter large enough to be an aneurysm). By computed tomography scan, there is a rind of tissue of variable thickness on the sides and the anterior surface of the aorta, which enhances with intravenous contrast material. Sometimes the outline of the inferior vena cava becomes indistinct but rarely does this result in obstruction of the cava. However, other types of retroperitoneal fibrosis can occlude the inferior vena cava.[11] The computed tomography appearance is somewhat like that of periaortitis, but the periphery of the inflammatory process is indistinct. The borders of the inferior vena cava become indistinct as encroachment and compression result in occlusion (Fig. 16.23).

Renal veins

The renal veins are large enough and opacify with sufficient density as to be easily studied by computed tomography scanning. The right one is usually oriented in an axial direction and somewhat parallels the course

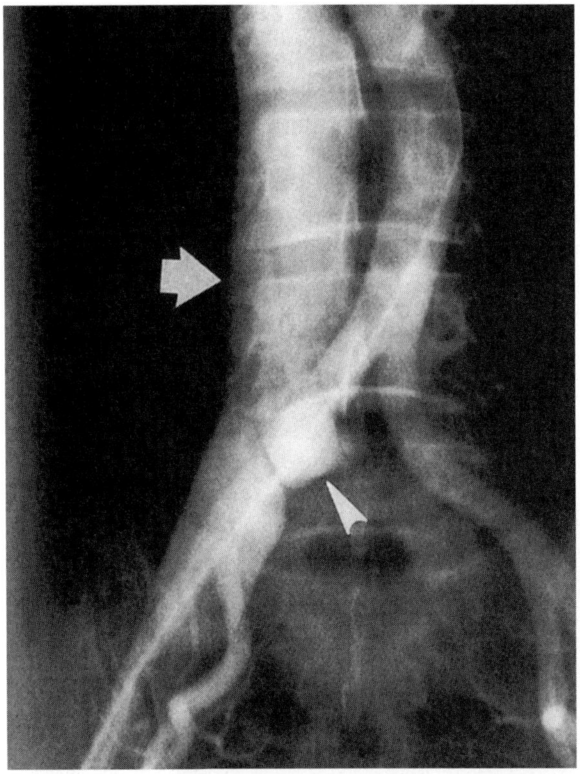

(a)

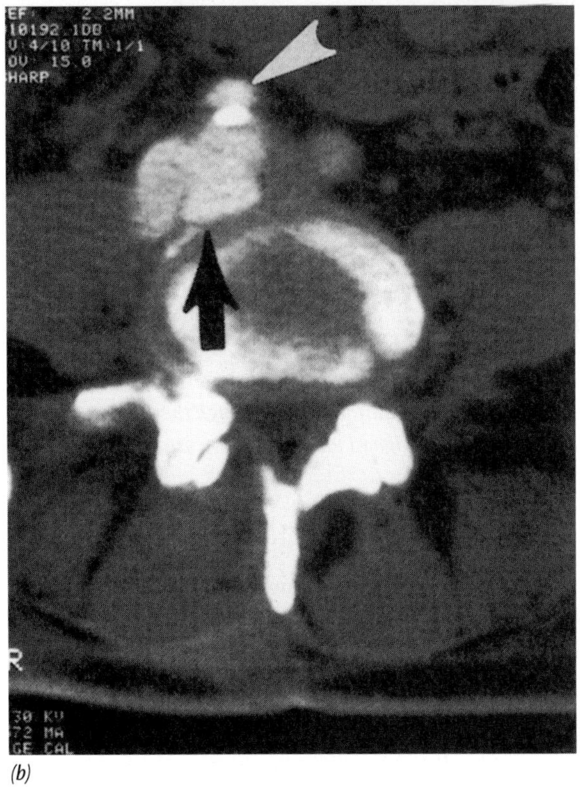

(b)

Figure 16.21 *Postoperative arteriovenous fistula between the right iliac artery and the low inferior vena cava. (a) Aortogram demonstrates rapid filling of the cava (arrow) from a fistula arising from the right common iliac artery (arrowhead). (b) Computed tomography scan taken through this level shows opacification of the right common iliac artery (arrowhead) and simultaneous filling of the inferior vena cava (arrow).*

of the inferior vena cava. The left one, however, has a horizontal orientation and crosses over the anterior surface of the aorta. At times there are double renal veins which can present a confusing picture. When the left one is double, the caudal one is posterior to the aorta. Sometimes, the single left renal vein may pass posterior to the aorta. In either case, there may be an associated large left gonadal vein, probably as remnant of a left inferior vena cava. The two major disease conditions of the renal veins are thrombosis, usually associated with membranous glomerulonephritis, and extension of tumor thrombus, usually from renal cell carcinoma.[9] In either case, the presence of the mass – thrombus or tumor – within the renal vein causes expansion of the diameter of the vein. There may or may not be contrast opacification outlining the thrombus depending upon its extent of involvement. Tumor thrombus may be very large and extend into the inferior vena cava, even into the right atrium (Fig. 16.24). The computed tomography scan can be used to identify the cephalad extension, which is important in planning surgery. When evaluating for the presence of caval involvement, one must remember that natural flow artifacts occur in the inferior vena cava adjacent to the inflow of the renal veins. The computed tomography image allows the diagnosis of tumor to be made and also allows staging of it.

Portal, mesenteric and hepatic veins

Computed tomography scanning provides a global view of the abdomen; the organs and their vessels are all within the field of view. Images can be timed to ensure that the arteries and veins are all opacified. Certainly, the central mesenteric and hepatic vessels will be seen. With a fast scanner and a cooperative patient, vessels as small as 4 mm diameter can be evaluated for thrombus if they are in axial orientation. In patients with Budd–Chiari syndrome (Fig. 16.25), the parenchyma of the liver will show an abnormal tissue perfusion on contrast scans with irregular mottling peripherally and more preservation of perfusion centrally, especially around the caudate lobe.[8,12] The location of the venous occlusion may not be detectable without an angiogram, but acute thrombus within the large hepatic veins or the high inferior vena cava will be identified. In portal hypertension (Fig. 16.26), atrophy of the liver, splenomegaly and varicose collateral venous drainage can be identified.[13] Occasionally calcifications in the walls of splanchnic veins can be found in patients with longstanding portal hypertension.[14] Acute thrombosis of the superior mesenteric and splenoportal veins (Fig. 16.27) may be an isolated finding with a benign clinical course[15,16] or accompanied by bowel wall thickening indicating inflammation or ischemia (see Chapter 25). Whilst many of these patients have venous thrombosis secondary to a primary coagulopathy, a search should be made on the computed

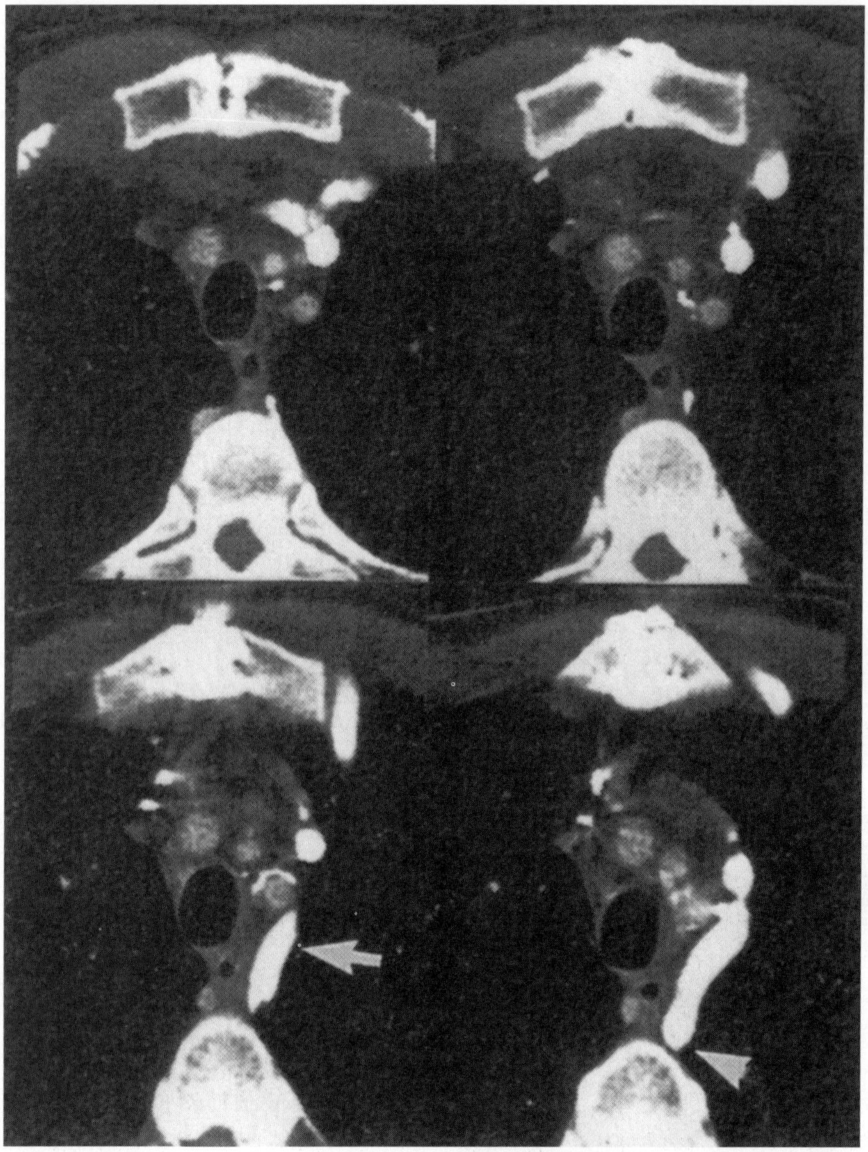

Figure 16.22 *Occlusion of the upper superior vena cava and the innominate veins from mediastinitis. The lowest portion of the superior vena cava is patent and fills from the azygos vein. (a) Computed tomography scans of four levels through the upper mediastinum show no evidence of opacification of the innominate veins. On the left, the highest intercostal vein (arrow) carries the majority of the contrast material to the left hemiazygos vein (arrowhead).*

tomography or magnetic resonance images for regional disease such as carcinoma of the abdominal organs, cirrhosis, or inflammatory bowel disease. These imaging modalities offer a global view of the abdomen, and they are a good method to monitor the course of thrombosis. Portal vein thrombosis may involve only some segments of the liver and cause parenchymal perfusion defects.[16] The thrombus and its extent are easily detected by computed tomography scanning if the contrast infusion is accurately matched to the scanning. A rare finding within the portal venous system is air. Computed tomography scanning is very sensitive to detect this whereas magnetic resonance imaging is not. Portal vein gas is usually associated with ischemic bowel, liver abscess, and other causes of sepsis, although trauma also may be the etiology.[17] Its presence is almost always a grave sign and is associated with a high mortality rate.

Pulmonary embolism

For several years we have been using the electron beam scanner for the diagnosis of acute and chronic pulmonary embolism. The initial feasibility study showed very encouraging results and a controlled, prospective study is underway. Emboli to major branches of the pulmonary arteries – segmental and larger – are almost always seen when present in the

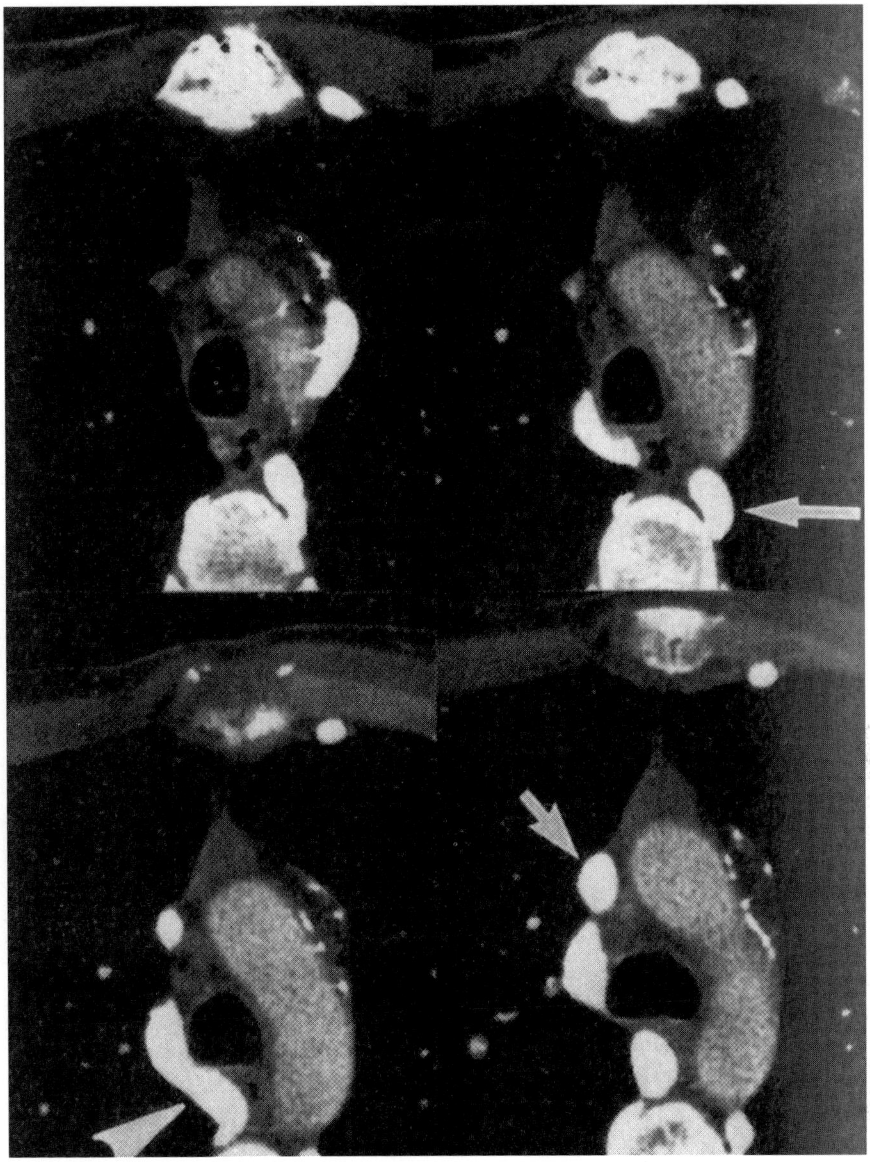

Figure 16.22(b) *Continuing sequence of computed tomography scans caudal to the level of (a) shows filling of the hemiazygos vein (arrow, right upper frame) and of the azygos vein (arrowhead) with subsequent filling of the low superior vena cava (arrow, right lower frame).*

upper and lower lobe arteries because of their vertical orientation (see Fig. 16.3). It is difficult to detect an embolus in a horizontally oriented segmental artery if its diameter is less than the thickness of the computed tomography slice. The distinction by computed tomography scans of acute and chronic embolism can usually be made on the appearance of the thrombus. If it is fresh, it occupies the center of the lumen and contrast surrounds it either completely or partially (see Fig. 16.3). Chronic embolism is organized and adherent to the wall of the pulmonary artery, usually as a plaque-like structure or circumferentially with contrast opacifying the center, recanalized area (Fig. 16.28). The horizontal segments of the right middle lobe arteries and the proximal lingular arteries are difficult to evaluate with the technical limitations of our current scanners. The procedure takes approximately 10 minutes and requires precise timing of the scanning with the contrast injection. The scans are gated to cardiac diastole using 0.1 s scan time. The utilization of this procedure may prove in the near future to have widespread acceptance. Our initial experience showed that the computed tomography study was more sensitive and specific than the ventilation/perfusion scan, and was almost as good as the angiogram.[18] An additional benefit of performing a computed tomography scan for a patient suspected of having pulmonary embolism is the ability to image the entire chest as a byproduct of studying the pulmonary

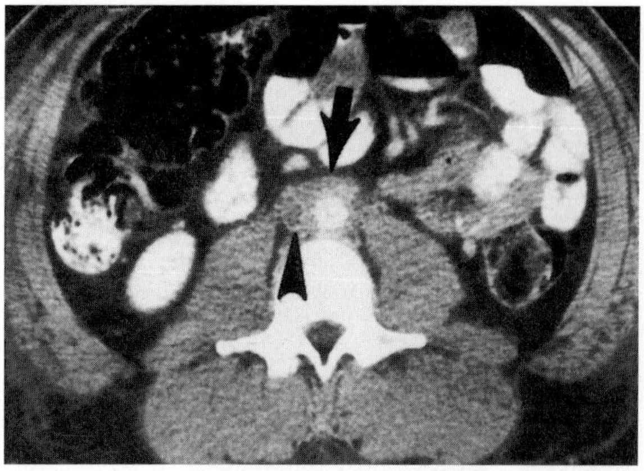

Figure 16.23 *Retroperitoneal fibrosis. Computed tomography scan through the infrarenal aorta shows a thick rind anteriorly (arrow) with occlusion of the inferior vena cava (arrowhead).*

arteries; atelectasis, pneumothorax, aortic aneurysm and dissection, and coronary artery calcification can all be detected with the same examination.

MAGNETIC RESONANCE IMAGING

The major advantage of magnetic resonance imaging over computed tomography and conventional venography in venous imaging is the ability to demonstrate flow and flow dynamics without the need for intravenous iodinated contrast material. There are few contraindications to magnetic resonance scanning with no known biological ill-effects at current clinical magnetic field strengths. Patients with certain cerebral aneurysm clips and various implanted electronic devices such as pacemakers and cardiac defibrillators represent the majority of instances of magnetic resonance incompatibility.

Despite all that magnetic resonance imaging can offer the patient with venous disorders, use in our practice is rather limited as compared with other modalities. There are various reasons why this very powerful technology is not commonly utilized. Ultrasonography provides most of the information required in the extremities and in certain abdominal applications. Contrast contraindications represent the most common situations when magnetic resonance imaging replaces contrast venography or computed tomography. The next most common usage is as a 'problem solver' role when other modalities do not or cannot provide diagnostic information. Pelvic deep venous thrombosis and flow quantification in grafts or in the portal system are typical examples where magnetic resonance imaging is clearly superior to other methods (Figs 16.29 and 16.30). Whilst magnetic resonance imaging is an excellent choice to image the vena cava, cavography is still frequently performed with stent or filter placement or with balloon angioplasty. It is seldom necessary to image the cava noninvasively before such interventions. Tumor involvement of the cava is beautifully demonstrated on coronal magnetic resonance imaging, but images performed with computed tomography scan are also frequently adequate (Figs 16.31 and 16.32). The cost of magnetic resonance imaging exceeds that of computed tomo-

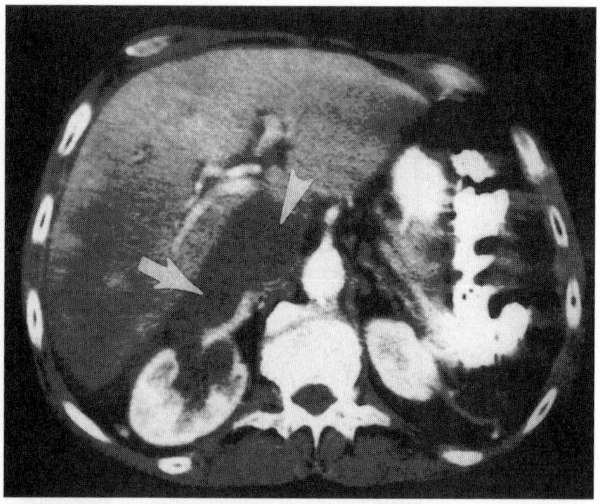

(a)

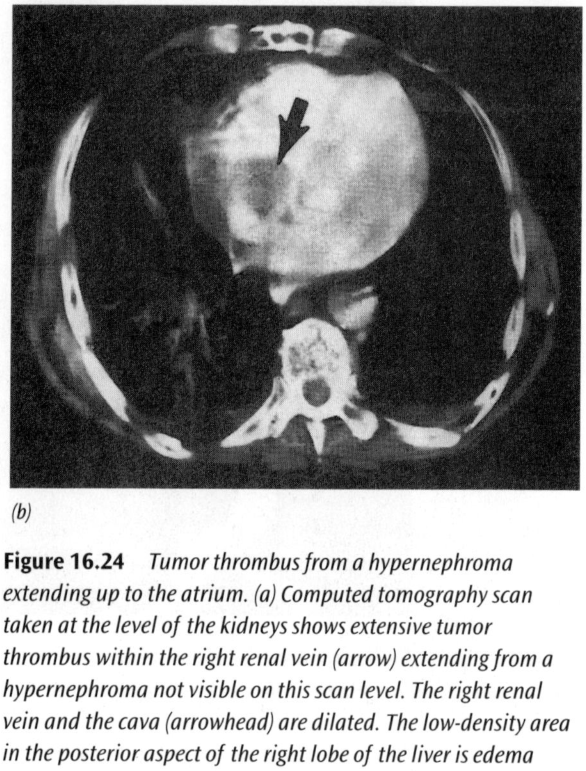

(b)

Figure 16.24 *Tumor thrombus from a hypernephroma extending up to the atrium. (a) Computed tomography scan taken at the level of the kidneys shows extensive tumor thrombus within the right renal vein (arrow) extending from a hypernephroma not visible on this scan level. The right renal vein and the cava (arrowhead) are dilated. The low-density area in the posterior aspect of the right lobe of the liver is edema secondary to obstruction of the right hepatic vein by the large tumor thrombus within the inferior vena cava (same patient as in Fig. 16.21). (b) Computed tomography scan taken through the heart shows cephalad extension of the tumor thrombus into the right atrium (arrow).*

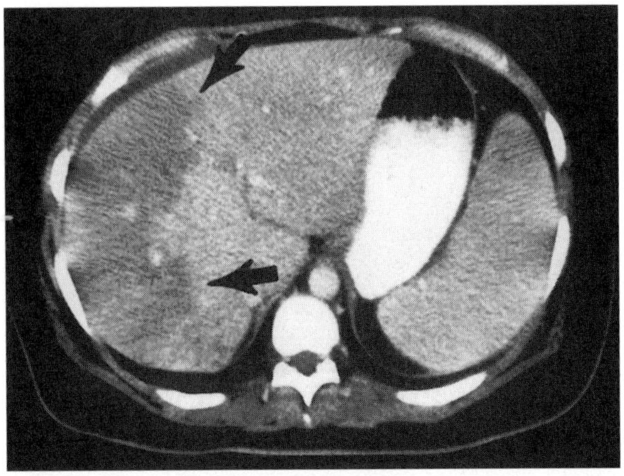

Figure 16.25 *Budd–Chiari syndrome: computed tomography scan through the liver – with contrast enhancement – shows mixed density parenchymal stain. The low-density zone in the right lobe (arrows) subtends the area of hepatic vein occlusion. The left lobe and caudate lobe are not involved and have normal density.*

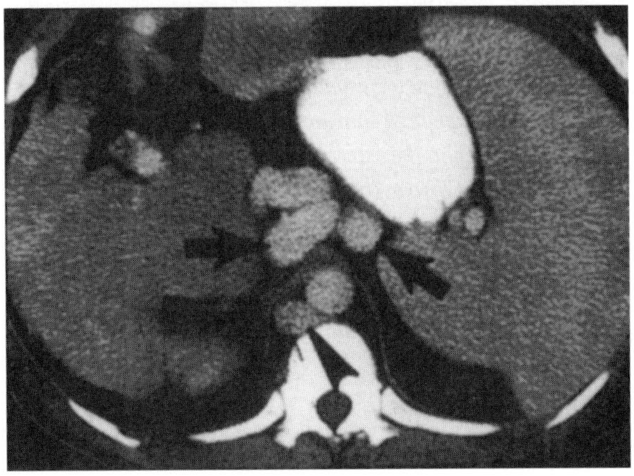

Figure 16.26 *Computed tomography scan through the upper abdomen shows huge varicosities of the left gastric vein (arrows) secondary to portal hypertension. Note the large azygos vein (arrowhead) posterior to the aorta. There is atrophy of the liver with enlargement of the caudate lobe and splenomegaly.*

graphy or ultrasonography. Interpretation of magnetic resonance vascular studies can be difficult for those not familiar with the various flow-related artifacts that are commonly present, whereas most clinicians are very comfortable with computed tomography and contrast venography. In addition, although noninvasive, magnetic resonance imaging is not an easy examination

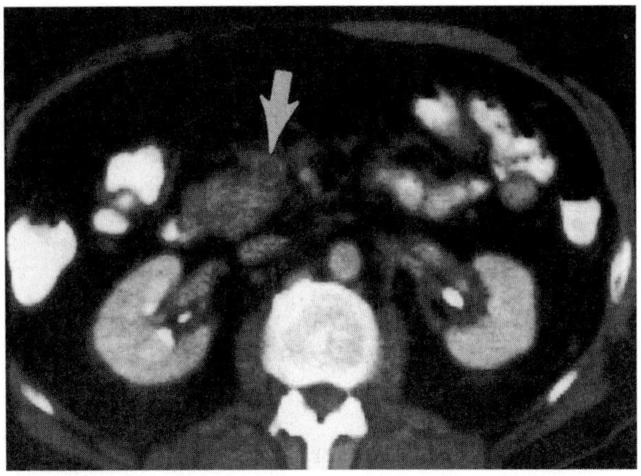

Figure 16.27 *Computed tomography scan of the mid-abdomen shows acute thrombus within the superior mesenteric vein (arrow).*

for many patients such as the obese, the elderly, and the very ill patient. Breath-hold and other fast-imaging sequences have shortened acquisition times, but patients are still required to remain motionless for several minutes for most applications.

Vena cava

Coronal magnetic resonance section through the cava can be striking in their clarity (Fig. 16.33). The wide field of view and natural contrast of flowing blood provided by magnetic resonance imaging demonstrate congenital anomalies, thrombosis, extrinsic compression, and tumor involvement noninvasively and without contrast.[19,20] Typically simple 'black blood' spin–echo imaging sequences are adequate and they provide the greatest anatomic detail in the abdomen of nonvascular structures. With this technique, the examinations are short and cost is limited. The addition of some type of gradient–echo sequence provides more sensitivity for flow demonstrating filling defects, stenoses, or arterio-venous communications.

Collateral formation in caval obstruction is often better demonstrated on gradient–echo and angiographic magnetic resonance images as compared to contrast venography or ultrasonography.[21,22] Detecting inferior vena cava thrombosis with the various caval filters in place can be done accurately and safely without concern of filter migration.[23]

Peripheral veins

Ultrasonography has dramatically reduced the need for contrast venography for the diagnosis of deep venous thrombosis in the extremities. However, detection of thrombus within calf veins and extension of deep venous

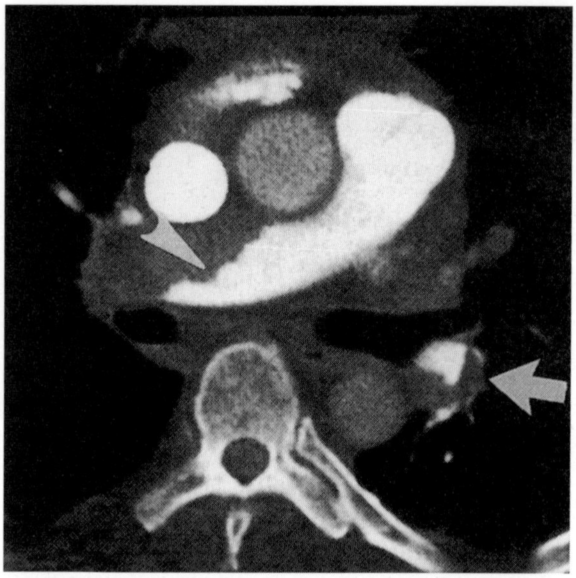

(a)

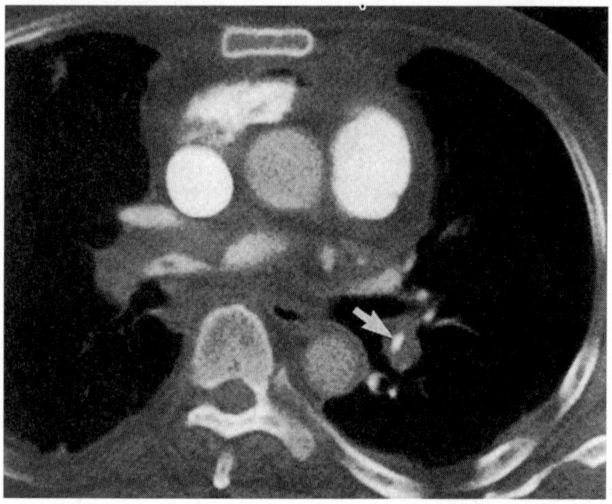

(b)

Figure 16.28 *Electron beam computed tomography scan showing chronic pulmonary embolism. (a) The scalloped border of the right pulmonary artery (arrowhead) represents laminated thrombus. There is also laminated thrombus (arrow) in the left lower lobe pulmonary artery. (b) Computed tomography scan 2 cm caudal to (b) shows a small, central recanalized lumen in the left lower pulmonary artery (arrow) with surrounding old laminated thrombus. This indicates recanalization of chronic pulmonary embolism.*

thrombosis into the pelvis and inferior vena cava are often unreliable. Magnetic resonance imaging, primarily utilizing gradient–echo imaging, can better image pelvic thrombus and has similar sensitivity and specificity for calf deep venous thrombosis when compared to contrast venography.[24] Magnetic resonance imaging has the added advantage in its ability to study both limbs simultaneously for the same cost and imaging time (Figs 16.34

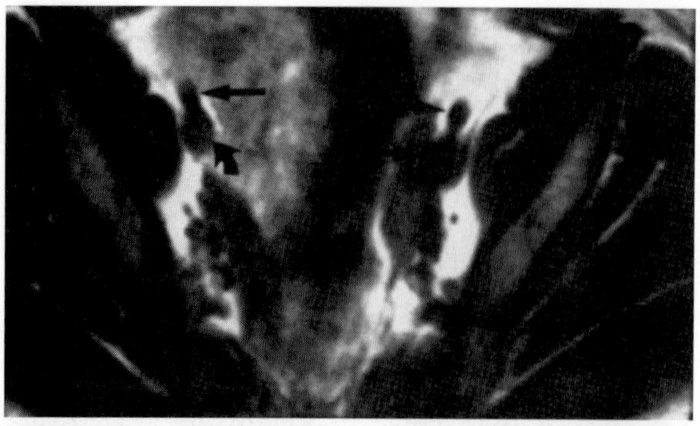

(a)

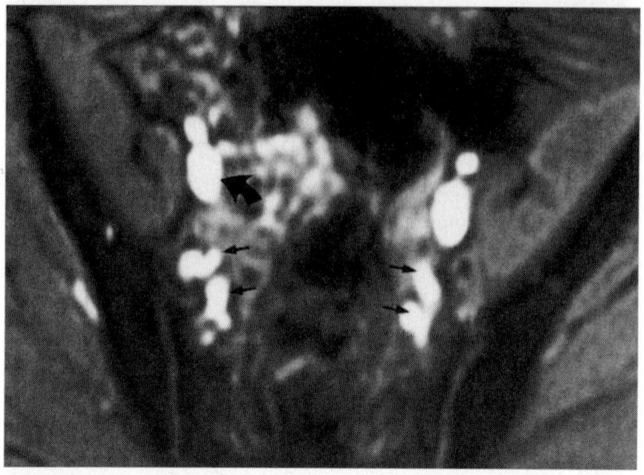

(b)

Figure 16.29 *Magnetic resonance image of the pelvic veins. (a) Standard T1-weighted spin–echo imaging demonstrates flow void phenomenon in the external iliac arteries and left external iliac vein (straight arrows) but with intermediate signal intensity in right external iliac vein (curved arrow), indicating possible thrombosis. (b) Gradient echo image demonstrates patency of the right external iliac vein (curved arrow) as well as numerous patent branches of the internal iliac venous and arterial systems (straight arrows).*

Figure 16.30 (opposite) *Left internal jugular vein–right atrial spinal vein graft. (a) Conventional venogram demonstrates patency of left internal jugular to right atrial appendage spiral vein graft (arrow). There is an occlude stent within the thrombosed superior vena cava (arrowhead). (b) Gradient echo image demonstrates the patency of the vein graft (arrow). There is signal loss in the superior vena cava which is an artifact caused by the metallic stent, resulting in the magnetic field disturbance (curved arrow). (c) Phase (top) and magnitude (bottom) images at the level of the lower neck demonstrate patency of the vein graft (arrow) located anterior to the left common carotid artery. The phase image contains both directional and velocity information. In this instance, flow toward the heart is set to give a high signal intensity. (d) Region of interest marker is placed around the vein graft and shows a typical venous flow plot and provides velocity and flow rates for future graft surveillance.*

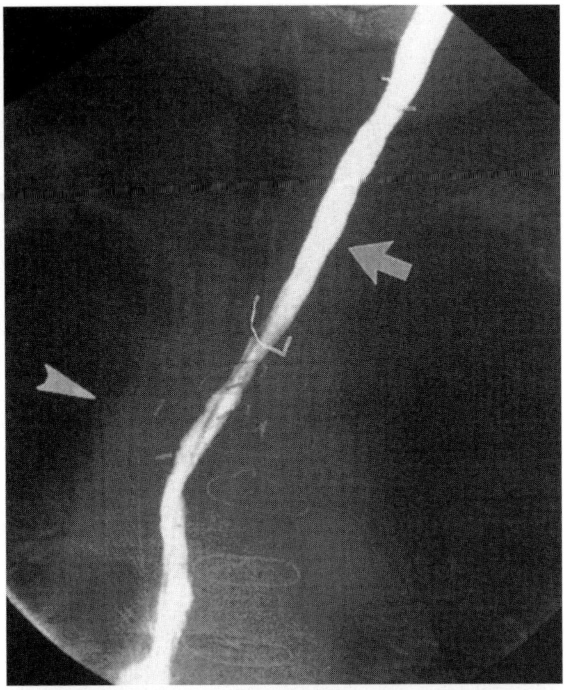

(a)

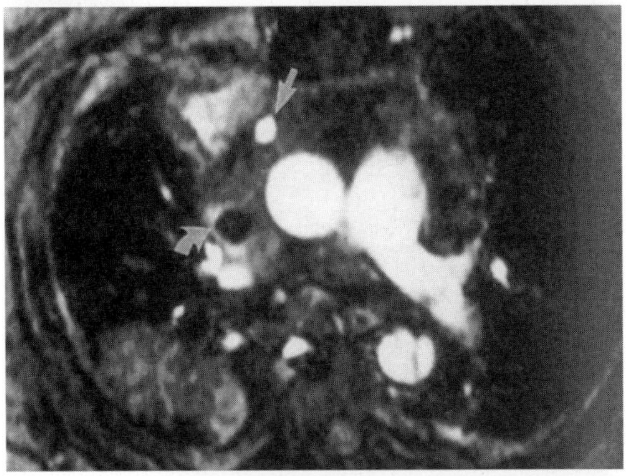

(b)

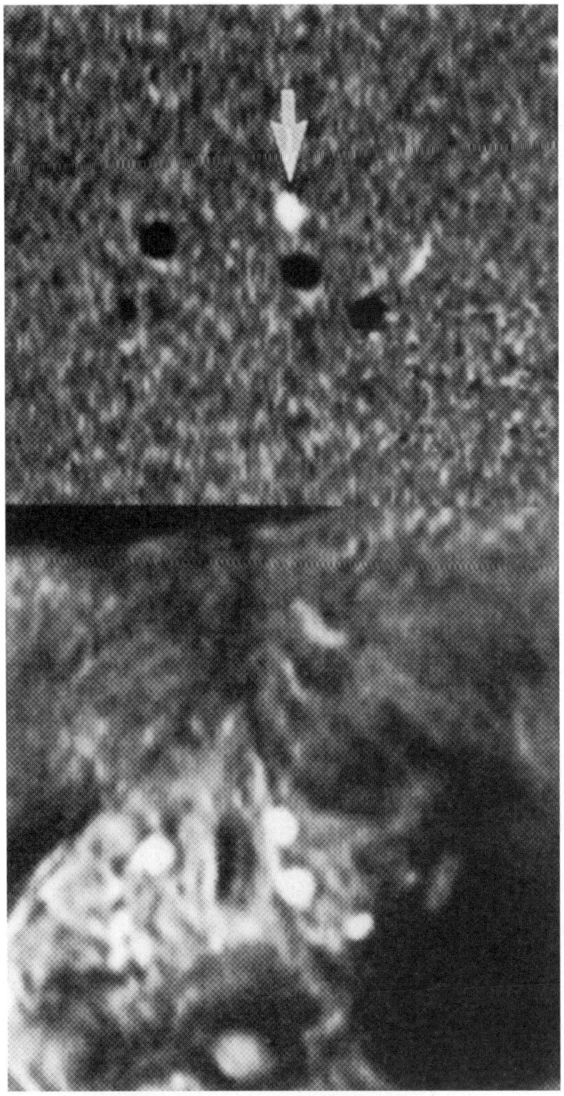

(c)

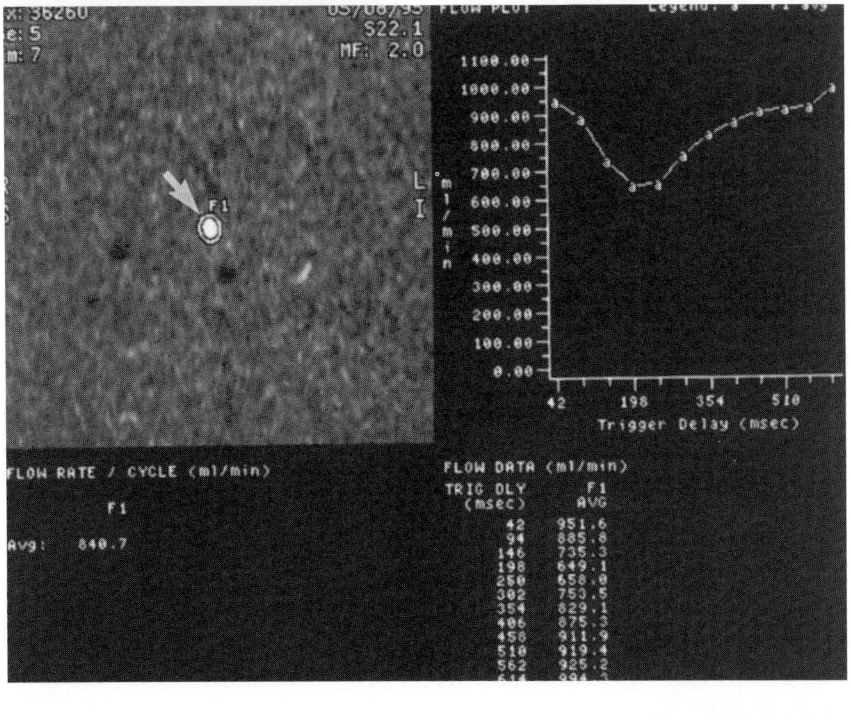
e: 5
m: 7
05/08/95
S22.1
MF: 2.0
FLOW PLOT
F1
1100.00
1000.00
900.00
800.00
700.00
600.00
500.00
400.00
300.00
200.00
100.00
0.00
ml/min
42
198
354
510
Trigger Delay (msec)
FLOW RATE / CYCLE (ml/min)
F1
Avg: 840.7
FLOW DATA (ml/min)
TRIG DLY (msec)
F1 AVG
42 951.6
94 885.8
146 735.3
198 649.1
250 658.0
302 753.5
354 829.1
406 875.3
458 911.9
510 919.4
562 925.2

(d)

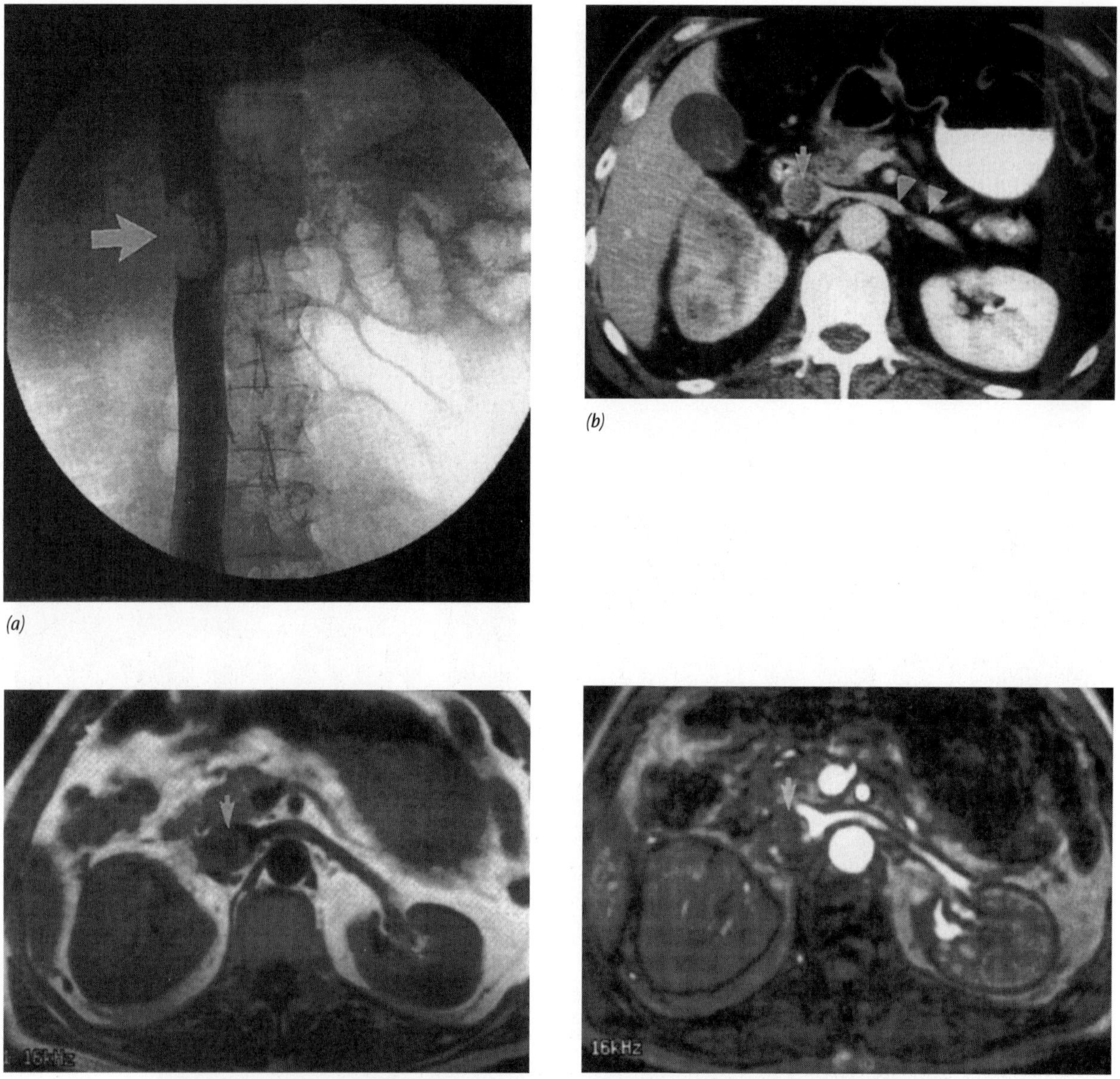

Figure 16.31 *Tumor thrombus in the inferior vena cava. (a) Cavogram demonstrates a filling defect at the level of the right renal vein entrance (arrow). (b) Computed tomography with contrast demonstrating right hypernephroma as well as filling defect in the inferior vena cava (arrow). The left renal vein is patent (arrowheads). (c) Spin–echo and (d) gradient–echo images demonstrate the tumor thrombus in the inferior vena cava (arrows).*

and 16.35). The thoracic inlet is a site of possible venous obstruction of the axillary and subclavian veins where magnetic resonance imaging can not only display the venous anatomy in coronal and sagittal planes but also the surrounding anatomic structures.[25]

KLIPPEL–TRENAUNAY SYNDROME

The value of magnetic resonance imaging for the study of patients with Klippel–Trenaunay syndrome is twofold; it identifies the venous drainage, and the presence and location of the venous malformations, and it displays the soft tissues of the extremities better than any other imaging modality. A magnetic resonance sequence of T2 weighting with second echo produces high signal intensity images of the venous network making it easy to identify (Fig. 16.36). The T1 sequences are better for soft tissue detail of the muscles and fat tissue although the veins are visible as flow voids (Fig. 16.37). This can be helpful in making the diagnosis of Klippel–Trenaunay syndrome in borderline cases. The typical findings are abnormally located, large veins in the

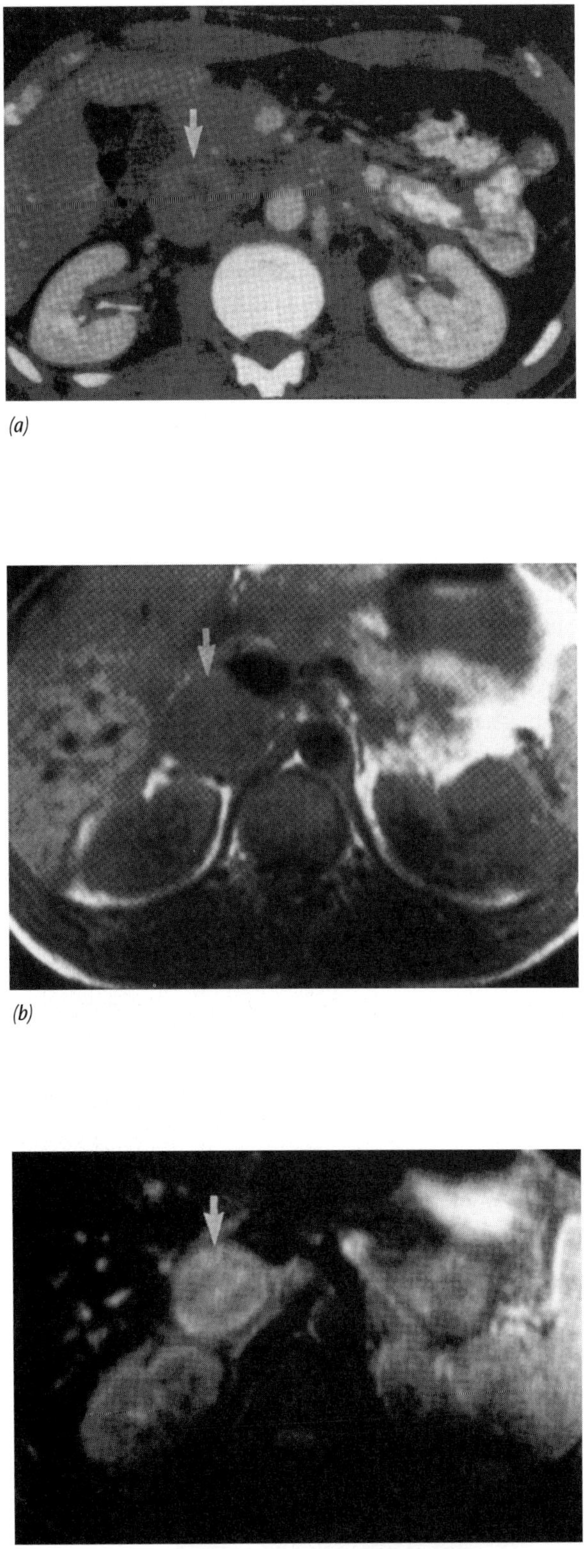

(a)

(b)

(c)

Figure 16.32 *Leiomyosarcoma. (a) Computed tomography scan with contrast demonstrating mixed density, tumor mass filling and expanding the inferior vena cava (arrow). (b) The typical magnetic resonance characteristics of tumor are demonstrated by the relatively low signal intensity (arrow) on T1-weighted images. (c) High signal intensity of tumor (arrow) is found on T2-weighted spin–echo images.*

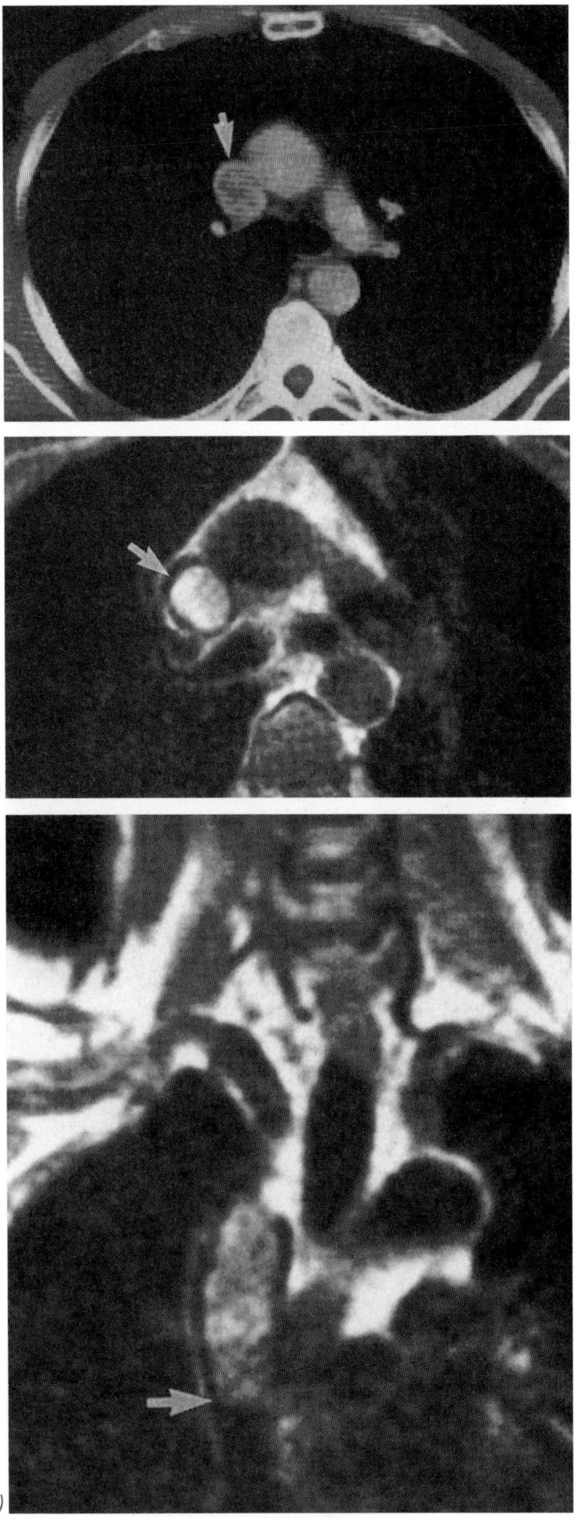

(a)

(b)

(c)

Figure 16.33 *Tumor thrombus in the superior vena cava. (a) Computed tomography with contrast but with poor vessel opacification demonstrates filling defect within the superior vena cava (arrow). (b) Axial spin–echo MR image better depicts the tumor thrombus seen within the superior vena cava. Note there is some signal void peripherally (arrow), indicating some residual patency. (c) Coronal spin–echo image demonstrating inferior aspect of the tumor thrombus (arrow). This was the result of metastatic renal cell carcinoma.*

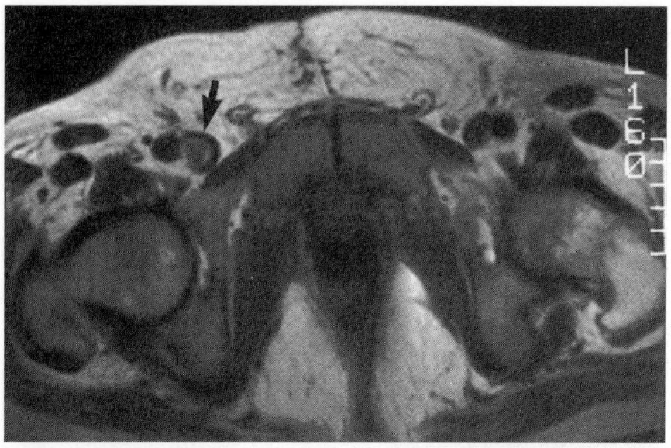

(a)

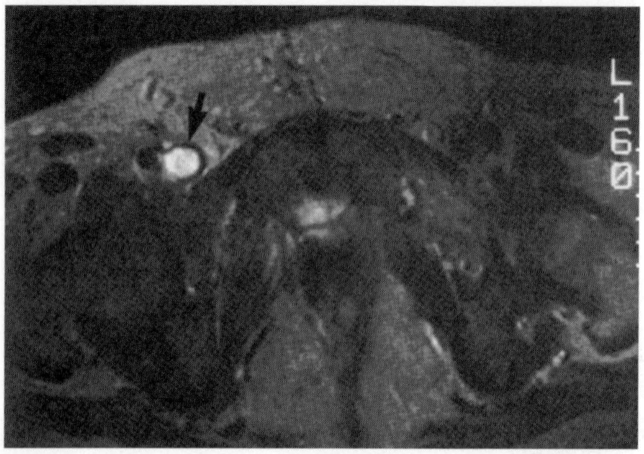

(b)

Figure 16.34 *Thrombus in the right femoral vein. (a) T1-weighted spin–echo image demonstrates high signal within the right common femoral vein (arrow) which is mildly dilated. (b) T2-weighted image also demonstrates high signal within the right common femoral vein, confirming the presence of thrombus (arrow). The remaining femoral vessels are patent.*

subcutaneous space, that is, large veins anteriorly and laterally or an extensive network. Diffuse networks of veins or venous malformations in the muscles of the extremity is another common finding.[26] This may result in increase in the diameter of the extremity, but the volume of the muscle is often reduced. Hypertrophy of the subcutaneous tissue is commonly found. In about one-third of the cases, persistent sciatic vein is found.[27] Phlebography of the extremity is still the best study for the deep venous system to be certain of its presence and continuity.

Portal, mesenteric and hepatic veins

Magnetic resonance imaging is ideally suited to demonstrate and quantitate venous flow within the abdomen.[28,29] Oblique imaging planes can be chosen to follow the course of the portal vein (Fig. 16.38). Magnetic resonance angiographic sequences can provide detailed projections of portal and hepatic branching patterns in preoperative preparation for liver resections or intrahepatic shunting.[30]

Pulmonary vessels

Anomalous venous connections, tumor invasion of the heart via pulmonary vein extension, and venous obstruction secondary to inflammatory or neoplastic conditions are readily demonstrated by magnetic resonance imaging.[7,18] It is also possible to identify pulmonary embolism if it is present in the large proximal arteries.

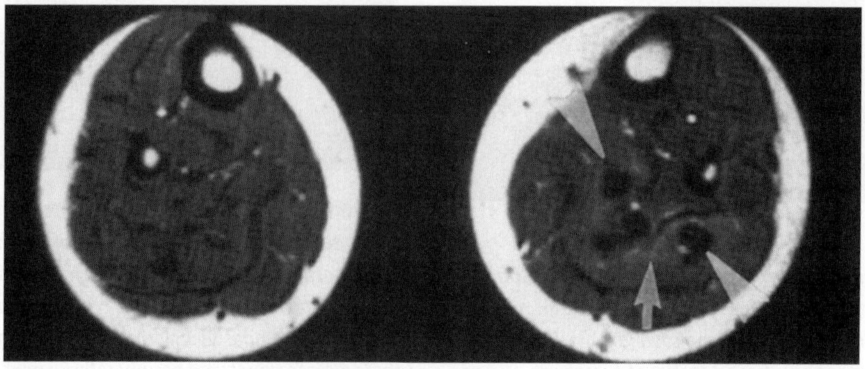

Figure 16.35 *Deep venous thrombosis of the left leg. Magnetic resonance imaging scan through the calf level shows dilated veins (arrowheads) in the left lower leg. The surrounding muscles are edematous as shown by the faint high intensity (arrow) compared to the normal tissue. Also, compare with the normal right leg.*

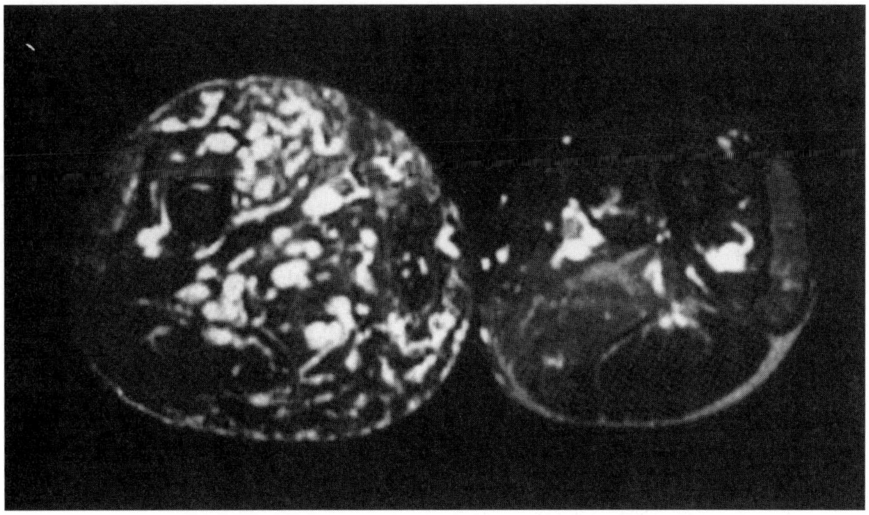

(a)

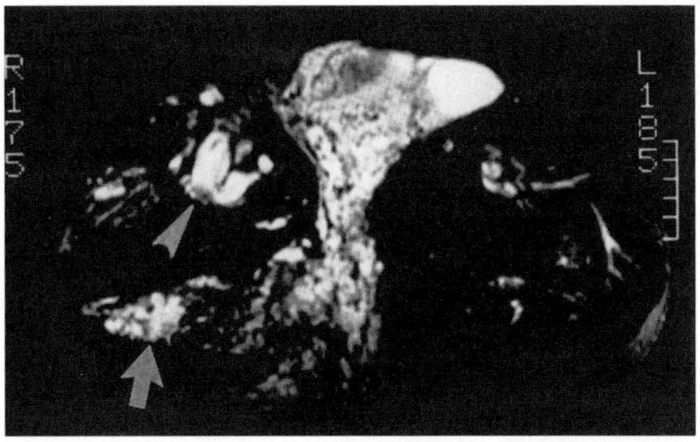

(b)

Figure 16.36 *Klippel–Trenaunay syndrome. (a) Magnetic resonance imaging scan taken through the mid-thigh level shows an extensive venous malformation throughout the muscles and in the subcutaneous space of the right thigh displayed as high signal (white) on the image. This thigh is also larger than the left. The left leg is only slightly involved. (b) Magnetic resonance imaging scan through the low pelvis shows extensive venous malformation of the right buttocks and the scrotum (the white areas of the scan). Note the cluster of dilated right sciatic veins (arrow). There are also dilated veins at the site of the proximal femoral vein (arrowhead).*

CONCLUSION

Magnetic resonance imaging is a powerful modality for imaging venous disorders throughout the body. While computed tomography is often adequate in most common clinical situations when ultrasonography is not diagnostic, the advantages of multiplanar acquisitions, sensitivity to flow, quantitative capabilities, and excellent spatial resolution without need for iodinated contrast or ionizing radiation make magnetic resonance imaging an ideal tool for comprehensive venous imaging. Its current utilization in medical practice largely depends upon practice habits and the available expertise. In the near future, the major determining factor of choosing an imaging modality is likely to become focused on cost-effectiveness.

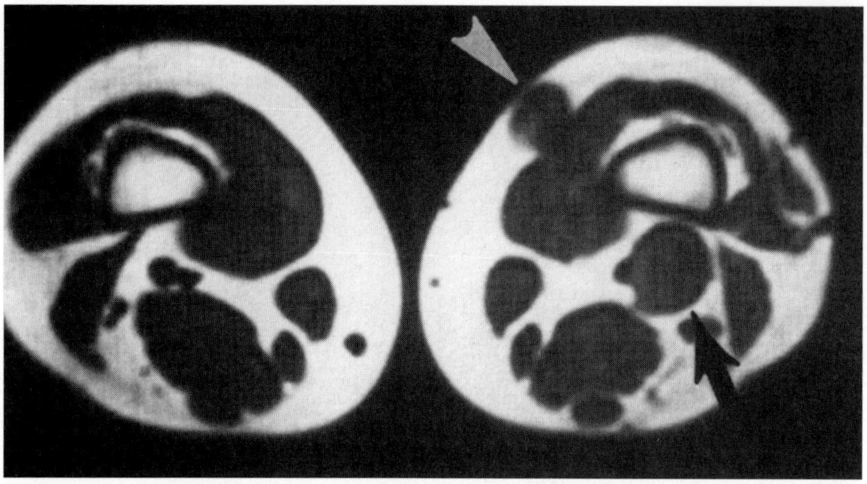

(a)

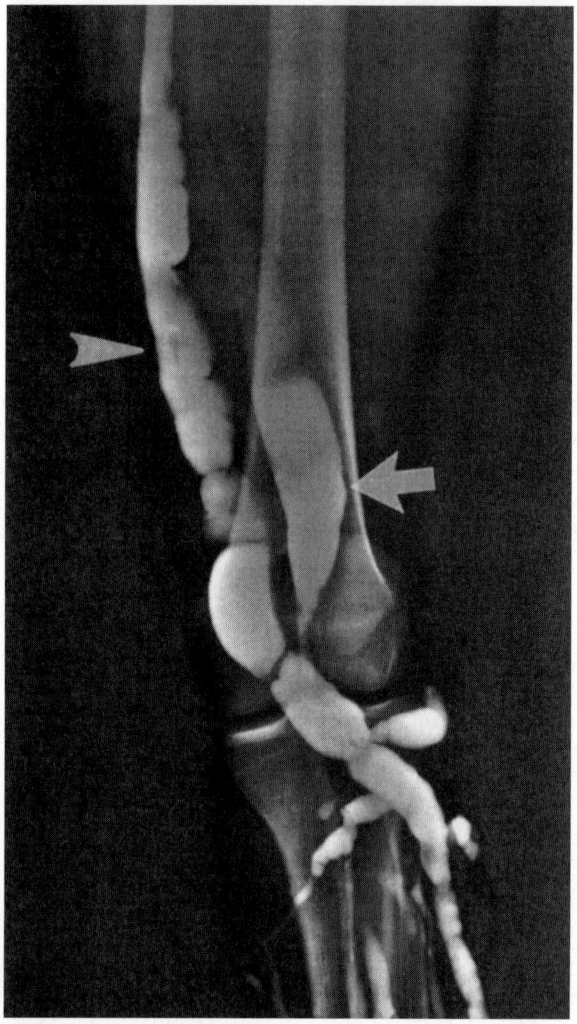

(b)

Figure 16.37 *Klippel–Trenaunay syndrome. (a) Axial magnetic resonance imaging scan through the distal thighs shows aneurysm of the left popliteal vein (arrow) and a dilated, anomalous vein in the subcutaneous tissue anteriorly (arrowhead). Note the slight muscle atrophy of the left leg compared with the right. (b) Venogram of the left leg shows the dilated popliteal vein (arrow) and the anomalous vein crossing the midline and ascending medially (arrowhead). Also note the stenotic zone of the popliteal vein at the knee joint level.*

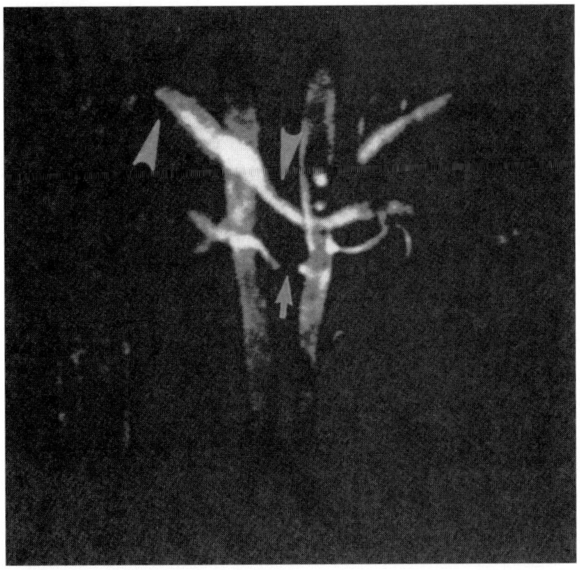

(a)

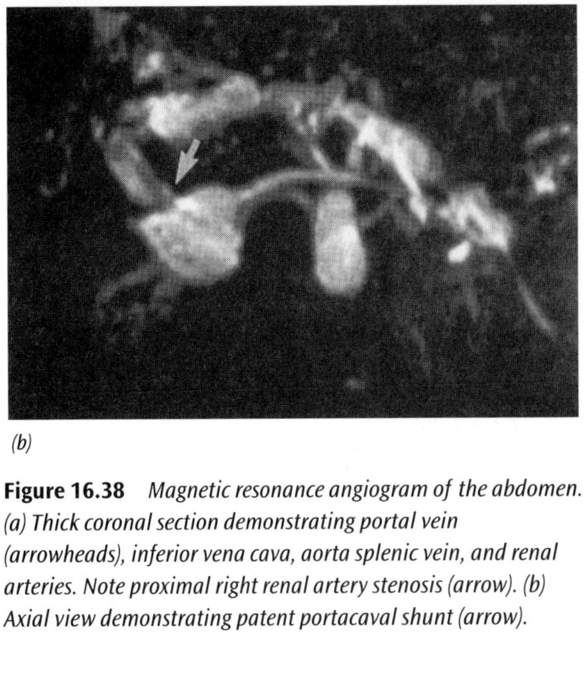

(b)

Figure 16.38 *Magnetic resonance angiogram of the abdomen. (a) Thick coronal section demonstrating portal vein (arrowheads), inferior vena cava, aorta splenic vein, and renal arteries. Note proximal right renal artery stenosis (arrow). (b) Axial view demonstrating patent portacaval shunt (arrow).*

REFERENCES

1. Ross CS, Hussey DH, Pennington EC, *et al.* Analysis of movement of intrathoracic neoplasms using ultrafast computerized tomography. *Int J Radiat Oncol Phys* 1990; **18**: 671–7.
2. Stanford W, Rooholamini SA, Gaivin JR. Ultrafast computed tomography in the diagnosis of aortic aneurysms and dissections. *J Thorac Imaging* 1990; **5**: 32–9.
3. Schwartz EE, Goodman LR, Haskin ME. Role of CT scanning in the superior vena cava syndrome. *Am J Clin Oncol* 1986; **9**: 71–8.
4. Moncada R, Demos TC, Marsan R, *et al.* CT diagnosis of idiopathic aneurysms of the thoracic systemic veins. *J Comput Assist Tomogr* 1985; **9**: 305–9.
5. Takada Y, Narimatsu A, Kohno A, *et al.* Anomalous left brachiocephalic vein: CT findings. *J Comput Assist Tomogr* 1992; **16**: 893–6.
6. Dudiak CM, Olson MC, Posniak HV. Abnormalities of the azygos system: CT evaluation. *Roentgenology* 1989; **24**: 47–55.
7. Choe YH, Lee HJ, Kim HS, *et al.* MRI of total anomalous pulmonary venous connections. *J Comput Assist Tomogr* 1994; **18**: 243–9.
8. Mori H, Maeda H, Fukuda T, *et al.* Acute thrombosis of the inferior vena cava and hepatic veins in patient with Budd–Chiari syndrome: CT demonstration. *AJR Am J Roentgenol* 1989; **153**: 987–91.
9. Didier D, Racle A, Etievent JP, Weill F. Tumor thrombus of the inferior vena cava secondary to malignant abdominal neoplasms: US and CT evaluation. *Radiology* 1987; **162**: 83–9.
10. Chen JC, Bongard F, Klein SR. A contemporary perspective on superior vena cava syndrome. *Am J Surg* 1990; **160**: 207–11.
11. Rhee RY, Gloviczki P, Luthra HS, *et al.* Iliocaval complication of retroperitoneal fibrosis. *Am J Surg* 1994; **168**: 179–83.
12. Vogelzang RL, Anschuetz SL, Gore RM. Budd–Chiari syndrome: CT observations. *Radiology* 1987; **163**: 329–33.
13. McCain AH, Bernardino ME, Sones PJ Jr, *et al.* Varices from portal hypertension: correlation of CT and angiography. *Radiology* 1985; **154**: 63–9.
14. Ayuso C, Luburich P, Vilana R, *et al.* Calcifications in the portal venous system: comparison of plain films, sonography, and CT. *AJR Am J Roentgenol* 1992; **159**: 321–3.
15. Vogelzang RL, Gore RM, Anschuetz SL, Blei AT. Thrombosis of the splanchnic veins: CT diagnosis. *AJR Am J Roentgenol* 1988; **150**: 93–6.
16. Marn CS, Francis IR. CT of portal venous occlusion. *AJR Am J Roentgenol* 1992; **159**: 717–26.
17. Aikawa H, Mori H, Miyake H, *et al.* Imaging and clinical significance of hepatic portal venous gas seen in adult patients. *Nippon Shokakibyo Gakkai Zasshi* 1994; **91**: 1320–7.
18. Teigen CL, Mans TP, Sheedy PF, *et al.* Pulmonary embolism: diagnosis with contrast-enhanced electron-beam CT and comparison with pulmonary angiography. *Radiology* 1995; **194**: 135–40.
19. Webb WR, Sostman HD. MR imaging of thoracic disease: clinical uses. *Radiology* 1992; **182**: 621–30.
20. Fisher MR, Hricak H, Higgins CB. Magnetic resonance imaging of developmental venous anomalies. *AJR Am J Roentgenol* 1985; **145**: 705–9.
21. Finn JP, Zisk JH, Edelman RR, *et al.* Central venous occlusion: MR angiography. *Radiology* 1993; **187**: 245–51.
22. Sonin AH, Mazer MJ, Powers TA. Obstruction of the inferior vena cava: a multiple-modality demonstration of causes, manifestations, and collateral pathways. *Radiographics* 1992; **12**: 309–22.

23. Liebman LE, Messersmith RN, Levin DN, *et al.* MR imaging of inferior vena caval filters: safety and artifacts. *AJR Am J Roentgenol* 1988; **150**: 1174–9.
24. Evans AJ, Sostman HD, Knelson MH, *et al.* Detection of deep venous thrombosis: prospective comparison of MR imaging with contrast venography. *AJR Am J Roentgenol* 1993; **161**: 131–9.
25. Weinreb JC, Mootz A, Cohen JM. MRI evaluation of mediastinal and thoracic inlet venous obstruction. *AJR Am J Roentgenol* 1986; **146**: 679–84.
26. Gloviczki P, Stanson AW, Stickler GB, *et al.* Klippel–Trenaunay syndrome: the risks and benefits of vascular interventions. *Surgery* 1991; **110**: 469–79.
27. Cherry KJ, Gloviczki P, Stanson AW. Persistent sciatic vein: the diagnosis and treatment of a rare condition. *J Vasc Surg* 1996; **23**: 490–7.
28. Arriv L, Menu Y, Dessarts I, *et al.* Diagnosis of abdominal venous thrombosis by means of spin-echo and gradient-echo MR imaging: analysis with receiver operating characteristic curves. *Radiology* 1991; **181**: 661–8.
29. Burkart DJ, Johnson CD, Ehman RL. Correlation of arterial and venous blood flow in the mesenteric system based on MR findings. *AJR Am J Roentgenol* 1993; **161**: 1279–82.
30. Rodgers PM, Ward J, Baudouin CJ, *et al.* Dynamic contrast-enhanced MR imaging of the portal venous system: comparison with x-ray angiography. *Radiology* 1994; **191**: 741–5.

PART 3

Management of acute venous disease

17

Superficial thrombophlebitis

ENRICO ASCHER AND ANIL HINGORANI

Although superficial venous thrombophlebitis (SVT) is a relatively common disorder and has potential morbidity from extension and pulmonary embolism (PE), it has received scant attention in the literature. It has been reported that acute SVT occurs in a recognized form in approximately 125 000 people in the USA.[1] However, the actual incidence is most likely far greater as many cases go unreported. Traditional teaching suggests that SVT is a self-limiting process of little consequence and small risk, leading some physicians to dismiss their patients with the clinical diagnosis of SVT and treat them with 'benign neglect'. In an attempt to dispel this misconception, the more current data regarding SVT and its treatment will be examined.

CLINICAL PRESENTATION

Approximately 35–46 % of patients diagnosed with SVT are males with an average age of 54 years old, while the average age for females is about 58 years old.[2,3] The most frequent predisposing risk factor for SVT is the presence of varicose veins which occurs in 62% of patients. Other factors associated with SVT include: age >60 years old, obesity, tobacco use and history of deep venous thrombosis (DVT) or SVT. Factors associated with extension of SVT include age >60 years old, male sex and history of DVT.

The physical diagnosis of superficial thrombophlebitis is based on the presence of erythematous streaking in the distribution of the superficial veins and tenderness with the thrombosis identified by a palpable cord. Pain and warmth are clinically evident and significant swelling may be present even without DVT. From time to time, a patient may present with erythema, pain and tenderness as a streak along the leg with a duplex ultrasound scan revealing no DVT or SVT. In these patients, the diagnosis of cellulitis or lymphangitis needs to be entertained.

ETIOLOGY

Blood flow changes, changes in the vessel walls and changes in the characteristics of the flow of blood, as cited by Virchow over 100 years ago, continue to play a recognized role in the etiology of SVT. Whilst stasis and trauma of the endothelium have been cited as a cause of SVT, a hypercoagulable state associated with SVT has been inadequately described. Furthermore, recent studies indicate that there is a 5–40% incidence of DVT which occurs in association with SVT, of which a substantial proportion be noncontiguous location with the SVT.[2,3] The presumed mechanism of DVT by direct extension of thrombosis from the superficial venous system to the deep venous system is therefore uncertain, and systemic factors in the pathophysiology of SVT should be explored.

In order to determine whether a hypercoagulable state contributes to the development of SVT, the prevalence of deficient levels of anticoagulants were measured in a population of patients with acute SVT.[4] Twenty-nine patients with SVT were entered into the study. All patients had duplex ultrasound scans performed on both the superficial and deep venous systems. Patients solely with SVT were treated with non-steroidal anti-inflammatory drugs whilst those with DVT were treated with heparin and warfarin. All patients had a coagulation profile performed that included:

- protein C antigen and activity;
- activated protein C (APC) resistance;
- protein S antigen and activity;
- antithrombin III (ATIII); and
- lupus-type anticoagulant.

Twelve patients (41%) were found to have abnormal results consistent with a hypercoagulable state. Five patients (38%) with combined SVT and DVT and seven patients (44%) with SVT alone were found to be hypercoagulable. Four patients had decreased levels of ATIII only and four patients had APC resistance identified. One patient had decreased protein C and protein S, and three patients had deficiencies of ATIII, protein C and protein S. The most prevalent anticoagulant deficiency was ATIII. Careful review of these findings suggests that patients with SVT are at an increased risk of having low levels of naturally occurring anticoagulants, particularly ATIII.

PATHOLOGY

While a great deal of literature exists describing the various changes that take place in the leukocyte–vessel wall interactions, cytokines/chemokines and various other factors involved with the development and resolution of DVT, data investigating the changes involved with SVT were not identified. Although some authors have alluded that the underlying pathology of SVT with DVT may be analogous, to date, this viewpoint remains mostly unsupported.

Trauma

The most common source of trauma associated with SVT is an intravenous cannula. This SVT may result in erythema, warmth and tenderness along its course. Treatment starts with removal of the cannula and warm compresses. The resultant lump may persist for months notwithstanding this treatment.

Suppurative thrombophlebitis

Suppurative SVT (SSVT) is also associated with the use of an intravenous cannula; however, SSVT may be lethal due to its association with septicemia. The associated signs and symptoms of SSVT include pus at an intravenous site, fever, leukocytosis and local intense pain.[5] Treatment begins with removal of the foreign body and intravenous antibiotics. Excision of the vein is rarely needed to clear infection.

Migratory thrombophlebitis

Migratory thrombophlebitis was first described by Jadioux in 1845,[6] as an entity characterized by repeated thrombosis developing in superficial veins at varying sites, but most commonly in the lower extremity. This entity may be associated with carcinoma and may precede diagnosis of the carcinoma by several years. Consequently, a work-up for occult malignancy may, in fact, be warranted when the diagnosis of migratory thrombophlebitis is made.

Lesser saphenous vein thrombophlebitis

Whilst the bulk of attention has been focused on SVT of the greater saphenous vein (GSV), SVT of the lesser saphenous vein (LSV) is also of clinical import. LSV SVT may progress into popliteal DVT. In a group of 56 patients with LSV SVT, 16% suffered from PE or DVT.[2] Therefore, it is crucial that patients with LSV SVT be treated similarly to those diagnosed with GSV SVT, employing the same careful duplex examination, follow-up and anticoagulation or ligation if the SVT approaches the popliteal vein.

Superficial thrombophlebitis with varicose veins

It has been reported that only 3–20% of SVT patients with varicose veins will develop DVT, as compared with 44–60% without varicose veins.[7–9] These findings suggest that patients with varicose veins have a different pathophysiology, such as a hypercoagulable state, as compared with those without varicose veins. In a more recent study, no increased incidence of extension to DVT or PE was noted when comparing patients with and without varicose veins in the 186 SVT patients identified.[2] Consequently, the question of whether the SVT patients with and without associated varicose veins should be thought of as separate classifications remains unclear.

Addressing those patients with SVT of varicose veins is essential. This type of SVT may remain localized to the cluster of tributary varicosities or may, from time to time, extend into GSV.[2] SVT of varicose veins may be without antecedent trauma. SVT is frequently found in varicose veins surrounding venous stasis ulcers. This diagnosis should be confirmed by duplex ultrasound examination as the degree of the SVT may be much greater than that based solely on clinical examination. Treatment consists of conservative therapy of warm compresses and non-steroidal anti-inflammatories.

Upper extremity SVT

Whilst not much appears in the literature on upper extremity SVT, it is considered to be the result of intravenous cannulation and infusion of caustic substances that damage the endothelium. Interestingly, the extension of upper extremity SVT into upper extremity

DVT or PE is a very rare occurrence as compared with lower extremity SVT.[10] Initial treatment of upper extremity SVT is catheter removal followed by conservative measures, such as warm compresses and non-steroidal anti-inflammatory medications.

DIAGNOSIS

Some authors believe that SVT is a benign common process that requires no further work-up unless symptoms fail to resolve quickly on their own.[11] This is in contrast to the findings that indicate DVT associated with SVT may not be clinically apparent.[2]

Duplex ultrasound scanning has become the test of choice for the diagnosis of DVT and the evaluation of SVT since first introduced by Talbot in 1982. The availability of reliable duplex ultrasonography of the deep and superficial venous systems has made routine determination of the location and incidence of DVT in association with SVT accurate and practical. Furthermore, the extent of involvement of the deep and superficial systems can be more accurately assessed utilizing this modality, as routine clinical examination may not be able to precisely evaluate the proximal extent of involvement of the deep or superficial systems. Duplex ultrasound imaging also offers the advantage of being inexpensive, noninvasive and can be repeated for follow-up examination. Since venography may cause the onset of phlebitis and an accurate diagnosis can be made solely by duplex imaging, venography is not recommended. Duplex imaging of patients with SVT has revealed the concomitant DVT to range from 5 to 40%.[2,12–15] It is important to note that up to 25% of these patients' DVTs may not be contiguous with the SVT or may be even in the contralateral lower extremity.[2]

THE NATURAL HISTORY OF SVT

The progression of isolated superficial venous thrombosis to deep vein thrombosis has been evaluated.[16] In one study, patients with thrombosis isolated to the superficial veins with no evidence of deep venous involvement by duplex ultrasound examination were assessed by follow-up duplex ultrasonography to determine the incidence of disease progression into the deep veins of the lower extremities. Initial and follow-up duplex scans evaluated the femoropopliteal and deep calf veins in their entirety with follow-up studies performed at an average of 6.3 days.

Two hundred sixty-three patients were identified with isolated superficial venous thrombosis. Thirty (11%) patients had documented progression to deep venous involvement. The most common site of deep vein involvement was the progression of disease from the greater saphenous vein in the thigh into the common femoral vein (21 patients, 70%), with 18 of these extensions noted to be nonocclusive and 12 having a free-floating component. Three patients had extended above-knee saphenous vein thrombi through thigh perforators to occlude the femoral vein in the thigh. Three patients had extended below-knee saphenous SVT into the popliteal vein and three patients had extended below-knee thrombi into the tibioperoneal veins with calf perforators. At the time of the follow-up examination, all 30 patients were being treated without anticoagulation. As a result of this type of experience, we recommend repeat duplex scanning for SVT of the GSV or LSV after 48 hours to assess for progression.[17]

TREATMENT

The location of the SVT determines the course of treatment. The therapy may be altered should the SVT involve tributaries of the GSV, distal GSV or GSV of the proximal thigh. Traditional treatment for SVT localized in tributaries of the GSV and the distal GSV has consisted of ambulation, warm soaks and non-steroidal anti-inflammatory agents.[1,18,19] Surgical excision may play a role in the rare case of recurrent bouts of thrombophlebitis in spite of maximal medical management. However, this type of management does not address the possibilities of clot extension or attendant DVT associated with proximal GSV SVT.

For SVT within 1 cm of the saphenofemoral junction, management with high saphenous ligation with or without saphenous vein stripping has been suggested to be the treatment of choice due to the recognized potential for extension into the deep system and embolization.[20–23] In a series of 43 patients who underwent ligation of the saphenofemoral junction with and without local CFV thrombectomy and stripping of the GSV, only 2 patients were found with postoperative contralateral DVT, of whom one had a PE.[3] Eighty-six percent of the patients were discharged within 3 days. Four patients developed a wound cellulitis that was treated with antibiotics. One patient had a wound hematoma requiring no treatment. Whilst satisfactory results were noted in these instances, several issues still remain unresolved. The question of whether or not to strip the GSV in addition to high ligation is not clearly addressed, although these patients do seem to experience less pain once the SVT is removed. Ligation was initially proposed to avert the development of deep venous thrombosis by preventing extension via the saphenofemoral junction. Stripping because of the extensive periphlebitis may not be possible or it might result in significant lymphatic injury. Since issues of non-contiguous DVT and post-ligation DVT with PE are not addressed by this therapy, alternative treatment options have also been explored.

A prospective nonrandomized study was conducted to evaluate the efficacy of a nonoperative approach of anticoagulation therapy to manage saphenofemoral junction thrombophlebitis (SFJT).[9] Over a 2-year period, 20 consecutive patients with SFJT were entered into the study. These patients were hospitalized and given a full course of heparin treatment. Duplex ultrasonography was performed before admission. Two to four days after admission, a follow-up duplex ultrasound scan was performed to assess resolution of SFJT and to reexamine the deep venous system. Patients with SFJT alone and resolution of SFJT as documented by duplex ultrasound scans were maintained on warfarin for 6 weeks. Those patients with SFJT and DVT were maintained on warfarin for 6 months. The incidence of concurrent DVT and its location were noted.

A 40% incidence (8 of 20 patients) of concurrent DVT with SFJT was found. Four patients had unilateral DVT, two had bilateral DVT, and two developed DVT with anticoagulation. DVT was contiguous with SFJT in five patients and noncontiguous in three patients. Of 13 duplex ultrasound scans obtained at 2–8 months follow-up, 7 demonstrated partial resolution of SFJT, 5 had complete resolution, and 1 demonstrated no resolution. There were no episodes of PE, or recurrent SFJT, and no anticoagulation complications occurred at maximum follow-up of 14 months. Anticoagulation therapy to manage SFJT was effective in achieving resolution, preventing recurrence and preventing PE within the follow-up period. The high incidence of DVT associated with SFJT suggests that careful evaluation of the deep venous system during the course of management is necessary.[9] It should be noted that the short-term effect of anticoagulation on progression to DVT or long-term effect on local recurrence of SVT had not been evaluated.

When comparing these two types of therapy, one group suggested that high ligation for SFJT would be more cost-effective than systemic anticoagulation for 6 months.[3] However, the question as to whether patients with SVT need to be treated for a 6-month period remains uncertain. Our treatment course of anticoagulation spans a period of 6 weeks and, over the last 10 years, we have noted no incidence of PE or complications of anticoagulation. Furthermore, significant cost savings could be realized if the low molecular weight heparins (LMWH) are used in an outpatient setting instead of unfractionated intravenous heparin.

This issue of anticoagulation versus surgical therapy was addressed in a prospective study. Four hundred forty-four patients were randomized to six different treatment plans [compression only, early surgery (with and without stripping), low-dose subcutaneous heparin, LMWH, and oral anticoagulant treatment] to treat superficial thrombophlebitis.[15] Patients presenting with SVT and large varicose veins without any suspected/documented systemic disorder were included in this study. Color duplex ultrasound scans were used to detect concomitant DVT and to evaluate the extension or reduction of SVT at 3 and 6 months.

The incidence of SVT extension was higher in the elastic compression and in the saphenous ligation groups ($P < 0.05$) after 3 and 6 months. There was no significant difference in DVT incidence at 3 months among the treatment groups. Stripping of the affected veins was associated with the lowest incidence of thrombus extension. The cost for compression solely was the lowest and was highest for treatment with LMWH. The highest social cost (lost working days, inactivity) was observed in subjects treated with stockings alone.

It is difficult to assess the results of this study, as the treatment protocols were not specifically identified. Furthermore, the exclusion criteria would eliminate many patients diagnosed with SVT in a clinical practice and the inclusion of almost any patient presenting with SVT, regardless of its location, made the remaining groups quite variable.

Although SVT occurs frequently, the best treatment regimen based on its underlying pathophysiology and resolution rate remains to be determined. The physician who diagnoses SVT should keep in mind that underlying coagulation abnormality, malignancy and associated DVT have been excluded. High SVT can be treated by both high ligation with or without stripping, once DVT is excluded or by anticoagulation. Follow-up with duplex to exclude progression is recommended.

REFERENCES

1. DeWeese MS. Nonoperative treatment of acute superficial thrombophlebitis and deep femoral venous thrombosis. In Ernst CB, Stanley JC, eds. *Current Therapy in Vascular Surgery.* Philadelphia: BC Decker, 1991: 952–60.
2. Lutter KS, Kerr TM, Roedersheimer LR, Lohr JM, Sampson MG, Cranley JJ. Superficial thrombophlebitis diagnosed by duplex scanning. *Surgery* 1991; **110**: 42–6.
3. Lohr JM, McDevitt DT, Lutter KS, Roedersheimer LR, Sampson MG. Operative management of greater saphenous thrombophlebitis involving the saphenofemoral junction. *Am J Surg* 1992; **164**: 269–75.
4. Hanson JN, Ascher E, DePippo P, *et al.* Saphenous vein thrombophlebitis (SVT): a deceptively benign disease. *J Vasc Surg* 1998; **27**: 677–80.
5. Hammond JS, Varas R, Ward CG. Suppurative thrombophlebitis: a new look at a continuing problem. *South Med J* 1988; **81**: 969–71.
6. Glasser ST. *Principles of Peripheral Vascular Surgery.* Philadelphia: FA Davis, 1959.
7. Bergqvist D, Jaroszewski H. Deep vein thrombosis in patients with superficial thrombophlebitis of the leg. *Br Med J* 1986; **292**: 658–9.

8. Prountjos P, Bastounis E, Hadjinikolaou L, Felekuras E, Balas P. Superficial venous thrombosis of the lower extremities co-existing with deep venous thrombosis. A phlebographic study on 57 cases. *Int Angiol* 1991; **10**: 263–5.
9. Ascer E, Lorensen F, Pollina RM, Gennaro M. Preliminary results of a nonoperative approach to saphenofemoral junction thrombophlebitis. *J Vasc Surg* 1995; **22**: 616–21.
10. Sassu GP, Chisholm CD, Howell JM, Huang E. A rare etiology for pulmonary embolism: basilic vein thrombosis. *J Emerg Med* 1990; **8**: 45–9.
11. Section XIII. Medical and surgical complications in pregnancy. In Cunningham FG *et al.*, eds. *Williams Obstetrics*, 20th edn. Stamford CT: Appleton & Lange, 1997: 1112.
12. Talbot SR. Use of real-time imaging in identifying deep venous obstruction: a preliminary report. *Bruit* 1982; **6**: 41–2.
13. Skillman JJ, Kent KC, Porter DH, Kim D. Simultaneous occurrence of superficial and deep thrombophlebitis in the lower extremity. *J Vasc Surg* 1990; **11**: 818–23.
14. Jorgensen JO, Hanel KC, Morgan AM, Hunt JM. The incidence of deep venous thrombosis in patients with superficial thrombophlebitis of the lower limbs. *J Vasc Surg* 1993; **18**: 70–3.
15. Belcaro G, Nicolaides AN, Errichi BM, *et al.* Superficial thrombophlebitis of the legs: a randomized, controlled, follow-up study. *Angiology* 1999; **50**: 523–9.
16. Chengelis DL, Bendick PJ, Glover JL, Brown OW, Ranval TJ. Progression of superficial venous thrombosis to deep vein thrombosis. *J Vasc Surg* 1996; **24**: 745–9.
17. Blumenberg RM, Barton E, Gelfand ML, Skudder P, Brennan J. Occult deep venous thrombosis complicating superficial thrombophlebitis. *J Vasc Surg* 1998; **27**: 338–43.
18. Hobbs JT. Superficial thrombophlebitis. In Hobbs JT, ed. *The Treatment of Venous Disorders.* Philadelphia: JB Lippincott, 1977: 414–27.
19. Ludbrook J, Jamieson GG. Disorders of veins. In Sabiston DC Jr, ed. *Textbook of Surgery*, 12th edn. Philadelphia: WB Saunders, 1981: 1808–27.
20. Husni EA, Williams WA. Superficial thrombophlebitis of lower limbs. *Surgery* 1982; **91**: 70–3.
21. Lofgren EP, Lofgren KA. The surgical treatment of superficial thrombophlebitis. *Surgery* 1981; **90**: 49–54.
22. Gjores JE. Surgical therapy of ascending thrombophlebitis in the saphenous system. *Angiology* 1962; **13**: 241–3.
23. Plate G, Eklof B, Jensen, Ohlin P. Deep venous thrombosis, pulmonary embolism and acute surgery in thrombophlebitis of the log saphenous vein. *Acta Chir Scand* 1985; **151**: 241–4.

18

Medical treatment of acute deep venous thrombosis

RUSSELL D HULL AND GRAHAM F PINEO

Unfractionated heparin, given by a continuous intravenous infusion with laboratory monitoring using the activated partial thromboplastin time (aPTT), with warfarin starting on day 1 or day 2 and continued for 3 months, has been the standard treatment of established venous thromboembolism. Heparin is used in a number of other clinical settings and constitutes one of the most frequently used agents in hospital medicine. Over the past 15 years, various low molecular weight heparins (LMWHs) have been evaluated against a number of different controls, including unfractionated heparin, for many of these clinical problems. In a number of countries, the LMWHs have replaced unfractionated heparin for both the prevention and treatment of venous thromboembolism. The optimal duration of oral anticoagulant therapy after an initial episode or recurrent episodes of venous thromboembolism is currently being studied in clinical trials. This chapter will review the medical management of venous thromboembolism with particular emphasis on the use of unfractionated heparin, low molecular weight heparin and oral anticoagulation.

TREATMENT OF VENOUS THROMBOEMBOLISM

The objectives of treatment in patients with venous thromboembolism are:

- to prevent death from PE;
- to prevent recurrent venous thromboembolism; and
- to prevent the postphlebitic syndrome.

Anticoagulant drugs heparin, low molecular weight heparin and warfarin constitute the mainstay of treatment of venous thrombosis. The use of graduated compression stockings for 24 months significantly decreases the incidence of the post-thrombotic syndrome. Furthermore, the incidence of the post-thrombotic syndrome is decreasing in recent years, suggesting that the more efficient treatment of venous thromboembolism and the prevention of recurrent deep vein thrombosis are having a positive impact on this complication.

Heparin therapy

The anticoagulant activity of unfractionated heparin depends upon a unique pentasaccharide which binds to antithrombin III (ATIII) and potentiates the inhibition of thrombin and activated factor X (Xa) by ATIII.[1–3] About one-third of all heparin molecules contain the unique pentasaccharide sequence, regardless of whether they are low or high molecular weight fractions.[1–3] It is the pentasaccharide sequence that confers the molecular high affinity for ATIII.[1–3] In addition, heparin catalyzes the inactivation of thrombin by another plasma cofactor (cofactor II) which acts independently of ATIII.[3]

Heparin has a number of other effects. These include the release of tissue factor pathway inhibitor, binding to numerous plasma and platelet proteins, endothelial cells, and leukocytes,[1] suppression of platelet function and an increase in vascular permeability.[3] The anticoagulant response to a standard dose of heparin varies widely between patients. This makes it necessary to monitor the anticoagulant response of heparin, using either the activated partial thromboplastin time (aPTT) or heparin levels and to titrate the dose to the individual patient.[3]

The accepted anticoagulant therapy for venous thromboembolism is a combination of continuous intravenous heparin and oral warfarin. The length of the initial intravenous heparin therapy has been reduced to 5 days, thus shortening the hospital stay and leading to significant cost saving.[4,5] The simultaneous use of initial heparin and warfarin has become clinical practice for all patients with venous thromboembolism who are medically stable.[4–6] Exceptions include patients who require immediate medical or surgical intervention, such as in thrombolysis or insertion of a vena cava filter, or patients at very high risk of bleeding. Heparin is continued until the INR has been within the therapeutic range (2–3) for two consecutive days.[6]

It has been established from experimental studies and clinical trials that efficacy of heparin therapy depends upon achieving a critical therapeutic level of heparin within the first 24 hours of treatment.[5,7,8] This finding was recently challenged in an overview of the available relevant literature where the authors were unable to find convincing evidence that the risk of recurrent venous thromboembolism was dependent on achieving a therapeutic aPTT result at 24–48 hours. However, data from three consecutive double-blind clinical trials indicate that failure to achieve the therapeutic aPTT threshold by 24 hours was associated with a 23.3% subsequent recurrent venous thromboembolism rate, compared with a rate of 4–6% for the patient group who were therapeutic at 24 hours.[8] The recurrences occurred throughout the 3-month follow-up period and could not be attributed to inadequate oral anticoagulant therapy.[7,8] The critical therapeutic level of heparin, as measured by the aPTT, is 1.5 times the mean of the control value or the upper limit of the normal aPTT range.[7] This corresponds to a heparin blood level of 0.2–0.4 U/ml by the protamine sulfate titration assay, and 0.35–0.70 by the anti-factor Xa assay.

However, there is a wide variability in the aPTT and heparin blood levels with different reagents and even with different batches of the same reagent. It is therefore vital for each laboratory to establish the minimal therapeutic level of heparin, as measured by the aPTT, that will provide a heparin blood level of at least 0.35 U/ml by the antifactor Xa assay for each batch of thromboplastin reagent being used, particularly if the reagent is provided by a different manufacturer.[3]

Although there is a strong correlation between subtherapeutic aPTT values and recurrent thromboembolism, the relationship between supratherapeutic aPTT and bleeding (aPTT ratio 2.5 or more) is less definite.[7] Indeed, bleeding during heparin therapy is more closely related to underlying clinical risk factors than to aPTT elevation above the therapeutic range. Recent studies confirm that weight and age >65 are independent risk factors for bleeding on heparin.

Numerous audits of heparin therapy indicate that administration of intravenous heparin is fraught with difficulty, and that the clinical practice of using an *ad hoc* approach to heparin dose-titration frequently results in inadequate therapy. For example, an audit of physician practices at three university-affiliated hospitals documented that 60% of patients failed to achieve an adequate aPTT response (ratio 1.5) during the initial 24 hours of therapy, and, further, that 30–40% of patients remained 'subtherapeutic' over the next 3–4 days.

The use of a prescriptive approach or protocol for administering intravenous heparin therapy has been evaluated in two prospective studies in patients with venous thromboembolism.[7,9] In one clinical trial for the treatment of proximal venous thrombosis, patients were given either intravenous heparin alone followed by warfarin, or intravenous heparin and simultaneous warfarin.[7] The heparin nomogram is summarized in Tables 18.1 and 18.2. Only 1 and 2% of the patients were undertreated for more than 24 hours in the heparin group and in the heparin and warfarin group, respectively. Recurrent venous thromboembolism (objectively documented) occurred infrequently in both groups

Table 18.1 *Heparin protocol*

Administer initial intravenous heparin bolus: 5000 U.

Administer continuous intravenous heparin infusion: commence at 42 ml/h of 20 000 U (1680 U/h) in 500 ml of two-thirds dextrose and one-third saline (a 24-hour heparin dose of 40 320 U), except in the following patients, in whom heparin infusion is commenced at a rate of 31 ml/h (1240 U/h, a 24-hour dose of 29 760 U):

- patients who have undergone surgery within the previous 2 weeks;
- patients with a previous history of peptic ulcer disease or gastrointestinal or genitourinary bleeding;
- patients with recent stroke (i.e. thrombotic stroke within 2 weeks previously);
- patients with a platelet count <150×10⁹/l;
- patients with miscellaneous reasons for a high risk of bleeding (e.g. hepatic failure, renal failure, or vitamin K deficiency).

Adjust heparin dose by use of the aPTT. The aPTT test is performed in all patients as follows:

- 4–6 hours after commencing heparin; the heparin dose is then adjusted;
- 4–6 hours after the first dosage adjustment;
- then, as indicated by the nomogram for the first 24 hours of therapy;
- thereafter, is once daily, unless the patient is subtherapeutic,* in which case the aPTT test is repeated 4–6 hours after the heparin dose is increased.

aPTT, activated partial thromboplastin time.
*Subtherapeutic, aPTT < 1.5 times the mean normal control value for the thromboplastin reagent being used.
Adapted from Hull RD *et al.*,[7] with permission.

Table 18.2 *Intravenous heparin dose titration nomogram according to the aPTT*

aPTT (s)	Rate change (ml/h)	Dose change (IU/24 h)[a]	Additional action
≤45	+6	+5760	Repeated aPTT[b] in 4–6 h
46–54	+3	+2880	Repeated aPTT in 4–6 h
55–85	0	0	None[c]
86–110	−3	−2880	Stop heparin sodium treatment for 1 h; repeated aPTT 4–6 h after restarting heparin treatment
>110	−6	−5760	Stop heparin treatment for 1 h; repeated aPTT 4–6h after restarting heparin treatment

[a] Heparin sodium concentration 20 000 IU in 500 ml = 40 IU/ml.
[b] With the use of Actin-FS thromboplastin reagent (Dade, Mississauga, Ontario, Canada).
[c] During the first 24 h, repeated aPTT in 4–6 h. Thereafter, the aPTT will be determined once daily, unless subtherapeutic.
aPTT, activated partial thromboplastin time.
Adapted from Hull RD *et al.*,[7] with permission.

(7%), rates similar to those previously reported. These findings demonstrated that subtherapy was avoided in most patients and that the heparin protocol resulted in effective delivery of heparin therapy in both groups.

In the other clinical trial, a weight-based heparin dosage nomogram was compared with a standard-care nomogram (Table 18.3).[9] Patients on the weight-adjusted heparin nomogram received a starting dose of 80 U/kg as a bolus and 18 U/kg/h as an infusion. The heparin dose was adjusted to maintain an aPTT of 1.5–2.3 times control. In the weight-adjusted group, 89% of patients achieved the therapeutic range within 24 hours compared with 75% in the standard-care group. The risk of recurrent thromboembolism was more frequent in the standard-care group, supporting the previous observation that subtherapeutic heparin during the initial 24 hours is associated with a higher incidence of recurrences. This study included patients with unstable angina and arterial thromboembolism in addition to venous thromboembolism, which suggests that the principles applied to a heparin nomogram for the treatment of venous thromboembolism may be generalizable to other clinical conditions. Continued use of the weight-based nomogram has been similarly effective.

Table 18.3 *Weight-based nomogram for initial intravenous heparin therapy: figures in parentheses show comparison with control*

	Dose (IU/kg)
Initial dose	80 bolus, then 18/h
aPTT <35 s (<1.2×)	80 bolus, then 4/h
aPTT 35–45 s (1.2–1.5×)	40 bolus, then 2/h
aPTT 46–70 s (1.5–2.3×)	No change
aPTT 71–90 s (2.3–3.0×)	Decrease infusion rate by 2/h
aPTT >90 s (>3.0×)	Hold infusion I h, then decrease infusion rate by 3/h

aPTT, activated partial thromboplastin time.
Adapted from Raschke RA *et al.*,[9] with permission.

Complications of heparin therapy

The main adverse effects of heparin therapy include bleeding, thrombocytopenia and osteoporosis. Patients at particular risk are those who have had recent surgery or trauma, or who have other clinical factors which predispose to bleeding on heparin, such as peptic ulcer, occult malignancy, liver disease, hemostatic defects, weight, age >65 years and female gender.

The management of bleeding on heparin will depend on the location and severity of bleeding, the risk of recurrent venous thromboembolism and the aPTT. Heparin should be discontinued temporarily or permanently. Patients with recent venous thromboembolism may be candidates for insertion of an inferior vena cava filter. If urgent reversal of heparin effect is required, protamine sulfate can be administered.[3]

Heparin-induced thrombocytopenia is a well-recognized complication of heparin therapy, usually occurring within 5–10 days after heparin treatment has started.[10–13] Approximately 1–2% of patients receiving unfractionated heparin will experience a fall in platelet count to less than the normal range or a 50% fall in the platelet count within the normal range. In the majority of cases, this mild-to-moderate thrombocytopenia appears to be a direct effect of heparin on platelets and is of no consequence. However, approximately 0.1–0.2% of patients receiving heparin develop an immune thrombocytopenia mediated by IgG antibody directed against a complex of PF4 and heparin.[12]

The development of thrombocytopenia may be accompanied by arterial or venous thrombosis, which may lead to serious consequences such as death or limb amputation.[12] The diagnosis of heparin-induced thrombocytopenia, with or without thrombosis, must be made on clinical grounds, because the assays with the highest sensitivity and specificity are not readily available and have a slow turnaround time.

When the diagnosis of heparin-induced thrombocytopenia is made, heparin in all forms must be stopped immediately. In those patients requiring ongoing anticoagulation, several alternatives exist.[12] The agents most extensively used recently include the heparinoid danaparoid,[13] hirudin[14] and, most recently, the specific antithrombin argatroban. Danaparoid is available for limited use on compassionate grounds and hirudin and argatroban have recently been approved for use in the USA and Canada. Warfarin may be used, but should not be started until one of the above agents has been used for three or four days to suppress thrombin generation. The defibrinogenating snake venom Arvin (ancrod) has been used quite extensively in the past but will be replaced by other agents. Insertion of an inferior vena cava filter is often indicated.

Osteoporosis has been reported in patients receiving unfractionated heparin in dosages of 20 000 U/day (or more) for more than 6 months. Demineralization can progress to the fracture of vertebral bodies or long bones, and the defect may not be entirely reversible.[3]

Low molecular weight heparin (LMWH)

Heparin currently in use clinically is polydispersed unmodified heparin, with a mean molecular weight ranging from 10 to 16 kDa. In recent years, low molecular weight derivatives of commercial heparin have been prepared that have a mean molecular weight of 4–5 kDa.[15,16]

The LMWHs commercially available are made by different processes (such as nitrous acid, alkaline, or enzymatic depolymerization) and they differ chemically and pharmacokinetically.[15,16] The clinical significance of these differences, however, is unclear, and there have been very few studies comparing different LMWHs with respect to clinical outcomes.[16] The doses of the different LMWHs have been established empirically and are not necessarily interchangeable. Therefore, at this time, the effectiveness and safety of each of the LMWHs must be tested separately.[16]

The LMWHs differ from unfractionated heparin in numerous ways. Of particular importance are the following: increased bioavailability[3,15,16] (>90% after subcutaneous injection), prolonged half-life and predictable clearance enabling once- or twice-daily injection, and predictable antithrombotic response based on body weight permitting treatment without laboratory monitoring.[3,15,16] Other possible advantages are their ability to inactivate platelet-bound factor Xa, resistance to inhibition by platelet factor IV and their decreased effect on platelet function and vascular permeability[3] (possibly accounting for less hemorrhagic effects at comparable antithrombotic doses).

There has been a hope that the LMWHs will have fewer serious complications such as bleeding[16,17] and heparin-induced thrombocytopenia,[10] when compared with unfractionated heparin. Evidence is accumulating that these complications are indeed less serious and less frequent with the use of LMWH. LMWH has not been approved for the prevention or treatment of venous thromboembolism in pregnancy. These drugs do not cross the placenta[3,16] and small case series suggest they may be both effective and safe. However, at the present time, the standard treatment for venous thromboembolism in pregnancy is twice-daily adjusted-dose subcutaneous unfractionated heparin.[6] The LMWHs all cross-react with unfractionated heparin and they can therefore not be used as alternative therapy in patients who develop heparin-induced thrombocytopenia. The heparinoid danaparoid possesses a 10–20% cross-reactivity with heparin and it can be safely used in patients who have no cross-reactivity.

Several different LMWHs and one heparinoid are available for the prevention and treatment of venous thromboembolism in various countries. Four LMWHs are approved for clinical use in Canada and three LMWHs and one heparinoid have been approved for use in the USA.

In a number of early clinical trials (some of which were dose finding), LMWH given by subcutaneous or intravenous injection was compared with continuous intravenous unfractionated heparin with repeat venography at day 7–10 being the primary end point. These studies demonstrated that LMWH was at least as effective as unfractionated heparin in preventing extension or increasing resolution of thrombi on repeat venography.

Subcutaneous unmonitored low molecular has been compared with continuous intravenous heparin in a number of clinical trials for the treatment of proximal venous thrombosis using long-term follow-up as an outcome measure.[18–24] (Table 18.4). These studies have shown that LMWH is at least as effective and safe as unfractionated heparin in the treatment of proximal venous thrombosis.[18–24] Pooling of the most methodologically sound studies indicates a significant advantage for LMWH in the reduction of major bleeding and mortality. More recent studies have indicated that LMWH used predominantly out of hospital was as effective and safe as intravenous unfractionated heparin given in hospital.[25–27] (Table 18.5) and three clinical trials showed that LMWH was as effective as intravenous heparin in the treatment of patients presenting with pulmonary embolism.[23,27,28] Economic analysis of treatment with LMWH versus intravenous heparin demonstrated that LMWH was cost-effective for treatment in hospital[29] as well as out of hospital. As these agents become more widely available for treatment, they have

Table 18.4 *Randomized trials of low molecular weight heparin vs unfractionated heparin for the in-hospital treatment of proximal deep vein thrombosis or acute pulmonary embolism: results of long-term follow up*

Reference	Treatment	Recurrent venous thromboembolism [no. (%)]	Major bleeding [no. (%)]	Mortality [no. (%)]
Hull *et al.*[18]	Tinzaparin	6/213 (2.8)	1/213 (0.5)	10/213 (4.7)
	Heparin	15/219 (6.8)	11/219 (5.0)	21/219 (9.6)
Prandoni *et al.*[19]	Nadroparin	6/85 (7.1)	1/85 (1.2)	6/85 (7.1)
	Heparin	12/85 (14.1)	3/85 (3.8)	12/85 (14.1)
Lopaciuk *et al.*[20]	Nadroparin	0/74	0/74	0/74
	Heparin	3/72 (4.2)	1/72 (1.4)	1/72 (1.4)
Simonneau *et al.*[21]	Enoxaparin	0/67	0/67	3/67 (4.5)
	Heparin	0/67	0/67	2/67 (3.0)
Lindmarker *et al.*[22]	Dalteparin	5/101 (5.0)	1/101	2/101 (2.0)
	Heparin	3/103 (2.9)	0/103	3/103 (2.9)
Simonneau *et al.*[23]	Tinzaparin	5/304 (1.6)	3/304 (1.0)	12/304 (3.9)
	Heparin	6/308 (1.9)	5/308 (1.6)	14/308 (4.5)
Decousus *et al.*[24]	Enoxaparin	10/195 (5.1)	7/195 (3.6)	10/195 (5.1)
	Heparin	12/205 (5.0)	8/205 (3.9)	15/205 (7.3)

Table 18.5 *Predominantly outpatient treatment of proximal deep vein thrombosis with low molecular weight heparin versus inpatient treatment with intravenous heparin*

Study	Treatment	Recurrent DVT	Major bleeding
Koopman *et al.*[25]	Nadroparin	14/202 (6.9%)	1/202 (0.5%)
	vs. heparin	17/198 (8.6%)	4/198 (2.0%)
Levine *et al.*[26]	Enoxaparin	13/247 (5.3%)	5/247 (2.0%)
	vs. heparin	17/253 (6.7%)	3/253 (1.2%)
Columbus study[27]	Reviparin	27/510 (5.3%)	16/510 (3.1%)
	vs. heparin	24/511 (4.9%)	12/511 (2.3%)

replaced intravenous unfractionated heparin in the initial management of patients with venous thromboembolism.

ORAL ANTICOAGULANT THERAPY

There are two distinct chemical groups of oral anticoagulants: the 4-hydroxycoumarin derivatives (e.g. warfarin) and the indanedione derivatives (e.g. phenindione). The coumarin derivatives are the oral anticoagulants of choice because they are associated with fewer non-hemorrhagic adverse effects than are the indanedione derivatives.

Warfarin

The anticoagulant effect of warfarin is mediated by the inhibition of the vitamin K-dependent γ-carboxylation of coagulation factors II, VII, IX and X.[30,31] This results in the synthesis of immunologically detectable but biologically inactive forms of these coagulation proteins. Warfarin also inhibits the vitamin K-dependent γ-carboxylation of proteins C and S.[31] Protein C circulates as a proenzyme that is activated on endothelial cells by the thrombin/thrombomodulin complex to form activated protein C. Activated protein C in the presence of protein S inhibits activated factor VIII and activated factor V activity.[30,31] Therefore, vitamin K antagonists such as warfarin create a biochemical paradox by producing an anticoagulant effect due to the inhibition of procoagulants (factors II, VII, IX and X) and a potentially thrombogenic effect by impairing the synthesis of naturally occurring inhibitors of coagulation (proteins C and S).[31] Heparin and warfarin treatment should overlap by 4–5 days when warfarin treatment is initiated in patients with thrombotic disease.

The anticoagulant effect of warfarin is delayed until the normal clotting factors are cleared from the circulation, and the peak effect does not occur until 36–72 hours after drug administration.[31] During the first few days of warfarin therapy the prothrombin time (PT) reflects mainly the depression of factor VII, which has a half-life of 5–7 hours. Equilibrium levels of factors II, IX and X are not reached until about 1 week after the initiation of therapy. The use of small initial daily doses (e.g. 5.0–7.5 mg) is the preferred approach for initiating warfarin treatment.

The dose–response relationship to warfarin therapy varies widely between individuals and, therefore, the dose must be carefully monitored to prevent under- or overdosing. A number of drugs interact with warfarin. Critical appraisal of the literature reporting such interactions indicates that the evidence substantiating many of the claims is limited.[31,32] Nonetheless, patients must be warned against taking any new drugs or natural compounds without the knowledge of their attending physician.

LABORATORY MONITORING AND THERAPEUTIC RANGE

The laboratory test most commonly used to measure the effects of warfarin is the one-stage PT test. The PT is sensitive to reduced activity of factors II, VII and X, but is insensitive to reduced activity of factor IX. Confusion about the appropriate therapeutic range has occurred because the different tissue thromboplastins used for measuring the PT vary considerably in sensitivity to the vitamin K-dependent clotting factors and in response to warfarin.

In order to promote the standardization of the PT for monitoring oral anticoagulant therapy, the World Health Organization (WHO) developed an international reference thromboplastin from human brain tissue and recommended that the PT ratio be expressed as the international normalized ratio, or INR. The INR is the PT ratio obtained by testing a given sample using the WHO reference thromboplastin. For practical clinical purposes, the INR for a given plasma sample is equivalent to the PT ratio obtained using a standardized human brain thromboplastin known as the Manchester Comparative Reagent, which has been widely used in the UK.[31]

Warfarin is administered in an initial dosage of 5.0–7.5 mg/day for the first 2 days. The daily dose is then adjusted according to the INR. Heparin therapy is discontinued on the fourth or fifth day following initiation of warfarin therapy, provided the INR is prolonged into the recommended therapeutic range (INR 2–3).[31] Because some individuals are either fast or slow metabolizers of the drug, the selection of the correct dosage of warfarin must be individualized. Therefore, frequent INR determinations are required initially to establish therapeutic anticoagulation.

Once the anticoagulant effect and patient's warfarin dose requirements are stable, the INR should be monitored at regular intervals throughout the course of warfarin therapy for venous thromboembolism. However, if there are factors that may produce an unpredictable response to warfarin (e.g. concomitant drug therapy), the INR should be monitored frequently to minimize the risk of complications due to poor anticoagulant control.[31,32] Several warfarin nomograms and computer software programs are now available to assist core givers in the control of warfarin therapy.

Also, there is increasing interest in the use of self-testing with portable INR monitors and in selective cases, self-management of oral anticoagulant therapy.

LONG-TERM TREATMENT OF VENOUS THROMBOEMBOLISM

Patients with established venous thrombosis or pulmonary embolism require long-term anticoagulant therapy to prevent recurrent disease. Warfarin therapy is highly effective and is preferred in most patients.[33] Adjusted-dose subcutaneous heparin is the treatment of choice where long-term oral anticoagulants are contraindicated such as in pregnancy. Adjusted-dose, subcutaneous heparin, or unmonitored low molecular weight heparin have been used for the long-term treatment of patients in whom oral anticoagulant therapy proves to be very difficult to control.[31]

In patients with proximal vein thrombosis, long-term therapy with warfarin reduces the frequency of objectively documented recurrent venous thromboembolism from 47 to 2%.[31,32] The use of a less intense warfarin regimen (INR 2–3) markedly reduces the risk of bleeding from 20 to 4%, without loss of effectiveness in comparison with more intense warfarin.[33] With the improved safety of oral anticoagulant therapy using a less intense warfarin regimen, there has been renewed interest in evaluating the long-term treatment of thrombotic disorders. In clinical trials in patients with atrial fibrillation, it has been shown that oral anticoagulant treatment can be given safely with a low risk of major bleeding complications (1–2% per year). In trials such as these, the safety of oral anticoagulant treatment depends heavily on the maintenance of a narrow therapeutic INR range. These and other studies have emphasized the importance of maintaining careful control of oral anticoagulant therapy, particularly with the use of anticoagulant management clinics if oral anticoagulants are going to be used for extended periods of time.

Data from clinical trials have documented an unacceptably high incidence of recurrent venous thromboembolism, including fatal pulmonary embolism, during the long-term clinical course of patients with proximal deep vein thrombosis who are treated according to the current practice with intravenous heparin for several days, followed by oral anticoagulant treatment for 3–6 months.[6,34–36] Three groups of patients who have a particularly poor prognosis have been identified: patients with idiopathic, recurrent venous thromboembolism, patients who are carriers of genetic mutations that predispose to venous thromboembolism, such as Factor V Leiden mutation, and patients with cancer.[6]

Duration of oral anticoagulants after a first episode of deep vein thrombosis

It has been recommended that all patients with a first episode of venous thromboembolism receive warfarin therapy for 3–6 months. Attempts to decrease the treatment to 4 weeks[37,38] or 6 weeks[35] resulted in higher rates of recurrent thromboembolism in comparison with either 12 or 26 weeks of treatment (11–18% recurrent thromboembolism in the following 1–2 years). Most of the recurrent thromboembolic events occurred in the 6–8 weeks immediately after anticoagulant treatment was stopped, and the incidence was higher in patients with continuing risk factors, such as cancer and immobilization.[36,38] Treatment with oral anticoagulants for 6 months reduced the incidence of recurrent thromboembolic events, but there was a cumulative incidence of recurrent events at 2 years (11%) and an ongoing risk of recurrent thromboembolism of approximately 5–6% per year.[35]

In patients with a first episode of idiopathic venous thromboembolism treated with intravenous heparin followed by warfarin for 3 months, continuation of warfarin for 24 months led to a significant reduction in the incidence of recurrent venous thromboembolism when compared with placebo.[39] The authors concluded that anticoagulant therapy for more than 3 months was required in such patients but the optimal duration of treatment remains undetermined. A recent study reported that the incidence of recurrent venous thromboembolism was lower in patients treated for 12 months compared with 3 months after a first episode of deep vein thrombosis but that at 2 years follow-up the recurrence rates were the same. This continued risk of recurrent thromboembolism even with 6 months of treatment after a first episode of deep vein thrombosis has encouraged the development of clinical trials evaluating the effectiveness of long-term anticoagulant treatment beyond 6 months.

Duration of oral anticoagulant treatment in patients with recurrent deep vein thrombosis

In a multicenter clinical trial, Schulman *et al.* randomized patients with a first recurrent episode of venous thromboembolism, to receive either 6 months or continued oral anticoagulants indefinitely, with a targeted INR of 2.0–2.85.[36] The analysis was reported at 4 years. In the patients receiving anticoagulants for 6 months, recurrent thromboembolism occurred in 20.7%, compared with 2.6% of patients on the indefinite treatment ($P < 0.001$). However, the rates of major bleeding were 2.7% in the 6 months group, compared with 8.6% in the indefinite group. In the indefinite group, two of the major hemorrhages were fatal, whereas there were no fatal hemorrhages in the 6 months group. This study showed that extending the duration of oral anticoagulants for approximately 4 years resulted in a significant decrease in the incidence of recurrent venous thromboembolism, but with a higher incidence of major bleeding. Without a mortality difference, the risk of hemorrhage versus the benefit of decreased recurrent thromboembolism with the use of extended warfarin treatment remains uncertain and will require further clinical trials.

Patients with reversible or time-limited risk factors should be treated with oral anticoagulants for 3–6 months. For patients experiencing a first episode of idiopathic venous thromboembolism, long-term anticoagulant therapy should be continued for at least 6 months using oral anticoagulants to prolong the prothrombin time to an INR of 2.0–3.0.[6] For patients with recurrent venous thromboembolism or a continuing risk factor such as immobilization, heart failure, cancer or the antiphospholipid antibody syndrome, anticoagulants should be continued for a longer period of time and possibly indefinitely, particularly for those patients with more than one recurrent episode of thrombosis.[6] Patients with the Factor V Leiden defect should probably receive indefinite anticoagulant treatment if they have recurrent disease or are homozygous for the gene. Recommendations for long-term anticoagulant therapy for the other thrombophilic conditions are less definite but constitute the topic for a number of epidemiologic studies.

Adverse effects

The major side-effect of oral anticoagulant therapy is bleeding.[31] Bleeding during well controlled oral anticoagulant therapy is usually due to surgery or other forms of trauma, or to local lesions, such as peptic ulcer or carcinoma.[31] Spontaneous bleeding may occur if warfarin sodium is given in an excessive dose, resulting in marked prolongation of the INR; this bleeding may be severe and even life-threatening. The risk of bleeding can be substantially reduced by adjustment of the warfarin dose to achieve a less intense anticoagulant effect than has traditionally been used in North America (INR 2.0–3.0; prothrombin time, 1.25–1.5 times control value obtained using a rabbit brain thromboplastin, such as Simplastin or Dade-C).[33]

Non-hemorrhagic side-effects of oral anticoagulant differ according to whether coumarin derivatives (e.g.

warfarin sodium) or indanediones are administered. Such side-effects are uncommon with coumarin anticoagulants, and the coumarins are therefore the oral anticoagulants of choice.

Coumarin-induced skin necrosis is a rare but serious complication that requires immediate cessation of oral anticoagulant therapy.[31] It usually occurs between 3 and 10 days after therapy has commenced, is commoner in women, and most often involves areas of abundant subcutaneous tissues, such as the abdomen, buttocks, thighs and breast. The mechanism of coumarin-induced skin necrosis, which is associated with microvascular thrombosis, is uncertain but appears to be related, at least in some patients, to depression of protein C level. Patients with congenital deficiencies of protein C may be particularly prone to the development of coumarin skin necrosis.

Management of patients on long-term oral anticoagulants requiring surgical intervention

Physicians are commonly confronted with the problem of managing oral anticoagulants in individuals who require temporary interruption of treatment for surgery or other invasive procedures.[40] In the absence of data from randomized clinical trials, recommendations can only be made based on cohort studies, retrospective reviews and expert opinions. The most common conditions requiring long-term anticoagulant therapy are atrial fibrillation, mechanical or prosthetic heart valve replacement, and venous thromboembolism.[40] For each of these conditions, the risk of arterial or venous thromboembolism, when anticoagulants have been discontinued, must be weighed against the risk of bleeding if intravenous heparin is applied before or after the surgical procedure, or if oral anticoagulant therapy is continued at the therapeutic level. The possible choices based on the risk/benefit assessment in the individual patient include:[40]

- discontinuing warfarin for 3–5 days before the procedure to allow the INR to return to normal and then restarting therapy shortly after surgery;
- lowering the warfarin dose to maintain an INR in the lower or subtherapeutic range during the surgical procedure; and
- discontinuing warfarin and treating the patient in hospital with intravenous heparin before and after the surgical procedure, until warfarin therapy can be reinstituted. Low molecular weight heparin is now being used in many of these circumstances.

Antidote to oral anticoagulant agents

The antidote to the vitamin K antagonists is vitamin K_1. If an excessive increase of the INR occurs, the treatment depends on the degree of the increase and whether or not the patient is bleeding. If the increase is mild and the patient is not bleeding, no specific treatment is necessary other than reduction in the warfarin dose. The INR can be expected to decrease during the next 24 hours with this approach. With more marked increase of the INR in patients who are not bleeding, treatment with small doses of vitamin K_1, given either orally or by subcutaneous injection (1.0–2.0 mg), could be considered. With very marked increase of the INR, particularly in a patient who is either actively bleeding or at risk of bleeding, the coagulation defect should be corrected.

Reported side-effects of vitamin K include flushing, dizziness, tachycardia, hypotension, dyspnea and sweating.[31] Intravenous administration of vitamin K_1 should be performed with caution to avoid inducing an anaphylactoid reaction. The risk of anaphylactoid reaction can be reduced by slow administration of vitamin K_1 at a rate no faster than 1 mg/min IV. In most patients, intravenous administration of vitamin K_1 produces a demonstrable effect on the INR within 6–8 hours and corrects the increased INR within 12–24 hours. Because the half-life of vitamin K_1 is less than that of warfarin sodium, a repeat course of vitamin K_1 may be necessary. If bleeding is very severe and life threatening, vitamin K therapy can be supplemented with concentrations of factors II, VII, IX and X.

Upper extremity deep vein thrombosis

The treatment of upper extremity deep vein thrombosis is the same as for proximal venous thrombosis, i.e. heparin or low molecular weight heparin plus warfarin for at least 3 months.[41] Patients with recent-onset upper extremity deep vein thrombosis have been treated with thrombolytic agents, but there is no evidence from clinical trials that this decreases long-term sequelae. The rare patient with thoracic outlet obstruction may benefit from surgery.

Recurrent venous thrombosis

The diagnosis of recurrent deep vein thrombosis is problematic, particularly if previous investigations are not available. Abnormalities persist on ultrasound studies for more than 12 months in the majority of patients and the impedance plethysmography remains abnormal at 3 months in approximately 30% of patients. If these tests have reverted to negative and become positive with a symptomatic recurrence or if a new defect is detected in the same leg or the contralateral leg, the diagnosis is quite evident. A new intraluminal filling defect on repeat venography is diagnostic. There is hope that the D-dimer assay may be of use in the exclusion of recurrent venous thrombosis, but this has not been adequately tested. The finding of a new defect on ventilation/perfusion lung scanning is helpful in making the diagnosis of pulmonary embolism. Otherwise, at the present time, if it is not possible to make a firm diagnosis of recurrent venous thromboembolism by objective tests, clinical judgment must be used.

Treatment of superficial thrombophlebitis

In the absence of associated deep vein thrombosis, the treatment of superficial thrombophlebitis is usually confined to symptomatic relief with analgesia and rest of the affected limb. The exception is the patient with superficial thrombophlebitis involving a large segment of the long saphenous vein, particularly when it occurs above the knee. These patients should be treated with heparin or low molecular weight heparin with or without oral anticoagulant therapy or superficial venous ligation. The presence of associated deep vein thrombosis requires the usual treatment with heparin or low molecular weight heparin along with warfarin for at least 3 months.

CONCLUSION

Based on a large number of level 1 clinical trials, the accepted medical treatment for acute deep venous thrombosis has been established. Until recently this consisted of unfractionated heparin given by continuous intravenous infusion with warfarin starting on day 1 or 2 and continued for 3 months with a targeted INR of 2.0–3.0. More recently a number of low molecular weight heparins have been shown to be at least as effective as unfractionated heparin in decreasing recurrent venous thromboembolism and, in fact, are associated with less major bleeding. Low molecular weight heparin has become the treatment of choice for both in-hospital and out-of-hospital treatment of deep venous thrombosis and, more recently, pulmonary embolism as well. Although warfarin has been used for years for the long-term treatment of patients suffering venous thromboembolism, the optimal duration of treatment after a first episode or recurrent episodes of venous thrombosis remains uncertain. Recent studies have indicated that patients with a first episode of idiopathic deep venous thrombosis require at least 6 months of long-term anticoagulant treatment and patients who have a first recurrence require at least 12 months of anticoagulant treatment. Because the risk of recurrent venous thromboembolism continues even after these extended periods of treatment, it is likely that future recommendations will be for even longer periods of treatment. These and other unanswered questions related to the management of acute deep venous thrombosis will be further clarified by the results of ongoing clinical trials.

REFERENCES

1. Lane DA. Heparin binding and neutralizing protein. In Lane DA, Lindahl U, eds. *Heparin, Chemical and Biological Properties, Clinical Applications.* London: Edward Amold, 1989: 363–91.
2. Rosenberg RD, Lam L. Correlation between structure and function of heparin. *Proc Natl Acad Sci USA* 1979; **76**: 1218–22.
3. Hirsh J, Warkentin TE, Shaughnessy SG, *et al.* Heparin and low-molecular-weight heparin: mechanisms of action, pharmacokinetics, dosing considerations, monitoring, efficacy and safety. *Chest* 2001; **119**(1): 654–945.
4. Gallus A, Jackaman J, Tillett J, *et al.* Safety and efficacy of warfarin started early after submassive venous thrombosis or pulmonary embolism. *Lancet* 1986; **2**: 1293–6.
5. Hull RD, Raskob GE, Rosenbloom D, *et al.* Heparin for 5 days as compared with 10 days in the initial treatment of proximal venous thrombosis. *N Engl J Med* 1990; **322**: 1260–4.
6. Hyers TN, Agnelli G, Hull RD, *et al.* Antithrombotic therapy for venous thromboembolic disease. *Chest* 2001; **119**(1): 1765–1935.
7. Hull RD, Raskob GE, Rosenbloom DR, *et al.* Optimal therapeutic level of heparin therapy in patients with venous thrombosis. *Arch Intern Med* 1992; **152**: 1589–95.
8. Hull RD, Raskob GE, Brant RF, Pineo GF, Valentine KA. The importance of initial heparin treatment on long-term clinical outcomes of antithrombotic therapy. *Arch Intern Med* 1997; **157**: 2317–21.
9. Raschke RA, Reilly BM, Guidry JR, *et al.* The weight based heparin dosing nomogram compared with a 'standard care' nomogram. *Ann Intern Med* 1993; **119**: 874–81.
10. Warkentin TE, Levine MN, Hirsh J, *et al.* Heparin induced thrombocytopenia in patients treated with low molecular weight heparin or unfractionated heparin. *N Engl J Med* 1995; **332**(20): 1330–5.
11. Keiton JG. Heparin-induced thrombocytopenia. *Haemostasis* 1986; **16**: 173–86.
12. Warkentin TE, Chong BH, Greinacher A. Heparin-induced thrombocytopenia: towards consensus. *Thromb Haemost* 1998; **79**: 1–7.
13. Magnani HN. Heparin-induced thrombocytopenia (HIT): an overview of 230 patients treated with orgaran (Org 10172). *Thromb Haemost* 1993; **70**: 554–61.
14. Greinacher A. Lepirudin for the treatment of heparin-induced thrombocytopenia: a prospective study. *Blood* 1998; **92**(10): 362a (abstract 1490).
15. Barrowcliffe TW, Curtis AD, Johnson EA, *et al.* An international standard for low molecular weight heparin. *Thromb Haemost* 1988; **60**: 1–7.
16. Weitz JI. Low molecular weight heparins. *N Engl J Med* 1997; **337**: 688–98.
17. Shaughnessy SG, Young E, Deschamps P, Hirsh J. The effects of low molecular weight and standard heparin on

calcium loss from fetal rat calvaria. *Blood* 1995; **86**: 1368–73.

18. Hull RD, Raskob GE, Pineo GF, *et al.* Subcutaneous low molecular weight heparin compared with continuous intravenous heparin in the treatment of proximal vein thrombosis. *N Engl J Med* 1992; **326**: 975–88.
19. Prandoni P, Lensing AW, Builer HR, *et al.* Comparison of subcutaneous low molecular weight heparin with intravenous standard heparin in proximal deep vein thrombosis. *Lancet* 1992; **339**: 441–5.
20. Lopaciuk S, Meissner AJ, Filipecki S, *et al.* Subcutaneous low molecular weight heparin versus subcutaneous unfractionated heparin in the treatment of deep vein thrombosis. A Polish multicentre trial. *Thromb Haemost* 1992; **68**: 14–18.
21. Simonneau G, Charbonnier B, Decousus H, *et al.* Subcutaneous low molecular weight heparin compared with continuous intravenous unfractionated heparin in the treatment of proximal deep vein thrombosis. *Arch Intern Med* 1993; **153**: 1541–6.
22. Lindmarker P, Holmstrom M, Granqvist S, Johnsson H, Locner D. Comparison of once-daily subcutaneous Fragmin with continuous intravenous unfractionated heparin in the treatment of deep venous thrombosis. *Thromb Haemost* 1994; **72**: 186–90.
23. Simonneau G, Sors H, Charbonnier B, *et al.* A comparison of low molecular weight heparin with unfractionated heparin for acute pulmonary embolism. *N Engl J Med* 1997; **337**: 663–9.
24. Decousus H, Leizorovicz A, Parent F, *et al.* A clinical trial of vena caval filters in the prevention of pulmonary embolism in patients with proximal deep vein thrombosis. *N Engl J Med* 1998; **338**: 409–15.
25. Koopman MMW, Prandoni P, Piovelia F, *et al.* Treatment of venous thrombosis with intravenous unfractionated heparin administered in the hospital as compared with subcutaneous low molecular weight heparin administered at home. *N Engl J Med* 1996; **334**: 682–7.
26. Levine M, Gent M, Hirsh J, *et al.* A comparison of low molecular weight heparin administered primarily at home with unfractionated heparin administered in the hospital for proximal deep vein thrombosis. *N Engl J Med* 1996; **334**: 677–81.
27. The Columbus Investigators. Low molecular weight heparin in the treatment of patients with venous thromboembolism. *N Engl J Med* 1997; **337**: 657–62.
28. Hull RD, Raskob GE, Brant RF, *et al.* Low-molecular-weight heparin versus heparin in the treatment of patients with pulmonary embolism. American-Canadian Thrombosis Study Group. *Arch Intern Med* 2000; **160**: 229–36.
29. Hull RD, Raskob GE, Rosenbloom D, *et al.* Treatment of proximal vein thrombosis with subcutaneous low molecular weight heparin vs. intravenous heparin. An economic perspective. *Arch Intern Med* 1997; **157**: 289–94.
30. Freedman MD. Oral anticoagulants: pharmacodynamics, clinical indications and adverse effects. *J Clin Pharmacol* 1992; **32**: 196–209.
31. Hirsh J, Dalen JE, Anderson DR, *et al.* Oral anticoagulants: mechanism of action, clinical effectiveness and optimal therapeutic range. *Chest* 2001; **119**(1): 85–215.
32. Wells PS, Holbrook AM, Crowther R, Hirsh J. Warfarin and its drug/food interactions; a critical appraisal of the literature. *Ann Intern Med* 1994; **121**: 676–83.
33. Hull R, Hirsh J, Jay R, *et al.* Different intensifies of oral anticoagulant therapy in the treatment of proximal vein thrombosis. *N Engl J Med* 1982; **307**: 1676–81.
34. Prandoni P, Lensing AWA, Cogo A, *et al.* The long term clinical course of acute deep venous thrombosis. *Ann Intern Med* 1996; **125**: 1–7.
35. Schulman S, Rhedin AS, Lindmarker P, *et al.* A comparison of six weeks with six months of oral anticoagulation therapy after a first episode of venous thromboembolism. *N Engl J Med* 1995; **332**: 1661–5.
36. Schulman S, Granqvist S, Holmstrom M, *et al.* The duration of oral anticoagulant therapy after a second episode of venous thromboembolism. *N Engl J Med* 1997; **336**: 393–8.
37. Research Committee of the British Thoracic Society. Optimum duration of anticoagulation for deep vein thrombosis and pulmonary embolism. *Lancet* 1992; **340**: 873–6.
38. Levine MN, Hirsh J, Gent M, *et al.* Optimal duration of oral anticoagulant therapy: a randomized trial comparing four weeks with three months of warfarin in patients with proximal deep vein thrombosis. *Thromb Haemost* 1995; **74**: 606–11.
39. Kearon C, Gent M, Hirsh J, *et al.* A comparison of three months of anticoagulation with extended anticoagulation for a first episode of idiopathic venous thromboembolism. *N Engl J Med* 1999; **340**(12): 901–7.
40. Stein PD, Alpert JS, Dalen JE, *et al.* Antithrombotic therapy in patients with mechanical and biological prosthetic heart valves. *Chest* 1998; **114**(5): 602S-10S.
41. Prandoni P, Polistena P, Bemardi E, *et al.* Upper-extremity deep vein thrombosis. *Arch Intern Med* 1997; **157**: 57–62.

19

Catheter-directed thrombolysis for the treatment of acute deep vein thrombosis

ANTHONY J COMEROTA

In the recent Fifth ACCP Consensus Conference on antithrombotic therapy, recommendations for the treatment of acute venous thromboembolic disease were published.[1] This report reflects a consensus of expert committees which reviewed the available literature and assigned grades to their recommendations based upon the quality of available clinical evidence, the best clinical evidence being the results of randomized trials. To date, the only randomized trials using thrombolytic therapy for the treatment of deep venous thrombosis used systemically delivered plasminogen activators. The shortcomings of systemic lytic therapy for the treatment of acute DVT have been recognized,[2] since very little of the delivered plasminogen activator reaches the thrombus occluding the vein. Since the basic mechanism of action of plasminogen activators is activation of fibrin-bound plasminogen (within the clot), systemic delivery often fails because very little of the infused plasminogen activator comes in contact with the clot. Despite the limitations of systemic delivery, it was recognized that thrombolytic therapy used early in the treatment of DVT decreases subsequent pain and swelling and reduces valvular dysfunction, thereby reducing the frequency and severity of the post-thrombotic syndrome.[3–5] The authors of the consensus statement recognized that the local delivery of thrombolytic agents was favored by many clinicians; however, they indicated that it appeared to offer no benefit in comparison to systemic infusion through a peripheral arm vein. Part of the confusion centers around the definition of 'local infusion' versus catheter-directed intra-thrombus infusion. Local infusion is systemic infusion with the venous access in the involved extremity. It has been shown that the 'local infusion' of plasminogen activators via a peripheral vein of the extremity with DVT is far less effective in clearing thrombus than intra-thrombus catheter-directed therapy.[6] The ACCP Consensus Committee concluded that 'the use of thrombolytic agents in the treatment of venous thromboembolism continues to be highly individualized and clinicians should have some latitude in using these agents. In general, patients with hemodynamically unstable pulmonary embolism or massive iliofemoral thrombosis are the best candidates'. To their credit, the authors of the ACCP consensus statement recognized the potential benefits of thrombolytic therapy; however, in the absence of level I evidence, the committee could not make firm recommendations regarding thrombolytic therapy.

Clinical justification for pursuing improved techniques for thrombolysis can be found from a review of clinical trials comparing systemic thrombolytic therapy to standard anticoagulation for the treatment of acute deep venous thrombosis.[7] It was found that 18% of patients treated with conventional anticoagulation had improvement or complete resolution of thrombus on post-treatment ascending phlebography compared with 63% of the patients treated with systemic thrombolysis. In a subsequent analysis, major bleeding complications were almost three times as prevalent in the thrombolysis group.[8] Because of the potential benefits of clearing the deep venous system of thrombus and restoring patency, techniques of improved delivery which would potentially increase efficacy and reduce complications have been pursued. The rationale for intra-thrombus delivery of thrombolytic agents is clear, since activation of fibrin-bound plasminogen is the underlying mechanism for efficient clot lysis. Widespread clinical experience has confirmed improved results with catheter-directed intra-thrombus delivery of plasminogen activators both on the arterial and venous side of the circulation.

Although randomized trials are not available, mounting clinical evidence and observational studies suggest that patients can be successfully treated with catheter-directed thrombolysis and that successful lysis is associated with improved quality of life. This chapter focuses on catheter-directed thrombolysis for the treatment of acute deep venous thrombosis, with emphasis on iliofemoral deep venous thrombosis.

RATIONALE FOR THROMBOLYTIC THERAPY

Extensive deep venous thrombosis presenting with a painfully swollen extremity often accompanied by cyanosis frequently results in debilitating post-thrombotic symptoms. It is commonly said that the post-thrombotic syndrome requires many years for its full manifestation; however, I have observed debilitating symptoms in active individuals from the time of the initial thrombotic event. While skin changes may take months to years to manifest, the painful swelling resulting from significant venous hypertension is immediate and often persistent.

Since the underlying pathophysiology of the post-thrombotic syndrome is ambulatory venous hypertension, and its components are venous obstruction and valvular incompetence, it is physiologically sound that restoring patency (avoiding obstruction) and/or preservation of valvular function will reduce venous hypertension and therefore reduce post-thrombotic sequelae. The combination of venous obstruction and valvular insufficiency has been shown to be particularly virulent.[9,10]

Prospective, natural-history studies have shown that patients develop progressive valvular incompetence over time, that valvular incompetence more commonly develops in patients with occlusive thrombosis compared with those with non-occlusive DVT, and that the more extensive the deep venous thrombosis, the more likely the patient is to develop valvular insufficiency.[11] Physiologic lysis of venous thrombosis occurs more effectively in some patients than others. In those who experience early recanalization (within months), venous valvular function is preserved more frequently than in patients with persistent thrombosis.[12] These natural-history studies demonstrate that persistent obstruction increases the severity of the post-thrombotic syndrome and that early lysis preserves valvular function. It is intuitive that treatment designed to eliminate thrombus will reduce post-thrombotic sequelae by eliminating obstruction and preserving valvular function.

If one were to use venous thrombectomy as a model to evaluate the outcome of thrombus removal on patients with acute iliofemoral DVT, one would observe that patients who had patency restored to their thrombosed venous segments had the lowest ambulatory venous pressures and the fewest post-thrombotic symptoms over the long term.[13–15] Patients with persistent venous obstruction had the most severe post-thrombotic symptoms, and the highest venous pressures. Therefore, it is apparent that long-term benefit of treatment is directly related to eliminating thrombus and maintaining a patent deep venous system.

Two prospective studies of systemic thrombolytic therapy for acute DVT followed patients from 1.6 to 6.5 years for the development of post-thrombotic symptoms.[3,4] Post-treatment evaluation demonstrated that the majority of patients who were free of post-thrombotic symptoms were treated with thrombolytic therapy, whereas the majority of patients with the severe symptoms of the post-thrombotic syndrome were treated with anticoagulation alone.

An important question is whether successful lysis of deep venous thrombi preserves valve function. In a long-term follow-up of a prospective, randomized study, Jeffery *et al.*[16] have shown significant functional benefit 5–10 years after successful lysis of acute DVT. It appears that in patients without a contraindication to thrombolytic therapy, lysis of extensive deep venous thrombosis is preferred and, if successful, preserves long-term venous function. Another important issue that has not yet been answered, is whether lytic therapy for acute DVT reduces the incidence of recurrent DVT?

The goals of treatment with catheter-directed thrombolysis for patients with iliofemoral DVT are:

- prevent pulmonary embolism;
- reduce/eliminate the acute symptoms of iliofemoral DVT; and
- reduce/avoid post-thrombotic consequences.

Patients who are successfully treated with catheter-directed thrombolysis will have patency restored to the venous segment treated. Efficient elimination of thrombus is likely to preserve valvular function, at least in some segments of the venous system. Additionally, many patients who are treated, especially those with left-sided iliofemoral DVT, are likely to have an underlying iliac vein stenosis, which will be uncovered after successful lysis. This underlying stenosis should be corrected to preserve long-term patency and to avoid recurrent thrombosis.

RESULTS OF CATHETER-DIRECTED THROMBOLYSIS

In 1992, Molina and colleagues reported their experience with catheter-directed thrombolysis for iliofemoral

DVT.[17] Ten of twelve patients were successfully treated, and six of the ten who had successful lysis required balloon dilation or stent placement to treat an underlying iliac vein stenosis.

Comerota *et al.*[18] have recommended a strategy of aggressive regional therapy for acute iliofemoral venous thrombosis which includes catheter-directed thrombolysis as the primary approach and venous thrombectomy for those who either fail catheter-directed thrombolysis or who have a contraindication to lytic therapy (Table 19.1).[6,19] Initial observations of success with proper catheter positioning have been confirmed over the long term. To date, we have treated 48 patients within the Temple University Health System for acute iliofemoral DVT with catheter-directed thrombolysis. Of the 48 patients, 39 (81%) had a successful lytic outcome. The catheter could not be properly positioned in three patients and one patient suffered perforation of the common femoral vein. Interestingly, two patients failed lysis with urokinase despite proper catheter positioning and two patients failed, presumably due to chronic venous occlusion. One patient suffered early rethrombosis of a successfully lysed iliofemoral venous segment due to an uncorrected common iliac vein stenosis. Avoidance of post-thrombotic symptoms was directly associated with restoration of patency in the deep venous system. Our currently preferred approach is an ultrasound-guided antegrade puncture and infusion through the ipsilateral popliteal vein or posterior tibial vein. Following thrombolysis, if an underlying iliac vein stenosis is present, angioplasty and/or stenting is performed.

At approximately the same time, Semba and Dake[20] reported their experience with 27 consecutive patients with iliofemoral DVT who underwent catheter-directed thrombolysis. Of the 27 patients, 20 had acute DVT whereas seven were classified as chronic. Patients were treated with an average of 4.9 million units of urokinase over 30 hours. Seventy-two percent of the patients had complete lysis and 20% partial lysis. Eight percent were considered failures. Sixteen of the 27 lower extremities treated had an underlying venous stenosis that was treated with angioplasty ($n = 2$) or angioplasty and stenting ($n = 14$). Overall, these authors reported a technical and clinical success rate of 85% in this difficult patient population. Bjarnason *et al.*[19] reported their experience

Table 19.1 *Outcome of catheter-directed thrombolysis for DVT from two large contemporary series*

Outcome	Bjarnason *et al.*[19] (n = 77)	Mewissen *et al.*[6] (n = 287)
Initial success	79%	83%
Iliac	86%	83%
Femoral	63%	79%
1° Patency at 1 year		
Iliac	63%	64%
Femoral	40%	47%
Success: thrombus age		
Acute	85% (1–21 days)	85% (1–10 days)
Chronic	42% (>21 days)	68% (>10 days)
Success: prior DVT		
+ Prior DVT	85%	20% (complete lysis)
– Prior DVT	87%	36% (complete lysis)
Success: malignancy		
Yes	79%	NA
No	89%	NA
Iliac stent: patent at 1 year		
+ Stent	54%	74%
– Stent	75%	53%
Duration of Rx (mean)	75 hours	48 hours
Dose of urokinase (mean)	1×10^7 IU	6.77×10^6 IU
Complications		
Major bleed	5%	11%
Intracranial (spontaneous)	0%	<1% (1 patient)
Pulmonary embolus	1% (1 patient)	1% (6 patients)
Fatal PE	0%	0.2% (1 patient)
Death 2° lysis	0%	0.4% (2 patients)

treating 87 lower extremities with iliofemoral DVT in 77 patients. The average duration of therapy was 75 hours at an average total dose of urokinase of 10 million units. They evolved from the right internal jugular vein approach to an ultrasound-guided popliteal vein or posterior tibial vein approach. The technical success rate was 79%. Acute DVT was treated more successfully than chronic. Patients treated within 21 days of acute symptoms had an 85% success rate compared with 42% of those having symptoms for more than 21 days. They also observed that iliofemoral DVT had a higher success rate (86%) than femoral-popliteal DVT (63%). The authors also made the interesting observation that the 2-year primary patency rate in patients with malignant disease was 41% compared with 75% in patients without malignancy.

Nineteen complications were reported, six of which were considered major. Two patients required blood transfusions, one as a result of bleeding from an arterial puncture site and the other from a gastrointestinal bleed. No patient suffered an intracranial bleed.

Mewissen *et al.*[6] reported the largest series of catheter-directed thrombolysis for lower extremity venous thrombosis to date. This is a report of a national multicenter registry of patients treated with lytic therapy for venous thrombosis. Two hundred and twenty-one patients with iliofemoral DVT and 79 with femoral-popliteal DVT were treated with urokinase infusions for a mean of 48 hours. An average dose of 6.77 million units of urokinase was used. After thrombolysis, 99 iliac and five femoral vein stenoses underwent angioplasty and stenting.

Complete lysis was observed in 31% of the infusions, 50–99% lysis in 52% and less than 50% in 17%. Thirty-four percent of patients with acute DVT had complete lysis whereas only 19% of patients with chronic DVT had complete patency restored. The degree of lysis was found to be a significant predictor of early and continued patency. Seventy-nine percent of limbs with complete lysis remained patent at 1 year compared with 58% of limbs with 50–99% lysis and 32% of limbs with less than 50% lysis.

Patients with iliofemoral DVT had significantly better 1-year patency (64%) compared with patients with femoral-popliteal DVT (47%). Interestingly, no patient who had isolated femoral-popliteal DVT for more than 10 days achieved complete lysis. It was apparent that adjunctive stent placement in iliac veins which had stenotic lesions improved patency rate. At 1 year, 74% of stented veins remained patent as compared to 53% of limbs without angioplasty or stenting. Stenting was not helpful in the femoral-popliteal segment. Four of the five stents placed in this location thrombosed within a mean of 42 days. The one patient with a femoral-popliteal vein stent remaining patent at 2 months was lost to follow-up.

Major bleeding complications were reported in 11%. Thirty-nine percent of the bleeding complications occurred at the venous puncture site and 13% were the result of a retroperitoneal bleed. Twenty-eight percent of patients had bleeding complications in other areas including the musculoskeletal, gastrointestinal, or genitourinary systems. There was one fatal intracranial hemorrhage and one patient suffered a subdural hematoma following blunt head injury, for a frequency of major neurologic complications of 0.4%. Pulmonary emboli during treatment occurred in six patients (1%), which is a frequency comparable to patients treated with anticoagulation. One patient suffered a fatal pulmonary embolism; therefore, two patients died as a result of catheter-directed thrombolysis for a mortality rate of 0.4% in this series.

Objective outcomes of patency were documented in the above-mentioned studies; however, only short-term radiographic evaluations were completed. Whilst it was the prevailing observation that successfully treated patients enjoyed sustained benefit from successful lysis, the question remained as to whether these patients enjoyed preservation of venous valve function or other objective measures of long-term benefit.

The venous registry patients provided an opportunity to evaluate whether catheter-directed thrombolysis for iliofemoral DVT had a beneficial effect on long-term outcome compared with patients with iliofemoral DVT who were treated with standard anticoagulation. A study assessing health-related quality of life was designed to evaluate whether catheter-directed thrombolysis for iliofemoral DVT is associated with improved health-related quality of life compared with standard anticoagulation, and whether health-related quality-of-life outcome in the thrombolysis group is related to lytic success.

To accomplish that purpose, an 80-item health-related quality-of-life questionnaire was developed which contained items assessing demographics, clinical history, clinical functioning, and well-being as well as specific DVT-related items. Mathias and colleagues[21] validated this instrument for use in this patient population. The validated questionnaire was then administered to 98 patients with iliofemoral DVT treated at least 6 months earlier.[22] Sixty-eight patients were identified through the national DVT registry and were treated with catheter-directed thrombolysis, and 30 patients were identified by their physician or medical record review and were treated with anticoagulation alone.

The majority of the patients were female (61%), Caucasian (95%), married (65%), and the mean time interval from their DVT to final follow-up was 22 months. The lytic group was younger (53 years) than the heparin group (61 years). Following treatment, patients treated with catheter-directed thrombolysis reported better overall physical functioning (P = 0.046), less stigma (P = 0.033), less health distress (P = 0.022), and fewer post-thrombotic symptoms (P = 0.006) compared with patients treated with anticoagulation alone. Within the lytic group, phlebographically successful lysis correlated with an improved health-related quality of life ($P = 0.038$). Interestingly, lytic failures and heparin treatment outcomes were similar. Failure of catheter-directed lysis did not adversely affect outcome compared with standard anticoagulation alone.

This health-related quality-of-life study objectively documented that patients with iliofemoral DVT treated with catheter-directed thrombolysis had an improved health-related quality of life compared with treatment with anticoagulation alone and that improved quality of life was directly related to successful lysis. Lytic failures and heparin treated patients reported a similar health-related quality of life at 22 months following treatment. It is important that future randomized trials comparing treatments for DVT include a health-related quality of life measure as part of their outcome analysis.

CURRENT TREATMENT APPROACH FOR ILIOFEMORAL DVT

The currently available literature and personal experience support catheter-directed thrombolysis as the preferred approach in patients with iliofemoral DVT who have no contraindication to thrombolytic therapy. In patients who fail catheter-directed thrombolysis or have a contraindication to lytic therapy, venous thrombectomy is recommended.

The algorithm in Fig. 19.1 summarizes the sequential decision making when treating these patients. Those who are not ambulatory or have a short life expectancy will be treated with anticoagulation alone. The remainder will be evaluated for either catheter-directed thrombolysis or venous thrombectomy. If the patient has a contraindication to thrombolysis, venous thrombectomy will be recommended. If there is no contraindication to lytic therapy, catheter-directed thrombolysis is the preferred approach (Fig. 19.2).

The FDA has recently restricted the distribution of urokinase. We have a growing experience with catheter-directed recombinant tissue plasminogen activator (rt-PA). Once the catheter is properly positioned, a bolus of 2–8 mg rt-PA is given followed by a continuous infusion of 2–4 mg/h. This appears to offer effective thrombolysis which is safe. The monitoring of lytic effect with sequential phlebograms at intervals of 8–12 hours is no different than those patients who were treated with urokinase (Fig. 19.3).

We have recently added mechanical clot extraction to lytic therapy. The percutaneous mechanical thrombectomy has been performed prior to and following infusions of thrombolytic agents. Preceding catheter-directed thrombolysis with mechanical venous thrombectomy reduces the thrombus load; however, initially infusing the thrombus with plasminogen

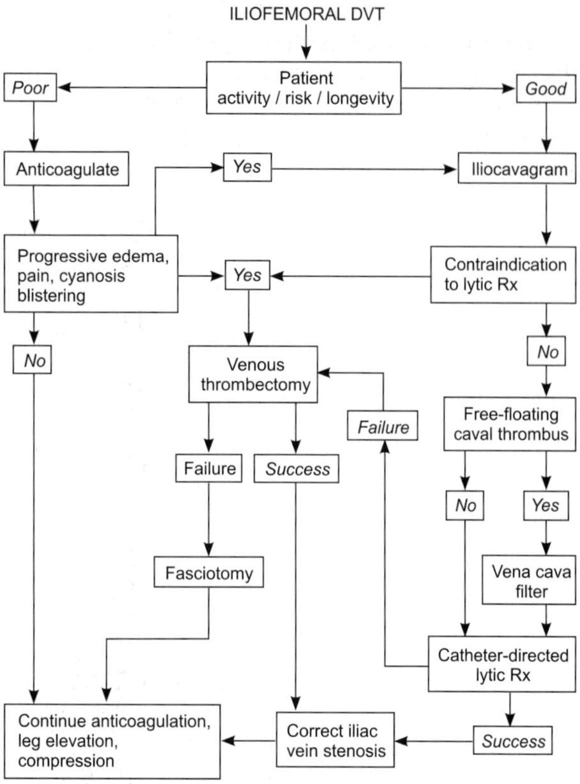

Figure 19.1 *Decision-making algorithm for the treatment of iliofemoral deep venous thrombosis.*

activators may soften and liquefy the clot to enhance the results of mechanical thrombectomy. The proper sequencing of catheter-directed lysis and mechanical thrombectomy has not been determined.

Once lytic therapy is complete and an underlying iliac lesion is corrected, patients are converted to full anticoagulation. In those patients requiring ongoing hospitalization, intravenous heparin can be used and the patient converted to oral anticoagulation with warfarin. If an IV line is no longer required or if patients can be ambulated and discharged, low molecular weight heparin is given subcutaneously using enoxaparin 1 mg/kg every 12 hours or dalteparin 100 U/kg every 12 hours. Oral anticoagulation with warfarin is initiated as lytic therapy is terminated. Oral anticoagulation is continued for no less than 1 year for an initial episode of DVT without an underlying hypercoagulable state.[23] If the patient has suffered a recurrent venous thrombosis or has an underlying hypercoagulable state, indefinite oral anticoagulation is recommended.

SUMMARY

Catheter-directed thrombolysis for iliofemoral venous thrombosis is recommended for patients who have no contraindication to thrombolytic therapy. The preferred approach is via an ipsilateral popliteal vein or posterior

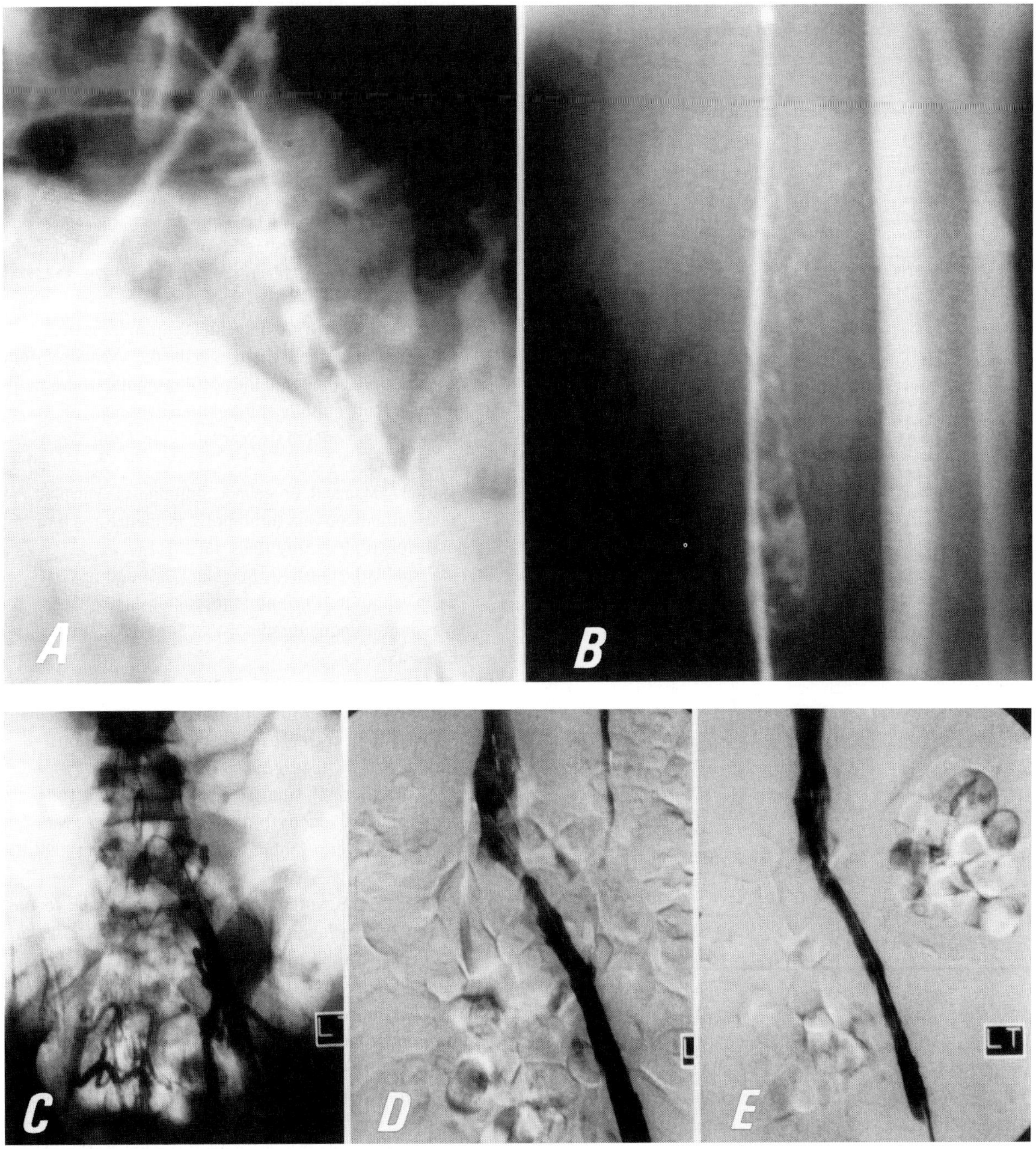

Figure 19.2 *An example of catheter-directed thrombolysis for iliofemoral DVT via the ultrasound-guided popliteal vein approach. (a) Ascending phlebogram demonstrating extensive iliofemoral DVT in a young woman who recently started taking estrogen. (b) Catheter traversing the left proximal superficial femoral vein (SFV) via a popliteal vein puncture extensive thrombosis is appreciated. (c) Phlebogram following thrombolysis demonstrates a patent iliofemoral system with a high-grade stenosis of the left common iliac vein. (d) Phlebogram post-balloon angioplasty of left common iliac vein showing residual stenosis of the left common iliac vein. (e) Phlebogram after stent deployment in the left iliac vein demonstrating a normal vein diameter and a fully patent iliofemoral venous system.*

tibial vein puncture with ultrasound guidance. rt-PA is currently used with an infusion of a 2–8 mg bolus followed by an infusion of 2–4 mg/h. Once lysis is complete, any residual iliac vein lesion is promptly corrected with balloon angioplasty and stenting if necessary. Anticoagulation is continued for at least 1 year if the patient is being treated for an initial venous thrombotic event, and indefinitely for a recurrent DVT or if a patient has an associated hypercoagulable state. Successful lysis is associated with a reduction in post-thrombotic morbidity and improved health-related quality of life.

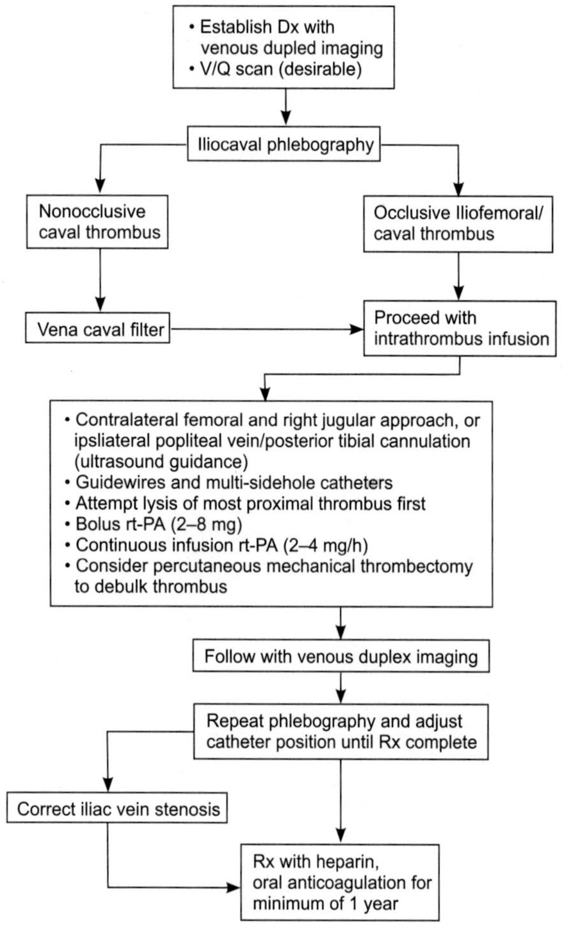

Figure 19.3 *Algorithm for catheter-directed thrombolysis for iliofemoral DVT.*

REFERENCES

1. Hyers TM, Agnelli G, Hull RD, *et al.* Antithrombotic therapy for venous thromboembolic disease. *Chest* 1998; **114**: 5615–785.
2. Comerota AJ. Thrombolytic therapy for acute deep vein thrombosis. In Comerota AJ, ed. *Thrombolytic Therapy for Peripheral Vascular Disease.* Philadelphia: JB Lippincott, 1995: 175–95.
3. Arnesen H, Hoiseth A, Ly B. Streptokinase or heparin in the treatment of deep vein thrombosis: follow-up results of a prospective study. *Acta Med Scand* 1982; **211**: 65–71.
4. Elliott MS, Immelman EJ, Jeffery P, *et al.* A comparative randomized trial of heparin versus streptokinase in the treatment of acute proximal venous thrombosis: an interim report of a prospective trial. *Br J Surg* 1979; **66**: 838–42.
5. Watz R, Savidge GF. Rapid thrombolysis and preservation of valvular venous function in high deep vein thrombosis. *Acta Med Scand* 1979; **205**: 293–8.
6. Mewissen MW, Seabrook GR, Meissner MH, Cynamon J, Labropoulos N, Houghton SH. Catheter-directed thrombolysis for lower extremity deep venous thrombosis: report of a national multicenter registry. *Radiology* 1999; **211**: 39–49.
7. Comerota AJ, Aldridge SA. Thrombolytic therapy for acute deep vein thrombosis. *Semin Vasc Surg* 1992; **5**(2): 76.
8. Comerota AJ, Aldridge SC. Thrombolytic therapy for deep venous thrombosis: a clinical review. *Can J Surg* 1993; **36**: 359–64.
9. Shull KC, Nicolaides AN, Fernandes E, Fernandes J. Significance of popliteal reflux in relation to ambulatory venous pressure and ulceration. *Arch Surg* 1979; **114**: 1304–6.
10. Johnson BF, Manzo RA, Bergelin RO, Strandness DE. Relationship between changes in the deep venous system and the development of the postthrombotic syndrome after an acute episode of lower limb deep vein thrombosis: a one- to six-year follow-up. *J Vasc Surg* 1995; **21**: 307–13.
11. Markel A, Manzo R, Bergelin R, Strandness E. Valvular reflux after deep vein thrombosis: incidence and time of occurrence. *J Vasc Surg* 1992; **15**: 377–84.
12. Meissner MH, Manzo RA, Bergelin RO, Strandness DE. Deep venous insufficiency: the relationship between lysis and subsequent reflux. *J Vasc Surg* 1993; **18**: 596–605.
13. Plate G, Einarsson E, Ohlin P, Jensen R, Qvsarfordt P, Eklöf B. Thrombectomy with temporary arteriovenous fistula: the treatment of choice in acute iliofemoral venous thrombosis. *J Vasc Surg* 1984; **1**: 867–76.
14. Plate G, Åkesson H, Einarsson E, Ohlin P, Eklöf B. Long-term results of venous thrombectomy combined with temporary arterio-venous fistula. *Eur J Vasc Surg* 1990; **4**: 483–9.
15. Plate G, Eklöf B, Norgren L, Ohlin P, Dahlstrom JA. Venous thrombectomy for iliofemoral vein thrombosis – 10 year results of a prospective randomized study. *Eur J Vasc Endovasc Surg* 1997; **14**: 367–71.
16. Jeffery P, Immelman E, Ammore J. Treatment of deep vein thrombosis with heparin or streptokinase: long-term venous function assessment. *Proceedings of the Second International Vascular Symposium, London*, abstract No. S20.3.
17. Molina JF, Hunter D, Yedlina JW. Thrombolytic therapy for iliofemoral venous thrombosis. *Vasc Surg* 1992; **26**: 630–7.
18. Comerota AJ, Aldridge SA, Cohen G, *et al.* A strategy of aggressive regional therapy for acute iliofemoral venous thrombosis with contemporary venous thrombectomy or catheter-directed thrombolysis. *J Vasc Surg* 1994; **20**: 244–54.
19. Bjarnason H, Kruse JR, Asinger DA, *et al.* Iliofemoral deep venous thrombosis: safety and efficacy outcome during 5 years of catheter-directed thrombolytic therapy. *J Vasc Interv Radiol* 1997; **8**: 405–18.
20. Semba CP, Dake MD. Iliofemoral deep venous thrombosis: Aggressive therapy with catheter directed thrombolysis. *Radiology* 1994; **191**: 487–94.

21. Mathias SD, Prebil LA, Patterman CG, Chmiel JJ, Throm RC, Comerota AJ. A health related quality-of-life measure in patients with deep vein thrombosis: a validation study. *Drug Inf J* 1999; **33**: 1173–87.
22. Comerota AJ, Throm RC, Mathias S, Haughton SH, Mewissen MW. Catheter-directed thrombolysis for iliofemoral deep vein thrombosis improves health-related quality of life. *J Vasc Surg* 2000; **32**: 130–7.
23. Kearon C, Gent M, Hirsh J, *et al.* A comparison of three months of anticoagulation with extended anticoagulation for a first episode of idiopathic venous thromboembolism. *N Engl J Med* 1999; **342**(12): 955–60.

20

Surgical treatment of acute iliofemoral deep venous thrombosis

BO EKLOF, ROBERT L KISTNER AND ELNA M MASUDA

There are data that indicate that early and quick removal of an acute venous thrombus may prevent the destruction of the venous wall and valve, i.e. stop the progress to the post-thrombotic syndrome (PTS):

- Wakefield *et al.*[1] have shown in an experimental venous thrombus model that the leukocyte adhesion molecule – P-selectin – activates the leukocytes emigrating into the venous wall, creating an inflammation that destroys the venous wall and the valves;
- Harris *et al.*[2] showed in their experimental model that if the thrombus was removed early, the inflammatory changes were reversible;
- Strandness *et al.*[3] have previously shown that the remaining proximal thrombotic occlusion in human leg veins will lead to progressive distal valvular incompetence.

We therefore recommend an aggressive treatment with rapid removal of the occluding thrombus in active patients with acute iliofemoral deep venous thrombosis (DVT).

The first line of treatment should be catheter-directed intra-thrombus thrombolysis (CDITT) with or without adjunct procedures such as angioplasty and stenting as described in Chapter 19. When there are contra-indications or failure of thrombolysis, thrombectomy (TE) with a temporary arteriovenous (AV) fistula is a valid alternative. Both interventions will be followed by anticoagulation. These aggressive interventions are not justified in chronically ill, bedridden, high-risk, or aged patients, or those with serious intercurrent disease and/or limited life expectancy. In this group of patients these interventions can only be justified for limb salvage in phlegmasia cerulea dolens where conservative treatment does not prevent the development of an acute compartment syndrome with venous gangrene.

Low molecular weight heparin (LMWH), as described in Chapter 18, is highly effective in the initial treatment of DVT but there are no long-term studies of LMWH regarding development of PTS. The uncritical use of LMWH in all cases of iliofemoral DVT is a step backwards, denying a large group of patients the opportunity of removal of the clot that potentially could relieve them from the disability following the PTS. The role of LMWH in acute iliofemoral DVT regarding the prevention of PTS should be tested in a prospective randomized trial compared with the aggressive approach.

THROMBECTOMY

Historical background

The history of venous TE in the USA is quite interesting. At the annual meeting of the New England Surgical Society at Poland Spring, Maine, on September 28, 1940, John Homans[4] from Tufts College Medical School presented the paper 'Exploration and division of the femoral and iliac veins in the treatment of thrombophlebitis of the leg'. Homans, who was an advocate for division of the femoral vein to prevent PE, raised many suggestions and questions that are pertinent today:

> I believe that in the future, instead of at once dividing the various femoral veins, it might be permissible to repair the vein and institute for the next few days a vigorous heparinization. Such a procedure is probably, in skilled hands, less hazardous than nonoperative treatment.

He also advocated division of the femoral or iliac veins following an old thrombophlebitis to prevent reflux. This 'will always do good, and never harm'. In this paper, Homans discussed indications for TE with or without ligation of the femoral vein, the technique, the complications and the importance to prevent reflux. The modern era of TE in the USA started with Howard Mahorner's paper,[5] 'New management for thrombosis of deep veins of extremities', in 1954, when he advocated TE followed by restoration of vein lumen and regional heparinization. He presented six patients, five of whom had an excellent result with rapid disappearance of leg swelling, very little late morbidity and minimum leg edema. There was no PE prior or subsequent to surgery. He claimed that this method restores vein function with preservation of the vein lumen and vein valves. In a paper in 1957,[6] he reported 16 patients in whom TE was performed in 14 legs and two arms with excellent results in 12, good in two and poor in two patients. The enthusiastic wave, created by the Mahorner blues and boosted specially by the report by Haller and Abrams in 1963,[7] was efficiently quelled by Lansing and Davis[8] in 1968 with their 5-year follow-up of Haller and Abrams' patients. Haller and Abrams presented 45 patients with iliofemoral venous thrombosis (IFVT) who underwent TE. In 34 patients with short history (<10 days), excellent bidirectional flow was established in 31 patients (91%). At follow-up after an average of 18 months, 26 of these 31 patients (84%) had normal legs, where ascending venography was permitted in 13 patients, showing normal patency of the deep venous system in 11 (85%). Lansing and Davis reported the 5-year follow-up results of the 34 patients with short history, where only 17 patients (50%) were interviewed: 16 patients were found to have swelling of the leg requiring stockings. One patient had developed an ulcer. Ascending venography in the supine position was performed in 15 patients, showing patent veins in most patients but 'the involved area of the deep venous system was found to be incompetent in all cases and there were no functioning valves'. This study is flawed because they did not study the iliac vein to prove patency and their interpretation of incompetence of the valves in the femoral and popliteal vein cannot reliably be drawn from only an ascending venographic study in the supine patient. The paper was presented at the annual meeting of the American Surgical Association in Boston April 18, 1968, where Rollins Hanlon thought it was 'an important paper despite the rather melancholy message which it brings, reversing some previous optimistic reports' and requested the need 'to have a series of patients followed objectively with clinical and radiographic data over a long period of time after two treatment regimens, operative and non-operative'. At the annual meeting of the Southern Surgical Association at Hot Springs, Virginia, December 8–10, 1969, William Edwards[9] presented a paper, 'Iliofemoral venous thrombosis: reappraisal of thrombectomy', in which he argued with Lansing's results and concluded that:

> venous TE offers an effective and safe method of restoring flow in the deep venous system; when the thrombus is less than 10 days in duration and is of the iliofemoral segment, TE is recommended; venograms at operation to determine the patency of the deep venous system will aid in complete removal of the thrombus and give a basis for later comparison and evaluation of long-term patency.

In the discussion, Lansing repeated his findings from the 5-year follow-up and questioned the value of TE. Haller stated that he was never consulted about the follow-up report. At a recent visit to Louisville, he had studied 17 patients in whom total removal of the thrombus had been possible, where none had any residual edema. Despite some optimism for TE at this meeting, the impact of Lansing's report was striking, and only few papers have since been published from the USA. They all, however, showed very good clinical results above 75%.

Two reports basically abolished venous TE in the USA: Karp and Wylie's[10] 1-page short paper on 10 patients, eight of whom had reocclusion of the femoral vein before discharge, and Lansing and Davis'[8] skewed paper based on a third of the original material, using questionable methods to reach their verdict without communication with the original investigators. There seems, however, to be renewed interest in venous thrombectomy judged from the current American textbooks in vascular surgery. This revival is mainly based on positive reports from Europe.

Modern venous reconstructive surgery using valvuloplasty can show good long-term results in primary venous disease with severe reflux, while the results of vein segment transfer and autologous vein transplantation in secondary (post-thrombotic) venous disease are much less promising.[11] It is, therefore, important to treat thrombosis of the leg early and successfully to avoid obstruction of the venous outflow tract and preserve valvular function in order to prevent the development of a severe post-thrombotic syndrome.

Surgical technique

The first TE for IFVT was performed by Lawen in Germany in 1937.[12] Surgery today is performed under intubation anesthesia; 10 cmH_2O PEEP is added during manipulation of the thrombus to prevent perioperative

PE. The involved leg and abdomen are prepared. A longitudinal incision is made in the groin to expose the long saphenous vein (LSV), which is followed to its confluence with the common femoral vein (CFV), which is dissected up to the inguinal ligament. The superficial femoral artery 3–4 cm below the femoral bifurcation is prepared for construction of the AV fistula. Further dissection depends upon the etiology of the IFVT. In primary IFVT (Fig. 20.1) with subsequent distal progression of the thrombus, a longitudinal venotomy is made in the CFV and a venous Fogarty TE catheter is passed through the thrombus into the IVC (Fig. 20.2). The balloon is inflated and repeated exercises with the Fogarty catheter are performed until no more thrombotic material is extracted. With the balloon inflated in the common iliac vein, a suction catheter is introduced to the level of the internal iliac vein to evacuate thrombi from this vein. Backflow is not a reliable sign of clearance since a proximal valve in the external iliac vein may be present in 25% of cases preventing retrograde flow in a cleared vein. On the other hand, backflow can be excellent from the internal iliac vein and its tributaries despite a remaining

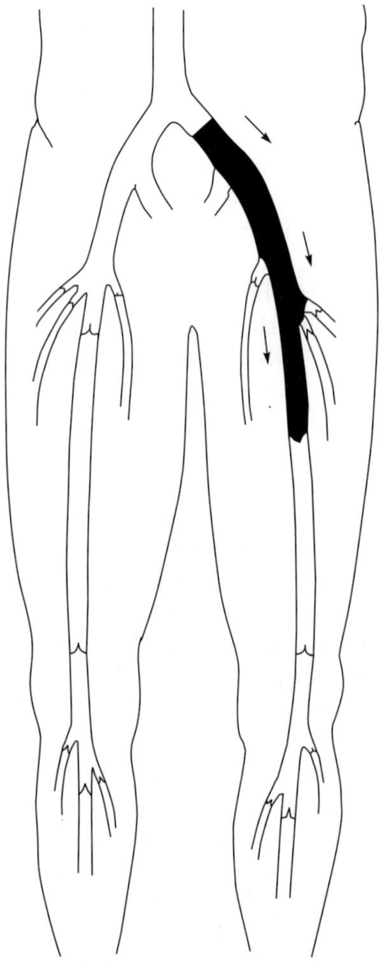

Figure 20.1 *Primary, descending iliofemoral DVT. The thrombus starts in the iliac vein and subsequently descends distally into the leg.*

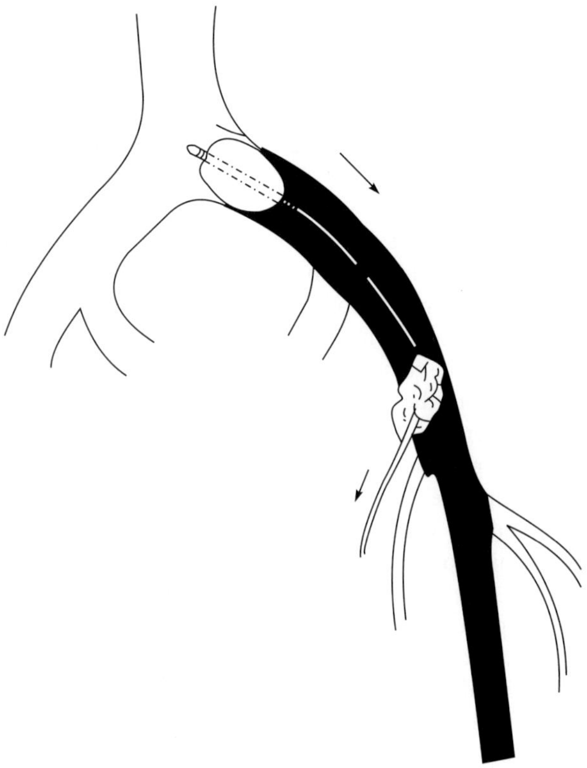

Figure 20.2 *In primary iliofemoral DVT, a longitudinal venotomy is made in the CFV and a venous Fogarty catheter is passed through the thrombus into the IVC. The balloon is inflated and repeated exercises with the Fogarty catheter are performed until no more thrombotic material is extracted.*

occlusion of the common iliac vein. Therefore, an intraoperative completion venogram is mandatory. An alternative is the use of an angioscope, which enables removal of residual thrombus material under direct vision. The distal thrombus in the leg is removed by manual massage of the leg starting at the foot. The Fogarty catheter can sometimes be gently advanced in retrograde fashion. The aim is to remove all fresh thrombi from the leg. In IFVT secondary to ascending thrombosis from the calf (Fig. 20.3), the thrombus in the superficial femoral vein (SFV) is often old and adherent to the venous wall and we have already lost the battle of the valves. The objective is to restore patency and preserve valvular function. If iliac patency is established but the thrombus in the femoral vein is too old to remove, then it is preferable to ligate the superficial femoral vein (Fig. 20.4). Recanalization will otherwise lead to valvular incompetence and subsequent reflux. In a 13-year follow-up after SFV ligation, Masuda *et al.*[13] found excellent clinical and physiologic results without post-thrombotic syndrome. If normal flow in the SFV cannot be re-established, we recommend extending the incision distally and exploring the orifices of the deep femoral branches. These are isolated and venous flow is restored with a small Fogarty catheter. The SFV is ligated. The

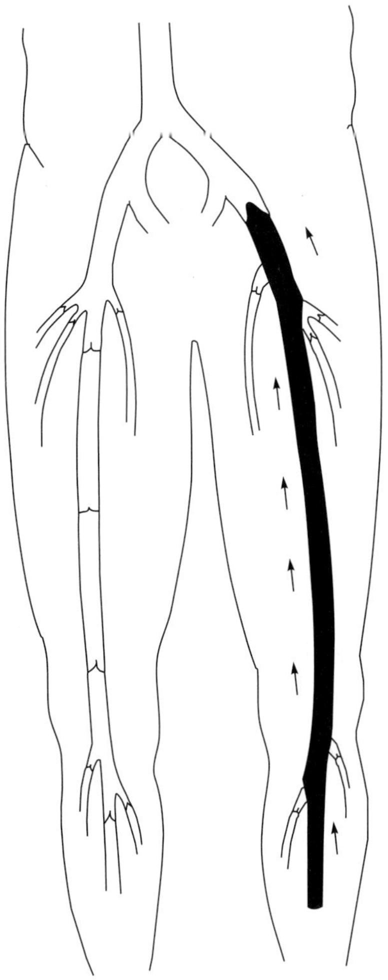

Figure 20.3 *Secondary ascending iliofemoral DVT. The thrombus usually starts in the calf veins, subsequently ascending up into the iliac vein. The thrombus in the SFV is often old and adherent to the venous wall and we have already lost the battle of the valves.*

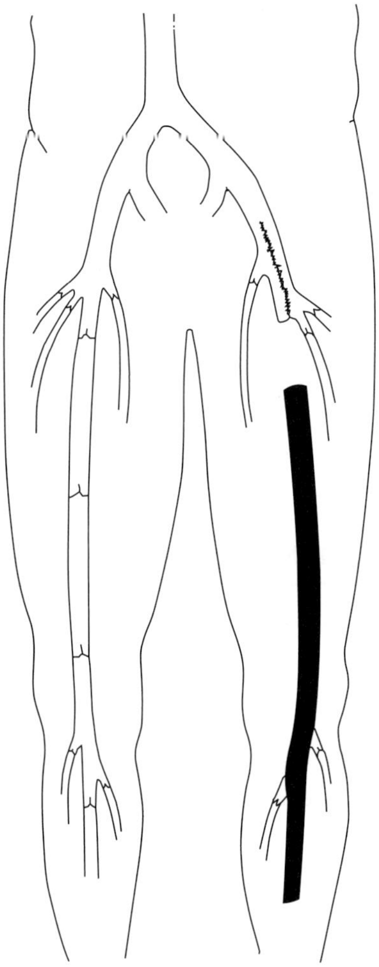

Figure 20.4 *In secondary iliofemoral DVT we start with thrombectomy of the iliac segment. If normal flow in the SFV cannot be established, we recommend extending the incision distally, restoring flow from the profunda branches, and ligating the SFV.*

venotomy is closed with continuous suture and an AVF created using the LSV, anastomosing it end to side to the superficial femoral artery. An intraoperative venogram is performed through a catheter inserted in a branch of the AVF. After a satisfactory completion venogram the wound is closed in layers without drainage. If there are signs of iliac vein compression, which can occur in about 50% of left-sided IFVT, we recommend intraoperative angioplasty and stenting.

If phlegmasia cerulea dolens or venous gangrene is present, we start the operation with fasciotomy of the calf compartments in order to release the pressure and re-establish the circulation. If there is extension of the thrombus into the IVC, the cava is approached transperitoneally through a subcostal incision. The IVC is exposed by deflecting the ascending colon and duodenum medially. Depending upon the venographic findings relative to the top of the thrombus, the IVC is controlled, usually just below the renal veins. The IVC is opened and the thrombus is removed by massage, especially of the iliac venous system. If the iliofemoral segment is involved, the operation is continued in the groin as described above. When laparotomy is contraindicated in patients in poor condition, a caval filter of the Greenfield type can be introduced before the TE to protect against fatal PE.

Heparin is continued at least 5 days postoperatively and warfarin is started the first postoperative day and continued routinely for 6 months. The patient is ambulant the day after the operation, wearing a compression stocking. The patient is usually discharged on the tenth postoperative day to return after 6 weeks for closure of the fistula. The objectives of a temporary AV fistula are to increase blood flow in the thrombectomized segment to prevent immediate re-thrombosis, to allow time for healing of the endothelium and to promote development of collaterals in case of incomplete clearance or immediate re-thrombosis of the iliac segment. A new percutaneous technique for fistula closure was developed by Endrys in Kuwait.[14] Through a puncture of the femoral artery on the opposite surgically untouched side, a catheter is inserted and positioned at the fistula level. Prior to inflation and release of the balloon or coil, an arteriovenogram can be performed to evaluate the patency of the iliac and caval veins, which is of prognostic value. More than 10% of patients have been shown to have remaining significant stenosis of the iliac vein despite initial successful surgery. A transvenous percutaneous angioplasty with stenting can be performed under the protection of the AV fistula, which is closed 4 weeks later after repeat arteriovenography.

COMPLICATIONS OF SURGICAL MANAGEMENT

Mortality

One of the reasons that induced surgeons to abandon TE in the 1960s was the high mortality. Surgery still bears a risk but with the present pre- and postoperative precautions, results have improved. In our series of over 300 patients, two died. One patient succumbed in an acute respiratory failure due to chronic pulmonary fibrosis. Autopsy did not reveal any fresh pulmonary emboli. The other patient had a preoperatively undetected cirrhosis of the liver. He also had an IVC extension of the thrombus. The patient died in multiorgan failure on the 32nd postoperative day following intra-abdominal hemorrhage and severe shock due to postoperative over-anticoagulation.

Pulmonary embolism

In our experience we have no case of fatal PE in the perioperative period. To avoid this problem it is of utmost importance to demand a preoperative venogram that can exclude an extension of the thrombus into the IVC, which can be fractured during manipulation with the Fogarty catheter. We do not use a separate balloon catheter to occlude the IVC but routinely ask the anesthetist to apply PEEP during the operative manipulation of the thrombotic vein. In a prospective randomized study from Sweden,[15] we found positive perfusion scans at admission in 45% of all patients with additional defects seen after 1 and 4 weeks in the conservatively treated group, in 11% and 12%, respectively, and in the thrombectomized group in 20% and 0%, respectively. Mavor[16] demonstrated that incomplete clearance of the thrombus in the iliac vein increased the incidence of re-thrombosis and PE. In the Swedish series, no additional perfusion defects developed after the first postoperative week following TE with AV fistula. Since the AV fistula effectively prevented re-thrombosis, it can be assumed the fistula was one reason for the low incidence of postoperative PE.

Earlier reports of high mortality due to fatal PE have not been borne out in our experience. Possible reasons for the decreased risk of developing significant symptomatic and fatal PE with the present technique are:

- careful selection of patients;
- preoperative demonstration by venography of the extension and level of the top of the thrombus, requiring an extended surgical approach if the IVC is involved;
- use of PEEP during surgery to decrease the risk for perioperative PE;
- intraoperative venography or venoscopy to prove clearance of the iliac vein;
- utilization of an AV fistula to decrease risk of immediate re-thrombosis with PE.

Early morbidity after thrombectomy

The rate of early re-thrombosis of the iliac vein varies. In a retrospective study from Hawaii,[17] it was 34% in primary IFVT (8/24) and 18% in secondary IFVT (6/33) without use of temporary AV fistula. In a prospective randomized study from Sweden[18] using an AV fistula, 13% had early re-thrombosis of the iliac vein. This low rate of early re-thrombosis using a temporary AV fistula is corroborated by a collected series of 555 patients[19] showing 12% re-thrombosis. Important factors to avoid this complication are:

- rarely operating if the symptoms of iliac obstruction are more than 7 days;
- use of the Fogarty catheter to clear the external and common iliac vein with special consideration of the internal iliac vein;
- direct caval approach when the IVC is involved;
- intraoperative venography or venoscopy to demonstrate clearance of the iliac vein;
- liberal and early indication for decompressive leg fasciotomy in patients with phlegmasia cerulea dolens;
- use of a temporary AV fistula;
- early ambulation wearing compression stockings;
- carefully monitored postoperative anticoagulant administration.

Postoperative bleeding with hematoma formation in the groin was not uncommon despite drainage of the wound, as full anticoagulation with heparin was continued for 5 days after operation. To avoid compression of the vein with risk of thrombosis and infection, the hematomas should be evacuated. Early re-thrombosis was previously common but with the use of the temporary AV fistula it is now 12%. If there is an immediate reocclusion of the liac vein, an immediate reconstruction with re-exploration followed by angioplasty and stenting or a femorofemoral crossover bypass graft is considered to prevent retrograde formation of thrombus and subsequent valve insufficiency. Venous gangrene is very rare and in most cases due to underlying malignancy. With liberal indications for fasciotomy in phlegmasia cerulea dolens, it can be prevented. Groin infection was very common until we improved preoperative hygiene and started prophylactic antibiotics. Still we see lymphatic drainage that usually stops after 2–3 weeks. In two patients in the Swedish series, the AV fistula did cause high-output cardiac failure which immediately reverted after closure of the fistula. Both operations were performed in elderly patients with previously known compromised cardiac function and can be avoided by careful selection of patients. One objection to the fistula has been the assumption of increased venous pressure leading to swelling of the lower limb. We did not find any increase of the iliac vein pressure if the outflow was normal. If there was a stenosis of the vein cardial to the fistula, the pressure was higher. This stresses the importance of clearing the proximal vein.

LATE RESULTS

There are few studies on long-term results after TE with AVF. There are eight studies of clinical results in 521 patients with more than 2 years of follow-up where 'clinical success' is claimed in 62%.[20] There are five studies on iliac vein patency in 247 patients with more than 2 years of follow-up showing 82% patency (range 77–88%).[19] There are five studies on femoropopliteal valvular competence in 259 patients with more than 2 years of follow-up showing 60% competency (range 36–84%).[19] In the prospective, randomized study from Sweden, we found a highly significant difference in the number of asymptomatic patients after 6 months, with 42% in the surgical group versus 7% in the conservatively treated group.[18] At 5 years, 37% of the operated patients were asymptomatic compared with 18% in the conservative group.[20] At 10 years, 54% in the surgical group were basically asymptomatic (class 0–2 new CEAP classification) compared with 23% in the conservative group; however, not a significant difference.[21] Iliac vein patency at 6 months was 76% in the surgical group compared with 35% in the conservative group, demonstrated by venography.[18] This significant difference was upheld after 5 and 10 years with 77% and 77% patency in the surgical group, respectively, versus 30% and 47% in the conservative group, respectively.[20,21] Femoropopliteal valvular competence at 6 months was 52% in the surgical group compared with 26% in the conservatively treated group, using descending venography with Valsalva, a significant difference.[18] After 5 years, the patients who underwent TE had significantly lower ambulatory venous pressures, improved venous emptying as shown by plethysmography, and a better calf pump function with less reflux as measured by foot volumetry. Combining the results of all functional tests, 36% of the surgical patients had normal venous function compared with 11% of the conservatively treated group. These differences were not statistically significant due to loss of patients.[20] At 10 years, using duplex scanning popliteal reflux was found in 32% in the surgical group compared with 67% in the conservative group. Six patients who had a successful TE 10 years before without obstruction of the iliac vein at the time of surgery were all asymptomatic with patent iliac veins, and 50% had competent popliteal veins.[21] Successful TE seems to be beneficial in the long term.

SUMMARY

The treatment of acute iliofemoral DVT should aim at

- prevention of fatal PE;
- decrease of pain and swelling of the involved leg, trying to stop the development of phlegmasia cerulea dolens and venous gangrene;
- prevention of the disabling post-thrombotic syndrome by early removal of the blood clot avoiding proximal venous obstruction and preserving normal, functioning valves preventing reflux.

The first choice to accomplish early and quick removal of the thrombus is catheter-directed intra-thrombus thrombolysis. When there are contraindications or failure of thrombolysis, thrombectomy with a temporary AV fistula is a valid alternative.

REFERENCES

1. Downing LJ, Wakefield TW, Strieter RM, *et al.* Anti-P-selectin antibody decreases inflammation and thrombus formation in venous thrombosis. *J Vasc Surg* 1997; **25**: 816–28.
2. See-Tho K, Harris EJJ. Thrombosis with outflow obstruction delays thrombolysis and results in chronic wall thickening of rat veins. *J Vasc Surg* 1998; **28**: 115–22.
3. Caps MT, Manzo RA, Bergelin RO, *et al.* Venous valvular reflux in veins not involved at the time of acute deep vein thrombosis. *J Vasc Surg* 1995; **22**: 524–31.
4. Homans J. Exploration and division of the femoral and iliac veins in the treatment of thrombophlebitis of the leg. *J Am Med Assoc* 1941; **224**: 179–86.
5. Mahorner H. New management for thrombosis of deep veins of extremities. *Am Surg* 1954; **20**: 487–98.
6. Mahorner H, Castleberry JW, Coleman WO. Attempts to restore function in major veins which are the site of massive thrombosis. *Ann Surg* 1957; **146**: 510–22.

7. Haller JAJ, Abrams BL. Use of thrombectomy in the treatment of acute iliofemoral venous thrombosis in forty-five patients. *Ann Surg* 1963; **158**: 561–9.
8. Lansing AM, Davis WM. Five-year follow-up study of iliofemoral venous thrombectomy. *Ann Surg* 1968; **168**: 620–8.
9. Edwards WH, Sawyers JL, Foster JH. Iliofemoral venous thrombosis: reappraisal of thrombectomy. *Ann Surg* 1970; **171**: 961–70.
10. Karp RB, Wylie EJ. Recurrent thrombosis after iliofemoral venous thrombectomy. *Surg Forum* 1966; **17**: 147.
11. Kistner RL. Valve repair and segment transposition in primary valvular insufficiency. In Bergan JJ, Yao JST, eds. *Venous Disorders*. Philadelphia: WB Saunders, 1991: 261–72.
12. Lawen A. Uber Thrombektomie bei Venenthrombose und Arteriospamus. *Zentralbl Chir* 1937; **64**: 961–8.
13. Masuda EM, Kistner RL, Ferris EB. Long-term effects of superficial femoral vein ligation: thirteen-year follow-up. *J Vasc Surg* 1992; **16**: 741–9.
14. Endrys J, Eklof B, Neglen P, Zyka I, Peregrin J. Percutaneous balloon occlusion of surgical arteriovenous fistulae following venous thrombectomy. *Cardiovasc Interv Radiol* 1989; **12**: 226–9.
15. Plate G, Ohlin P, Eklof B. Pulmonary embolism in acute iliofemoral venous thrombosis. *Br J Surg* 1985; **72**: 912–15.
16. Mavor GE, Galloway JMD. The iliofemoral venous segment as a source of pulmonary emboli. *Lancet* 1967; **22**: 871–4.
17. Kistner RL, Sparkuhl MD. Surgery in acute and chronic venous disease. *Surgery* 1979; **85**: 31–43.
18. Plate G, Einarsson E, Ohlin P, Jensen R, Qvarfordt P, Eklof B. Thrombectomy with temporary arteriovenous fistula: the treatment of choice in acute iliofemoral venous thrombosis. *J Vasc Surg* 1984; **1**: 867–76.
19. Eklof B, Kistner RL. Is there a role for thrombectomy in iliofemoral venous thrombosis? *Semin Vasc Surg* 1996; **9**: 34–45.
20. Plate G, Akesson H, Einarsson E, Ohlin P, Eklof B. Long-term results of venous thrombectomy combined with a temporary arterio-venous fistula. *Eur J Vasc Surg* 1990; **4**: 483–9.
21. Plate G, Eklof B, Norgren L, *et al.* Venous thrombectomy for iliofemoral vein thrombosis. 10-year results of a prospective randomized study. *Eur J Vasc Endovasc Surg* 1997; **14**: 367–74.

21

Endovascular and surgical management of acute axillary-subclavian venous thrombosis

YARON STERNBACH AND RICHARD M GREEN

Acute thrombosis of the axillary-subclavian vein is an infrequent event, encompassing less than 4% of all deep venous thromboses.[1,2] Initially described by Paget as a constellation of upper extremity swelling and pain, its correlation with venous thrombosis of the affected arm was subsequently postulated by von Schroetter. The resultant *Paget–von Schroetter syndrome* was ultimately found to be associated with exertion of the affected arm in a repetitive pattern and became synonymous with *effort thrombosis.* It is widely acknowledged that, in patients without obvious risk factors for venous thrombosis, extrinsic compression of the subclavian vein within the thoracic outlet is an important etiologic factor. This manifestation may therefore also be referred to as the *vasculogenic thoracic outlet syndrome.*

Since Hughes' initial review of the world experience with axillary-subclavian deep venous thrombosis (ASDVT) in 1949,[3] an explosion of catheter-based therapies and techniques have profoundly altered the landscape of this entity. Contemporary medical practice employs the subclavian vein for long-term antibiotic infusions, parenteral hyperalimentation, administration of chemotherapy, invasive cardiac monitoring, placement of pacemakers or automatic defibrillators and access for hemodialysis. Screening venography studies have demonstrated that up to 40%[4] of patients with indwelling subclavian venous catheters develop thromboses with high variability in the number that becomes symptomatic. In accordance with these changes, a shift has been observed to a preponderance of catheter-associated thrombosis in contemporary series. The incidence of pulmonary emboli (PE) in patients with effort thrombosis may be as high as 15% in patients assessed prospectively though symptoms are rare.[5] However, patients with catheter-associated thrombosis had an even higher incidence of PE with recurrent massive emboli, causing death in spite of adequate anticoagulation.[6]

Classification of ASDVT is generally according to the underlying cause. The *primary* form comprises approximately one-quarter of all ASDVT and is applied when no obvious cause may be identified at initial evaluation. This group includes patients with effort thrombosis and the associated anatomic abnormalities of the thoracic outlet. Those diagnosed with *secondary* ASDVT have an indwelling venous catheter or device, or are known to be hypercoagulable due to inherited disorders or existing co-morbid conditions.

This chapter focuses primarily on the management of patients with thromboses that are not catheter-related and the applicable endovascular and surgical therapies. Regardless of cause, the natural history of ASDVT patients left untreated is similar with varying degrees of functional impairment related directly to the extent of thrombus and the associated venous hypertension in the affected extremity.

DIAGNOSIS

Almost regardless of cause, evaluation is sought due to varying degrees of abnormal swelling of one upper extremity that may be accompanied by venous distension in the hand and forearm and the emergence of prominent veins along the anterior chest wall. Other typical signs of deep venous thrombosis may also be present including bluish discoloration and a tender, palpable cord in the arm, axilla or neck. Patients with primary ASDVT typically describe arm tightness or an aching pain in the dominant extremity that is exacerbated by exercise. In this group, young, active males predominate. A history of repetitive strenuous activity is noted and is most often associated with manual labor or sports. Occasionally, numbness or tingling of the arm and hand may be reported as well. This does not necessarily implicate nerve involvement. Rather than suffering from a concomitant neurogenic thoracic outlet syndrome, the symptoms may be due to edema and its effect on the peripheral nerves.

The diagnosis of axillo-subclavian venous thrombosis is usually suggested by the clinical history and the initial physical examination. After clinical suspicion has been established, evaluation by venous color Doppler and ultrasound (duplex) is performed. Duplex is a generally inexpensive and readily available diagnostic modality. Although limited by the clavicle in its ability to image the medial third of the subclavian vein, adjunctive use of indirect criteria such as poorly augmentable flow and asymmetric venous distension with limited venous compression may enhance accuracy. Additional information may also be gained about the status of the adjacent internal jugular veins, which may contain thrombus but cannot be effectively assessed by extremity venography.[7] Duplex scanning is the primary imaging modality employed in patient follow-up after treatment. Although magnetic resonance techniques and computed tomography have been used to confirm ASDVT, these studies tend to be less readily available, significantly more expensive and subject to a variety of artifacts. Radionuclide scans may detect thrombus but offer little additional anatomic information.

Angiographic diagnosis remains the gold standard. When meticulously performed, superior accuracy may be obtained and access for catheter-based interventions is afforded. In addition, one may gain an appreciation of the venous collaterals present. Although adequate diagnostic studies may be obtained by cannulation of a distal arm vein, antecubital venous access is generally readily available. Occasionally, ultrasound guidance will prove a useful adjunctus in an edematous arm. Initial imaging may be performed with the arm in the anatomic position (abduction of 30°) and should allow imaging of the entire axillary-subclavian venous system. Visualization of the basilic vein is imperative as the cephalic vein may join the subclavian vein proximally, bypassing the affected venous segment. Although ASDVT may be readily diagnosed, a complete examination entails multiple injections of contrast with the arm externally rotated and variably abducted at 90 and 180° in order to provoke venous compression that may otherwise be missed. If the medial third of the subclavian vein is not well imaged at its confluence with the superior vena cava, additional views may be obtained with contrast injected through a catheter that has been advanced proximally. A typical study is shown in Fig. 21.1.

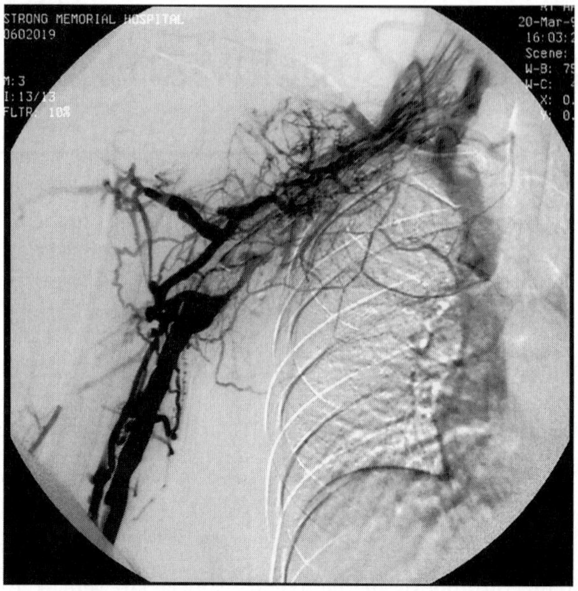

(a)

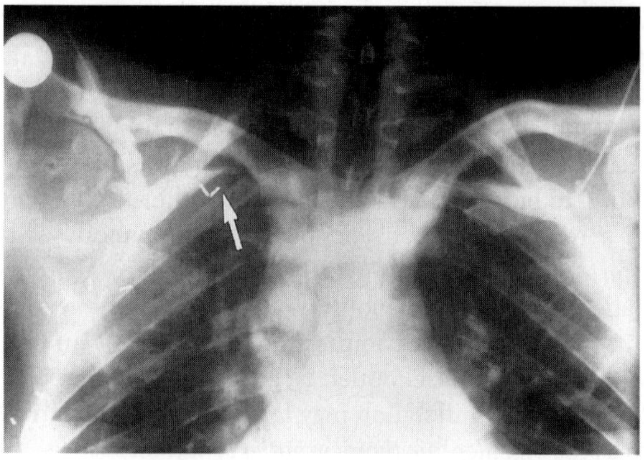

(b)

Figure 21.1 *(a) Venogram used to identify occlusive axillo-subclavian venous disease. (b) Site of venous compression identified at venogram with the arm abducted and externally rotated.*

MANAGEMENT

In spite of the understanding gained regarding ASDVT in recent years, single institution experiences remain relatively small, as this is an infrequent disease process. Level I data are not available as prospective randomized clinical trials have not been performed to compare various treatment regimens for acute thrombosis. Consequently, the clinician is most often guided by institutional expertise, outcomes reported in small series, and personal or local biases.

ANTICOAGULATION

Regardless of treatment initiated, anticoagulation has generally been regarded as the mainstay of therapy once the diagnosis of acute ASDVT has been made, both for relief of extremity symptoms and for prophylaxis against pulmonary embolism. Conservative measures, typically limited to rest and arm elevation, have been advocated by some,[8] though they appear to result in a greater incidence of residual symptoms and associated functional impairment.[9,10] In a meta-analysis of 17 studies published over a 40-year period, Becker *et al.* attempted to analyze treatment outcomes for 329 patients.[11] After stratification based on ASDVT etiology, the review concluded that anticoagulation with heparin and warfarin is less likely to be associated with significant residual symptoms (36%) as compared with those patients who were not anticoagulated (64%). Although the incidence of PE in patients with ASDVT appears to be substantially lower than patients with iliofemoral deep vein thrombosis, it certainly poses a significant risk, particularly in catheter-associated ASDVT where fatal PEs have been reported. Therefore, unless significant contraindications exist, patients diagnosed with symptomatic ASDVT should be therapeutically anticoagulated.

Whether prophylactic anticoagulation is indicated to prevent secondary ASDVT has been investigated in patients with indwelling subclavian vein catheters. Bern *et al.* noted that low-dose (1 mg/day) warfarin reduced the incidence of ASDVT from 37.5% in controls to 9.5% in those in the anticoagulated group.[12] A similar outcome was noted more recently by Boraks *et al.*, who prospectively followed a cohort of high-risk patients and compared them with historical controls. Of the treatment group, 5% developed symptomatic ASDVT confirmed by duplex or venography at a median of 72 days from the time of catheter insertion whilst 15% of controls had developed similar findings at a median of 16 days.[13] Such findings lend credence to a more aggressive approach in warfarin prophylaxis for catheter-associated thrombosis.

THROMBOLYSIS

The recent emergence of thrombolytic therapy in cardiovascular disease has in many ways altered the approach to both peripheral arterial and venous occlusion. For patients with acute primary ASDVT, it is difficult to argue against restoration of venous flow. Operative thrombectomy has been largely supplanted by thrombolysis as the initial intervention. It aims to restore venous patency and identify the underlying venous lesion as well as the dynamic subclavian venous compression at the thoracic outlet characteristic of Paget–von Schroetter syndrome (Fig. 21.2). With advances in imaging technology and catheter-based techniques, there has been a trend away from systemic thrombolysis and toward catheter-directed lytic therapy administration. Such techniques allow for direct deposition of the lytic agent within the thrombus and provide a means of immediately assessing the efficacy of the treatment. It is postulated that less time is necessary to achieve the optimal result and systemic lytic effects are dampened. Whilst most of the initial experience accrued has been with Urokinase (Abbott Pharmaceuticals), a single report appears to confirm the efficacy and safety of recombinant tissue plasminogen activator (t-PA).[14] Comparison of the thrombolysis experience detailed in multiple reports is problematic due to variability in patient populations and duration of symptoms. However, it seems reasonable to expect recanalization rates of 70–80% for patients with new onset of symptoms. In Adelman's report of patients with effort thrombosis, complete lysis was achieved in 14 of 17 patients (82.4%), all but one of whom obtained treatment within 8 days of symptom onset.[15]

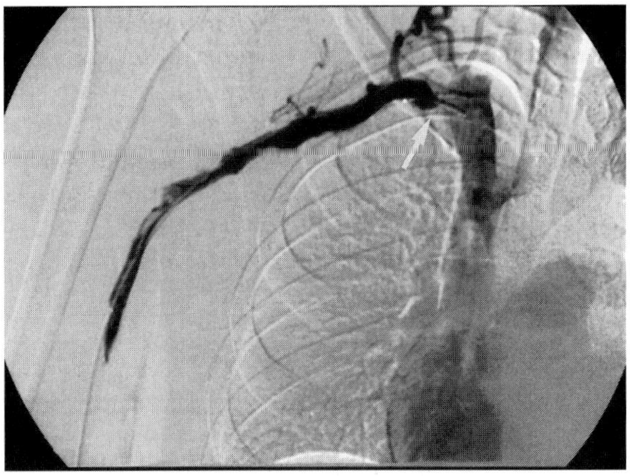

Figure 21.2 *Recanalization of occluded subclavian vein following thrombolysis, allowing for identification of the underlying occlusive lesion (arrow).*

As access to Urokinase has been curtailed in recent months, it seems reasonable to substitute other lytic agents in this clinical situation. Such procedures should still be approached with caution as experience with many of the other agents for non-coronary indications is limited.

It is, however, important to remain critical of the result after successful venous recanalization. An occasional patient may experience complete clot lysis with resolution of symptoms. If no angiographic abnormality can be identified, it may be reasonable to conclude treatment with anticoagulation alone. More commonly, extrinsic venous compression may be demonstrated in the thoracic outlet or incomplete lysis with residual thrombus is seen with intrinsic venous lesions such as stenoses or webs. Such findings underscore the limitations of thrombolysis as an isolated therapy in treating primary ASDVT gave rise to the concept of multimodal therapy.

ENDOVASCULAR INTERVENTION

Beyond thrombolysis, advances in catheter-based technologies have prompted some practitioners to apply a variety of procedures to improve outcome whilst limiting the use of surgery and its inherent risks. Percutaneous transluminal balloon angioplasty (PTA) alone or in conjunction with stent deployment has been viewed as an attractive option for patients with venous stenosis. Sharp needle recanalization of central venous occlusions has also been performed.[16] Glanz *et al.* attempted PTA in a series of 19 patients with primary ASDVT and residual stenosis after thrombolysis who did not undergo thoracic outlet decompression.[17] They reported a technical success rate of 76% with primary patency rates of 35% at 1 year and 6% at 2 years. Such disappointing outcomes were substantiated by others with a more limited experience and led to the empiric use of stents for prevention of elastic recoil of the vessel wall and restenosis. Although multiple small experiences report the use of a variety of stents, both rigid balloon-expandable devices (Palmaz, Cordis/Johnson and Johnson) and even flexible self-deploying stents (Wallstent, Schneider/Boston Scientific) have been deformed or fractured.[18] These results highlight extrinsic vein compression as the dominant pathologic process and point to the need for adjunctive surgical intervention. What remains unclear is the long-term patency associated with such procedures, even when the thoracic outlet is decompressed. Extrapolation from the PTA and stenting experience with dialysis patients suggests inadequate long-term results for a generally young healthy patient population.

SURGICAL TREATMENT FOR EXTRINSIC COMPRESSION

A thorough understanding of the relevant anatomy is crucial to selecting the optimal operative approach and effecting an appropriate surgical solution (Fig. 21.3). The axillary vein becomes the subclavian vein as it passes into the costoclavicular space. Centrally, the innominate vein is formed at the confluence with the internal jugular vein en route to the superior vena cava. The costoclavicular space is bounded inferiorly by the first rib and superiorly

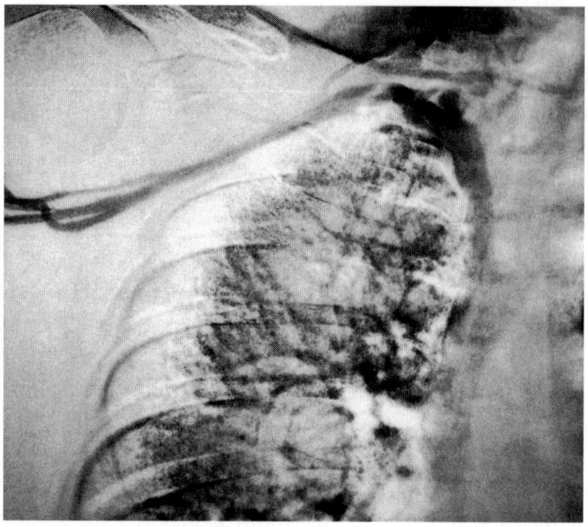

Figure 21.3 *Axillo-subclavian venous reconstruction employing the ipsilateral internal jugular vein.*

by the clavicle. The subclavian vein is located medially within this space between the subclavius tendon on the medial aspect and the anterior scalene muscles laterally. External rotation of the arm with abduction causes clavicular rotation with resultant compression of the vein. A similar effect is created by the military position with the chest projected forward and the shoulders held back. This position is reproduced repeatedly by lifting weights on a bench press apparatus. Therefore, although onset of the patient's symptoms may be fairly recent, the vein involved has likely been chronically traumatized with resultant scarring and occasionally stricture formation. For patients with classic effort thrombosis, decompression of the subclavian vein within the thoracic outlet after thrombolysis appears crucial to attaining long-term asymptomatic, functional upper extremities as demonstrated by Machleder.[19] This parallels DeWeese's experience in the need to supplement operative thrombectomy with medial claviculectomy or first rib resection for optimal long-term outcomes.[20] Whereas some consensus has evolved as to the utility of first rib resection, greater variability remains as to the optimal operative approach. In addition, the surgeon must consider whether intrinsic venous disease with residual obstruction merits intraoperative attention as well.

Decompression of the thoracic outlet essentially requires resection of either the clavicle or the first rib. Division of the anterior scalene muscle fibers at their insertion, division of the subclavius tendon and local venolysis must supplement each of these procedures. Failure to complete any of these adjuncts may lead to persistent obstruction or trauma, with either failure of management or late recurrence. First rib resection has most commonly been accomplished from a transaxillary approach. This exposure leaves little obvious scarring and generally does not deform the chest wall. It allows for resection of the rib and completion of the aforementioned adjunctive procedures; however, true control of the vein is difficult if adjunctive venous procedures are needed due to residual thrombus or stricture. Certainly, balloon occlusion techniques may facilitate use of this approach, although access to the internal jugular vein remains problematic. More recently, Molina[21] has demonstrated success in treating acute and subacute effort thrombosis patients after thrombolysis with an infraclavicular first rib resection which was accompanied by vein patch angioplasty in patients with residual stenoses. At the University of California/San Francisco, a supraclavicular approach to the first rib is preferred although in two-thirds of patients, it is accompanied by an infraclavicular or transaxillary counterincision.[22] Their follow-up at a mean of 31 months reported by Azakie *et al.* suggests a complete resolution of symptoms with unimpeded resumption of activity in 24 of 25 patients with acute ASDVT or symptomatic stenosis with positional occlusion.

Resection of the medial third of the clavicle successfully decompresses the subclavian vein at the thoracic outlet. This approach, although thought by some to produce excessive chest wall deformity with scarring and functional impairment, affords complete exposure of the relevant anatomy and allows for venous reconstruction or bypass as needed. In a review of the experience with this approach at the University of Rochester[23] that included follow-up of 3–9 years, all 11 patients had returned to their pre-thrombosis vocations without limitations including two patients who regularly perform heavy physical labor. Although two of 11 patients are bothered by local scar appearance and one mechanic complains of ipsilateral shoulder aching with overuse, all are completely satisfied from a functional standpoint. Such outcomes indicate that successful treatment of ASDVT is possible with restoration of the premorbid functional status.

THE VEIN WITH AN INTRINSIC NARROWING

Venous reconstruction has been performed in patients undergoing anatomic decompression of the thoracic outlet if residual thrombus is present or venous stenosis or occlusion has been documented. Today, an additional emerging indication is the failure of preoperative endovascular measures aimed at treating such lesions. Acute shorter lesions (<2 cm) may be successfully treated by operative thrombectomy with vein patch venoplasty. Longer narrowings do not respond as favorably. Other bypasses have been described. Most commonly, a patent ipsilateral internal jugular vein is dissected for a variable length cephalad and ligated distally. The vein is then turned down and anastomosed to the patent distal axillary or subclavian vein segment. Advantages of this approach include a single anastomosis and dissection within a single operative field. Greater saphenous and cephalic veins have also been used as bypass grafts to the internal jugular vein or as crossovers. Temporary distal arteriovenous fistulae for up to 3 months are useful adjuncts recommended by most authors including Sanders.[24] The use of PTFE bypasses to the internal jugular vein or the vena cava has been less frequent but should probably be accompanied by an arteriovenous fistula that is left intact.

Although endovascular interventions have thus far achieved suboptimal results when performed preoperatively, they may yet prove beneficial adjuncts in addressing intrinsic venous stenoses when performed after first rib resection, either intraoperatively or in a combined imaging suite or shortly afterward.

TIMING THE OPERATION

All practitioners recognize that any vessel that has recently undergone thrombolysis is at risk for recurrent thrombosis. In the axillary-subclavian venous system, venous narrowing with the attendant hemodynamic effects and possible endothelial changes may contribute to such risk. This forms one basis for anticoagulation of all such patients, regardless of outcome or planned procedure. For those with clear indications for an adjunctive surgical intervention, the timing of the procedure has been a source of debate. Intuitively, immediate surgery should lessen the risk of recurrent thrombosis. In addition, a more rapid return to premorbid function should be achieved. However, Machleder's work appears to refute such a hypothesis. The experience of Urschel[25] and a more recent paper by Lee *et al.*[26] attest to the success of operative decompression of the thoracic outlet within hours or days. Certainly if endovascular intervention such as PTA is to play a role in post-thrombolytic intervention, one may consider leaving a guidewire in place across highly stenotic or diseased vein segments to facilitate the intraoperative procedure.

REFERENCES

1. Prescott SM, Tikoff G. Deep venous thrombosis of the upper extremity: a reappraisal. *Circulation* 1979; **59**(2): 350–5.
2. Lindbald B, Tengborn L, Berquidt D. Deep vein thrombosis of the axillary-subclavian veins. *Eur J Vasc Surg* 1988; **2**(3): 161–5.
3. Hughes ESR. Venous obstruction in the upper extremity

(Pagett–Schroetter syndrome). *Int Abstr Surg* 1949; **88**: 89–127.
4. Horne MK, May DJ, Alexander HR, *et al.* Venographic surveillance of tunneled central venous access devices in adult oncology patients. *Ann Surg Oncol* 1995; **2**(2): 174–8.
5. Monreal M, Lafoz E, Ruiz J, *et al.* Upper extremity deep venous thrombosis and pulmonary embolism. *Chest* 1991; **99**(2): 280–3.
6. Monreal M, Raventos A, Lerma R, *et al.* Pulmonary embolism in patients with upper extremity DVT associated with central venous lines – a prospective study. *Thromb Haemost* 1994; **72**(4): 548–50.
7. Kroger K, Gocke C, Schelo C, *et al.* Association of subclavian and jugular venous thrombosis: color doppler sonograhic evaluation. *Angiology* 1998; **49**(3): 189–91.
8. Ameli FM, Minas T, Weiss M, Provan JL. Consequences of conservative conventional management of axillary vein thrombosis. *Can J Surg* 1987; **30**(3): 167–9.
9. AbuRahma AF, Short YS, White JF 3rd, Boland JP. Treatment alternatives for axillary-subclavian vein thrombosis: long-term follow-up. *Cardiovasc Surg* 1996; **4**(6): 783–7.
10. Tilney NL, Griffiths HFG, Edwards EA. Natural history of major venous thrombosis of the upper extremity. *Arch Surg* 1970; **101**: 792–6.
11. Becker DM, Philbrick JT, Walker FB. Axillary and subclavian venous thrombosis: prognosis and treatment. *Arch Intern Med* 1991; **151**(10): 934–43.
12. Bern MM, Lokich JJ, Wallach SR, *et al.* Very low doses of warfarin can prevent thrombosis in central vein catheters. *Ann Intern Med* 1990; **112**(6): 423–38.
13. Boraks P, Seale J, Price J, *et al.* Prevention of central venous catheter associated thrombosis using minidose warfarin in patients with haematological malignancies. *Br J Haematol* 1998; **101**(3): 483–6.
14. Chang R, Horne MK, Mayo DJ, *et al.* Pulse-spray treatment for subclavian and jugular venous thrombi with recombinant tissue plasminogen activator. *J Vasc Interv Radiol* 1996; **7**(6): 845–51.
15. Adelman MA, Stone DH, Riles TS, Lamparello PJ, Giangola G, Rosen RJ. A multidisciplinary approach to the treatment of Paget Schroetter syndrome. *Ann Vasc Surg* 1997; **11**(2): 149–54.
16. Farrell T, Lang EV, Barnhart W. Sharp recanalization of central venous occlusion. *J Vasc Interv Radiol* 1999; **10**(2 Pt 1): 149–54.
17. Glanz S, Gordon DH, Butt KMH, *et al.* Axillary and subclavian vein stenosis: percutaneous angioplasty. *Radiology* 1988; **168**(2): 371–3.
18. Meier GH, Polack JD, Rosenblatt M, *et al.* Initial experience with venous stents in exertional axillary-subclavian vein thrombosis. *J Vasc Surg* 1996; **24**(6): 974–81.
19. Machleder HI. Evaluation of a new treatment strategy for Paget-Schroetter syndrome: spontaneous thrombosis of the axillary-subclavian vein. *J Vasc Surg* 1993; **17**(2): 305–15.
20. DeWeese JA, Adams JT, Gaiser DI. Subclavian venous thrombectomy. *Circulation* 1970; **41**(5 Suppl II); 156–64.
21. Molina JE. Need for emergency treatment in subclavian vein effort thrombosis. *J Am Coll Surg* 1995; **181**(5): 414–20.
22. Azakie A, McElihnney DB, Thompson RW, *et al.* Surgical management of subclavian-vein effort thrombosis as a result of thoracic outlet compression. *J Vasc Surg* 1998; **28**(5): 777–86.
23. Green RM, Waldman D, Ouriel K, Riggs P, Deweese JA. Claviculectomy for subclavian venous repair: long term functional results. *J Vasc Surg* 2000; **32**: 315–21.
24. Sanders RJ, Cooper MA. Surgical management of subclavian venous obstruction, including six cases of subclavian vein bypass. *Surgery* 1995; **118**(5): 856–63.
25. Urschel HC, Razzuck MA. Improved management of the Paget-Schroetter syndrome secondary to thoracic outlet compression. *Ann Thorac Surg* 1991; **52**(6): 1217–21.
26. Lee MC, Grassi CJ, Belkin M, *et al.* Early operative intervention after thrombolytic therapy for primary subclavian vein thrombosis: an effective treatment approach. *J Vasc Surg* 1998; **27**(6): 1101–7.

22

Pulmonary embolism

H BROWNELL WHEELER AND FREDERICK A ANDERSON, JR

Pulmonary embolism (PE) is the third leading cause of death from cardiovascular disease, exceeded only by ischemic heart disease and stroke.[1] The exact number of deaths due to PE in the USA each year is unknown because of the low autopsy rate, and because most deaths due to PE are never diagnosed. Estimates of the number of PE deaths each year in the USA range from 50 000[2] to 200 000.[3] PE is recognized as one of the leading causes of death in North America and Europe, and may be the most common preventable cause of death in hospitals.

In recent years, there has been a gradual decline in non-fatal cases of PE diagnosed in the USA. Data from the National Hospital Discharge Survey[4] show a 37% decline in the number of PE diagnosed in acute care hospitals from 133 000 diagnoses in 1982 to 84 000 in 1992. It should be kept in mind that the number of cases that are clinically diagnosed is significantly less than the true incidence.

During the same time period, there was a 108% increase in the diagnosis of deep vein thrombosis (DVT) (from 92 000 diagnoses to 192 000). Since PE is a direct consequence of DVT, these opposing trends seem paradoxical. However, it is reasonable to speculate that improved methods of diagnosis and more effective treatment of DVT may have reduced the incidence of PE. More widespread use of prophylaxis may also have played a role, since numerous studies have demonstrated that the incidence and mortality from PE can be reduced by prophylaxis.[5,6] In short, it seems likely that the reduction in clinically diagnosed PE in recent years may be due to improved clinical management, at least in part. Consequently, it is important for all clinicians to be familiar with the diagnosis, treatment and prophylaxis of PE in order to reduce still further its significant morbidity and mortality.

HISTORICAL OVERVIEW

In 1846, Rudolf Virchow performed 76 autopsies in which large ante-mortem thrombi obstructed the pulmonary arteries and were presumed to be the cause of death in 11 patients (14.5%). Venous thrombi were found in 10 of these 11 patients. Virchow correctly surmised that large fragments of thrombi had broken off and been carried through the bloodstream until they lodged in the pulmonary arteries, occluding the outflow tract of the right ventricle and causing the patient's death. Subsequent autopsy studies documented a similar 10–15% incidence of fatal PE until the 1970s, but the incidence seems to be somewhat lower now. In a Scandinavian autopsy study of over 5000 deaths following surgery, PE was found in 24% of cases, but was deemed to be the principal cause of death in only 6.4%.[7]

No effective treatment was available for over a century after Virchow's seminal observations on the pathophysiology of PE. Heparin was identified by Maclean and Howell as early as 1916, but it was not until 1960 that Barritt and Jordan conducted the first randomized clinical trial using heparin for the treatment of acute PE.[8] This trial was concluded prematurely because no fatalities had been observed in 16 patients treated with heparin, whereas there had been five deaths from recurrent PE in the 19 control patients. In addition, there were five non-fatal recurrences of PE in the control group, whereas there were none in the treatment group.

Despite the small number of patients, the results were so striking that no similar controlled trial has been undertaken since. Heparin has become widely established as the standard treatment for PE, with a recurrence rate of roughly 5% and a mortality of less than 2% when the patient is adequately anticoagulated.

Sporadic attempts at prophylaxis of PE through the use of anticoagulants were reported in the 1940s, but the major impetus to anticoagulant prophylaxis came from the work of two British pathologists in the late 1950s. Sevitt and Gallagher documented that 40–50% of elderly patients who died after a fractured femur, tibia or pelvis succumbed to PE. They postulated that this high mortality could be reduced by anticoagulant prophylaxis at the time of hospital admission. A randomized prospective trial of oral anticoagulation in patients with fractured hips was therefore undertaken. No deaths were observed in 150 patients with fractured hips who were treated with oral anticoagulants, except for two patients in whom the anticoagulants had been discontinued. On the other hand, there was a 10% mortality from PE in 150 control patients.[9] These dramatic results stimulated many other studies of prophylaxis for DVT/PE, especially in patients with fractured hips or elective total hip replacement. Kakkar organized a multicenter European trial of low-dose heparin prophylaxis for PE in general surgical patients. Sixteen deaths from PE occurred in the control group, but only two deaths occurred in patients who received low-dose heparin.[6] Many subsequent reports confirmed the value of prophylaxis for PE, which has become standard practice for high-risk patients in most hospitals (see Chapter 15).

CLINICAL MANIFESTATIONS

The clinical presentation of PE depends upon its magnitude. Any sudden and otherwise unexplained hypotension, chest pain or respiratory distress should suggest the possibility of PE. Massive PE causes acute cor pulmonale, with sudden cardiovascular collapse, syncope or sudden death. The typical patient is hypotensive, cyanotic and has distended neck veins. On auscultation of the heart, the pulmonic second sound is often accentuated.

Unfortunately, the majority of patients who die suddenly from PE never have the diagnosis suspected. Goldhaber reported that only 30% of all patients with autopsy-proved PE had the clinical diagnosis suspected prior to post-mortem examination.[10] Similar figures have been reported by others. The diagnosis is unsuspected in at least two-thirds of the patients who die from PE.

Patients with moderately large, but less than massive PE typically complain of sudden dyspnea and have a rapid respiratory rate. They often complain of chest pain as well. In a recent study, 94% of all patients with documented PE were found to have either dyspnea or chest pain as presenting symptoms. Other early symptoms may include palpitations and sweating.[11]

When the embolus obstructs an end artery, it may lead to pulmonary infarction. When the infarct has been present long enough to cause pleural inflammation, chest pain may be exacerbated by breathing and a friction rub may be present on auscultation. Rales may also be present. Patients often develop a cough and occasionally have hemoptysis as well (see Tables 22.1 and 22. 2).

Table 22.1 *The frequency of symptoms in 97 patients with confirmed PE**

Symptom	Percentage
Dyspnea	79
Chest pain	65
Sudden-onset dyspnea	59
Sweating	41
Cough	39
Palpitations	31
Pleuritic pain	28
Hemoptysis	13
Syncope	11

*Adapted from Manganelli *et al.*[11]

Table 22.2 *The frequency of physical signs in 97 patients with confirmed PE**

Sign	Percentage
Respiratory rate >25/min	59
Heart rate >100/min	41
Increased pulmonic second sound	40
Decreased breath sounds	38
Neck vein distension	31
Hypotension	24
Rales	24
Pleural rub	23
Cyanosis	18

*Adapted from Manganelli *et al.*[11]

Small PE in the pulmonary parenchyma are quite common, but usually asymptomatic. They may not be important clinically, except to indicate the increased possibility of recurrent PE. Perfusion lung scans have shown presumptive evidence of postoperative PE in up to 58% of general surgical patients, with an average incidence of roughly 25%. Virtually all these patients are asymptomatic and have good clinical outcomes, even without treatment.[12] In the absence of pulmonary infarction, symptoms may not occur until 50% or more of the pulmonary outflow tract has been obstructed by PE, unless the patient has significant other cardiac or pulmonary disease as well. However, in patients with severe cardiopulmonary disease, even a small PE can cause distressing symptoms or prove fatal.

The likelihood of PE is greater in patients who have clinical signs and symptoms of DVT. However, DVT is often asymptomatic. Even extensive DVT may have no symptoms or signs in a patient at bed rest. Only 25% of patients with documented PE have any clinical indication of underlying DVT, even though over 90% of PE come from the pelvic or leg veins.[13] In addition to looking for clinical signs and symptoms of DVT, the physician should also try to identify underlying risk factors. The likelihood of PE increases in proportion to the number of risk factors for DVT that are present.

Because of the nonspecific nature of its symptoms, the diagnosis of PE cannot be made conclusively on clinical grounds alone. Nevertheless, it is useful to estimate the probability of PE on the basis of clinical evaluation. Classifying patients according to the probability of disease can enhance the predictive value of diagnostic procedures.[14] A knowledgeable clinician can classify patients as to their probability of PE (low, moderate or high) on the basis of a careful clinical evaluation, which should include both identification of risk factors for DVT and a search for other possible causes of the clinical findings.[15] Several studies[16,17] have demonstrated that the predictive value of diagnostic tests for PE, especially the perfusion lung scan, is greatly enhanced when the test result is correlated with the clinical probability of disease.

DIAGNOSTIC TESTS

In critically ill patients who are suspected of PE, it is important to utilize diagnostic procedures which can be done rapidly at the bedside. These include electrocardiogram (ECG), chest x-ray, arterial blood gases, and noninvasive tests for DVT.

Both the chest x-ray and ECG may suggest the presence of PE, but their primary value is in identifying other cardiac or pulmonary pathology which might cause a similar clinical picture. In a patient with PE, the chest x-ray may show enlargement of the right ventricle, which is best seen in a lateral view. The pulmonary hilum may be distended, whereas the lung markings (which are primarily blood vessels) may be strikingly diminished in the area supplied by the obstructed artery. In the remainder of the lung, the markings may appear unusually prominent due to vascular congestion. When a pulmonary infarct is present, the chest x-ray may show a triangular or wedge-shaped defect with its base on the pleural surface. Blunting of the costophrenic angle or frank pleural effusion may be observed. Nearly 80% of patients with PE have some abnormality on chest x-ray, but x-ray findings alone are rarely a sufficient basis to establish the diagnosis.

The ECG is useful primarily to identify myocardial infarction, arrhythmias, or other cardiac causes of the patient's symptoms. In the presence of PE, it may show a pattern of acute right heart strain. However, the S1 Q3 T3 pattern which has been described as characteristic of PE is present in only 16% of patients with confirmed PE.[11]

A low arterial P_{O_2} is highly suspicious for PE, especially when the chest x-ray does not reveal any obvious pulmonary cause for hypoxia. On the other hand, a normal arterial P_{O_2} makes a clinical diagnosis of PE much less likely.

Demonstration of DVT by duplex ultrasound or impedance plethysmography (IPG) increases the probability of PE. More importantly, it may avoid the need to transport a critically ill patient for a lung scan or a pulmonary angiogram, since the treatment for DVT is usually appropriate for PE as well.

Pulmonary angiography is the ultimate reference standard for the diagnosis of PE. When the angiogram shows an internal filling defect in the pulmonary arteries, the diagnosis is confirmed (see Figs 22.1a, 22.2a).

Although angiography can demonstrate PE clearly, several factors limit its clinical utility. It is an invasive procedure requiring injection of contrast material. It is associated with some risk, particularly in patients with severe pulmonary hypertension, right heart failure or respiratory failure. Transporting a critically ill patient to the angiography suite can be difficult and even dangerous. Sophisticated radiographic equipment and a high level of technical expertise are required to demonstrate PE clearly. Because of lack of suitable x-ray equipment or skilled personnel, pulmonary angiography is unavailable in some hospitals. Even large hospitals may not be able to carry out pulmonary angiography on nights or weekends. In addition, the high cost of pulmonary angiography precludes its routine use for screening patients without a high clinical probability of PE. For all these reasons, pulmonary angiography is not suitable for routine use to establish the diagnosis of PE, although it remains the accepted reference standard.

The most commonly employed diagnostic test for PE is the perfusion lung scan. It is less invasive, has lower risk and is less expensive than pulmonary angiography. A normal perfusion scan essentially rules out the diagnosis of PE. Unfortunately, an abnormal scan does not necessarily establish the diagnosis. In patients with abnormal perfusion scans and suspected PE, the diagnosis of PE is confirmed in less than 50% of patients when compared with pulmonary angiography.[18] Reduced pulmonary blood flow can occur from a variety of conditions other than PE. Atelectasis, pneumothorax, emphysema and chronic pulmonary disease are some of the more common conditions that can cause abnormal perfusion scans.

A chest x-ray is useful in interpreting an abnormal perfusion lung scan, since it can rule out other

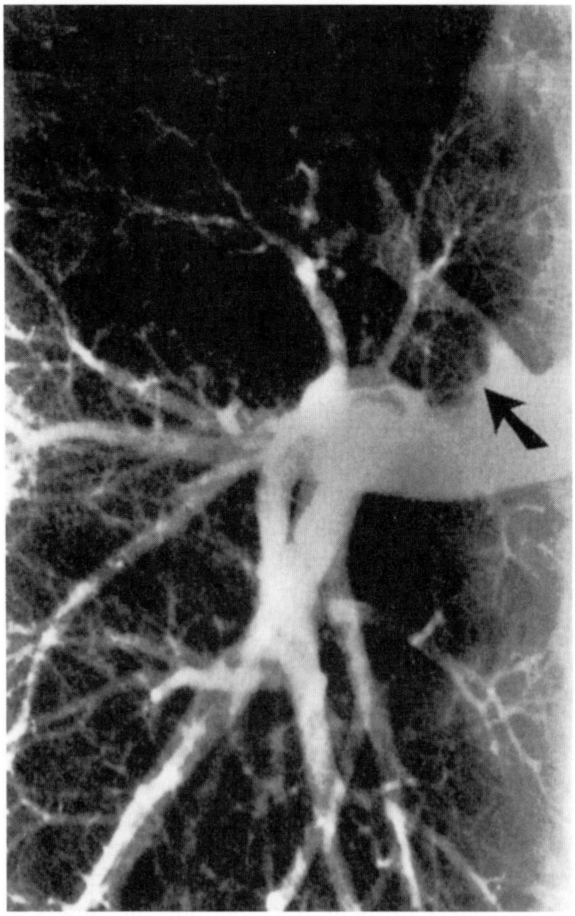

(a)

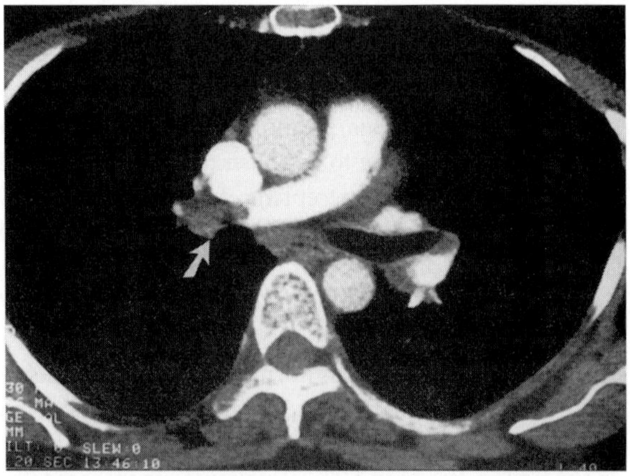

(b)

Figure 22.1 *Acute pulmonary embolism. (a) Pulmonary angiography shows an acute embolus (arrow) partially obstructing the right pulmonary artery. (b) A CT scan with intravenous contrast material, obtained on an electron beam scanner, was the initial diagnostic study that identified embolism. Notice the filling defect (arrow) due to embolus in the right pulmonary artery.*

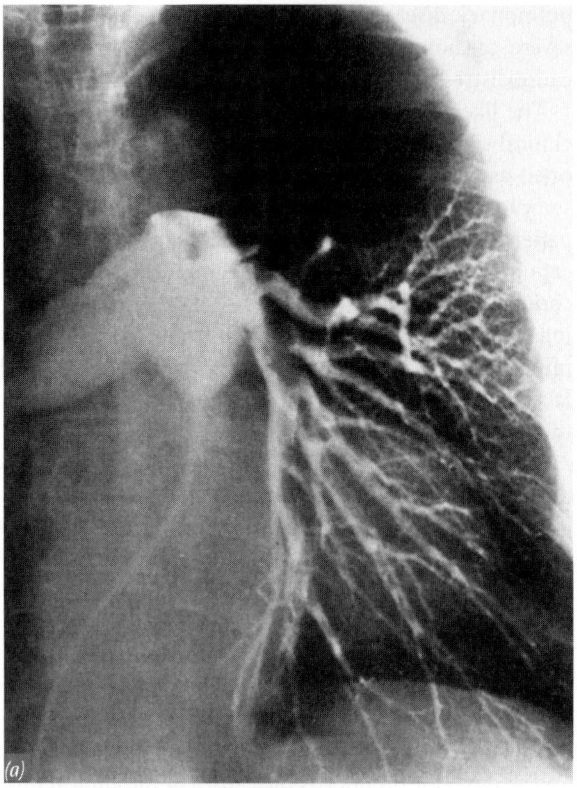

(a)

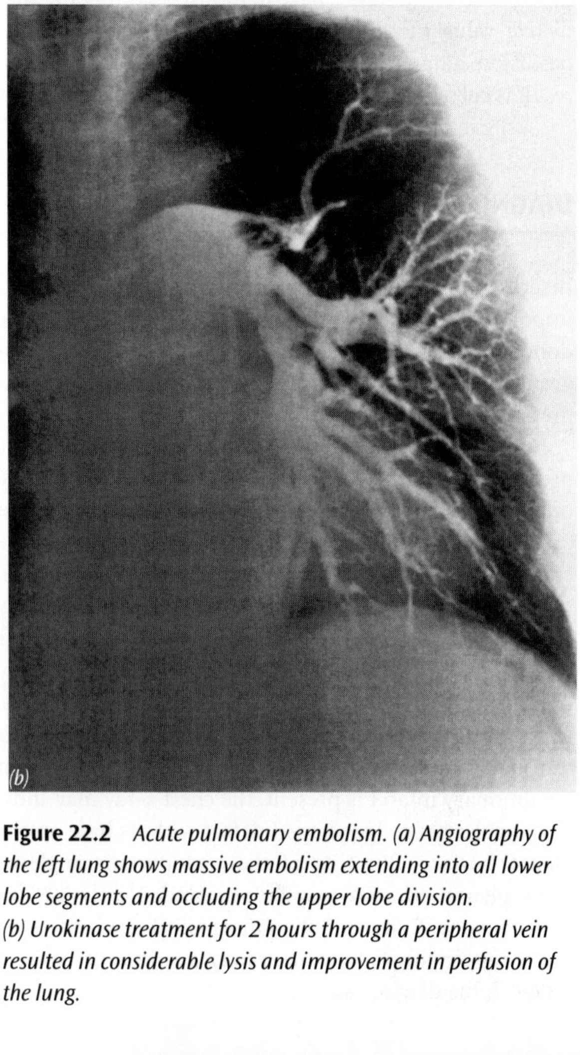

(b)

Figure 22.2 *Acute pulmonary embolism. (a) Angiography of the left lung shows massive embolism extending into all lower lobe segments and occluding the upper lobe division. (b) Urokinase treatment for 2 hours through a peripheral vein resulted in considerable lysis and improvement in perfusion of the lung.*

pulmonary causes of reduced blood flow. The chest x-ray may also show findings suggestive of PE (as described above). When the chest x-ray is normal, or when its findings are not suggestive of other pulmonary pathology, an abnormal perfusion lung scan has a much higher probability of reflecting PE.

Ventilation scans with radioactive gases or aerosols are also helpful in the evaluation of perfusion scans. Comparison of the ventilation scan with the perfusion scan can help to differentiate between perfusion defects due to PE and perfusion defects due to pulmonary causes (which are likely to impair ventilation as well). Unfortunately, the ventilation scan is not a simple or inexpensive procedure. Nevertheless, a normal ventilation scan in the presence of an abnormal perfusion scan is associated with a high probability of PE (see Fig. 22.3).

When the ventilation/perfusion lung scan is read as indicating a high probability of PE, and when the clinical probability of PE is also high, the diagnostic accuracy as compared to pulmonary angiography is 96%.[18] Similarly, when the lung scan demonstrates a low probability of PE, and when the clinical probability of PE is also low, the likelihood of demonstrating PE by angiography is only 2–9%.[18] Unfortunately, many patients do not fall

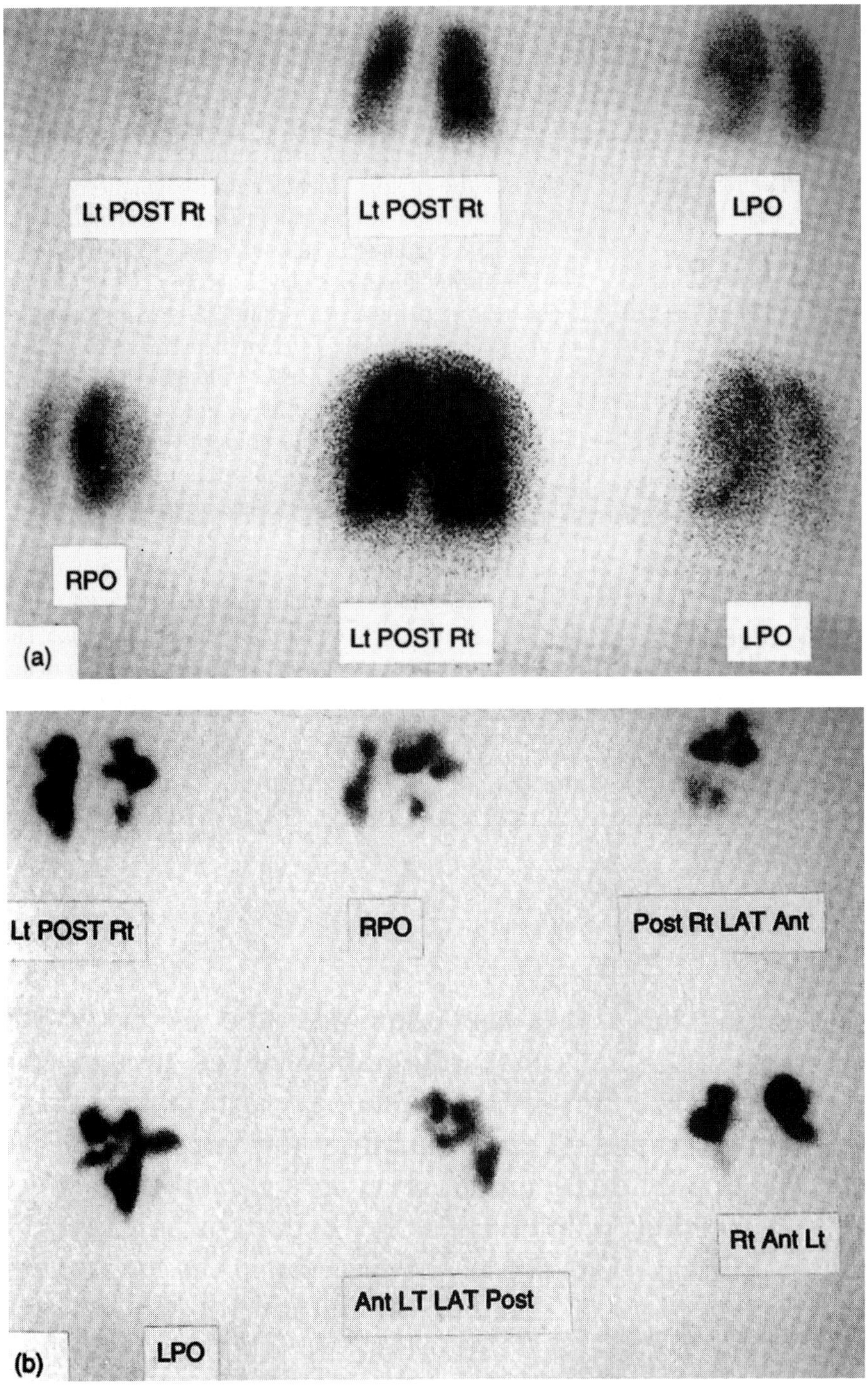

Figure 22.3 *Ventilation and perfusion isotope lung scans showing high probability of pulmonary embolism. (a) Ventilation scan shows normal distribution of the isotope throughout the lungs. (b) Perfusion scan shows multiple segmental defects bilaterally.*

into either of these two clear-cut categories. They require pulmonary angiography or other diagnostic testing because the predictive value of the lung scan results is too low to allow treatment decisions to be made (see Fig. 22.4).[18]

Pulmonary emboli have also been demonstrated by echocardiography (including transesophageal echocardiography), even though echocardiography cannot visualize most of the pulmonary arterial tree. The greatest use of echocardiography is in evaluating the presence of acute cor pulmonale. When PE causes greater than 50% pulmonary arterial obstruction, pulmonary artery hypertension causes distension of the right ventricle. The degree of distension can be quantitated by echocardiography. Since a decrease in outflow obstruction leads to a decrease in right ventricular distension as well, the effectiveness of fibrinolytic agents has been monitored in this fashion.[19]

Computer-assisted tomography has also been employed for the diagnosis of PE. The diagnosis can be quite striking when the CT scan is obtained on an electron beam scanner following the injection of IV contrast material (see Fig. 22.1b). Magnetic resonance imaging can also make the diagnosis of PE in selected patients, but it is neither practical in critically ill patients nor cost-effective.

TREATMENT

Nonspecific supportive measures should be undertaken immediately. The patient may breathe more comfortably if the head of the bed is elevated slightly, although this may exacerbate cerebral hypoperfusion if the patient is in shock. Oxygen should be administered by bi-pronged nasal catheter, face tent or both. In patients who are critically ill, endotracheal intubation and assisted respiration may be required. However, the major cause of hypoxia is lack of perfusion of the pulmonary parenchyma. Oxygen inhalation alone can do little to correct this defect. Pain and apprehension may be minimized by small doses of intravenous narcotics (for example, 2–4 mg morphine sulfate), but large doses of narcotics may cause respiratory depression. An intravenous line should be placed for rapid delivery of medication, but intravenous fluid administration should be restricted because it may exacerbate the elevated right ventricular pressure.

Heparin has been the cornerstone of treatment for PE ever since the classic study by Barritt and Jordan.[8] Adequate anticoagulation stops further progression of thrombosis and is associated with less than 5% recurrence rate of PE in most series. In heparinized patients, emboli typically undergo dissolution over a period of several days as a result of the natural fibrinolytic mechanisms of the body. Pulmonary emboli undergo lysis much more commonly than thrombi in the pelvis or legs. Because of this, adequate anticoagulation usually results in a favorable clinical outcome with respect to the pulmonary circulation. However, incomplete lysis may lead to chronic pulmonary hypertension (see Fig. 22.4).

In treating patients with acute PE, it is important to establish a therapeutic level of heparin as rapidly as possible. Patients with massive PE may require large amounts of heparin to achieve adequate PTT levels (1.5–2.5×/control). An initial bolus of 5000–10 000 units of heparin should be given intravenously, followed by 1000–2000 units/h thereafter, depending on the patient's weight and last PTT result. The necessary daily dose may reach 40 000 units or more.

The patient must be carefully monitored by PTT after the first 48 hours to avoid over-anticoagulation. The initial requirement for high doses of heparin with major PE usually decreases after the first 24–72 hours. Continuing the dose necessary to achieve a therapeutic PTT level initially may result in major bleeding later in the patient's hospital course. On the other hand, worry

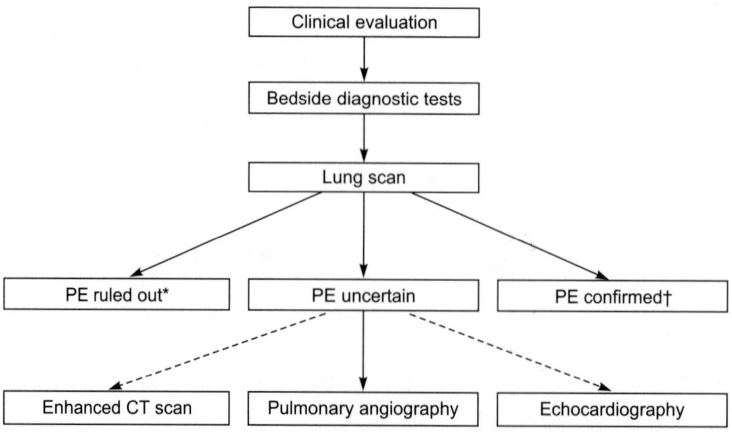

Figure 22.4 *Algorithm for the diagnosis of acute pulmonary embolism. *Normal/low probability lung scan and low clinical probability; †high probability lung scan and high clinical probability.*

about possible over-anticoagulation early in the patient's course may result in failure to achieve a therapeutic level of heparinization, leading to recurrent, and sometimes fatal, PE. It has been demonstrated that 10% of patients with venous thromboembolic disease never achieve a therapeutic level of heparin during the entire course of their hospital treatment.[20] The typical mistake of an inexperienced clinician is to give too little heparin early in the patient's course, when the heparin requirement is high, and too much heparin later, when the heparin requirement is low. Unfortunately, the consequence of such errors may be recurrent PE early in the patient's treatment or major bleeding complications later.

Heparin is usually continued for 7–10 days, during which time the patient is converted to oral anticoagulation, usually with warfarin. The starting dose of warfarin is 10 mg daily for the first 2 days, continued thereafter at the estimated daily maintenance dose for an INR of 2.0–3.0. Oral anticoagulation should be continued for a minimum of 3 months, and sometimes indefinitely, if the patient has ongoing risk factors. Shorter periods of heparin treatment (usually 5 days) have recently been employed successfully for the treatment of DVT, with a corresponding reduction in the length of hospital stay. Shorter periods of heparin treatment for PE may be employed in the future as well.

Fibrinolytic agents have been utilized to increase the rate of lysis of PE, particularly when the patient's life appears to be threatened. Immediate clot lysis may be life saving when the patient may not survive long enough for spontaneous lysis of an embolus to occur. The most rapid clot dissolution has been reported with tissue plasminogen activator (t-PA).[19] Urokinase (UK) has also been used effectively for the lysis of PE (see Fig. 22.2), but a definite advantage has been shown for t-PA (versus UK) in the rate of clot lysis during the first few hours following PE.[19] Both agents have a distinct advantage with respect to the rapidity of clot lysis over heparin treatment alone, as does streptokinase (SK), which was the first thrombolytic agent employed for the lysis of PE and is the least expensive. However, SK is less rapid than t-PA or UK in its rate of lysis and is more likely to be associated with pyrexia.

The following thrombolytic regimens for PE have been approved by the FDA:

- streptokinase: 250 000 units as a loading dose over 30 minutes followed by 100 000 units/h for 24 hours;
- urokinase: 4400 IU/kg as a loading dose over 10 minutes, followed by 4400 IU/kg/h for 12–24 hours (drug not currently available);
- t-PA: 100 mg as a continuous intravenous infusion administered over 2 hours.

None of these regimens employs concomitant heparin therapy because of the increased danger of bleeding. If heparin has been started, it should be stopped. The PTT should be 1.5 times control or less before starting infusion of thrombolytic agents. After lytic therapy, it is important to wait until the PTT is less than 80 seconds before starting or resuming IV heparin infusion.[19]

The most serious complication of lytic agents is intracranial bleeding, which occurs in approximately 1% of patients. Retroperitoneal hemorrhage can also be life threatening. Despite concerns about such major bleeding complications, thrombolysis has been utilized more widely in recent years, particularly since it has been found to be effective for up to 14 days after the onset of PE.[19] Bleeding complications can be minimized by taking a careful neurologic history, by minimizing venipunctures or arterial punctures, and by a careful history designed to identify other potential causes of bleeding. Short infusions of fibrinolytic agents are less apt to be associated with bleeding. They do not require an ICU bed, unless the patient's condition is unstable from the PE itself.

Early fibrinolytic therapy for PE was usually carried out as an emergency procedure as soon as the diagnosis was established, often in the middle of the night. It was associated with a high rate of bleeding complications, despite aggressive laboratory monitoring of hematologic tests; and it was extremely expensive. Current thrombolysis is more apt to be carried out during the usual working day, at any time up to 2 weeks after the onset of symptoms. It can be administered as a brief IV infusion through a peripheral vein, and there are no special laboratory tests required. When the long-term outcome after fibrinolytic therapy of PE is compared with heparin treatment alone, right ventricular function and pulmonary perfusion have been improved. Consequently, the indications for fibrinolytic therapy have been expanded to include patients with PE who are clinically stable. In a randomized controlled trial of 100 patients with PE, there were three non-fatal and two fatal recurrent PEs among patients assigned to heparin alone, compared with none among patients who received t-PA followed by heparin ($P < 0.06$).[21] If these results are confirmed by others, fibrinolysis may become the standard treatment for PE, even in patients who are hemodynamically stable. However, at present, because of the high cost of fibrinolytic agents and the potential risk of bleeding, fibrinolytic agents are indicated primarily in patients with PE who are critically ill.

In patients who do not receive fibrinolytic therapy, placement of an IVC filter should be considered in those who are critically ill. These patients might succumb to a recurrent PE, even if it is relatively small. Indications for IVC filters are covered in more detail in Chapter 16.

When a patient with acute PE appears preterminal, or when fibrinolytic therapy is unavailable, emergency pulmonary embolectomy should be considered. This procedure can be life saving, but is now rarely indicated. Most patients with massive PE either succumb before they can be moved to the operating room (OR), or else they stabilize hemodynamically so that a hazardous emergency operation is no longer indicated. Such patients are often candidates for lytic treatment or insertion of an IVC filter instead. Nevertheless, on infrequent occasions, a patient with massive PE, who would otherwise have died, will survive long enough to undergo successful pulmonary embolectomy (see Fig. 22.5). However, in most critically ill patients who have PE demonstrated by pulmonary angiography, it is more expeditious to start lytic therapy at the time of angiography, rather than to take the patient to the OR for pulmonary embolectomy.

Some patients who survive PE fail to undergo lysis of the embolus and may develop chronic pulmonary hypertension (see Fig. 22.6.). Elective pulmonary embolectomy at a later date has proved helpful for such patients.

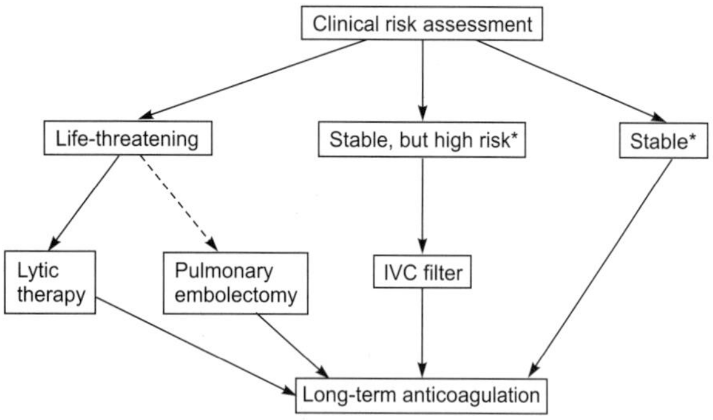

Figure 22.5 *Algorithm for the treatment of acute pulmonary embolism. *Lytic therapy may also be considered.*

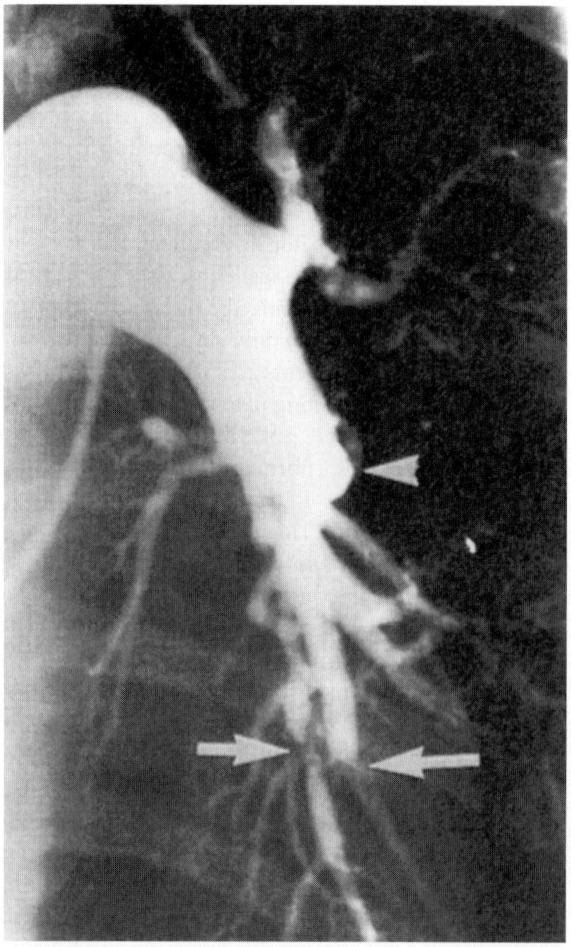

Figure 22.6 *Chronic pulmonary embolism: angiography of the left lung shows multiple sites of arterial stenosis (arrows) and one segmental arterial occlusion (arrowhead).*

SUMMARY

Pulmonary embolism remains a leading cause of death, but its mortality can be reduced by improved medical management. Prevention of PE is particularly important. This can be accomplished both through prophylaxis of patients at high risk and through early diagnosis and appropriate treatment of DVT, which is the precursor of PE. Early diagnosis and treatment of PE can also reduce its mortality.

A high level of clinical suspicion for PE should be maintained in patients with recognized risk factors for DVT. When signs and symptoms of PE are observed, especially sudden and unexplained dyspnea or chest pain, clinical evaluation is useful in determining the probability of PE and in evaluating the predictive value of diagnostic tests. Bedside diagnostic tests, such as ECG, chest x-ray and arterial blood gases, can often identify other causes for the patient's symptoms or strengthen the clinical suspicion of PE.

Perfusion lung scan is the primary diagnostic procedure for PE. Pulmonary angiography, enhanced CT chest scans and echocardiography are used selectively. Once the diagnosis is established, the cornerstone of treatment is adequate and long-term anticoagulation. Lytic agents have also proved useful, especially in critically ill patients. Their use is increasing, despite worries about bleeding complications and costs. Pulmonary embolectomy is an infrequent, but sometimes life-saving emergency operation for patients near death. Insertion of an IVC filter is indicated in patients who cannot receive adequate anticoagulation, or in whom anticoagulation has failed, or in selected patients at particularly high risk from recurrent PE.

ACKNOWLEDGMENT

The pulmonary angiograms and lung scans were kindly provided by Dr Anthony W Stanson, Department of Diagnostic Radiology, Mayo Clinic, Rochester, Minnesota.

REFERENCES

1. Giuntini C, DiRicco G, Marini C, Melillo E, Palla A. Epidemiology. *Chest* 1995; **107**: 3S–9S.
2. Anderson FA, Jr, Wheeler HB, Goldberg RJ, *et al.* A population-based perspective of the hospital incidence and case-fatality rates of deep vein thrombosis and pulmonary embolism: the Worcester DVT Study. *Arch Intern Med* 1991; **151**: 933–8.
3. Dalen JE, Alpert JS. Natural history of pulmonary embolism. *Prog Cardiovasc Dis* 1975; **17**: 257–70.
4. Graves EJ. National Hospital Discharge Survey: annual summary, 1982 (–1992). In *Vital and Health Statistics.* National Center for Health Statistics.
5. Collins R, Scrimgeour A, Yusuf S, Peto R. Reduction in fatal pulmonary embolism and venous thrombosis by perioperative administration of subcutaneous heparin. Overview of results of randomized trials in general, orthopedic and urologic surgery. *N Engl J Med* 1988; **318**: 1162–73.
6. Prevention of fatal postoperative pulmonary embolism by low doses of heparin. An international multicentre trial. *Lancet* 1975; **2**: 45–51.
7. Bergqvist D, Lindbald B. A 30-year survey of pulmonary embolism verified at autopsy: an analysis of 1274 surgical patients. *Br J Surg* 1985; **72**: 105–8.
8. Barritt DW, Jordan SC. Anticoagulant drugs in the treatment of pulmonary embolism. A controlled trial. *Lancet* 1960; **1**: 1309–12.
9. Sevitt S, Gallagher NG. Prevention of venous thrombosis and pulmonary embolism in injured patients: a trial of anticoagulant prophylaxis with phenindione in middle-aged and elderly patients with fractured necks of femurs. *Lancet* 1959; **2**: 981–9.
10. Goldhaber SZ, Hennekens CH, Evans DA, Newton EC, Godleski JJ. Factors associated with an antemortem diagnosis of major pulmonary embolism. *Am J Med* 1982; **73**: 822–6.
11. Manganelli D, Palla A, Donnamaria V, Giuntini C. Clinical features of pulmonary embolism: doubts and certainties. *Chest* 1995; **107**: 25S–32S.
12. Bergqvist D. *Postoperative Thromboembolism.* New York: Springer, 1983.
13. Browse NL, Thomas ML. Source of nonlethal pulmonary emboli. *Lancet* 1974; **1**: 258–9.
14. Wheeler HB, Hirsh J, Wells P, Anderson FA, Jr. Diagnostic tests for deep vein thrombosis: clinical usefulness depends on probability of disease. *Arch Intern Med* 1994; **154**: 1921–8.
15. Gallus A, Salzman EW, Hirsh J, Marder VJ. Prevention of venous thrombosis. In Colman RW, Hirsh J, Marder VJ, Salzman EW, eds. *Hemostasis and Thrombosis.* Philadelphia: Lippincott, 1994: 1331–45.
16. Hull RD, Raskob GE, Coates G, Panju AA, Gill GJ. A new noninvasive management strategy for patients with suspected pulmonary embolism. *Arch Intern Med* 1989; **149**: 2549–55.
17. Dalen JE. When can treatment be withheld in patients with suspected pulmonary embolism? *Arch Intern Med* 1993; **153**: 1415–18.
18. PIOPED Investigators. Value of the ventilation/perfusion scan in acute pulmonary embolism. Results of the prospective investigation of pulmonary embolism diagnosis (PIOPED). *J Am Med Assoc* 1990; **263**: 2753–9.
19. Goldhaber SZ. Contemporary pulmonary embolism thrombolysis. *Chest* 1995; **107**: 45S–51S.
20. Wheeler AP, Jaquiss RD, Newman JH. Physician practices in the treatment of pulmonary embolism and deep vein thrombosis. *Arch Intern Med* 1988; **148**: 1321–5.
21. Goldhaber SZ, Haire WD, Feldstein ML. Alteplase versus heparin in acute pulmonary embolism: randomized trial assessing right-ventricular function and pulmonary perfusion. *Lancet* 1993; **341**: 507–11.

23

Current recommendations for prevention of deep venous thrombosis

JOHN A HEIT

Venous thromboembolism (VTE) is a major health problem, with at least 201 000 first-lifetime cases per year in the USA.[1,2] Of these patients, 25% die within 7 days of venous thromboembolism onset, and for 20%, death is so rapid that there is insufficient time for intervention.[3] Observed survival after either deep vein thrombosis (DVT) or pulmonary embolism (PE) is significantly less than expected (Fig. 23.1). Moreover, after controlling for other co-morbid diseases, survival after PE is significantly reduced for up to 3 months compared with survival after DVT alone.[3] Consequently, prevention of VTE is essential in order to improve survival. However, despite improved prophylaxis regimens,[4] the incidence of VTE has been relatively constant at about 1 per 1000 since 1979 (Fig. 23.2).[2] The failure to reduce the incidence of VTE may be due to several factors, including an increased number of persons at risk, failure to recognize persons at risk, and failure to modify risk factors or provide prophylaxis.[5,6]

The aims of this chapter are to outline the risk factors for VTE among hospitalized patients, review the efficacy and safety of alternative prophylaxis regimens, and provide recommendations regarding the most suitable prophylaxis regimens based on the estimated risk. The primary goal of VTE prophylaxis is to prevent fatal PE. It is important to appreciate the relationship between DVT

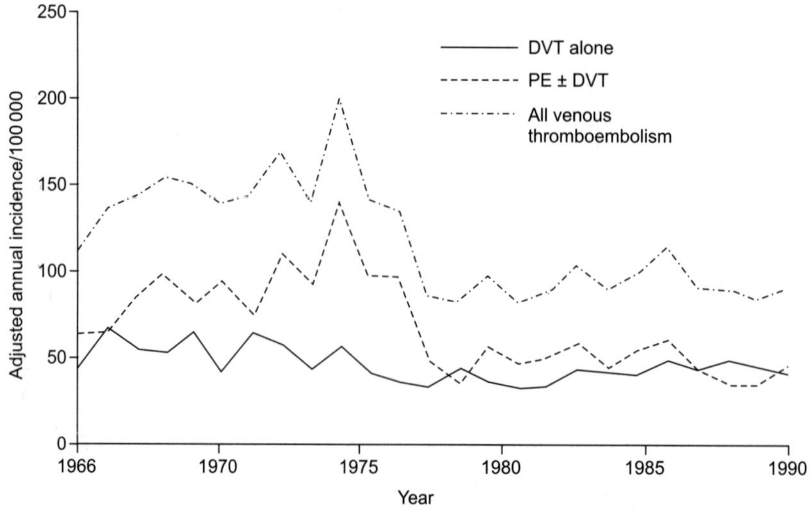

Figure 23.1 *Annual incidence of venous thromboembolism among Olmsted County, Minnesota residents, 1966–90, by age and gender.*

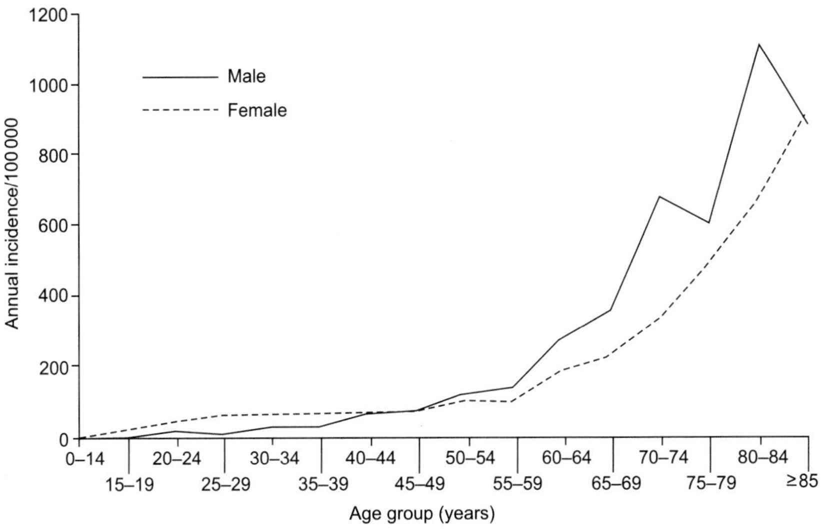

Figure 23.2 *Age- and sex-adjusted annual incidence of all venous thromboembolism, deep vein thrombosis (DVT) alone, and pulmonary embolism with or without deep vein thrombosis (PE ± DVT) among Olmsted County, Minnesota residents, by calendar year, 1966–90.*

and PE. Pulmonary embolism is a frequent and often silent complication of venous thromboembolism. At least 50% of patients with symptomatic proximal (popliteal or iliofemoral) DVT have asymptomatic PE. Factors which determine whether a PE becomes symptomatic include the size and location of the embolus, and the patient's underlying cardiopulmonary reserve. Healthy patients are more likely to tolerate a relatively large embolus whereas patients with chronic cardiopulmonary disease may become significantly hypoxemic or hypotensive with even small emboli. Typically, thrombi arise in the calf veins and propagate proximally to the deep veins of the thigh. Because thrombi within the proximal leg deep veins are larger, proximal DVT is associated with symptomatic PE more often than are isolated calf thrombi. However, isolated calf vein thrombi not only can embolize but, depending on the factors listed above, can lead to clinically significant PE. To achieve the goal of fatal PE prevention, prophylaxis regimens should maximize the risk reduction for total DVT (isolated calf DVT as well as proximal DVT).

RISK FACTORS FOR VENOUS THROMBOEMBOLISM

Several patient characteristics have been identified as independent risk factors for VTE. Increasing age is a major risk factor; VTE incidence increases markedly with age for both men and women (Fig. 23.3).[1,2] Pulmonary embolism accounts for an increasing proportion of VTE with increasing age for both genders (Fig. 23.4), which has important implications for the future. As the average US population age increases, VTE mortality is likely to increase because of the significantly worse survival after PE. Venous thromboembolism incidence also varies by ethnic ancestry; the incidence is highest among Caucasian- and African-Americans, intermediate among Hispanic-Americans, and lowest among Asian-Americans, whilst the incidence among native-Americans is unknown.[7] Other important and independent risk factors for VTE include surgery, trauma, hospital or nursing home confinement, malig-

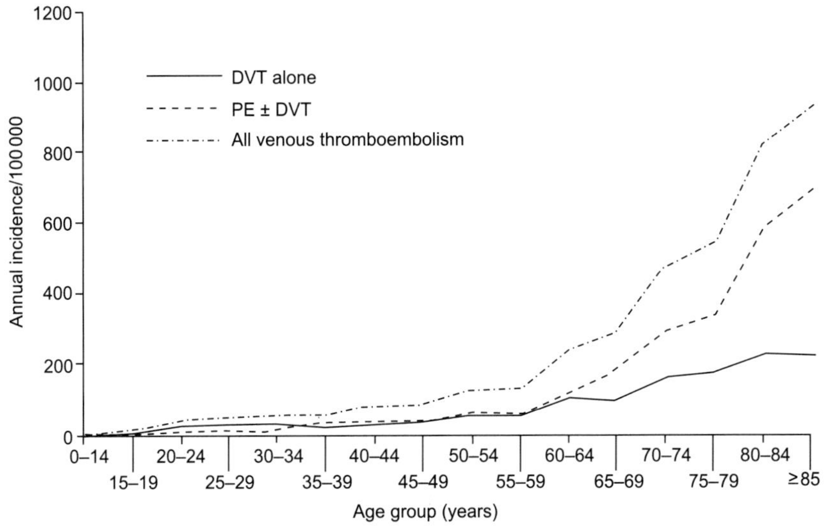

Figure 23.3 *Annual incidence of all venous thromboembolism, deep vein thrombosis (DVT) alone, and pulmonary embolism with or without deep vein thrombosis (PE ± DVT) among Olmsted County, Minnesota residents, 1966–90, by age.*

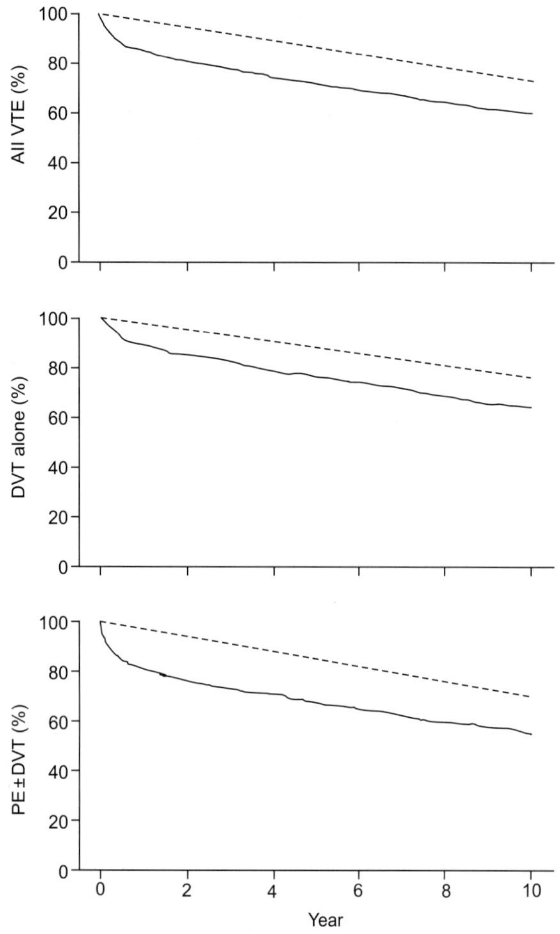

Figure 23.4 *Observed survival (3/4) after all venous thromboembolism (VTE), deep vein thrombosis (DVT) alone, and pulmonary embolism with or without deep vein thrombosis (PE ± DVT), conditional upon surviving for 7 days, among Olmsted County residents with first lifetime venous thromboembolism during the study period, 1966–90, compared to expected survival (- - -) based on Minnesota Caucasians of like age and gender.*

Table 23.1 *Clinical risk factors for venous thromboembolism*

General risk factors
Increasing age
Trauma
Surgery
Leg immobilization or paralysis
Central venous catheter or transvenous pacemaker
Hospital or nursing home confinement
Prior superficial vein thrombosis
Varicose veins
Acquired or secondary thrombophilia
Malignancy
Myeloproliferative disorders
Heparin-induced thrombocytopenia
Nephrotic syndrome
Disseminated intravascular coagulation (DIC)
Oral contraceptives and estrogen therapy
Lupus anticoagulant/anticardiolipin antibody
Pregnancy/postpartum state
Paroxysmal nocturnal hemoglobinuria
Anticancer drugs
Inflammatory bowel disease
Thromboangiitis obliterans (Buerger's disease)
Behçet's syndrome
Primary or familial thrombophilia
Antithrombin III deficiency
Protein C deficiency
Protein S deficiency
Activated protein C resistance
Factor V R506Q (Leiden) mutation
Prothrombin 20210G→A mutation
Dysfibrinogenemia
Hypoplasminogenemia
Hyperhomocystinemia

nancy (with and without concurrent chemotherapy), prior central vein catheterization or transvenous pacemaker (for upper extremity deep vein thrombosis), prior superficial vein thrombosis, varicose veins, and neurologic disease with extremity paresis.[8] Serious liver disease is associated with a significantly reduced risk of VTE, while the risk associated with varicose veins varies with age; the risk is highest among younger patients and diminishes with age. Among women, pregnancy and the puerperium, oral contraceptive use and estrogen replacement therapy, are additional important risk factors. Table 23.1 lists the general risk factors for VTE as well as acquired and familial disorders associated with thrombosis (thrombophilia). In general, these risk factors are additive; the risk of VTE is compounded by an increasing number of concurrent risk factors. Patients with acquired or familial thrombophilia who have additional general risk factors (such as surgery, trauma, or immobilization) are at particularly high risk. Acute myocardial infarction and congestive heart failure patients (especially with concurrent atrial fibrillation, cardiac chamber enlargement, or reduced ejection fraction) are at risk for intracardiac thrombi and systemic embolization in addition to VTE.[9] In the absence of other contraindications, these patients receive systemic anticoagulation rather than prophylaxis. Patients with central venous catheters frequently develop axillary/subclavian vein thrombosis, which may be associated with PE. Prophylaxis is warranted for patients requiring chronic central venous catheters (e.g. chronic parenteral nutrition or chemotherapy patients). In the absence of prophylaxis, acute stroke or spinal cord injury patients have a 40% DVT prevalence in the paretic lower extremity.

Patients with recent surgery requiring anesthesia have a 22-fold increased risk for VTE.[8] Table 23.2 summarizes the postoperative prevalence of isolated calf DVT, proximal DVT, symptomatic PE, and fatal PE in the absence of prophylaxis[4] and categorizes patients into low, moderate, high, or very high risk based on this VTE

Table 23.2 *Deep vein thrombosis prevalence in the absence of prophylaxis by type of surgery*[4]

Type of surgery	Total DVT prevalence (%)	95% CI
General surgery*	19	17–21
Abdominal/pelvic surgery for malignant disease*	29	25–33
Total hip replacement†	51	47–55
Total knee replacement†	61	52–70
Hip fracture surgery†	48	43–53
Neurosurgery*	24	20–28
Multiple trauma patients†	53	49–57

*As detected by the radiolabeled fibrinogen uptake test.
†As detected by ascending venography.

prevalence. Major surgery on patients of advanced age (>70 years) or patients with previous VTE, malignancy, or paralysis is associated with very high risk. In addition, patients requiring abdominal or pelvic surgery for malignancy or major orthopedic surgery of the leg (total hip or knee replacement surgery, or surgery for hip fracture), and multiple trauma patients also are at very high risk (Table 23.3). Other factors that may affect risk include the type and duration of anesthesia, intra-operative blood loss with associated hypotension, patient body mass index, and the degree and duration of postoperative immobilization.

VENOUS THROMBOEMBOLISM PROPHYLAXIS METHODS AND REGIMENS

Venous thromboembolism prophylaxis may be divided into two general strategies: primary (non-pharmacological or pharmacological) and secondary or 'surveillance' prophylaxis. Surveillance prophylaxis is defined as a strategy of serially screening for asymptomatic DVT, usually with noninvasive diagnostic tests [e.g. impedance plethysmography (IPG) or duplex ultrasonography]; only patients discovered to have DVT are treated. Unfortunately, color duplex ultrasonography and impedance plethysmography are insensitive to asymptomatic DVT (both proximal and isolated calf DVT). Screening for asymptomatic DVT with color duplex ultrasonography at the time of hospital discharge is ineffective in preventing VTE after discharge.[10,11] Consequently, withholding primary prophylaxis in lieu of surveillance prophylaxis with duplex ultrasonography or impedance plethysmography is inadequate.

Non-pharmacological prophylaxis methods

Non-pharmacological prophylaxis methods include elastic compression stockings, intermittent external pneumatic leg compression (IPC), leg elevation, and early patient mobilization. All are useful as either primary prophylaxis or as an adjunct combined with anticoagulant prophylaxis. IPC is especially effective for patients receiving total knee replacement or radical retropubic prostatectomy for prostate cancer. In addition, IPC is an attractive prophylaxis option for multiple trauma patients or medical patients in whom anticoagulant-based prophylaxis is contraindicated due to active bleeding, or surgery in which even minimal bleeding could be catastrophic (i.e. neurosurgery or spinal surgery). The data are insufficient to recommend intermittent pneumatic plantar compression. IPC should be initiated preoperatively if possible, and continued until the patient is fully ambulatory. The utility of IPC is limited by patient intolerance and non-compliance, non-use during periods of physical therapy, and unsuitability for continued home use after hospital discharge.

The postoperative DVT prevalence may be reduced in total hip or knee replacement patients who receive regional (spinal or epidural) rather than general anesthesia.[12] However, due to the very high risk, these patients still warrant primary prophylaxis. Data are insufficient to assess the effect of cemented versus non-cemented prostheses for total hip or knee replacement, or continuous passive motion devices for total knee replacement on postoperative DVT prevalence.

Table 23.3 *Classification of thromboembolism risk by postoperative venous thromboembolism prevalence*[4]

Thromboembolism event	Thromboembolism risk*			
	Low	Moderate	High	Very high
Calf vein thrombosis	2	10–20	20–40	40–80
Proximal leg vein thrombosis	0.4	2–4	4–8	10–20
Symptomatic pulmonary embolism	0.2	1–2	2–4	4–10
Fatal pulmonary embolism	0.002	0.1–0.4	0.4–1.0	1–5

*Examples: low risk – uncomplicated surgery, age = 40, no other clinical risk factors; moderate risk – major surgery, age > 40, no other clinical risk factors; high risk – major surgery, age > 40, additional risk factors or myocardial infarction; very high risk – major surgery, age > 40, previous venous thromboembolism, malignancy, orthopedic surgery of the lower limb, trauma, hip fracture, stroke, or spinal cord injury.

Preoperative prophylactic inferior vena cava (IVC) filter placement should be discouraged since in most cases IPC is an effective alternative with no increase in bleeding risk. IVC filter placement should be reserved for patients with clear indications (i.e. acute pulmonary embolism in the presence of active bleeding or therapeutic anticoagulation). An IVC filter may be suitable prophylaxis for the multiple trauma patient who has leg injuries which preclude use of IPC.

Pharmacological prophylaxis methods

Pharmacological prophylaxis modalities include low-dose unfractionated heparin, adjusted-dose unfractionated heparin, low molecular weight heparin and heparinoids (LMWH), adjusted-dose oral anticoagulants (e.g. warfarin sodium; INR = 2.0–3.0), and 'two-step' warfarin (Table 23.4).[4] Unfractionated heparin is a mixture of glycosaminoglycan molecules with a wide range of molecular weights (average molecular weight = 40 000 Da). Unfractionated heparin catalyzes antithrombin III inhibition of activated procoagulant factors IIa (thrombin), IXa, Xa, XIa and XIIa. Unfractionated heparin is poorly absorbed after subcutaneous injection and binds nonspecifically to endothelial cells and many other non-anticoagulant proteins. These two factors account for the inter-individual variation in the anticoagulant response to the same unfractionated heparin dose. Nevertheless, subcutaneous low-dose (e.g. 'mini-dose', 5000 U) unfractionated heparin prophylaxis is safe and effective prophylaxis for moderate-risk general surgery patients (Table 23.2). For high- and very-high-risk patients, low-dose unfractionated heparin is effective, but provides inadequate risk reduction. In these higher-risk patients, the postoperative increase in 'acute phase reactant' plasma proteins causes an increase in heparin nonspecific binding and a reduction in the heparin effect on the activated partial thromboplastin time (aPTT). Realization of this problem led to the development of the 'adjusted-dose' unfractionated heparin regimen, whereby the postoperative dose of heparin is increased to maintain the aPTT in the upper normal range (Table 23.3). While this regimen has proven very effective in high-risk patients, it has not been adopted widely due to the inconvenience of monitoring and repeated dose adjustment. Low-dose heparin is associated with an increased incidence of postoperative wound hematoma. In addition, there is a small but definite risk of heparin-induced thrombocytopenia and thrombosis (HITT), a potentially devastating thrombotic complication.[13] Consequently, the platelet count should be monitored at least every other day and the heparin stopped if the platelet count decreases by 30–50% of the baseline count.

Low molecular weight heparins are derived from standard unfractionated heparin by enzymatic or chemical depolymerization and have an average molecular weight of 5000–6000 Da. The reduced molecular weight favorably alters the pharmacological characteristics of LMWH such that absorption after subcutaneous injection is virtually complete and nonspecific plasma protein binding is markedly reduced. Consequently, the anticoagulant response after a LMWH subcutaneous injection is predictable and reproducible such that laboratory monitoring and dose adjustment are unnecessary. Low molecular weight heparinoids (e.g. danaparoid sodium) consist of heparan sulfate, dermatan sulfate, and chondroitin sulfate, and have pharmacological characteristics similar to LMWH. Low molecular weight heparins or heparinoids are very effective prophylaxis for high- and very-high-risk surgical patients.[14] Although the mode of action is similar, the pharmacology of available low molecular weight heparins and heparinoids differs sufficiently that the dose of each drug must be individualized. Because no rigorous trials have been performed in which one LMWH was compared to another, one LMWH cannot be recommended over

Table 23.4 *Pharmacological venous thromboembolism prophylaxis regimens*

Modality	Regimen
Adjusted-dose unfractionated heparin	3500 U SC q.8 hours, started 2 h before surgery; after surgery, dose adjusted to maintain the aPTT within the upper normal range
Low molecular weight heparin	
Ardeparin sodium (Normiflo®)	50 anti-Xa IU/kg SC b.i.d., started 12–24 h after surgery
Dalteparin sodium (Fragmin®)	5000 anti-Xa IU SC q.d., started 12 h before surgery
Danaparoid sodium* (Orgaran®)	750 U SC b.i.d., started 2 h before surgery
Enoxaparin sodium (Lovenox®)	30 mg SC b.i.d., started 12–24 h after surgery, or 40 mg SC q.d., started 10–12 h before surgery
Tinzaparin sodium (Innohep®)	75 anti-Xa IU/kg SC q.d., started 12–24 h after surgery
rHirudin (desirudin, Revasc®)	15 mg SC b.i.d., started 30 min before surgery (but after regional anesthesia, if used)

*Heparinoid.

another. In North America, the initial LMWH dose usually is given 12–24 hours after surgery, whilst in Europe a dose is given 10–12 hours before surgery. A recent review comparing preoperative versus post-operatively initiated LMWH concluded that any difference in efficacy was likely to be small,[15] and this has been confirmed in a recent large randomized clinical trial.[16]

At similar antithrombotic doses, LMWH causes less bleeding compared with unfractionated heparin. However, among patients receiving total hip and knee replacement, LMWH causes more bleeding than adjusted-dose warfarin.[17,18] While the incidence of HITT is less frequent with LMWH compared with unfractionated heparin,[13] there is substantial cross-reactivity and HITT patients cannot be switched safely to LMWH. Currently, the LMWH cost per dose is approximately 10-fold greater than unfractionated heparin.

Epidural or spinal hematoma after neuraxial blockade (e.g. spinal or epidural) anesthesia is a rare complication of anticoagulation therapy or prophylaxis.[19,20] A December 1997 FDA Public Health Advisory Committee called attention to safety reports describing 43 US patients who developed epidural or spinal hematoma or bleeding after receiving enoxaparin sodium. Of these patients, 28 underwent emergency decompressive laminectomy and 16 were left with permanent paraplegia.[21] Where reported, 78% of the patients were women and the median age was 78 years (range 28–90). Three patients had a history of either ankylosing spondylitis or vertebral compression fractures.

Nearly 90% of these cases occurred in patients receiving enoxaparin as prophylaxis after surgery, primarily total knee or hip replacement surgery with spinal or epidural anesthesia, epidural analgesia, or attempted analgesia, or spinal surgery. Only two patients had spontaneous spinal hematomas while receiving enoxaparin prophylaxis. Factors suspected of predisposing patients to spinal hematoma included enoxaparin overdose, commencing enoxaparin prior to establishment of hemostasis, use of epidural catheters, use of concurrent medications known to increase bleeding, vertebral column abnormalities, older age and female gender.[19–21] In a review of neuraxial complications associated with concurrent low molecular weight heparin or heparinoid prophylaxis and regional anesthesia or analgesia, the following recommendations were provided for patients receiving an initial low molecular weight dose before surgery:

- regional anesthesia should be avoided in patients with a clinical bleeding disorder or in patients receiving other drugs which potentially may impair hemostasis (e.g. aspirin or non-steroidal anti-inflammatory drugs, platelet inhibitors, or other anticoagulants);
- insertion of the spinal needle should be delayed for 10–12 hours after the initial low molecular weight heparin injection;
- regional anesthesia should be avoided in patients with a hemorrhagic aspirate (e.g. 'bloody tap') during the initial spinal needle placement;
- a single-dose spinal anesthetic is preferred over continuous epidural anesthesia;
- for patients receiving continuous anesthesia, the epidural catheter should be left indwelling overnight and removed the following day; and
- low molecular weight heparin injections should be delayed for at least 2 hours after spinal needle placement or catheter removal.[20]

For patients in whom prophylaxis is started after surgery, the initial low molecular weight heparin injection should be delayed for at least 2 hours after catheter removal. All patients should be monitored carefully and frequently for early signs of cord compression (e.g. progression of lower extremity numbness or weakness, or bowel or bladder dysfunction). For patients in whom spinal hematoma is suspected, diagnostic imaging and definitive surgical therapy must be performed as rapidly as possible in order to avoid permanent paresis.

Oral anticoagulants (e.g. warfarin sodium) inhibit vitamin K-mediated post-translational modification of factors II (prothrombin), VII, IX, X, and proteins C and S. Whilst warfarin rapidly inhibits vitamin K activity, prolongation of the prothrombin time is delayed in proportion to the normal circulating plasma half-lives of the preformed vitamin K-dependent clotting factors. When administered the night before surgery, therapeutic warfarin anticoagulation (INR = 2.0–3.0) is not achieved until the second or third postoperative day.[17] The 'two-step' warfarin regimen was developed to circumvent the delay in warfarin anticoagulant effect and yet avoid the excess bleeding associated with fully therapeutic warfarin anticoagulation during surgery (Table 23.4).[22] This warfarin regimen is effective in high- and very-high-risk surgery patients but has not been adopted widely.

Aspirin probably provides only modest benefit as VTE prophylaxis. Consequently, aspirin is not recommended as primary prophylaxis.

PROPHYLAXIS RECOMMENDATIONS

General surgery[4]

For low-risk general surgery patients (e.g. minor surgery, age 40 years, no other concomitant risk factors), only early ambulation is recommended. For moderate-risk general surgery patients (e.g. major surgery, age = 40 years, no other concomitant risk factors), either elastic compression stockings, low-dose heparin or IPC provide adequate risk reduction. High-risk general surgery patients (e.g. major surgery in patients = 40 years of age who have other concomitant risk factors) warrant elastic

Table 23.5 *Prophylaxis recommendations by indication and level of risk*

Indication	Prophylaxis recommendations
General surgery	
Low risk	Early ambulation
Moderate risk	ES*, IPC†, or low-dose heparin‡ (every 12 h)
High risk	Low-dose heparin (every 8 h) or LMWH¶
Very high risk	Low-dose heparin or LMWH, combined with IPC
Total hip replacement	Warfarin,§ adjusted-dose heparin, LMWH, or desirudin
Total knee replacement	Warfarin, LMWH, or IPC
Hip fracture surgery	Warfarin or LMWH
Neurosurgery	IPC or LMWH
Multiple trauma	IPC or LMWH
Acute spinal cord injury with paralysis	Adjusted-dose heparin, LMWH, or IPC
Stroke with lower extremity paralysis	IPC combined with low-dose heparin, or LMWH
Acute myocardial infarction	Therapeutic heparin; low-dose heparin or IPC for prophylaxis
High-risk general medical patients	Low-dose heparin or LMWH

*Elastic compression leg stockings.
†Intermittent external pneumatic leg compression.
‡Unfractionated heparin, 5000 U SC.
¶Low molecular weight heparin.
§Dose adjusted to provide a target INR = 2.0–3.0.

compression stockings in combination with either low-dose heparin or IPC. In very-high-risk general surgery patients with multiple concomitant risk factors, combined elastic compression stockings, low-dose heparin or LMWH, and IPC may be appropriate. LMWH is effective in the very-high-risk general surgery population.[23]

Vascular surgery

In general, the same general surgery categorizations and prophylaxis recommendations apply to the patient undergoing vascular surgery. However, these patients are unique in that they frequently receive systemic heparin anticoagulation during the course of their surgery. Consequently, preoperative low-dose heparin or intra-operative IPC are unwarranted. Nevertheless, patients undergoing thoracic or thoracoabdominal aortic reconstructions or other complicated vascular surgery (i.e. ruptured aortic aneurysm repair, major vascular amputations, major venous reconstructions) frequently require extended intensive care unit (ICU) support. The mobility of these patients is limited and they often suffer multi-organ system failure. Although there are no vascular surgery-specific data, extrapolation from other ICU patients suggests that the VTE risk is high and warrants prophylaxis. For patients in whom the risk of bleeding is high, IPC combined with elastic compression stockings is an excellent prophylaxis choice. Elastic compression stockings combined with either low-dose heparin or LMWH are appropriate pharmacologic prophylaxis strategies.

Total hip and knee replacement surgery

Meta-analysis has shown that low-dose heparin is effective prophylaxis for total hip replacement surgery; however, the risk reduction is inadequate compared with other prophylaxis methods. Adjusted-dose unfractionated heparin is safe and effective but inconvenient. Two trials have demonstrated the safety and efficacy of 'two-step' warfarin prophylaxis after total hip replacement, and several cohort studies have demonstrated that adjusted-dose warfarin anticoagulation is safe and effective prophylaxis after both total hip or knee replacement surgery. Multiple trials have shown that LMWH is safe and effective prophylaxis after total hip or knee replacement; LMWH is more effective than warfarin but causes more bleeding. Consequently, the choice of LMWH or adjusted-dose warfarin depends on the estimated VTE and bleeding risks. Recombinant hirudin prophylaxis is more effective than LMWH for total hip replacement patients.[24] IPC is the most effective non-pharmacological prophylaxis for total knee replacement patients. IPC may provide a risk reduction that is similar to LMWH.

The optimal duration of prophylaxis following total hip or knee replacement surgery is uncertain. Most trials continued prophylaxis for at least 7–10 days. However, the current duration of postoperative hospitalization is often 4 days or less, which may provide an inadequate duration of prophylaxis. Based on studies in which a venogram was performed about 6 weeks after surgery, the incidence of asymptomatic DVT after hospital discharge is substantial (Table 23.6).[25–28] However, large studies of total hip and total knee replacement patients

Table 23.6 *Deep vein thrombosis (DVT) prevalence as determined by venography*, versus symptomatic DVT or pulmonary embolism (PE) cumulative incidence† after total hip replacement (THR) or total knee replacement (TKR) surgery*

Author	Operation	No.	Prophylaxis type [in-hospital (out-of-hospital)]	Duration of prophylaxis [days (days)]‡	Venographic DVT [*n* (%)] Proximal	Venographic DVT [*n* (%)] Distal	PE [*n* (%)]	Fatal PE [*n* (%)]
Planes[25]*¶	THR	90	LMWH (LMWH)	14 (21)	6 (5.9)	1 (1.2)	0	0
		89	LMWH (placebo)	14 (21)	7 (7.9)	10 (11.4)	0	0
Bergqvist[26]*¶	THR	117	LMWH (LMWH)	11 (19)	8 (7.0)¶	13 (11.0)	0	0
		116	LMWH (placebo)	10 (18)	28 (24.0)	15 (13.0)	2 (2.0)	0
Dahl[27]*¶	THR	114	LMWH-Dextran (LMWH)	7 (28)	10 (8.8)	12 (10.5)	0	0
		104	LMWH-Dextran (placebo)	7 (28)	14 (13.5)	19 (18.3)	3 (2.8)	1 (0.5)
Hull[28]*¶	THR	174	Preop LMWH (LMWH)	6 (29)	5 (3.1)	25 (14.1)		
		171	Postop LMWH (LMWH)	6 (29)	3 (2.0)	35 (20.2)		
		188	Warfarin (placebo)	6 (29)	14 (9.2)	55 (27.5)		
					Symptomatic DVT or PE			
Robinson[10]†	THR	249	Warfarin (none)	9.8 (0)	3 (1.2)			0
	TKR	257	Warfarin (none)	9.8 (0)	2 (0.8)			0
Leclerc[11]†	THR	1142	LMWH (none)	9 (0)	49 (4.3)			0
	TKR	842	LMWH (none)	9 (0)	33 (3.9)			3 (0.4)
Colwell[18]†	THR	1516	LMWH (none)	7.5 (0)	55 (3.6)			2 (0.1)
		1495	Warfarin (none)	7.0 (0)	56 (3.7)			2 (0.1)
					Symptomatic DVT or PE, or all cause death			
Heit[29]†	THR/TKR	607	LMWH (LMWH)	7.3 (41)	9 (1.5)			0
		588	LMWH (placebo)	7.3 (41)	12 (2.0)			0

‡Number of days of in-hospital prophylaxis (number of days of out-of-hospital prophylaxis).
¶For Planes *et al.*,[25] 35-day total DVT prevalence: LMWH (LMWH) = 7.1%, LMWH (placebo) = 19.3%; *P* = 0.018 (proximal DVT, *P* = NS; distal DVT, *P* = 0.006); for Bergqvist *et al.*,[26] 28–29-day total DVT or PE prevalence: LMWH (LMWH) = 18%, LMWH (placebo) = 39%; *P* <0.001 (proximal DVT, *P* <0.001; distal DVT, *P* = NS); for Dahl *et al.*,[27] 35-day total DVT prevalence: LMWH-Dextran (LMWH) = 19.3%, LMWH-Dextran (placebo) = 31.7%; *P* = 0.034; and for Hull *et al.*,[28] 35-day total DVT prevalence: preop LMWH (LMWH) = 17.2%, postop LMWH (LMWH) = 22.2%, warfarin sodium (placebo) =36.7% (total DVT, *P* <0.001 for preop LMWH vs warfarin and *P* = 0.003 for postop LMWH vs warfarin; proximal DVT, *P* = 0.02 for preop LMWH vs warfarin and *P* = 0.007 for postop LMWH vs warfarin).

who received only in-hospital prophylaxis with LMWH or adjusted-dose warfarin found the 3–6-month incidence of symptomatic venous thromboembolism and fatal PE was much lower. This finding suggests that most asymptomatic DVT present at or developing after hospital discharge resolve spontaneously (Table 23.6).[10,11,18] In a recent clinical trial, total hip or total knee replacement patients with no clinical evidence of VTE after 4–10 days of LMWH were randomly allocated to either continued once-daily LMWH or placebo.[29] After a mean 7.3 days of in-hospital LMWH prophylaxis, 1.5% of 607 patients receiving extended out-of-hospital LMWH, and 2.0% of 588 patients receiving placebo, developed symptomatic DVT or PE, or died, during the interval from hospital discharge to 12 weeks after surgery (OR = 0.7, 95% CI: 0.3, 1.7, *P* = 0.5; absolute difference = –0.56 %, 95% CI: –2.22%, 1.10%). Although the possibility of a small difference (as much as 2.2%) in favor of continued outpatient LMWH prophylaxis cannot be excluded, most total hip and total knee replacement patients do not benefit from extending LMWH prophylaxis after hospital discharge. Nevertheless, of all symptomatic DVT and PE occurring within 3–6 months after total hip or total knee replacement surgery, about 45–80% occur after hospital discharge.[11,18,29–31] All patients should receive 4–10 days of LMWH prophylaxis, or 7–10 days of warfarin prophylaxis. Patients with continuing VTE risk factors (e.g. a previous history of VTE, obesity, continued immobilization, bilateral simultaneous total knee replacement) should be considered for extended out-of-hospital prophylaxis with either once-daily LMWH or adjusted-dose warfarin (INR = 2.0–3.0).

Hip fracture surgery

Prophylaxis of hip fracture patients remains a major challenge due to the risk of bleeding associated with recent trauma. The risk of DVT is increased if hospital admission is delayed for more than 2 days after hip fracture.[32] Moreover, the risk of fatal pulmonary embolism is reduced if hip fracture patients are operated within 24 hours of their injury.[33] Either adjusted-dose warfarin or LMWH prophylaxis is recommended and should be administered as soon as the patient is clinically stable. A recent study found a modest (15%) reduction in the risk for all vascular events in hip fracture patients receiving concurrent aspirin (132 mg/day) prophylaxis.[34]

Neurosurgery

IPC, with or without elastic compression stockings, has been the prophylaxis of choice for elective neurosurgery patients since even minimal bleeding could be catastrophic. Low-dose heparin is an acceptable alternative, and for high-risk patients, combination IPC and low-dose heparin appears particularly effective. A recent study found LMWH plus elastic stockings was more effective than elastic stockings alone.[35]

Acute spinal cord injury with leg paralysis

The period of greatest risk for VTE is the first 2 weeks after injury, with symptomatic PE rarely occurring beyond 3 months. Consequently, the prophylaxis duration in the absence of other risk factors should be 3 months from the date of injury. Based on the available evidence, adjusted-dose heparin and LMWH are effective prophylaxis for patients with acute spinal cord injury and paralysis, while low-dose heparin and IPC are inadequate. However, the combination of IPC, elastic compression stockings, and low-dose heparin is effective.

Multiple trauma

Asymptomatic DVT is common in trauma patients (injury severity score >9). Using venography, one study found a high DVT prevalence after lower extremity fractures (69%), spinal cord injury (62%), or isolated injury to the face, chest, or abdomen (50%).[36] In a large clinical trial, LMWH was more effective than low-dose heparin prophylaxis with no difference in major bleeding.[37] By extrapolation from other high-risk populations, IPC is recommended for multiple trauma patients with active bleeding. If IPC is not feasible due to leg trauma, prophylactic IVC filter placement may be appropriate in selected patients who cannot tolerate any of the other three recommended modalities.

Acute stroke with lower extremity paralysis

Low-dose heparin and LMWH are effective as prophylaxis after acute stroke with paresis or paralysis.[4] IPC combined with low-dose heparin is more effective prophylaxis than low-dose heparin alone.[38] In the patient with stroke associated with cerebral hemorrhage in whom anticoagulation is contraindicated, IPC is an appropriate alternative.

Other medical conditions

Low-dose heparin is safe and effective prophylaxis for hospitalized patients with other general medical conditions (Table 23.1). For bleeding patients, IPC would be expected to provide similar prophylaxis efficacy. A recent clinical trial found LMWH to be more effective than placebo among hospitalized patients with acute medical illnesses.[39] Whether LMWH is more effective than low-dose heparin is unknown. Extrapolating from other clinical trial data, combination prophylaxis with IPC, elastic compression stockings, and low-dose heparin, or LMWH prophylaxis is appropriate for patients with multiple concomitant risk factors.

CONCLUSION

Recognition of the patient at risk and delivery of appropriate prophylaxis is imperative in order to reduce the incidence of VTE (including fatal PE) in hospitalized patients. This chapter provides estimates of risk and a summary of effective prophylaxis methods such that physicians can tailor an individual patient's prophylaxis regimen to maximize DVT risk reduction in the safest and most cost-effective manner.

REFERENCES

1. Anderson F, Wheeler H, Goldberg R, *et al.* A population-based perspective of the hospital incidence and case-fatality rates of deep vein thrombosis and pulmonary embolism. *Arch Intern Med* 1991; **151**: 933–8.
2. Silverstein MD, Heit JA, Mohr DN, Petterson TM, O'Fallon WM, Melton LJ III. Trends in the incidence of deep vein thrombosis and pulmonary embolism: a 25-year population-based study. *Arch Intern Med* 1998; **158**: 585–93.
3. Heit JA, Silverstein MD, Mohr DN, Petterson TM, O'Fallon WM, Melton LJ III. Predictors of survival after deep vein thrombosis and pulmonary embolism. *Arch Intern Med* 1999; **159**: 445–53.
4. Clagett GP, Anderson FA Jr, Geerts W, *et al.* Prevention of venous thromboembolism. *Chest* 1998; **114**: 531S–60S.
5. Anderson F, Wheeler H, Goldberg R, *et al.* Physician practices in the prevention of venous thromboembolism. *Ann Intern Med* 1991; **115**: 591–5.
6. Bratzler DW, Raskob GE, Murray CK, Bumpus LJ, Piatt DS. Underuse of venous thromboembolism prophylaxis for general surgery patients: physician practices in the community hospital setting. *Arch Intern Med* 1998; **158**(17): 1909–12.

7. White RH, Zhou H, Romano PS. Incidence of idiopathic deep venous thrombosis and secondary thromboembolism among ethnic groups in California. *Ann Intern Med* 1998; **128**: 737–40.
8. Heit JA, Silverstein MD, Mohr DN, Petterson TM, O'Fallon WM, Melton LJ III. Risk factors for deep vein thrombosis and pulmonary embolism: a population-based case-control study. *Arch Intern Med* 2000; **160**: 809–15.
9. Cairns J, Théroux P, Lewis HD Jr, Ezekowitz M, Meade TW, Sutton GC. Antithrombotic agents in coronary disease. *Chest* 1998; **114**: 611S–33S.
10. Robinson KS, Anderson DR, Gross M, *et al.* Ultrasonographic screening before hospital discharge for deep venous thrombosis after arthroplasty: the Post-Arthroplasty Screening Study. *Ann Intern Med* 1997; **127**: 439–45.
11. Leclerc JR, Gent M, Hirsh J, Geerts WH, Ginsberg JS, Members of the Canadian Collaborative Group. The incidence of symptomatic venous thromboembolism during and after prophylaxis with enoxaparin: a multi-institutional cohort study in patients who underwent hip or knee arthroplasty. *Arch Intern Med* 1998; **158**: 873–8.
12. Prins M, Hirsh J. A comparison of general anesthesia and regional anesthesia as a risk factor for deep vein thrombosis following hip surgery: a critical review. *Thromb Haemost* 1990; **64**: 497–500.
13. Warkentin T, Levine M, Hirsh J, *et al.* Heparin-induced thrombocytopenia in patients treated with low-molecular-weight heparin or unfractionated heparin. *N Engl J Med* 1995; **332**: 1330–5.
14. Green D, Hirsh J, Heit J, *et al.* Low molecular weight heparin: a critical analysis of clinical trials. *Pharmacol Rev* 1994; **46**: 89–109.
15. Kearon C, Hirsh J. Starting prophylaxis for venous thromboembolism postoperatively. *Arch Intern Med* 1995; **155**: 366–72.
16. Pineo GF, Hull RD, for the NAFT Investigators. A comparison of pre-operative dalteparin with post-operative dalteparin and with warfarin sodium for prophylaxis against deep vein thrombosis after total hip replacement during the acute hospital stay. *Thromb Haemost* 1999; **abstr 1194**: 376.
17. Francis CW, Pellegrini VD Jr, Totterman S, *et al.* Prevention of deep-vein thrombosis after total hip arthroplasty. Comparison of warfarin and dalteparin. *J Bone Joint Surg* 1997; **79A**: 1365–72.
18. Colwell CW, Collins DK, Paulson R, *et al.* Comparison of enoxaparin and warfarin for the prevention of venous thromboembolic disease after total hip arthroplasty. *J Bone Joint Surg* 1999; **81A**: 932–40.
19. Vandermeulen EP, Van Asken H, Vermylen J. Anticoagulants and spinal-epidural anesthesia. *Anesth Analg* 1994; **79**: 1165–77.
20. Horlocker T, Heit JA. Low molecular weight heparin: biochemistry, pharmacology, perioperative prophylaxis regimens, and guidelines for regional anesthetic management. *Anesth Analg* 1997; **85**: 874–85.
21. Wysowski DK, Talarico L, Bacsanyi J, Botstein P. Spinal and epidural hematoma and low-molecular-weight heparin. *N Engl J Med* 1998; **338**: 1774–5.
22. Francis CW, Pellegrini VD, Marder VJ, *et al.* Comparison of warfarin and external pneumatic compression in prevention of venous thrombosis after total hip replacement. *J Am Med Assoc* 1992; **267**: 2911–15.
23. ENOXACAN Study Group. Efficacy and safety of enoxaparin versus unfractionated heparin for prevention of deep vein thrombosis in elective cancer surgery: a double-blind randomized multicentre trial with venographic assessment. *Br J Surg* 1997; **84**: 1099–103.
24. Eriksson BI, Wille-Jørgensen P, Kälebo P, *et al.* A comparison of recombinant hirudin with a low-molecular-weight heparin to prevent thromboembolic complications after total hip replacement. *N Engl J Med* 1997; **337**: 1329–35.
25. Planes A, Vochelle N, Darmon J-Y, Fagolla M, Bellaud M, Huet Y. Risk of deep-venous thrombosis after hospital discharge in patients having undergone total hip replacement: double-blind randomized comparison of enoxaparin and placebo. *Lancet* 1996; **348**: 28–31.
26. Bergqvist D, Benoni G, Björgell O, *et al.* Low-molecular-weight heparin (enoxaparin) as prophylaxis against venous thromboembolism after total hip replacement. *N Engl J Med* 1996; **335**: 696–700.
27. Dahl OE, Andreassen G, Aspelin T, *et al.* Prolonged thromboprophylaxis following hip replacement surgery-results of a double-blind, prospective, randomized, placebo-controlled study with dalteparin (Fragmin). *Thromb Haemost* 1997; **77**: 26–31.
28. Hull RD, Pineo GR, for the NAFT Investigators. A double blind, randomized comparison of extended out-of-hospital prophylaxis using dalteparin versus placebo in patients undergoing elective hip replacement. *Thromb Haemost* 1999; **abstr 17**: 6.
29. Heit JA, Elliott CG, Trowbridge AA, Morrey BF, Gent M, Hirsh J for the Ardeparin Arthroplasty Study Group. The need for extended out-of-hospital prophylaxis against venous thromboembolism after hip or knee replacement. A randomized, double-blind, placebo-controlled trial. *Ann Intern Med* 2000; **132**: 853–61.
30. Warwick D, Williams MH, Bannister GC. Death and thromboembolic disease after total hip replacement. *J Bone Joint Surg* 1995; **77B**: 6–10.
31. White RH, Romano PS, Zhou H, Rodrigo J, Bargar W. Incidence and time course of thromboembolic outcomes following total hip or knee arthroplasty. *Arch Intern Med* 1998; **158**(14): 1525–31.
32. Hefley WF Jr, Nelson CL, Puskarich-May CL. Effect of delayed admission to the hospital on the preoperative prevalence of deep-vein thrombosis associated with fractures about the hip. *J Bone Joint Surg* 1996; **78A**: 581–3.
33. Perez JV, Warwick DJ, Case CP, Bannister GC. Death after proximal femoral fracture – an autopsy study. *Injury* 1995; **26**: 237–40.

34. Prentice CRM, Collins R, Rodgers A, MacMahon S, for the PEP trial investigators. The Pulmonary Embolism Prevention (PEP) Trial: effects of low-dose aspirin on major vascular events in patients with hip fracture. *Thromb Haemost* 1999; **abstr 608**: 193.
35. Agnelli G, Piovella F, Buoncristiani P, *et al.* Enoxaparin plus compression stockings compared with compression stockings alone in the prevention of venous thromboembolism after elective neurosurgery. *N Engl J Med* 1998; **339**: 80–5.
36. Geerts WH, Code KI, Jay RM, *et al.* A prospective study of venous thromboembolism after major trauma. *N Engl J Med* 1994; **331**: 1601–6.
37. Geerts WH, Jam RM, Code KI, *et al.* A comparison of low-dose heparin with low-molecular-weight heparin as prophylaxis against venous thromboembolism after major trauma. *N Engl J Med* 1996; **335**: 701–7.
38. Kamran SI, Downey D, Ruff RL. Pneumatic sequential compression reduces the risk of deep vein thrombosis in stroke patients. *Neurology* 1998; **50**: 1683–8.
39. Samama MM, Cohen AT, Darmon J-Y, *et al.* A comparison of enoxaparin with placebo for the prevention of venous thromboembolism in acutely ill medical patients. *N Engl J Med* 1999; **341**: 793–800.

24

Indications and techniques of inferior vena cava interruption

LAZAR J GREENFIELD AND MARY C PROCTOR

John Hunter introduced one of the earliest techniques for prevention of pulmonary embolism (PE) when he ligated the femoral vein at the level of the thrombus. Later Homans addressed the problem by ligating both femoral veins. When these techniques failed to prevent recurrent PE, vena caval interruption was performed which involved a laparotomy under general anesthesia. These procedures added significant morbidity from lower extremity edema, stasis ulceration and the post-thrombotic syndrome. In addition, collateral vessels opened, allowing recurrent PE in up to 15% of patients, thus negating the purpose of the procedure. Mortality following ligation was unacceptably high, ranging from 4% in low-risk patients to 39% in patients with significant cardiac disease.[1]

Suture or staple grids and external caval clips were used in an effort to provide channels for blood flow while preventing PE. These procedures also required laparotomy and general anesthesia. Whilst a clipping procedure was simpler than ligation or plication, it still presented a major risk from general anesthesia. More significantly, the final outcome of all these procedures was often the same; lower extremity stasis sequelae and recurrent PE. Rarely, vena caval clips are applied in patients already undergoing an abdominal procedure but ligation and plication are purely of historical interest.

In the late 1960s, methods were developed that allowed caval interruption devices to be placed directly into the vena cava through the femoral or jugular vein. These procedures were conducted under local anesthesia and required only a small surgical incision. More recently, filters are placed percutaneously. Over the last 30 years, intracaval devices have undergone significant improvement with respect to efficacy, patency and ease of insertion and are widely used as both treatment and prophylaxis of thromboembolic disease.

COMMON INDICATIONS

Six indications have frequently been used as guidelines when selecting patients for caval interruption. These are described below. Table 24.1 demonstrates the changes in the percentage of placements for each indication over the past 22 years. The most recent review demonstrates an increase in prophylactic placement.

Contraindication to anticoagulation

The most frequently cited reason for selecting caval interruption versus anticoagulation is the presence of a

Table 24.1 *Indications for placement of Greenfield vena caval filters: a summary of 642 placements over a 27-year period*

Indication	Year of publication					
	1977	1981	1984	1988	1993	1999
Contraindication	23*	30	35	38	45	39
Complication	16	16	18	17	16	14
Failure	38	30	31	27	20	10
Embolectomy	8	10	9	8	5	2
Prophylaxis	11	17	18	17	13	32
Other	4	0	1	2	1	<1

* Percent of placements.

contraindication to anticoagulation. Hull and Raskob separated these contraindications into absolute and relative groups.[2] There is no consensus as to what comprises each category and further study is warranted. Serious active bleeding, recent spinal cord injury, hemorrhage, stroke and recent operation or trauma are important contraindications. Advanced age, malignancy and pregnancy have also been offered as relative contraindications but remain controversial. Many contraindications are reversed over time, allowing anticoagulation to be started at a later time. Relative contraindications may become more commonly accepted by some if temporary filters are approved for use by the FDA.

Complications of anticoagulation

Patients who suffer a complication while being treated with anticoagulants are also candidates for caval interruption. The major complication associated with anticoagulation is bleeding. Five to 10% of patients treated with intravenous heparin will develop a bleeding complication during the duration of therapy. The severity of bleeding is variable. The risk of bleeding while on heparin appears to be dose dependent and varies with the patient's inherent risk, i.e. prior surgery or trauma, predisposing clinical factors or underlying hemostatic conditions.[3,4]

In addition to bleeding complications, heparin-induced thrombocytopenia develops in 1.1–2.9% of patients.[5] Should this occur, all heparin must be discontinued, even that used for flushing lines and catheters as the condition responds to cessation of therapy. Rarely, patients may develop a sensitivity to heparin with development of a cutaneous rash or anaphylaxis. Osteoporosis has also been found in a small number of patients and may develop when heparin is used during pregnancy.[6]

Bleeding may also occur in up to 10% of patients treated with warfarin. The degree of bleeding is most often associated with the inactivation of the clotting cascade as indicated by the international normalized ratio (INR). Patients with significantly elevated INRs are more likely to develop major hemorrhagic complications than those with mildly elevated levels.[7] Routine monitoring and dietary counseling will help to prevent such complications. Monitoring should also be undertaken when there has been a change in concomitant medications. Several drugs have either a synergistic or antagonistic interaction with warfarin resulting in decreased efficacy or increased risk of adverse events.

In addition to bleeding complications, a small number of patients develop warfarin-associated skin necrosis which usually is seen early and in the absence of adequate heparinization. It is most likely to occur in areas of increased subcutaneous fat and may also be associated with the 'blue toe' syndrome. Should this develop, the drug must be discontinued.[8]

Failure of anticoagulation

Failure of anticoagulation to prevent recurrent thromboembolic events is another indication for filter placement. Prior to determining that anticoagulation has failed, it should be established that the patient was adequately anticoagulated. Many times, failures of anticoagulation are failures to reach therapeutic drug levels. The patient who develops recurrence or extension of thromboembolism while anticoagulated may, in fact, not be adequately anticoagulated. In order to reduce this risk, patients should be monitored closely during the initiation of therapy with heparin to assure they are therapeutic within the first 24 hours. Nomograms have been developed to ensure that this takes place.[9,10]

Pulmonary embolectomy

Patients who suffer massive PE and become hemodynamically unstable may benefit from an open or transvenous catheter pulmonary embolectomy. While this procedure significantly improves the patients' clinical situation, they remain at risk for recurrent pulmonary embolism. Two of the earliest patients who underwent a catheter pulmonary embolectomy died of recurrent PE prior to being able to undergo caval interruption. These deaths provided the impetus for development of the original Greenfield stainless steel filter that could be inserted transvenously at the completion of the embolectomy (Fig. 24.1). From that time, vena caval filters have been placed following embolectomy, resulting in a reduced incidence of postoperative mortality from PE.[11]

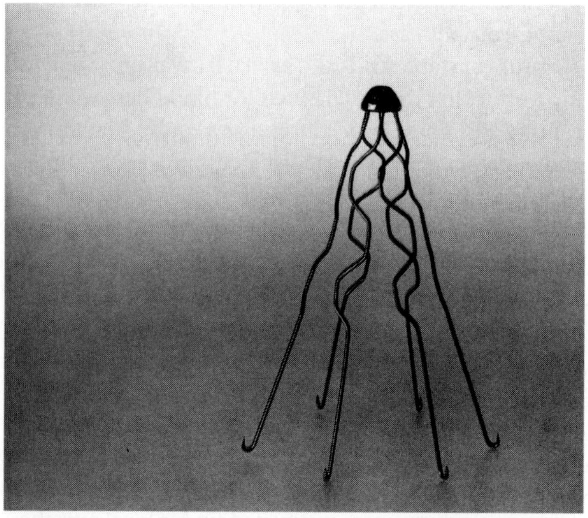

Figure 24.1 *The original stainless steel Greenfield filter first used in 1972. (Used with permission from Rutherford RB, ed.* Vascular Surgery, *4th edition, WB Saunders Company, 1995)*

Prophylaxis

The use of filters for prophylaxis of PE represents the fastest growing indication for placement. This is especially true since the introduction of the reduced profile percutaneous filters, which can be placed without operative intervention, lowering both the risk to the patient and the cost of the procedure.

Vena caval filters are being used prophylactically in patients at high risk of thromboembolism who are scheduled for major elective orthopedic surgical procedures.[12,13] Some physicians believe that the risk of placing the filter is significantly less than the risk of developing deep venous thrombosis (DVT) and having to undergo anticoagulant therapy. Other orthopedic surgeons are electing to place filters in postoperative patients who develop DVT rather than anticoagulate them because the risk of a bleeding complication while on heparin is high and a significant bleed may jeopardize the new joint.[13,14] These practices present a major departure from the earlier 'prophylactic' indication.

Patients who sustain major trauma, including long bone or pelvic fractures, major venous injuries, or head and spinal cord injuries, have an excessive risk of thromboembolism as a result of the injury.[15,16] In addition, other iatrogenic factors or underlying medical conditions can increase this risk. In many cases, the need for emergency surgery or the suspicion of major organ injury precludes the use of anticoagulation. In these instances, many trauma surgeons have recommended the use of a vena caval filter.[17–19] In a retrospective cohort study, Rodriguez *et al.* demonstrated a significant risk reduction in PE and PE-related mortality when filters were placed prophylactically as compared with comparable patients treated with standard methods of prophylaxis (OR = 8.27; 95% CI = 1.4–48.8).[20] These retrospective findings need to be evaluated in a large randomized clinical trial. Rogers *et al.* have published long-term follow-up of these patients and found no significant adverse events.[21]

In a more traditional context, a prophylactic indication referred to patients with an underlying cardiac or pulmonary condition such as congestive heart failure, chronic obstructive pulmonary disease and pulmonary hypertension. The purpose of the filter is to provide additional protection from potentially fatal embolism, in addition to the use of standard anticoagulation.

The prophylactic use of a Greenfield vena caval filter in patients with malignancy has generated controversy and it is difficult to reach conclusions based upon the literature. Some investigators have suggested that placing a filter as the primary method of prophylaxis is the most effective method of treating these patients.[22] Retrospective reviews such as by Ihnat support a conservative use of filters which apply the same indications as used with other patients.[23] Other prospective studies have demonstrated that the life span following filter placement is too short to justify its placement. The significant factors that need to be evaluated are the issues of quality of life and the cost/effectiveness of the filter in these situations.[24]

Recurrent PE

Recurrent PE is a standard indication for filter placement[25] which is used both in situations where the patient has a vena caval device in place that failed and when no device had been used. The risk from further embolism is considered sufficient to warrant filter placement.

Table 24.1 compares the indications as identified in the major reports of patient outcomes published over the 27 year history of the Greenfield filter.

TECHNIQUES

In the late 1960s, the Mobin-Uddin umbrella was introduced and became widely used because of its efficacy and ease of placement. Whilst it effectively prevented pulmonary embolism, it did so at the expense of caval patency.[26] The incidence of occlusion was reported to be as high as 65%. In addition, there were significant problems with migration of the device into the right heart or pulmonary artery. As a result, it was later withdrawn from the market. The Greenfield filter was first used in 1972 to provide protection against PE. As a result of its unique cone geometry, the long-term patency rate has been above 95% over the past 27 years.[27] Mathematical modeling and *in vitro* studies have proved that the unique design allows up to 70% of the cone volume to be filled with thrombus before significant reductions in blood flow occur. The original 24F stainless steel filter was developed for operative insertion via a femoral or jugular venotomy under local anesthesia. The operative procedure was preceded by a venacavogram to determine the shape and size of the vena cava to rule out caval anomalies and to allow identification of the appropriate site for placement. This required both a radiological and surgical procedure for each case resulting in two separate charges.

Using the Seldinger technique for access to the vascular system, interventional radiologists attempted percutaneous placement of the original 24F filter through a sheath in the femoral vein. Whilst filters were able to be placed successfully in the majority of cases, there was a high rate of insertion-site thrombosis secondary to the large 28F access sheath. Pais reported the incidence to be over 30%; however, Dorfman found a much lower incidence.[28] The procedures required a large puncture site with a high risk of bleeding complications. As a result, devices with smaller delivery systems were developed. These devices are reviewed later. In addition to a reduction in the size of the delivery system, these devices no longer required surgical insertion and could be placed percutaneously in the radiology suite at the time of venacavography, thus eliminating the need for surgical intervention. By eliminating the need for the surgeon and the surgical suite, the cost of the procedure could be reduced. With the new-found ease of insertion and reduced procedural cost, the use of vena caval filters increased significantly. Interestingly though, the saving was short-lived. In a 1992 review, no difference was found between the charges for radiologic versus surgical placement.[24]

With the advent of percutaneous techniques, several new permanent vena caval filters were introduced. These devices include the Bird's Nest filter (Cook, Bloomington, IN), the Vena Tech filter (Braun, Evanston, IL), and the Simon Nitinol filter (Nitinol Medical Technologies, Woburn, MA) (Fig. 24.2). Table 24.2 summarizes current outcomes.

Placement techniques for each of the filters differs and the most appropriate step-by-step guide for placement can be found in the operator's instructions provided by the manufacturers. These directions should be followed carefully to ensure the safety of the patient.

Percutaneous devices can be placed from the right femoral or jugular vein as well as the left femoral vein. The Simon Nitinol filter has the smallest delivery system, 9F, which can reportedly be placed via the antecubital vein.[29] The reduced profile delivery systems have significantly reduced the incidence of insertion-site thrombosis associated with the original 24F Greenfield filter. The significance of thrombi at the insertion site is not well understood but it is feared that they may have a potential for propagation. To the contrary, in a recent database review of nearly 180 patients with follow-up after percutaneous Titanium Greenfield filter placement, there were no long-term problems in the 9% of patients who initially developed insertion-site thrombosis.

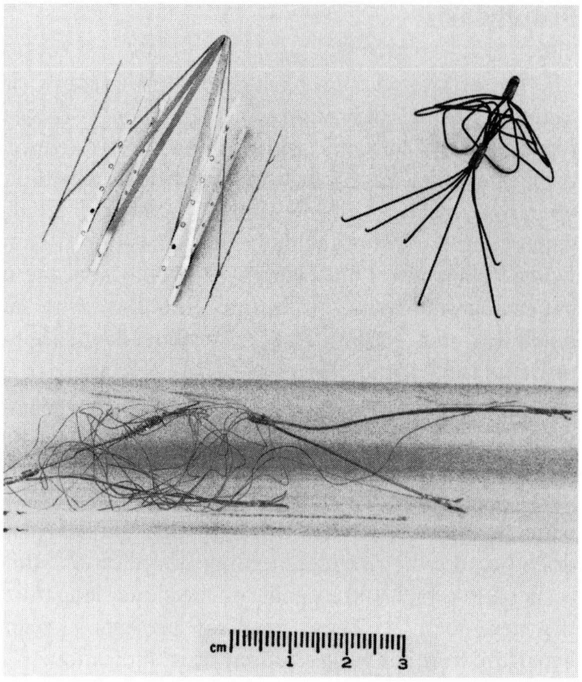

Figure 24.2 *Vena caval filters currently available in addition to the Greenfield filter. Top row, left to right: Vena Tech, Simon Nitinol; bottom row: Bird's Nest filter. (Used with permission from Lotke PA, ed.* Seminars in Arthroplasty, *WB Saunders Company, 1992).*

In general, inferior vena caval filters are typically placed with the apex near the level of the lowest renal vein, in the vicinity of L2–3. This offers protection from emboli originating in the lower extremities and the iliac veins. There are situations when the filter is positioned above this level. Early in our experience, a few patients had Greenfield filters inadvertently as well as intentionally placed in the suprarenal IVC. These patients were

Table 24.2 *Summary of the most recent published outcome studies of the marketed vena caval filters*

Source	Greenfield SGF 24F Greenfield[51]	Greenfield TGF-MH Greenfield[32]	Vena Tech Crochet[41]	Bird's Nest Lord[52, 53]	Simon Nitinol McCowan[45]
Number placed	642	173	142	61	20
Number followed	246	113	137	37	16
Recurrent PE (%)	4	4	4	5	0
Caval patency (%)	96	99	70	1–85	75
Filter patency (%)	96	99	*	95	*
Insertion-site DVT (%)	1	2	8	*	*
Migration (%)	*	7	18	0	6
Penetration (%)	*	<1	0	*	31
Follow-up period (years)	20	4	6	3.5	2
Follow-up tests	AP & lateral x-ray Duplex ultrasound Venacavography	AP & lateral x-ray Duplex ultrasound Venacavography CT	AP x-ray Duplex ultrasound Venacavography	AP x-ray Duplex ultrasound Venacavography	AP x-ray Duplex ultrasound

*Not reported.

followed and found to have similar outcomes to those patients with infrarenal filters. There was no obstruction of the renal vein or loss in renal function. Based upon this experience, a larger series of patients have had intentional suprarenal Greenfield filter placements with similar results.[27] Indications include suprarenal placement in women of childbearing potential and those with an embolic source at a higher level within the IVC or in the ovarian vein. While several women have had event-free pregnancies with a filter in the standard position, given the opportunity, suprarenal placement should be considered in an attempt to keep the gravid uterus from contact with the filter.

The Greenfield filter is the only one of the marketed filters that has been demonstrated to maintain IVC patency and avoid renal vein occlusion during sequential follow-up studies. The most recent report of patients with suprarenal filters that spans nearly 20 years supports these conclusions.[30] In a few rare cases where the source of emboli is found in the upper extremities, a Greenfield filter has also been placed in the superior vena cava. The filter functions well in this location but it is extremely important to remember that placement in the superior vena cava requires a jugular carrier system to be placed through a femoral access or vice versa. In this manner, the filter is oriented correctly to trap emboli from the upper extremities with maximal efficacy.[31,32]

One of the difficulties experienced when comparing vena caval filter devices is the variability in types of follow-up that have been reported. Five major reports of objectively documented Greenfield filter patient outcomes have been published.[33–37] The follow-up included abdominal radiographs to determine the position of the filter and either venographic or ultrasound studies to determine the patency of the filter. In addition, reports on subgroups of patients have also been published.[38,39] These reports have covered 27 years of experience with the stainless steel and the titanium devices. In all, the patency rate has remained at 96% and the rate of recurrent PE has been between 3 and 5%.[1]

Long-term reports are currently becoming available for the Vena Tech filter. These objective studies coming from more than one center have revealed a higher degree of caval occlusion than suggested by the earlier reports.[40] The initial studies suggested a 2% incidence of recurrent PE and a 4% incidence of caval occlusion. The long-term results have shown a occlusion rate of 30%.[41,42]

The initial reports on the efficacy and safety of the Bird's Nest filter were based upon a limited number of objective studies and a larger number of telephone follow-ups.[43] There have been no reports of large series of patients. The major indication for this filter is the infrequent occurrence of a mega cava. The other devices can be used in cavas up to 28 mm diameter after correcting for radiographic magnification. The Bird's Nest devices can be used for patients with up to a 40 mm cava. Early patency and efficacy data from these reports suggest the rates are comparable to the Greenfield filter; however, the reports are based upon incomplete data, and proximal migration has been seen in some series (Table 24.2). While Savin and Goldberg have suggested that the Greenfield titanium and percutaneous stainless steel filters could be placed in larger cavas, this position is not supported by the manufacturer.[44]

The Simon Nitinol filter has a reported 2% incidence of recurrent PE and caval occlusion rate of 19%. There have not been any published long-term follow-up reports of this device. In a few small series, there have been a number of caval occlusions and migrations.[45]

There is a misconception that because the published data for vena caval filters is similar, they are equivalent. Outcomes from a recent *in vivo* animal study demonstrated that this is not true. Figure 24.3 shows that thrombus resolution in the Bird's Nest, Simon Nitinol and Vena Tech filters results in heavy layers of fibrin webbing, whilst Fig. 24.4 demonstrates the absence of webbing associated with the stainless steel, titanium and an investigational device.

Two of the earliest caval interruption devices were designed for temporary use. These include the Eichelter

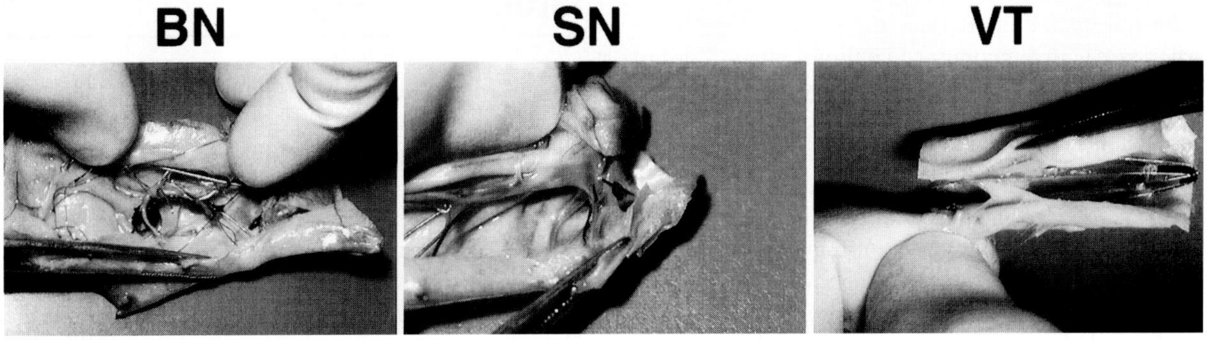

Figure 24.3 *Results of experimental thromboembolism to the Birds Nest (BN), Simon Nitinol (SN) and Vena Tech (VT) filters in sheep allowing sufficient time (30 days) for thrombus resolution. All filters show fibrous webbing.*

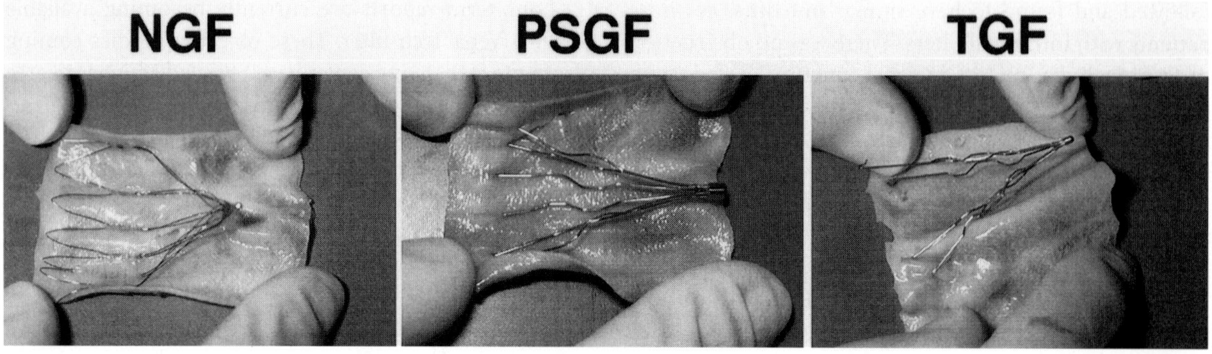

Figure 24.4 *Results of experimental thromboembolism to the experimental filter (NGF), the percutaneous stainless steel Greenfield filter (PSGF) and the titanium Greenfield filter (TGF) in sheep with the same protocol as in Fig. 24.3. All filters were clear of any residual fibrous tissue.*

sieve and the Moser balloon. These were soon abandoned in response to concern for the fate of a trapped embolus.[1]

There has been some renewed interest on the part of orthopedic and trauma surgeons to have a temporary vena caval filter available for use in patients who have a time-limited risk of developing thromboembolism. Several issues concerning the use of such devices need to be examined such as:

- correctly identifying the window during which the patient is at risk;
- how to handle a filter that has trapped a large embolus;
- the cost of replacing temporary devices in patients who become septic, etc.

There are no currently approved temporary filters available in the USA. However, FDA approval has been obtained for a catheter called 'Protect', which is designed for delivery of thrombolytic therapy. This catheter opens into a filter at the base, which is designed to trap any large emboli that may be released during the course of lysis. This device received approval as a catheter but not as a filter and no clinical trials were required. Close inspection of this new device suggests a striking similarity to the Eichelter catheter, which was withdrawn during the late 1960s as permanent devices were felt to offer superior protection.

Investigators from Europe and Canada have wider experience with temporary and optional filters. Milward has published an excellent review of potential indications for use of these devices and a description of filters that have been evaluated.[46] Zwaan *et al.* reported experience with three different systems, the Cook Tulip filter, the Angiocor and Antheor filter in 67 cases. They found one fatal PE and seven trapped emboli, six insertion-site hematomas, two subclavian thromboses, one infection, one air embolism and one filter fracture. They conclude that as 'none of the complications are long term their use seems sensible'.[47] This rate of adverse events is considerably higher than that reported for permanent devices. The focus of their conclusion is on ease of insertion but the device they selected, the Antheor filter, has been withdrawn from the market due to its high failure rate.

Like permanent filters, the temporary and optional devices differ significantly in design and function[48] and carefully controlled studies are needed before they are made available in the USA.

For many years, filter placement was in the hands of general or vascular surgeons who evaluated the need for a filter, placed the device and then provided continual follow-up. With the introduction of interventional radiographic techniques, many physicians elected to refer these patients to radiologists for placement. Recently, there is some indication that the pendulum is swinging back.

It has been demonstrated that vena caval filters can be safely placed at the bedside using a combination of fluoroscopy and ultrasound or ultrasound alone. This is especially useful for critically ill patients, those who are pregnant or have a contraindication to contrast, or patients who exceed the safe weight limits of standard radiographic equipment.[49,50] This technique has been shown to be safe and cost-effective.

FOLLOW-UP

Patients with vena caval filters should undergo follow-up on an annual basis. The purpose of the examination is to evaluate the mechanical stability of the filter and to determine the patency of the vena cava. In addition, the condition of the lower extremities is evaluated to monitor the ongoing risk for recurrent thrombosis. Because so many of these devices are placed by radiologists, it is important that information about the filter placement be passed along to the patient's local physician so arrangements for the appropriate studies can be made.

Follow-up should include physical examination of the lower extremities to observe for edema, hyperpigmentation, tissue loss and other signs of the post-thrombotic syndrome. The patient should be questioned regarding the need for and use of support hose. The use of anticoagulants and any adverse events associated with them should be investigated. In addition, information concerning recent hospitalizations and operations should be obtained. The patient should be questioned regarding the possible recurrence of thrombosis or pulmonary embolism since the last evaluation. Anteroposterior and lateral radiographs of the filter should be obtained and compared to previous studies. If there is any question of filter leg crossing, a 30° cranial-caudal radiograph should be obtained. These radiographs will demonstrate the mechanical stability and physical integrity of the device. Patients should also undergo a venous ultrasound examination to determine the patency of the filter and the vena cava. These studies should be done early in the day when there is less interference from bowel gas and with the patient fasted overnight. If the study is indeterminate and the patient is symptomatic, a venacavogram should be obtained.

Emergent follow-up should be obtained if the patient develops new bilateral lower extremity edema. Should this occur, a duplex scan of the vena cava should be performed to look for thrombus in the filter or IVC. If the results of the ultrasound study are indeterminate, the patient should undergo a venacavogram to look for caval obstruction. If occlusion is documented, and felt to be of recent origin (<7 days) and the patient's medical condition allows, thrombolytic therapy may be attempted. Patients who present with signs or symptoms of PE should also undergo venacavogram to determine the patency of the filter and the presence of trapped or propagating emboli. Rare propagation of thrombus above the level of the filter may be an indication for a second suprarenal filter rather than lytic therapy. The *Journal of Vascular and Interventional Radiology* and *Journal of Vascular Surgery* are jointly publishing a guide for reporting standards for vena caval filters. Once implemented, this guidance should result in outcome reports that allow improved comparison of devices.

SUMMARY

The current cost constraints of medical care mandate that we study the cost/benefit ratio of medical interventions. The tendency to employ technology when it becomes available rather than undertake well designed trials must be resisted. Failure to do this over time can lead to overuse. This may be the case with vena caval filters. Before some of the newer indications for vena caval filters become a standard of care, it is important to question and confirm those situations in which the filter provides the most cost-effective intervention. If evidence is lacking, then clinical trials ought to be conducted to test the question. Two major areas that currently require study are the use of filters in patients with various stages of malignancy and victims of multiple major trauma.

As the market for vena caval filters expands, new devices will be developed. The method of evaluation and the objective end points for performance need to be thoughtfully defined. Given the large sample size required to demonstrate a statistical difference between devices, randomized clinical trials do not appear to be feasible. Yet, it is not sufficient to approve new devices on the basis that they perform 'like a previously approved device'. An example is the Vena Tech filter, which was approved on a 510 K to the Greenfield filter because it shared a conical design. Yet over time, it has become clear that it does not perform like the Greenfield filter, having an occlusion rate of 30% versus 4% for the Greenfield filter. The different types of wire and the addition of stabilizing limbs may reduce the long-term patency of the device.

Vena caval filters provide protection against pulmonary embolism without many of the adverse events associated with surgical interruption. They are intended for use in patients who are at risk for PE but for whom anticoagulation is contraindicated or not thought to be sufficient. The record of the Greenfield filter over a 27-year period supports its therapeutic benefit with few, if any, sequelae. As improved techniques for delivery of these devices and new materials and designs are developed, it is essential to keep in focus the indications and appropriate use of these devices. Rather than focusing on the differences among the various devices (which will be sorted out over time) the major effort ought to be directed toward identifying those patients who are at highest risk for significant pulmonary embolism. Efforts must also continue to be directed to improved methods of thromboprophylaxis since no filter can influence the development or course of the underlying disorder. This is clearly a case where a well-planned offense is the best defense against this unnecessary source of morbidity and mortality.

REFERENCES

1. Greenfield LJ, Wakefield T. Prevention of venous thrombosis and pulmonary embolism. In Tompkins R, Cameron J, Langer B, *et al.*, eds. *Advances in Surgery.* Chicago: Year Book Medical Publishers, 1989: 301–23.
2. Hull RD, Raskob GE. Pulmonary thromboembolism. In Kelley WN, ed. *Textbook of Internal Medicine.* New York: JB Lippincott, 1989: 1943–51.
3. Hirsh J. Oral anticoagulant drugs. *N Engl J Med* 1991; **324**(26): 1865–75.

4. Harrington R, Ansell J. Risk-benefit assessment of anticoagulant therapy. *Drug Safety* 1991; **6**(1): 54–69.
5. Schmitt BP, Adelman B. Heparin-associated thrombocytopenia: a critical review and pooled analysis. *Am J Med Sci* 1993; **305**: 208–15.
6. Greaves M. Anticoagulants in pregnancy. *Pharmacol Ther* 1993; **59**: 311–27.
7. Landefeld CS, Beyth RJ. Anticoagulant-related bleeding: clinical epidemiology, prediction, and prevention. *Am J Med* 1993; **95**: 315–28.
8. Eby CS. Warfarin-induced skin necrosis. *Hematol Oncol Clin North Am* 1993; **7**: 1291–300.
9. Hull RD, Raskob GE, Brant RF, Pineo GF, Valentine KA. The importance of initial heparin treatment on long-term clinical outcomes of antithrombotic therapy. *Arch Intern Med* 1997; **137**: 2317–21.
10. Hull RD, Raskob GE, Rosenbloom D, *et al.* Optimal therapeutic level of heparin therapy in patients with venous thrombosis. *Arch Intern Med* 1992; **152**: 1589–95.
11. Greenfield LJ, Peyton M, Brown P, Elkins R. Transvenous management of pulmonary embolic disease. *Ann Surg* 1974; **180**(4): 461–8.
12. Webb LX, Rush P, Fuller S, Meredith JW. Greenfield filter prophylaxis of pulmonary embolism in patients undergoing surgery for acetabular fracture. *J Orthop Trauma* 1992; **6**(2): 139–45.
13. Emerson RH Jr, Cross R, Head WC. Prophylactic and early therapeutic use of the Greenfield filter in hip and knee joint arthroplasty. *J Arthroplasty* 1991; **6**: 129–35.
14. Golueke PJ, Garrett WV, Thompson JE, Smith BL, Talkington CM. Interruption of the vena cava by means of the Greenfield filter: expanding the indications. *Surgery* 1988; **103**(1): 111–17.
15. Rogers FB, Shackford SR, Ricci MA, Wilson JT, Parsons S. Routine prophylactic vena cava filter insertion in severely-injured trauma patients decreases the incidence of pulmonary embolism. *J Am Coll Surg* 1995; **180**(6): 641–7.
16. Wilson JT, Rogers FB, Wald SL, Shackford SR, Ricci MA. Prophylactic vena cava filter insertion in patients with traumatic spinal cord injury: preliminary results. *Neurosurgery* 1994; **35**: 234–9.
17. Rogers FB, Shackford SR, Wilson J, Ricci MA, Morris CS. Prophylactic vena cava filter insertion in severely injured trauma patients: indications and preliminary results. *J Trauma* 1993; **35**(4): 637–42.
18. Collins D, Barnes C, McCowan T, *et al.* Vena caval filter use in orthopaedic trauma patients with recognized preoperative venous thromboembolic disease. *J Orthop Trauma* 1992; **6**: 135–8.
19. Rosenthal D, McKinsey JF, Levy AM, Lamis PA, Clark MD. Use of the Greenfield filter in patients with major trauma. *Cardiovasc Surg* 1994; **2**(1): 52–5.
20. Rodriguez JL, Lopez JM, Proctor MC, *et al.* Early placement of prophylactic vena caval filters in injured patients at high risk for a pulmonary embolism. *J Trauma* 1996; **40**(5): 797–804.
21. Rogers FB, Strindberg G, Shackford SR, *et al.* Five-year follow-up of prophylactic vena cava filters in high-risk trauma patients. *Arch Surg* 1998; **133**: 406–12.
22. Cohen J, Grella L, Citron M. Greenfield filter instead of heparin as primary treatment for deep venous thrombosis or pulmonary embolism in patients with cancer. *Cancer* 1992; **70**: 1993–6.
23. Ihnat DM, Mills JL, Hughes JD, Gentile AT, Berman SS, Westerband A. Treatment of patients with venous thromboembolism and malignant disease: should vena cava filter placement be routine. *J Vasc Surg* 1998; **28**: 800–7.
24. Magnant JG, Walsh DB, Juravsky LI, Cronenwett JL. Current use of inferior vena cava filters. *J Vasc Surg* 1992; **16**: 701–6.
25. Greenfield LJ. Intraluminal techniques for vena caval interruption and pulmonary embolectomy. *World J Surg* 1978; **2**: 45–59.
26. Mansour M, Chang AE, Sindelar WF. Interruption of the inferior vena cava for the prevention of recurrent pulmonary embolism. *Am Surg* 1985; **51**: 375–80.
27. Greenfield LJ, Proctor MC. Suprarenal filter placement. *J Vasc Surg* 1998; **28**: 432–8.
28. Dorfman GS, Cronan JJ, Paolella LP, *et al.* Iatrogenic changes at the venotomy site after percutaneous placement of the Greenfield filter. *Radiology* 1989; **173**(1): 159–62.
29. Kim D, Schlam B, Porter DH, Simon M. Insertion of the Simon Nitinol caval filter: value of the antecubital vein approach. *Am J Roentgenol* 1991; **157**: 521–2.
30. Greenfield LJ, Cho KJ, Proctor MC, Sobel M, Shah S, Wingo J. Late results of suprarenal Greenfield vena cava filter placement. *Arch Surg* 1992; **127**: 969–73.
31. Greenfield LJ, Cho KJ, Proctor MC, *et al.* Results of a multicenter study of the modified hook titanium Greenfield filter. *J Vasc Surg* 1991; **14**: 253–7.
32. Greenfield LJ, Proctor MC, Cho KJ, *et al.* (1994) Extended evaluation of the titanium Greenfield vena caval filter. *J Vasc Surg* **20**: 458–65.
33. Greenfield LJ, Proctor MC. Current treatment and prevention of pulmonary embolus with the Greenfield filter. In Braverman MH, Tawes RL, eds. *Surgical Technology II*. San Francisco: Surgical Technology International, 1993: 289–91.
34. Greenfield LJ, Michna BA. Twelve-Year clinical experience with the Greenfield vena caval filter. *Surgery* 1988; **104**(4): 706–12.
35. Greenfield LJ. Current indications for and results of Greenfield filter placement. *J Vasc Surg* 1984; **1**(3): 502–4.
36. Greenfield LJ, Peyton R, Crute S, Barnes RW. Greenfield vena caval filter experience: late results in 156 patients. *Arch Surg* 1981; **116**: 1451–5.
37. Greenfield LJ, Zocco J, Wilk J, Schroeder T, Elkins R. Clinical experience with the Kim-Ray Greenfield vena caval filter. *Ann Surg* 1977; **185**(6): 692–8.

38. Jarrell B, Szentpetery S, Mendez-Picon G, Lee H, Greenfield LJ. Greenfield filter in renal transplant patients. *Arch Surg* 1981; **116**: 930–2.
39. Hux C, Wapner R, Chayen B, Rattan P, Jarrell B, Greenfield LJ. Use of the Greenfield filter for thromboembolic disease in pregnancy. *Am J Obstet Gynecol* 1986; **155**: 734–7.
40. Millward S, Peterson R, Moher D, *et al.* LGM (Vena Tech) vena caval filter: experience at a single institution. *J Vasc Interv Radiol* 1994; **5**: 351–6.
41. Crochet DP, Stora O, Ferry D, *et al.* Vena Tech-LGM filter: long-term results of a prospective study. *Radiology* 1993; **188**: 857–60.
42. Crochet DP, Brunel P, Trogrlic S, Grossetete R, Auget JL, Dary C. Long-term follow-up of vena tech-LGM filter: predictors and frequency of caval occlusion. *J Vasc Interv Radiol* 1999; **10**: 137–42.
43. Roehm J, Johnsrude I, Barth M, Gianturco C. The Bird's Nest inferior vena cava filter: progress report. *Radiology* 1988; **168**(3): 745–9.
44. Savin MA, Shlansky-Goldberg RD. Greenfield filter fixation in large venae cavae. *J Vasc Interv Radiol* 1998; **9**: 75–80.
45. McCowan TC, Ferris EJ, Carver DK, Molpus WM. Complications of the nitinol vena caval filter. *J Vasc Interv Radiol* 1992; **3**: 401–8.
46. Millward SF. Temporary and retrievable inferior vena cava filters: current status. *J Vasc Interv Radiol* 1998; **9**: 381–7.
47. Zwaan M, Lorch H, Kulke C, *et al.* Clinical experience with temporary vena caval filters. *J Vasc Interv Radiol* 1998; **9**: 594–601.
48. Lorch H, Zwaan M, Kulke C, Weiss H. In vitro studies of temporary vena cava filters. *Cardiovasc Interv Radiol* 1998; **21**: 146–50.
49. Sing RF, Smith CH, Miles WS, Messick WJ. Preliminary results of bedside inferior vena cava filter placement. Safe and cost-effective. *Chest* 1998; **114**: 315–16.
50. Van Natta TL, Morris JA, Eddy VA, *et al.* Elective bedside surgery in critically injured patients is safe and cost-effective. *Ann Surg* 1998; **227**: 618–26.
51. Greenfield LJ, Proctor MC. Twenty-year clinical experience with the Greenfield filter. *Cardiovasc Surg* 1995; **3**(2): 199–205.
52. Lord R, Benn I. Early and late results after Bird's Nest filter placement in the inferior vena cava: clinical and duplex ultrasound follow-up. *Aust N Z J Surg* 1994; **64**(2): 106–14.
53. Mohan CR, Hoballah JJ, Sharp WJ, Kresowik T, Lu CT, Carson JD. Comparative efficacy and complications of vena caval filters. *J Vas Surg* 1995; **21**(2): 235–46.

25

Acute mesenteric venous thrombosis

ROBERT Y RHEE, PETER GLOVICZKI, COREY JOST, C MICHAEL JOHNSON AND KENNETH J CHERRY, JR

Mesenteric venous thrombosis (MVT) is an uncommon but often lethal form of intestinal ischemia. First described by Fagge in 1876, it was characterized as a clinical entity by Warren and Eberhard in 1935.[1,2] It comprises 5–15% of all cases with acute mesenteric ischemia.[3–5] Patients with mesenteric venous thrombosis often present with nonspecific signs and symptoms. Despite modern diagnostic tools and methods, delay in diagnosis is still frequent and is a significant contributory factor to the reported 13–50% mortality.[6–13] Recently, the disease has been recognized more readily because of the increased use of computed tomography (CT), ultrasonography and magnetic resonance imaging (MRI) in the evaluation of abdominal pathology.[14–19] In addition, an increased awareness of the complications of coagulation abnormalities has also contributed to earlier recognition and treatment of this disease.[6–12]

In a comprehensive review of the world's literature from 1911 to 1984, Abdu *et al.* found 372 patients with MVT.[6] We reported on the Mayo Clinic experience that included 72 patients treated for MVT between 1972 and 1993.[7] Of the 72 patients, 53 had acute MVT, presenting with symptoms of less than 4 weeks' duration. Those with symptoms greater than 4 weeks' duration, but without bowel infarction, or those with MVT diagnosed as incidental and clinically insignificant finding on abdominal imaging were classified as having chronic MVT. In this chapter, we focus on acute MVT, and discuss etiology, clinical presentation, diagnosis and treatment of this disease.

ETIOLOGY

Mesenteric vein thrombosis classically has been classified as primary MVT if it occurred spontaneously as an idiopathic thrombosis of mesenteric veins not associated with any other disease or etiologic factor. All other MVT that had known associated pathologic processes were classified as secondary MVT. Predisposing conditions resulting in secondary MVT are hypercoagulability, cirrhosis, splenomegaly, cancer, infection, trauma, recent operative intervention, pancreatitis and diverticular disease. The number of patients with primary, idiopathic MVT is continuously decreasing, as more patients are now diagnosed with secondary MVT as the result of increased awareness of predisposing disorders, particularly newly defined hypercoagulable states.[6,7,10,11] In a classic autopsy study from 1948, Johnson and Baggenstoss[20] from the Mayo Clinic identified 99 cases of MVT. All but eight (12%) in their series had etiologic factors associated with mesenteric venous thrombosis. Abdu *et al.*[6] found that 81% of all cases of MVT were secondary. In our series, the prevalence of secondary MVT was also high (79%).[7] Besides previous abdominal surgery, deficiency of physiologic anticoagulants (antithrombin III, protein C, protein S, factor V Leiden, and plasminogen activator),[11,21–26] hematological disorders (polycythemia vera, thrombocytosis, hyperfibrinogenemia, myeloproliferative disorders, hyperhomocystinemia, antiphospholipid and anticardiolipin antibodies)[27–30] and estrogen-related hormonal changes[31] have been implicated as major risk factors (Table 25.1). Twenty of 53 patients (38%) in our review had a documented hypercoagulable state, with polycythemia vera being the most common disorder. Other hematologic problems included myeloproliferative disorders, hyperfibrinogenemia and deficiencies in antithrombin III, protein C and protein S.

Table 25.1 *Conditions associated with acute mesenteric venous thrombosis in 53 patients treated at the Mayo Clinic between 1972 and 1993*

Condition	No. patients (%)
Previous abdominal surgery	28 (53)
Hypercoagulable state	20 (38)
Previous MVT	17 (32)
Smoking	15 (28)
Previous DVT	15 (28)
Alcohol abuse	8 (15)
Malignant tumor	10 (19)
Cirrhosis	10 (19)
Oral contraceptives	4 (8)

DVT, deep venous thrombosis; MVT, mesenteric venous thrombosis.

PRESENTATION

The symptoms of acute MVT are generally nonspecific. Similar to patients with arterial mesenteric ischemia, Abdu *et al.* found that the only constant finding of MVT was pain out of proportion to the physical findings.[6] However, unlike acute arterial mesenteric ischemia, the progression of this disease appears to be slow, often presenting with steady low-grade symptoms for greater than 48 hours' duration. In our study, only three patients (7%) had symptoms requiring surgical intervention within 24 hours of admission, 16% had symptoms for 24–48 hours and 75% had them for longer than 48 hours. The most common presenting symptom was diffuse, nonspecific abdominal pain (83%) (Table 25.2). Abdominal distension and blood found during rectal examination were the most common signs on admission (Table 25.3). Peritoneal signs were present in only 36% and fever in 25% of the patients.

Table 25.2 *Symptoms of acute mesenteric venous thrombosis in 53 patients*

Symptom	No. patients (%)
Abdominal pain	44 (83)
Anorexia	28 (53)
Diarrhea	23 (43)
Nausea & vomiting	22 (42)
Upper GI bleeding	15 (28)
Lower GI bleeding	12 (23)
Constipation	7 (13)

GI, gastrointestinal.

Table 25.3 *Signs of acute mesenteric venous thrombosis in 53 patients*

Sign	No. patients (%)
Abdominal distension	27 (51)
Blood on rectal examination	17 (32)
Peritonitis	19 (36)
Ascites	5 (9)
Hypotension (<90 mmHg)	3 (6)
Tachycardia (>110/min)	11 (21)
Fever (>38°C)	13 (25)
Leukocytosis (>10.0 × 10^9/l)	26 (49)
Lactate (>1.65 mmol/l)	15 (28)
Amylase (>115 U/l)	10 (18)
Creatine kinase (>350 U/l)	4 (8)

LABORATORY TESTS

Generally, serum laboratory tests are not helpful in making the diagnosis of acute MVT. While abnormal laboratory tests support the diagnosis of mesenteric ischemia, negative tests do not exclude MVT. Boley *et al.* reported that a white blood cell count greater than 12 × 10^9/l and bandemia were present in two-thirds of their patients.[10] In our series, leukocytosis was present in only half of patients. Other classic signs of ischemic bowel such as elevated serum lactate level or increased amylase were found in 28% and 19% of the patients, respectively. Coagulation profile, fibrinogen levels and platelet counts were normal in most of our patients.

RADIOGRAPHIC DIAGNOSIS

Plain abdominal films are usually obtained as the initial diagnostic test in most patients presenting with abdominal complaints. In acute MVT, however, abdominal films were generally nonspecific and are of limited value in diagnostic process. A nonspecific ileus pattern is seen in 90% of patients and less than 5% demonstrate evidence of ischemic bowel such as air in the bowel wall or the portal system, or free air in the abdominal cavity, confirming perforation.

Computed tomography has become the test of choice in the diagnosis of acute MVT. This is supported by Harward *et al.*[8] when they reported 90% sensitivity. In our series, it was performed in 20 patients. None had peritonitis at the time when the CT scan was performed. The most common positive finding on CT was the demonstration of thrombus in the superior mesenteric vein (55%) (Fig. 25.1). Thrombus may also be noted in the portal or splenic veins. Abnormal bowel characteristics on CT (i.e. bowel wall thickening, pneumatosis, 'streaky' mesentery) were found in 70% of patients. When evidence for bowel ischemia and presence of venous thrombosis were considered together, sensitivity of the CT in showing an abnormality was 100%. Ultrasonography with or without color duplex evaluations of the mesenteric veins can also be diagnostic if obtained early (Fig. 25.2a,b). It had 80% sensitivity in our study in demonstrating a thrombus or the absence of flow in the mesenteric veins. Abdominal duplex scanning was similar in diagnostic value to CT scanning in a study reported by Miller *et al.*[32]

Mesenteric arteriography, however, continues to be the standard diagnostic test in patients with a clinical suspicion for arterial cause of mesenteric ischemia or if the CT is equivocal or non-diagnostic of suspected venous thrombosis. In our material the presence of thrombus or non-filling of the superior mesenteric vein (Fig. 25.3a,b) was diagnostic of MVT in five of seven patients studied (sensitivity = 71%). Sluggish filling of large mesenteric veins or prolonged blushing in the region of the superior mesenteric vein are other findings suggestive of mesenteric venous thrombosis.

Magnetic resonance imaging and magnetic resonance angiography have also been used to diagnose mesenteric venous thrombosis. Gehl *et al.*[33] identified abdominal venous obstruction in 15 patients and found the results of magnetic resonance imaging to be comparable to those obtained with computed tomography.

Unfortunately, despite increased use of more sophisticated diagnostic modalities, delay in diagnosis was still frequent. In the group of patients we treated, the median delay in diagnosis was 48 hours. Indeed, of the 53 patients in our study, the correct diagnosis of MVT was established before laparotomy only in 37 patients.

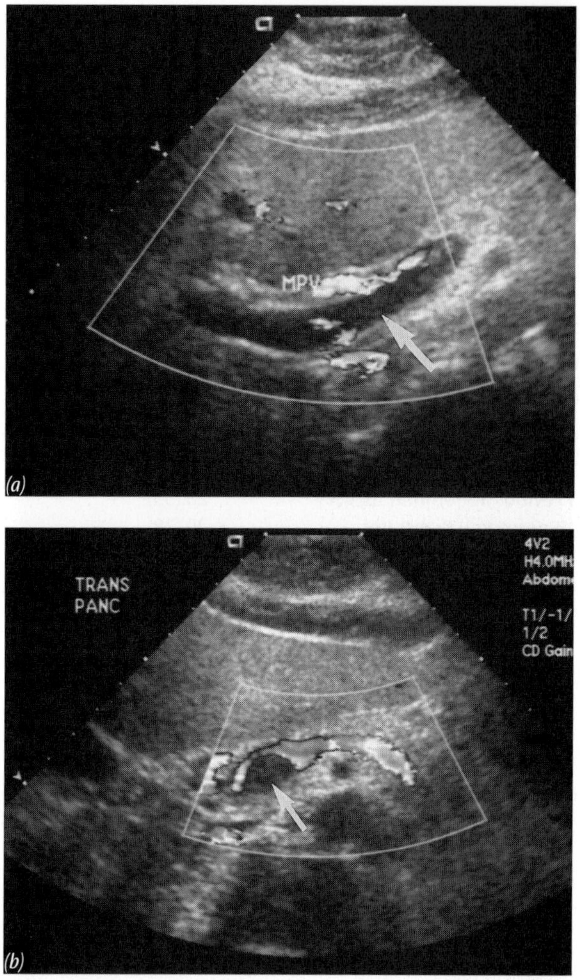

Figure 25.2 *Duplex ultrasonogram of an 82-year-old female with acute mesenteric thrombosis. (a) Arrow denotes thrombus in the superior mesenteric vein at its confluence with the portal vein. (b) Arrow indicates nonocclusive thrombus projecting into the portal vein. (With permission of the Mayo Foundation).*

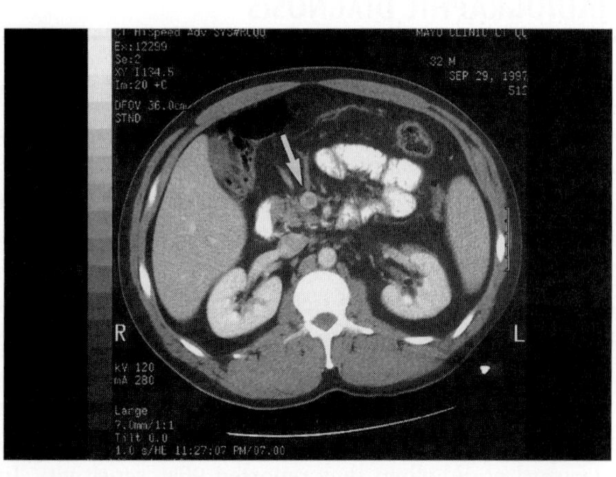

Figure 25.1 *Computed tomography scan of a 35-year-old male with acute mesenteric venous thrombosis. Arrow shows thrombus in the superior mesenteric vein. (With permission of the Mayo Foundation).*

TREATMENT

The management of patients with acute MVT should be based on clinical presentation and on the severity of symptoms. The goals of treatment are to prevent bowel necrosis or, if bowel necrosis had already occurred, to resect the nonviable bowel. An equally important goal is to restore the fluid and electrolyte imbalance of the body, to prevent infection and further propagation of thrombosis. The cornerstone of all forms of treatment is anticoagulation with heparin, started as early as possible, once the diagnosis of acute MVT is established. Thrombolysis has the potential to become an effective treatment in patients without bowel infarction.

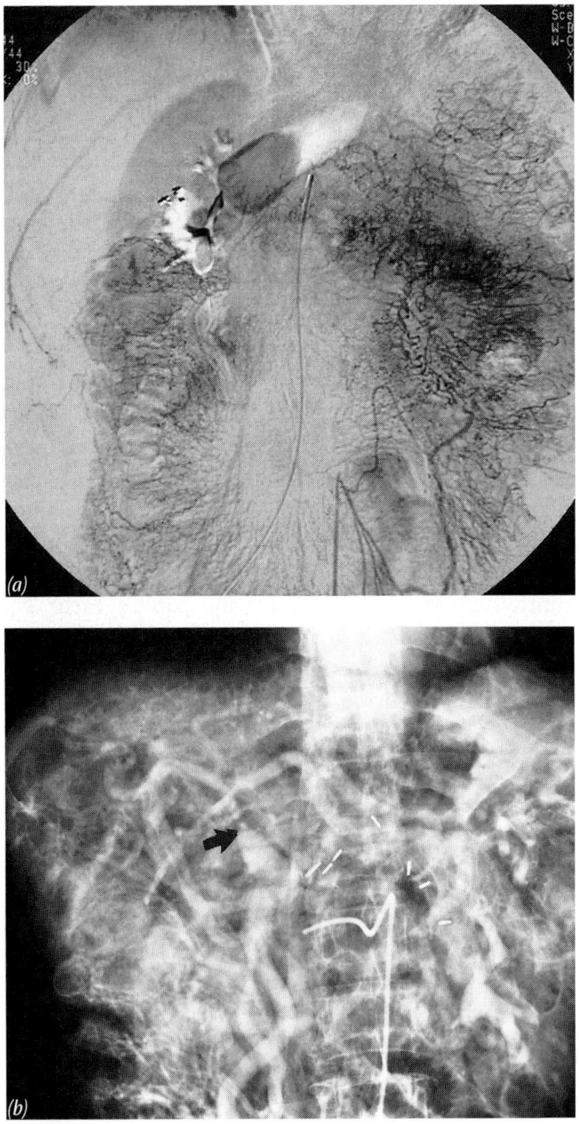

Figure 25.3 *Mesenteric arteriography with venous phase. (a) Acute mesenteric venous thrombosis in a 79-year-old male. Note lack of contrast in the superior mesenteric or portal veins on late images. (With permission of the Mayo Foundation). (b) Chronic mesenteric venous thrombosis. Arrow indicates portal and superior mesenteric venous occlusion. Note the abundant venous collateralization around the occlusion. (From Rhee* et al.[7]*)*

Surgical management

In general, all patients with localized or diffuse peritonitis undergo prompt laparotomy (Fig. 25.4). Normal or only mildly abnormal blood tests should not deter surgical exploration, and radiographic findings should supplement, not replace, clinical indication for exploration. Fluid resuscitation with intravenous crystalloids is started and broad-spectrum antibiotics are given during preparation for the operation. In our

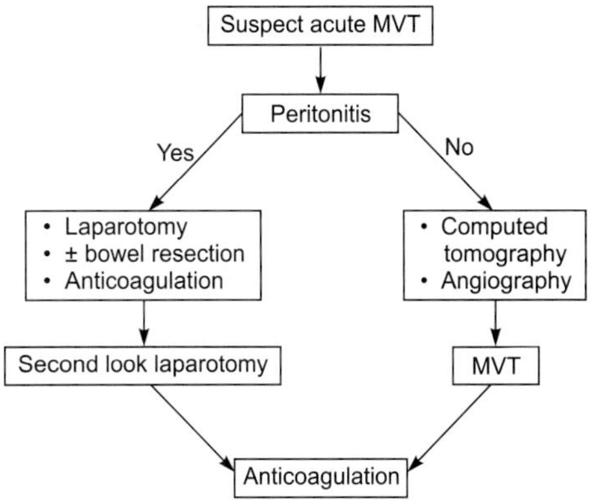

Figure 25.4 *Management algorithm for acute mesenteric venous thrombosis. (From Rhee* et al.[7]*)*

material, 34 of 52 patients (64%) required abdominal exploration. Intraoperative findings included an intact arterial supply with pulsatile flow palpable in the superior mesenteric artery in all but one patient. Examination of the superior mesenteric vein reveals fresh and frequently old thrombus in the vein and there is thrombus in the smaller, distal mesenteric veins (Fig. 25.5). Edema and cyanotic discoloration of the mesentery and bowel wall were characteristic findings. The incidence of transmural bowel necrosis requiring resection in our patients was high (88%). Twenty-one percent of patients who underwent exploration had bowel perforation.

We favor resection of only the obviously nonviable portion of the bowel and perform end-to-end anastomosis, if possible. In one of four patients, however, we had to perform a diverting ileostomy or colostomy. A second-look laparotomy should be performed liberally, and this should be decided during the first operation, based on the question on the viability of the remaining bowel. We routinely use intravenous fluorescein (with Wood's light illumination) intraoperatively to confirm perfusion to the bowel.

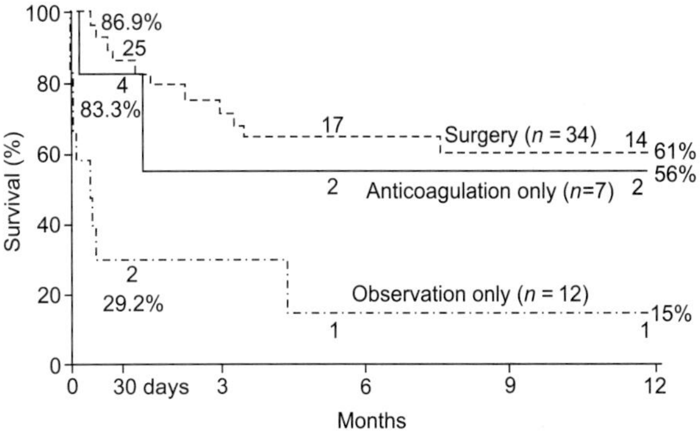

Figure 25.5 *Survival curves of acute mesenteric venous thrombosis treated with surgery and anticoagulation, anticoagulation alone and observation. (From Rhee* et al.[7]*)*

Of the 14 patients who underwent a second-look operation in our series, bowel resection was required in all. The average length of the resected bowel was extensive despite efforts to minimize resection: 109 cm of the small bowel was resected during the initial operation and 45 cm at the second operation (121 cm total). In four patients, extensive necrosis of the entire jejunoileum was found and bowel resection was not performed.

Although successful thrombectomy of the superior mesenteric vein has been described,[34,35] only one patient in our series underwent thrombectomy. However, rethrombosis occurred, requiring further bowel resection. We have not encountered a patient with a fresh proximal thrombus in the superior mesenteric vein without mechanical cause of the venous thrombosis (i.e. tumor) suitable for thrombectomy. Most patients with acute MVT have diffuse venous thrombosis with distal extension not suitable for venous thrombectomy.

If heparin was not started preoperatively, heparin infusion must be initiated during the operation, and full anticoagulation is maintained perioperatively, in spite of the increased risk of bleeding complications. Perioperative anticoagulation decreases the risk of rethrombosis and, as discussed later, improves survival.[10]

Nonoperative management

Anticoagulation with intravenous heparin is the mainstay of medical treatment. We follow the recommendations of Boley[10] and begin heparin at the time of diagnosis (5000 units given as an initial bolus, followed by an intravenous infusion of 1000 units/hour). Low molecular weight heparin can also be used as initial treatment in patients who do not have peritonitis warranting immediate exploration. Unless there is a definite contraindication, such as bleeding esophageal varices, we maintain most patients on lifelong anticoagulation with warfarin sodium to decrease chances of recurrence. Intravenous hydration and close observation of all patients is necessary. To relieve mesenteric vasospasm in those patients who were diagnosed with mesenteric arteriogram, intra-arterial papaverine, as suggested by Boley *et al.*[10] can be considered. Nineteen of our patients did not develop peritonitis and were managed nonoperatively with anticoagulation and observation.

The use of thrombolytic therapy in patients with acute MVT is still controversial, although successful outcome has been reported.[24,36] The thrombolytic agent, like streptokinase, urokinase or tissue plasminogen activator, has been delivered through transhepatic puncture or by direct transcatheter perfusion into the superior mesenteric artery. If bleeding complications can be decreased, thrombolysis may emerge as a first-line treatment option for many patients. Still, surgical treatment is required for those with bowel infarction with peritonitis.

OUTCOME

Patients with acute mesenteric venous thrombosis continue to have elevated mortality and an increased number of postoperative complications. The 30-day mortality of our patients was 27% and this was comparable to mortality rates published in other series.[2–6,8–14] It has decreased slightly from 32% during the early part of our study to 24% in the last decade (Fig. 25.6). Twenty of our 53 patients (38%) had relentless progression of MVT with the venous thrombosis ultimately resulting in their death. Eight patients (15%) died of other causes: malignant tumor (three patients), pulmonary embolism (two patients), liver failure, gastrointestinal bleeding and multisystem organ failure, in one patient each. The patients hospitalized for MVT typically had a long clinical course (22 days), and in-hospital complications of treatment occurred in 55% of our patients (Table 25.4). Short bowel syndrome as a result of extensive bowel resection developed in 40% of the patients.

Anticoagulation significantly prolonged survival in our series and in other studies (Table 25.5).[6,7,10,13]

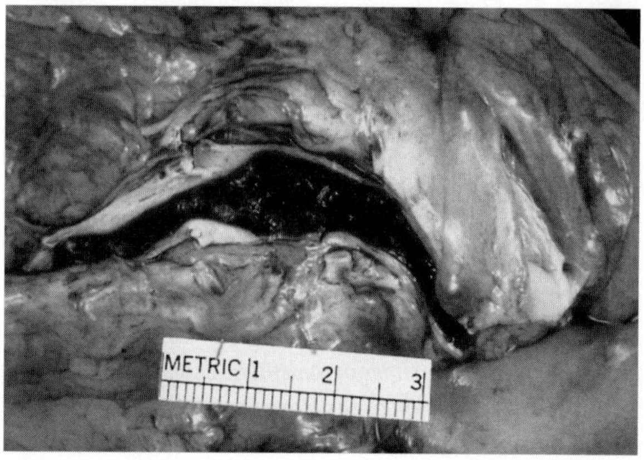

Figure 25.6 *Pathology specimen of the small bowel mesentery showing a thrombus in the superior mesenteric vein. (From Rhee et al.[7])*

Table 25.4 *Complications of surgical treatment for acute mesenteric venous thrombosis in 53 patients*

Complication	No. patients (%)
Short bowel syndrome	12 (23)
Wound infection	11 (21)
Sepsis	9 (17)
Pneumonia	7 (13)
Pulmonary embolus	5 (9)
Renal failure	5 (9)
Gastrointestinal bleeding	3 (6)

Table 25.5 *Management and early mortality of 164 patients with acute mesenteric venous thrombosis*

1st Author (year)	No. patients	Surgical treatment		Nonoperative treatment only	Anticoagulation	Mortality no. (%)
		Bowel resection	Laparotomy only			
Sack (1982)[9]	9	9	0	0	6	2 (22)
Wilson (1987)[11]	16	10	3	3	6	8 (50)
Clavien (1988)[12]	12	12	0	0	12	5 (42)
Harward (1989)[8]	16	5	0	11	7	3 (19)
Levy (1990)[13]	21	19	2	2	17	8 (38)
Grieshop (1991)[14]	15	5	0	10	9	2 (13)
Boley (1992)[10]	22	22	0	0	22	7 (32)
Rhee (1994)[7]	53	30	4	19	33	14 (27)
Totals	164	112	9	45	112	

Anticoagulation improved survival in both the surgical and nonsurgical groups (Fig. 25.7). The recurrence rate of acute MVT was high and occurred in 36% of our patients. The majority of the recurrences occurred during the same hospitalization or within 30 days (74%). Our analysis did not reveal any differences in. survival among patients with documented hypercoagulable states, pancreatitis, obesity or any other associated conditions. The number of patients in the different subgroups, however, was small.

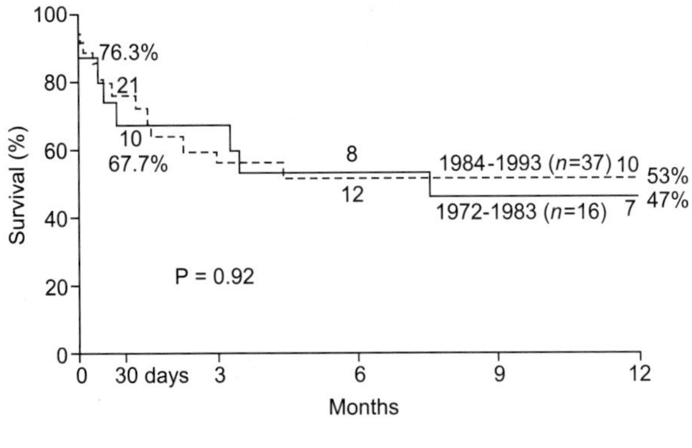

Figure 25.7 *Survival curves of patients with acute mesenteric venous thrombosis during the early (1972–1983) and late (1984–1993) periods of the study. (From Rhee* et al.[7]*)*

CONCLUSIONS

Mesenteric venous thrombosis continues to be uncommon but it should be suspected in patients with acute visceral ischemia. Presenting abdominal signs and symptoms are usually nonspecific; however a history of previous venous thrombosis or known thrombotic disorder should be helpful clues to the diagnosis. Computed tomography with intravenous contrast appears to be the most sensitive diagnostic test and should be obtained if MVT is suspected. Duplex scanning and magnetic resonance venography are also helpful to confirm the diagnosis. Patients with peritonitis require prompt abdominal exploration to resect the nonviable portion of the bowel, with liberal use of second-look procedures. Early anticoagulation with heparin and intravenous hydration are the most important components of the medical treatment, although in patients without peritonitis thrombolysis can also be considered. Most patients are maintained on lifelong treatment with oral anticoagulants. Despite improved diagnostic tests and an increased awareness of acute MVT, the rate of mortality, complications and recurrent disease remains high.

REFERENCES

1. Fagge M. Mesenteric venous thrombosis. *Trans Pathol Soc Lond* 1876; **27**: 124–5.
2. Warren S, Eberhard TP. Mesenteric venous thrombosis. *Surg Gynecol Obstet* 1935; **61**: 102–21.
3. Ottinger LW, Austen WG. A study of 136 patients with mesenteric infarction. *Surg Gynecol Obstet* 1967; **124**: 251–61.
4. Hansen HJB, Christoffersen JK, Occlusive mesenteric infarction: a retrospective study of 83 cases. *Acta Chir Scand* 1976; **472**: 103–8.
5. Kairaluoma IVff, Karkola P, Heikkinen E, *et al.* Mesenteric infarction. *Am J Surg* 1977; **133**: 188–93.
6. Abdu R, Zakhour BJ, Dallis DJ. Mesenteric venous thrombosis – 1911 to 1984. *Surgery* 1987; **101**: 383–8.
7. Rhee RY, Gloviczki P, Mendonca CT, *et al.* Mesenteric venous thrombosis: still a lethal disease in the 1990s. *J Vasc Surg* 1994; **20**: 688–97.
8. Harward TRS, Green D, Bergan JJ, Rizzo RJ, Yao JST. Mesenteric venous thrombosis. *J Vasc Surg* 1989; **9**: 328–33.

9. Sack J, Aldrete JS. Primary mesenteric venous thrombosis. *Surg Gynecol Obstet* 1982; **154**: 205–8.
10. Boley SJ, Kaleya RN, Brandt U. Mesenteric venous thrombosis. *Surg Clin North Am* 1992; **72**: 183–201.
11. Wilson C, Walker ID, Davidson JF, Imrie CW. Mesenteric venous thrombosis and antithrombin III deficiency. *J Clin Pathol* 1987; **40**: 906–8.
12. Clavien PA, Harder F. Mesenteric venous thrombosis. *Helv Chir Acta* 1988; **55**: 29–34.
13. Levy PJ, Krausz NK, Manny I. The role of second-look procedure in improving survival time for patients with mesenteric venous thrombosis. *Surg Gynecol Obstet* 1990; **170**: 287–91.
14. Grieshop RJ, Dalsing MC, Ckirit DF, Lalka SG, Sawchuk AP. Acute mesenteric venous thrombosis: revisited in a time of diagnostic clarity. *Am Surg* 1991; **57**: 573–8.
15. Rahmouni A, Mathieu D, Golli M, *et al.* Value of CT and sonography in the conservative management of acute splenoportal and superior mesenteric venous thrombosis. *Gastrointest Radiol* 1992; **17**: 135–40.
16. Carr N, Jamison MH. Superior mesenteric venous thrombosis. *Br J Surg* 1981; **68**: 343–4.
17. Kispert JF Jr, Kazmers A. Acute intestinal ischemia caused by mesenteric venous thrombosis. *Semin Vasc Surg* 1990; **3**: 157–71.
18. Kitchens CS. Evolution of our understanding of the pathophysiology of primary mesenteric venous thrombosis. *Am J Surg* 1992; **163**: 346–8.
19. Dada FS, Balan AD. Recurrent primary mesenteric venous thrombosis. *South Med J* 1987; **80**: 1329–30.
20. Johnson CC, Baggenstoss AH. Mesenteric vascular occlusion I. Study of 99 cases of occlusion of the veins. *Proc Staff Meet Mayo Clin* 1949; **24**: 628–36.
21. Bemelman WA, Butzelaar RMJK, Khargi Y, Keeman JN. Mesenteric venous thrombosis caused by deficiency of physiologic anti-coagulants: report of a case. *Neth J Surg* 1990; **42–1**: 16–19.
22. Tollefson DFJ, Friedman KD, Marlar RA, Bandyk DF, Towne JB. Protein C deficiency; a cause of unusual or unexplained thrombosis. *Arch Surg* 1988; **123**: 881–4.
23. Inagaki I-L, Sakakibara O, Miyaike IL, Eimoto T, Yura I. Mesenteric venous thrombosis in familial free protein S deficiency. *Am J Gastroenterol* 1993; **88**: 134–8.
24. Ludwig DJ, Hauptmann E, Rosoff L Jr, Neuzil D. Mesenteric and portal vein thrombosis in a young patient with protein S deficiency treated with urokinase via the superior mesenteric artery. *J Vasc Surg* 1999; **30**: 551–4.
25. Leebeek FW, Lameris JS, van Buren HR, *et al.* Budd–Chiari syndrome, portal vein and mesenteric vein thrombosis in a patient homozygous for factor V Leiden mutation treated by TIPS and thrombolysis. *Br J Haematol* 1998; **102**(4): 929–31.
26. Boyko OB, Pizzo SV. Mesenteric vein thrombosis and vascular plasminogen activator. *Arch Pathol Lab Med* 1983; **107**(10): 541–2.
27. Ostermiller W Jr, Carter R. Mesenteric venous thrombosis secondary to polycythemia vera. *Am Surg* 1969; **35**: 407–9.
28. Lee HJ, Park JW, Chang JC. Mesenteric and portal venous obstruction associated with primary antiphospholipic antibody syndrome. *J Gastroenterol Hepatol* 1997; **12**(12): 822–6.
29. Marie I, Levesque H, Lecam-Duchez V, *et al.* Mesenteric venous thrombosis revealing both factor II G20212A and hyperhomocysteinemia related to pernicious anemia. *Gastroenterology* 2000; **118**(1): 237–8.
30. Blanc P, Barki J, Fabre JM, *et al.* Superior mesenteric vein thrombosis associated with anticardiolipin antibody without autoimmune disease. *Am J Hematol* 1995; **48**(2): 137.
31. Nesbit RR Jr, DeWeese JA. Mesenteric venous thrombosis and oral contraceptives. *South Med J* 1977; **70**: 360–2.
32. Miller VE, Berland LL. Pulsed doppler duplex sonography and CT of portal vein thrombosis. *Am J Roentgenol* 1985; **145**: 73–7.
33. Gehl BB, Bohndorf Y, Klose KC, Gunther RW. Two-dimensional MR angiography in the evaluation of abdominal veins with gradients refocused sequences. *J Comput Assist Tomogr* 1990; **14**: 619–24.
34. Inahara T. Acute superior mesenteric venous thrombosis: treatment by thrombectomy. *Ann Surg* 1971; **174**: 956–61.
35. Bergentz SE, Ericsson B, Hedner U, Leandoer L, Nilsson IM. Thrombosis in the superior mesenteric and portal veins: Report of a case treated with thrombectomy. *Surgery* 1974; **76**: 286–90.
36. Robin P, Gurel Y, Lang K, Lagarrigue F, Scotto JM. Complete thrombolysis of mesenteric vein occlusion with recombinant tissue-type plasminogen activator. *Lancet* 1988; **1**(2): 1391.

PART 4

Management of chronic venous disease

26

Sclerotherapy guidelines

J LEONEL VILLAVICENCIO*

BRIEF HISTORICAL REVIEW

It is generally recognized that the operation introduced by Trendelenburg in 1860 and published in 1890 was the beginning of modern surgery for varicose veins.[1] Intraluminal stripping as a surgical procedure was first reported by Keller in the USA in 1905,[2] even though Charles Mayo had performed an operation for varicose veins in Rochester, Minnesota in 1888 and reported the results of his operation with an external stripper in 1904 and 1906.[3,4] Babcock, in 1907,[5] reported stripping of the saphenous vein with an instrument that was the prototype of all intraluminal strippers currently used. The Mayo and the Babcock operations were extensively utilized by American surgeons for more than two decades. Surgery had been accompanied by considerable morbidity. Sepsis and pulmonary embolism were frequent in the pre-antibiotic era when patients were recommended bed rest for 8–10 days. Sclerotherapy was received with great expectations after many years of experience in Europe and replaced surgery as the treatment of choice. It was introduced in 1927 by McPheeters and Dixon[6–8] of the Mayo Clinic, using a solution of quinine and urethane. Sodium morrhuate was introduced in 1931 and was extensively used in the USA during the next two decades. Failure of the injection treatment of varicose veins was recognized early by McPheeters and De Takats,[8,9] and later by Smith[10] who published one of the largest clinical series emphasizing the poor long-term results obtained with the method.

The reports of these investigators were confirmed and expanded in the publications by Ochsner[11] and Waugh.[12] The latter reported a recurrence rate of nearly 60% at 5 years using sclerotherapy either alone or in combination with high ligation. These experiences have been later confirmed by Hobbs[13] and Einarsson and Eklof[14] in randomized controlled studies. The failure of sclerotherapy rekindled the interest in the surgical treatment of varicose veins when, in 1957, Myers reported the excellent results obtained by an extensive operation for varicose veins utilizing new instrumentation.[15]

With the introduction of new sclerosing agents, less toxic and highly effective, there has been a wave of enthusiasm for sclerotherapy in the USA that has made it necessary to reassess our knowledge on this form of treatment and establish guidelines for the training and practice of sclerotherapy.

The physician should be familiar with the following aspects of sclerotherapy: indications, contraindications, diagnostic methods to identify the etiology of the varices, its distribution and the points of reflux. The physician should also become familiar with the available sclerosing agents, their modes of action, materials, techniques, compression methods, complications and long-term results.

*The collaboration of members of the American Venous Forum Ad Hoc Committee on Sclerotherapy – Mitchel P Goldman, Joanne M Lohr, John R Pfeifer, Robert Cranley and Richard Spence – is gratefully acknowledged.

The opinions or assertions contained herein are the private one of the author and are not to be construed as official or as reflecting the view of the Department of Defense, Department of the Army or the Uniformed Services University of the Health Sciences.

TRAINING OF THE PHYSICIAN

Optimally, during his training, the physician should have received instruction in the nonoperative and operative management of venous diseases, including stasis dermatitis, venous ulceration, varicose veins and telangiectasias, and preferably have had exposure to sclerotherapy procedures either during his training or by attending sclerotherapy courses which may include video tape and live demonstrations. In addition, it is desirable that the training is complemented by specific instruction in centers of sclerotherapy recommended by recognized professional societies. Sclerotherapy is taught to residents and vascular fellows at the Venous and Lymphatic Teaching Clinics at Walter Reed Army and National Naval Medical Centers in Washington, DC. Despite its therapeutic possibilities, unfortunately, sclerotherapy is not taught in any formal residency program, either surgical or medical.

DIAGNOSIS AND EXAMINATION

Diagnosis

A complete clinical history and physical examination should be performed during the initial visit. Symptoms relative to menses, activity, presence of pain, edema, heaviness and type of work should be investigated. During the initial visit, it is determined if the patient is a candidate for sclerotherapy or for surgery, or for both. After the interview, the physical examination will confirm the clinical impression. Noninvasive vascular examination and/or invasive testing (Doppler ultrasound, duplex scanning, air plethysmography, photoplethysmography, phlebography) should be judiciously employed to obtain information about the etiology of the varicose veins and the hemodynamic assessment of the superficial and deep systems. This is important because in cases of severe reflux, sclerotherapy will be only temporarily successful. On the other hand, if the varices are secondary to arteriovenous fistula, sclerotherapy is not indicated because of the risk of the sclerosing agent passing into the arterial system, producing serious complications.

Informed consent

Patients considered for sclerotherapy should be informed of the nature of the treatment that they will receive, the results that may be expected, and the side-effects that may reasonably be expected from the treatment, such as skin necrosis, pigmentation, thrombophlebitis, etc. All patients should sign an Informed Consent Form. Pre-injection photography is strongly recommended. (Patient's consent should always be obtained.)

Clinical history

The etiology of the varicose veins should be determined. Each one of the following four groups of varicosities has a different etiology, pathophysiology and treatment:

- familial or primary: telangiectasias are considered in this group;
- post-thrombotic or secondary;
- congenital malformations of venous predominance; and
- post-traumatic or acquired arteriovenous fistula.

In most patients, the diagnosis can be made during the initial interview. Special emphasis should be placed on obtaining a history of diseases which may modify the therapeutic approach, such as asthma, allergic diseases, tendency to keloids or pigmentation, bleeding diathesis, history of deep venous thrombosis, and hypercoagulable states.

The intake of medications that may interfere with the clotting mechanism, such as aspirin, anticoagulants and certain non-steroidal anti-inflammatory agents, should be investigated. The use of oral contraceptives, estrogens and other hormonal agents whose role in the coagulation mechanisms is well known should also be investigated.

Physical examination

The patient should be examined in the upright position under good illumination. Tangential lighting is excellent for demonstration of the bulging varicose veins. The distribution of the varicosities should be carefully noticed. The physician should be familiar with the indications and use of the noninvasive vascular techniques.

Primary varicose veins appear early in life and are usually present in one or more members of the family. 'Venous spiders' (telangiectasia), venous lakes and other skin blemishes appear, especially in women, on the medial, posterior and lateral aspects of the thigh and less often in the lower leg and calf. These blemishes have a striking familial tendency (Fig. 26.1).

Varicose veins may appear in the extremities as a sequela of a post-thrombotic episode. In these cases, edema, pigmentation, eczema and venous ulcers may also be present. (Fig. 26.2) It is recognized that primary deep and superficial venous insufficiency may produce similar manifestations. Patients with congenital malformations of venous predominance may have varicose veins, 'port-wine stains', hypertrophy of soft tissues and bone overgrowth of the extremity. In these patients, the presence of congenital arteriovenous fistulae should be ruled out. Patients with predominantly venous malformations may benefit with sclerotherapy (Fig. 26.3). The presence of arteriovenous fistulae is a contraindication for sclerotherapy.

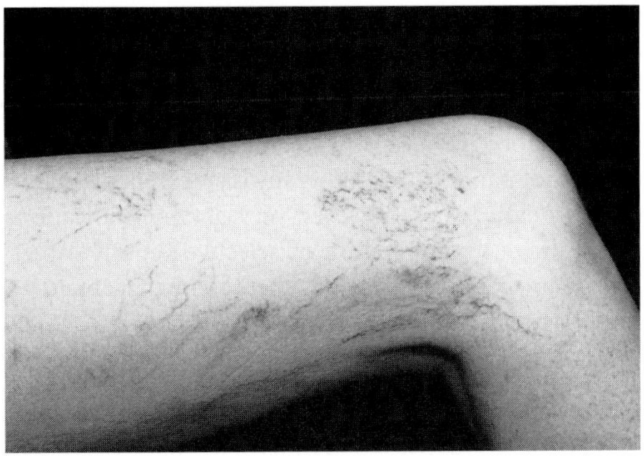

Figure 26.1 *Diffuse venous lakes and 'spider veins' on the lateral aspect of the leg and knee of a 19-year-old patient. Telangiectasias have a striking familial tendency.*

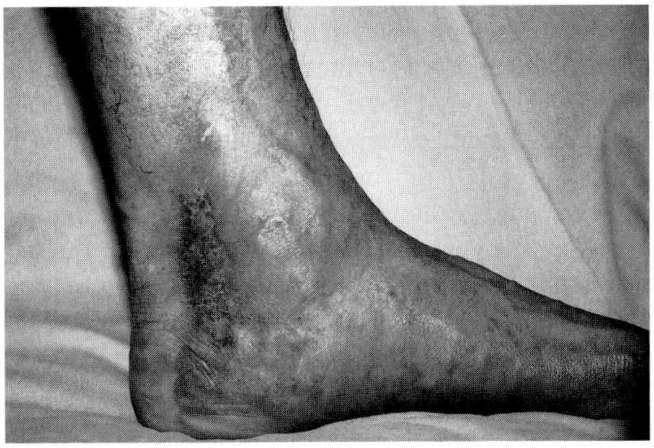

Figure 26.2 *Post-thrombotic varicose veins. Sequelae of a deep venous thrombosis are clearly observed in the medial aspect of the retromalleolar area in this patient. Deep venous thrombosis occurred 12 years before. Sclerotherapy and compression are valuable adjuncts in the management of these challenging problems.*

Varicose veins may also appear as a manifestation of traumatic arteriovenous fistula. The hemodynamic effects on the venous system will depend on the location, size and duration of the fistula. Acquired arteriovenous fistulae are treated surgically or by endovascular techniques. Sclerotherapy may be used only after the arteriovenous shunt has been corrected.

The venous tributaries of the internal iliac vein may be a pathway for varicose veins. The internal pudendal, obturator and gluteal veins are tributaries of the internal iliac vein and drain the venous areas of the buttocks, upper and medial aspects of the thigh and perineum. Any intrapelvic source of venous hypertension must be investigated. This includes ovarian reflux. Sclerotherapy is useful in mild cases of vulvar varices.

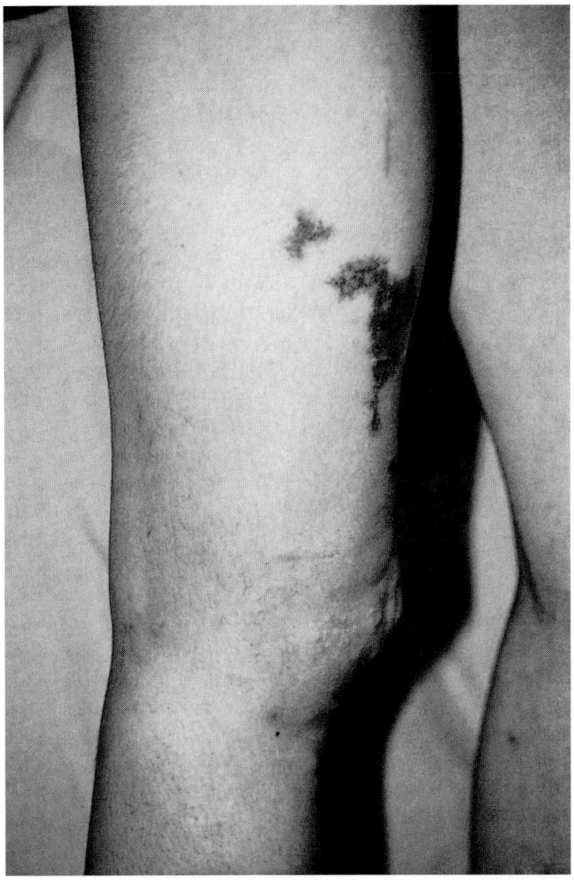

Figure 26.3 *A port-wine stain on the anterolateral aspect of the right thigh and a spongy hemangioma at the knee, are present in this patient with Klippel–Trenaunay syndrome. After surgery (surgical scars are visible), sclerotherapy followed by compression are essential steps in the management of this condition.*

Laboratory examination

The clinical history and the physical examination need to be supplemented by laboratory data on an individual basis. Appropriate blood tests should be performed in patients with hypercoagulability or other manifestations of systemic disease. These include, but are not limited to, protein S, protein C, antithrombin III, and lupus anticoagulant.

Noninvasive vascular examination

Doppler ultrasound examination is valuable to assess reflux at the saphenofemoral and saphenopopliteal junctions and other areas of perforators (Fig. 26.4). Air plethysmography, photoplethysmography and color duplex scanning are the most widely used noninvasive tests. Noninvasive vascular testing should be utilized to assess the hemodynamics of the superficial and deep venous systems, detection of incompetent perforators

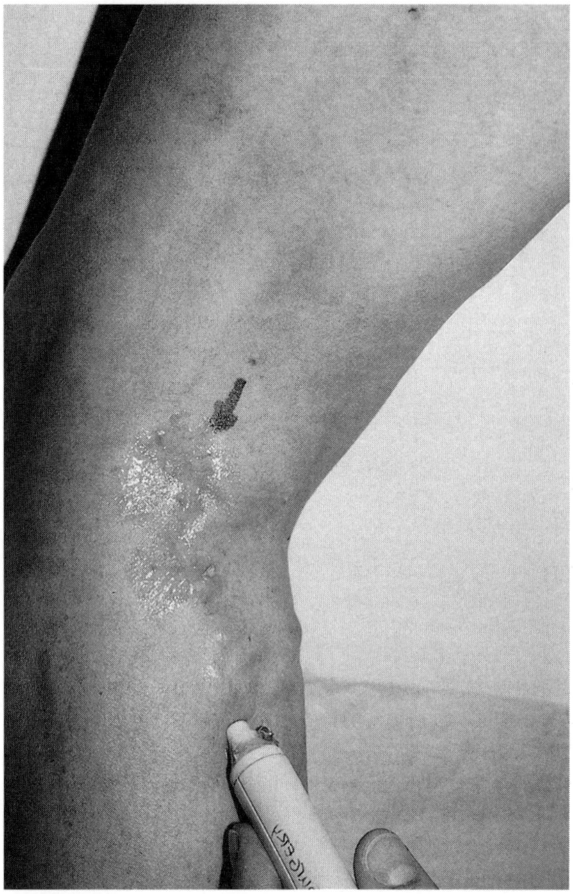

Figure 26.4 *An 8 MHz continuous-wave Doppler probe is shown to document the connection between a large perforator in the distal third of the thigh (black arrow) with grossly dilated clusters of varicose veins extending to the popliteal area and posterior aspect of the calf. This perforator was the only anomaly in this patient who otherwise had competent saphenous systems.*

and to rule out venous thrombosis. These tests are rarely indicated in cases of telangiectasia. In general, the routine use of these expensive vascular examinations in sclerotherapy patients should be discouraged. Echo-sclerotherapy (the use of ultrasound-guided injections) is discussed later.

Invasive studies such as ascending or descending phlebography are indicated in complex cases of venous disorders such as congenital malformations, pelvic varices and recurrent varicose veins to guide the physician in selecting a therapeutic option.

In all patients with venous disease, a complete examination of the arterial system is essential. Assessment of peripheral pulses should be done in all patients. Ankle/brachial index determinations should be done when considered appropriate.

INDICATIONS FOR SCLEROTHERAPY

Surgical techniques carefully tailored for each type of venous problem have provided lasting relief to a large number of patients. Sclerotherapy is an excellent method of treatment. It has, however, very definite indications. The judicious combination of selective venous surgery and sclerotherapy constitutes the best management for most types of varicose veins. The following are the indications for sclerotherapy:

- superficial venules, 'venous spiders' (veins under 1 mm), venous lakes, and other small venous blemishes. The treatment of these superficial varicosities is mainly cosmetic, even though some of them may be symptomatic (Fig. 26.1).
- varicosities of 1–3 mm in diameter in the absence of detectable valvular reflux by Doppler duplex.
- postoperative residual veins are veins under 3 mm in diameter that the surgeon chose not to excise in order to limit the number of incisions. They may be treated by sclerotherapy when the superficial ecchymoses have disappeared and the incisions are healed (usually after the second postoperative month).
- varicosities 3–4 mm in diameter observed during the postoperative follow-up period. These veins should be treated by sclerotherapy when they are not secondary to a missed incompetent perforator. Residual and/or recurrent incompetent perforators 4 mm or larger should be surgically divided under local anesthesia, although sometimes they can also be sclerosed with varying degrees of success. Once the reflux is eliminated, remaining varicosities may be treated by sclerotherapy.
- small congenital vascular malformations of venous predominance, such as the so-called cavernous hemangiomas. These may be successfully eliminated by sclerotherapy. In extensive venous malformations where surgery is not indicated, sclerotherapy may offer palliative relief, such as the case of certain variants of the Klippel–Trenaunay syndrome, where there is hypoplasia or aplasia of the deep venous system.
- bleeding varicosities (varicorrhage). These can be controlled by the injection of a concentrated sclerosing agent. The agent should be injected following the empty vein technique. Adequate compression is used for 1 week or longer (30–40 mmHg). This treatment produces immediate thrombosis of the vein and temporarily controls the problem.
- incompetent perforators. Sclerotherapy of incompetent perforators requires special expertise. According to most reports, it is accompanied by a high incidence of recurrence, and may lead to deep venous thrombosis. Injection of 'duplex guided' (echo-sclerotherapy) sclerosing agents at the

saphenofemoral or saphenopopliteal junction is not recommended. In most published series, the recurrence rate is high and the risks involved are real and should not be considered lightly.[16] Incompetent, large perforators (>4 mm) properly identified, are best treated surgically.

- large varices surrounding a leg ulcer. In this situation, sclerotherapy enhances the ulcer healing by eliminating temporarily the venous hypertension present in the ulcer area (Fig. 26.5).

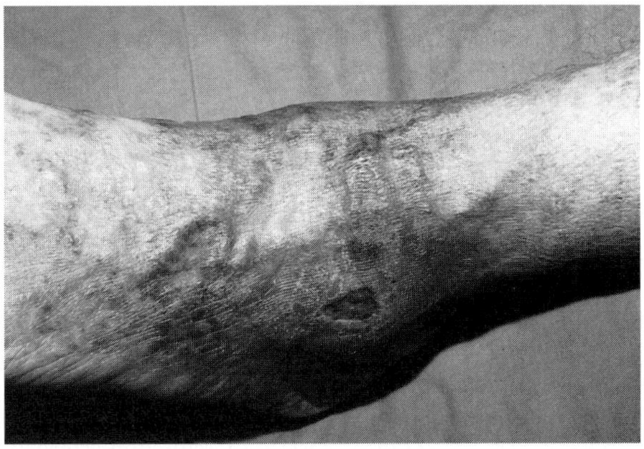

Figure 26.5 *Sclerotherapy of the large veins surrounding a leg ulcer enhances healing by decreasing the venous hypertension in the area. This is a temporary measure while a definitive treatment is planned.*

CONTRAINDICATIONS FOR SCLEROTHERAPY

The list of contraindications for sclerotherapy varies in different countries and in different medical specialties. In several European countries, it is common to inject large varicose veins and perforators. In Austria, France, Switzerland, Germany, and the UK, there are phlebologists who practice the injection of large varicose veins, disregarding the presence of reflux points. Several randomized prospective studies have demonstrated that sclerotherapy as a single form of treatment for all forms of varicose veins has a high incidence of recurrence. For this reason, most vascular surgeons will not inject large varicose veins connected to an important source of reflux. These patients are best treated by surgery. The following conditions are contraindication for sclerotherapy:

- Pregnancy. Pregnant women should preferably not be injected. In cases of vulvar varices, threatening rupture, or large varicose veins in the neighborhood of a leg ulcer, a localized injection can be performed in a pregnant woman to temporarily solve an important clinical problem.
- Elderly and sedentary patients. Sclerotherapy in the elderly (70 years) should be individualized. There are some elderly patients with normal skin and in good physical condition who may be submitted to sclerotherapy without problems. On the other hand, there are elderly and debilitated patients who are not good candidates for sclerotherapy due to their lack of mobility and increased risk for deep venous thrombosis.
- Generalized, severe systemic disease (diabetes, cardiac, renal, hepatic, pulmonary, collagen diseases and malignancies).
- Advanced rheumatic disease, orthoarthritis or any disease of the musculoskeletal system that interferes with the patient's mobility.
- Arterial insufficiency of the lower extremities as evidenced by intermittent claudication, coldness, skin atrophy, and weak or absent pulses, is a contraindication. In questionable cases, ankle brachial index should be determined. Patients with A–B index below 0.8 should preferably not be injected.
- Patients with history of severe allergic disease or bronchial asthma should be carefully evaluated. Even with the newer sclerotherapy agents, serious anaphylactic reactions have been reported on rare occasions. In cases of history of severe allergic disease, the safest sclerosing agents are 65% dextrose or hypertonic saline 11.7–23.4%.
- Acute febrile illnesses as manifested by fever (38°C or higher) with signs and symptoms of acute systemic disease.
- Acute superficial or deep thrombophlebitis.
- Obesity. Mobility is restricted in obese individuals (greater than 25% of ideal weight) and external compression is difficult to apply. Treatment under these conditions should be individualized and the risk-benefit of the procedure should be carefully considered.
- Varicose veins in communication with a source of venous reflux demonstrated by bidirectional Doppler ultrasound and/or duplex scanning studies have an unacceptable high incidence of recurrences.
- Patients on anticoagulants. Because of the risk of extensive ecchymosis secondary to the venipuncture, patients on anticoagulants, aspirin or anti-inflammatory drugs should stop treatment 1 week before the injections.

TREATMENT

General measures

Patients with chronic venous insufficiency will benefit with the following measures:

- Elevation. If there are no contraindications of elevation of the extremity (hiatal hernia), the patient

should be advised to sleep with the foot of the bed elevated 6–8 inches (2.5–3 cm), placing wooden blocks between the floor and foot of the bed.
- External compression. This may be in the form of elastic bandages, elastic stockings or nonelastic compression systems. It is recognized that compression is the mainstay in the treatment of venous disease.
- Hygiene of the extremity. Cleansing and lubrication of the extremity should be recommended to every patient.

Treatment by injection of sclerosing agents

All currently employed sclerosing agents produce a similar histological effect. The endothelial cells swell and become disrupted immediately after the injection. The acute inflammatory reaction forms a red thrombus. Depending on the agent concentration, the reaction may range from a complete lack of effect to a strong periphlebitic reaction. According to their mode of action, the sclerosing agents may be classified into osmotic, detergent, or corrosive. Examples of osmotic agents are sodium chloride 23.4%, glucose 65% and sodium salicylate. The detergent agents are sodium tetradecyl sulfate (Sotradecol), polidocanol (Aethoxysklerol) and sodium morrhuate. Corrosive agents are sodium and potassium iodide with the addition of benzyl alcohol, and chromated glycerin (Scleremo).

Selection of the sclerotherapy agent

Each sclerotherapy agent has a unique safety and efficacy profile. The agent, concentration and quantity of the solution injected will be determined by the type and size, as well as for the site of the varicose vein to be injected. The Food and Drug Administration has approved sodium tetradecyl sulfate, sodium morrhuate and ethanolamine oleate. A phase III multicenter trial of polidocanol has been completed to provide the basis for approval of this sclerosing agent, which is widely used in other parts of the world. Hypertonic saline is not approved by the FDA as a sclerosant agent.

Concentration of sclerosant for different vein sizes

TELANGIECTASIAS (VENOUS SPIDERS)

Veins measuring 1 mm or less in diameter are best treated with a concentration of 0.125–0.250% sodium tetradecyl sulfate, or 0.5% polidocanol. Hypertonic saline in strengths of 11.7–23.4%, mixed with a small amount of lidocaine (lignocaine) to decrease the burning sensation, has been extensively used in the treatment of small venous blemishes and telangiectasias (Table 26.1). It should be noted that some of the telangiectatic webs appear to be connected to larger feeding veins. The presence of these communications makes it necessary to treat the larger veins first, as recommended by the French School of Sclerotherapy. Polidocanol, 0.5%, may on occasion be injected paravascularly without producing necrosis. One of us (JLV) used this form of therapy extensively during the early years of his practice.

VEINS MEASURING 1–3 MM IN DIAMETER

In these veins, concentrations of 23.4% hypertonic saline, 0.50–0.75% sodium tetradecyl sulfate or 0.75–1% polidocanol are usually successful in achieving sclerosis. The lower concentration (0.50%) should be used for the smaller vein size (near 1 mm). As the vein approaches 3 mm in diameter, the higher concentration may be utilized (0.75%).

VARICOSE VEINS 3–6 MM IN DIAMETER

These veins are best treated with concentrations of 1–3% sodium tetradecyl sulfate or 2–3% polidocanol. These concentrations are also useful in some small congenital vascular lesions of venous predominance with vessels ranging from 3 to 4 mm in diameter. Again, the lower concentrations should be used for the veins of smaller size.

LARGE VEINS SURROUNDING ULCERS OF THE LEGS

Sclerosis of these veins with 3% sodium tetradecyl sulfate or 3–4% polidocanol is successful in inducing thrombosis of the varix and is especially useful to control

Table 26.1 *Guidelines for surgery and sclerotherapy*

Vein size	Concentration of sclerosant		
	Hypertonic saline	Sodium tetradecyl sulfate (Sotradecol)	Polidocanol (Aethoxysklerol)
Telangiectasia (under 1 mm)	11.7–23.4%* + lidocaine	0.125–0.25%	0.5%
Veins 1–3 mm	15–23.4% + lidocaine	0.5–0.75%	0.75–1%
Veins 3–6 mm	–	1–3%	2–3%
Veins >6 mm	–	Surgical treatment	–
Saphenofemoral and saphenopopliteal junctions	–	Surgical treatment	–

*Smaller concentrations are used for smaller caliber veins.

an episode of bleeding. This method enhances healing of the ulcer while definitive measures for its treatment are considered (Fig. 26.5).

VARICOSITIES ASSOCIATED TO CONGENITAL VASCULAR ANOMALIES

Small hemangiomas or varicosities accompanying malformations such as the Klippel–Trenaunay syndrome may be treated with high concentrations of sclerotherapy agents such as 3% sodium tetradecyl sulfate or 4% polidocanol. Sclerotherapy in these cases is performed either to supplement surgery or as a sole form of treatment, when surgery cannot be performed and the patient needs some form of palliation (Fig. 26.6).

Sclerotherapy agents, particularly the detergent sclerosants, have recently been utilized in the form of foam. Even though this physical form of a sclerosant has been known as the air block technique since 1944, it is not until now that foam-sclerotherapy has been reintroduced.[17] Sadoun[17] states that the administration of sclerosing agents as microfoam into dilated varicose veins using a specific type of microbubbles, modifies the current conditions for sclerotherapy because the echogenicity of the microbubbles renders them visible using ultrasound color flow. In addition, the amount of active agent is greatly reduced and therefore its toxicity is diminished. The microfoam is injected and its course followed by echo-duplex. The volume injected varies between 20 and 80 ml of sodium tetradecyl sulfate or polidocanol. The real amount of the active agent delivered is 4–5 ml.

Cabrera *et al.* has had impressive results in the management of extensive congenital vascular malformations using microfoam sclerosants.[18]

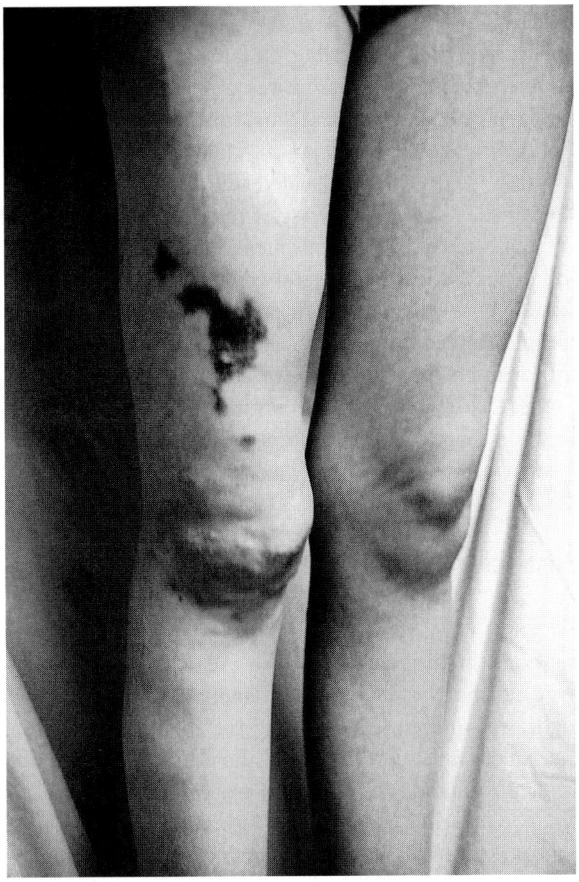

Figure 26.6 *Circumscribed venous dilatations (hemangiomas) often present in patients with congenital malformations of venous predominance, such as illustrated here, can be successfully treated by serial treatments with 2–3% sodium tetradecyl sulfate. Post-treatment compression for 1–2 weeks brings relief and decreases the venous hypertension in these patients.*

Materials

The following materials should be available:

- disposable 1–3 ml syringes (non-luer-lock);
- fine hypodermic needles 1/2 inch in length, short bevel, 27, 30 or 33 gauge;
- skin antiseptic agent;
- sterile gauze (10×10 cm), and other items for local compression such as dental rolls, foam rubber cushions, felt pad, etc.
- sclerosing agent. The syringes should be properly labeled with the concentration and nature of the material utilized;
- clear light source;
- magnifying loops (magnification × 2–3);
- caliper for vessel diameter measurement;
- external compression material, which may be in the form of elastic stockings (20–30 mm pressure), elastic bandages, or low-stretch material;
- no. 65 Beaver surgical blades with handle (for microthrombectomy);
- an emergency kit should be available in every room where sclerotherapy is performed. It should contain epinephrine solution 1:1000, injectable corticoids (Solu-Cortef, Solu-Medrol), heparin, diphenhydramine (Benadryl), Alupent inhaler and oxygen;
- a photographic camera with synchronized flash. A photo should be taken before and at least 16 weeks after the treatment. Patients often forget the pretreatment appearance. The photographic documentation may clear any misunderstandings.

TECHNIQUES OF SCLEROTHERAPY

General principles

Successful sclerotherapy is based first on the elimination of the reflux points. Often, this is best accomplished surgically. Once the reflux points have been controlled, the treatment should proceed as follows:

- large varices should be treated first and the small ones, last;
- from the most proximal varices to the most distal ones.

The small caliber veins should always be injected with minimal concentration of the sclerotherapy agent. Large veins are best treated with higher concentrations of the agent. The use of sclerosing solutions that are too strong for the size of the vein is still one of the most common errors and a potential source of complications.

Techniques for small veins (telangiectasia or spider veins)

Good lighting and magnification (× 2–3) are essential. Patients should be injected in the recumbent position beginning with injections on the area that the patient considers the 'worst area'. The technique of the 'air block' is useful in small veins and telangiectasia (Fig. 26.7). The tiny air bubbles will produce immediate blanching of the vein when the needle is correctly placed. The technique of air block may be abandoned when enough experience has been acquired. Small volumes of the agent minimize patient discomfort and prevent complications. Each injection should deliver from 0.25 ml to 0.5 ml. Immediately after the injection, the veins appear reddish and swollen as a consequence of local inflammation. A total volume of sclerosing agent of 2–4 ml may be injected during the first session, distributed among different areas. The total volume of hypertonic saline may be up to 10 ml. The injected area is compressed with a thick piece of gauze, foam rubber cushions, or dental rolls. Firm external compression is applied over the entire leg, care being taken to protect the flexion areas of the ankle and behind the knee. Thigh-high elastic stockings are more comfortable than elastic bandages, which tend to dislodge with patient activity. The compression is kept in place for a minimum of 3 days. One week later, the leg is examined and any thrombus is evacuated with a no. 65 Beaver blade. In small veins, a no. 22 needle is also effective. External compression is applied again for 3 days and the extremity is re-examined 1 week later. Patients are instructed to ambulate as much as possible and avoid prolonged standing or sitting positions.

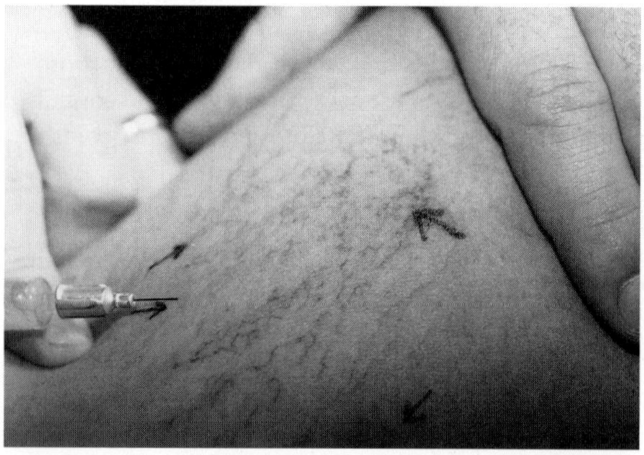

Figure 26.7 *The 'air-block' technique is illustrated here. The arrows point to areas of initial treatment. Slightly larger veins connecting with a rich network of telangiectasias should be first injected. A small amount of air mixed with a sclerosing agent (in this case, sodium tetradecyl sulfate), produces tiny air bubbles which can be readily seen during the slow injection of the sclerosing agent. A no. 30 needle is essential in the puncture of these tiny veins.*

Injection of veins 3–6 mm in diameter

The veins should be examined with the patient in the upright position. Injection is performed in the recumbent position. A tilting table is ideal for sclerotherapy. For larger veins, a quarter of an inch long, a 26–27 gauge needle is best. In this technique, the vein is punctured, the tilted table elevated and the injection performed into an empty vein. Aspiration of blood confirms the intravascular position of the needle. The volume injected depends on the caliber of the vessel. An amount of 0.5 ml is usually sufficient per vein site. Several sites along the course of the same vein may need to be injected. The total volume injected in different sites will depend on the sclerosing agent used and the manufacturer's specifications. After the injection has been completed, pressure is applied over the injected veins with a thick piece of gauze or a foam rubber cushion. Compression (20–30 mm pressure) should be applied at least for 1 week and should not be removed at all during this period.

Post-sclerotherapy compression

External compression may be applied by several methods including the use of elastic bandages, local padding and elastic stockings. Graduated compression is highly recommended, applying the higher pressures at the ankle and the lower at the knee. Compression applied by bandages can be of the elastic or nonelastic type. For sclerotherapy, the most commonly used bandages are elastic. The patient must be instructed to apply the bandage correctly and to identify any source of problems secondary to the improper application of the bandage. The correct application of an elastic bandage is an art and must be taught to the health professional. Additional compression may be applied in special areas by using rubber cushions or folded gauze. The aim is to produce apposition of the inflamed vein walls and avoid thrombus formation.

COMPRESSION STOCKINGS

Graduated compression stockings are available in below-the-knee, above-the-knee, mid-thigh, thigh-high and other styles. The type of stocking to be recommended will be determined by the anatomy of the extremity, as well as by the type of varicosity injected. Compression stockings are available as class I (10–20 mmHg), class II (20–30 mmHg), class III (30–40 mmHg) and class IV (40–50 mmHg). The stockings should be worn during the entire period of treatment.

Post-injection thrombectomy

Following the injection of a sclerosing agent into veins of any size, it is common that, despite adequate compression, a thrombus forms within the injected veins. When left *in situ*, the thrombus organizes and the blood turns into hemosiderin, transforming the blue vein into a brownish cord. This is an adverse event called pigmentation. It occurs in approximately 20% of cases and usually fades away in 80% of the patients within 2 years.

The thrombus or intravascular hematoma, as it is also known, may be easily evacuated during the first 2–3 weeks after the injection, thus diminishing the amount of trapped blood and consequently the amount of hemosiderin. It has been the experience of many investigators that the early evacuation of the thrombus leads to decreased incidence and severity of pigmentation. There has been, however, no randomized study proving or disproving this observation. Even though the ideal time to evacuate the thrombus is during the first 2–3 weeks when the material has not become organized, evacuation of thrombus has been successful in some cases even after 8 weeks post-injection.

TECHNIQUE

Veins 1 mm or less

Thrombectomy of veins of this size can be successfully performed using loop magnification and the tip of a no. 65 Beaver blade or a microsurgical knife. A 22 gauge needle may be used for telangiectasia. The Beaver scalpel is an extremely sharp instrument, superior to the no. 11 blade. After skin asepsis, a quick needle puncture or mini-stab incision (1.5 mm) is performed. Anesthesia is not necessary since the procedure is relatively painless. A good rule of thumb is to make one puncture or mini-stab incision every 3 mm along the entire length of the thrombosed vein (Fig. 26.8). Once the incision has been made, gentle extrusion of the thrombus can be performed between two cotton swabs. Efforts to extrude the trapped blood through two or three mini-stab incisions or needle punctures in a long segment of vein usually result in incomplete evacuation of the thrombus.

Veins larger than 1 mm

Larger veins need to be thrombectomized through 2 mm mini-stab incisions placed 3 mm apart along the axis of the vein. Incisions should be made with the no. 65 Beaver blade. Satisfactory thrombus extrusion cannot be obtained through needle punctures. In large veins (3–5 mm in diameter), gentle extrusion of the thrombus is performed between the tips of the gloved fingers. Gloves should be utilized in all microthrombectomy procedures.

At the end of the procedure, compression is applied with a folded sterile 10×10 cm gauze. A Kerlix gauze bandage secures the compression pads in place. External compression is applied with an elastic stocking or elastic bandage. In the case of veins under 1 mm, compression is used only for 24 hours. In larger veins, it is recommended that compression be maintained for a minimum

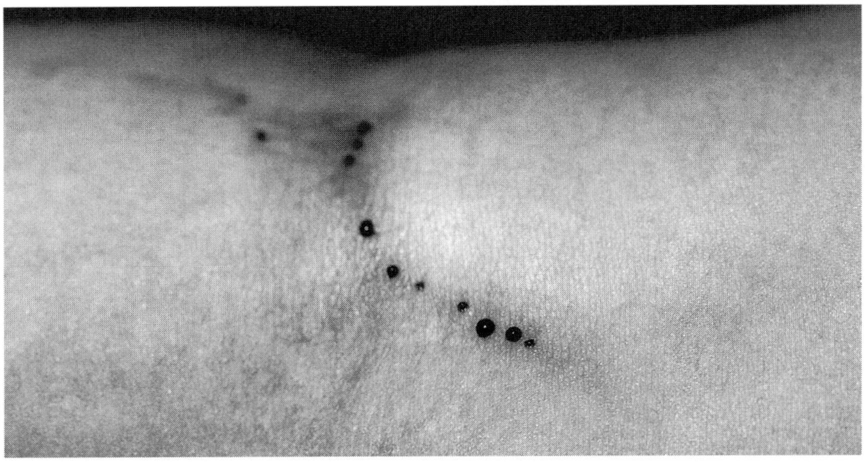

Figure 26.8 *A thrombus forms quite frequently after the sclerosing injection of any size vein. The thrombus turns into hemosiderin, which may transform the blue vein into a brownish cord. Microthrombectomy, using a microsurgical blade and 'Q' tips, clears the veins of thrombus and diminishes the possibilities for pigmentation.*

of 3 days. A follow-up 'retouch' visit to clear any remaining thrombus is scheduled for 1 week later. Photographs of the treated areas should be obtained before and 12–16 weeks after the procedure.

COMPLICATIONS

Every sclerosing agent may have undesirable reactions. The most common complications and side-effects of sclerotherapy are as follows.

PIGMENTATION

Brown streaks develop in 10–30% of all patients treated for essential telangiectasia (Fig. 26.9); in 80% of the cases, they resolve spontaneously between 6 and 24 months. Pigmentation can be observed with any of the sclerotherapy agents described, including saline. Microthrombectomy, by removing the thrombus that contains the mixture of red cells and sclerosing agent, may diminish the incidence of pigmentation. A prospective randomized study comparing thrombectomized versus non-thrombectomized areas is underway.

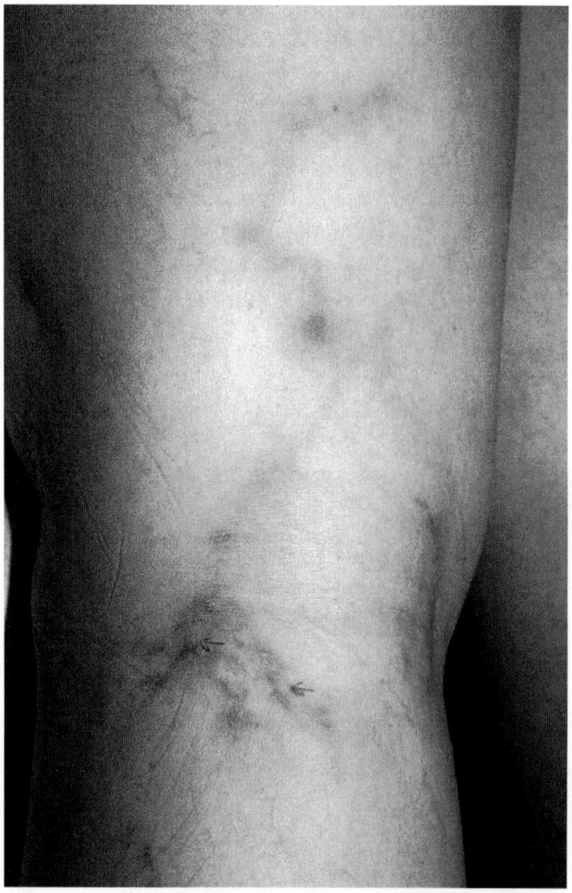

Figure 26.9 *A common post-sclerotherapy adverse event is the development of pigmentation in the injected veins. In 80% of the cases, it fades spontaneously between 1 and 2 years. In other cases, it may be permanent.*

TRANSIENT EDEMA AND SWELLING

This complication occurs in almost every patient and begins shortly after injection. This is an expected inflammatory reaction that produces mild discomfort during the first 5–10 minutes post-injection.

ECCHYMOSIS

Ecchymosis occurs in about 20% of the patients, especially in older individuals with fragile skin. It usually fades after the second or third week.

PAIN, TENDERNESS AND DISCOMFORT

The injection of most sclerosing agents produces a certain degree of pain and discomfort, which gradually disappears and is greatly relieved by compression.

THROMBOPHLEBITIS

The injection of a sclerosing agent produces acute inflammation of the vein. Often a thrombus is formed at the injected site and may involve veins located several inches away from the site of the injection. To prevent this occurrence, the amount of substance injected should be small (usually 0.5 ml or less) and compression should be applied on the injected vein immediately after the injection.

SKIN NECROSIS

Skin necrosis (Fig. 26.10) is usually the result of the following:

- too high concentration of a sclerosing agent for the size of selected vein;
- extravasation;
- excessive pressure in the syringe;
- fast injection;
- injection into a skin arteriole (red spider veins).

INEFFECTIVE INJECTION

This is usually the result of an inadequate concentration of the sclerosing agent for the size of the vein chosen. The physician observes that the vein persists at the injected site. A second injection with a higher concentration is usually effective.

DEEP VENOUS THROMBOSIS

This complication is rare. However, it has been reported by several authors and is associated with injections into large segments of varicose veins ranging in size from 8 mm or more, using high concentration agents. Difficulty in mobilization of the patient, bed rest, or sitting for prolonged periods of time contributes to increase the

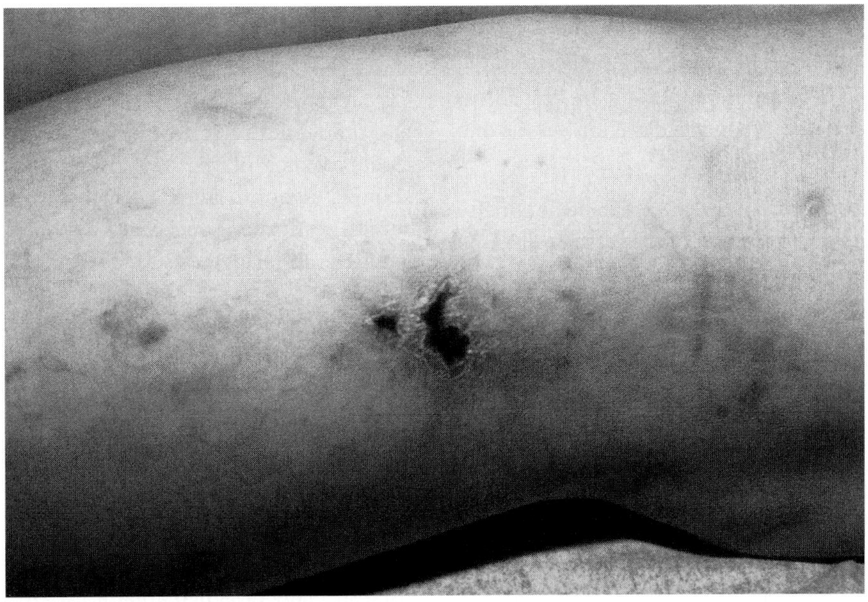

Figure 26.10 *Skin necrosis following an extravascular injection of a sclerosing agent. Concentration of the agent should be in direct relationship with the caliber of the vein. This complication may also occur if the injection is performed into the so-called 'red telangiectasias' which may be in connection with skin arterioles.*

incidence of this complication. If unusual swelling or pain develops after the injection, the deep system should be examined with duplex scanning as soon as possible.

ANAPHYLACTIC REACTIONS

This complication has been greatly reduced with the use of the modern and more purified sclerotherapy agents. However, any physician performing sclerotherapy should be prepared to manage a major anaphylactic reaction. A kit containing oxygen, epinephrine and injectable steroids should be available at all times.

MATTING

Matting is the development of a reddish area of very fine vessels that appear in the surroundings of the injected vein. It occurs in 10–30% of all patients treated for telangiectasia and in about 15% of all patients treated for larger vessels (Fig. 26.11). Matting often resolves spontaneously within a year. Sometimes the problem may be permanent. Hormone therapy and obesity contribute to a higher incidence of matting. Laser treatment seems to be beneficial in some cases.

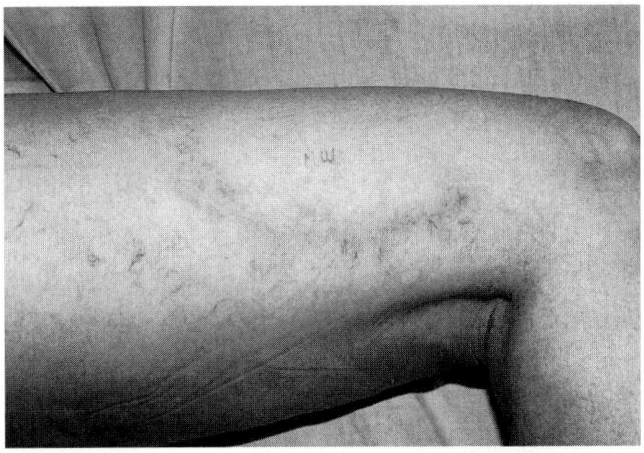

Figure 26.11 *A rare complication of sclerotherapy, especially in 'overtreated' areas is the presence of a fine reddish network of extremely small veins in the area of the treated varicosities. This adverse event is called matting and may occur after treating spider veins or larger varicosities, as was the case in this patient.*

VISUAL MANIFESTATIONS

Bright lights, migraine headaches, dizziness and hypotension are rare manifestations, but the physician should be aware of its occurrence. They occur usually after injection of relatively large volumes of sclerosant.

INTRA-ARTERIAL INJECTION

This complication is serious and often leads to gangrene. There are certain dangerous areas that should be avoided. The posterior tibial artery is susceptible to this complication because of its superficial position. The saphenofemoral and saphenopopliteal junctions are high-risk areas and should always be approached surgically.

COMPRESSION AFTER SCLEROTHERAPY

Although there are physicians who do not use compression after a session of sclerotherapy, there are reasons to suggest that compression is beneficial even in vessels of a small diameter:[19]

- A more effective fibrosis of the vessel can be obtained when there is direct apposition of the vessel walls.
- Compression will decrease the extent of thrombus formation in the injected vessel. When the thrombus is minimized there is a lesser degree of pigmentation.
- Good compression will improve the efficiency of the calf muscle pump and will prevent the extension of the thrombi into the deep system.
- Compression decreases the amount of discomfort secondary to the injection. The duration of compression for veins other than telangiectasia must be for a minimum of 1 week. In most European centers that follow the schools of Sigg and Fegan, compression is applied for 3 weeks.

RESULTS

Excellent results can be obtained when the principles and guidelines of sclerotherapy are followed. Complete disappearance of the varicosities may be observed as soon as a month after a single treatment. Most often, several sessions are necessary to eliminate the unsightly venules and telangiectasias (Fig. 26.12).

THE ROLE OF LASER AND ELECTRODESICCATION IN THE MANAGEMENT OF TELANGIECTASIA

Electrodesiccation has been used extensively by our group in the management of telangiectasias and other venous blemishes, from 1968 to 1982. Even though we used specially designed apparatuses to vary the intensity of the electrical current necessary to destroy the tiny

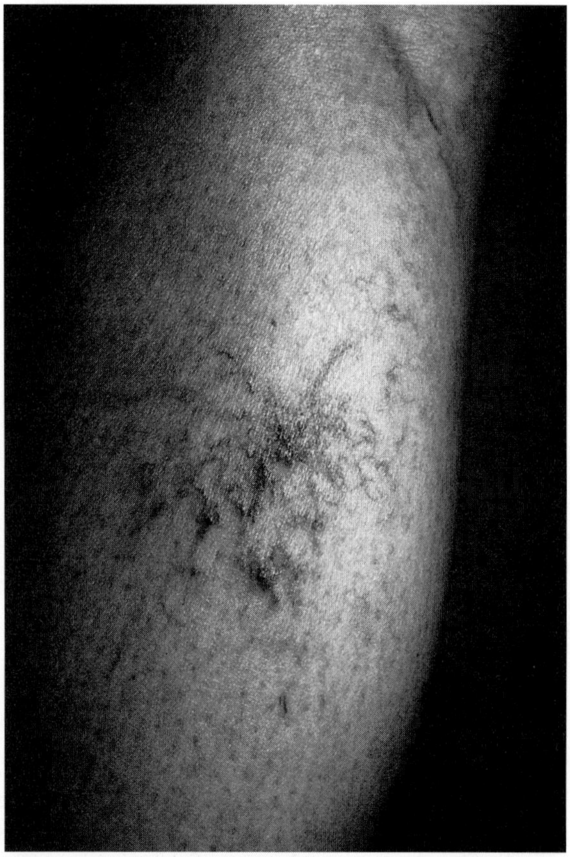

(a)

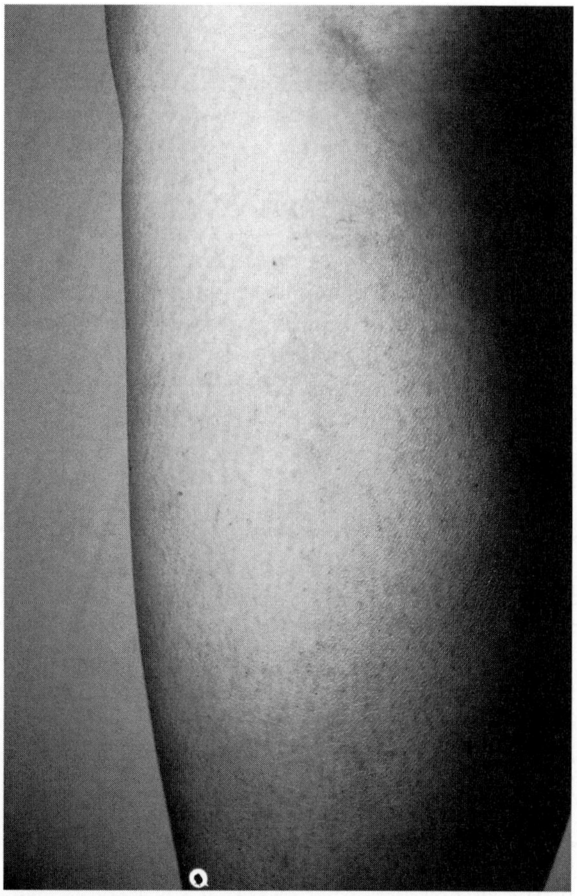

(b)

Figure 26.12 *(a) Typical cluster of venous lakes, telangiectasias and small venules in the posterior aspect of the calf. Surgery is completely ineffective in these cases. (b) After 5 sessions and 11 months, excellent results can be observed. (Courtesy Dr D Duffy)* cutaneous vessels, the procedure produced varying degrees of pain and small hypopigmented scars. In an effort to decrease or prevent the dermal necrosis induced by electrodesiccation, special insulated superfine needles were developed by the electromedical industry. The needles have an insulated shaft which leaves bare 1 mm at the tip. This allows the needle to be introduced, producing minimal dermal scarring. Since the procedure produces varying degrees of pain, and patients have different tolerance levels to the electrical stimuli, we choose to utilize a light epidural anesthesia in patients with extensive telangiectasias on both extremities. In this manner, with the assistance of a second operator, in one single session, both extremities can be treated simultaneously. The attractiveness of this modality of treatment is that it saves the patient a considerable amount of time, decreases the amount of office visits and, especially, eliminates completely the pain factor.

Lasers were received with great enthusiasm in 1975 and many centers acquired the costly machines that promised to be the solution for the problem of telangiectasias and other skin blemishes. However, laser's adverse effects, such as cutaneous necrosis, varying degrees of pain similar to electrodesiccation, hypo- or hyperpigmentation, and its relative ineffectiveness compared with sclerotherapy, have been powerful reasons to abandon this method for the management of the blue telangiectasias. Recently, new forms of lasers have been introduced as effective treatment for capillary hemangiomas, such as the port-wine stain of some congenital vascular malformations, and in the management of red telangiectasias, post-sclerotherapy pigmentation, and other adverse effects of sclerotherapy.[20,21] Laser and pulsed light are used to treat smaller spider veins, especially on the face and upper body. Red spider veins, also called telangiectasias, respond well to laser treatment on the face. Even though there are promising newer lasers in development, at the present time, this procedure is of limited value for the treatment of lower-extremity spider veins. It should be recognized that laser and pulsed light treatments also may cause scarring.[22]

DISCLAIMER

These guidelines represent the consensus of a group of physicians with expertise in sclerotherapy. They should not be considered, however, as the only manner to practice sclerotherapy. It is recognized that there are alternative techniques that render acceptable results. The statements and recommendations contained in these guidelines are general in nature. Every patient needs to be considered and treated on an individual basis. The final decision on the procedure of choice rests on the physician after he has analyzed the needs of the patient.

REFERENCES

1. Trendelenburg FV. Uber Die Unterbindung Der Vena Saphena Magna Bei Unterschenkel Varizen. *Beitr Klin Chir* 1890; **7**:195.
2. Keller WL. A new method of extirpating the internal saphenous and similar veins in varicose conditions: a preliminary report. *N Y Med J* 1905; **82**: 385.
3. Mayo CH. The surgical treatment of varicose veins. *St Paul Med J* 1904; **6**: 695.
4. Mayo CH. Treatment of varicose veins. *Surg Gynecol Obstet* 1906; **2**: 385.
5. Babcock WW. A new operation for the extirpation of varicose veins of the leg. *N Y Med J* 1907; **86**: 153.
6. McPheeters HO. Injection treatment of varicose veins by the use of sclerosing solutions. *Surg Gynecol Obstet* 1927; **45**: 541–7.
7. Dixon FC. The results of injection treatment of varicose veins. *Proc Staff Meet Mayo Clin* 1930; **5**: 42.
8. McPheeters HO. Injection treatment of varicose veins. *Am J Surg* 1930; **10**: 19–31.
9. De Takats G. Causes of failure in the treatment of varicose veins. *J Am Med Assoc* 1931; **96**: 1111–14.
10. Smith FL. Varicose veins, complications and results of treatment of 5,000 patients. *Milit Surg* 1939; **85**: 514.
11. Ochsner A, Mahorner HR. The modern treatment of varicose veins. *Surgery* 1937; **2**: 889.
12. Waugh JM. Ligation and injection of great saphenous veins. *Proc Staff Meet Mayo Clin* 1941; **16**: 832.
13. Hobbs JT. Surgery and sclerotherapy in the treatment of varicose veins. *Arch Surg* 1974; **109**: 793–6.
14. Einarsson E, Eklof B, Neglen P. Sclerotherapy or surgery for varicose veins: a prospective, randomized study. *Phlebology* 1993; **8**: 22–6.
15. Myers TT. Results and technique of a stripping operation for varicose veins. *J Am Med Assoc* 1957; **163**: 87.
16. Bishop CCR, Fronek HS, Fronek A, Dile RB, Bernstein EF. Real time color duplex scanning sclerotherapy of the greater saphenous vein. *J Vasc Surg* 1991; **14**: 505–8.
17. Sadoun S, Benigni JP. La Mousse de sclerosant: etat de l'art. In Rabe E, Gerlach H, Lechner W, eds. *Phlebology 1999*. Cologne: Viavital Verlag GmbH, 1999: 146.
18. Cabrera GJ, Garcia-Olmedo MA, Cabrera J Jr. Microfoam sclerotherapy. A new concept in sclerotherapy. Long-term results. [Escleroterapia en microespuma: Nuevo Concepto En Escleroterapia. Resultados a Largo Plazo] *Rev Panam Flebologia y Linfol* 1999; **34**: 29–37.
19. Weiss RA, Sadick NS, Goldman MP, Weiss MA. Post-sclerotherapy compression: controlled comparative study of duration of compression and its effects on clinical outcome. *Dermatol Surg* 1999; **25**: 105–8.
20. Goldman MP, Fitzpatrick RE. Pulsed dye laser treatment of leg telangiectasia: with and without simultaneous sclerotherapy. *J Dermatol Surg Oncol* 1990; **16**: 338–44.
21. Goldman MP. Post-sclerotherapy hyperpigmentation: treatment with a flashlamp excited pulsed dye laser. *J Dermatol Surg Oncol* 1992; **18**: 417–22.

22. Villavicencio JL, Lohr J, Pfeifer JR, Duffy D, Weiss R. Getting a leg up on varicose vein treatment choices. Ad Hoc Committee on Sclerotherapy. The American Venous Forum. Federal Trade Commission brochure, November 1999.

SUGGESTED READING

Bergan JJ, Goldman MP, eds. *Varicose and Telangiectatic Leg Veins: Diagnosis and Treatment.* St Louis, MO: Quality Medical Publishing, 1993.

Bergan JJ, Yao JST. *Venous Disorders.* Philadelphia: WB Saunders, 1991.

Bodian EL. Techniques of sclerotherapy for sunburst venous blemishes. *J Dermatol Surg Oncol* 1985; **11**: 696–704.

Bohler-Sommeregger K, Karnel F, Schuller-Petrovic S, *et al.* Do telangiectasia communicate with the deep venous system? *J Dermatol Surg Oncol* 1992; **18**: 403–6.

Browse NL, Burnand KG, Thomas ML. *Diseases of the Veins: Pathology, Diagnosis and Treatment.* Baltimore: Edward Arnold, 1988.

Carlin MC, Ratz JL. Treatment of telangiectasia: comparison of sclerosing agents. *J Dermatol Surg Oncol* 1987; **13**: 1181–4.

Dodd H, Cockett FB. *Pathology and Surgery of the Veins of the Lower Limb*, 2nd edn. Edinburgh: Churchill Livingstone, 1976: 106.

Duffy DM. Small vessel sclerotherapy: an overview. *Adv Dermatol* 1988; **3**: 221–42.

Fegan GW. Treatment of varicose veins by injection compression: a method practiced in Eire. In Hobbs JT, ed. *The Treatment of Venous Disorders.* Philadelphia: JB Lippincott, 1977: 99–112.

Fegan WG. Continuous compression technique of injecting varicose veins. *Lancet* 1963; **2**: 109–12.

Goldman MP. *Sclerotherapy Treatment of Varicose and Telangiectatic Leg Veins*, 2nd edn. St Louis, MO: Mosby Yearbook, 1995.

Goldman MP, Bennett RG. Treatment of telangiectasia: a review. *J Am Acad Dermatol* 1987; **17**: 167–82.

Goldman MP, Weiss RA, Bergan JJ. Diagnosis and treatment of varicose veins, a review. *J Am Acad Dermatol* 1994: **31**: 393–413.

Goren G. Injection sclerotherapy for varicose veins; history and effectiveness. *Phlebology* 1991; **6**: 7–11.

Green D. Mechanism of action of sclerotherapy. *Semin Dermatol* 1993; **12**: 88–97.

Hobbs JT. The management of varicose veins. *Surg Annu* 1980; **12**: 169.

Imhoff E, Stemmer R. Classification and mechanism of action of sclerosing agents. *Phlebologie* 1969; **22**: 145–8.

Neglen P, Einarsson E, Eklof B. High tie with sclerotherapy for saphenous vein insufficiency. *Phlebology* 1986; **1**: 105–11.

Sadick NS. Sclerotherapy of varicose and telangiectatic leg veins: minimal sclerosant concentration of hypertonic saline and its relationship to vessel diameter. *J Dermatol Surg Oncol* 1991; **17**: 65–70.

Villavicencio JL, Gomez ER, Coffey JA, Lauer CG, Rich NM. What the vascular surgeon should know about sclerotherapy in the management of varicose veins. In Veith FJ, ed. *Current Critical Problems in Vascular Surgery*, Vol 3. St Louis, MO: Quality Medical Publishing, 1991: 128–34.

Weiss RA, Weiss MA. Doppler ultrasound findings in reticular veins of the thigh, subdermic lateral venous system, and implications for sclerotherapy. *J Dermatol Surg Oncol* 1993; **19**: 947–52.

27

Sclerotherapy of telangiectasia

ROBERT A WEISS AND MARGARET A WEISS

Sclerotherapy, when performed properly, is not only a markedly effective treatment for telangiectasia but a highly effective adjunct to venous surgery. Sclerotherapy allows rapid treatment of large networks of reticular varicose veins that branch from and coexist with axial varicosities. Although surgery by the ambulatory stab avulsion technique may be performed on reticular veins,[1] it is time consuming, requires multiple sessions and may require extensive amounts of local anesthesia in patients with reticular extensive networks (Fig. 27.1).

Treating extensive reticular networks is important as the volume of blood sequestered and stagnant in these reticular veins and associated telangiectatic webs may produce symptoms of venous hypertension. In a survey of 350 patients, it was reported that the most common symptom of telangiectasias was a sensation of muscle fatigue in the affected legs with localized pain or burning in the region of telangiectasias and/or small reticular varicosities.[2] Symptoms were worsened by prolonged standing or sitting as reported by flight attendants and these symptoms are significantly relieved by the wearing of ready-to-wear support hose.[3]

Vein size alone does not predict the presence of symptoms.[4] The size of the vessels causing symptoms

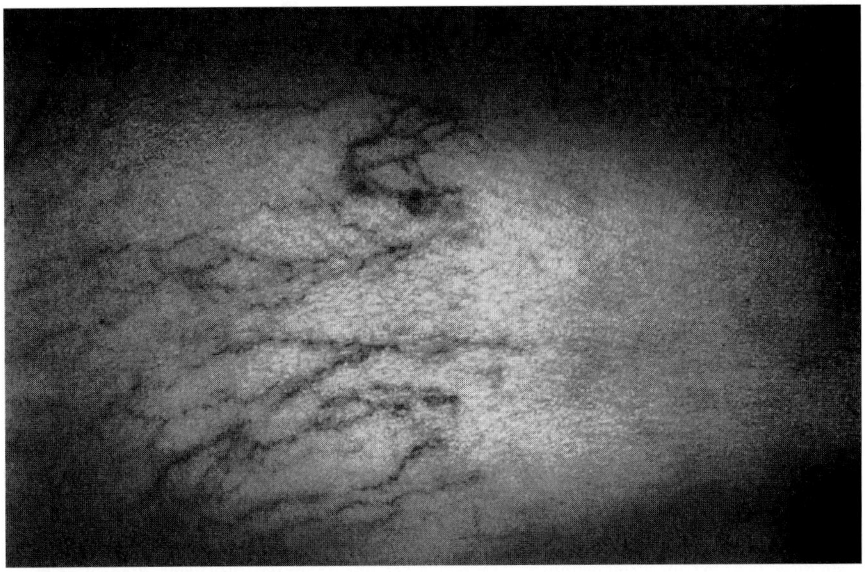

Figure 27.1 *Extensive network of reticular veins. Patient has multiple reticular veins associated with webs of telangiectasia. This clinical situation is not very amenable to surgery.*

may be very small, even 1–2 mm in diameter or less. Lofgren observed that veins of small caliber may give rise to surprising pain, whilst larger varicosities often caused no symptoms of pain.[5] It is our belief from observation of nearly 14 000 patients that reticular varicosities associated with telangiectatic webs are highly unrecognized causes of leg pain in young and middle-aged women.

In addition, the appearance of the telangiectatic veins may be so disturbing to females that they will not bare their legs in public, foregoing major outdoor activities and thus limiting lifestyle. Sclerotherapy not only offers the possibility of remarkable cosmetic results but is likely to yield an 85% reduction in symptoms when performed properly.[2]

The assumption that experience with venipuncture confers expertise in sclerotherapy is a common error. Successful treatment not only requires the proper technique but is dependent on knowledge of concentrations of sclerosing solutions and proper use of compression. Although reported techniques for sclerotherapy of different types and sizes of varicose and telangiectatic leg veins vary greatly, there are basic principles which are universal.[6–9] Expertise in sclerotherapy is best attained by not only reviewing written accounts of proper technique but by direct observation.

Patients may present with telangiectatic webs with or without associated axial varicosities due to junctional or large perforator incompetence. Therefore a detailed history with physical examination will be useful to select those patients requiring further noninvasive diagnostic evaluation prior to treatment.[10] Detection and elimination of the larger sources of reflux must be accomplished prior to undertaking treatment of telangiectasias. This is to prevent treatment failure by recanalization in a higher flow setting and to minimize post-sclerosis pigmentation, which occurs when treated telangiectasia become packed with red blood cells from high-pressure reflux into a treated site.[9] Duplex study of patients presenting for treatment of 'cosmetic' leg veins demonstrated a relatively high incidence of early associated axial reflux.[11]

This may be explained by arborizing networks of telangiectasias being dilated cutaneous venules with intrinsic connections to underlying larger veins.[12,13] Valves may be found throughout the postcapillary venous system regulating flow within the smallest of venules.[14] Thus increased venous pressure could be transmitted directly in a cascade effect, with the increased pressure causing increased diameter and incompetence of venous valves from the reticular veins to telangiectasias.

The microanatomy responsible for the transmission of venous hypertension into telangiectasias via reticular varicosities was recently diagrammed with the use of high-resolution duplex ultrasound by Somjen (Fig. 27.2).[15] The reticular vein is a thin-walled blue superficial venulectasia thought to be part of a network of subcuticular veins communicating with the venous system via direct connections to the saphenous system or by small perforating veins that can course through superficial and/or deep fascia. These reticular veins are commonly called 'feeder' veins since the assumption is that reflux through them causes the groups of telangi-

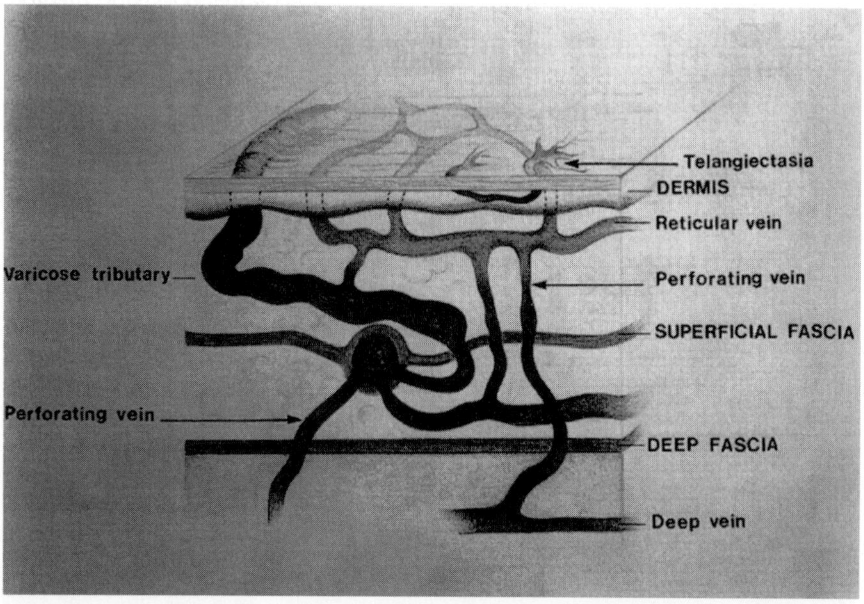

Figure 27.2 *Schematic of reticular anatomy. Microanatomy of telangiectasias associated with reticular veins demonstrating connection to deep vein directly or to superficial venous system by way of normal or varicose veins. (Reprinted by permission of Elsevier from Somjen GM, Ziegenbein R, Johnston AH, Royle JP. Anatomical examination of leg telangiectases with duplex scanning [see comments].* J Dermatol Surg Oncol *1993;* ***19****: 940–5).*

ectasias. Tretbar has shown by Doppler studies that free reflux with augmentation is usually heard through the reticular veins, and sometimes in an upwards pattern against the flow of gravity.[16] In approximately 50% of these patients, the reticular veins appear to be tributaries of larger calf incompetent perforators.

CLASSIFICATION AND ANATOMY

In order to diagnose and treat telangiectasias in a logical way, a precise classification is helpful (Table 27.1). A discussion of painful and cosmetic telangiectasias includes telangiectasias (type 1), venulectasias (type 2) and associated blue reticular veins (type 3). For the purposes of sclerotherapy of telangiectasias, it will be assumed that the major primary varicose veins of type 4 (branch) and type 5 (truncal) have already been eliminated by other means or are absent.

Table 27.1 *Classification of veins*

Type I	Telangiectasia (spider veins); 0.1–1 mm diameter; usually red
Type IA	Telangiectatic matting (red network)
Type II	Venulectasia; 1–2 mm diameter; violaceous
Type IIA	Venulectatic matting (violaceous network)
Type III	Reticular varicosities (feeder veins); 2–4 mm diameter; cyanotic blue to blue green
Type IV	Nonsaphenous varicosities (saphenous tributary); 3–8 mm diameter; blue to blue-green or colorless if deeper
Type V	Saphenous varicosities (truncal or axial varicosities); 5 mm diameter or greater; blue to blue-green, colorless if deeper, may be palpable and not visible

Adapted from Weiss RA, Weiss MA. Sclerotherapy. In Wheeland RG, ed. *Cutaneous Surgery*. Philadelphia, WB Saunders, 1994: 951–81.

LATERAL VENOUS SYSTEM

Originally described by Albanese,[17] the lateral venous system consists of reticular veins at a depth just below the dermis, longitudinally traversing the lateral and posterior thigh and calf often having more complex communications at the lateral knee (Fig. 27.3). This system may become varicose often in the absence of saphenous system varicosities. In our experience, these lateral minor varicosities present initially at a younger age (teens through thirties), typically several decades before the onset of the 'major' varicosities. Onset earlier than most varicosities may be apparent from study of the embryology of the venous system of the leg.

Based on the studies of Hochstetter,[18] during the earliest stages of formation of the venous system of the leg, the predominant system is a network of superficial veins from which the lateral venous system is derived. During the next phase the deep venous system develops in a rudimentary way and the superficial external saphenous vein is dominant, connected by small perforators to the deep system. When the deep veins become predominant, the external saphenous vein disintegrates at the thigh but not without leaving a few thigh perforators intact. Albanese speculates that in areas where the superficial veins do not involute, the superficial embryonic veins remain and may become easily and prematurely varicose.[17] This occurs for three reasons:

- these veins are poorly supported by surrounding connective tissue because of their superficial location;
- direct transfascial perforators continue to connect them with the deep system; and
- many of these perforators rely on support of surrounding fascia which becomes loosened by the large movements of the knee.

With perforators at the lateral knee serving as a direct source of transmission of high pressure from the deep venous system accompanied by a lack of structural support, 'reticular' veins may easily become stretched and distended. The term minor varicose vein is fully justified for these lateral thigh reticular veins.

Our continuous-wave (CW) Doppler findings confirm that reflux through the lateral subdermic venous system is very frequently responsible for large areas of telangiectatic webs on the lateral and posterior thighs.[15,19] This reticular plexus also extends down the calf and is often responsible for telangiectatic webs on the lateral and posterior calf as well. Both CW Doppler and duplex findings concur that perforating veins in the region of the knee allow communications between the lateral subdermic reticular system and the deep venous system, particularly the popliteal and femoral veins.[19] In addition, there are mid-lateral thigh perforators and mid-lateral calf perforators which are connected to the lateral venous system and may contribute reflux as well.

The great importance of heredity as a factor in the development of thigh reticular varicose veins is confirmed by an epidemiologic study of the female Japanese population.[20] Intradermal venectasia, colored red-purple, often located on the thigh or knee, were included as a separate category. These 'web-type' varicosities were not reported to increase in frequency with age as did the saphenous types. The conclusion was that pre-existing factors were most important.

STEPS PRIOR TO TREATMENT

Every patient must initially be evaluated by detailed history with regards to contraindications such as a history of venous thrombosis and diabetes. Previous venous surgery may warrant further testing before

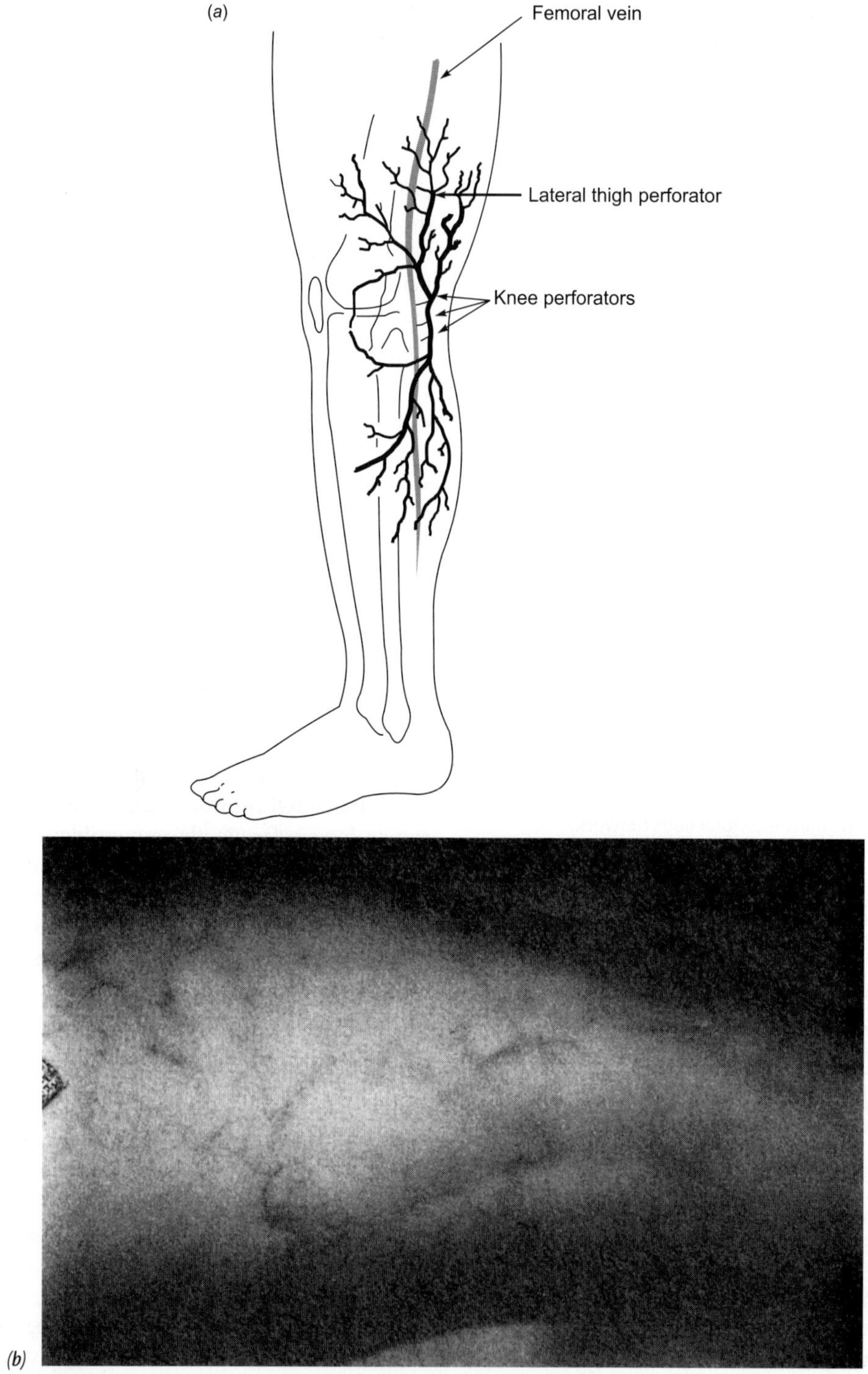

Figure 27.3 *(a) Schematic of lateral venous system. (Reprinted by permission from Mosby in Goldman MP, Weiss RA, Bergan JJ. Diagnosis and treatment of varicose veins – a review [review].* J Am Acad Dermatol *1994;* ***31****(Part 1): 393–413) (b) Clinical appearance of varicose lateral venous system in a 25-year-old female on the right lateral thigh gradually enlarging since age 16. One telangiectatic web is associated with a dominant reticular venous system. This patient had symptoms of aching, fatigue, burning and night cramps which disappeared when the varicosity was eliminated by sclerotherapy.*

proceeding. Family history is also influential as those patients with a family history of large varicose veins are more likely to have early axial reflux even when presenting with telangiectasias alone.[10,21,22]

Physical examination is performed by viewing the patient's legs in a 360° rotation so that common sites of major reflux are observed. Palpation is sometimes performed along the saphenous veins to rule out early varicosities which cannot be seen. Based on the history and physical examination, noninvasive diagnostic vascular tests, including Doppler, plethysmography and duplex ultrasound, are performed as necessary.[23] Once the patient is judged to be a candidate for sclerotherapy, it is necessary to obtain informed consent. This consists of a detailed discussion of the potential complications such as hyperpigmentation, matting and ulceration. We now show a video which graphically depicts the common side-effects. The necessity for multiple treatment sessions is emphasized. Once the patient understands the risks and signs the consent form, photographs or digital images of the areas to be treated are taken. These serve to evaluate treatment progress and allow the patient to recognize improvement.

Patients are told to wear shorts and not to use moisturizers or shave their legs on the day of treatment. Shaving the leg may cause erythematous streaks, making it difficult to visualize patterns of reticular and telangiectatic veins. Use of moisturizers causes poor adhesion of tape used to secure compression following injections and causes slower evaporation of alcohol. More alcohol retention on the skin will cause increased stinging with skin puncture.

Patients are encouraged to eat at least a small meal beforehand in order to minimize vasovagal reactions. The room in which sclerotherapy is performed is kept cool to minimize vasovagal reactions. The first treatment session is usually limited to one or two sites in order to observe the patient for allergic reactions, ability to tolerate the burning or cramping of a hypertonic solution, judge the effectiveness of a particular concentration and class of sclerosing agent, and to observe any reactions to the tape used for compression. The patient returns in 4–6 weeks to compare the test site with pretreatment photographs or digital images. At each session, all sites treated are noted in anatomic diagrams in the chart (Fig. 27.4).

TREATMENT OF RETICULAR VEINS

The basic principle of treatment from the largest to the smallest varicosities should be applied to all sizes of veins. Treatment begins with injection of the reticular veins, then venulectasias, then telangiectatic webs or networks and finally to the smallest and most isolated telangiectasias.

The CW Doppler findings have been used to identify sources of reflux into telangiectatic groups.[9] For example, a group of telangiectasias on the lateral thigh are known to have associated reticular veins which are part of a varicose lateral subdermic venous system; the loudest Doppler flow signal can often be traced between the lateral femoral condyle and superior to the fibular head.[9] Knowledge of this anatomy of perforating veins suggests that injections be initiated at this site of the knee and continued every 3–4 cm following the course of the reticular vein. Usually no more than 0.5 ml sclerosing solution per injection site is necessary, although some longer reticular veins may require up to 1 ml of solution.

A frequently asked question is whether injection of solution into a reticular vein in association with telangiectasias obviates the need to inject the telangiectasias directly. The answer is that sclerosing solution is invariably diluted in the process of flowing from the reticular into the telangiectatic vein, thus becoming less potent. Sclerosant may also be inactivated by binding or interacting with blood proteins. Furthermore, sclerosant may be lost by leakage through damaged endothelium. If insufficient concentration or quantity of sclerosing solution contacts the wall of a telangiectasia, then it may not respond. A poor response by telangiectasias may be seen even with a good response with decrease in size or disappearance of injected reticular veins.[24] Thus even though reflux through a reticular vein may be eliminated by its destruction with sclerotherapy, the associated telangiectasias may no longer have the elasticity to contract without elimination by effective sclerosis. The telangiectasias must therefore be injected in addition.

The next question that arises is if telangiectasias are treated separately, should they be treated during a subsequent visit? The French phlebologists prefer to treat reticular veins at a separate session so that they may observe the effects of treatment. They argue that unless the reticular vein has been properly eliminated, the telangiectasia is unlikely to respond properly even if treated by the correct technique. We believe that results will be seen sooner if the end point of a sclerotherapy session is contraction of the reticular veins and swelling, loss of distinctive boundaries and/or darkening of the telangiectasias. Therefore treatment is performed of both at the same session until the proper end point is observed. When no clear feeder vessel is seen or identified by Doppler, then the point at which the telangiectasias begin to branch out is the site at which to begin injection.

INJECTION TECHNIQUE

Injection of reticular veins is very similar to large varicose veins, although the concentrations, strength and volume of sclerosing solutions are decreased (Table 27.2). The patient is recumbent and a 3 ml syringe with a 27–30 gauge needle bent to an angle of 10–30° is inserted into the reticular vein, which is usually superficial and visibly blue, and therefore usually does not require preliminary marking by pen. When the sensation of piercing the vein is felt, the plunger is pulled back with the thumb of the dominant hand gently until blood is seen beginning to back up into the transparent plastic hub (Fig. 27.5a,b) This is possible even with a 30 gauge needle. If the wall of the reticular vein is very thin, the

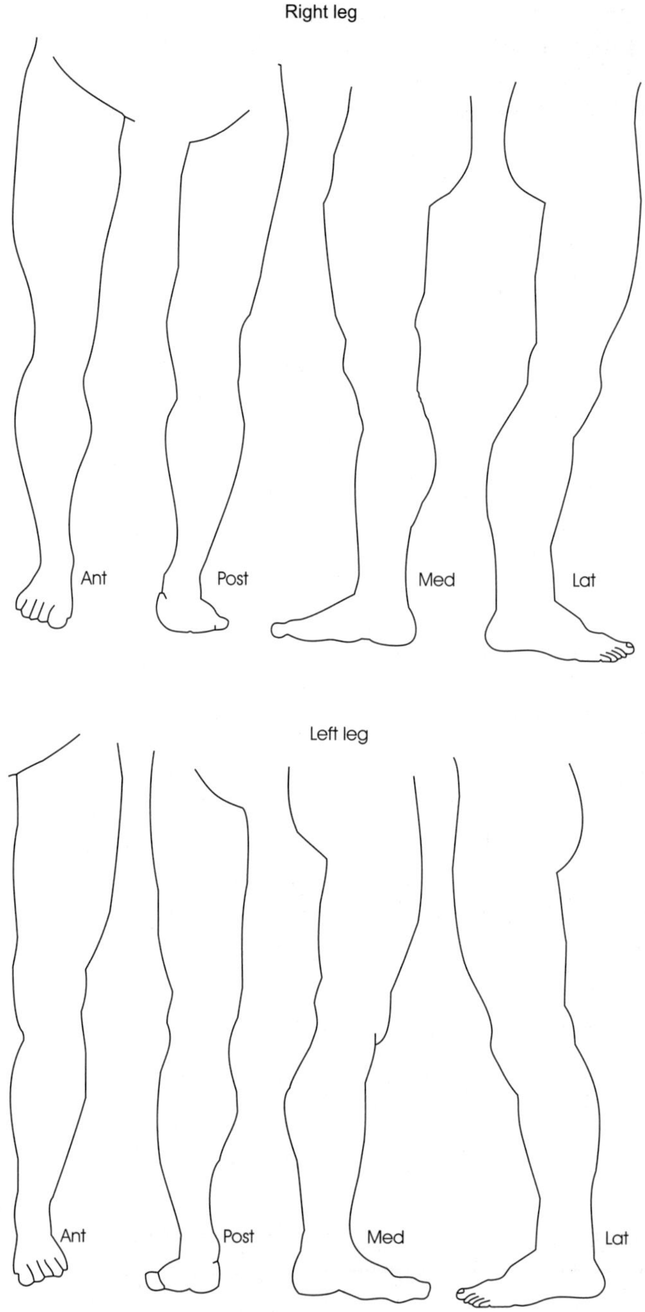

Figure 27.4 *Anatomic diagrams to document treatment sites at each visit.*

suction created by pulling back on the syringe may cause the wall to adhere to the needle bevel and prevent aspiration of blood. In this case one can move the needle gently forward and backward and if no resistance is felt, the vein has probably been cannulated and the injection may proceed very cautiously. The authors have also observed the reticular vein to spasmodically shrink and virtually disappear from view following a cannulation attempt. When this occurs, another injection site along the reticular vein must be sought. The cannulation of a reticular vein can be more difficult than a protuberant venulectasia or telangiectasia.

Usually the volume per injection site is no more than 0.5 ml but the capacity of long reticular veins may be large so that under certain circumstances injection volume may exceed 1 ml. The progress of solution may be followed visually and the injection stopped when the entire reticular vein has cleared of blood. Within 30–60 seconds, the reticular vein will undergo a muscular contraction as well.

Sclerosant concentrations are less than for varicose veins, recommended solutions and concentrations are: 0.2–0.5% sodium tetradecyl sulfate (STS; Sotradecol), 0.5–1% polidocanol (not FDA approved), or 23.4%

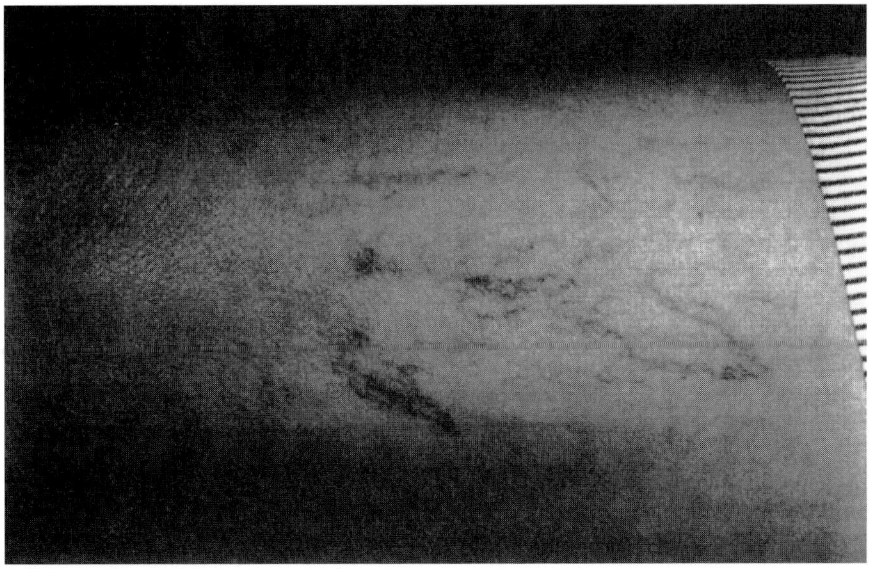

(a)

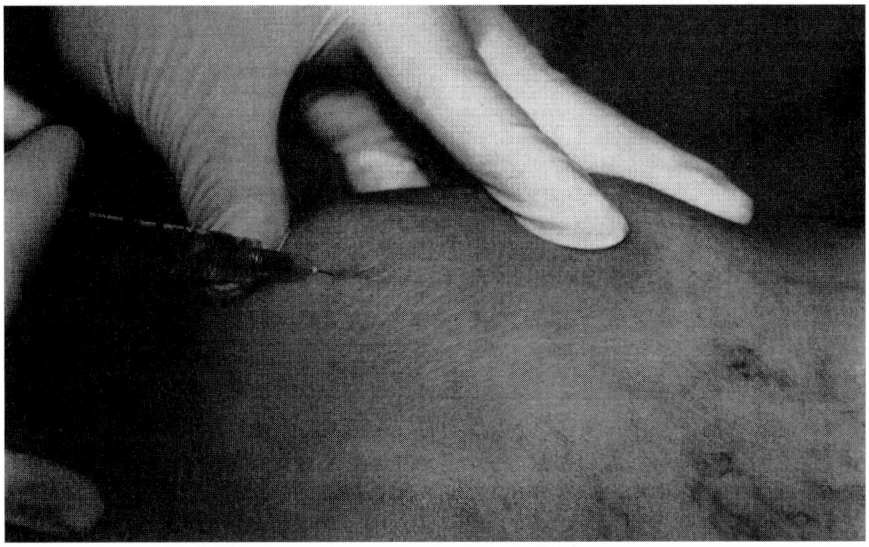

(b)

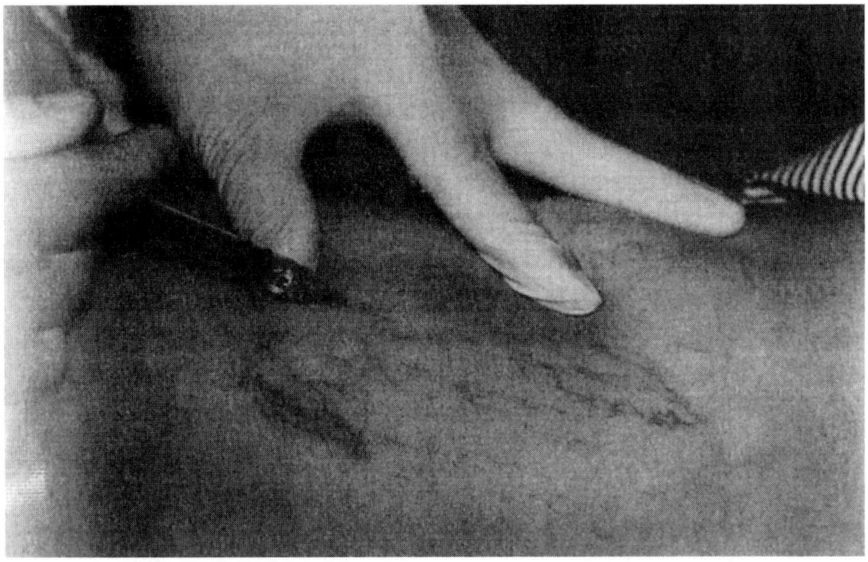

(c)

Figure 27.5 *Injection of a reticular vein. (a) Telangiectatic webs associated with a reticular vein on the medial thigh of a 38-year-old female. (b) Injection is started at origin of reticular vein medial to patella. Aspiration of blood confirms intravascular position of needle, even with 30 G needle. The thumb of the nondominant hand helps to support the needle hub to better enable minute adjustments of depth and angle of needle. Approximately 0.5 ml 0.5% sodium tetradecyl sulfate is injected. Immediate spasm of the reticular vein was noted. (c) Injection of a telangiectasia. After the reticular vein is adequately treated, the associated telangiectatic webs require injection. No blood is aspirated but the intravascular cannulation is appreciated by touch and the effortless filling of the telangiectatic web. A portion of the web is seen filled with sclerosing solution and maintaining spasm. Approximately 0.2 ml 0.1% sodium tetradecyl sulfate has been injected. No bleb formation at the site of injection has yet occurred. The moment a bleb is seen, the injection is stopped. Two more injections were required to complete the treatment of the telangiectasias.*

Table 27.2 *Commonly employed sclerosing solutions for telangiectasias, venulectasias and reticular veins – classification, usage, concentrations*

Sclerosing solution	Classification	Usage	Concentration
Sodium tetradecyl sulfate (Sotradecol)	Detergent	Telangiectasia	0.1–0.2%
		Venulectasia	0.2–0.3%
		Reticular	0.2–0.5%
Hypertonic saline	Hypertonic	Telangiectasia, venulectasia	11.7–23.4%
Hypertonic saline (10%) and dextrose (25%)	Hypertonic	Telangiectasia, venulectasia, reticular	Full strength
Non-FDA approved			
Polidocanol (Aethoxysklerol)	Detergent	Telangiectasia	0.25–0.5%
		Venulectasia	0.5–1.0%
		Reticular	1.0–2.0%
72% glycerin with 6% chromium salt (Scleremo)	Chemical irritant	Telangiectasia	Diluted 50%
		Venulectasia	Undiluted
		Reticular	Not used

Other solutions, such as sodium morrhuate, polyiodinated iodide and ethanolamine oleate are usually reserved for larger varicose veins.

hypertonic saline (HS) or hypertonic saline and dextrose (Sclerodex; not FDA approved). Until the physician gains experience cannulating reticular veins, cautious injection with the FDA-approved sclerosants cannot be overemphasized. A bruise will usually occur almost immediately and resistance to injection will be felt when the reticular vein has not been properly cannulated. For the inexperienced physician, polidocanol will be the safest solution to begin with. The minimal sclerosant concentration known to be effective for a certain diameter should be utilized.[25]

Injection of telangiectasias

The sclerotherapy tray is prepared with the necessary equipment:

- cotton balls soaked with 70% isopropyl alcohol
- protective gloves
- 3 ml disposable syringes
- 30 g disposable transparent hub needles
- cotton balls or STD pads for compression
- Transpore™ and/or paper tape
- nitroglycerine (2%) paste (for prolonged blanching)
- sclerosing solutions:
  - sodium tetradecyl sulfate (ranging concentrations 0.1–0.5%) (polidocanol when available)
  - hypertonic saline (11.7–23.4%)
  - hypertonic saline (10%) and dextrose (25%)(mixed by local pharmacy).

The patient is placed in either the prone or supine position on a hydraulic motorized table with height adjustment allowing easy access to all regions of the leg. The areas are repeatedly cleansed with cotton balls heavily saturated with 70% isopropyl alcohol. This allows better visualization of the vessels by increasing light transmission through otherwise reflective white scale on the epidermal surface. Following complete evaporation of the alcohol, a 30 gauge needle, bent to an angle of 10–30° with the bevel up, is placed on the skin so that the needle is parallel to the skin surface. A 3 ml syringe filled with 1.5–2 ml solution is held between the index and middle fingers while the fourth and fifth finger support the syringe against the leg in a fixed position, facilitating accurate penetration of the vessel.

The nondominant hand is used to stretch the skin around the needle and may offer additional support for the syringe (Fig. 27.5c). The firmly supported needle is then moved slowly 1–2 mm forward, piercing the vein just sufficiently to allow infusion of solution with the most minimal pressure on the plunger. Magnifying lenses on the order of 2–3× may help visualization of cannulation of the smallest telangiectasias.

The technique requires a gentle, precise touch, as one learns to appreciate the subtle sensation one feels on entering the vessel. Similarly, one learns to recognize the appearance of the bevel of the needle within the lumen of the telangiectasia. Sometimes minimal withdrawal of the needle may allow the easy flow of sclerosing solution. A very sharp needle is critical for this fine touch; the needle is changed as often as every three to four punctures to minimize tearing of the vessel. The use of 32–33 gauge needles is not advised because they easily veer off course.

Injection of a tiny bolus of air (<0.05 ml) may be helpful to establish that the needle is within the vein, as slight clearing 1–3 mm ahead of the bevel can be seen. Bodian claims that a larger air bolus allows the arborizing vessels to clear instantly, allowing greater spread of the sclerosing solution.[26] Others have found this to occur infrequently and generally find a larger air bolus not necessary.[2] The sclerosing solution is refrigerated in 2 ml aliquots to enhance vasoconstriction by cold and to sequester the solutions so that the possibility of accidental injection of a sclerosing solution during routine procedures in the treatment room is minimized. Solutions of STS greater than 0.5% cannot be stored in syringes but are stored in glass vials until just prior to injection. STS will dissolve some of the rubber of the syringe plunger, causing difficulty moving the plunger and contaminating the sclerosing solution with rubber breakdown products (personal communication, Wyeth-Ayerst Laboratories). For added safety, we now employ latex-free syringes as the incidence of latex allergy is rapidly increasing.[27] It is possible for STS to make soluble the latex from the syringe prior to injection. This raises the question of whether STS allergic reactions may be due to latex but this remains to be proven.

Concentrations of sclerosants utilized for telangiectasias are less than for reticular veins; successfully employed solutions and concentrations are: 0.1–0.2% sodium tetradecyl sulfate (STS; Sotradecol), 0.1–0.5% polidocanol (not FDA approved), or 11.7–23.4 % hypertonic saline (HS) or hypertonic saline and dextrose (Sclerodex; not FDA approved). The initial treatment of telangiectatic webs begins with the minimal effective concentration (FDA approved) of sclerosing solution which is usually the lowest concentration listed above.[25] When ineffective sclerosis occurs judged at a subsequent visit, the concentration not the volume of sclerosing solution is increased.

The injection of telangiectasias is performed extremely slowly using drops of sclerosant (0.1– 0.2 ml or less), and with minimal or no pressure on a 3 ml syringe to maintain filling of the veins and contact with the vessel wall for approximately 10–15 seconds. Rapid flushing of the vessels with large volumes of sclerosant causes unnecessarily large quantities to be utilized, increasing the risks for allergic reactions. Particularly when using a hypertonic solution, the injection of sclerosant is stopped when blanching in a radius of 2 cm has occurred or when 15 seconds has passed, thus minimizing the cramping and burning. When using painless detergent sclerosants, small volumes with small amounts of short duration blanching will minimize side-effects such as telangiectatic matting. Occasionally no blanching occurs at the site of injection and the sclerosing solution flows easily through the telangiectasia or can even be seen flowing through adjacent telangiectasias or reticular veins several centimeters away from the injection site. In this case the injection is stopped after no more than 0.5 ml sclerosant has been injected. Following the injection, immediate manual compression is applied. As a general rule no more than 0.5 ml is injected into any single site.

By minimizing volume, pressure and duration of injection, not only is pain minimized, but the risks of extravasation are minimized as well. Multiple areas (for example, at least 10 areas of 2–4 cm of telangiectasias on one thigh) can be treated with as little as 2–3 ml sclerosant. Maximum amount of sclerosants per session in our clinic include: 4 ml of 3% STS, 10 ml hypertonic saline and, when FDA approved, 5 ml of 3% polidocanol.

To minimize skin necrosis, extravasation must be avoided. If resistance to the easy injection of sclerosant or the beginning of any 'bleb' at the injection site is noted, the injection is stopped immediately. The physician needs to keep an eye on the injection site at all times in order to notice the 'bleb' at the moment of its occurrence. Some physicians keep a syringe of 5–10 ml normal saline nearby to flush and dilute any areas of extravasation that may develop. Sclerosant thought to have extravasated may also be diluted with 0.5–1.0% lidocaine without epinephrine (further vasoconstriction must be minimized).

Immediately after injection, the treated area is gently massaged, usually in the desired direction of further spread of sclerosant. This may help to reduce pain and hasten the spread of the sclerosant through the targeted vessels. Any vessel larger than approximately 0.5 mm or, more importantly, any size that protrudes above the surface of the skin, benefits from compression. After spreading the solution by massage for 5–10 seconds, cotton balls are then secured over the injection sites by paper tape or Transpore™ tape. This is followed with compression stockings for 2 weeks. Cosmetic telangiectasias receive 15–20 mmHg ready-to-wear compression for 2 weeks. For more extensive reticular networks, graduated 20–30 mmHg compression hose is worn for 2–3 weeks.[28] Patients are encouraged to walk, and not restrict their activities, with the exception of heavy weightlifting with the legs or any activity which results in sustained forceful muscular contraction leading to venous pressure elevation.

Treatment intervals vary; allowing 4–8 weeks between treatments helps to minimize the number of necessary sessions. Often telangiectasias will ultimately clear after exhibiting no initial response within the first 2 weeks. Typically a patient will undergo three to five treatments separated by 1 month each. After the initial series of treatments, a 'rest' period of 4–6 months will allow pigmentation and matting to clear and cause remaining reticular veins to establish 'new' routes of drainage. Approximately 80% of patients will clear satisfactorily during the first course of treatment. The physician may then judge and re-evaluate any remaining telangiectatic webs or new telangiectasias for the best approach for another round of treatment.

When patients have had a poor response to sclerotherapy after the initial series of treatments, the following may be considered. If one class of sclerosant achieves poor results, switch to another class, such as from hypertonic to detergent or vice versa. One must reassess whether the source of reflux from a reticular vein into a group of telangiectasias was adequately treated both by physical examination, CW Doppler or duplex if necessary. The question of larger areas of reflux from axial varicosities that might have been overlooked must be considered. The patient must be carefully questioned about proper compliance with compression since many patients abandon compression within several days after sclerotherapy.

The age of the patient must be considered as well, since younger patients respond more quickly and thoroughly than older individuals. Some post-menopausal women taking high doses of estrogen and progesterone may improve the results of sclerotherapy by temporarily suspending hormonal supplementation.

ROLE OF LASERS FOR TREATMENT OF TELANGIECTASIAS

Recent reports of lasers for telangiectasias show significant progress over the last 2 years. While the mainstay has been the pulsed dye laser for facial telangiectasias, newer wavelengths are being explored. Most recently, the near infrared 1064 nm laser has been rediscovered with pulse durations of up to 16 ms. Success rates with this 1064 nm laser have been reported up to 75% with little or no epidermal injury.[29] Improved delivery systems allow for longer pulse durations (up to 50 ms), associated cooling of the epidermis for less risk of burning the epidermis and longer wavelengths of light for deeper penetration. Laser therapy still remains an adjunctive therapy, however.

SUMMARY

In summary, sclerotherapy of telangiectasias is highly effective when approached in a systematic logical way. Clearing rates of 90% have been reported. Experience gained over time greatly enhances results. Every patient should be approached with knowledge of the venous anatomy, understanding of the principles of reflux, thorough informed consent, photographic documentation, and familiarity with different sclerosing solution volumes and concentrations. Treatment based on this foundation is highly likely to be successful.

REFERENCES

1. Ramelet AA. La phlebectomie ambulatoire selon Mueller: Technique, avantages, desavantages. *J Mal Vasc* 1991; **16**: 119–22.
2. Weiss RA, Weiss MA. Resolution of pain associated with varicose and telangiectatic leg veins after compression sclerotherapy. *J Dermatol Surg Oncol* 1990; **16**: 333–6.
3. Weiss RA, Duffy D. Clinical benefits of lightweight compression: reduction of venous- related symptoms by ready-to-wear lightweight gradient compression hosiery. *Dermatol Surg* 1999; **25**(9): 701–4.
4. Weiss RA, Heagle CR, Raymond-Martimbeau P. The bulletin of the North American Society of Phlebology. Insurance Advisory Committee Report. *J Dermatol Surg Oncol* 1992; **18**: 609–16.
5. Lofgren KA. Varicose veins: their symptoms, complications, and management. *Postgrad Med* 1979; **65**(6): 131–9.
6. Goldman MP, Bennett RG. Treatment of telangiectasia: a review. *J Am Acad Dermatol* 1987; **17**: 167–82.
7. Goldman PM. Sclerotherapy for superficial venules and telangiectasias of the lower extremities. *Dermatol Clin* 1987; **5**: 369–79.
8. Weiss RA, Weiss MA. Sclerotherapy. In Wheeland RG, ed. *Cutaneous Surgery.* Philadelphia: WB Saunders, 1994: 951–81.
9. Weiss RA, Weiss MA. Painful telangiectasias: diagnosis and treatment. In Bergan JJ, Weiss RA, Goldman MP, eds. *Varicose Veins and Telangiectasias: Diagnosis and Treatment*, 2nd edn. St Louis, MO: Quality Medical Publishing, 1999: 389–406.
10. Goldman MP, Weiss RA, Bergan JJ. Diagnosis and treatment of varicose veins – a review. *J Am Acad Dermatol* 1994; **31**(3, Part 1): 393–413.
11. Thibault P, Bray A, Wlodarczyk J, Lewis W. Cosmetic leg veins: evaluation using duplex venous imaging. *J Dermatol Surg Oncol* 1990; **16**: 612–18.
12. deFaria JL, Moraes IN. Histopathology of telangiectasias associated with varicose veins. *Dermatologica* 1963; **127**: 321.
13. Wokalek H, Vanscheidt W, Martay K, Leder O. Morphology and localization of sunburst varicosities: an electron microscopic and morphometric study. *J Dermatol Surg Oncol* 1989; **15**: 149–54.
14. Braverman IM, Keh-Yen A. Ultrastructure of the human dermal microcirculation. IV. Valve-containing collecting veins at the dermal-subcutaneous junction. *J Invest Dermatol* 1983; **81**(5): 438–42.
15. Somjen GM, Ziegenbein R, Johnston AH, Royle JP. Anatomical examination of leg telangiectases with duplex scanning. *J Dermatol Surg Oncol* 1993; **19**(10): 940–5.
16. Tretbar LL. The origin of reflux in incompetent blue reticular/telangiectasia veins. In Davy A, Stemmer R, eds. *Phlebologie '89.* Paris, France: John Libby Eurotext Ltd, 1989: 95–6.
17. Albanese AR, Albanese AM, Albanese EF. Lateral subdermic varicose vein system of the legs. Its surgical treatment by the chiseling tube method. *Vasc Surg* 1969; **3**: 81–9.
18. Hochstetter F. *Morphologishes Jahrbuch* 1891; **17 Bd**.
19. Weiss RA, Weiss MA. Doppler ultrasound findings in reticular veins of the thigh subdermic lateral venous system and implications for sclerotherapy. *J Dermatol Surg Oncol* 1993; **19**(10): 947–51.
20. Hirai M, Naiki K, Nakayama R. Prevalence and risk factors of varicose veins in Japanese women. *Angiology* 1990; **41**: 228–32.

21. Komsuoglu B, Goldeli O, Kulan K, Cetinarslan B, Komsuoglu SS. Prevalence and risk factors of varicose veins in an elderly population. *Gerontology* 1994; **40**(1): 25–31.
22. Schultz-Ehrenburg U, Weindorf N, Matthes U, Hirche H. New epidemiological findings with regard to initial stages of varicose veins (Bochum study I–III). In Raymond-Martimbeau P, Prescott R, Zummo M, eds. *Phlebologie '92.* Paris: John Libbey Eurotext, 1992: 234–6.
23. Weiss RA. Vascular studies of the legs for venous or arterial disease. *Dermatol Clin* 1994; **12**(1): 175–90.
24. Tretbar LL. Injection sclerotherapy for spider telangiectasias: a 20-year experience with sodium tetradecyl sulfate. *J Dermatol Surg Oncol* 1989; **15**: 223–5.
25. Sadick NS. Sclerotherapy of varicose and telangiectatic leg veins. Minimal sclerosant concentration of hypertonic saline and its relationship to vessel diameter. *J Dermatol Surg Oncol* 1991; **17**: 65–70.
26. Bodian EL. Sclerotherapy: a personal appraisal. *J Dermatol Surg Oncol* 1989; **15**: 156–61.
27. Cheng L, Lee D. Review of latex allergy. *J Am Board Fam Pract* 1999; **12**(4): 285–92.
28. Weiss RA, Sadick NS, Goldman MP, Weiss MA. Post-sclerotherapy compression: controlled comparative study of duration of compression and its effects on clinical outcome. *Dermatol Surg* 1999; **25**(2): 105–8.
29. Weiss RA, Weiss MA. Early clinical results with a multiple synchronized pulse 1064nm laser for leg telangiectasias and reticular veins. *Dermatol Surg* 1999; **25**(5): 399–402.

28

Complications of sclerotherapy

MITCHEL P GOLDMAN

Sclerotherapy treatment of varicose and telangiectatic leg veins is a safe procedure with few adverse sequelae. However, as with any therapeutic technique, sclerotherapy carries with it a number of potential adverse sequelae and complications. Fairly common, and often self-limiting, side-effects include perivascular cutaneous pigmentation, edema of the injected extremity, a flare of new telangiectasias, pain with injection of certain sclerosing solutions, localized urticaria over injected sites, blisters or folliculitis caused by post-sclerosis compression, recurrence of previously treated vessels, stress-related problems, and localized hirsutism. Relatively rare complications include localized cutaneous necrosis; systemic allergic reactions; thrombophlebitis of the injected vessel; arterial injection with resultant distal necrosis; deep venous thrombosis, which may result in chronic venous insufficiency or pulmonary emboli. This chapter addresses the pathophysiology of the most common of these reactions, methods for reducing their incidence, and treatment of their occurrence.

POST-SCLEROTHERAPY HYPERPIGMENTATION

Cutaneous pigmentation to some degree is relatively common after sclerotherapy of veins. The incidence appears to depend on technique and strength of sclerosing solution. Fortunately, when it occurs it usually resolves within 6–12 months. A recent evaluation of patients in one practice found a 1% incidence of pigmentation persisting after 1 year.[1] When using detergent types of sclerosing solutions, pigmentation is usually linear along the course of the treated blood vessel (Fig. 28.1). Osmotic sclerosing solutions may produce punctate pigmentation at points of injection, which may be related to their mechanism of action through an osmotic gradient that produces maximal osmolality and resultant endothelial destruction at the injection site (Fig. 28.2).

The etiology of this pigmentation is secondary to hemosiderin staining of the dermis.[2] In addition, defects in iron storage or transport mechanisms or both have also been found in a significant number of patients who developed post-sclerotherapy pigmentation.[3] This phenomenon probably occurs when red blood cells extravasate into the dermis after the rupture of treated vessels. In addition, perivascular inflammation promotes degranulation of perivascular mast cells, releasing histamine which leads to endothelial cell contraction, widening endothelial gaps through which extravasation of red blood cells can occur. Thus, injecting a sclerosing solution dilates the vessel both directly through pressure generated by the syringe and indirectly through histamine-induced endothelial cell contraction. Perivascular phagocytosis of red blood cells occurs by macrophages, which produces hemosiderin, an indigestible residue of hemoglobin degradation. Pigmentation resolves from a gradual resorption of ferritin particles by macrophages.

Treatment technique should limit the degree of intravascular pressure to prevent extravasation of red blood cells. Larger feeding varices, incompetent varices,

This chapter is an abbreviated version of Goldman MP. Complications and adverse sequelae. In *Sclerotherapy Treatment of Varicose and Telangiectatic Leg Veins*, 3rd edn. St Louis: CV Mosby, 2001.

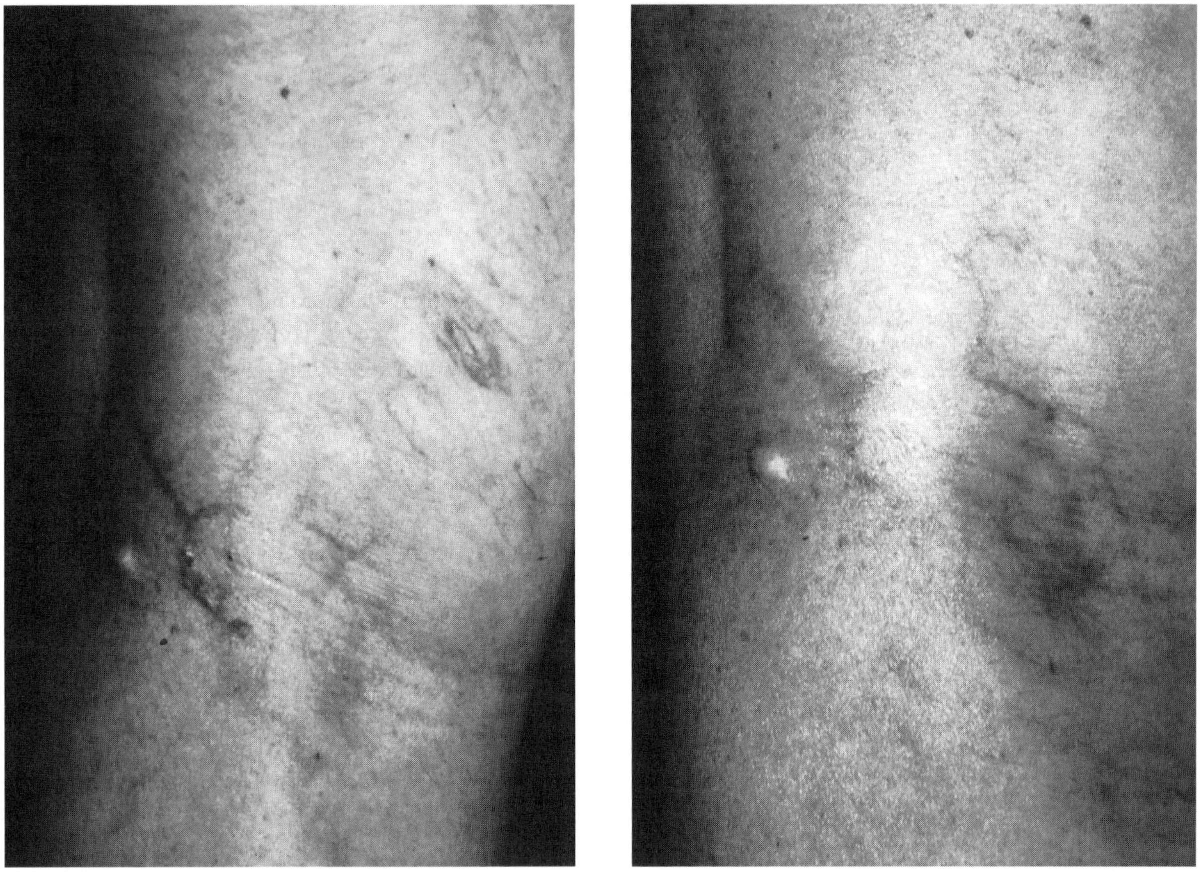

(a) (b)

Figure 28.1 *Linear pigmentation along the course of the treated blood vessel. (a) Before treatment. (b) Eight weeks after treatment with polidocanol 0.5%. (Reproduced with permission from Goldman MP, ed.* Sclerotherapy Treatment of Varicose and Telangiectatic Leg Veins, *3rd edn. St Louis: CV Mosby, 2001: 192)*

and points of high-pressure reflux should be treated first. Doing so minimizes the extent of proximal intravascular pressure.

Because telangiectasia and small venules are composed essentially of endothelial cells with a thin (if any) muscular coat and basement membrane, excessive intravascular pressure from injection may cause vessel rupture. In addition, endothelial pores and spaces between cells in the vascular wall will dilate in response to pressure, leading to extravasation of red blood cells. It is therefore important to inject intravascularly with minimal pressure. Since injection pressure is inversely proportional to the square of the piston radius, using a syringe with a larger radius will result in less pressure. The average piston radius is 8 mm for a 2 ml syringe and 5 mm for a 1 ml syringe. The calculated pressure with an implied force of 250 g is 180 mmHg for a 2 ml syringe and more than 300 mmHg for a 1 ml syringe. This is one reason I recommend using a 2–3 ml syringe for sclerotherapy.

Removal of post-sclerotherapy coagula may decrease the incidence of pigmentation. Thrombi are thought to occur to some degree after sclerotherapy of all veins, regardless of size, because of the inability to occlude the vascular lumen completely with external pressure. Persistent thrombi are thought to produce a subacute perivenulitis that can persist for months. The perivenulitis favors extravasation of red blood cells through a damaged endothelium or by increasing the permeability of treated endothelium. In addition, intratissue fixation of hemosiderin may occur. This provides a rationale for drainage of all foci of trapped blood 2–4 weeks after sclerotherapy. Sometimes blood can be released even 2 months after sclerotherapy.

To prevent the development of pigmentation, sclerotherapy should produce limited endothelial necrosis and not total vessel destruction with its resulting diapedesis of red blood cells. This may be achieved by using meticulous technique, avoiding excessive injection pressures, selecting the appropriate solution concentration, and treating areas of reflux venous return in a proximal-to-distal manner.

Treatment of pigmentation, once it occurs, is often unsuccessful. Because this pigmentation primarily is caused by hemosiderin deposition and not melanin incontinence, bleaching agents that affect melanocytic

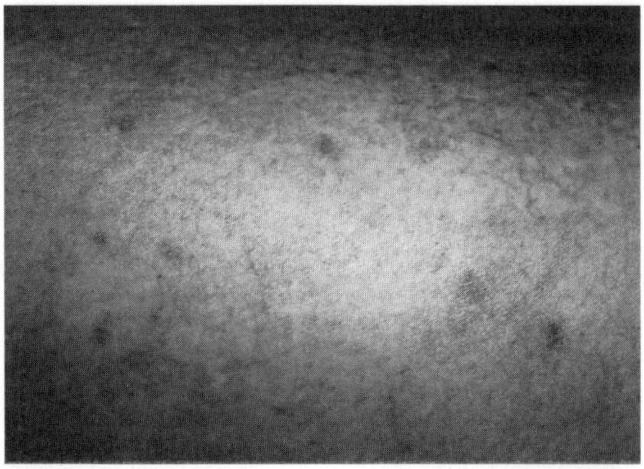

Figure 28.2 *Punctate pigmentation 8 weeks after treatment with Sclerodex. (Reproduced with permission from Goldman MP. Adverse sequela of sclerotherapy treatment of varicose and telangiectatic leg veins. In Bergan JJ, Goldman MP, eds.* Varicose Veins: Diagnosis and Treatment. *St Louis: Quality Medical Publishing, 1993)*

function are usually ineffective. Exfoliants (trichloroacetic acid) may hasten the apparent resolution of this pigmentation by decreasing the overlying cutaneous pigmentation, but they carry a risk of scarring, permanent hypopigmentation, and post-inflammatory hyperpigmentation.

Continuing graduated compression after development of pigmentation may hasten resorption of hemosiderin. Compression also improves lipodermatosclerotic skin changes, including hyperpigmentation. Therefore, it seems reasonable to promote wearing graduated support stockings after treatment. Laser treatment has been demonstrated as efficacious in 45–69% of patients with pigmentation of 12 or 6 months' duration, respectively.[4] Hemosiderin has an absorption spectrum that peaks at 410–415 nm, followed by a gradually sloping curve throughout the visible spectrum. The copper vapor laser at 511 nm in a continuous air-brush technique and the flashlamp-excited pulsed dye laser at 510 nm should interact relatively specifically with the hemosiderin absorption spectrum. These lasers are thought to result in physical fragmentation of pigment granules, which are later removed by phagocytosis. However, penetration of laser energy at 510 and 511 nm is limited to 1 mm below the granular layer. Since hemosiderin may occur up to 2.8 mm below the granular layer, non-thermal effects may result in clinical resolution. An inflammatory reaction from thermal and/or photoacoustic effects may stimulate hemosiderin absorption. I have also had fair success in treating persistent pigmentation with the Q-switched ruby, alexandrite, and Nd:YAG lasers.[5,6] These lasers were developed to treat tattoos and do so with great efficacy. Since hemosiderin can be considered a tattoo of sorts, it is not surprising that this treatment modality is efficacious.

TELANGIECTATIC MATTING

Fine red telangiectasias occur in a number of patients after either sclerotherapy or surgical ligation of varicose veins and leg telangiectasias (Fig. 28.3). The reported incidence of telangiectatic matting is approximately 16%.[7,8] Telangiectatic matting may appear anywhere on the leg, but most commonly appears on the medial ankle and medial thighs.

The etiology of telangiectatic matting is unknown but is believed to be related either to angiogenesis or to a dilation of existing subclinical blood vessels by the promotion of collateral flow through arteriovenous anastomoses. One or both of these mechanisms may occur. Probable risk factors for the development of telangiectatic matting in patients with leg telangiectasia include obesity, use of estrogen-containing hormones, pregnancy, and a family history of telangiectatic veins. Excessive post-sclerotherapy inflammation may also predispose toward development of telangiectatic matting.

The development of new vessels can occur in 2–3 days. Observations of mammalian systems have demonstrated the development of a vein from a capillary, an artery from a vein, a vein from an artery, or from either back to a capillary. Angiogenic factors either act directly on the endothelium to stimulate locomotion and mitosis or indirectly by mobilization of host helper cells (mast cells and macrophages) with release of endothelial growth factors. Endothelial damage and obstruction of blood flow are both factors that promote angiogenesis. Endothelial damage leads to the release of heparin and other mast cell factors that both promote the dilation of existing blood vessels and stimulate angiogenesis. It is remarkable that a greater incidence of post-sclerosis telangiectatic matting does not occur.

Sclerotherapy produces some degree of perivascular inflammation. Inflammation may be considered a hypermetabolic state, with new vessel growth occurring as a result of increased metabolic demand. One should therefore try to limit the degree of inflammation as much as possible. This is achieved by choosing an appropriate solution concentration for each type of vessel treated and limiting the quantity of solution to the amount that will not produce excessive endothelial damage.

Treatment modalities for telangiectatic matting are limited. Reinjection with hypertonic solutions may be helpful. Injection of any feeding reticular veins or venulectasias is also helpful. In addition, the pulsed dye laser at 585, 595 or 610 nm, the Photoderm VL or 1064 nm Vasculite laser (Energy Systems Corporation, Waythan, MA), the Versapulse laser at 532 nm using a long-pulsed mode from 15 to 30 ms (Coherent Inc., Santa Clara, CA), or the Cool Touch-Varia 1064 nm laser (Cool Touch Corporation, CA) may be useful in treating these vessels.[9–11] Unfortunately, telangiectatic matting may be resistant to treatment.

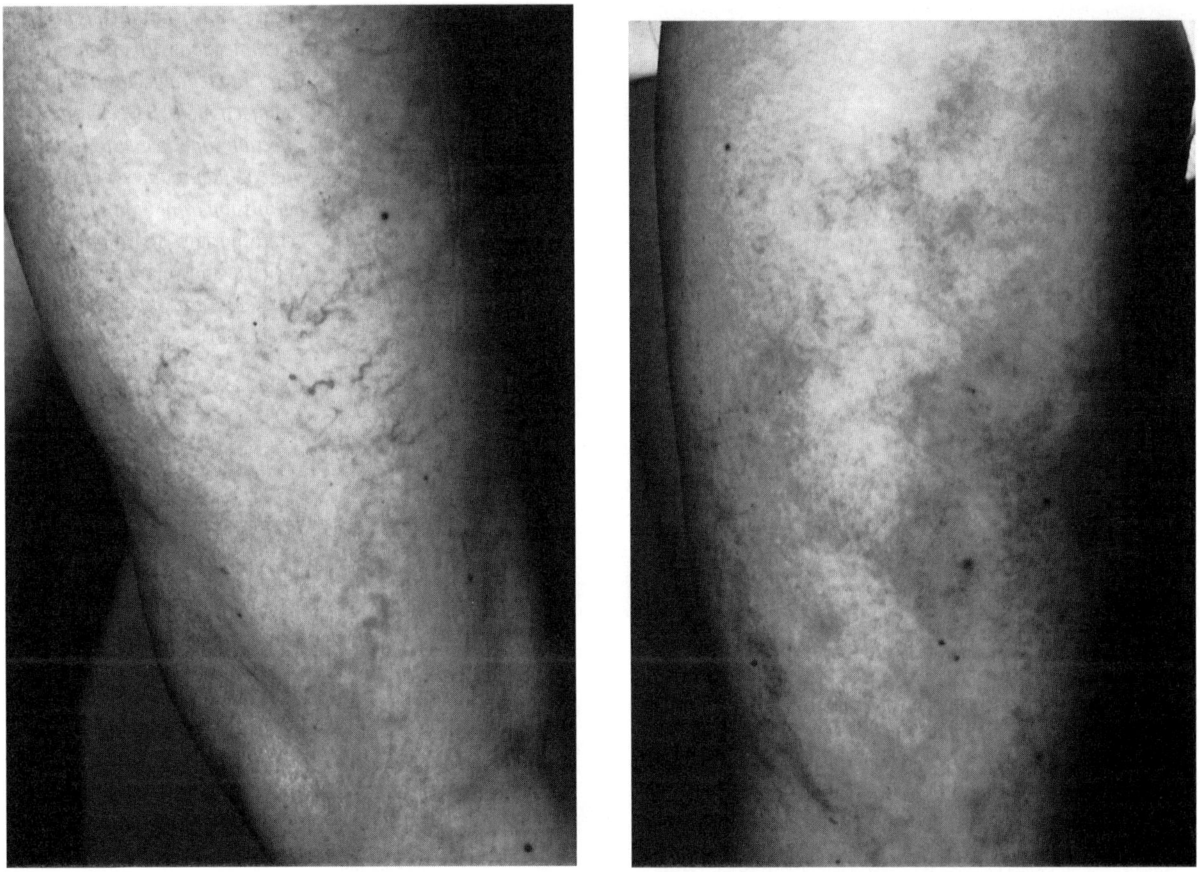

(a) (b)

Figure 28.3 *Typical telangiectatic matting in a 36-year-old woman. (a) Before sclerotherapy treatment, left lateral thigh. (b) Six weeks after treating telangiectatic veins with polidocanol 0.5%. Note development of extensive telangiectatic matting. (Reproduced with permission from Goldman MP. Adverse sequela of sclerotherapy treatment of varicose and telangiectatic leg veins. In Bergan JJ, Goldman MP, eds.* Varicose Veins: Diagnosis and Treatment. *St Louis: Quality Medical Publishing, 1993)*

CUTANEOUS NECROSIS

Cutaneous necrosis may occur with the injection of any sclerosing agent even under ideal circumstances and does not necessarily represent physician error. Fortunately, its occurrence is both rare and usually of limited sequelae. It may be the result of:

- extravasation of a sclerosing solution into the perivascular tissues;
- injection into a dermal arteriole or an arteriole feeding into a telangiectatic or varicose vein;
- a reactive vasospasm of the vessel;
- excessive cutaneous pressure created by compression techniques (Fig. 28.4).

Extravasation of caustic sclerosing solutions may directly destroy tissue. The final clinical appearance of the skin may not be apparent for several days; thus therapeutic intervention must be undertaken as soon as possible in all cases.

During injection of an abnormal vein or telangiectasia, even the most adept physician may inadvertently inject a small quantity of sclerosing solution into the perivascular tissue. A tiny amount of sclerosing solution may be left in the tissue when the needle is withdrawn, and sclerosing solution may leak out of the injected vessel, which has been traumatized by multiple or through-and-through needle punctures. Rarely, the injection of a strong sclerosing solution into a fragile vessel may lead to endothelial necrosis and rupture, producing a 'blow-out' of the vessel and perivascular extravasation of sclerosing solution. Therefore injection technique is an important but not foolproof factor in avoiding this complication, even under optimal circumstances.

Hyperosmotic agents with an osmolality greater than that of serum (281–289 mosmol/l) can cause tissue damage as a result of osmotic factors. Epidermal necrosis has even occurred from extravasation of solutions containing 10% dextrose. Hypertonic saline 23.4% is a caustic sclerosing agent, as demonstrated in intradermal injection experiments. Clinically, small punctate spots of superficial epidermal damage occur at points of injection, especially when a small bleb of the solution escapes from the vein.

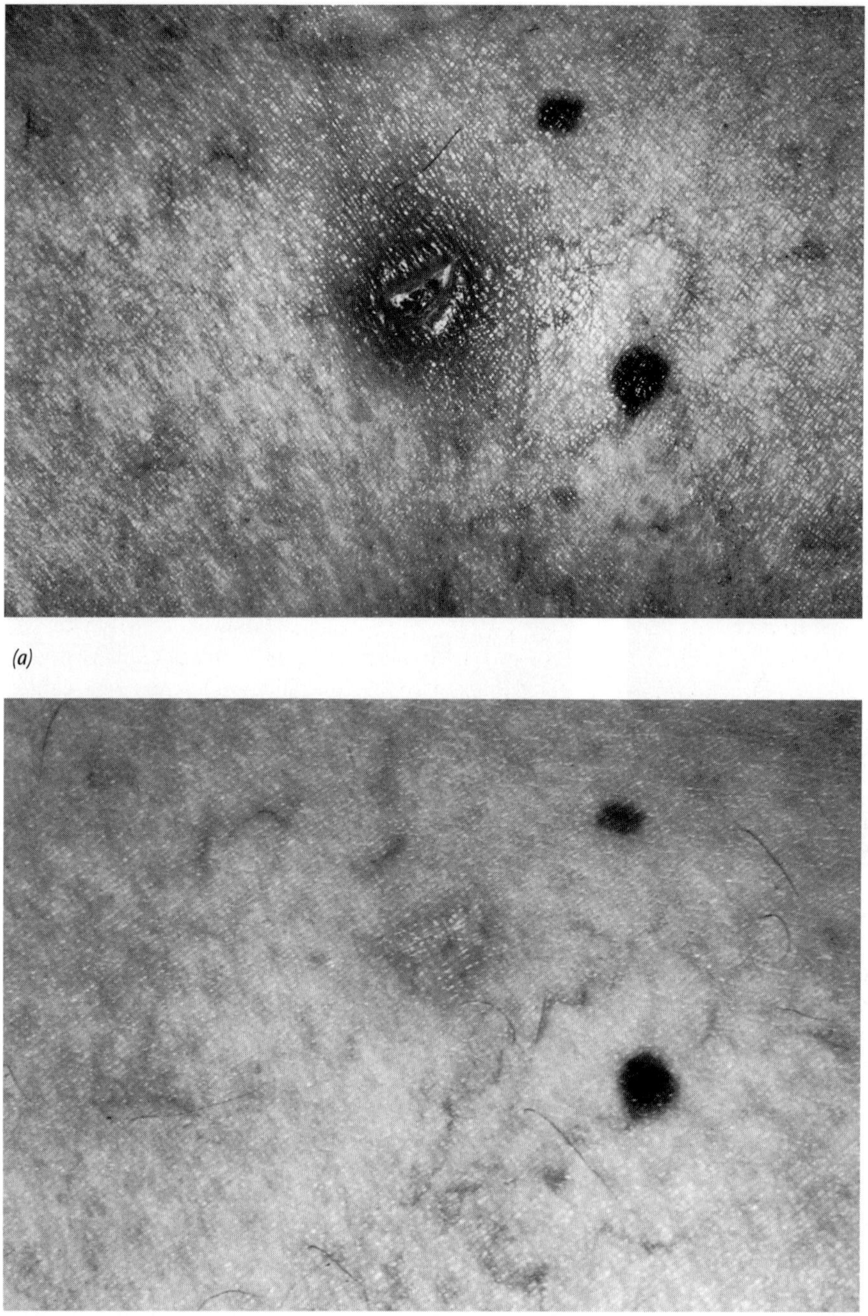

(a)

(b)

Figure 28.4 *Cutaneous necrosis after injection with polidocanol 0.5% into telangiectasia. (a) Preinjection; (b) 5 weeks after injection superficial ulceration is present. (Reproduced with permission from Goldman MP, ed.* Sclerotherapy Treatment of Varicose and Telangiectatic Leg Veins, *3rd edn. St Louis: CV Mosby, 2001: 203)*

Experimentally, polidocanol is minimally toxic to subcutaneous tissue. Although some physicians advocate the use of intradermal polidocanol 0.5% to treat tiny telangiectatic leg veins, polidocanol in sufficient concentration will cause cutaneous necrosis. Solutions of polidocanol greater than 1.0% may produce superficial necrosis with intradermal injection.

Even when sclerotherapy is performed with expert technique, using the safest sclerosing solutions and concentrations, cutaneous ulceration may occur. Therefore it appears that extravasation of caustic sclerosing solutions alone is not totally responsible for this complication. De Faria and Moraes have observed that one in 26 leg telangiectasias is associated with a dermal arteriole.[12] It is my opinion that inadvertent injection into or near this communication is the most common cause of cutaneous ulcerations.

I have noted the development of 3–6 mm diameter ulcerations in approximately 0.0001% of injections with polidocanol 0.5%. Five consecutive ulcerations that appeared over the course of 12 months were excised. In these patients, each cutaneous ulceration developed as the result of the occlusion of the feeding dermal arteriole.[13] This produced a classic wedge-shaped arterial ulceration.

Rarely, after injection of the sclerosing solution an immediate porcelain-white appearance to the skin is noted at the site of injection. A hemorrhagic bulla usually forms over this area within 2–48 hours and progresses to an ulcer. This cutaneous reaction might represent an arterial spasm. In an attempt to reverse the spasm, vigorous massage when the white macule appears has sometimes averted ulceration. However, prevention of the ulceration with massage alone is not always successful. Massaging in nitroglycerin ointment 2% may prevent the development of ulcerations in this setting.

If extravasation of sclerosing solution occurs, the solution must be diluted as soon as possible. Hypertonic solutions should be diluted with copious amounts of physiological saline solution. At least 10 times the volume of extravasated solution should be injected to limit osmotic damage. Detergent sclerosing solutions of adequate strength may also be toxic to tissues. Dilution is again of paramount importance.

It seems prudent to dilute the concentration of a caustic solution with hyaluronidase (Wydase, lyophilized, 150 USP units/ml) in the diluent. Hyaluronidase enzymatically breaks down connective tissue hyaluronic acid. This is hypothesized to disrupt the normal interstitial fluid barrier to allow rapid diffusion of solution through tissues, thereby increasing effective absorption. In addition to accelerated dilution, cellular stabilization and wound repair properties of hyaluronidase appear useful in preventing cutaneous necrosis from inadvertent sclerosing solution extravasation. I recommend injecting 300 USP units of hyaluronidase diluted in 5 ml 0.9% sodium chloride solution into multiple sites around the extravasated area. Studies have demonstrated that hyaluronidase solution must be injected within 60 minutes of extravasation to be effective.

ALLERGIC REACTION

Systemic reactions caused by sclerotherapy treatment occur very rarely. Minor reactions such as urticaria are easily treated with an oral antihistamine such as diphenhydramine (Benadryl), 25–50 mg by mouth. Rarely, the addition of corticosteroids is needed if the reaction does not subside readily. A short course of prednisone, 40–60 mg/day for 1 week, in conjunction with systemic antihistamine every 6–8 hours is helpful. Suppression of the adrenal axis is not a problem with this short course, so a tapering schedule is not necessary.

Bronchospasm is estimated to occur after sclerotherapy in 0.001% of patients. It usually responds to the addition of an inhaled bronchodilator or intravenous aminophylline, 6 mg/kg over 20 minutes, or to the antihistamine-corticosteroid regimen already noted.

Anaphylaxis is a systemic hypersensitivity response caused by exposure or, more commonly, re-exposure to a sensitizing substance. Since the risk of anaphylaxis increases with repeated exposures to the antigen, one should always be prepared for this reaction in every patient. The signs and symptoms of anaphylaxis initially may be subtle and often include anxiety, itching, sneezing, coughing, urticaria and angioedema. Wheezing may be accompanied by hoarseness of the voice and vomiting. Shortly after these presenting signs, breathing becomes more difficult, and the patient usually collapses from cardiovascular failure resulting from systemic vasodilatation. One helpful clue toward distinguishing between anaphylaxis and vasovagal reactions is heart rate. Sinus tachycardia is almost always present in a patient with anaphylaxis, whereas bradycardia or cardiac rhythm disturbances are commonplace in vasovagal reactions.

The recommended treatment is to give epinephrine (adrenaline) 0.2–0.5 ml 1:1000 subcutaneously. This can be repeated three or four times at intervals of 5–15 minutes to maintain a systolic blood pressure above 90–100 mmHg. This should be followed with establishment of an intravenous line of 0.9% sodium chloride solution. Diphenhydramine hydrochloride 50 mg is given next along with cimetidine 300 mg; both the intravenous solution and oxygen are given at 4–6 l/min. An endotracheal tube or tracheotomy is necessary for laryngeal obstruction. For asthma or wheezing, intravenous theophylline, 4–6 mg/kg, is infused over 15 minutes. At this point it is appropriate to transfer the patient to hospital. Methylprednisolone sodium succinate 60 mg is given intravenously and repeated every 6 hours for four doses. Corticosteroids are not an emergency medication since their effect appears only after 1–3 hours. They are given to prevent the recurrence of symptoms 3–8 hours after the initial event. The patient should be hospitalized overnight for observation.

Vasovagal reactions may also require treatment if they do not respond to the Trendelenburg position. The administration of atropine (0.4 mg/U subcutaneously) may be necessary.[13] Reports of death with the potential for induction of arrhythmia exist.[14]

Sodium morrhuate

Sodium morrhuate causes a variety of allergic reactions, ranging from mild erythema with pruritus to generalized urticaria to gastrointestinal disturbances with abdominal pain and diarrhea to anaphylaxis. It has been estimated that unfavorable reactions when treating varicose leg veins occur in 3% of patients. The reason for the high number of allergic reactions with this product may be related to the inability to remove all the fish proteins that are present in sodium morrhuate. In fact, 20.8% of the fatty acid composition of the solution is unknown. Many cases of anaphylaxis have occurred within a few minutes after the drug is injected or more commonly when therapy is re-instituted after a few weeks. Most of these cases occurred before 1950. Rarely, anaphylaxis has resulted in fatalities, many of which have not been reported in the medical literature.

Ethanolamine oleate

Ethanolamine oleate is a synthetic mixture of ethanolamine and oleic acid with an empirical formula of C20H41NO3. Anaphylactic reactions, some of which have been fatal, have been reported with its use. Generalized urticaria occurs in approximately one in 400 patients.

Sodium tetradecyl sulphate (STS)

A comprehensive review of the medical literature (in multiple specialities and languages) until 1987 disclosed a total of 47 cases of nonfatal allergic reactions in a review of 14 404 treated patients. This included six case reports.[15] Fegan has reviewed his experience with STS in 16 000 patients. He reported 15 cases of 'serum sickness, with hot stinging pain in the skin, and an erythematous rash developing 30 to 90 minutes after injection'.[16] A recent review on the treatment of 2686 patients with STS over 2 years found a 0.22% incidence of urticaria and/or anaphylactoid reactions.[17] If one were to combine only those reviews of over 1000 patients, the incidence of nonfatal allergic reactions would be <0.3%.

Polidocanol (POL)

Allergic reactions to polidocanol have been reported in four patients in a review of the world's literature up to 1987, with an estimated incidence of 0.01%.[15] Guex reported seven cases of minor general urticaria in nearly 11 000 patients treated over 12 years. Kreussler and Company, the product manufacturer in Germany, has documented 37 cases of suspected sensitivity from 1987 to 1993 (personal correspondence, January 1995). Of these reports, most were either vasovagal events or unproven allergic reactions. Nine patients were given repeat challenges with POL, with only three demonstrating an allergic reaction (urticaria or erythematous dermatitis). One patient died of anaphylactic shock 5 minutes after injection with 1 ml despite maximal intervention. The Australian Polidocanol Open Clinical Trial at 2 years, with over 8000 treated patients, reported nine local urticarial reactions and three generalized reactions, with two patients developing a rash, for a frequency of approximately 0.2%. There were no cases of anaphylaxis.[18] In short, POL appears to be no less allergenic than STS with both sclerosing solutions having an excellent safety record.

Chromated glycerin

Chromated glycerin 72% is a sclerosing solution whose incidence of side-effects is very low. Hypersensitivity is a very rare complication although contact sensitivity to chromium occurs in approximately 5% of the population. This effect occurs because chromium needs to bind to skin proteins to become an effective antigen. This may be related to the necessity for epidermal Langerhans' cells to produce an allergic response, whereas T-lymphocyte accessory cooperation is not optimal with intravenous injection and its resulting endothelial necrosis.

Polyiodide iodine

Polyiodide iodine is a stabilized water solution of iodide ions, sodium iodine, and benzyl alcohol. Sigg[19] reported on their experience in over 400 000 injections with polyiodide iodine with an incidence of 0.13 allergic cutaneous reactions per 1000. No systemic allergic reactions were observed. Obvious contraindications to the use of polyiodide iodine are hyperthyroidism and allergies to iodine and benzyl alcohol.

Hypertonic saline

Hypertonic saline solution shows no evidence of allergenicity or toxicity. Complications that may arise from its specific use include hypertension that may be exacerbated in predisposed patients when an excessive sodium load is given, sudden hypernatremia, central nervous system disorders, extensive hemolysis, and cortical necrosis of the kidneys. Sometimes blood appears in the urine after one to two acts of micturition and sometimes at additional times throughout the day. There are usually no other ill-effects, and the hematuria resolves spontaneously. Hematuria probably occurs because of hemolysis of red blood cells during sclerotherapy.

SUPERFICIAL THROMBOPHLEBITIS

Superficial thrombophlebitis appears 1–3 weeks after injection as a tender erythematous induration over the injected vein. In my experience this complication occurs to some degree in approximately 0.01% of patients. Severe cases requiring treatment with compression and anti-inflammatory agents occur very rarely (0.001% of patients totalling more than 10 000 separate injections).

An inadequate degree or length of compression results in excessive intravascular thrombosis. Thus to avoid this complication, one should prevent or minimize the development of post-sclerosis thrombosis by using compression pads and hosiery.

Thrombophlebitis is not a complication that should be taken lightly. If untreated, the inflammation and thrombus may spread to perforating veins and the deep venous system, which leads to valvular damage and possible pulmonary embolic events. When thrombophlebitis occurs, the thrombus should be evacuated and adequate compression and frequent ambulation should be maintained until the pain and inflammation resolve. Aspirin or other non-steroidal anti-inflammatory agents may be helpful in limiting both the inflammation and pain. In addition, depending on the extent of superficial thrombosis and its proximity to the saphenofemoral junction, ligation and stripping of the greater saphenous vein and/or anticoagulation with delayed surgery may be beneficial.[20]

ARTERIAL INJECTION

The most feared complication in sclerotherapy is inadvertent injection into an artery. Fortunately, this complication is very rare. Five examples of this complication had been reported to the Medical Defence Union in Great Britain by 1985.[21] Cockett has reported 18 cases, including those reported to the two medical protection societies in the UK over a 10-year period.[22] However, Cockett believes even this number is too low because many cases occur that never reach the courts or the medical literature. Biegeleisen *et al.* have reported seven cases in their practice history of more than 10 years.[23] From France 40 cases have been reported over 17 years.[24]

Arterial injection of a sclerosing solution causes the development of an embolus. This has been experimentally confirmed in the canine femoral artery. These experiments demonstrate little effect on the artery itself with injection. The sclerosing solution acts to denature blood in smaller arteries, producing a sludge embolus that obstructs the microcirculation. Stagnant blood flow, secondary thrombosis, and necrosis soon follow.[25]

The most common location for arterial injection to occur is in the posterior or medial malleolar region, particularly when an effort is made to inject the internal ankle perforator vein, specifically in the posterior tibial artery. The patient will usually, but not always, note immediate pain. The pain slowly propagates down into the foot and outer toes over the following 2–6 hours. During this time, arterial pedal pulses are palpable; 10–12 hours later the four outer toes are white, with the sole of the foot becoming painful. Cutaneous blanching of the injected area usually occurs in an arterial pattern associated with a loss of pulse and progressive cyanosis of the injected area.

Another area in which the artery and veins are in close proximity is the junction of the femoral and greater saphenous veins. In this location the external pudendal artery bifurcates and may surround the greater saphenous vein shortly after the location of its connection with the femoral vein. In addition, the junction of the greater saphenous vein with the popliteal vein has been demonstrated to have a tortuous and variably located satellite arteriole. Because these collateral arteries vary anatomically in these locations, duplex scanning may be useful before sclerosing these vessels but does not guarantee absolute safety.

With the onset of duplex-assisted sclerotherapy, small arteries in superficial and deep aspects of the thigh and calf have been inadvertently injected. As described previously, the usual sequelae are both loss of tissue (cutaneous and subcutaneous) and nerve damage, which may result in muscle atrophy and/or necrosis. Color-flow duplex scanning and the use of open needles when sclerosing these very tricky areas are recommended. A physician should be present at all times to give immediate treatment if needed.

Arterial injection is a true sclerotherapy emergency. The extent of cutaneous necrosis is usually related to the amount of solution injected. Therapeutic efforts to treat this complication are usually unsatisfactory but should be attempted. On realization of arterial injection, blood and sclerosing solution should be aspirated back into the syringe to empty the artery as rapidly and completely as possible. The needle should not be withdrawn, but the syringe should be replaced with one containing 10 000 units of heparin, which should be injected slowly into the artery. Unfortunately, this maneuver is difficult to accomplish since the patient is usually in considerable pain and may find it difficult to hold still. In addition, some patients have no complaints of pain and only demonstrate a mild, sharply demarcated erythema that becomes dusky and cyanotic after a few hours.

Other treatments include periarterial infiltration with procaine 3%, 1 ml, which will form a complex with sodium tetradecyl sulphate and render it inactive. The foot should be cooled with ice packs to minimize tissue anoxia. Immediate heparinization (continued for 6 days) and administration of intravenous dextran 10%, 500 ml per dose, for 3 days is recommended. Use of intravenous thrombolytic agents such as streptokinase, urokinase, t-PA and the like also may be considered if there are no contraindications for its use. Finally, use of oral prazosin, hydralazine, or nifedipine for 30 days should be considered.

Use of intravenous heparin followed by subcutaneous heparin has been found to avert skin necrosis. The protective effect of heparin may be unrelated to its anticoagulant activity. Post-ischemic endothelial cell dysfunction was prevented with heparin perfusion in the rat hind limb model. It is postulated that direct interactions of heparin with the endothelium, inducing maintenance of a strong luminal charge, may produce beneficial membrane-stabilizing effects. Heparin may also modulate the activity of tumor necrosis factor, contributing to this effect.

Prevention of this dreaded complication is best accomplished by visualization of the blood emanating from the needle. If it is pulsatile and continues to flow after the leg is horizontal, injection should not be attempted at this site. Theoretically, visualization of arteries and veins with duplex-assisted sclerotherapy should negate this risk. Indeed, newer color-flow duplex imagery allows visualization of minute arteries and veins. However, a number of arterial ulcerations have occurred with this technique, even when injecting posterior calf, gastrocnemius and saphenofemoral junctional varicose veins. Thus no technique is completely free from this complication.

DEEP VENOUS THROMBOSIS AND PULMONARY EMBOLISM

Pulmonary emboli and deep venous thrombosis occur very rarely after sclerotherapy. The literature contains many case reports but does not permit an exact estimate of the incidence of post-sclerotherapy deep venous thrombosis or pulmonary embolism. A review by Feied summarizes the major reports and risk factors for deep venous thrombosis.[26]

The diagnosis of deep venous thrombosis is often clinically difficult, with up to 50% of cases going unnoticed. Embolization of a thrombus occurs in more than 50% of patients and is not diagnosed in up to 70% of cases, with a mortality rate approaching 35% without treatment. Both the use of preventive measures and maintaining clinical suspicion are important in preventing this complication. Thus the reported incidence of deep venous thrombosis post-sclerotherapy treatment is greatly underestimated.

In the 1930s and 1940s, clinically evident pulmonary embolism after sclerotherapy of varicose veins occurred in, at most, 0.14% of patients. In a review of 28 cases of pulmonary embolism after sclerotherapy, most cases occurred in patients at bed rest. Pulmonary embolism occurred 1–21 days after the treatment session. The incidence in this series was estimated as one case of pulmonary embolism per 10 000 patients.

The cause of deep venous thrombosis, with or without pulmonary embolism, after sclerotherapy is unclear. The three major factors responsible for deep venous thrombosis were first elucidated more than 100 years ago by Virchow:

- endothelial damage
- vascular stasis
- changes in coagulability.

Sclerotherapy treatment always produces the first two causes in the triad, with coagulability changes related to the unique properties of sclerosing solutions in addition to the predisposing factors of the patient. Chemical endophlebitis produced by sclerotherapy should anchor the thrombus to the site of injection. Histologic examination of treated varicose veins has demonstrated that firm thrombosis occurs only on the damaged endothelium. Nonadherent thrombosis occurs on normal endothelium. Therefore the most logical explanation for the development of emboli is damage to the deep venous system by migration of sclerosing solution or a partly attached thrombosis into deep veins from treated superficial veins. This may occur as a result either of injection of excessive volumes of sclerosing solution or physical inactivity after injection. An additional possibility concerns injection of tributary perforator veins, which may directly communicate with the deep venous system. In this situation, inadequate compression or injection of even 0.5 ml of sclerosing solution may force nonadherent thrombi into the deep circulation with muscle contraction. Ascending venography and digital subtraction phlebography in women with leg telangiectasia found that 0.7 ml of contrast medium injected into telangiectatic branches spread into the saphenous system in eight of 15 patients. Two of the eight patients had telangiectasia as the only clinically perceptible abnormality.[27] Therefore it is possible that up to 13% of patients with telangiectatic veins are at risk for the spread of sclerosing solution directly into the deep venous system. This further emphasizes the importance of limiting injection volumes.

A report on massive pulmonary embolism following high ligation combined with sclerotherapy reinforces the above-mentioned recommendations.[28] One should consider not performing sclerotherapy in a patient who is unable to ambulate or is predisposed to hypercoagulation by coexistent systemic illness or surgical trauma.

The inappropriate tourniquet effect of an excessively tight wrap on the thigh is a rare cause for the development of deep venous thrombosis. Occlusion of deep venous flow results in popliteal vein thrombosis, which can be resolved with conservative treatment. The adverse effects of non-graduated compression emphasize the importance of using properly fitted graduated support stockings in sclerotherapy treatment.

A number of primary and secondary hypercoagulable states exist that can be ruled out through the use of an appropriate patient history and a review of systems in the presclerotherapy treatment evaluation. The prevalence of inherited thrombotic syndromes in the general population is one in 2500–5000 but increases to 4% in patients with a past history of thrombosis. In addition, a past history of deep venous thrombosis raises the likelihood of new postoperative venous thrombosis from 26% to 68%, whereas a past history of both deep venous thrombosis and pulmonary embolism gives a near 100% incidence of thrombosis. Thus sclerotherapy should be undertaken cautiously in patients with previous deep venous thrombosis. Further detail on all hypercoagulable states is beyond the scope of this chapter.

Because of the potentially lethal nature of excessive thrombosis, all attempts should be made to minimize its occurrence. The sclerosing solution quantity should be limited to 0.5–1 ml per injection site to prevent leakage of the solution into the deep venous system. Other techniques that minimize damage to the deep venous system include rapid compression of the injected vein with a 30–40 mmHg pressure stocking, followed by immediate ambulation or calf movement of the injected extremity and frequent ambulation thereafter to promote rapid dilution of the solution from the injected area. Full dorsiflexion of the ankle empties all deep leg veins, including muscular and soleal sinuses. Using these recommendations, Fegan reported no cases of deep venous thrombosis or pulmonary emboli in 13 352 patients when the sclerosing solution quantity was limited to 0.5 ml and rapid compression was used.

The critical time period for thrombus formation in sclerotherapy-treated vessels is approximately 9 hours after treatment. Therefore compression stockings or bandages are of most benefit during the night after sclerotherapy treatment and during other periods of relative vascular stasis when an intravascular thrombus is being formed.

Consideration must be given to treating elderly patients, since they have a reportedly increased risk for deep venous thrombosis. It is hypothesized that the major cause for this increased risk is the relative pooling of blood in the soleal venous sinuses, which occurs from decreased calf muscle pump infusion. In the elderly population it may be best to perform small treatments, with calf pumping given manually immediately after injection.

Since deep venous thrombosis is a potentially life-threatening complication, its treatment must be rapid and decisive. After effective anticoagulation with intravenous heparin has been achieved, oral anticoagulation with warfarin and other inhibitors of vitamin K metabolism should begin. Alternatively, patients may continue receiving subcutaneous heparin. Intravenous heparin should be continued for 3–5 days after initiation of warfarin to prevent an early reduction in anticoagulant protein C and protein S function before procoagulant activity is affected.

Peripheral infusions of lytic agents may be superior to anticoagulation in the rapidity of clot resolution, in the reduction of late symptoms, and in the reduction of the risk of recurrent thrombosis. If peripheral systemic lytic therapy is ineffective, direct infusion of lytic agents into the thrombus may be useful. To prevent recurrence, thrombolytic therapy should be followed by the use of antiplatelet agents such as aspirin or warfarin, or both. A more complete discussion of the various lytic agents is beyond the scope of this chapter.

REFERENCES

A complete list of references can be found in Goldman.[5]

1. Georgiev M. Postsclerotherapy hyperpigmentations: a one-year followup. *J Dermatol Surg Oncol* 1990; **16**: 608–10.
2. Goldman MP, Kaplan RP, Duffy DM. Postsclerotherapy hyperpigmentation: a histologic evaluation. *J Dermatol Surg Oncol* 1987; **13**: 547–50.
3. Thibault P, Wlodarczyk J. Correlation of serum ferritin levels and postsclerotherapy pigmentation: prospective study. *J Dermatol Surg Oncol* 1994; **20**: 684–6.
4. Goldman MP. Postsclerotherapy hyperpigmentation: treatment with a flashlamp excited pulsed dye laser. *J Dermatol Surg Oncol* 1992; **18**: 417–22.
5. Goldman MP. Complications and adverse sequelae of sclerotherapy. In Goldman MP, Weiss RA, Bergan JJ, eds. *Varicose Veins and Telangiectasias: Diagnosis and Treatment*, 2nd edn. St Louis, MO: Quality Medical Publishing, 1999: 300–79.
6. Kilmer SL, Goldman MP, Fitzpatrick RE. Treatment of benign pigmented cutaneous lesions. In Goldman MP, Fitzpatrick RE, eds. *Cutaneous Laser Surgery: the Art and Science of Selective Photothermolysis.* St Louis, MO: Mosby, 1999: 179–212.
7. Weiss RA, Weiss MA.) Incidence of side effects in the treatment of telangiectasias by compression sclerotherapy: hypertonic saline vs polidocanol. *J Dermatol Surg Oncol* 1990; **16**: 800–4.
8. Davis LT, Duffy DM. Determination of incidence and risk factors for post-sclerotherapy telangiectatic matting of the lower extremity: a retrospective analysis. *J Dermatol Surg Oncol* 1990; **16**: 327–30.
9. Dover JS, Sadick NS, Goldman MP. The role of lasers and light sources in the treatment of leg veins. *Dermatol Surg* 1999; **25**: 328–36.
10. Goldman MP. Laser and non-coherent pulsed light treatment of leg telangiectasias and venules. In Goldman MP, Bergan JJ, eds. *Ambulatory Treatment of Venous Disease.* St Louis, MO: Mosby, 1996: 89–98.
11. Goldman MP, Fitzpatrick RE. Laser treatment of cutaneous vascular lesions. In Goldman MP, Fitzpatrick RE, eds. *Cutaneous Laser Surgery: the Art and Science of Selective Photothermolysis.* St Louis, MO: Mosby, 1999: 19–178.
12. de Faria JL, Moraes IN. Histopathology of the telangiectasias associated with varicose veins. *Dermatologia* 1963; **127**: 321–9.
13. Fisher DA. Treatment of vasovagal reactions. *J Am Acad Dermatol* 1998; **38**: 287–8.
14. Tijel R. Cardiac arrest following routine venipuncture. *J Am Med Assoc* 1976; **236**: 1845–7.
15. Goldman MP, Bennett RG. Treatment of telangiectasia: a review. *J Am Acad Dermatol* 1987; **17**: 167–8.
16. Fegan WG. The complications of compression sclerotherapy. *Practitioner* 1971; **207**: 797–9.

17. Thibault PK. Sclerotherapy of varicose veins and telangiectasias: a 2-year experience with sodium tetradecyl sulphate. *Aust N Z J Phlebol* 1999; **3**: 25–30.
18. Conrad P, Malouf GM. The Australian polidocanol (Aethoxysklerol) open clinical trial results at two years. Presented at the Annual Meeting of the North American Society of Phlebology, Maui, Hawaii, 21 February 1984.
19. Sigg K. The treatment of varicosities and accompanying complications. *Angiology* 1952; **3**: 355–79.
20. Belcaro G, Nicolaides AN, Errichi BM, *et al.* Superficial thrombophlebitis of the legs: a randomized, controlled, follow-up study. *Angiology* 1999; **50**: 523–9.
21. British Medical Journal. From our legal correspondent: hazards of compression sclerotherapy. *Br Med J* 1975; **3**: 714–15.
22. Cockett FB. Arterial complications during surgery and sclerotherapy of varicose veins. *Phlebology* 1986; **1**: 3–6.
23. Biegeleisen K, Neilsen RD, O'Shaughnessy A. Inadvertent intra-arterial injection complicating ordinary and ultrasound-guided selerotherapy. *J Dermatol Surg Oncol* 1993; **19**: 953–8.
24. Natali J, Maraval M, Carrance F. Recent statistics on complications of sclerotherapy. Presented at the Annual Meeting of the North American Society of Phlebology, Maui, 21 February 1984.
25. Staubesand J, Seydewitz V. Ultrastructural changes following perivascular and intra-arterial injection of sclerosing agents: an experimental contribution to the problem of iatrogenic damage. *Phlébologie* 1991; **44**: 16–22.
26. Feied CF. Deep vein thrombosis: the risks of sclerotherapy in hypercoagulable states. *Semin Dermatol* 1993; **12**: 135–49.
27. Bohler-Sommeregger K, Karnel F, Schuller-Petrovic S, *et al.* Do telangiectasias communicate with the deep venous system? *J Dermatol Surg Oncol* 1992; **18**: 403–6.
28. Biegeleisen K, Neilsen RD, O'Shaughnessy A. Inadvertent intra-arterial injection complicating ordinary and ultrasound-guided sclerotherapy. *J Dermatol Surg Oncol* 1993; **19**: 953–8.

29

Surgical management of primary and recurrent varicose veins

JOHN J BERGAN

Whether varicose veins are a disease or a disorder has been argued, but this is of no importance to the patient who has the condition. For her, and sometimes him, the dilated veins are undesirable. Often when the patient seeks advice, this is poorly given because the physician's perception, like that of society, is that varices are not a major problem. Yet, they occur frequently with an acknowledged incidence as low as 10%[1] and as high as 50% of a given population.[2] Epidemiologic studies which report such a wide variation in incidence could be looked upon as flawed.[3] However, another explanation lies in the definition of a varicose vein. Dodd and Cockett said that, 'a varicose vein is one which has permanently lost its valvular efficiency. . . . As a result of continuous dilation under pressure in the course of time, a varicose vein becomes elongated, tortuous, pouched, and thickened'.[4] Others, including the Widmers in their much-quoted studies, include intradermal (hyphenweb veins) (telangiectasias) and subcutaneous (reticular) veins.[5] These differences in definition are sufficient to explain discrepancies in incidence studies without denying the importance of the varicosities to the individual who is afflicted by them.

We have chosen to adopt the definition of Arnoldi because it lays the groundwork for a unified theory of causation which is in agreement with observed facts. He stressed that varicosities were '. . . any dilated elongated, or tortuous veins, irrespective of size'.[6]

Combining the observations of Dodd and Cockett with those of Arnoldi allows an understanding that elongated, dilated, tortuous, pouched, and thickened veins with incompetent valves are physiologically identical despite their differences in size. This leads to the logical conclusion that they are derived from the same hereditary/hormonal influences and respond to the same hydrostatic and hydrodynamic forces. The telangiectasias of the skin, the blue-green reticular varicosities under the skin and large grape-like varicosities, which lie even deeper, all conform to the appropriate definition and respond to the appropriate forces.

ETIOLOGY

Planning treatment of the abnormalities mentioned above demands some understanding of the etiology of primary venous insufficiency. Whilst many complex and differing influences have already been discovered and many others remain to be elucidated, it is only necessary to focus on the four factors previously named when advising patients about their condition. The four main influences are heredity, female sex hormones, gravitational hydrostatic force, and hydrodynamic muscular compartment forces.

A familial tendency toward development of varicose veins is understood by physicians and patients. It is felt by some to be dominant;[7] others believe that it is a recessive trait.[8] It is postulated that the inherited defect is alteration in vein wall collagen and/or elastin.[9] Dilation of the vein wall in varices is frequently focal and, therefore, a specific defect in that location is responsible for the asymmetric abnormality.

Female hormonal influences on the veins are profound.[10] For example, varicose veins develop in pregnancy. In 70–80% of cases, they appear in the first trimester, often within 2–3 weeks of gestation. As this is a time when the corpus luteum is elaborating progesterone, it is of interest that an increased venous capacitance is found in women taking high-dose progesterone contraceptive pills. Also, venous distensibility is greatest during the luteal phase as compared with the follicular phase of the menstrual cycle. The alteration in distensibility correlates closely with progesterone levels.

Two forces act on the hereditary/hormonal substrate to produce dilation and elongation of veins. The first, the weight of the blood column from the right atrium to the affected vein through valveless conduits or incompetent valves, is a constant, gravitational force and may be referred to as hydrostatic (Fig. 29.1). The second is the pressure exerted by contracting muscles on adjacent veins. This may be called a hydrodynamic force. The first captured the attention of Paul of Aegina and Trendelenburg whose observations were separated by 1200 years but both of whom suggested interruption of the gravitational force by ligating affected veins in the thigh. The second, or hydrodynamic, force was the subject of Carl Arnoldi's research.[11,12] He emphasized the transmission of compartmental force through failed perforating vein valves to subcutaneous veins as a cause of venous varicosities (Fig. 29.2).

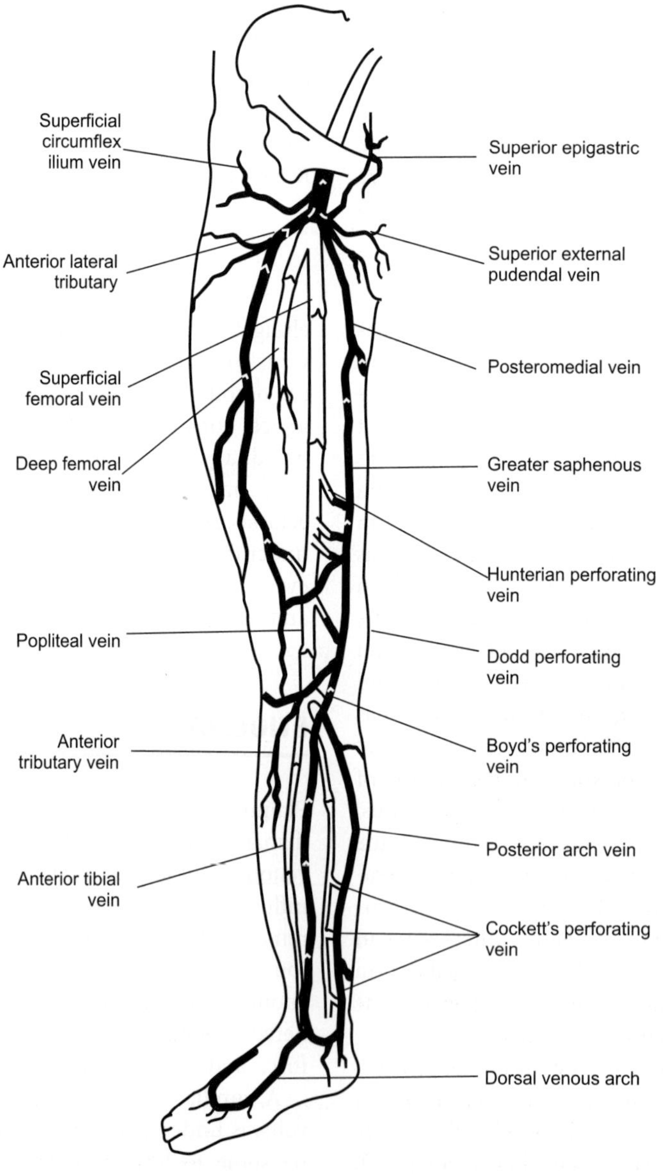

Figure 29.1 *This diagram of the superficial venous system of the lower extremity shows clearly why the theory of descending incompetence of veins – the centrifugal theory – is believed to cause varicosities. Note the relationship of major named perforating veins to the saphenous vein and the posterior arch vein.*

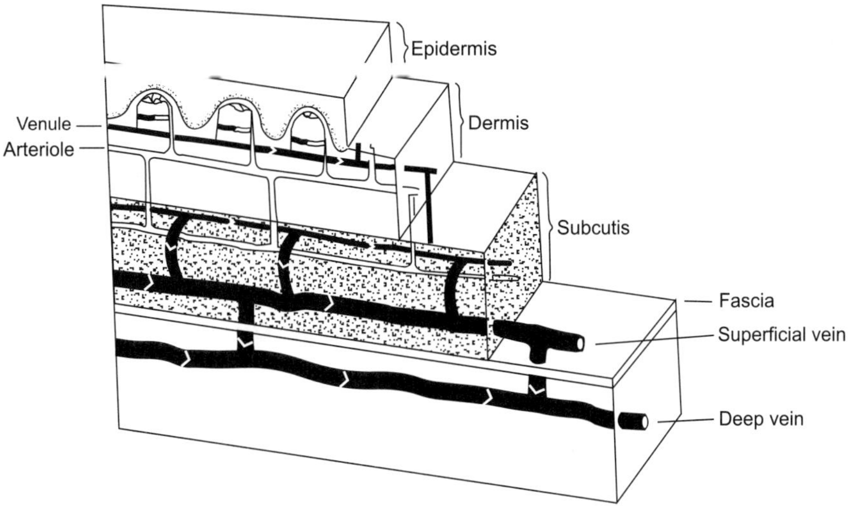

Figure 29.2 *As seen in this diagram, check valves between the deep and superficial venous system protect veins in the subcutis and dermis from muscular compartment pressure. Sudden failure of these allows new telangiectatic blemishes to appear quickly. Chronic failure causes elongation and dilation of larger subcutaneous veins.*

PRACTICAL APPLICATION OF ETIOLOGIC PRINCIPLES

As progesterone inhibits smooth muscle contractility, it provides stability for the pregnant uterus. Unfortunately, it inhibits smooth muscle contractility in the venous wall and allows dilation of subcutaneous veins so that they expand against the dense subdermal somatic nerve network and cause characteristic symptoms. These are maximal on the first day of a menstrual period when the effects of progesterone-stimulated venous dilation may cause sudden giving way of a competent valve. This explains the phenomenon of a sudden appearance of a cluster of varicosities or a telangiectatic blemish. This may occur on the leg of a pregnant woman during the first trimester of pregnancy, a time of minimal uterine enlargement. Considering the power of hydrodynamic compartmental forces which regularly exceed 150 mmHg, it is not surprising that the sudden appearance of such primary venous cutaneous blemishes corresponds to locations of named and unnamed, but familiar, perforating veins.

Hydrostatic forces causing progressively descending valvular insufficiency is an easily understood concept and no doubt accounts for some varicose vein progression. This has been termed the centrifugal theory of venous incompetence. However, progression of varicosities from distal to proximal has been noted by many physicians and recorded by several interested investigators.[13,14] Putting together the facts that muscular compartmental forces are powerful, blood is an incompressible fluid and perforating veins may lose their check valve function, explains the distal-to-proximal progression of valvular incompetence, the centripetal theory of progressive venous insufficiency (Fig.29.3).[15]

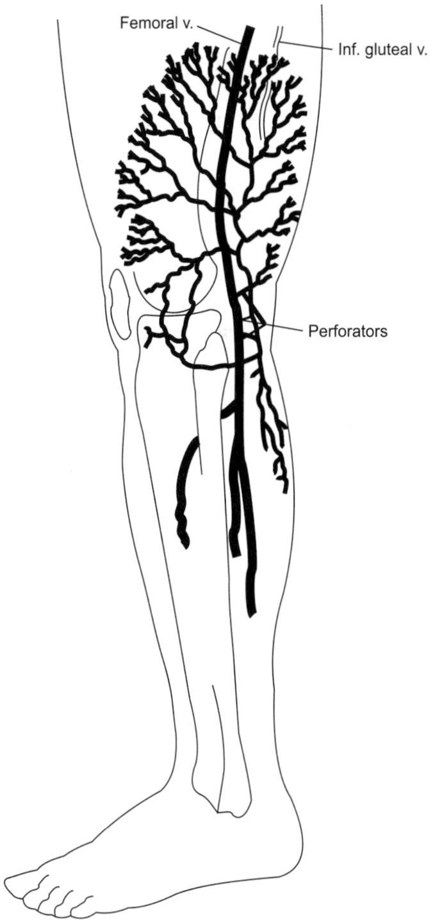

Figure 29.3 *Careful use of the Doppler and high-resolution duplex scanning has shown that this diagram produced by Weiss is accurate. Unnamed perforators lose check valve function and unsupported subcutaneous and intracutaneous veins enlarge. This explains the fan-like distribution of telangiectasias and the tree-like arborization of reticular veins.*

SURGICAL INDICATIONS

Indications for surgical intervention in treatment of primary venous insufficiency are listed in Table 29.1. Actually, the very appearance of telangiectatic blemishes and protuberant, saccular varicosities may stimulate the afflicted individual to seek consultation. Ultimately, this may be the only indication for intervention. Unfortunately, negative physician perception regarding availability and efficacy of treatment of varices may deny the patient the precise care which is sought.[16] Furthermore, symptoms of primary venous insufficiency may be present but not recognized by the patient until asked for during thorough history taking. The characteristic symptoms include aching pain, easy leg fatigue and leg heaviness, all worsening as the day progresses so that the patient sits down in the afternoon and elevates the legs for some relief. These symptoms will be maximal on the first day of a menstrual period when progesterone-related vein dilation is amplified by estrogen. The symptoms may not be recognized by the patient as being due to the varicose veins so they must be asked for by the interested physician. Neither the patient nor the physician may understand that these symptoms arise from telangiectatic blemishes as well as venous varicosities. However, this is true and some 50% of patients with telangiectasias will have such symptoms and 85% will be relieved of them by appropriate therapy.[17]

Other indications for intervention for venous varicosities include superficial thrombophlebitis in varicose clusters, external bleeding from high-pressure venous blebs, or advanced changes of chronic venous insufficiency. These include server ankle hyperpigmentation, subcutaneous lipodermatosclerosis, atrophie blanche, or frank ulceration.

Specific findings on physical examination, which lead toward surgical intervention rather than sclerotherapy, include the finding of axial reflux in the greater saphenous vein or lesser saphenous vein. Experience teaches that sclerotherapy of varicosities in the presence of saphenous reflux will fail. Also, large varices of the medial thigh lend themselves to surgical removal rather than sclerotherapy for two reasons. First, large varices respond better to removal because they are subject to superficial thrombophlebitis after injection. Second, large varices in this location are frequently associated with large perforating veins in the Hunterian or Dodd location and these may be difficult to obliterate by injection.

Table 29.1 *Varicose veins: indications for intervention*

General appearance
Aching pain
Leg heaviness
Easy leg fatigue
Superficial thrombophlebitis
External bleeding
Ankle hyperpigmentation
Lipodermatosclerosis
Atrophie blanche
Venous ulcer

SURGICAL OPTIONS

Options available for surgical treatment of varicose veins are listed in Table 29.2. Objectives of surgical treatment should be ablation of the hydrostatic forces of axial, saphenous vein reflux and removal of the hydrodynamic forces of perforator vein reflux. These should be combined with extraction of the varicose vein clusters in as cosmetic a fashion as possible.

Ligation of the saphenous vein at the saphenofemoral junction has been practiced widely in the belief that this would control gravitational reflux while preserving the vein for subsequent arterial bypass. It is true that the saphenous vein is largely preserved after proximal ligation.[18] However, reflux continues and hydrostatic forces are not controlled.[19] Recurrent varicose veins are more frequent after saphenous ligation than after stripping.[20] Recurrent varicose veins are more frequent after saphenous ligation and sclerotherapy than after stripping and sclerotherapy.[21] A prospective, randomized trial comparing proximal saphenous ligation and stab avulsion of varices to stripping of the thigh portion of the saphenous vein and stab avulsion of varices has shown superior results with the latter procedure.[22]

In the past, few of the randomized trials of saphenous vein surgery reported late results. These have finally appeared.[23] Routine saphenous vein stripping reduced the rate of varicosity recurrence and the need for reoperation for recurrent saphenofemoral incompetence at 6 years from 21% in limbs subjected to saphenous ligation to 6% in limbs having saphenous stripping, giving a relative risk of 0.28, a confidence interval of 0.13–0.59. Although there are arguments in favor of retaining the long saphenous vein for possible arterial bypass grafting, a reoperation rate of more than 20% makes this strategy

Table 29.2 *Surgical procedures used in treatment of varicose veins*

Ankle-to-groin saphenous vein stripping (with stab avulsion)
Segmental saphenous vein stripping (with stab avulsion)
Saphenous vein ligation, high, low, both
Saphenous vein ligation and sclerotherapy
Saphenous vein ligation and stab avulsion of varices
Stab avulsion of varices without saphenous stripping (phlebectomy)

undesirable. Almost three-quarters of the limbs that had undergone ligation of the saphenous vein alone had an incompetent long saphenous vein on duplex imaging.

Although modern saphenous vein stripping extends only from groin to knee, it should be noted that one-fourth of the limbs subjected to saphenous vein stripping in this study still had incompetence in the residual distal long saphenous vein below the knee. Counterbalancing that was the fact that many of these patients had minimal evidence of varicosities. The authors of this definitive report stated: 'Until future studies show an advantage for retaining the long saphenous vein in selected patients, stripping should be a routine part of primary long saphenous varicose vein surgery.'

In studying recurrent varicose veins, preservation of patency of the saphenous vein and continued reflux in the saphenous vein have been found to be the most frequent elements in such recurrence.[24–26] In patients presenting for surgical relief of recurrent varicosities, Ruckley's group found that two-thirds required removal of the saphenous vein as part of the repeat procedure.[24]

Before accurate delineation of sites of origin of varicosities, groin-to-knee stripping of the saphenous vein was considered to be the standard operation that should be done in every operated case. Turn-of-the-century publications had conveyed the belief that reflux was uniformly distributed over the entire length of the saphenous vein.[27–29] The object of excision of the saphenous vein is to remove its gravitational reflux and detach its perforator vein tributaries. Therefore, it has been found unnecessary to remove the below-knee portion. While perforating veins of the medial thigh are largely a part of the saphenous system, this is not true in the leg. Below the knee, important perforating veins are part of the posterior arch circulation. A further argument against routine removal of the saphenous vein below the knee was the discovery of saphenous nerve injury associated with the operation. This occurred in the upper third of the leg as well as adjacent to the ankle incision.[30]

SURGICAL PROCEDURE

As indicated above, knowledge of the pathophysiologic hydrodynamics, relevant venous anatomy, and results of the various surgical procedures allows precise prescription of the proper surgical procedure for each patient and each limb to be benefited by surgical intervention. In surgical patients,[31] groin-to-knee stripping will be part of the operation chosen. In nearly all patients, this will be supplemented by stab avulsion of clusters of varicose veins. Table 29.3 shows the most common patterns of clusters of varicosities and indicates which perforating veins will be detached from the superficial venous circulation by removal of the varices. In one-third of the patients, the saphenofemoral junction will be found to be competent and, therefore, can be left intact. However, stab avulsion of clusters of varicosities derived from reflux from Hunterian or Dodd perforating veins may also remove segments of the greater saphenous vein. Finally, approximately 15% of patients will be found to have lesser saphenous venous incompetence and the operation will need to include careful removal of some or all of that structure (Fig. 29.2).

Table 29.3 *Sites of origin of common patterns of varicose clusters*

Location of cluster	Perforator
Medial thigh, mid-third	Hunterian
Medial thigh, distal third	Dodd
Medial leg, upper third	Boyd
Ankle, posteromedial	Cockett
Ankle, anteromedial	Sherman
Posterolateral knee crease	Unnamed

Greater saphenous stripping

In principle, incisions at groin and ankle are transverse and placed within skin lines. Experience has revealed that best cosmetic results are obtained with vertical incisions throughout the leg and thigh, and these allow preservation of lymphatics as well. Transverse incisions are used in knee creases, and oblique incisions in skin lines are appropriate over the patella. Preoperative marking must be accurately done so as to outline extent of varicose clusters, clinical points of control of varices, and clinically identified location of perforating veins.

In the groin, an oblique variation of the transverse incision will be appropriate. This should be placed 1 cm above, not below, the visible inguinal skin cease. This allows accurate and direct identification of the junction. Anatomy of the named tributaries is infinitely variable, but there is a general theme whose nomenclature is found in Fig. 29.1.

In order not to leave a network of interanastomosing inguinal tributaries behind, a special effort should be made to draw into the groin incision each of the saphenous tributaries. They should be placed on traction until their primary or even secondary tributaries can be controlled. The importance of this maneuver is underscored by Ruckley's description of the residual inguinal network as an important cause of varicose recurrence.[24]

A major cause of discomfort and occasional permanent skin pigmentation is blood extravasated subcutaneously during and after saphenous stripping. This can be minimized (Table 29.4):

- by use of an hemostatic tourniquet;
- by leg elevation prior to and during the actual stripping;

***Table 29.4** Maneuvers to decrease blood loss during saphenous stripping*

Orthopedic tourniquet
Leg elevation during stripping
Internal hemostatic packing*

*A 5 cm wide roller gauze, soaked in lidocaine 0.5%, with added epinephrine.

- by internal packing of the stripper track, using 5 cm wide roller gauze, soaked in lidocaine (lignocaine) 0–0.5% with added epinephrine (adrenaline).

The disposable plastic Codman stripper can be introduced from above downward, as Doppler and duplex studies will have confirmed saphenous junctional incompetence. Examination of the saphenous vein angioscopically has revealed remarkably few valves in those saphenous veins that have come to surgery.[32] Valves which have been observed to be present have been monocuspid, deformed, or even perforated. The reasons for these deformities have not been elucidated but could be due to leukocyte trapping and activation in valve cusps. As the valves consist of only collagen and epithelium,[33] elaboration of collagenase by activated leukocytes could explain all the valve damage that has been observed.

The vein stripper, introduced from above, can be exposed distally with a short transverse incision in the knee skin crease at the medial edge of the popliteal space. This is one of the three places where the saphenous vein is anatomically constant, and it is helpful to mark this location preoperatively with the patient standing. The skin incision in this location will be cosmetically acceptable.

Should the stripper pass relatively unobstructed to the ankle, it can be exposed there with an exceedingly small skin incision placed in a carefully chosen skin line. Passage of the stripper from above downward to the ankle has proved absence of functioning valves, and stripping of the vein from above downward is unlikely to cause nerve damage (Fig. 29.4). At the ankle, the vein should be very cleanly dissected to free it from surrounding nerve fibers before the actual stripping is done.

Stripping of the saphenous vein has been shown to produce profound distal venous hypertension. This can be seen in virtually every such operation. Therefore, if considerable stab avulsion is to be done, it is best to proceed to this directly before actual downward stripping is done. The stab avulsion, assisted by the Varady dissector, Müller hooks, or other such devices will successfully detach perforating veins from their tributary varicose clusters. Dissection of each perforator at fascial level is neither necessary nor cosmetically acceptable. Neither is it necessary to ligate or clip

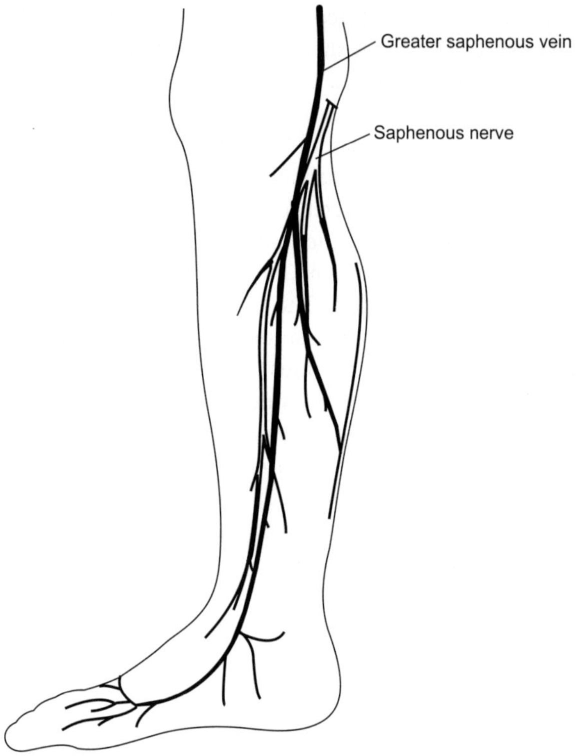

Figure 29.4 *This diagram emphasizes the course of the saphenous nerve in the leg. It illustrates why ascending ankle-to-groin stripping made the nerve vulnerable to injury and why groin-to-knee stripping is less of a hazard.*

retained vein ends after stab avulsion. The elevated leg, trauma-induced venospasm, and direct pressure will assure adequate hemostasis.

Techniques of phlebectomy have been markedly refined by experienced workers in Europe.[34] The size of the incision depends on the size of the varicose vein, the thickness of the vein wall, and its adherence to perivenous tissues. Incisions are made 1–2 mm in length. They are oriented vertically except in areas where skin lines are obviously horizontal. The varicosity is exteriorized by hook or forceps technique, divided, and then avulsed as far as is possible. Subsequent incisions are made as widely spaced as possible. Following avulsion of the varicosity, skin edges can be approximated with tape or with a single absorbable suture.

Surgery of the lesser saphenous vein

Surgery of the lesser saphenous vein is very little like surgery of the greater saphenous vein. There is one similarity. The anatomy of the saphenopopliteal junction is just as irregular as anatomy of the saphenofemoral junction. Indications for surgery of the lesser saphenous vein are similar to those of the greater saphenous vein, that is, reflux in the lesser saphenous vein accompanied by symptomatic varices tributary to that system.

Anatomically, the lesser saphenous vein begins at the lateral end of the dorsal venous arch of the foot (Fig. 29.5). It terminates irregularly in the popliteal fossa. Unlike the greater saphenous vein, it perforates the deep fascia in the middle third of the calf and lies deep to the deep fascia between that level and the termination at the popliteal space.

While earlier surgeons described a normal, low, or high termination of the saphenous vein, this has now been more carefully defined by duplex ultrasonography. Now it is known that a very low termination below the knee joint occurs in only 2% of cases, whereas 42% of the time, the termination is within 5 cm of the knee joint crease. This is its only termination in those cases. However, the lesser saphenous vein may continue up into the thigh and terminate elsewhere. For example, it terminates in the Giacomini vein in about 15% of cases, half of which also have a standard saphenopopliteal junction. The lesser saphenous vein may terminate higher into a femoropopliteal vein or posterior subcutaneous thigh vein. In nearly half these cases, the femoropopliteal vein may enter into a thigh perforating vein or, more rarely, split into two or more branches which may reach the gluteal area. One-third of these also have a standard saphenopopliteal junction.[34]

Further differences between the lesser saphenous vein and the greater saphenous vein include the fact that, in the posterior leg, the lesser saphenous vein has segmental reflux in most cases. Paul van Bemmelen found that the proximal part of the vein was incompetent in 36% of cases while the mid-calf portion was incompetent in 31%.[35] In more than half of the affected lesser saphenous veins, the incompetence was limited to only one segment and it is important to note that in the distal half of the leg, the lesser saphenous vein was normal in 26% of cases. The importance of this derives from the fact that

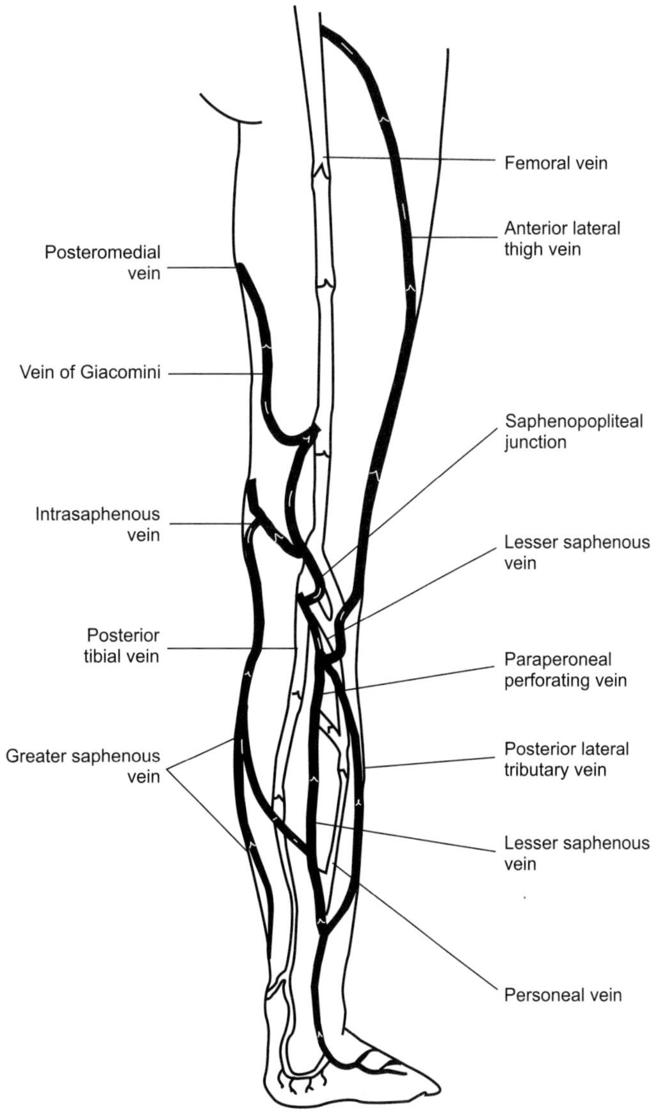

Figure 29.5 *This diagram of the superficial venous system of the posterior leg and thigh serves to identify the accepted patterns of named veins. In practice, variation, not conformity, is the rule.*

the sural nerve is vulnerable to injury in the retromalleolar space on the lateral aspect of the ankle.

Because of the variability of the anatomy and the limited nature of lesser saphenous reflux, it is essential that the continuous-wave hand-held Doppler examination be supplemented by duplex examination. The objective of the duplex examination is to confirm lesser saphenous reflux and identify the termination of the lesser saphenous vein. This can be marked on the skin if the examination is done immediately preoperatively, but more often, as the examination is remote from the operative procedure, the distance from the sole of the foot to the termination of the saphenous vein is carefully measured and recorded in the report of duplex examination. Should that examination be absent, it may be possible to locate the termination of the lesser saphenous vein by careful continuous-wave, hand-held Doppler evaluation, that is, assessing location of reflux and the proximal extent of reflux will locate the lesser saphenous termination.

Hobbs recommends on-table lesser saphenous varicography.[36] Many of his observations were made before the days of duplex examination. Saphenous varicography on table is performed by cannulating a varicose cluster on the posterior aspect of the calf, placing the leg in a lateral position with the x-ray film below the knee joint, skin creases in the popliteal spaces marked by steel hypodermic needles, and the film exposed during injection of 20 ml contrast solution.

The surgical procedure is done with the patient prone and the popliteal space relaxed by knee flexion. The incision is made over the termination of the lesser saphenous vein and centered on the junction between the middle and lateral thirds of the popliteal space. This can be made 5 cm in length to expose the deep fascia. This structure can be further relaxed by more knee flexion. The incision in the deep fascia can be made parallel to the skin incision or longitudinally to effect more exposure. Should the tibial nerve and common peroneal nerve be in the exposed area, these should be carefully preserved. Similarly, the sural nerve should be identified and preserved. Frequently, the lesser saphenous vein or tributaries to it will encircle one or more of these nerve structures. When the encircling veins are varicose, the dissection may be tricky indeed.

Division of the tributaries and especially the proximal tributary to the vein of Giacomini will mobilize the lesser saphenous termination. The vein can be divided and suture ligated near its termination in the popliteal vein. Distally, stripping can be carried out with the disposable plastic Codman stripper or, better, with the Oesch stripper. As there are no equivalents to the Hunterian or Dodd perforating vein in the posterior calf, the stripping can be limited to the proximal lesser saphenous vein to above mid-calf in most cases. A concise description of this technique has been provided by Goren.[37]

After ligation, we have followed the original Oesch technique, which dictates that after the saphenous vein is divided, the stainless steel stripper is passed with its angled tip in a downward direction. It will usually pass only to the varicose cluster in the posterior calf. There the angled tip of the stripper can be palpated through the skin and skin pressure will allow the stripper to perforate the vein wall and become subcutaneous. A 3 mm stab incision exposes the tip of the stripper and the actual vein which has been penetrated is not visualized. A strong, nonabsorbable suture is tied to the end of the stainless steel stripper and this suture, in turn, is fixed to the end of the vein so that it can be inverted into itself as the stripper is removed distally. Once the inverted vein appears in the distal incision, it can be grasped directly with the hemostat and traction placed on the vein as close to the skin as possible to avoid tearing the relatively fragile lesser saphenous vein. Gastrocnemius veins should be searched for in the proximal incision as their persistence will contribute to recurrent varicosities in the posterior calf.

RESULTS OF VARICOSE VEIN SURGERY

In the 5-year period ending January 1, 2000, 595 patients were operated upon for primary venous insufficiency and in all, 702 limbs were operated upon. All operations were performed on an outpatient basis and only three patients required hospitalization, one for seizure disorder and two for significant pain. The most common complication was ecchymosis in the medial thigh in its proximal third. None of these ecchymoses required treatment but in five patients, hyperpigmentation occurred either in that area of ecchymosis or distally in the calf. Ecchymosis was occasionally seen in the retromalleolar area, indicating that bleeding had occurred beneath the deep fascia of the leg.

The next most frequent complication was unexpected. This was the appearance of lymphoceles in 18 cases. These were usually along the path of stripping of the greater saphenous vein, although one appeared in the supramalleolar portion of the saphenous vein removal at the ankle. None of the lymphoceles required treatment and all spontaneously resolved. The last of these mentioned required 2.5 months for complete resolution. There were two wound infections, both in the groin. Neither required surgical debridement or secondary closure. Both healed with institution of antibiotic coverage.

Transient numbness in the saphenous nerve distribution was present in 46 cases. This was invariably traced to a site of stab avulsion.[38] In a report from Innsbruck, 454 limbs in 276 patients were operated upon using four different operative techniques. Statistically, there was no difference in the frequency of saphenous nerve lesions whether the long saphenous vein of the lower leg was stripped in a retrograde or orthograde fashion or using non-invaginating or invaginating techniques.

Two unusual complications occurred. One was a posterior tibial nerve injury at the ankle, which caused significant disability and required physiotherapy for resolution. This did resolve after 7 months and was occasioned by surgery on a retromalleolar perforating vein in order to diminish the effects of a corona phlebectatica. The other unusual complication was a cutaneous area of skin loss appearing under the hard rubber wedge of a Löfqvist tourniquet. It was later learned in correspondence with Löfqvist that this complication occurs when the wedge has been autoclaved, cooled in saline, and handed to the surgeon in a cooled state only to rewarm from the effects of heat retained in the core of the wedge. When rewarming occurs under the pressure of the tourniquet, cutaneous loss can be expected. The loss in this case required full-thickness skin grafting.

SURGERY OF RECURRENT VARICOSE VEINS

Precise study of recurrent saphenous veins by varicography, phlebography, continuous-wave Doppler, and duplex Doppler examination has now clarified their patterns. Lessons learned in study of such recurrent varicosities has influenced the performance of the primary operation. The figure of 20% has been quoted as the incidence of recurrent varicosities after apparent adequate surgery.[25]

The most useful classification of recurrent varicosities following operation on the greater saphenous vein has been provided by Ruckley's group.[24] They divide the types of recurrence into two types (Fig. 29.6). In the first, the saphenofemoral venous complex is intact in one way or another. This implies that a direct operation on the groin will be required. Reflux is encountered to a retained greater saphenous vein either through main-stem recurrence or through tributaries which then anastomose to the retained greater saphenous vein in the proximal thigh. Another cause is neovascularization through the hematoma caused by groin exploration. The second type of recurrence, implying that no groin exploration will be required, is through mid-thigh perforating veins into the retained saphenous system. Ruckley's group calls attention to the fact that in two-thirds of the cases of recurrence, the retained greater saphenous vein was implicated.

Quigley in Australia found varicose recurrence rates of 64% within the greater saphenous system when such recurrences were studied by duplex techniques.[39] Redwood and Lambert, studying patients who had previous groin exploration, found that 58% of the limbs had saphenofemoral junction incompetence.[40] These findings support Ruckley's and it is apparent that recurrent varicosities in two-thirds of cases are associated

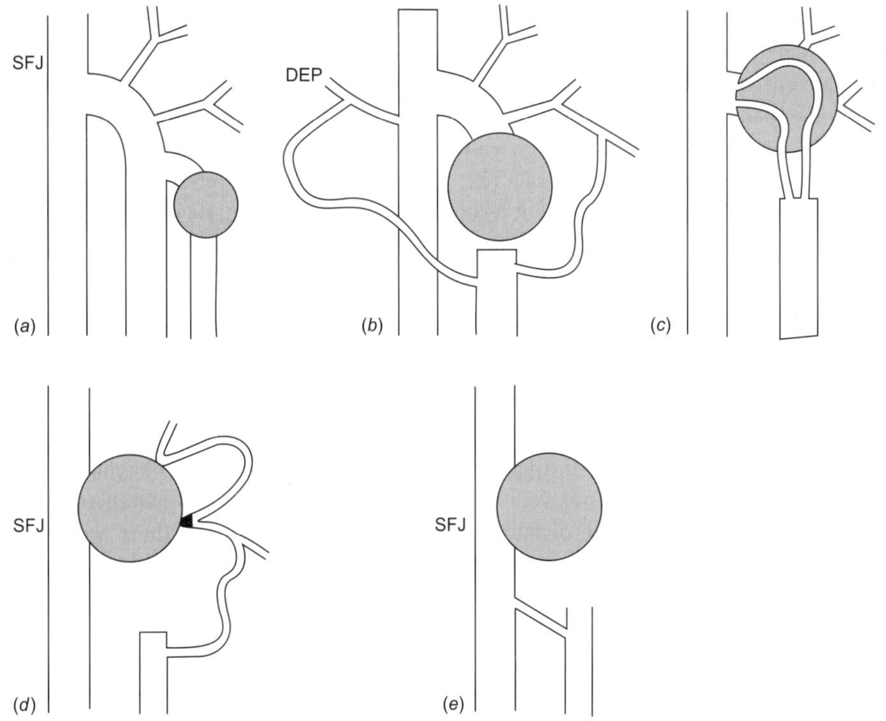

Figure 29.6 *Recurrent varicosities may require a groin re-exploration (type 1, saphenous venous complex intact) or they may not (type 2, saphenous venous complex obliterated). Careful preoperative imaging will define the cause of recurrence of varicosities. In roughly two-thirds of cases, a retained saphenous vein segment is implicated.*

with proximal saphenofemoral ligation and that this would be impossible following groin-to-knee stripping.

Indications for operation for recurrent varicose veins are similar to those for primary varicose veins, that is, symptomatic clusters of varicose veins associated with saphenous or perforator reflex. In those cases in which there is no groin communication to the recurrent veins, groin exploration will not be required. In this situation, the varicosities emanate from incompetent perforating veins. The most common of these has been found to be the mid-thigh or Hunterian group of perforating veins.

It is essential that patients be studied either with duplex imaging or varicography in order that all sites of recurrence be identified and dealt with at the time of surgical re-exploration.

OPERATIVE TECHNIQUE

Re-exploration of the saphenofemoral junction for recurrent varicose veins can be difficult. The caput medusa of collateral veins or neovascularization consists of thin-walled, elongated, dilated, tortuous vessels under high venous pressure with all of this encased in scar from the previous surgical dissection. It can be presumed that if reflux has been found across the saphenofemoral junction by preoperative examination, a significant saphenous stump has been left. This may receive any number of tributaries whose reverse flow is coursing distally to feed the recurrent varices by gravitational pressure.

Whilst each surgeon may have developed his or her own approach to recurrent varices, the lateral technique of Li can be recommended.[41] This subscribes to the surgical maxim that in performing repeat surgery, you should proceed from the normal to the abnormal. The surgical incision may simply reopen the old if it was placed correctly high in the thigh. Otherwise, the new incision should be placed 1 cm above the inguinal skin crease. This should be carried laterally so as to expose the femoral artery. Opening the femoral sheath so that the anterior surface of the common femoral artery is seen will allow the medial dissection to proceed in a proper plane. The proximal common femoral vein below the inguinal ligament can be exposed in this way through an undamaged field. After the common femoral vein has been exposed, the dissection can proceed distally to expose the stump of the saphenous vein. This is usually long enough to free up circumferentially, apply clamps, and transect the main trunk of the vessel. The new stump can be flush ligated at the femoral vein at this point in the operation. Resection of the distal saphenous vein, its tributaries, accompanying lymphatic vessels, scar, and entangled fat can be done with assurance that a complete operation will be accomplished without hazard to the femoral vein.

Although some have advocated only saphenous religation in treatment of varicose recurrences,[42] this seems illogical now that the unsatisfactory natural history of primary proximal saphenous ligation has been defined. For this reason, we have chosen to remove the residual refluxing saphenous vein as part of the re-operation. The purpose of this maneuver is to detach those perforating veins that are connected to the saphenous vein. As the greater saphenous vein has a constant location at the medial border of the popliteal space, an inconspicuous transverse incision in skin lines can be placed to expose the vein in this location. This is facilitated by preoperative marking, identifying the vein by palpation or the continuous-wave Doppler instrument. Depending upon the length of the residual proximal saphenous vein, either the intraluminal or the extraluminal stripper can be used to resect the vein. Sometimes use of the angioscope with its illumination turned full up will allow accurate identification of the location of the proximal end of the residual saphenous vein. Distally, if the stripper passes to the ankle, that incompetent portion of the residual vein can be removed by the invagination technique. Otherwise, the remaining portion of the procedure is performed as a phlebectomy by stab avulsion.

In the 24-month period ending 1 January 1995, 29 patients (two men) were operated upon for recurrent varicose veins. All operations were done on an outpatient basis, and no patient required hospitalization. A total of 33 limbs were operated upon. Multiple sources of the recurrent varices were present in most limbs but an attempt was made to identify the most important cause in each instance. Saphenofemoral incompetence following presumed proximal saphenous ligation was present in 14 limbs. Two limbs had prior groin-to-knee saphenous stripping. Seven limbs demonstrated lesser saphenous incompetence but this had not been the target of the primary operation in any of them. Eight limbs had identifiable perforator vein origin of the major recurrence. Four were from mid-thigh, two from distal thigh, and two from posterior calf perforating veins. Multiple sources of varix recurrence were present in the remaining limbs.

Surgical complications were fewer than expected. Significant thigh ecchymosis was present in seven limbs and this was thought to be related to use of the external vein stripper in several instances. No wound infections were encountered but there was one lymphocele. No nerve deficits were recorded.

HEMODYNAMIC IMPROVEMENT AFTER VEIN STRIPPING

Investigations of venous pathophysiology in continental Europe are influenced by the observations of Friedrich

Trendelenburg, Professor of Surgery in Bonn in the 1880s. In his 1891 publication advocating greater saphenous vein ligation, he coined the term 'private circulation' to describe the gravitational reflux down the saphenous vein which returns proximally through perforating veins and the deep venous system.[43] Later observers have noted that this private circulation is associated with primary deep venous valvular incompetence and that this is the most importance consequence of saphenous reflux.[44] Before the advent of duplex scanning, this was chiefly a phlebographic diagnosis.[45] Careful study of phlebograms confirmed correlation of increased deep vein diameter with severity of reflux.[46] Normal femoropopliteal venous junction diameter was found to be 12 mm in 75 limbs. This increased to 17 mm in limbs with saphenous reflux to the ankle. Furthermore, the increased volume of flow in the affected veins was associated with increased tortuosity of these vessels so that the angle of the femoropopliteal junction (ideally 180°) decreased from an observed 158° in normals to 142° in limbs with severe reflux. Earlier study of phlebograms had shown that deep venous diameter was greatest in limbs with superficial venous reflux. Deep veins in limbs with proven prior deep venous thrombosis were actually found to be thinner in diameter than normal and those limbs with superficial reflux.[47] Doppler ultrasonography has shown that deep venous reflux in limbs with varicose veins proven not to have been the site of previous thrombosis is a startling 20.6%. Such deep venous reflux correlates with the severity of superficial reflux.[48]

Using indirect parameters of venous pathophysiology, hemodynamics of the deep venous system were observed to improve after treatment of superficial venous incompetence.[45] Normalization was not achieved in all cases, and it was felt that earlier intervention might prevent postoperative continuing development of superficial incompetence.

Hemodynamic improvement of global limb venous function as measured by mercury strain gauge and photoplethysmography has been demonstrated following groin-to-ankle saphenous stripping combined with stab avulsion of varicose cluster.[49] This bettering, detected immediately postoperatively, was further improved 6 months after operation but deterioration of venous function was seen after 1 year. By contrast, using the same techniques, Struckmann found persisting decrease in venous reflux and increase in expelled volume 5 years after radical venous stripping and venous avulsions.[50] Differences in these observations could be accounted for by differences in duration of the preoperative venous insufficiency because, as suggested above, earlier operation could produce more long-lasting hemodynamic improvement. Measurement of foot volumetry has also shown improvement of venous function after correction of superficial reflux.[51]

In the severest form of lower limb venous insufficiency, the post-thrombotic state, measurements have been done using mercury strain gauge.[52] After open subfascial perforator vein interruption, no changes were seen in arterial flow, venous capacity, or venous emptying. However, venous reflux flow and venous volume were decreased significantly.

When considering the indirect observations mentioned above, it is not surprising that direct observation of deep venous reflux shows postoperative bettering. We documented preoperative reflux in the superficial femoral vein in 29 limbs, three of which also showed popliteal venous reflux. Though these were patients with relatively short duration of symptoms, all had sufficient greater saphenous reflux to indicate groin-to-knee saphenous stripping and stab avulsion of varicose clusters.[53] In 27 limbs, superficial femoral reflux was abolished, and in two, popliteal reflux disappeared. These observations have been extended to 38 limbs with similar results, and this experience has been duplicated by others (Stiles C, Ballard J, personal communication).

Alternative techniques in varicose vein removal

Surgical treatments never remain static. Two changes in saphenous vein surgery have occurred in recent years. The first is directed towards saving the saphenous vein and the second towards ablating this structure with minimal invasion. Banding of the subterminal saphenous vein valve has taken an international flavor.[54,55]

The best studied group of patients comes from Korea where 10 men and 69 women (42 right limbs, 37 left limbs) had external banding valvuloplasty of the subterminal saphenous vein valve. Clinical and Doppler information postoperatively was augmented by air plethysmography results.[56] A total of 63 limbs (79.7%) showed no saphenous vein reflux but 14 limbs (17.7%) showed reverse flow on duplex scanning. Two limbs exhibited thrombus within the greater saphenous vein after surgery. Thus, more than 20% of the limbs were in acute failure. Air plethysmographic data revealed that saphenous vein diameter was reduced postoperatively. The calf venous volume was similarly reduced as was the venous filling index. The ejection fraction was improved as was the residual venous volume. These preliminary data show that external banding valvuloplasty can correct valvular reflux and abnormal venous hemodynamics. Thus, the saphenous vein can be saved for future use. However, the 20% acute failure rate should be kept in mind when patients are being selected for this procedure.

The second technique designed to ablate the saphenous vein utilizes the principle of direct-contact radio frequency energy application to the lumen of the saphenous vein. The end result is endovenous shrinkage or occlusion of the vein as collagen contracts under the heat generated by the radio frequency energy. In practice, the electrode can be introduced percutaneously at knee level in a suitable popliteal crease. The electrode, under duplex guidance, can be placed at the saphenofemoral junction and then the radio frequency generator activated as the electrode is withdrawn very slowly.[57]

The earliest significant report on this procedure has now appeared.[58] A total of 301 limbs in CEAP clinical classes 2 and 3 were treated in 206 women and 67 men. Endovenous obliteration was combined with saphenofemoral junction ligation in 67 limbs and, in 181 limbs, stab avulsion phlebectomy was also done. Acute occlusion of the saphenous vein was achieved in 290 limbs (96%). The 11 obliteration failures were treated by subsequent saphenous stripping or managed expectantly. Complications included paresthesias in 15%, thermal injuries in eight limbs, and recanalization in 21 limbs, 11 of which had Doppler-detectable saphenous reflux. The 91 patients followed for more than 6 months showed significant improvement in CEAP classification and progressive relief from clinical symptoms. Ninety-four percent of the patients treated rated themselves as being symptom free or substantially improved.

These early results suggest that ablation of the saphenous vein by radio frequency energy may be as effective as surgical stripping. A question remains about the necessity of proximal saphenofemoral ligation and similarly, the need for radical removal of the tributaries to the saphenofemoral junction as this is not achieved by the technique. Further experience should reveal the value of this form of treatment.

Noting that removal of varicosities done in Roman times with hook phlebectomy has changed little in 2000 years, Spitz in Aurora applied an original technique to this portion of the varicose vein operation.[59] The technical system that he used has been termed the TriVex® system developed by Smith & Nephew Endoscopy of Andover, Massachusetts. The device in practice is a rotating tubular inner blade encased in a protective stationary outer sheath. The working opening is placed adjacent to varicosities, which are then morcellated, aspirated, and removed by suction irrigation. Control of the procedure is through a handpiece which directs the vein fragments into a container connected to a hospital wall suction. Blade speed is 800–1000 r.p.m. for forward, and reverse and oscillation of the tip can be added at 800–1000 r.p.m.

Following development of the technique, Spitz studied operations on 51 women and 5 men. There were 58 unilateral procedures and one bilateral operation. The operative time ranged from 23 to 58 minutes but averaged 41 minutes. The number of incisions per limb averaged 5.6. Complications such as cellulitis, small hematoma formation, swelling or bruising beyond that to be expected occurred in four limbs (6.7%). Objective analog pain scores, cosmetic scores, and satisfaction scores were favorable compared with a historical control group of 109 similar patients who underwent stab avulsion hook phlebectomy.

CONCLUSION

Varicose vein surgery continues to progress and the application of new minimally invasive techniques shows some promise. Available information now allows a unified explanation for the occurrence of telangiectatic blemishes, reticular varicosities, and varicose veins. An understanding of their hemodynamic cause and appropriate pre-intervention evaluation allows precise prescription of appropriate treatment. Such treatment can be on an outpatient basis and, in the case of saphenous insufficiency, this should include at least a groin-to-knee stripping. It is expected that this will decrease incidence of varicose recurrences and allow the most optimal hemodynamic improvement.

REFERENCES

1. Burkitt DP. Varicose veins, deep vein thrombosis, and hemorrhoids: epidemiology and suggested etiology. *Br Med J* 1972; **2**: 556.
2. Bland L, Widmer LK. Varicose veins and chronic venous insufficiency. *Acta Chir Scand Suppl* 1988; **544**: 9–11.
3. Evans CJ, Fowkes FR, Hajivassiliou CA, *et al.* Epidemiology of varicose veins. *Int Angiol* 1944; **13**: 263–70.
4. Dodd H, Cockett F. *The Pathology and Surgery of the Veins of the Lower Limb.* Edinburgh: ES Livingston, 1956.
5. Widmer LK. *Peripheral Venous Disorders: Prevalence and Sociomedical Importance: Observations in 4,529 Apparently Healthy Persons. Basle Study III.* Bern: Hans Huber, 1978.
6. Arnoldi CC. The aetiology of primary varicose veins. *Dan Med Bull* 1957; **4**: 102–7.
7. Ottley C. Hereditary and varicose veins. *Br Med J* 1934; **1**: 528.
8. Trosier J, Le B. Etude genetique des varices. *Ann Med (Fr)* 1937; **41**: 30–3.
9. Rose SS, Ahmed A. Some thoughts on the aetiology of varicose veins. *Int J Cardiovasc Surg* 1985; **27**: 584–93.
10. Bergan JJ. Causes of venous varicosities and telangiectasias: implications for treatment. *J Vasc Biol Med* 1995; **85**: 1101–6.
11. Arnoldi CC. Venous pressure in the leg of healthy human subjects at rest and during muscular exercise in the nearly erect position. *Acta Chir Scand* 1965; **130**: 570.
12. Arnoldi CC. Venous pressure in patients with valvular incompetence of the veins of the lower limb. *Acta Chir Scand* 1966; **132**: 427–30.

13. Fegan WG. Continuous compression technique of injecting varicose veins. *Lancet* 1963; **2**: 109–12.
14. Chant ADB, Jones HO, Townsend JCF, Edmund-Williams J. Radiologic demonstration of the relationship between calf varices and saphenofemoral incompetence. *Clin Radiol* 1972; **23**: 519–23.
15. Cotton LT. *Pathology and Aetiology of Varicose Veins.* Oxford: Oxford University Press, 1957.
16. Weiss RA, Weiss MA, Goldman MP. Physicians' negative perception of sclerotherapy for venous disorders: review of a 7-year experience with modern sclerotherapy. *South Med J* 1992; **85**: 1101–6.
17. Weiss RA, Weiss MA. Resolution of pain associated with varicose and telangiectatic leg veins after compression sclerotherapy. *J Dermatol Surg Oncol* 1990; **16**: 333–6.
18. Rutherford RB, Sawyer JD, Jones DN. The fate of residual saphenous vein after partial removal or ligation. *J Vasc Surg* 1990; **12**: 422–8.
19. McMullin GM, Coleridge Smith PD, Scurr JH. Objective assessment of high ligation without stripping the long saphenous vein. *Br J Surg* 1991; **78**: 1139–42.
20. Munn SR, Morton JB, MacBeth WAAG, McLeish AR. To strip or not to strip the long saphenous vein? A varicose veins trial. *Br J Surg* 1981; **68**: 426–8.
21. Neglen P. Treatment of varicosities of saphenous origin: comparison of ligation, selective excision, and sclerotherapy. In Bergan JJ, Goldman MP, eds. *Varicose Veins and Telangiectasias: Diagnosis and Management.* St Louis, MO: Quality Medical Publishing, 1993: 148–65.
22. Sarin S, Scurr JH, Coleridge Smith PD. Assessment of stripping the long saphenous vein in the treatment of primary varicose veins. *Br J Surg* 1992; **79**: 889–93.
23. Dwerryhouse S, Davies B, Harradine K, Earnshaw JJ. Stripping the long saphenous vein reduces the rate of reoperation for recurrent varicose veins: five-year results of a randomized trial. *J Vasc Surg* 1999; **29**: 589–92.
24. Stonebridge PA, Chalmers N, Beggs I, *et al.* Recurrent varicose veins: a varicographic analysis leading to a new practical classification. *Br J Surg* 1995; **82**: 60–2.
25. Darke SG. The morphology of recurrent varicose veins. *Eur J Vasc Surg* 1992; **6**: 512–17.
26. Conrad P. Groin-to-knee down stripping of the long saphenous vein. *Phlebology* 1992; **7**: 20–2.
27. Mayo CH. Treatment of varicose veins. *Surg Gynecol Obstet* 1906; **2**: 385–8.
28. Babcock WW. A new operation for extirpation of varicose veins. *N Y Med J* 1907; **86**: 1553.
29. Keller WL. A new method for extirpating the internal saphenous and similar veins in varicose conditions: a preliminary report. *N Y Med J* 1905; **82**: 385–9.
30. Bergan JJ. *Surgery of the Veins of the Lower Extremity.* Philadelphia: WB Saunders, 1990.
31. Goren G, Yellin AE. Primary varicose veins: topographic and hemodynamic correlations. *J Cardiovasc Surg* 1990; **31**: 672–7.
32. Gradman WS, Segalowitz J. Grundfest W. Venoscopy in varicose vein surgery: initial experience. *Phlebology* 1993; **8**: 145–50.
33. Butterworth DM, Rose SS, Clark P, *et al.* Light microscopy, immunohistochemistry, and electron microscopy of the valves of the lower limb veins and jugular veins. *Phlebology* 1992; **7**: 1–3.
34. Ricci S, Georgiev M, Goldman MP. *Ambulatory Phlebectomy: a Practical Guide for Treating Varicose Veins.* St Louis, MO: CV Mosby, 1995.
35. Van Bemmelen PS, Bedford G, Beach K, Strandness DE Jr. Quantitative segmental evaluation of venous valvular reflux with ultrasound scanning. *J Vasc Surg* 1989; **10**: 425–31.
36. Hobbs JT. Perioperative venography to ensure accurate saphenopopliteal vein ligation. *Br Med J* 1980; **280**: 1578.
37. Goren G. Yellin AE. Invaginated axial saphenectomy by a semirigid stripper: perforate-invaginate stripping. *J Vasc Surg* 1994; **20**: 970–7.
38. Gasser BG, Pohl P, Mildner A. Läsionen des Nervus saphenus in Abhängigkeit von der Technik des strippings. *Phlebologie* 1995; **24**: 76–7.
39. Quigley FG, Raptis S, Cashman M. Duplex ultrasonography of recurrent varicose veins. *Cardiovasc Surg* 1994; **2**: 775–7.
40. Redwood NFW, Lambert D. Patterns of reflux in recurrent varicose veins assessed by duplex scanning. *Br J Surg* 1994; **81**: 1450–1.
41. Li AKC. A technique for reexploration of the saphenofemoral junction for recurrent varicose veins. *Br J Surg* 1975; **62**: 745–6.
42. Belardi P, Lucerti G. Advantages of the lateral approach for reexploration of the saphenofemoral junction for recurrent varicose veins. *Cardiovasc Surg* 1994; **2**: 772–4.
43. Trendelenburg F. Über die Unterbindung der Vena saphena magna bei unterschenkel varicen. *Beitr Z Klin Chir* 1891; **7**: 195.
44. Hach-Wunderle V. Die secundare popliteal und femoralveneninsuffizienz. *Phlebologie* 1992; **21**: 52–8.
45. Stranzenbach W, Hach W. Phlebographische verlaufsbeobach-tungen der sekundaren popliteal und femoral veneninsuffizienz bei stannvarikose. *Phlebologie* 1991; **20**: 25–9.
46. Hach W, Schirmers U, Becker L. *Mikrozirkulation und Blutrheologic.* Baden Baden: Witzstrock, 1980: 468–70.
47. Fischer H, Siebrecht H. Das kaliber den tiefen unterschenkelvenen bei der primaren varicose und beim postthrombotischen syndrome (eine phlebographische studie). *Der Hautarzt* 1970; **5**: 205–11.
48. Almgren B, Eriksson I. Primary deep venous incompetence in limbs with varicose veins. *Acta Chir Scand* 1989; **155**: 455–60.
49. Hirai M. Naiki K. Hemodynamic evaluation of venous function after surgical treatment of varicose veins. *Vasc Surg* 1992; **26**: 345–50.

50. Struckmann JR. Assessment of venous muscle pump function by ambulatory calf volume strain gauge plethysmography after surgical treatment of varicose veins: a prospective study of 21 patients. *Surgery* 1987; **103**: 347–53.
51. Norgren L. Foot volumetry before and after surgical treatment of patients with varicose veins. *Acta Chir Scand* 1975; **141**: 129.
52. Perhoniemi V, Salo JA, Haapianinen R, Salo H. Strain gauge plethysmography in the assessment of venous reflux after subfascial closure of perforating veins: a prospective study of 20 patients. *J Vasc Surg* 1990; **12**: 34–7.
53. Walsh JC, Bergan JJ, Beeman S, Comer TP. Femoral venous reflux is abolished by greater saphenous vein stripping. *Ann Vasc Surg* 1994; **8**: 566–70.
54. Lane RJ, McMahon C, Cuzzilla M. The treatment of varicose veins using the venous valve cuff. *Phlebology* 1994; **9**: 136–45.
55. Corcos L, Procaci T, Penruzzi G, Dini M, De Anna D. Saphenofemoral valves: histopathological observation and diagnostic approach before surgery. *Dermatol Surg* 1996; **22**: 873–80.
56. Ik Kim D, Boong Lee B, Bergan JJ. Venous hemodynamic changes after external banding valvuloplasty with varicosectomy in the treatment of primary varicose veins. *J Cardiovasc Surg* 1999; **40**: 567–70.
57. Weiss RA, Goldman MP. Controlled radiofrequency-mediated endovenous shrinkage and occlusion. In Goldman MP, Weiss RA, Bergan JJ, eds. *Varicose Veins and Telangiectasias: Diagnosis and Management*, 2nd edn. St Louis, MO: Quality Medical Publishing, 1999: 217–24.
58. Chandler JG, Pichot O, Sessa C, Bergan JJ. Treatment of primary venous insufficiency by endovenous saphenous vein obliteration. *J Vasc Surg*, in press.
59. Spitz GA, Braxton JM, Bergan JJ. Outpatient varicose vein surgery with transilluminated powered phlebectomy. *Vasc Surg* 2000; **34**: 547–55.

30

Compression treatment of chronic venous insufficiency

ALEXANDER D NICOLOFF, GREGORY L MONETA AND JOHN M PORTER

Despite recent interest in surgical strategies to manage chronic venous insufficiency and venous ulceration, nonoperative therapy remains overwhelmingly the primary mode of treatment worldwide. While strict bed rest and limb elevation have been known for decades to be effective therapy for venous insufficiency and ulceration, this is impractical for most patients. The goals of nonoperative management in chronic venous insufficiency are to control symptoms, promote healing of ulcers, and prevent ulcer recurrence while permitting normal ambulatory status. Compression therapy continues to be the mainstay of nonoperative management of chronic venous insufficiency and venous ulceration. This chapter discusses the theories behind the mechanism of compression therapy and reviews the various modalities employed.

COMPRESSION THERAPY: THEORIES OF MECHANISM

Compression therapy is the current 'gold standard' treatment for chronic venous insufficiency. The mechanism of benefit of compression therapy in patients with chronic venous insufficiency and/or venous ulceration remains unknown. Most investigation has yielded conflicting results. The effect of compression therapy on deep venous hemodynamics has been the topic of multiple studies. We and other investigators, using both invasive and noninvasive techniques, have been unable to demonstrate significant changes in ambulatory venous pressure or venous recovery times with compression therapy,[1] whereas other researchers have described modest trends toward normal in these parameters with compression stockings.[2–4]

Improvements in skin and subcutaneous tissue microcirculatory hemodynamics may contribute to the benefits of compression therapy. Laser Doppler flowmetry demonstrates a dependency-induced resting cutaneous hyperemia in patients with chronic venous insufficiency but not in normals.[5] Using this technique, impairment of the so-called venoarteriolar reflex appears to improve with 40 mm Hg (measured compression at the ankle) compression stockings,[3] but is unchanged with 20 mm Hg compression bandages.

Another plausible mechanism for compression therapy is a direct effect on subcutaneous pressure. Clinically, edema reduction is the rule in patients with chronic venous insufficiency who wear elastic compression hosiery. Cutaneous metabolism may improve following edema resorption due to enhanced diffusion of oxygen and other nutrients to the cellular elements of the skin and subcutaneous tissues. Supine perimalleolar subcutaneous pressures increase with elastic compression in limbs with chronic venous insufficiency.[6] This rise in subcutaneous tissue pressure should act to counter transcapillary Starling forces which favor leakage of fluid out of the capillary. Videomicroscopy techniques also demonstrate increased skin capillary density with edema resolution.[7] Kolari *et al.*[8] have also demonstrated an increase in skin tcP_{O_2} following edema reduction.

ELASTIC COMPRESSION STOCKINGS

Conrad Jobst introduced gradient ambulatory compression therapy in the 1950s. He designed the first ambulatory gradient compression stockings to mimic the hydrostatic forces exerted by water in a swimming pool. Over 40 years later, ambulatory compression hosiery remains the most widely accepted treatment for chronic venous insufficiency. Currently, elastic compression stockings of varying compositions, strengths and lengths are manufactured. Multiple clinical reports have demonstrated the benefits of compression stockings in the treatment of chronic venous insufficiency and venous ulceration.[9–11]

In our practice, patients with venous ulceration are treated almost exclusively with local wound care and elastic compression therapy. The Oregon protocol for the treatment of venous stasis ulceration[12] is summarized below:

- initial period of bed rest with limb elevation either at home or in the hospital;
- systemic antibiotics to treat any associated cellulitis;
- daily ulcer cleansing and dry gauze dressing changes;
- corticoid ointment to areas of stasis dermatitis surrounding the ulcer as needed;
- continued use of elastic compression stockings for life following ulcer healing.

Patients initially undergo an assessment of lower extremity edema and possible infection associated with their venous ulcer. In patients with severe edema, 5–7 days of bed rest are prescribed to aid in initial edema resolution. Cellulitis is treated with short-term intravenous or oral antibiotics in conjunction with local wound care (soap and water scrubbing followed by dry gauze dressings changed every 12 hours). No topical agents are applied directly to the ulcer, but 0.1% hydrocortisone cream is applied twice daily to areas of surrounding stasis dermatitis. When the edema and cellulitis have resolved, patients are fitted with below-knee 30–40 mmHg elastic compression stockings. Two pairs are prescribed to permit laundering on alternate days. Patients are instructed to wear the stockings at all times while ambulatory and to remove them upon going to bed. Wound care throughout the course of compression therapy consists of a simple daily soap and water washing of the ulcer. The ulcer is covered with a dry gauze and held in place by the compression stocking. A 'shorty' nylon stocking may be used as a liner under the compression stocking. This serves to hold the dressing in place and facilitates placement of the compression stocking. Foam wedges are used in limb areas where the ankle topography makes uniform compression unlikely (Fig. 30.1). Once the ulcer has healed, ambulatory compression therapy is continued for life. Stockings are replaced at intervals of 3–6 months as needed to maintain compression strength.

Our results with elastic compression management of venous ulcers in 113 patients treated over 15 years have been reported.[13] One hundred and two patients (90%) were compliant with stocking use and 105 (93%) experienced complete ulcer healing. Mean time to ulcer healing was 5.3 months. Complete ulcer healing occurred in 99 of 102 patients (97%) who were compliant with stocking use versus 6 of 11 patients (55%) who

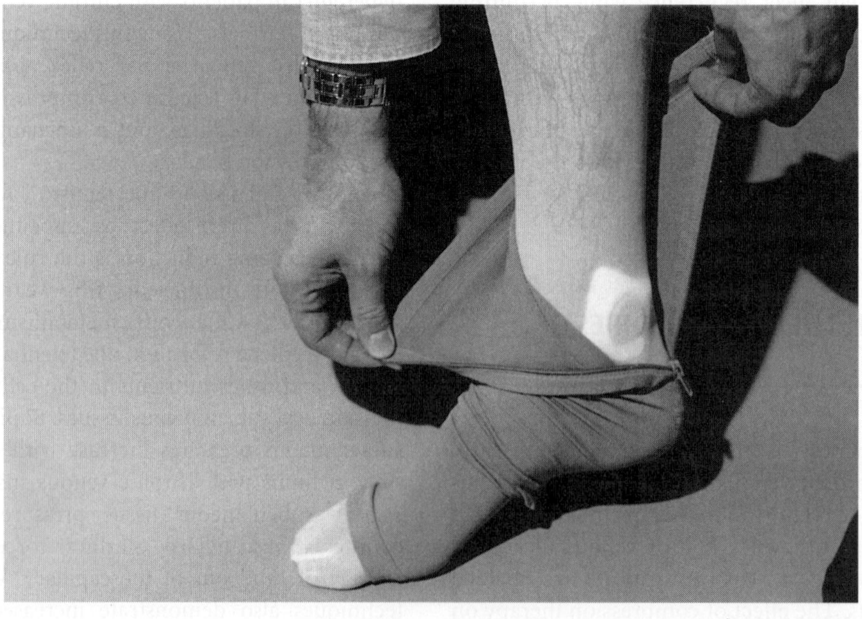

Figure 30.1 *Dry gauze dressing with foam wedge overlying ulcer to help provide uniform compression. A 'shorty' nylon stocking is then placed over the dressing and wedge to help hold them in place. The nylon also facilitates compression stocking placement. Note the side-zippered compression stocking, an alternative that may also allow easier application of the elastic stocking (see text).*

were noncompliant ($P<0.0001$). Long-term follow-up (mean 30 months) was available in 73 patients. Fifty-eight (79%) continued to be compliant with ambulatory compression therapy after initial ulcer healing. Ulcer recurrence in this group was 16% during the follow-up period and 29% by 5-year life table analysis. In patients noncompliant with long-term elastic compression therapy, recurrence was 100% by 36 months. These patients represented a cross-section of venous ulcer patients. Their mean age was 59 years (range, 19–90 years) and 27% of ulcers were recurrent. A population of older patients with a larger percentage of recurrent or long-standing would be expected to do less well.

The major criticism of the use of compression therapy for the treatment of venous ulceration is patient compliance with the use of stockings. Clearly, many patients are often initially intolerant of compression in areas of hypersensitivity adjacent to an active ulcer or at sites of previously healed ulcers. We initially instruct patients to wear their stockings only as long as is easily tolerable. This may be only 10–15 minutes. With patience and persistent physician encouragement, almost all patients will gradually increase the time they can tolerate elastic stockings. Another strategy is to fit the patient with lesser strength stockings (20–30 mmHg) initially, followed by greater strength elastic stockings when they are able to be tolerated.

Many elderly patients will have difficulty applying elastic stockings. Silk inner toe liners, stockings with zippered sides, and devices that assist in the application of the stockings are commercially available (Fig. 30.2a,b). The Butler device in particular is useful in the frequent situation in which the patient cannot flex or bend enough to reach his or her feet. The use of these devices and gradual adaptation to the tactile sensation of elastic compression ultimately leads to excellent compliance in most patients. On rare occasions, however, a patient will still be unable to wear elastic compression stockings. These infrequent patients can be managed with alternative forms of compression therapy (see below).

Exacerbation of underlying arterial insufficiency is cited as another potential hazard with elastic compression. One survey found 49 of 154 community general surgeons (32%) had anecdotal experience with clinical deterioration of leg ulcers using compression therapy, with 12 resultant amputations. Callam and associates[14] analyzed 600 patients with 827 leg ulcers of multiple etiologies and found an ankle to brachial systolic blood pressure ratio less than 0.9 in 176 limbs (21%) and recommended against compression therapy in patients with evidence of arterial insufficiency. Presently we recommend arterial reconstruction for the occasional patient with a venous ulcer and ankle-brachial index (ABI) less than 0.6 when the ulcer fails to make reasonable progress with elastic compression therapy alone. In patients with critical leg ischemia (ABI <0.4) arterial

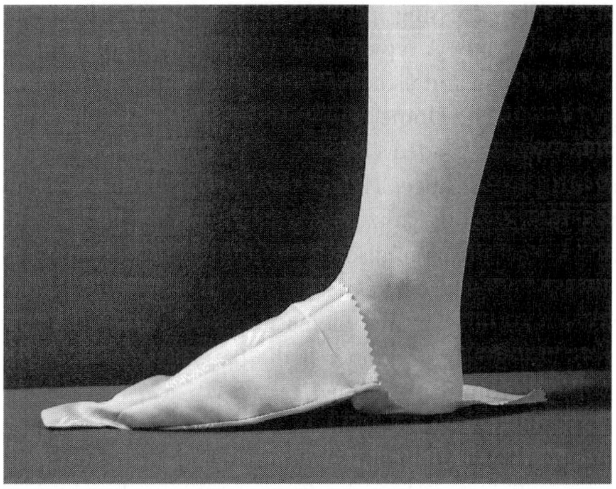

(a)

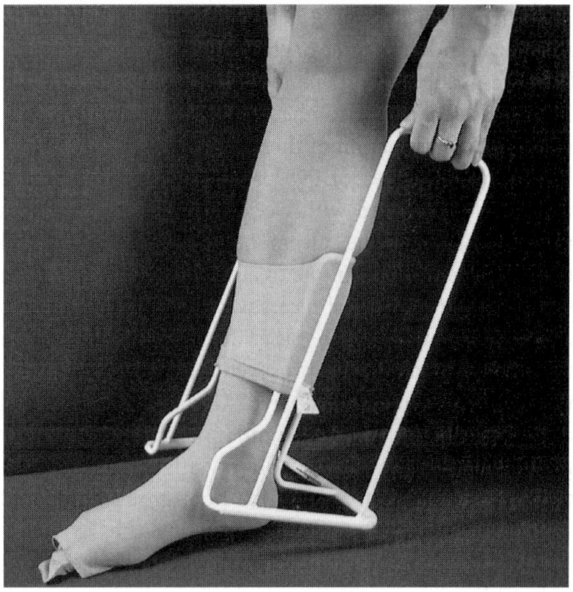

(b)

Figure 30.2 *(a) Inner silk liner fitted on the toe for easier stocking placement. (b) The Butler device which holds stocking open allowing patient to step into same facilitating placement. (Reproduced with permission from Mayberry JC, Moneta GL, Taylor LM, Porter JM. Nonoperative treatment of venous stasis ulcer. In Bergan JJ, Yao JST, eds.* Venous Disorders. *Philadelphia: WB Saunders, 1991: 381–95)*

reconstruction is performed as part of the initial management of venous ulceration.

PASTE GAUZE BOOTS

The German dermatologist Unna developed the paste gauze compression dressing in 1896. The current version of the dressing (Dome-Paste) contains calamine, zinc oxide, glycerin, sorbitol, gelatin, and magnesium aluminum silicate and is still popularly called an Unna boot. The dressing provides both compression and topical therapy. A typical Unna boot consists of a three-layer dressing and usually requires application by trained personnel. The Dome-Paste rolled gauze bandage is first applied with graded compression from the forefoot to just below the knee. The next layer consists of a 10-cm wide continuous gauze dressing followed by an outer layer of elastic wrap also applied with graded compression. The bandage becomes stiff after drying. Its rigidity may aid in preventing edema formation. Bandages are changed weekly or sooner if the patient has significant drainage from the ulcer bed.

Although Unna boots do not require patient education and participation in application, they are uncomfortable to wear. This can adversely affect compliance. In addition, the physician is unable to monitor the ulcer after the boot is applied, the technique is labor intensive and therefore expensive, and the degree of compression provided by the bandage is operator dependent. Occasionally, contact dermatitis secondary to the paraben preservative may require discontinuation of therapy.

A 15-year review[15] of 998 patients with one or more venous ulcers treated with weekly Unna boot bandages revealed 73% of the ulcers healed in patients who returned for more than one treatment. The median time to healing for individual ulcers was 9 weeks. Unna boots have been compared to other forms of compression treatment. A randomized prospective trial of 21 patients[16] with venous ulcers compared Unna boots to mild compression stockings (24 mmHg at the ankle). Both groups healed 70% of their ulcers with average healing times of 7.3 weeks for the Unna boot group compared with 18.4 weeks (11.8 weeks excluding the 78 weeks required by a single patient with extensive calf ulcerations to heal) for the compression stockings patients.

Another randomized study compared Unna boots to polyurethane foam dressings and elastic compression wraps in 26 patients with chronic venous insufficiency and venous ulcers.[17] After 12 months, patients treated with Unna boots had faster healing rates and greater overall wound healing. Unna boots have also been compared to hydrocolloid dressings (Duoderm) in a 6-month trial treating 87 venous ulcers in 84 patients.[18] Seventy percent of the ulcers treated with Unna boots healed by 6 months compared with 38% of those treated with hydrocolloid dressings alone. An additional study comparing Unna boots to hydrocolloid dressings and elastic compression bandages found no statistical difference in healing rates after 12 weeks.[19] A prospective but non-randomized trial of 28 patients with venous ulcers compared ulcer healing times in patients treated with Unna boots alone versus those treated with Unna boots and injection sclerotherapy of Doppler-determined venous channels adjacent to the ulcer.[20] Mean ulcer healing time was 4.3 weeks in the adjunctive sclerotherapy treated group compared with 6.1 weeks in the group treated with Unna boots alone.

Recently there has been growing interest in skin substitutes as adjuncts to venous ulcer therapy. Falanga *et al.*[21] performed a prospective, randomized trial comparing Unna boot compression therapy alone to treatment with an allogeneic cultured human skin equivalent (HSE) in addition to Unna boot compression. HSE is an allogeneic cultured bilayer of human skin origin containing both epidermal and dermal components. Significantly more patients with HSE had healed ulcers at 6 months (63% versus 49%). Median time to complete ulcer closure was significantly shorter in the group treated with HSE (61 days versus 181 days), particularly in patients with larger and deeper ulcers. These data suggest that skin substitutes may improve ulcer healing results with compression therapy, especially with respect to those ulcers that are particularly difficult to heal.

OTHER FORMS OF COMPRESSION

Additional forms of elastic compression include simple elastic wraps and multilayered wrapped dressings. Achieving and maintaining appropriate pressure gradients with elastic wraps is highly operator dependent. Despite this, satisfactory and effective dressings can be applied. One study[22] employed a four-layer dressing (multilayer wrap of orthopedic wool, crepe bandages, and elastic cohesive wraps; Coban) for treatment of 126 consecutive patients (148 ulcerated limbs) who had been refractory to simple elastic wraps. Seventy-four percent of ulcers healed by 12 weeks and measurements of compressive pressures at the ankle demonstrated only a 10% decline after one week. The multilayer wraps, such as the Profore® multilayer compression bandage system are purported to retain their compression longer, distribute the compression more evenly over the affected leg, and allow better absorption of wound exudate than simple wraps (Fig. 30.3). We use this type of dressing as an alternative in patients whose ulcers are refractory to simple graded compression stocking therapy and/or a legging orthosis (see below). In general, however, the above results are an exception as the results of most studies of elastic wraps for the treatment of venous ulceration have shown them to be inferior to compression stockings or Unna boots.[23,24]

The legging orthosis (CircAid) (Fig. 30.4a, b) consists of multiple pliable adjustable compression bands that are held in place with Velcro tape. The orthosis wraps around the leg from the ankle to the knee. The device provides firm compression similar to an Unna boot but with increased ease of application. The adjustable nature of the bands allows it to be individually tailored and adjusted as limb edema resolves. A trial of 13 patients with 15 venous ulcers who were unable to wear elastic

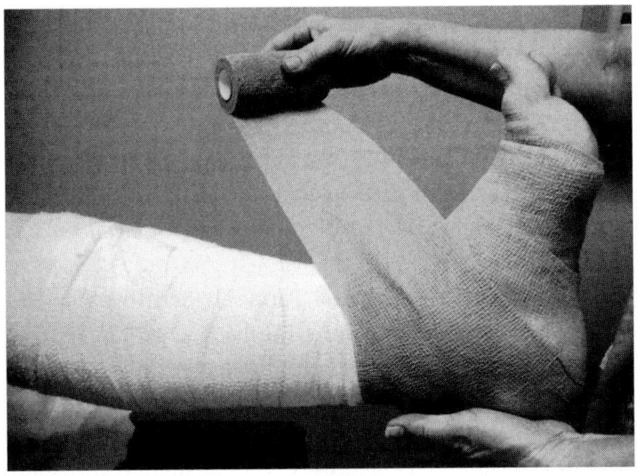

Figure 30.3 *The Profore® multilayerd bandage system is an example of a four layered elastic compression bandage. The various layers are designed for better absorption and maintenance of compression strength compared to simple wraps.*

stockings and who were treated with the CircAid device found that 53% of ulcers were healed at 12 months.[25] Although these results are modest, our anecdotal experience with the orthosis in a small number of patients has been favorable with respect to both edema resolution and ulcer healing. We currently employ it in patients who are unable or unwilling to wear compression stockings.

ADJUNCTIVE COMPRESSION DEVICES

External pneumatic compression devices providing sequential, gradient, intermittent pneumatic compression have received the most attention as adjunctive compression devices. They are used widely for prophylaxis of deep venous thrombosis in nonambulatory hospitalized patients. Several reports describe the use of intermittent pneumatic compression devices in the treatment of venous ulcers. One group[26] treated eight patients with phlebographically documented chronic venous insufficiency and venous ulcers that had been present from 1 to 60 months with intermittent pneumatic compression for 45 minutes, 5 days a week for a total of 2 weeks. It was then continued twice weekly until the ulcer healed. Between intermittent pneumatic compression treatments the ulcers were dressed with wet to dry saline dressings and the limbs were bandaged with elastic compression wraps. All ulcers healed (mean time, 5 weeks). The authors compared this to a mean healing time of 13 weeks in earlier patients with elastic compression bandages alone and concluded the addition of intermittent pneumatic compression therapy led to more rapid ulcer healing.

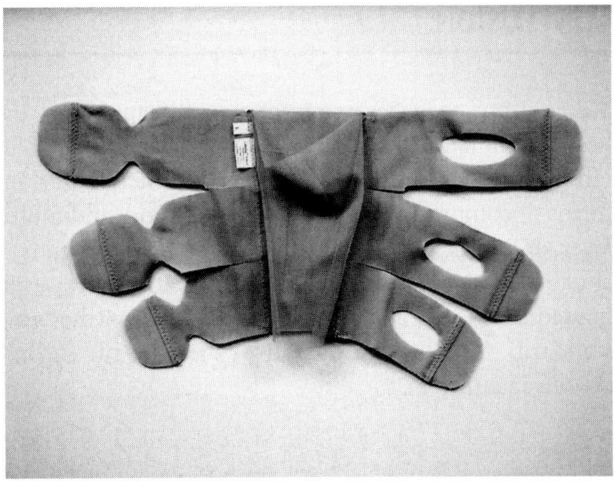

(a)

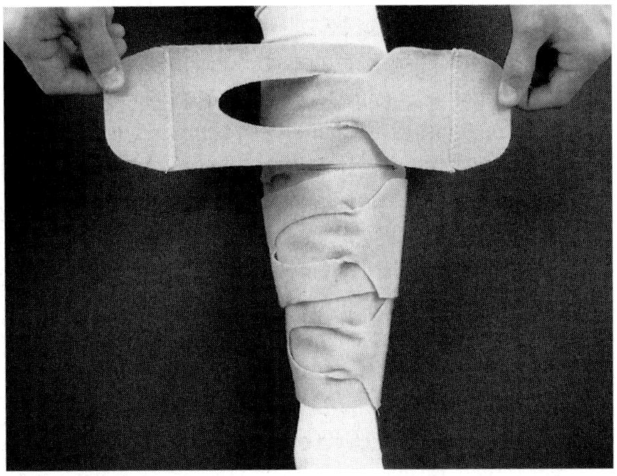

(b)

Figure 30.4 *(a) The CircAid device demonstrating the multiple nonelastic straps. (b) The device in place on a patient, with the top circumferential band being adjusted. (Reproduced with permission from Nehler MR, Moneta GL, Chitwood RW, Porter JM. The lower extremity venous system. Part III: Nonoperative treatment of chronic venous insufficiency. In Goldstone J, ed.* Perspectives in Vascular Surgery, *vol 5. St Louis, MO: Quality Medical Publishing, 1992: 100–13)*

A randomized study[27] of 45 patients, with chronic venous insufficiency and venous ulcers of at least 12 weeks' duration, compared treatment with intermittent pneumatic compression and 30–40 mmHg ambulatory compression stockings with compression stockings alone for 3 months or until ulcer healing. Only one of the 24 patients treated with stockings alone healed their ulcer, while 10 of 21 patients in the intermittent pneumatic compression group healed. Thus, while the use of adjunctive intermittent compression has not gained widespread acceptance, the results of the few available studies indicate it may be useful in the treatment of venous ulcers refractory to ambulatory compression therapy alone.

CONCLUSION

We continue to believe compression therapy offers the best combination of simplicity, efficacy, and cost effectiveness in the healing of venous ulcers. Various forms of compression including elastic, rigid, and multilayer dressings are available depending on the clinical situation and needs of the individual patient. However, graded elastic compression hosiery remains the 'gold standard' for the nonoperative therapy of chronic venous insufficiency.

REFERENCES

1. Mayberry JC, Moneta GL, DeFrang RD, Porter JM. The influence of elastic compression stockings on deep venous hemodynamics. *J Vasc Surg* 1991; **13**: 91–100.
2. Christopoulos DG, Nicolaides AN, Szendro G, Irvine AT, Bull M, Eastcott HHG. Air-plethysmography and the effect of elastic compression on venous hemodynamics of the leg. *J Vasc Surg* 1987; **5**: 148–59.
3. Christopoulos DG, Nicolaides AN, Belcaro G, Kalodiki E. Venous hypertensive microangiopathy in relation to clinical severity and effect of elastic compression. *J Dermatol Surg Oncol* 1991; **17**: 809–13.
4. Nilsson L, Austrell CH, Norgen L. Venous function during late pregnancy, the effect of elastic compression hosiery. *Vasa* 1992; **21**: 203–5.
5. Abdulsalam AA, Scurr JH, Coleridge Smith PD. Assessment of microangiopathy of the skin in chronic venous insufficiency by laser Doppler fluxmetry (Abstract). *J Vasc Surg* 1993; **17**: 429.
6. Nehler MR, Moneta GL, Woodard DM, *et al.* Perimalleolar subcutaneous pressure effects of elastic compression stockings. *J Vasc Surg* 1993; **18**(5): 783–8.
7. Mahler F, Chen D. Intravital microscopy for evaluation of chronic venous incompetence. *Int J Microcirc Exp (Suppl)* 1990; **106**: 1.
8. Kolari PJ, Pekanmaki K. Effects of intermittent compression treatment on skin perfusion and oxygenation in lower legs with venous ulcers. *Vasa* 1988; **16**: 312–17.
9. Dinn E, Henry M. Treatment of venous ulceration by injection sclerotherapy and compression hosiery: a 5-year study. *Phlebology* 1992; **7**: 23–6.
10. Anning ST. Leg ulcers – the results of treatment. *Angiology* 1956; **7**: 505–16.
11. Kitahama A, Elliot LF, Kerstein MD, Menendez CV. Leg ulcer: conservative management or surgical treatment? *J Am Med Assoc* 1982; **247**: 197–9.
12. Nehler MR, Kim YW, Moneta GL, Porter JM. Nonoperative therapy for patients with chronic venous insufficiency. In Callow AD, Ernst CB, eds. *Vascular Surgery: Theory and Practice.* Norwalk, CT: Appleton & Lange, 1995.
13. Mayberry JC, Moneta GL, Taylor LM, Porter JM. Fifteen-year results of ambulatory compression therapy for chronic venous ulcers. *Surgery* 1991; **109**: 575–81.
14. Callam MJ, Harper DR, Dale JJ, Ruckley CV. Arterial disease in chronic leg ulceration: an underestimated hazard? Lothian and Forth Valley leg ulcer study. *Br Med J* 1987; **294**: 929–31.
15. Lippmann HI, Fishman LM, Farrar RH, Bernstein RK, Zybert PA. Edema control in the management of disabling chronic venous insufficiency. *Arch Phys Med Rehabil* 1994; **75**: 436–41.
16. Hendricks WM, Swallow RT. Management of stasis leg ulcers with Unna's boots versus elastic support stockings. *J Am Acad Dermatol* 1985; **12**: 90–8.
17. Rubin JR, Alexander J, Plecha EJ, Marman C. Unna's boot vs. polyurethane foam dressings for the treatment of venous ulceration. *Arch Surg* 1990; **125**: 489–90.
18. Kitka MJ, Schuler JJ, Meyer JP, *et al.* A prospective, randomized trial of Unna's boots versus hydroactive dressing in the treatment of venous stasis ulcers. *J Vasc Surg* 1988; **7**: 478–86.
19. Cordts PR, Hanrahan LM, Rodriguez AA, Woodson J, LaMorte WW, Menzoian JO. A prospective, randomized trial of Unna's boot versus Duoderm CGF hydroactive dressing plus compression in the management of venous leg ulcers. *J Vasc Surg* 1992; **15**: 480–6.
20. Queral LA, Criado FJ, Lilly MP, Rudolphi D. The role of sclerotherapy as an adjunct to Unna's boot for treating venous ulcers: a prospective study. *J Vasc Surg* 1990; **11**: 572–5.
21. Falanga V, Margolis D, Auletta O, *et al.* and the Human Skin Equivalent Investigators Group. Rapid healing of venous ulcers and lack of clinical rejection with an allogeneic cultured human skin equivalent. *Arch Dermatol* 1998; **134**: 293–300.
22. Blair SD, Wright DD, Backhouse LM, Riddle E, Mcollum CN. Sustained compression and healing of chronic venous ulcers. *Br Med J* 1988; **297**: 1159–61.
23. Ormiston MC, Seymour MT, Venn GE, Cohen RI, Fox JA. Controlled trial of Iodosorb in chronic venous ulcers. *Br Med J* 1985; **291**: 308–10.
24. Backhouse CM, Blair SD, Savage P, Walton J, McCollum CN. Controlled trial of occlusive dressings in healing chronic venous ulcers. *Br J Surg* 1987; **74**: 626–7.
25. Spence RK, Hardesty WH, Brown AS, *et al.* Experience with the 'CircAid' garment in the treatment of the nonhealing venous stasis ulcer. Presented at the 16th Annual World Congress of the International Union of Angiology in Paris, 1992.
26. Pekanmaki K, Kolari PJ, Kiistala U. Intermittent pneumatic compression treatment for post-thrombotic leg ulcers. *Clin Exp Dermatol* 1987; **12**: 350–3.
27. Coleridge Smith P, Sarin S, Hasty J, Scurr JH. Sequential gradient pneumatic compression enhances venous ulcer healing: a randomized trial. *Surgery* 1990; **108**: 871–5.

31

The drug treatment of chronic venous insufficiency and venous ulceration

PHILIP D COLERIDGE SMITH

The management of venous diseases has relied on compression treatments and surgical interventions for many years. The growth of drug treatment in some sectors of medicine has been considerable. However, I think that it is fair to say that no huge advance has been made in the drug treatment of patients with venous disease to match those in many other medical specialities where revolutions in management have occurred with advances in pharmacology. In many countries, drugs remain widely used in patients with venous diseases as adjunctive treatments. The aim of this chapter is to discuss these for patients with varicose veins and chronic venous diseases leading to skin changes and leg ulceration. Which drugs should be used in treating venous diseases and when?

VARICOSE VEINS

In patients with varicose veins compression treatment, sclerotherapy or surgical removal of veins remain the most effective therapeutic measures in achieving relief of symptoms. No drug has so far been shown to result in the resolution of varicose veins, other than when used as part of a regimen of sclerotherapy. This is true of truncal varices as well as telangiectasias and reticular varices. However, varicose veins are often associated with two groups of symptoms that commonly trouble patients. These include edema and unpleasant feelings in the legs such as aching in the region of varices, 'restless legs' or a feeling of swelling of the lower limbs. These may be addressed by treatment of the underlying condition using compression stockings, sclerotherapy or surgery. However, in many countries 'venotonic' drugs are used to manage these problems. Patients living in regions of hot weather find wearing compression stockings unbearable at some times of the year and surgeons may abandon surgical treatment during the summer season. This has opened a long-established market for the use of drugs. Many of the drugs used for this purpose are derived from plants, although more recently synthetic drugs have been developed. This groups of drugs was originally developed during the 1960s and 1970s when lesser standards of scientific proof were required than is the case today. The studies that supported the use of these drugs did not use hard clinical end points, since the symptoms which they were designed to treat were highly subjective. More recently, double-blind studies have confirmed the efficacy of some of these drugs against the symptoms of venous disease.

'Venoactive drugs'

A classification of the venoactive drugs based on published literature is shown in Table 31.1.[1,2] A wide range of compounds is shown here and by no means all of these are available as drugs in every country.

The mechanisms by which this class of drugs act remain unclear. As various possible causes of venous disease have been advanced with scientific advance, the possibility that these mechanisms are modified by these drugs has been suggested. Until recently, very little work had been done to assess how venoactive drugs modify the physiology of the microcirculation of the leg to reduce edema and symptoms related to venous disease.

Table 31.1 *Classification of venotonic drugs*

Natural products
Benzopyrones
α-Benzopyrones (coumarins)
  Coumarin (1,2-benzopyrone; 5,6-α-benzopyrone), melitot coumarinic derivatives
  Esculetin (6,7-dihydrooxycoumarin)
  Umbelliferone (7-hydroxycoumarin)
  Dicoumarols (dimers of 4-hydroxycoumarins): oral anticoagulants
γ-Benzopyrones (flavonoids)
  Flavone and flavonols
    Diosmin, kaempferol, diosmetin, quercetin,
    Rutine and derivatives, troxerutin, *O*-(β-hydroxyethyl) rutosides (hydroxyethylrutosides or oxerutins)
  Flavanes and flavanones
    Hesperetin, hesperidene, catechin, methylchalcone, flavonoic acid, etc.
Saponosides
  Escin, horse-chestnut extracts (protoescigenin, barringtogenol, α- and β-escin, cryptoescin)
  Extracts of *Ruscus* (ruscosides), *Centella asiatica*
Other plant extracts
  Anthocyanosides: blueberry extract
  Pycnogenols: leucocianidol, procyanidolic oligomeres: grape seed extracts
  Ginkgo biloba
  Ergot derivatives: dihydroergotamine, dihydroergocristine, dihydroergocryptine

Synthetic products
Adenosine phosphate
Benzarone
Calcium dobesilate
Chromocarb diethylamine
Heptaminol
Naftazone
Tribenoside

HYDROXYRUTOSIDES

Hydroxyrutosides are a class of flavonoid drug derived from plant glycosides (Figs 31.1, 31.2). They initially gained favor 30 years ago when experimental studies indicated that they reduced capillary permeability following burns in dogs. A number of clinical studies evaluating their effect on symptoms associated with CVI followed.[3,4] In general, these indicated that hydroxyrutosides appeared to be more effective than placebo in reducing aching, tiredness, muscle cramps and other symptoms which are difficult to evaluate objectively.

Hydroxyrutosides are commonly used to treat edema and several clinical trials and other studies have been reported. Treatment with doses between 1 and 2 g/day have been studied in detail. Calf circumference, a measurement prone to substantial variability, has been used as an assessment of leg edema. Four weeks treatment with hydroxyrutosides resulted in a mean reduction in calf circumference of 2.1–2.5 mm greater in the rutoside compared with the placebo group.[5,6] The mean reduction was 6.1 mm greater in the rutoside group after 8 weeks of treatment, with a similar trend in the reduction of ankle circumference. Pitting edema was also reduced more by rutosides than by placebo.[7]

The water-displacement method is a more reliable method of assessing calf volume. The leg volume measured by this technique increased significantly during a 4-week period of placebo, but this increase was not observed during rutoside treatment.[8] A similar trend was observed in another investigation which employed electrical conductivity to assess the amount of extracellular fluid in the limb.[7] In a study carried out in 40 patients undergoing surgery for varicose veins, there was no difference in leg volume between the placebo and rutosides treatment groups in the first 6 postoperative weeks. Compression stockings were worn during the study, and the effect of these on leg edema hid any additional effect of the drug treatment.[9]

The change in leg edema has also been assessed by strain-gauge plethysmography.[10] A single intravenous bolus of rutosides increased the reserve venous volume and decreased capillary filtration rate as compared with placebo. In the same study, oral treatment increased the reserve venous volume and venous emptying, but did not change the capillary filtration rate.

The influence of hydroxyrutosides on the microcirculation has been assessed in one study, in which capillary filtration was assessed by a strain-gauge method.[11] Forty patients with ankle edema due to mild-to-moderate venous hypertension were assigned to receive either rutosides 2000 mg/day or placebo for 4 weeks. No differences were observed between the two treatment groups in the microcirculatory parameters assessed in this 4-week trial. Our own investigations of capillary filtration using a similar technique showed little difference between patients with venous disease and control subjects. Therefore, assessment of capillary filtration by this method may not be an appropriate method of measuring of the effects of treatment for venous disease.

The use of hydroxyrutosides in venous disease appears to have significant symptomatic value,[12–14] reducing swelling cramps and edema. Its use could be considered in patients suffering these symptoms in whom compression treatments are contraindicated or not tolerated by the patient.

CALCIUM DOBESILATE

This synthetic drug has also been investigated in its effects on edema. Two randomized clinical trials in which a total of 275 patients were included have been published.[15,16] Calcium dobesilate decreased the maximum circumference of the calf and the minimum circumference of the ankle to a greater extent than placebo at day 28, whereas calf circumference was also

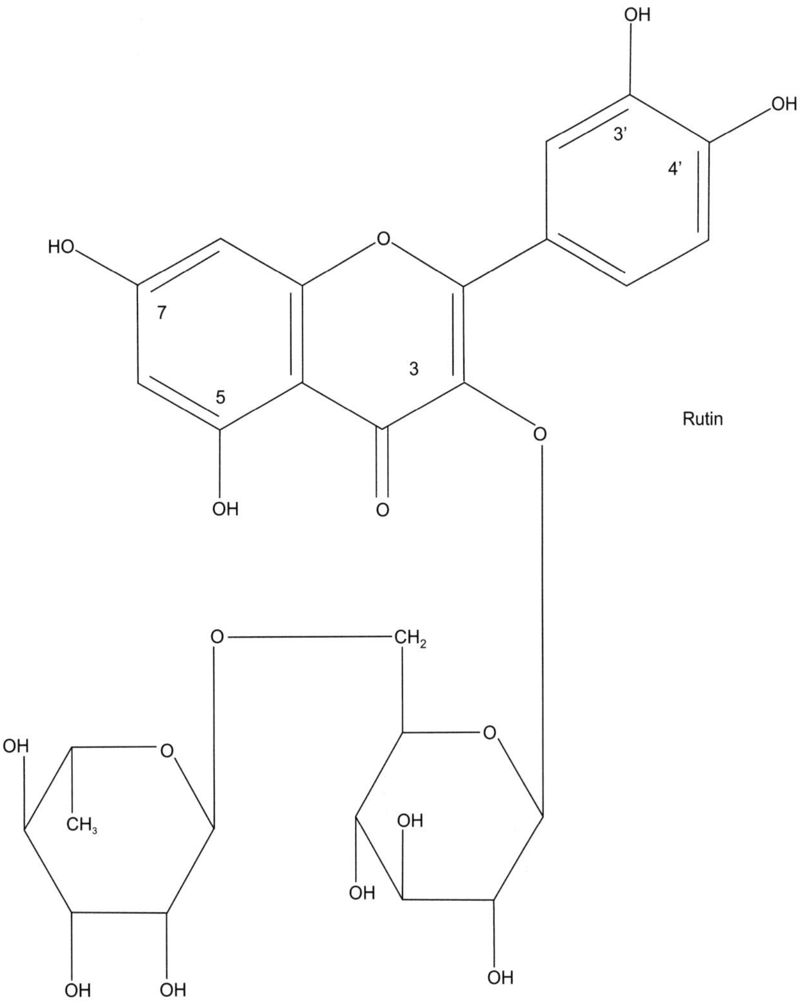

Figure 31.1 *The molecular structure of rutin.*

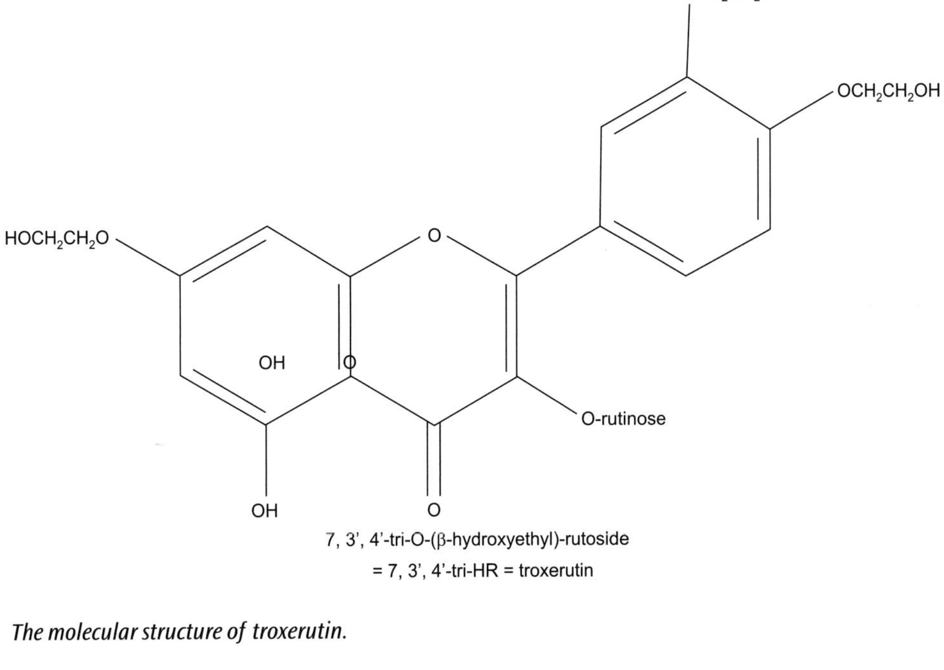

Figure 31.2 *The molecular structure of troxerutin.*

significantly reduced at day 14. Relative leg volume was reduced by 3.8% with calcium dobesilate and 1.2% with placebo (P <0.001). A 'malleolar swelling' clinical score ranging from −3 (total relief) to +1 (deterioration) was reported to be −1.70 with calcium dobesilate and −0.48 with placebo (P <0.001). This 'malleolar swelling' matched strain-gauge plethysmography measures of limb circumference.

This drug has a measurable effect on the edema and symptoms attributable to venous disease.

HORSE-CHESTNUT EXTRACT (ESCIN)

Little objective evidence of efficacy is available for horse chestnut extract. In 125 female patients with chronic venous insufficiency, neither horse chestnut extract nor placebo reduced ankle circumference after 2 months of treatment. The rate of improvement of swelling was identical in both groups.[17] There is no published evidence that horse chestnut extract assists ulcer healing or prevents recurrence. Escin continues to be widely used in medicines sold for the purpose of treating the symptoms of venous disease.

DIOSMIN

Diosmin is a member of the flavonoid family (Fig 31.3). It has been shown that the intestinal absorption and therefore bioavailability of this drug may be increased by micronization.[18] This is a high-tech process in which the particle size of the active ingredient is reduced from 60 μm to less than 2 μm. The clinical efficacy of micronized diosmin (Daflon 500 mg, Detralex, Arvenum 500, Capiven, Venitol, Variton, Ardium, Servier, Courbevoie, France) is significantly reinforced by this process.[19,20] Several studies indicate its efficacy on edema and the symptoms of venous disease. The symptoms that have been investigated include heaviness, discomfort, itching, cramps, pain and swelling. These must be quantified using scores or a visual analog scale rather than objective measurements, but these data tend to result in considerable variance of data. Consequently, large numbers of patients must be included in studies based on this type of measurement to be confident of conclusions reached. Laurent[21] examined the efficacy of micronized diosmin in 200 patients in a double-blind, placebo-controlled trial lasting 2 months. Outcome measures assessed the symptoms of venous disease using visual analog scales. Micronized diosmin improved functional and organic venous insufficiency (symptoms of venous disease not associated with major venous valvular incompetence) by 71% and 66%, respectively, compared with 36% and 38% for placebo. However, although symptomatic improvement is important to patients, objective evidence of efficacy on measures of severity of venous disease are more reassuring! Micronized diosmin has also been investigated in the context of edema reduction. In Laurent's study, the mean difference in the reduction of supramalleolar circumference was 6.7 mm (right limb) and 6.1 mm (left limb) in favor of micronized diosmin in patients with functional symptoms. In patients with varicose veins or post-thrombotic syndrome, the reduction was 6.8 mm (right limb) and 6.5 mm (left limb). The supramalleolar circumference remained unchanged in the placebo group.

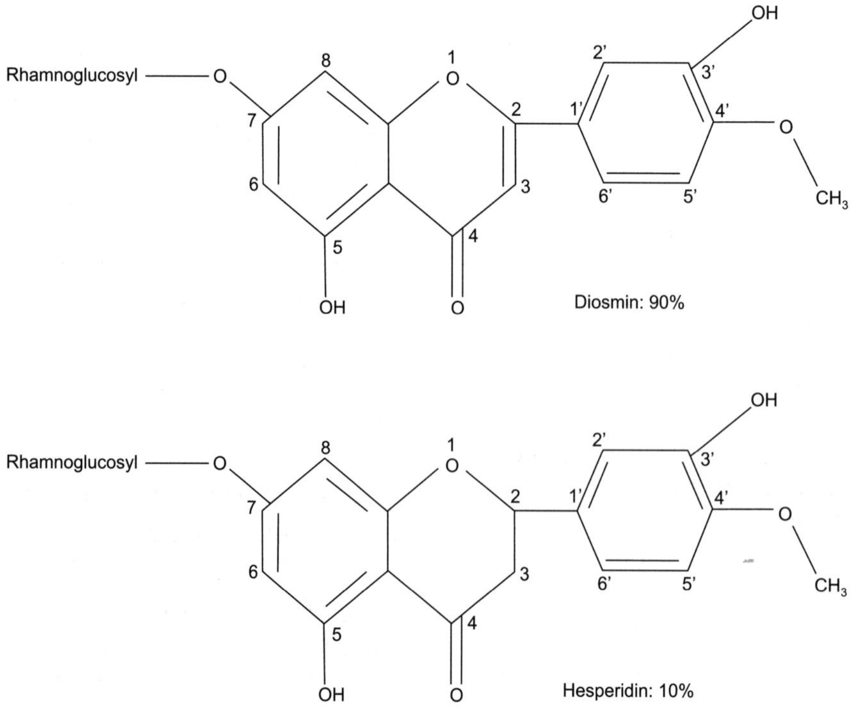

Figure 31.3 *The molecular structure of dosmin and hesperidine.*

The mode of efficacy of this drug is incompletely understood. Studies have shown that it increases venous tone[22,23] and lymphatic flow.[24–26] It also decreases hyper-permeability[27] and increases capillary resistance.[28] A recent paper has shown that it modifies the interaction of leukocytes with endothelium in a hamster skin-fold model used to investigate the effect of Daflon 500 mg on the microcirculation following ischemia-reperfusion. The group of animals pretreated with Daflon 500 mg exhibited less neutrophil adhesion in the postcapillary venules at 30 minutes, 2 hours and 24 hours after reperfusion, compared with the control group.[29] In another model of the microcirculation, small bowel and cremaster of rats, Korthuis showed that Daflon 500 mg inhibits leukocyte adhesion and migration induced by ischemia/reperfusion.[30] Bouskela has also confirmed this in the hamster cheek pouch model of the microcirculation.[31] The mechanism by which this is achieved has not been defined, although these are important observations since they imply that Daflon 500 mg may protect the tissues in experimental models of ischaemia. Bouskela has reported further findings in the hamster cheek pouch.[32] Fluorescein-isothiocyanate-labeled dextran was used to study the microcirculation. The number of microvascular 'leakage points' was identified in the cheek pouch using fluorescence microscopy. Histamine, bradykinin and leukotriene B_4 were applied topically to cause microvascular disturbance. These increased the number of leakage points. This effect could be prevented by pretreating the animals with Daflon 500 mg. Daflon 500 mg appears to protect the microcirculation against inflammatory mediators in this model.

The effect of Daflon 500 mg on the microcirculation in man has been investigated in a study in which laser Doppler fluxmetry, transcutaneous oxygen and carbon dioxide levels were assessed in the skin.[33] Patients with mild venous disease (no skin changes) were randomized to receive 500 mg, 1 g or 2 g Daflon per day. Small increases in tc$P\text{O}_2$ and decreases of tc$P\text{CO}_2$ were observed in all groups after 3 months of treatment, with no difference seen between the different dosage regimens. No changes in laser Doppler flux were found. Since patients without skin changes show only minor disturbances in tc$P\text{O}_2$ and tc$P\text{CO}_2$ levels, the scope for improvement in these measures of mild venous disease is limited. It is only in liposclerotic skin that these parameters show large changes and where improvement would be expected following effective treatment. No study has so far been reported in which Daflon 500 mg has been used in this patient group with transcutaneous oximetry used as an outcome measure.

Diuretics

Generalized leg edema is a feature of proximal large vein obstruction, while localized edema is commonly associated with areas of lipodermatosclerosis (LDS).[34] Simple diuretics are not generally used in edema due to venous disease, since the increased permeability to proteins seen in venous hypertension leads to a protein rich edema which is unsuitable for such treatment.[35] In addition, hemoconcentration may occur, leading to reduced capillary blood flow and the risk of deep venous thrombosis.

Edema reduction *per se* is probably not an important consideration in the treatment of venous ulcers. Myers *et al.* have shown that healing of ulcers is unrelated to the amount of leg swelling; in their words, 'the edema and the ulcer are due to the same cause, probably venous stasis, and any therapy which does not improve venous drainage is probably doomed to failure'.[36] Although the concept of venous stasis is now thought to be unsound, the second half of their statement is likely to remain true.

Other treatments

Advertisements have appeared in newspapers in the USA and in the UK in recent months promoting vitamin K containing creams as useful in the treatment of telangiectasias of the leg. I can find no published literature to support the claims made in these advertisements. One published item mentions these treatments[37] and dismisses them as useless in view of the lack of supporting scientific evidence! A clinical trial has now confirmed the lack of efficacy of vitamin K creams in the treatment of telangiectasias of the legs.[38]

Venoactive drugs summary

In summary, venoactive drugs remain widely used against the common symptoms of varicose veins and have clear efficacy in some areas, particularly in addressing edema. They do not influence the progress of the development of varicose veins themselves. The mechanism of action of these drugs remains to be explained fully. There is reasonable evidence that flavonoids influence the process of leukocyte–endothelial interaction which probably modifies many other inflammatory events that may be the cause of symptoms experienced by patients with venous disease.

CHRONIC VENOUS DISEASE RESULTING IN SKIN CHANGES AND LEG ULCERATION

Venous ulceration and the skin changes which precede ulceration are best managed by careful objective evaluation of the venous system of the lower limb followed by compression bandaging or stockings and surgical treatment where appropriate. Systemic drugs and topical applications are widely used in the management of leg ulceration, but what should we use and when? Surgical intervention is appropriate where leg ulceration is attributable mainly to superficial venous incompetence alone in a patient fit enough for this procedure. In some studies this would apply to as many as half the patients presenting with venous ulceration.[39,40] A number of studies show that healing usually progresses well in such patients and recurrent ulceration is not a common problem.[41] A relatively small proportion of patients are suitable for deep vein reconstructive procedures, many excluded because of age and infirmity or medical unfitness for a large vascular procedure. In general, such patients are best managed by compression treatments alone. Unfortunately whilst compression treatment can usually achieve healing if high enough levels of compression are used, recurrence is a common problem with an annual recurrence rate of 25% per year.[42] Perhaps drugs can speed healing or prevent recurrence. Many clinical studies published over the years have studied this problem and examination of them is informative and revealing!

Antibiotics

'Virtually every antibiotic that has ever been produced has been used to treat venous ulcers but there is very little evidence that they help healing unless the ulcer is contaminated by a single pathogenic organism'.[34] This quotation from Browse *et al.* summarizes the present position regarding systemic antibiotic treatment in venous ulceration. Naturally, clinical infection of an ulcer must be treated, but this is best done by local ulcer toilet, unless cellulitis or septicemia supervene. The possible exception to this rule is the use of metronidazole. There is some evidence that this compound, given orally, increases the rate of healing of both venous and pressure ulcers when they are infected with *Clostridium* and other anaerobes.[43] Even then, systemic treatment may not be superior to topical application; Jones *et al.* have demonstrated the rapid effectiveness of metronidazole soaked dressings in such cases.[44] In general, systemic antibiotics do not play a role in the management of the uncomplicated venous ulcer.

Zinc

Adequate nutrition is essential for leg ulcer healing as it is for wound healing of other types. For a number of years, special attention was given to the concept that, in particular, zinc levels were depressed in patients with venous ulcers and that supplementation might speed healing. Greaves and Skillen, in an old but widely quoted paper, reported complete healing in 13 of 18 patients with previously intractable ulceration after a 4-month course of 220 mg zinc sulphate three times daily.[45] During this period they continued with their previous conservative treatment as outpatients. Pretreatment serum zinc levels were found to be significantly lower in the patient group than in controls. In a later report, Greaves and Ive published their results over a longer period, in a double-blind trial of oral zinc in 38 patients with venous ulcers.[46] They were unable to confirm their initial good results, with only three of the treated group and two of the placebo group showing complete healing after 4 months. Serum zinc levels were not measured in this study. These negative results were confirmed by Myers and Cherry[47] in a study of 40 ulcer patients and by Phillips *et al.*[48] in 42 patients; in both studies, healing occurred at the same rate in zinc-treated and control patients.

More recently, Schraibmann and Stratton have compared the nutritional status of venous ulcer patients with that of age- and sex-matched controls.[49] Of 11 indices thought to represent nutritional deficiency, only one (hemoglobin) was significantly lower in patients with venous ulcers. Serum zinc was, in fact, slightly higher on average in this group than in controls. It would seem, therefore, that zinc supplements to the diet are unlikely to be of much benefit to the majority of patients, although they may have a role in the management of those few patients with severe nutritional problems. No subsequent publication has studied zinc as a therapeutic treatment in venous ulceration.

Fibrinolytic therapy

The concept of an oxygen diffusion barrier causing skin hypoxia was first proposed by Browse and Burnand in 1982.[50] This theory led to attempts to reverse the damaging cutaneous effects of venous hypertension by enhancing fibrinolysis. The effect of stanozolol, an anabolic steroid with profibrinolytic properties, was evaluated in 14 patients with long-standing LDS, without active ulceration.[51] After 3 months, all showed clinical improvement both subjectively and objectively (by mapping the area of LDS). Serum parameters of fibrinolytic activity improved in all cases. One might criticize the study for including three patients in whom the LDS was not associated with any venous abnormality. However, this pilot study justified a larger trial of fibrinolytic treatment in CVI.

This was performed as a 6-month double-blind crossover trial on 23 patients with long-standing LDS which had not responded to compression hosiery.[52] All patients continued with stockings during the trial. The area of liposclerotic skin fell during treatment with both stanozolol and placebo. The rate at which it fell was faster on stanozolol than on placebo, although this difference did not reach statistical significance. Leg volume as measured by plethysmography increased on the steroid, presumably as a result of fluid retention. Skin biopsy analysis suggested but did not prove that tissue fibrin was reduced by stanozolol treatment; foot vein pressure reduction on exercise was improved to the same extent on both active and placebo treatment. All but one patient described subjective improvement during the trial but were unable to differentiate between the active and placebo periods. The exception to this was in pain relief, which was significantly better while taking the steroid.

A further double-blind study of 60 patients was performed to evaluate the efficacy of this drug.[53] Stanozolol combined with compression stockings caused a reduction of liposclerotic skin area of 28% over 6 months. However, when the separate contributions of the two treatment elements (compression and stanozolol) were calculated using multivariate analysis of variance, the effect attributable to stanozolol alone was not statistically significant.

One of the problems in evaluating the response of LDS to treatment is the paucity of hard end points that can be measured; how does one quantify, for example, lightening of pigmentation, or reduction of induration? Treatment of venous ulceration, by contrast, allows the simple question to be asked: healed or not healed? Fibrinolytic treatment for venous ulceration has been evaluated in one trial of 75 patients.[54] Patients were allocated to receive either stanozolol or placebo for up to 420 days, with conventional compression treatment in all cases. In an interim report, the authors found complete healing in 26 of 40 ulcers in the stanozolol group and 27 of 44 in the placebo group, indicating no benefit from active over placebo treatment.

In summary, one may say that fibrinolytic enhancement may be of minor benefit in the symptomatic treatment of LDS, but that it does not appear to improve ulcer healing. Before dismissing the concept, one must note that only one agent, stanozolol, has been extensively studied for this purpose, and it is possible that more potent, less toxic fibrinolytic agents could be more effective. Stanozolol has now been withdrawn from use in the UK for the treatment of patients with venous disease.

Drugs which modify leukocyte metabolism

Disappointment with existing pharmacological treatments, together with some theoretical objections to the notion of impaired oxygen diffusion in LDS,[55,56] has led to the search for alternative lines of drug treatment on venous skin damage. The discovery of the involvement of leukocytes in the development of venous ulceration has opened new avenues of investigation in this area.[57] A number of drugs which modify white cell activation have been evaluated in patients with venous ulceration with interesting results.

PROSTAGLANDIN E_1

Prostaglandin E_1 (PGE_1) has a number of profound effects on the microcirculation, including reduction of white cell activation, platelet aggregation inhibition, small vessel vasodilatation and reduction of vessel wall cholesterol levels.[58] It has been evaluated in the treatment of various aspects of arterial disease; less work has been done on its use in venous ulceration. An early trial of the use of intravenous PGE_1 in ulcers of both arterial and venous aetiology reported improvement in four of five venous ulcers on PGE_1 as opposed to four of seven on placebo – hardly a dramatic result.[59] A recent trial has yielded rather more impressive findings.[60] Forty-four patients with proven venous ulceration took part in a double-blind, placebo-controlled trial. Each received an infusion of PGE_1 (or placebo) over 3 hours daily for 6 weeks, in addition to standard dressings and compression bandaging. Those on PGE_1 showed a significant improvement in such parameters as edema reduction, symptoms and 'ulcer score', based on depth, diameter, etc. Perhaps more importantly, 8 of 20 patients on active treatment healed their ulcers completely within the trial period, whereas only 2 of 22 controls did so.

The reason for the different outcomes in these two trials probably relates to the dose of PGE_1 given. In Beitner *et al.*'s study, only two infusions were given. These consisted of 360 μγ PGE_1 in 3 liters of isotonic saline over 72 hours, a month apart. In the second trial, 60 μg were given over 3 hours every day for 6 weeks – a total dose 3.5 times bigger than that in the earlier study. Although this rather intensive way of treating ulcers is not, at first sight, attractive, the cost of such treatment must be weighed against the many millions of pounds spent each year in the UK on the outpatient care of unhealed ulcers.

Unfortunately no further studies have been published and the regular use of PGE_1 in the management of leg ulceration has proceeded no further.

Prostacyclin analogs

Iloprost (Schering, Berlin), a synthetic prostacyclin analog, has been used with success in the treatment of arterial and diabetic ulcers.[61] The mechanism of action of prostacyclin includes increased fibrinolytic activity;[62] the drug also has profound effects on leukocyte activity by reducing aggregation and adherence to endothelium,[63,64] in addition to its better known effects on platelet behavior.[65] However, a study in which this was applied topically to venous ulcers was disappointing.[66] The trial design was a randomized, double-blind, placebo-controlled study in 11 centers in Germany with 49 patients allocated to placebo, 49 patients to 0.0005% iloprost and 50 patients to 0.002% iloprost. The study solutions were applied twice weekly for a period of 8 weeks on the ulcer edge and ulcer surrounding. This study failed to show any statistically significant reduction in the ulcer size as a result of the iloprost treatment compared with the placebo treatment. Perhaps this was true failure of efficacy of this drug, or perhaps the drug delivery system did not achieve therapeutic levels in the tissues. No further data has been published concerning iloprost in the management of venous disease and it is not in common use in the management of leg ulceration.

PENTOXIFYLLINE

Pentoxifylline has been used for the treatment of claudication for a number of years, with moderate success.[67] It was thought that it may act by improving red cell deformability and thus improve oxygen delivery to ischemic tissue. Recent work on the drug indicates that it actually has a potent effect on inhibition of cytokine-mediated neutrophil activation.[68] The same workers also showed it to reduce white cell adhesion to endothelium and to reduce the release of superoxide free radicals produced in the so-called respiratory burst characteristic of neutrophil degranulation. Theoretically, therefore, it should be of benefit in venous disease if the white cell activation model described above is valid.

Weitgasser evaluated the effect of the drug in a double-blind, placebo-controlled trial of 59 patients with venous ulcers.[69] Of 30 patients on active treatment, 26 'improved'; this was assessed by comparing photographs of the ulcer before and after treatment. Only 13 of 29 patients on placebo improved, a statistically significant difference. Unfortunately, no firm data are given regarding the numbers of healed and unhealed ulcers at the end of the trial, which rather dilutes its impact. Herger subsequently studied the effect of the drug on 73 patients with ulceration, in 42 of whom the cause was venous insufficiency.[70] The protocol of drug administration was rather vague; the dosages 'in most cases' were 400 mg three or four times a day, and some patients also received pentoxifylline infusions. Treatment lasted for 8 weeks. 62 of the 73 ulcers healed; we do not know how many of the specifically venous ulcers are included in this figure. The trial was not placebo-controlled.

A Greek study in 1989 examined the effect of 1200 mg pentoxifylline per day on ten patients with proven venous ulcers, with partial or complete healing in eight after 6 weeks.[71] Unfortunately, this trial did not use a control group. A more rigorous trial has been reported by Colgan *et al.*[72] This was a multicenter, placebo-controlled, double-blind prospective study of 80 patients with venous ulcers. After 6 months of treatment with 1200 mg/day of pentoxifylline or placebo, 23 of 38 patients in the active arm had a healed ulcer, whilst 12 of 42 in the placebo-treated arm had the same result. This difference was statistically significant. (In both trials, patients continued with conventional hosiery and general ulcer care).

A further study in 200 patients has now been completed and the results published.[73] This was a complex study of 2 × 2 × 2 factorial design, testing pentoxifylline against placebo, hydrocolloid dressing against a viscose dressing, and a single-layer bandage against four-layer bandaging. In essence, half the patients received high levels of compression and half received much lower levels of compression. There was a trend towards more rapid healing in the pentoxifylline group, but this did not reach statistical significance. Perhaps the use of higher levels of compression concealed any effect of pentoxifylline. Clearly this is a treatment with some efficacy, but of small magnitude. Its exact role in the management of patients with venous ulceration remains unclear.

ASPIRIN

The use of aspirin has been reported in a number of patients undergoing treatment for leg ulceration.[74] The authors describe a measurable effect of aspirin on the rate of ulcer healing. However, this study includes 20 patients of whom only 4 healed their ulcers after 4 months of treatment. This is extremely preliminary data on which to base any conclusions concerning treatment of patients. One paper proposes that abnormalities in coagulation measurements [fibrinogen, factor VIII related antigen, von Willebrand antigen and plasminogen activator inhibitor-1 (PAI-1)], which are perturbed in patients with venous disease, may be modified by the therapeutic use of aspirin.[75] Currently the mode of action of aspirin and the extent of its efficacy in the management of venous ulceration remain to be shown. Since 1995, no further paper has been published that addresses the efficacy of aspirin in venous leg ulceration, so the actual effect of aspirin on leg ulceration has never been reliably established. This is clearly because of the lack of possible commercial exploitation should any positive effect be discovered, but perhaps other platelet antagonists could be studied.

Ifetroban

Effects of the oral thromboxane A_2 receptor antagonist ifetroban (250 mg daily) on healing of chronic lower-extremity venous stasis ulcers has been studied. This drug has a profound inhibitory effect on platelet activation and therefore could be a commercially viable successor to aspirin should efficacy be shown. In a prospective, randomized, double-blind, placebo-controlled multicenter study,[76] 165 patients were randomized to ifetroban ($n = 83$) versus placebo ($n = 82$) for a period of 12 weeks. Both groups were treated with sustained graduated compression and hydrocolloid dressings for the ulcers. Complete ulcer healing was achieved after 12 weeks in 55% of patients receiving ifetroban and in 54% of those taking a placebo with no significant differences; 84% of ulcers in both groups achieved greater than 50% area reduction in size. This was a well-conducted study with a clear primary end point (complete ulcer healing in a patient). The findings strongly refute the suggestion that platelet inhibition will lead to leg ulcer healing.

Venoactive drugs in leg ulceration

Far less has been written about the efficacy of this group in the management of leg ulceration than in the management of the symptoms of varicose veins. Interest in this field has increased in recent years and a few studies have been published.

A study on the effect of rutosides on symptoms in 112 patients with venous insufficiency included four with ulceration. All four took rutosides for 8 weeks; only one showed any evidence of improvement.[77] Other studies have shown no evidence that hydroxyrutosides improve venous ulcer healing or prevent its recurrence. In 138 patients with recently healed venous ulcers, Wright[78] compared the efficacy of below-the-knee elastic stockings combined with hydroxyrutosides (Paroven 500 mg b.d.) or placebo. The recurrence rates at 12 months were 23% with hydroxyrutosides and 22% with placebo. After 18 months, the figures were 34% and 32%. These results show no evidence that hydroxyrutosides prevent ulcer recurrence when combined with elastic compression. It is clear that rutosides have a measurable effect on edema in patients with venous disease. Unfortunately, they do not have any effect on preventing venous leg ulcer recurrence. A possible extension of this conclusion is that treatment of edema alone (where rutosides have efficacy) is insufficient to treat leg ulceration. Some additional factor must be influenced in order to speed ulcer healing (in which rutosides have not been tested) or to prevent recurrence of ulceration.

FLAVONOIDS

The effect of Daflon 500 mg in a venous ulcer healing study has been recently reported.[79] Patients were randomized to receive Daflon 500 mg or placebo combined with standard compression bandaging during an 8-week follow-up period. In 91 patients with an ulcer diameter of 10 cm or less, 14 of 44 (32%) patients receiving Daflon 500 mg compared with 6 of 47 (13%) receiving placebo healed their ulcers ($P = 0.028$, chi square) after 8 weeks of treatment. The time to achieve healing was shorter in the Daflon 500 mg group than in the placebo group ($P = 0.037$). This is the only member of the 'edema-protective' drug group which has been shown to modify ulcer healing. Despite the fact that the study was relatively small and the duration of treatment was short (8 weeks), the results are encouraging. A larger clinical trial is currently in progress in which more patients are followed for 6 months in order to confirm the promising results already obtained. The possible mechanism of action of this drug is not yet clear, although several of its effects have been described above in the section on treatment of varicose veins.

A recent pilot study has been conducted[80] using micronized purified flavonoid fraction (MPFF) (Daflon 500 mg, Servier, Paris, France). Twenty patients with chronic venous disease (CEAP clinical stage 2–4) were treated for 60 days with Daflon 500 mg twice daily taken orally. There was no placebo control group in this pilot study. Blood samples before and after the treatment were collected from a foot vein. Plasma levels of the soluble endothelial adhesion molecules sVCAM-1, sICAM-1, sP-selectin and sE-selectin were determined. In addition, the endothelial-derived von Willebrand factor (vWF), the neutrophil secondary granule enzyme lactoferrin and vascular endothelial growth factor (VEGF) levels were determined using a standard sandwich ELISA method. In addition, the neutrophil and monocyte surface adhesion molecules CD11b and L-selectin (CD62L) were assessed by a flow cytometric technique.

The expression of the leukocyte adhesion molecule CD62L was substantially decreased on monocytes and neutrophils by MPFF treatment; however, CD11b expression was not modified. This finding suggests that leukocyte L-selectin interaction with endothelial selectins responsible for the initial stages of adhesion may be modulated by MPFF treatment, reducing the likelihood of leukocyte adhesion and presumably acting as an anti-inflammatory mechanism.

Significant downregulation of plasma levels of sVCAM-1 and sICAM-1 activity following therapy was observed indicating that endothelial damage which ensues in venous disease from chronic venous hypertension was mitigated by MPFF treatment. More detailed study is required to determine whether these measurable anti-inflammatory effects of flavonoids are central to the efficacy of flavonoids in the management of venous disease.

Topically applied preparations

A wide range of preparations is applied to venous leg ulcers in an attempt to heal them. A review of these would constitute a chapter in itself! A particular feature of patients with chronic venous disease of the leg and leg ulceration is their ability to become sensitized to many topically applied compounds. In most leg ulcer clinics, extreme care is used in topical applications since many commonly used drugs can produce skin sensitization. Antibiotics are common culprits. Aminoglycoside antibiotics commonly present in preparations for topical use may cause skin sensitization. They have no effect on the healing of venous leg ulcers and should never be used! Topical steroids are often invaluable in the management of skin eczema resulting from sensitivity to one of the many chemicals used in the treatment of leg ulcers.

Sometimes sensitization occurs to one of the components of steroid creams and occasionally to the steroids themselves.

'Active' treatments which might be applied topically include antiseptics such as cadexomer iodine. Cadexomer iodine paste has been compared to hydrocolloid dressings or paraffin gauze dressings and been found to lead to more rapid reduction in ulcer surface area.[81] However, this paper did not assess time to complete healing of ulcers and therefore falls short of modern levels of proof of efficacy. The use of local antiseptic agents might address the bacterial colonization of ulcers but since it seems unlikely that infection is the main cause of the continuation of a leg ulcer the effect of this type of treatment might be limited.

The work of Knighton suggested to many that venous leg ulcer healing could be speeded by the use of growth factors derived from platelets.[82] This has led to preparations of platelet growth factors being licenced in the USA for use in non-healing leg and foot ulcers in patients with diabetes.[83] However, there is little convincing evidence of the efficacy of this type of compound in venous leg ulcers. Some authors have investigated granulocyte-macrophage colony stimulating factor (GM-CSF) in the treatment of venous leg ulcers.[84] However, no large-scale leg ulcer healing study has been published showing an advantage of this type of treatment. A number of problems present themselves with this method of management. First, it makes the assumption that venous leg ulceration is the result of faulty healing as well as the mechanisms which resulted in leg ulceration in the first place. It presumably makes the assumption that levels of growth factors in healing ulcers are pathologically reduced. There is no published evidence to support this assumption. Studies investigating the levels of tissue growth factors in ulcers mainly show greatly increased levels of tissue growth factors. Finally, there are the logistics of delivering a drug to an ulcer at a dose that is sustained and effective. This is especially difficult since ulcer dressings may remain in place for several days. To me it seems highly improbable that such an approach will be effective in patients with venous leg ulcers.

CONCLUSIONS

To return to the original question that I posed, what should we use and when? In the case of varicose veins, no drug will remove or diminish the varices except when used as sclerosant during sclerotherapy for varices. Where mitigation of symptoms is required, compression stockings are very effective in temperate countries. In hot countries and where it is desirable to treat edema, venoactive drugs should be considered if they are available. Hydroxyrutosides and drugs containing diosmin and herperidine are effective.

In the management of leg ulceration, the following systemically administered drugs are ineffective at achieving healing of ulcers: aspirin, ifetroban, stanozolol, antibiotics, hydroxyrutosides. Topical growth factors have yet to be shown to have efficacy in this context. The following drugs have some efficacy in achieving ulcer healing when given systemically: pentoxifylline, flavonoids. It is clear that the available pharmacological treatments for venous disease are less effective than compression treatments or surgery in achieving healing of ulcers and that drug treatments should always be used as part of a regimen of management rather than as an isolated treatment.

REFERENCES

1. Modified from Ramelet AA, Monti M. *Phlebologie*, 3rd edn. Paris, France: Masson, 1994: 71–7.
2. The management of chronic venous disorders of the leg: an evidenced-based report of an international task force. *Phlebology* 1999; **14**(Suppl 1:92): 67.
3. Balmer A, Limoni C. A double-blind placebo-controlled trial of VENORUTON on the symptoms and signs of chronic venous insufficiency. *Vasa* 1980; **9**: 76–82.
4. Pulvertaft TB. General practice treatment of symptoms of venous insufficiency with oxerutins. Results of a 660 patient multicentre study in the UK. *Vasa* 1983; **12**: 373–6.
5. De Jongste AB, Jonker JJC, Huisman MV, *et al.* A double blind three center clinical trial on the short-term efficacy of O-(β-hydroxyethyl)-rutosides in patients with post-thrombotic syndrome. *Thromb Haemost* 1989; **62**: 826–9.
6. Bergqvist D, Hallboeok T, Lindblad B, Lindhagen A. A double-blind trial of O-(β-hydroxyethyl)-rutosides in patients with chronic venous insufficiency. *Vasa* 1981; **10**: 253–60.
7. Prerovsky I, Roztocil K, Hlavova A, *et al.* The effect of hydroxyethylrutosides after acute and chronic oral administration in patients with venous diseases. A double-blind study. *Angiologica* 1972; **9**: 408–14.
8. Cloarec M, Clement R, Griton P. A double-blind clinical trial of hydroxyethylrutosides in the treatment of the symptoms and signs of chronic venous insufficiency. *Phlebology* 1996; **11**: 76–82.
9. Kranendonk SE, Koster AM. A double-blind clinical trial of the efficacy and tolerability of O-(β-hydroxyethyl)-rutosides and compression stockings in the treatment of leg oedema and symptoms following surgery for varicose veins. *Phlebology* 1993; **8**: 77–81.
10. Bergqvist D, Hallböök T, Lindblad B, Lindhagen A. A double-blind trial of O-(hydroxyethyl)-rutoside in patients with chronic venous insufficiency. *Vasa* 1981; **10**: 253–60.
11. Renton S, Leon M, Belcaro G, Nicolaides AN. The effect of hydroxyethylrutosides on capillary filtration in moderate venous hypertension. *Int Angiol* 1994; **13**: 259–62.

12. Neumann HAM, van den Broek MJTB. Evaluation of O-(β-hydroxyethyl)-rutosides in chronic venous insufficiency by means of non-invasive techniques. *Phlebology* 1990; **5**(Suppl 1): 13–20.
13. de Jongste AB, Jonker JJC, Huisman MV, ten Cate JW, Azar AJ. A double-blind trial on the short-term efficacy of HR in patients with the post-thrombotic syndrome. *Phlebology* 1990; **5**(Suppl 1): 21–2.
14. Nocker W, Diebschlag W, Lehmacher W. Clinical trials of the dose-related effects of O-(β-hydroxyethyl)-rutosides in patients with chronic venous insufficiency. *Phlebology* 1990; **5**(Suppl 1): 23–6.
15. Hachen HJ, Lorenz P. Double-blind clinical and plethysmographic study of calcium dobesilate in patients with peripheral microvascular disorders. *Angiology* 1982; **33**: 480–8.
16. Widmer L, Biland L, Barras JP. Doxium® 500 in chronic venous insufficiency: a double-blind placebo. Controlled multicentre study. *Int Angiol* 1990; **9**: 105–10.
17. Zuccarelli F, Ducros JJ, Egal G, *et al.* Efficacitè clinique du Veinotonyl 75® dans l'insuffisance veineuse des membres inférieurs. *Artères Veines* 1993; **XII**: 375–9.
18. Johnston AM, Paul HJ, Young CG. Effects of micronization on digestive absorption of diosmin. *Phlebology* 1994; **9**(Suppl 1): 4–6.
19. Cospite M, Cospite V. Treatment of haemorrhoids with Daflon 500 mg. *Phlebology* 1992; **7**(Suppl 2): 53–6.
20. Cospite M, Dominici A. Double blind study of the pharmacodynamic and clinical advantages of 5682SE in venous insufficiency. Advantages of the new micronized form. *Angiology* 1989; **8**(Suppl 4): 61–5.
21. Laurent R, Gilly R, Frileux C. Clinical evaluation of a venotropic drug in man. Example of Daflon 500 mg. *Int Angiol* 1988; **7**(Suppl to no. 2): 39–43.
22. Juteau N, Bakri F, Pomies JP, *et al.* The human saphenous vein in pharmacology: effect of a new micronized flavonoidic fraction (Daflon 500 mg) on norepinephrine induced contraction. *Int Angiol* 1995; **14**(3 Suppl 1): 8–13.
23. Ibegbuna V, Nicolaides AN, Sowade O, Leon M, Geroulakos G. Venous elasticity after treatment with Daflon 500 mg. *Angiology* 1997; **48**: 45–9.
24. Cotonat A, Cotonat J. Lymphagogue and pulsatile activities of Daflon 500 mg on canine thoracic lymph duct. *Int Angiol* 1989; **8**(4 Suppl): 15–18.
25. Gargouil YM, Perdrix L, Chapelain B, Gaborieau R. Effects of Daflon 500 mg on bovine vessels contractility. *Int Angiol* 1989; **8**(4 Suppl): 19–22.
26. McHale NG, Hollywood MA. Control of lymphatic pumping: interest of Daflon 500 mg. *Phlebology* 1994; **9**(Suppl 1): 23–5.
27. Behar A, Lagrue G, Cohen-Boulakia F, Baillet J. Study of capillary filtration by double labelling I^{131} albumin and Tc^{99m} red cells. Application to the pharmacodynamic activity of Daflon 500 mg. *Int Angiol* 1988; **7**(2 Suppl): 35–8.
28. Galley P, Thiollet M. A double blind, placebo controlled trial of a new venoactive flavonoid fraction (S 5682) in the treatment of symptomatic capillary fragility. *Int Angiol* 1993; **12**: 69–72.
29. Friesenecker B, Tsai AG, Intaglietta M. Cellular basis of inflammation, oedema and the activity of Daflon 500 mg. *Int J Microcirc* 1995; **15**: 17–21.
30. Korthuis RJ, Gute DC. Post-ischaemic leucocyte-endothelial cell interactions and microvascular barrier dysfunction in skeletal muscle: cellular mechanisms and effect of Daflon 500 mg. *Int J Microcirc Clin Exp* 1997; **17**(Suppl 1): 11–17.
31. Bouskela E, Donyo K. Effects of oral administration of purified micronized flavonoid fraction on increased microvascular permeability induced by various agents and on ischemia-reperfusion in the hamster cheek pouch. *Angiology* 1997; **48**: 391–9.
32. Bouskela E, Donyo KA, Verbeuren TJ. Effects of Daflon 500 mg on increased microvascular permeability in normal hamsters. *Int J Microcirc* 1995; **15**: 22–6.
33. Belcaro G, Cesarone MR, De Sanctis MT, *et al.* Laser Doppler and transcutaneous oximetry: modern investigations to assess drug efficacy in chronic venous insufficiency. *Int J Microcirc* 1995; **15**(Suppl 1): 45–9.
34. Browse NL, Burnand KG, Lea Thomas ML. *Diseases of the Veins*. London: Arnold, 1988.
35. Felix W. Treatment of venous diseases by drugs. In Davy A, Stemmer R, eds. *Phlebologie '89*. London: John Libbey, 1989: 698–702.
36. Myers MB, Rightor M, Cherry G. Relationship between edema and the healing rate of stasis ulcers of the leg. *Am J Surg* 1972; **124**: 666–8.
37. Robb-Nicholson C. I have a number of spider veins on my legs and have had unsuccessful treatments for them – both injection and laser therapy. I recently read an ad for a cream called Dermal-K, which is supposed to alleviate the condition. How effective is this cream? *Harv Womens Health Watch* 1998; **6**: 8.
38. McCoy S, Evans A, Tiller A, Malouf GM. A blinded prospective comparative trial of a topical vitamin K cream for the treatment of leg telangiectases. *Aust N Z J Phlebol* 2000; **4**.
39. Scriven JM, Hartshorne T, Thrush AJ, Bell PR, Naylor AR, London NJ. Role of saphenous vein surgery in the treatment of venous ulceration. *Br J Surg* 1998; **85**: 781–4.
40. Shami SK, Sarin S, Cheatle TR, Coleridge Smith PD, Scurr JH. Venous ulcers and the superficial venous system. *J Vasc Surg* 1993; **17**: 487–90.
41. Ghauri AS, Nyamekye I, Grabs AJ, Farndon JR, Whyman MR, Poskitt KR. Influence of a specialised leg ulcer service and venous surgery on the outcome of venous leg ulcers. *Eur J Vasc Endovasc Surg* 1998; **16**: 238–44.
42. Franks PJ, Oldroyd MI, Dickson D, Sharp EJ, Moffatt CJ. Risk factors for leg ulcer recurrence: a randomized trial of two types of compression stocking. *Age Ageing* 1995; **24**: 490–4.
43. Baker PG, Haig G. Metronidazole in the treatment of chronic pressure sores and ulcers. *Practitioner* 1981; **225**: 569–73.

44. Jones PH, Willis AT, Ferguson IR. Treatment of anaerobically infected pressure sores with topical metronidazole. *Lancet* 1978; **1**: 214.
45. Greaves MW, Skillen AW. Effects of long-continued ingestion of zinc sulphate in patients with venous leg ulceration. *Lancet* 1970; **2**: 889–91.
46. Greaves MW, Ive FA. Double-blind trial of zinc sulphate in the treatment of chronic venous leg ulceration. *Br J Dermatol* 1972; **87**: 632–4.
47. Myers MB, Cherry G. Zinc and the healing of chronic leg ulcers. *Am J Surg* 1970; **120**: 77–81.
48. Phillips A, Davidson M, Greaves MW. Venous leg ulceration: evaluation of zinc treatment, serum zinc and rate of healing. *Clin Exp Dermatol* 1977; **2**: 395–9.
49. Schraibmann IG, Stratton FJ. Nutritional status of patients with leg ulcers. *J R Soc Med* 1985; **78**: 39–42.
50. Browse NL, Burnand KG. The cause of venous ulceration. *Lancet* 1982; **2**: 243–5.
51. Browse NL, Jarrett PEM, Morland M, Burnand K. Treatment of liposclerosis of the leg by fibrinolytic enhancement: a preliminary report. *Br Med J* 1977; **2**: 434–5.
52. Burnand K, Lemenson G, Morland M, Jarrett PEM, Browse NL. Venous lipodermatosclerosis: treatment by fibrinolytic enhancement and elastic compression. *Br Med J* 1980; **280**: 7–11.
53. McMullin GM, Watkin GT, Coleridge Smith PD, Scurr JH. Efficacy of fibrinolytic enhancement in the treatment of venous insufficiency. *Phlebology* 1991; **6**: 233–9.
54. Layer GT, Stacey MC, Burnand KG. Stanozolol and the treatment of venous ulceration – an interim report. *Phlebology* 1986; **1**: 197–203.
55. Dodd HJ, Gaylarde PM, Sarkany I. Skin oxygen tension in venous insufficiency of the lower leg. *J R Soc Med* 1985; **78**: 373–6.
56. Michel CC. Aetiology of venous ulceration (letter). *Br J Surg* 1990; **77**: 1071.
57. Coleridge Smith PD, Thomas P, Scurr JH, Dormandy JA. Causes of venous ulceration: a new hypothesis. *Br Med J* 1988; **296**: 1726–7.
58. Sinzinger H, Virgolini I, Fitscha P. Pathomechanisms of atherosclerosis beneficially affected by prostaglandin E1 (PGE1) – an update. *Vasa Suppl* 1989; **28**: 6–13.
59. Beitner H, Hamar H, Olsson AG, Thyresson N. Prostaglandin E1 treatment of leg ulcers caused by venous or arterial incompetence. *Acta Dermatovener (Stockh)* 1980; **60**: 425–30.
60. Rudofsky G. Intravenous prostaglandin E1 in the treatment of venous ulcers – a double-blind, placebo-controlled trial. *Vasa Suppl* 1989; **28**: 39–43.
61. Muller B, Krais T, Sturzebacher S, Witt W, Schillinger E, Baldus B. Potential therapeutic mechanisms of stable prostacyclin (PGI2) mimetics in severe peripheral vascular disease. *Biomed Biochim Acta* 1988; **47**: S40–4.
62. Musial J, Wilczynska M, Sladek K, Ciernewski CS, Nizankowski R, Szczeklik A. Fibrinolytic activity of prostacyclin and iloprost in patients with peripheral arterial disease. *Prostaglandins* 1986; **31**: 61–70.
63. Belch JJF, Saniabadi A, Dickson R, Sturrock RD, Forbes CD. Effect of iloprost (ZK 36374) on white cell behaviour. In Gryglewski RJ, Stock G, eds. *Prostacyclin and its Stable Analogue Iloprost.* Berlin: Springer-Verlag, 1987: 97–102.
64. Muller B, Schmidtke M, Witt W. Adherence of leucocytes to electrically damaged venules in vivo. *Eicosanoids* 1988; **1**: 13–17.
65. Sturzebecher CS, Losert W. Effects of iloprost on platelet activation in vitro. In Gryglewski RJ, Stock G, eds. *Prostacyclin and its Stable Analogue Iloprost.* Berlin: Springer-Verlag, 1987: 39–45.
66. Werner-Schlenzka H, Kuhlmann RK. Treatment of venous leg ulcers with topical iloprost: a placebo controlled study. *Vasa* 1994; **23**: 145–50.
67. Roekkaerts F, Deleers L. Trental 400 in the treatment of intermittent claudication: results of long-term, placebo-controlled administration. *Angiology* 1984; **35**: 396–406.
68. Sullivan GW, Carper HT, Novick WJ, Mandell GL. Inhibition of the inflammatory action of interleukin-1 and tumour necrosis factor (alpha) on neutrophil function by pentoxifylline. *Infect Immunol* 1988; **56**: 1722–9.
69. Weitgasser H. The use of pentoxifylline ('Trental' 400) in the treatment of leg ulcers: results of a double-blind trial. *Pharmatherapeutica* 1983; **3**(Suppl 1):143–51.
70. Herger R. The significance of the microcirculation in the treatment of leg ulcers. *Therapiewoche* 1986; **36**: 3818–28.
71. Angelides NS, Weil von der Ahe, CA. Effect of oral pentoxifylline therapy on venous lower extremity ulcers due to deep venous incompetence. *Angiology* 1989; **40**: 752–63.
72. Colgan M-P, Dormandy JA, Jones PW, Schraibman IG, Shanik DG, Young RAL. Oxpentifylline treatment of venous ulcers of the leg. *Br Med J* 1990; **300**: 972–5.
73. Dale JJ, Ruckley CV, Harper DR, Gibson B, Nelson EA, Prescott RJ. A randomised double-blind placebo controlled trial of oxpentifylline in the treatment of venous leg ulcers. *Phlebology* 1995; **Suppl 1**: 917–18.
74. Layton AM, Ibbotson SH, Davies JA, Goodfield MJ. Randomised trial of oral aspirin for chronic venous leg ulcers. *Lancet* 1994; **344**: 164–5.
75. Ibbotson SH, Layton AM, Davies JA, Goodfield MJ. The effect of aspirin on haemostatic activity in the treatment of chronic venous leg ulceration. *Br J Dermatol* 1995; **132**: 422–6.
76. Lyon RT, Veith FJ, Bolton L, Machado F. Clinical benchmark for healing of chronic venous ulcers. Venous Ulcer Study Collaborators. *Am J Surg* 1998; **176**: 172–5.
77. Pulvertaft TB. Paroven in the treatment of chronic venous insufficiency. *Practitioner* 1979; **223**: 838–41.
78. Wright DD, Franks PJ, Blair SD, Backhouse CM, Moffatt C, McCollum CN. Oxerutins in the prevention of recurrence in chronic venous ulceration: randomised controlled trial. *Br J Surg* 1991; **78**: 1269–70.
79. Guilhou JJ, Dereure O, Marzin L, *et al.* Efficacy of Daflon

500 mg in venous leg ulcer healing: a double-blind, randomised, controlled versus placebo trial in 107 patients. *Angiology* 1997; **48**: 77–85.

80. Shoab SS, Porter J, Scurr JH, Coleridge smith PD. Endothelial activation response to oral micronised flavonoid therapy in patients with chronic venous disease – a prospective study. *Eur J Vasc Endovasc Surg* 1999; **17**: 313–18.
81. Hansson C, Persson L-M, Stenquist B, *et al.* The effects of cadexomer iodine paste in the treatment of venous leg ulcers compared with hydrocolloid dressing and paraffin gauze dressing. *Int J Dermatol* 1998; **37**: 390–6.
82. Knighton DR, Ciresi K, Fiegel VD, Schumerth S, Butler E, Cerra F. Stimulation of repair in chronic, nonhealing, cutaneous ulcers using platelet-derived wound healing formula. *Surg Gynecol Obstet* 1990; **170**: 56–60.
83. Steed DL, Webster MW, Ricotta JJ, *et al.* Clinical evaluation of recombinant human platelet-derived growth factor for the treatment of lower extremity diabetic ulcers. *J Vasc Surg* 1995; **21**: 71–81.
84. Marques da Costa R, Jesus FM, Aniceto C, Mendes M Double-blind randomized placebo-controlled trial of the use of granulocyte-macrophage colony-stimulating factor in chronic leg ulcers. *Am J Surg* 1997; **173**: 165–8.

32

Advances in the local treatment of venous ulcers using bioengineered skin

GAIL DE IMUS AND VINCENT FALANGA

Two new advances have emerged in the last decade that have ushered in an exciting era in the treatment of chronic venous ulcers – bioengineered skin substitutes and topical growth factors. Prior to this, therapy focused mainly on different systems of compression and specialized wound dressings. With a limited armamentarium to manage chronic nonhealing wounds, investigators raced to discover the magic bullet that would stimulate wound healing and hasten re-epithelialization; provide a permanent wound coverage; decrease morbidity and contractures; ameliorate pain; and improve the patients' quality of life. The ideal form of therapy would be widely available with minimal wait time, easy to use (preferably in an office or home care setting), available for multiple and repeated applications, painless, and cost-effective. This chapter concentrates on the role of bioengineered skin in revolutionizing the local treatment of venous ulcers.

BIOENGINEERED LIVING SKIN SUBSTITUTES

Historical perspective: the path towards a living bilayered skin equivalent

Advances in cell and tissue culture techniques have paved the way for scientists to 'bioengineer' human tissue equivalents[1–5] that have properties as close to those of natural skin as possible. The pioneering work that triggered this revolution came from Rheinwald and Green in 1975,[6] who were able to reliably grow human epidermal cells in culture for the first time. Based on their techniques and variants, numerous investigators followed suit and developed cultured autologous keratinocyte grafts, cultured allogeneic keratinocyte grafts, autologous/allogeneic composites, acellular collagen matrices, and cellular matrices,[5] all of which are precursors to our present living skin construct. Some of the disadvantages encountered with the autologous and allogeneic keratinocyte models included the required 3–4 week interval between biopsy and grafting autologous sheets, the difficulty in handling the fragile sheets on gauze, short-term stability, and the lack of a dermal component leading to wound contracture and blistering.[5,7,8] Autologous/allogeneic composites derived from cadaveric skin did contain a dermal component;[9] however, it only provided an extracellular matrix and lacked viable fibroblasts.[5] More advanced acellular collagen matrices such as Alloderm® (Lifecell Corporation, The Woodlands, TX, USA) and Integra® (Life Sciences Corporation, Plainsboro, NJ, USA) provided a more stable dermal matrix. Later on, dermal and epidermal cells were ultimately added to Integra,[5] converting it from an acellular to a cellular collagen matrix.

Silastic® (Dow-Corning Corporation, Midland, MI, USA), developed in 1981 by Burke *et al.*,[10] was the first of the 'bilayered' skin substitutes. The 'epidermis' was composed of the temporary silastic membrane, which was later replaced by epidermal grafts once the dermis became vascularized. The 'dermis' was composed of a sponge of porous bovine collagen and shark chondroitin crosslinked with glutaraldehyde. Though this bilayered graft did result in significant improvement in wound closure, it required a cumbersome two-step application. Proper drainage of wound fluid was also hampered by the nonporous Silastic membrane – leading to an increased risk of infection, graft dehiscence, and hematoma formation.[5]

Second-generation bilayered grafts incorporated cellular components such as cultured autologous keratinocytes supported by a collagen-glycosaminoglycan (GAG) base. Autologous fibroblasts were also added to the dermal matrix.[11] This 'open-matrix' collagen had a 70% graft failure rate due to enzymatic degradation by collagenase and increased susceptibility to bacterial infection.[7,9] Boyce *et al.*[12] improved on this model by replacing the collagen-GAG base to a base similar to Silastic's bovine collagen and chondroitin 6-sulfate. Moreover, unlike its predecessor, this base contained dermal fibroblasts, which was thought to be clinically beneficial.

Further progress occurred. Once the components of the skin matrices were laid down, it was now time to breathe life into the product in order for it to mimic the dynamic nature of natural skin. Fibroblasts were cultured from neonatal foreskin and grown *in vitro* within a polyglactin 910 or polyglycolic acid bioabsorbable mesh – similar to that used in manufacturing suture material. These living fibroblasts proliferate and secrete human dermal collagen, fibronectin, GAGs, growth factors and other dermal matrix proteins.[13] Named Dermagraft® (Advanced Tissue sciences, La Jolla, CA, USA), this living, metabolically active, immunologically inert dermal substitute[13] laid under a split-thickness skin graft, led to complete wound closure within just 14 days of graft take.[14] It was suggested that the living fibroblasts respond to the recipient's tissue and subsequently modulate the secretion of growth factors.[14]

These advances did not occur sequentially, but there has been a natural evolution to more complex constructs. Now that the dermis contained viable, reproducing cells, it was time to incorporate a living epidermis into a bilayered skin equivalent. Doing so would obviate the need to harvest a top-layer split-thickness skin graft to lay over the living dermis. Bell *et al.*[15] derived fibroblasts from human neonatal foreskin and incorporated it into a bovine type 1 collagen lattice. Viable keratinocytes were then seeded on top to produce a graft that contained both a viable dermis and epidermis. Modifying Bell's procedure, Parenteau *et al.*[16] manufactured the living construct we now know as Graftskin® (Organogenesis, Canton, MA, USA) and licenced as Apligraf™ by Novartis Pharmaceutical Corporation (East Hanover, NJ, USA).

Graftskin: redefining the treatment of venous leg ulcers

Graftskin, the generic name of Apligraf, was approved by the Food and Drug Administration (FDA) in May of 1998 after pivotal trials by Falanga *et al.*[2,17] proved its efficacy in the treatment of venous leg ulcers. Two hundred and ninety-three patients with nonhealing venous ulcers were enrolled in this, the largest prospective, randomized, multicentered, controlled study of venous ulcers to date.[2] The treatment group (n = 127) received Apligraf and compression therapy with an elastic bandage alone (Coban; 3M, Minneapolis, MN, USA), while the control group (n = 106) was treated with the standard inelastic zinc oxide impregnated bandage (Unna boot) followed by Coban. During the clinical trial, the treatment group required an average of 2.3 applications of Graftskin – receiving an additional Apligraf when less than 50% re-epithelialization was achieved over the wound bed within the designated 3-week period. Healing was assessed by physical examination and computerized planimetry. Patients were followed weekly for 8 weeks, then at 3, 6 and 12 months. No adverse events were noted and there were no clinical signs of rejection. The fact that Graftskin does not show any signs of rejection both *in vitro* and *in vivo* may be due to the lack of professional antigen-presenting cells, such as endothelial and Langerhans cells, in the construct.[2,17] However, further studies are needed to evaluate the possibilities of subclinical rejection and its role in the performance of this product.

Results of the study showed that Graftskin was able to heal venous ulcers, especially chronic, nonhealing ones, more effectively and faster than standard compression therapy. Complete healing was achieved in 78 patients treated with Apligraf and in 39 patients treated with Unna boot alone (P = 0.012).[18] The average time required for complete wound closure was 57 days for the treatment group and 181 days for the control group (P = 0.0066).[18] Another interesting observation was made in a subgroup of 120 patients whose 'difficult-to heal' ulcers were present for more than a year. At the 6-month follow-up visit, Graftskin healed more ulcers than placebo (47% versus 19%; P = 0.002) and in less time (181 days versus not attained; P = 0.0038).[2]

The exact mechanism by which Apligraf accelerates healing is currently under investigation. One postulate is that it delivers new cell to a chronic wound trapped in a nonhealing mode due to its unresponsiveness to certain cell signals and growth factors.[2,19] It has been shown that fibroblasts cultured from venous ulcers are no longer responsive to the stimulatory effects of TGF-β_1 and may have decreased expression of TGF-β_1 type II receptors.[17] By delivering neonatal fibroblasts, we may be 'jump-starting' the process to a healing mode by providing the cells, growth factors and other stimulatory substances in the right sequence and concentration necessary for the stimulation of keratinocyte migration and the synthesis of essential matrix materials. Acting initially as merely a form of skin replacement, Graftskin then becomes 'smart' and adjusts the wound microenvironment in order to stimulate healing, possibly from the wound edge or appendages within the bed.[5,18,20] This is also a good argument for 'dosing' Apligraf in more difficult-to-heal wounds. The ideal intervals between each application and the question regarding the persistence of product in the wound bed is still under investigation.

Indications of Graftskin in venous ulcers: choosing the right patient at the right time

From the clinical trials outlined above, Graftskin has been proven effective for venous ulcers that have not healed for more than a month. In fact, it has been shown to be even more effective for long-standing, difficult-to heal, venous ulcers of more than a year's duration. Faced with a patient with a new ulcer, it is difficult to determine whether or not their venous ulcers will heal quickly or whether they will benefit from the application of Graftskin. Modifying a formula by Margolis, Tallman *et al.*[21] have proposed an equation which predicts complete ulcer healing of venous ulcers based on observing the initial rate of healing after 4 weeks of treatment with standard compression. Ulcers healing at a rate greater than 0.1 cm/week were observed to undergo complete healing, whereas those that healed at a rate of less than 0.05 cm/week failed to heal. Using this model, one can treat patients with standard compression for an initial period of 1 month. If they heal at a rate less than 0.5 cm/week, the decision to re-evaluate the wound and to apply bioengineered skin or other treatments may be the most appropriate course of action. Figure 32.1 outlines our proposed algorithm for the local treatment of venous ulcers using Graftskin. Other factors that may help determine nonhealing wounds are the initial size and duration of the ulcer, the patient's age, the amount of adjacent lipodermatosclerosis, and the ulcer's location. The bigger and more circumferential the ulcer, the less likely it is to heal. More chronic wounds in older patients carry a poorer prognosis. The more fibrosis surrounding the wound bed, the less likely it is to re-epithelialize. Because of the difficulty in applying proper degrees of compression, ulcers located below the lateral or medial malleolus are also less likely to heal. Moreover, in the elderly and in patients with substantial difficulty in dealing with a chronic wound and loss of quality of life, it may be more ethical to treat the ulcer effectively from the start.

The pretreatment phase: optimizing the wound bed

Having first determined the right candidate ulcer for Graftskin, it then becomes important to determine the optimum time of application. The wound bed has to be 'primed' in order to increase the chances of initial graft take and by eliminating existing infection (i.e. cellulitis), decreasing the bacterial burden, reducing the amount of exudate and necrotic tissue, and ensuring minimal bleeding at the time the graft is laid.

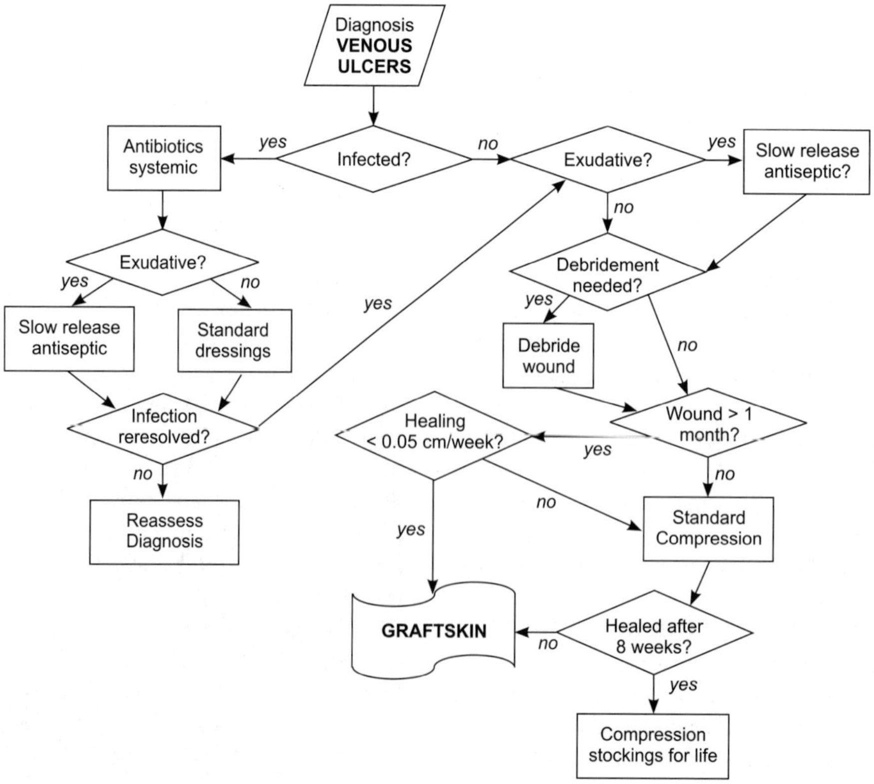

Figure 32.1 *Algorithm for the treatment of venous ulcers using Graftskin.*

Multiple methods have been used to achieve these goals. One method that we have found very useful is the application of cadexomer iodine (Iodoflex or Iodosorb; Smith & Nephew, York, UK). This slow-release iodine preparation is manufactured in the form of microbeads, which are capable of absorbing 70% of their weight. Cadexomer iodine has been found to be nontoxic and effective, particularly in wounds with moderate-to-high amounts of exudate. Treatment is applied every 2–3 days (sometimes daily), depending on the amount of exudate present. This topical treatment may need to be combined with the administration of the appropriate systemic antibiotics in order to decrease the bacterial burden. If the patient's infection is not responsive to oral medications, we may opt for a short course of intravenous antibiotics prior to the application of the graft.

Debridement is recommended for ulcers that have more necrotic wound beds and steep hyperproliferative edges indicative of the 'nonhealing' mode. The wound bed is initially scored with a scalpel. The necrotic material is then scraped off with a large curette until as much as possible of the fibrotic tissue and exudate is removed. The edges may also be saucerized – with removal of a rim of tissue a few millimeters from the margins of the ulcer.[1] Pain is managed with either topical anesthetics or local infiltration with lidocaine. Though not often necessary, debridement of larger ulcers may require general anesthesia.

The correct timing of the debridement procedure is crucial to the success of graft take. Ideally, debridement of severely necrotic wounds should be done 1–2 days before the application of Graftskin. This is to decrease the amount of fresh bleeding under the Graftskin that may cause it to be lifted off the wound bed. A 'floating graft', which is not directly adherent to the bed, has a smaller chance of taking. In cases where debridement has to be done on the same day, one may consider anchoring the graft with basting sutures and using bolsters to increase graft-to-wound bed contact.

On the day of the procedure, the wound again undergoes extensive irrigation with sterile normal saline in order to minimize the bacterial load that may have accumulated after the initial debridement procedure. A metal irrigation tray hooked to a suction mechanism and placed under the patient's leg may facilitate this step.

The technique of applying Graftskin: a step-by-step algorithm

The procedure of applying Graftskin is simple and can be done in an office or surgical outpatient setting (Fig. 32.1). It requires no anesthesia lest debridement or suturing is required. In general, no hospitalization is necessary. Patients are discharged to home after the 30–45 minute procedure is completed.

APLIGRAF PREPARATION: FROM THE TISSUE CULTURE WELL TO THE WOUND BED

Graftskin is shipped in a sealed, sterile plastic bag and stored in an incubator or viability unit especially provided by the company for its use. This maintains the temperature at around 31°C. Shelf-life studies indicate that it can be stored for up to 5 days.[21] One should verify the expiration date on the package prior to applying the graft.

Once the surgeon is ready to apply the graft, the bag is taken out of the incubator. The seal is broken by cutting the bag with a pair of scissors. Each unit of Graftskin, measuring 7.5 cm in diameter, is packaged in a plastic transwell insert that sits on top of a well of pink nutrient agarose. This nutrient media sustains the graft, which is separated from it by a thin clear porous disc.

Prior to removing the graft from its casing, it is helpful to moisten the surface of the graft with a few drops of normal saline. This will facilitate smoother handling of the graft. Then, using the wooden end of a cotton applicator, a portion of the edge of the Graftskin is gently teased towards the center until 20–25% of it is peeled away from the edge. One should try not to puncture the agar material below, as its effects on wound healing have not yet been studied. Also, one should avoid abrading the surface of Graftskin with the cotton applicator so as not to disturb the stratum corneum.

Using both hands, one can easily lift the graft from the transwell. Moist gloves may ease the handling of the product. Keeping in mind the orientation of the graft, the product is laid on to the meshing plate or carrier with the epidermal side up. The dermis has a glistening surface compared to the duller epidermal side.

Using a standard mesher, the graft is then meshed with a ratio of 1:1.5 (Fig. 32.2). At times, in order to cover a larger surface area, Graftskin has been meshed at a ratio of 1:3 to allow for more expansion. When using a mesher, one should take care not to allow the graft to stick to the mesher's roller. Moistening the graft with a few drops of normal saline prior to meshing often avoids

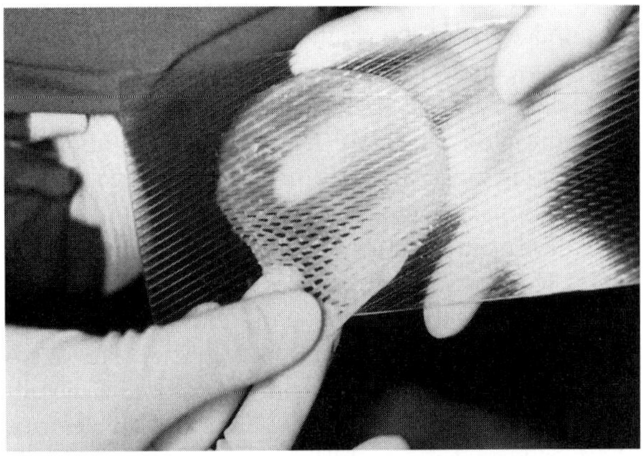

Figure 32.2 *Graftskin meshed to a ratio of 1:1.5.*

this problem. The graft is 'received' at the other end, flat on the plastic carrier.

Another option is to fenestrate the graft using a scalpel. Slits are made randomly or perpendicular to each other in order to ensure that tissue fluid or exudate from the wound bed will be allowed to escape through. This will lessen the likelihood of causing a 'floating graft', as previously discussed.

Once meshed, the Graftskin is then laid directly over the wound bed with the epidermal (dull) side up (Fig. 32.3). Using the cotton end of a cotton-tipped applicator, one positions the graft to cover the entire surface of the wound. It is useful to overlap the graft over the wound edges, as this may later prove helpful in the removal of the dressing. Some physicians opt to trim the edges of the graft using scissors, allowing for a 1–1.5 cm overlap with the margins. In cases where more than one site needs to be covered, the graft may be cut to the appropriate size required.

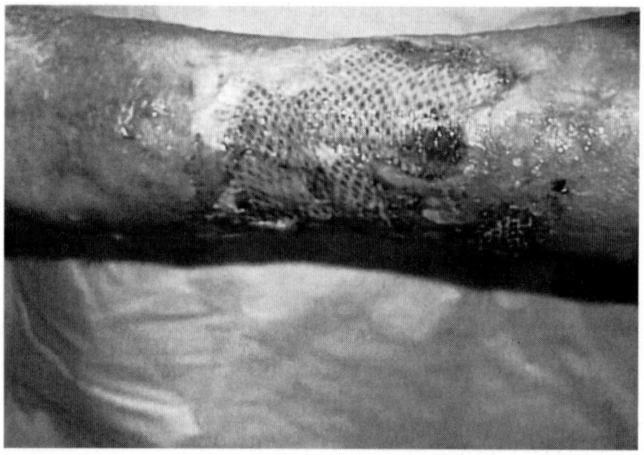

Figure 32.3 *Graftskin laid over the circumferential venous ulcers of several years' duration in a 93-year-old woman who did not respond to compression therapy.*

Anchoring and dressing techniques: the 'sandwich wrap'

Once the graft is in place, care should be taken so as not to dislodge it from the wound bed. In order to secure the graft, some clinicians opt to suture the edges using 4.0 or 5.0 nylon placed at each quadrant, about 0.5–1.0 cm from the ulcer edge.[1] We have found that this is not necessary in most cases. In order to anchor the graft into place and maximize its contact with the wound bed, we have developed what we have coined a 'foam sandwich wrap'. This dressing is composed of a layer of Xeroform gauze laid directly over the graft, followed by strips of foam dressing (Allevyn; Smith & Nephew). The size of the strips depends on the size of the wound. Generally, the length of the strips should be just a little smaller than the length of the ulcer bed. This type of nonadherent foam was chosen because it is able to absorb any extra wound fluid. By cutting the foam into strips, one does not occlude the graft completely. Another alternative is to puncture the foam dressing using 2 mm or 3 mm punch biopsy instruments to allow the escape of fluid. This may be cut to fit within the wound bed over the primary dressing.

The third layer of the primary dressing (foam sandwich wrap) is composed of another piece of Xeroform gauze. This should be cut bigger than the previous piece in contact with Graftskin in order to better anchor the entire dressing and facilitate the removal of the dressing on follow-up.

Obviously, other dressings can be used depending on the operator's preference. Some clinicians recommend using Mepitel (SCA; Molnlycke, Goteborg, Sweden), a non-adherent silicone dressing. This product is unique in that it initially sticks to the surface, but is easily stripped off its base once it is removed – much like the phenomenon of 'stick-on' paper pads. This is advantageous as it decreases the risk of lifting the graft off with the dressing. One disadvantage is that it is not as conformable as Xeroform. Clearly, there is a need for a generation of wound dressings which are optimal for bioengineered skin products. Once the primary dressing is in place, the leg is then wrapped using a compression wrap. We generally use Profore (Smith & Nephew), a four-layer compression dressing. The patients are instructed to strictly avoid disturbing the dressing.

Evaluating Graftskin take: post-treatment protocol

Unless they complain of pain, excessive exudate, or have problems with their compression dressing, patients are seen 1 week after the procedure. Occasionally, especially for ulcers that have been very exudative, the compression bandage and secondary wraps are changed after 2 or 3 days. During this initial follow-up visit, the primary dressing is left undisturbed unless there are clinical signs of infection. Only the top layer of Xeroform and the foam dressing are carefully stripped away from the primary dressing. If some portions are adherent and are not easily removed, the primary dressing should be left alone in order to minimize the risks of dislodging the graft.

On the second-week visit, the primary dressing is carefully removed, taking care not to strip off the Apligraf along with the dressing. Waiting an additional week allows for sufficient contact time between the graft and the wound bed. Healing is stimulated leading to early re-epithelialization. Upon removal of the primary dressing, the hydrated Apligraf often appears yellow. This appearance should not be mistaken for a sign of infection.

On subsequent follow-up visits, usually every 2–3 weeks, the degree of re-epithelialization can be gauged by the 'wrinkle test'.[22] With a use of a cotton applicator, one gently presses on the surface of the wound. Areas that are already re-epithelialized will produce a fine wrinkling radiating from the area of contact with the wound. Coarse wrinkling is noted when applying firm pressure on fibrous tissue and non-re-epitheliazed wounds. This simple test is an easy, inexpensive and reliable way of gauging epidermal healing.

At times, there has been a need to 'dose' Apligraf in order to restimulate the healing process. Once the wound shows signs of being dormant, another piece can be applied to the wound bed. Usually, we wait about 6 weeks after the last application before a second application is contemplated,[1] but this is a matter of clinical judgment.

Once the ulcer is completely re-epithelialized, Profore compression bandages are continued for another month, until the patient is able to obtain graded compression stockings delivering 30 mmHg pressure at the ankle.[1]

CONCLUSION

A type of bioengineered skin (Graftskin) has revolutionized the treatment of nonhealing venous ulcers. It is an ideal form of therapy in that it is easy to use, available with minimal wait time, painless and cost-effective. It may be applied on multiple ulcers repeatedly without the limitation of available donor sites. It has been proven to stimulate wound healing and hasten re-epithelialization after initially providing wound coverage. It has been reported to improve the patient's quality of life by ameliorating pain, decreasing morbidity and minimizing contractures, possibly by dermal remodeling. Whether the graft persists in the wound bed after several weeks or whether the epidermis within the wound comes from the Graftskin or is a result of epidermal migration from the wound edges is still under investigation. For now, this therapy gives physicians another useful tool in the treatment of difficult-to-heal venous ulcers. This novel therapy needs to be combined with compression therapy, proper wound care, topical growth factors and, if possible, surgical correction of the underlying venous insufficiency.

Figures 32.4 and 32.5 exemplify accelerated healing of venous ulcers using Graftskin.

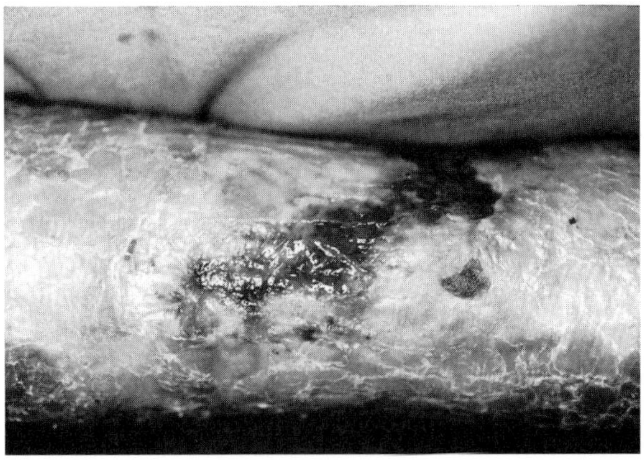

Figure 32.4 *The appearance of the ulcer 1 month after therapy with Graftskin.*

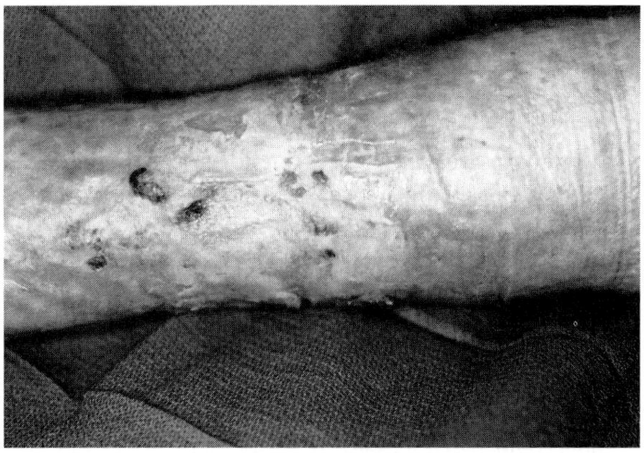

Figure 32.5 *Near-complete healing 4 months after treatment with Graftskin.*

REFERENCES

1. Falanga V. How to use Apligraf to treat venous ulcers. *Skin Aging* 1999; **Feb**: 30–6.
2. Falanga V. Apligraf treatment of venous ulcers and other chronic wounds. *J Dermatol* 1998; **25**(12): 812–17.
3. Skin Substitute Consensus Development Panel. Nonoperative management of venous leg ulcers: evolving role of skin substitutes. *Vasc Surg* 1999; **33**(2): 197–210.
4. Falanga V. Iodine-containing pharmaceuticals: a reappraisal. In *Proceedings of the 6th European Conference on Advances on Wound Management, Oct. 1–4, 1996, Amsterdam.* London: Macmillan Magazines Ltd, 1997: 191–4.
5. Eaglestein W, Falanga V. Tissue engineering and the development of Apligraf, a human skin equivalent. *Clin Ther* 1997; **19**(5): 894–905.
6. Rheinwald, JG, Green H. Serial cultivation of strings of human epidermal keratinocytes: the formation of keratinizing colonies from single cells. *Cell* 1975; **6**: 331–44.
7. Phillips TJ. Keratinocyte grafts for wound healing. *Clin Dermatol* 1994; **12**: 171–81.
8. Myers S, Navsaria H, Sanders R, Green C, Leigh I. Transplantation of keratinocytes in the treatment of wounds. *Am J Surg* 1995; **170**: 75–83.
9. Nanchahal J, Ward CM. New grafts for old? A review of alternatives to autologous skin. *Br J Plast Surg* 1992; **45**: 354–63.

10. Burke JF, Yannas IV, Quinby WC, *et al.* Successful use of a physiologically acceptable artificial skin in the treatment of extensive burn injury. *Ann Surg* 1981; **194**: 413–28.
11. Hansbrough JF, Boyce ST, Cooper ML, Foreman TJ. Burn wound closure with cultured autologous keratinocytes and fibroblasts attached to a collagen glycosaminoglycan substrate. *J Am Med Assoc* 1989; **262**: 2125–30.
12. Boyce ST, Glatter R, Kitsmiller WJ. Treatment of chronic wounds with cultured skin substitutes: a pilot study. *Wounds* 1995; **7**: 24–9.
13. Gentzkow GD, Iwasaki SD, Hershon KS, *et al.* Use of Dermagraft, a cultured human dermis, to treat diabetic foot. *Diabetes Care* 1996; **19**: 350–4.
14. Hansborough JF, Dore C, Hansborough WB. Clinical trials of a living dermal tissue replacement placed beneath a meshed, split-thickness skin grafts on excised burn wounds. *J Burn Care Rehabil* 1992; **13**: 519–29.
15. Bell E, Ehrlich HP, Buttle DJ, *et al.* Living tissue formed in vitro and accepted as skin-equivalent tissue of full thickness. *Science* 1981; **211**: 1052–4.
16. Parenteau NL, Nolte CM, Bilbo P, *et al.* Epidermis generated in vitro: practical considerations and applications. *J Cell Biochem* 1991; **45**: 245–51.
17. Falanga V, Margolis D, Alvarez O, *et al.* Healing of venous ulcers and lack of clinical rejection with an allogeneic cultured human skin equivalent. *Arch Dermatol* 1998; **134**: 293–300.
18. Sabolinski ML, Alvarez O, Auletta M, *et al.* Cultured skin as a 'smart material' for healing wounds: experience in venous ulcers. *Biomaterials* 1996; **17**(3): 311–20.
19. Hasan A, Murata H, Falabella A, *et al.* Dermal fibroblasts from venous ulcers are unresponsive to the action of transforming growth factor-β1. *J Dermatol Sci* 1997; **6**: 59–66.
20. Tallman P, Muscare E, Carson P, Eaglstein WH, Falanga V. Initial rate of healing predicts complete ulcer healing of venous ulcers. *Arch Dermatol* 1997; **133**: 1231–4.
21. Investigator's Brochure. *Graftskin Lining Skin Equivalent.* Organogenesis, Inc.
22. Falanga V. The 'wrinkle test': clinical use for detecting early epidermal resurfacing (letter). *J Dermatol Surg Oncol* 1993; **19**: 172–3.

33

Surgical repair of incompetent venous valves

RYAN D NACHREINER, AMARDIP S BHULLER AND MICHAEL C DALSING

INTRODUCTION AND HISTORY

The sequelae of chronic venous insufficiency (CVI) have been recognized for over 2000 years, and have been responsible for significant patient suffering and economic loss.[1] Treatment was originally medical, and focused on control of the patient's symptoms. Surgical innovation was avoided for fear of postoperative thrombosis, which would destroy the surgical repair and place the patient at risk of deep venous thrombosis.[2] The lack of accurate tools with which to make the proper diagnosis also hampered any progress. However, with advances in diagnostic imaging, surgical technology, and anticoagulation, our understanding and ability to approach venous disease has greatly increased over the past 40 years.

The development of ascending and descending venography in the 1940s was a critical breakthrough allowing visual confirmation of the causes of CVI by an accurate, reproducible, yet invasive method.[3] Plethysmography and venous duplex ultrasonography have added noninvasive, easily reproducible methods for the sequential quantification and anatomic classification of venous disease.

During the early part of this century, several investigators studied vein valve reconstruction and replacement in canine models.[4–6] However, treatment in humans was still limited to compressive therapy until Linton introduced the concept of ligating grossly incompetent veins.[7,8] Ligation continued as the mainstay of surgical treatment for the next 30 years. In 1968, Kistner first reported using a method of internal valvuloplasty to address venous reflux resulting from a primary etiology.[9] The development of external and angioscopic-assisted valvuloplasty operations followed much later. In addition, valve replacement was established as a feasible option when valve repair was not possible. The topic of this chapter will be limited to surgical repair of primary venous valvular disease.

ANATOMY AND PATHOLOGY

As discussed in more detail in Chapter 2, the lower extremity veins are arranged into three systems: superficial, perforating, and deep.[8] The superficial and deep systems are essentially parallel systems, whilst perforating veins connect the two at various points along the leg. Valves are distributed throughout each system and, in general, maintain superficial to deep and caudad to cephalad flow. Blood flow is generated by hydrostatic means whilst at rest and by muscular contraction during exercise.[10] The calf muscle pump is primarily responsible for contraction induced venous flow. Breakdown of any of the conduits or the pump can lead to CVI. Venous valvular reflux resulting in clinically significant insufficiency can be isolated to a single system, or involve multiple systems. The resultant venous hypertension initiates a sequence of events which eventually manifests as edema, pain, hyperpigmentation, and/or ulceration (the hallmarks of CVI). The complex interaction of the components of the venous system, not to mention the local end-organ effects, mandates a comprehensive approach when considering surgery for the treatment of CVI.

Chronic venous insufficiency can result from two distinct pathologic processes. The more common etiology is the post-thrombotic syndrome (PTS) accounting for an estimated 60–85% of patients with

CVI.[11–13] It is the end result of thrombosis and the subsequent inflammation of the valve cusps and vein wall during the process of recanalization. This leads to scarring and shortening of the cusps. Failure of the cusps to achieve normal coaptation results in reflux. Reflux secondary to the PTS is not amenable to direct surgical repair of the now destroyed valve.

Primary reflux is the result of structural abnormalities in the vein wall and valve itself. Although the precise etiology has not been characterized, it is presumed to be congenital in origin.[12] Redundant, malopposed cusps and venous dilation permit valve prolapse and reflux. Unlike the PTS, there is no evidence of previous thrombosis or inflammation near the valve.[13] It is possible, however, to have both proximal primary reflux and distal PTS in the same leg.[14] A rare cause of primary reflux is the complete absence of valves secondary to agenesis.[12] With the exception of valvular agenesis, primary reflux is amenable to direct surgical repair of the venous valve.

SELECTION OF PATIENTS

Patients with clinical evidence of CVI require a thorough evaluation prior to consideration for valve repair. This should begin with a complete history and physical examination. Assessment of the clinical status should comply with the reporting standards laid out in the CEAP classification system.[15] Initial imaging should be noninvasive, including venous duplex ultrasonography and air plethysmography. Others may substitute an alternative hemodynamic test. Duplex scanning differentiates refluxive from obstructive disease and identifies which systems and what levels demonstrate reflux. Air plethysmography assesses the physiologic status of the leg by evaluating venous emptying and filling, as well as the efficiency of the calf muscle pump.

After documenting that CVI exists, all patients should be given a trial of optimal medical management. In addition, patients with superficial venous reflux and/or perforator incompetence should have these problems addressed prior to consideration of a deep venous reconstruction.

Surgical correction of the deep venous system should only be considered for those patients who have persistent, severe manifestations of CVI. This usually means patients with clinical class 5 or 6 disease, although occasionally patients with a lower class of disease and disabling symptoms will be considered candidates. The decision to operate should be based on the clinical status of the patient, not the noninvasive data, since the patient's symptoms may not correlate directly with the laboratory findings.[16] In addition to meeting the clinical criteria, patients selected for surgery should be highly motivated to participate in their recovery since ultimate success is dependent on their compliance with postoperative management.

Prior to operation, all patients undergo ascending and descending venography. Ascending venography confirms the patency of the venous systems, eliminates venous obstruction as a problem that would be addressed by an alternative surgery, and defines the venous anatomy. It is our practice to obtain ambulatory venous pressure measurements during the performance of the ascending venogram to corroborate the noninvasive findings. Descending venography demonstrates the location of valves, if present, and the degree of reflux. In addition, descending venography can distinguish the typical elongated, redundant valves responsible for primary reflux from the shortened, retracted valves typical of the PTS.[13] Patients with reflux down the thigh and past the knee during a Valsalva maneuver (grade 3 or 4 reflux) with intact valve cusps are considered potential candidates for primary valve repair.[17]

It is critical to determine the reflux status of the profunda femoris vein (PFV). When dealing with primary reflux, repair of the most proximal valve in the superficial femoral vein (SFV) will usually suffice if the PFV is competent.[2,11] However, repair of more than one valve must be entertained when SFV and PFV reflux coexist, as several authors have documented the detrimental impact of persistent PFV reflux following repair of the SFV valve alone.[14,18] The popliteal valve provides an alternative repair location. This valve is touted as a 'gate keeper' for the distal deep venous system. It is a location more commonly considered in valve transplant procedures, but some interest has been demonstrated in utilizing it for valve repairs in primary reflux conditions.[19] Even more distal valves can be approached but are seldom treated.[19]

SURGICAL OPTIONS

Internal valvuloplasty

The diligent long-term follow-up by Kistner and his colleagues has established internal valvuloplasty as the standard of care in the surgical correction of primary reflux.[14] They have demonstrated that valve repair is possible and successful in properly selected patients.

Intermittent pneumatic compression begins at the time of anesthetic induction if feasible. The usual surgical approach utilizes a standard groin incision to access the most proximal SFV valve. The major veins including, when appropriate, the greater saphenous, common femoral, superficial femoral, profunda femoris veins, and all venous branches are isolated and individually controlled. A sufficient length is needed to allow both exposure of the valve cusps and optimal proximal and distal control. A strip test confirms valve incompetence (Fig. 33.1). The patient should be fully anticoagulated with heparin prior to valve repair. There are several options for gaining valve exposure. Kistner proposes a longitudinal venotomy bisecting the leaflets at the commissure (Fig. 33.2). Raju advocates a supravalvular, transverse venotomy (Fig. 33.3),[20] whilst Sottiurai utilizes a hybrid 'T'-shaped, supravalvular incision with extension to but not through the valve sinus (Fig. 33.4).[21] The redundant valve cusp is plicated to the vein wall using multiple interrupted 7-0 prolene reefing sutures. It has been estimated that plication of approximately 20% of the leaflet length should restore competence,[22] although the best gauge is visual inspection. A 'no touch' technique should be employed when dealing with the leaflets. Inadvertent tears in the leaflets can be repaired with 9-0 suture, but adds dramatically to the difficulty of the case. Valve competence should be re-evaluated with a strip test and Doppler examination for reflux once the valve repair is complete and the venotomy has been closed. Drainage of the wound is optional but should be considered due to the need for postoperative anticoagulation. Wound closure is routine.

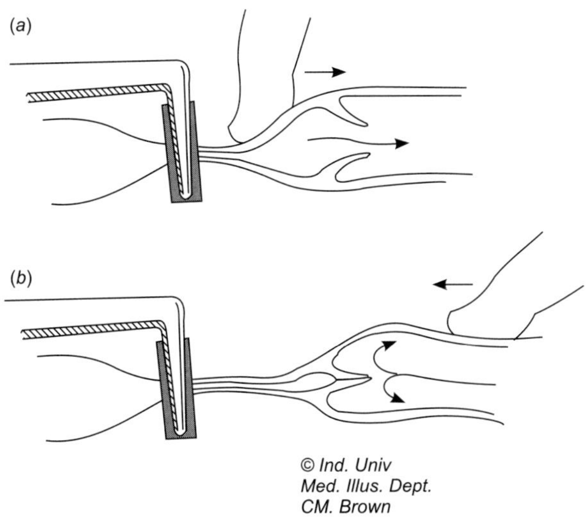

Figure 33.1 *Blood is stripped through the valve in the antegrade direction (a) and then forced back against the valve (b). An incompetent valve will allow blood to reflux into the distal segment, while a competent valve (shown) prevents reflux.*

Postoperative anticoagulation with heparin should be continued until long-term anticoagulation with warfarin can be instituted. Long-term anticoagulation is continued for at least 3 months. Intermittent pneumatic compression prevents venous stasis and minimizes the risk of postoperative thrombosis until patients are ambulatory. Other measures that aid in postoperative recovery include elevation of the legs while resting and diligent use of compression stockings until complete healing is achieved. Once valve competence is restored, symptomatic treatments such as compression stockings can sometimes be discarded but this must be tailored to the individual patient's situation. Kistner has found that approximately one-third of his patients can discard the lower extremity support.[14] Long-term follow-up consists of clinical examination, duplex scanning, and plethysmography to confirm valve competence and provide a meaningful clinical outcome score.[15]

Several alternative procedures for primary valve repair have been devised as experience has been gained in patient care and as advancements have been made in surgical technology. However, the surgical approach is generally similar to that for internal valvuloplasty in terms of preoperative preparation, intraoperative care, exposure of the vessels, and postoperative care. Each procedure is further outlined below.

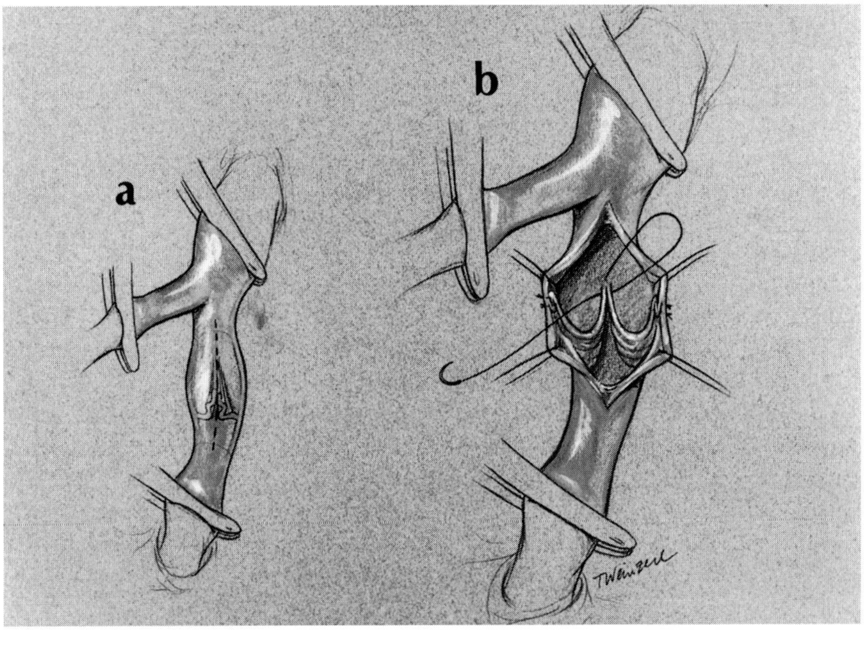

Figure 33.2 *Kistner developed the longitudinal venotomy to visualize the venous valve. A carefully performed incision through the commissure prevents damage to the valve cusps and provides excellent exposure throughout the procedure. The vein segment and valve prior to venotomy (a) and during valve repair (b) are illustrated in this drawing. (Adapted from Dalsing MC. Chronic venous disease. In Greenfield* et al. Surgery: Scientific Principles and Practice, *3rd edn. New York: Lippincott Williamson and Wilkins, 2001: Chapter 94).*

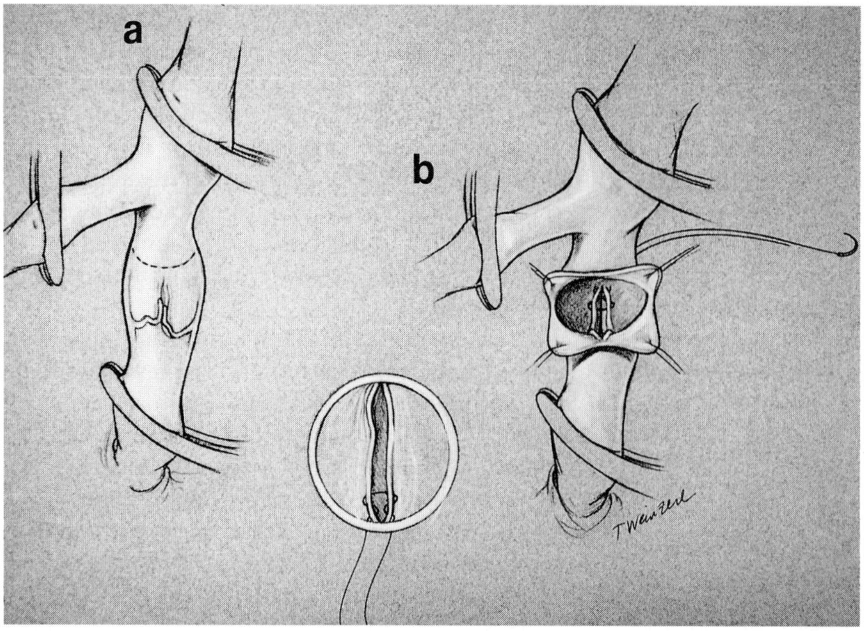

Figure 33.3 *Raju advocates a supravalvular venotomy to minimize the chance of damaging the valve cusps. The vein and valve are shown prior to (a) and during valvuloplasty (b).*

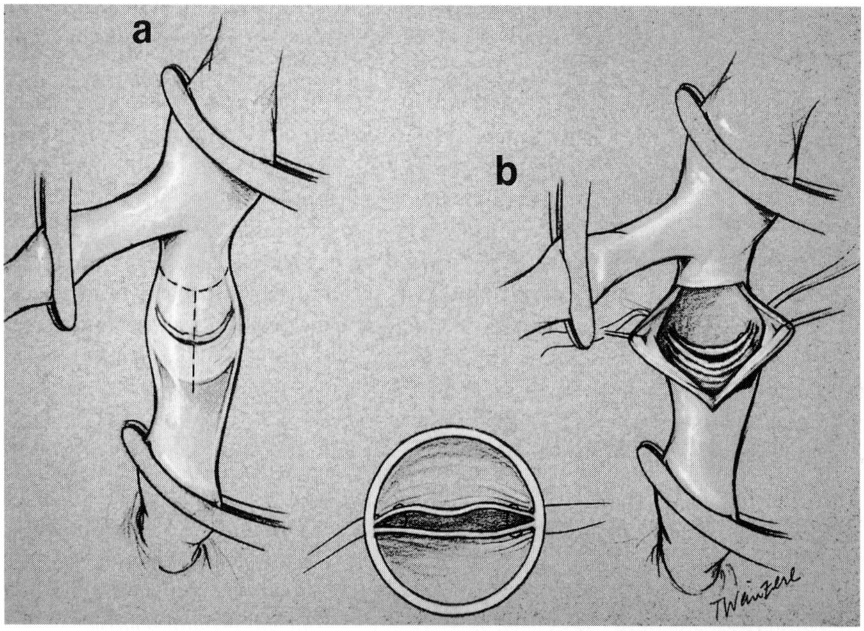

Figure 33.4 *Improved visualization of the valve can be achieved by a supravalvular incision with a 'T'-shaped extension into the valve sinus. This approach was developed by Sottiurai. The valve is shown before venotomy (a) and during valvuloplasty (b). (Adapted from Hahn TL, Dalsing MC. Chronic venous disease. In Faley VA, ed.* Vascular Nursing. *Philadelphia: WB Saunders, 1999: 364–87)*

External valvuloplasty

Kistner introduced external valvuloplasty in 1990, which is performed without the use of a venotomy.[23] The plicating sutures are placed from outside the lumen to tighten the commissural angle (Fig. 33.5). The chief advantages are less venous trauma, primarily due to the lack of a venotomy, and shorter operative times. In addition, blood flow does not need to be interrupted, so anticoagulation is not mandatory. The disadvantages include the lack of direct visualization and, possibly, a less precise reapproximation of the cusps. Limited anterior plication has been proposed as a variation in technique, which further minimizes dissection by utilizing limited exposure and repair of the anterior commissure alone.[24]

Angioscopic-assisted valvuloplasty

Angioscopic-assisted valvuloplasty was initially reported by Gloviczki in 1991 (Fig. 33.6).[25] It shares some of the advantages associated with external valvuloplasty since a large venotomy is avoided. However, systemic heparinization is mandatory. An angioscope is introduced through a side branch and advanced into the proximal SFV. It is positioned directly above the valve. Blood is cleared from the field by irrigation with

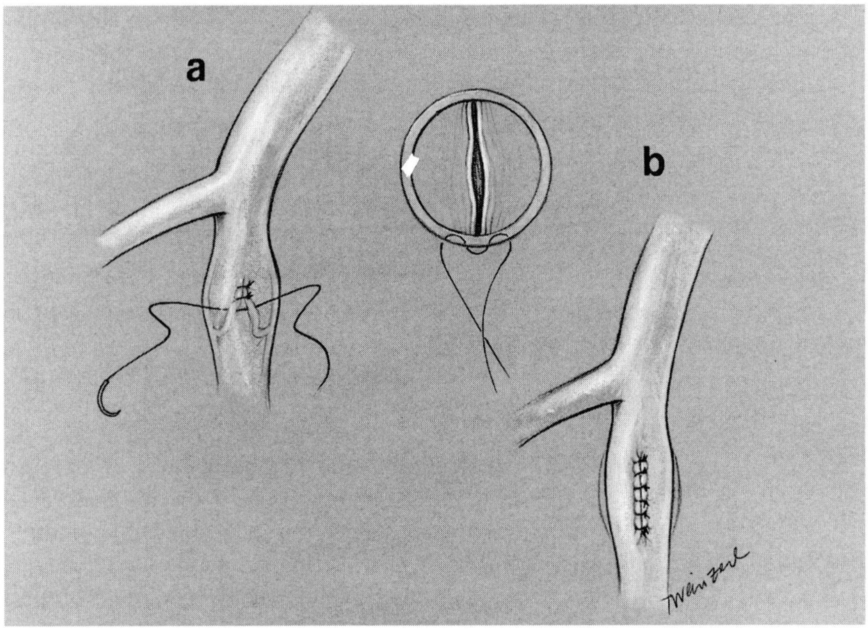

Figure 33.5 *External valvuloplasty does not require a venotomy (a). Sutures are placed so as to narrow the commissure and decrease the vein diameter, thus restoring valve competence (b).*

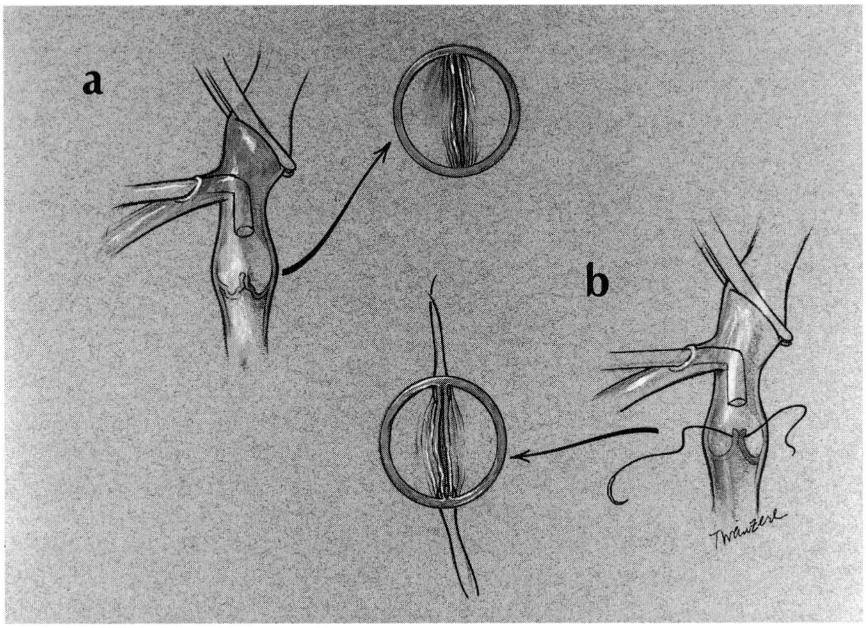

Figure 33.6 *In angioscopic-assisted valvuloplasty, the angioscope is introduced through a side branch and positioned directly above the valve (a). Sutures are passed from outside the lumen, but precise intraluminal placement and valve competence are guided by angioscopic visualization (b).*

heparinized saline solution, while vascular control prevents reintroduction of blood. Valve competence can be assessed by the rapid, retrograde infusion of heparinized irrigant whenever desired during valve repair. Prolene sutures (7-0) are passed from outside to inside the lumen. Intraluminal placement is directed by video-enhanced, magnified angioscopic visualization allowing for very precise reapproximation of the valve cusps. After the repair is complete, the angioscope is withdrawn, the side branch is ligated, and blood flow is restored.

External banding

An increased luminal diameter secondary to progressive dilation of the vein wall results in reflux simply because the valve cusps do not meet. Several authors have noted that valve competence is occasionally restored merely by the venospasm caused during dissection.[22,26] This observation prompted the use of an external band to reduce the diameter of the vein and maintain valve competence. Dacron, polytetrafluoroethylene (PTFE), and fascial sleeves have been used to create the vein cuffs

(Fig. 33.7). A 1–1.5 cm wide cuff is wrapped around the vein at the level of the valve and sutured to itself to re-establish the diameter required to maintain valve competence. The cuff is then anchored in place by suturing it to the adventitia. Alternatively, there is a commercially available Venocuff that can be gently tightened around the vein until competence is restored,[27] then sutured in place as noted above. As with external valvuloplasty, anticoagulation is not mandatory.

RESULTS

The efficacy of internal valvuloplasty in short-term follow-up is well established.[28–32] Good results, defined as a freedom from ulcer recurrence and the reduction of pain to mild levels, have been achieved in 60–80% of the patients in most series (Table 33.1). Valve competence is usually predictive of the clinical result, and direct imaging has demonstrated this to be present in approximately 70% of the repairs (Table 33.1). Long-term data are becoming available, with good clinical outcomes reported by Kistner in 73% of patients up to 21 years after repair.[14]

Raju *et al.* ranked repair durability in 316 primary valve repairs as assessed by venous duplex in a 1996 study.[19] Internal valvuloplasty and external banding appeared to be the most durable. Angioscopic repair was not ranked due to a lack of sufficient long-term data. However, angioscopic-assisted valvuloplasty appears to be a promising technique. In a small series, all patients experienced ulcer healing and hemodynamic improvement which was sustained for a period of 2–51 months.[30] External valvuloplasty does not seem to be as reliable in providing long-term valve competence or ulcer-free survival.[19] Nevertheless, long-term studies are needed to corroborate these preliminary results.

Complications are a component of any surgical procedure. The operative mortality for primary valve repair is minimal with most series reporting no operative deaths.[14,19,32] The need for postoperative anticoagulation has resulted in hematoma formation, generally isolated to the wound and reported in 2–11% of patients.[14,30,32] Wound infection (2–4%) and seroma formation (2–4%) are reported sporadically.[14,22] The previous fear of widespread deep venous thrombosis following valve repairs has not been realized with only a 0–11 % incidence reported in multiple series.[22,30,32]

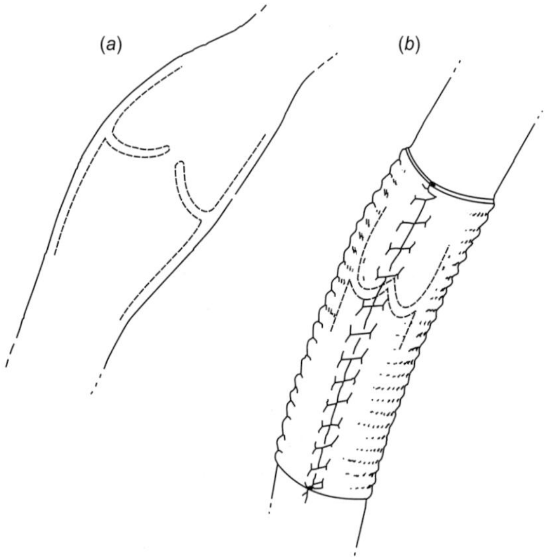

Figure 33.7 *The vein shown prior to (a) and following (b) placement of the external synthetic support which decreases the vein wall diameter and allows proper coaptation of the cusps to prevent reflux. (Adapted from Dalsing MC. Venous valvular insufficiency: pathophysiology and treatment options. In Trerotola SO, Savader SJ, Durham JD, eds.* Venous Interventions. *Fairfax: Society of Cardiovascular and Interventional Radiology, 1995: 225–38)*

SUMMARY

Chronic venous insufficiency due to primary reflux is amenable to direct surgical repair of the incompetent valve. Patients should be carefully selected on the basis of preoperative testing, and surgery should be considered only after optimal medical management and less aggressive surgical procedures have failed to control their symptoms. Internal valvuloplasty remains the 'gold

Table 33.1 *Follow-up data for internal valvuloplasty procedures*

Author	Year	No. limbs	Follow-up (months)	Clinical success (%)*	Valve competence (%)†
Eriksson and Almgren[28]	1988	17	6–84	62	–
Masuda and Kistner[14]	1994	32	48–252	73	77
Raju[31]	1997	68	12–144	62	–
Sottiurai[29]	1997	143	9–168	–	75
Lurie[31]	1997	52	36–108	73	–
Perrin[31]	1997	75	24–96	75	73

*Percentage of patients with good to excellent results defined by sustained ulcer healing and absent or minimal symptoms.
†Percentage of patients with minimal to no reflux assessed by ultrasound or venography.

standard' for surgical correction and has proven to be a durable repair resulting in long-term symptomatic improvement. Promising new techniques such as angioscopic-assisted valvuloplasty, external banding and external valvuloplasty appear to be effective in properly selected patients, but long-term follow-up is lacking. Overall, good results can be expected in approximately 70% of properly selected patients if diligent follow-up and patient compliance are achieved.

REFERENCES

1. Kistner RL, Eklof B. Operative procedures and their results in managing chronic venous insufficiency. In Callow A, Ernst C, eds. *Vascular Surgery: Theory and Practice.* Norwalk, CT: Appleton & Lange, 1995: 1547–71.
2. Kistner RL, Sparkuhl MD. Surgery in acute and chronic venous disease. *Surgery* 1979; **85**: 31–43.
3. Bauer G. The etiology of leg ulcers and their treatment by resection of the popliteal vein. *J Int Chir* 1948; **8**: 937–61.
4. Carrel A, Guthrie CC. Uniterminal and biterminal venous transplantation. *Surg Gynecol Obstet* 1906; **2**: 266–86.
5. Eiseman B, Malette W. An operative technique for the construction of venous valves. *Surg Gynecol Obstet* 1953; **97**: 731–4.
6. De Weese JA, Niguidula F. The replacement of short segments of veins with functional autogenous venous grafts. *Surg Gynecol Obstet* 1960; **110**: 303–8.
7. Linton RR. The communicating veins of the lower leg and the operative technique for their ligation. *Ann Surg* 1938; **107**: 582–93.
8. Linton RR. The post-thrombotic ulceration of the lower extremity: its etiology and surgical treatment. *Ann Surg* 1953; **138**: 415–32.
9. Kistner R. Surgical repair of a venous valve. *Straub Clin Proc* 1968; **24**: 41–3.
10. Wilson NM, Rutt DL, Browse NL. Repair and replacement of deep vein valves in the treatment of venous insufficiency. *Br J Surg* 1991; **78**: 388–94.
11. Cheatle TR, Perrin M. Venous valve repair: early results in fifty-two cases. *J Vasc Surg* 1994; **19**; 404–13.
12. Raju S. Operative management of chronic venous insufficiency. In Rutherford RB, ed. *Vascular Surgery.* Philadelphia: WB Saunders, 1995: 1851–62.
13. Kistner RL. Surgical repair of the incompetent femoral vein valve. *Arch Surg* 1975; **110**: 1336–42.
14. Masuda EM, Kistner RL. Long-term results of venous valve reconstruction: a four- to twenty-one year follow up. *J Vasc Surg* 1994; **19**: 391–403.
15. Porter JM, Moneta GL. An International Consensus Committee on Chronic Venous Disease. Reporting standards in venous disease: an update. *J Vasc Surg* 1995; **21**: 643–45.
16. Iafrati MD, Welch H, O'Donnell TF, Belkin M, Umphrey S, McLaughlin R. Correlation of venous noninvasive tests with the Society for Vascular Surgery clinical classification of chronic venous insufficiency. *J Vasc Surg* 1994; **19**: 1001–7.
17. Kistner RL, Ferris EB, Randhawa G, Kamida C. A method of performing descending venography. *J Vasc Surg* 1986; **4**: 464–8.
18. Eriksson I, Almgren B. Influence of the profunda femoris vein on venous hemodynamics of the limb. *J Vasc Surg* 1986; **4**: 390–5.
19. Raju S, Fredericks RK, Neglen PN, Bass JD. Durability of venous valve reconstruction techniques for 'primary' and postthrombotic reflux. *J Vasc Surg* 1996; **23**: 357–67.
20. Raju S. Venous insufficiency of the lower limb and stasis ulceration. *Ann Surg* 1983; **197**: 688–97.
21. Sottiurai VS. Technique in direct venous valvuloplasty. *J Vasc Surg* 1988; **8**: 646–8.
22. Raju S, Fredericks R. Valve reconstruction procedures for nonobstructive venous insufficiency: rationale, techniques, and results in 107 procedures with two- to eight-year follow-up. *J Vasc Surg* 1988; **7**: 301–10.
23. Kistner RL. Surgical technique of external venous valve repair. *Straub Found Proc* 1990; **55**: 15.
24. Belcaro G. Femoral vein valve repair with limited anterior plication. *J Cardiovasc Surg* 1993; **34**: 395–8.
25. Gloviczki P, Merrell SW, Bower TC. Femoral vein valve repair under direct vision without venotomy: a modified technique with use of angioscopy. *J Vasc Surg* 1991; **14**: 645–8.
26. Camilli S, Guarnera G. External banding valvuloplasty of the superficial femoral vein in the treatment of primary deep valvular incompetence. *Int Angiol* 1994; **13**: 218–22.
27. Jessup G, Lane R. Repair of incompetent venous valves: a new technique. *J Vasc Surg* 1988; **8**: 569–75.
28. Eriksson JI, Almgren B. Surgical reconstruction of deep vein valves. *Uppsala J Med Sci* 1988; **93**: 139–43.
29. Sottiurai VS. Surgical correction of recurrent venous ulcer. *J Cardiovasc Surg* 1991; **32**: 104–9.
30. Welch H, McLaughlin RL, O'Donnell TF. Femoral vein valvuloplasty: intraoperative angioscopic evaluation and hemodynamic improvement. *J Vasc Surg* 1992; **16**: 694–700.
31. Perrin MR, Lurie F, Sottiurai VS, Raju S. Proceedings of the Second Pacific Vascular Symposium: Advances in Venous Disease. *Vasc Surg* 1997; **31**: 268–83.
32. Jamieson WG, Chinnick B. Clinical results of deep venous valvular repair for chronic venous insufficiency. *Can J Surg* 1997; **40**: 294–9.

34

Venous valve transplantation and vein transposition for valvular incompetence of deep veins

THOMAS F O'DONNELL JR

Since our chapter on deep venous reconstruction was published in the *Handbook* 4 years ago, several factors have developed that have influenced the volume of two deep venous reconstructive procedures, vein valve transplant and venous segment transposition, that are carried out for post-thrombotic disease.[1] The first factor, the widespread use of the minimally invasive subfascial interruption of perforating veins (SEPS), has reduced the use of deep venous reconstruction. Presently many surgeons have employed SEPS as their initial surgical approach to venous ulcer, even in the face of deep venous involvement.[2] The second factor, the direct repair of damaged valves by techniques used for correcting primary valvular incompetence (PVI), has expanded the available procedures for post-thrombotic disease.[3] The third factor is that post-thrombotic disease may have different long-term results from those following treatment of PVI. The poorer surgical results with post-thrombotic syndrome are probably related to the more extensive damage of the deep venous system as well as an inherent susceptibility to further thrombosis, which can jeopardize venous reconstruction.[4,5] Finally, most high-volume venous reconstructive centers now favor vein valve transplantation as the operation of choice for post-thrombotic deep venous reflux.[6] This chapter discusses patient selection, preoperative evaluation and operative techniques and reviews the available results in the literature.

PATIENT SELECTION

Indications

Traditionally, deep venous reconstruction (DVR) for post-thrombotic disease has been reserved for patients in CEAP class C5 (healed ulcer) or C6 (open ulcer).[7] The restriction of DVR to the most advanced stages of chronic venous insufficiency is related to the magnitude of the operation, as well as to the potential for long-term relief of patients' symptoms and clinical state. Whilst some surgeons have performed DVR for either pain or for edema, we have restricted this complex procedure to patients with advanced subcutaneous and cutaneous sequelae of venous hypertension. If the long-term efficacy of this procedure is proven and accepted, it may be extended to patients with CEAP class 4 in order to prevent the development of ulcers. As mentioned above, patients with PVI seem to do better than those with post-thrombotic disease and, in addition, the surgical procedure for PVI is less complex. Therefore, some surgeons have been more willing to offer DVR to a selected group of patients with PVI at stage 4 rather than to patients with post-thrombotic syndrome at that stage.

Contraindications

There are several relative contraindications to DVR that become apparent during the preoperative evaluation of the patient (Table 34.1). The first of the anatomic considerations is the lack of an available donor valve to use in the deep venous circuit. For venous segment transposition, an absence of a valve at the saphenofemoral junction or of the saphenous vein itself, would dictate selection of the profunda femoris valve. Absence of a saphenous valve is quite common, because in the majority of these patients the saphenous vein has been stripped previously. If the profunda femoris vein has been damaged by the thrombotic process, this finding would limit its use in venous segment transposition. More frequently, the profunda femoris valve may be incompetent so that at the time of surgery an external valvuloplasty is required. For patients undergoing vein valve transplantation, we prefer to use a segment of axillary vein containing a functioning valve and as a second choice a brachial vein segment.[8] The anatomic absence of venous segment which contains a functioning valve is a contraindication to DVR in our mind.

Table 34.1 *Contraindication to deep venous reconstructive surgery*

Lack of available donor valve
Hemodynamically significant proximal obstruction
Concomitant ischemic arterial occlusive disease
Laboratory-defined hypercoagulable state

Patients with concomitant obstruction of large veins pose an interesting challenge. We usually do not advocate simultaneous surgical treatment of obstruction and reflux, but in rare instances, a sequential operation with relief of both obstruction and reflux has been carried out. First, the arm–foot vein pressure measurements of Raju are particularly useful in patients with both reflux and obstruction to determine if the obstruction is of hemodynamic significance.[9] If left uncorrected, hemodynamically significant obstruction may be associated with failure of a downstream vein valve transplant or venous segment transposition due to either valve disruption or dilation of the valve containing venous segment. Certainly, the presence of concomitant arterial disease in so-called 'mixed ulcers' is not uncommon. When arterial vascular laboratory studies indicate significant ischemia, i.e. Doppler ankle/brachial ratio less than 0.4 and an ankle PVR less than 5 mm, then arterial surgery should be carried out rather than DVR in an attempt to heal the ulcer. Whilst some surgeons have offered DVR for patients with hypercoagulable state, this has not been our common practice. Despite postoperative anticoagulation, the risk of thrombosis of the transplanted segment and subsequent failure may be too great.

Management of the patient with venous ulcer (C5, C6 disease)

The introduction of a minimally invasive method for interrupting incompetent perforating veins has altered most surgeons' management of patients with venous ulcer. In the early 1980s, the appreciable morbidity associated with the open approach to ligation of incompetent perforating veins (ICPVs), combined with the questionable value of ICPV ligation alone or combined with saphenous stripping in patients with post-thrombotic deep venous disease, turned many surgeons away from this form of treatment for venous ulcer.[2] In a randomized prospective trial, Pierick confirmed the advantages of subfascial endoscopic perforator vein ligation (SEPS) over the standard open approach in regards to decreased wound morbidity.[10] Others, including ourselves, had noted the superiority of SEPS based on retrospective comparisons with our previous non-contemporaneous open series.[11] The availability of this low-morbidity procedure has led to a resurgence of ICPV ligation for venous ulcer.

From a critical point of view, there are flaws, however, to this approach. No randomized prospective studies exist which compare ICPV ligation alone or combined with saphenectomy to saphenectomy alone.[2] Several physiologic studies suggest that ligation and stripping of the incompetent greater saphenous vein is the most important procedure and that ICVP ligation adds little physiologically. Indeed, in a study with a unique design by Akesson, no improvement in ambulatory venous pressure and foot volume plethysmography was observed by the addition of ICPV ligation 3 months following a saphenectomy alone.[12] The problem is a particularly real one for patients with post-thrombotic deep venous disease. The North American SEPS Vascular Registry data of Gloviczki and associates has demonstrated a 46% ulcer recurrence rate by life-table method at 2 years following SEPS ± ligation and stripping in this patient cohort.[13] The recurrence rate of the post-thrombotic group is double that of patients with primary valvular incompetence. It is still our practice, however, to offer SEPS combined with ligation and stripping as the initial procedure for a patient with C5/C6 disease and post-thrombotic deep venous involvement, because the patient has a one in two chance of avoiding a more extensive operation. We reserve DVR for patients whose ulcers have failed conservative management with elastic compression and recur after superficial venous surgery.

PREOPERATIVE EVALUATION

Duplex assessment

Following clinical staging – the C of the CEAP evaluation – duplex scanning is used to determine the etiology (E), anatomy (A) and physiology (P) of these C5/C6 patients.[14] Duplex scanning is employed not only in its hemodynamic mode, but also in its anatomic mode. The latter function allows one to discriminate PVI from post-thrombotic disease. Typically, patients with post-thrombotic disease demonstrate thickened vein walls and the absence of valve structures on duplex scanning. The vein's lumen is irregular, while segmental occlusion and extensive collateral vessel formation may be observed.[7] Assessment of reflux is carried out by the van Bemellen technique which employs a pressure cuff to produce reactive hyperemia.[15] We feel that this is a more reproducible technique than the manual calf compression method. Assessment of reflux is performed at the femoral, popliteal and tibial vessel levels for the deep system and at similar levels for the saphenous system. Both the extent of reflux and valve closure time increase with the clinical severity of the limb. Generally, patients who are candidates for DVR have valve closure times in excess of 4–5 seconds (normal less than 0.5 seconds) and the reflux extends to or beyond the popliteal level.

In addition to assessment of the deep venous system, duplex scanning can demonstrate missed branch veins, reduplicated saphenous veins as well as incompetent perforating veins, which may be recurrent following the initial SEPS procedures. Moreover, it is not uncommon to see extensive lesser saphenous reflux at the popliteal vein, which should be corrected at the time of DVR. We rarely elect to repeat superficial venous surgery and thereby delay DVR unless the patient has had his surgery performed at another institution. In that situation, we may not be confident that the patient has had a 'full run' at superficial venous surgery. Particular attention is paid to the operative note to determine whether a paratibial fasciotomy has been performed so that the deep posterior compartment has been explored. It is well recognized that the majority of the Cockett 2 and 3 perforators reside in the deep posterior compartment.[13] Unless this compartment is explored, complete surgical treatment of incompetent perforating veins has not been carried out.

Duplex scanning is also helpful in the anatomic planning for DVR. For venous transposition, duplex scanning may demonstrate a competent proximal valve(s) in the saphenous vein in rare instances that can be transposed into the deep venous system. More usually the profunda femoris valve is assessed for competence and that segment of vein examined for absence of wall thickening. Finally, duplex scanning of the axillary vein and brachial vein segments determines whether there is a segment containing a functioning valve, which can be used for transplantation. Occasionally ascending phlebography of the arm may be required to detail the presence of venous valves, preferably at the axillary, or alternatively at the brachial level.

The role of phlebography

Although we do not use routine phlebography for patients who are undergoing surgery of the superficial venous system, it is essential for performing DVR, particularly in the post-thrombotic limb.[7] The patient undergoes ascending phlebography at the same setting as descending phlebography. Duplex scanning correlates quite well with the level of reflux as we have demonstrated previously so that descending phlebography is confirmatory.[16] Patients with Kistner grade III or IV reflux are candidates for surgery. Ascending phlebography provides a road map to help the surgeon determine exactly where the valve containing venous segment will be placed. As is discussed subsequently, the above-knee popliteal segment is the preferential site for vein valve transplantation because of physiologic and anatomic considerations.[17] Several anatomic variances which may not always be evident on duplex scanning can be revealed by ascending phlebography. Duplication of the superficial femoral vein or more frequently axial transformation of the profunda femoris vein following extensive thrombosis of the superficial femoral vein is important to detect for proper siting of the transplanted segment. Duplication of the popliteal vein is quite frequent, which dictates transplantation above the duplication or ligation of one of the circuits. The presence of a large collateral network from the profunda femoris to the popliteal vein is also important, because the surgeon must place the transplanted segment below the entry of the collateral. It has been our practice to place the transplanted segment as close to the calf muscle pump as possible. Therefore, it is unusual for us to site a transplanted segment proximally in the superficial femoral vein. Extensive damage of the popliteal vein with severe recanalization changes and a non-usable lumen is our usual indication for a proximal reconstruction. Ascending phlebography confirms the etiology of the deep venous reflux as post-thrombotic occluded segments, recanalization changes, avalvular segments and extensive collateral networks.

Finally, ascending phlebography provides the exact location of incompetent perforating veins. Metallic rulers are placed on the x-ray film, which allow confirmation of the ICPV at concomitant SEPS and DVR. As we have demonstrated in a previous study, ascending phlebography is quite specific – if no ICPVs are seen on phlebography in that anatomic region, they are unlikely to be there.[11]

Medical evaluation

The usual age of the patient considered for DVR is in the late forties. Therefore, evaluation for occult coronary artery disease is important, even though this is not a hemodynamically stressful operation. All patients undergo a hypercoagulable screen, which includes measurement of the Leiden factor. As mentioned previously, it is unusual for us to offer DVR to patients with hypercoagulable state.

OPERATIVE PROCEDURES

Preoperative preparation

Surgery is not restricted solely to C5 cases (healed ulcers). Since the reconstructive procedure is distant from the site of ulceration, SEPS, if required, can be performed well above the ulcer (C6). The sole contra-indication to surgery is whether the ulcer is actively infected. Antibiotics, which are directed by deep culture (biopsy), are administered in these latter cases until the infection subsides. Since the surgical approach is carried out medially at the popliteal level or proximally at the inguinal area, division of bacteria-laden lymphatics should be avoided. Active wet-to-dry debridement of the ulcer is carried out and in rare cases formal debridement in the operating room may be required a week or so prior to DVR. On call to the operating room, the patient receives prophylactic antibiotics, usually a cephalo-sporin, and aspirin is administered the day before surgery for its antiplatelet effect.

Venous segment transfer

This procedure was devised by Kistner for patients with a competent saphenous or profunda femoris valve and deep venous reflux due to post-thrombotic changes.[18] The purpose of venous segment transfer is to transpose a competent valve-bearing venous segment into the main deep venous system at the groin level. Several surgical variations of venous segment transfer have been employed. The most straightforward technique involves ligation of the proximal incompetent superficial femoral vein and anastomosis of the transected distal end of the superficial femoral vein to the end of the competent ipsilateral saphenous vein. If the saphenous vein is incompetent or surgically absent, as is frequently the case in patients with advanced chronic venous insufficiency, the superficial femoral vein can be anastomosed end to side to the competent profunda femoris vein or end to end to its first branch.

PROCEDURE

The superficial femoral, saphenous, and profunda femoris veins are exposed in the usual manner (Fig. 34.1). Generally, there is a dense perivenous reaction to previous episodes of deep venous thrombosis. After at least 2 or 3 cm of superficial femoral, greater saphenous, and profunda femoris veins have been exposed and isolated, valvular function is assessed intraoperatively. The preoperative descending phlebogram usually has determined which valves are competent, but intra-operative confirmation should be carried out. Kistner has restricted the donor valve segment somewhat and now prefers to transfer the superficial femoral vein to the profunda femoris vein rather than to the greater saphenous vein. He stated that: 'late fatigue in the greater saphenous vein valve causes recurrence of clinical symptoms.'[18] Rather than attach the superficial femoral vein end to side to the profunda femoris vein, the superficial femoral vein may be anastomosed end to end to the first branch of the profunda femoris vein. With the patient heparinized, the superficial femoral vein is

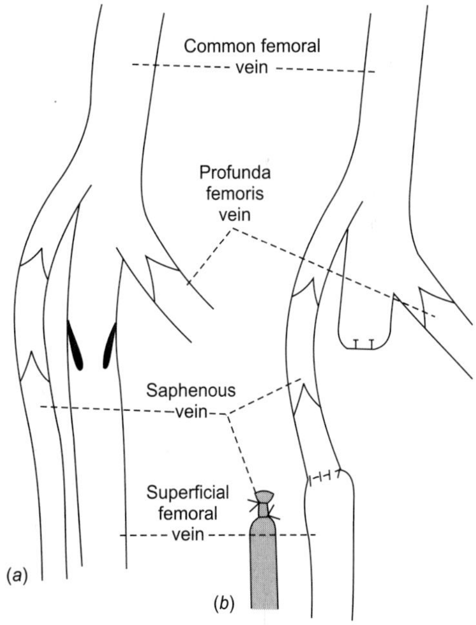

Figure 34.1 *Venous segment transfer. (a) The proximal valve of the superficial femoral vein is noted to be incompetent. The distal superficial femoral vein is transposed to the proximal greater saphenous vein to provide the latter's competent valves. Alternatively, the superficial femoral vein may be joined end to side, thereby utilizing the competent valves of the profunda femoris vein. (Reproduced with permission from O'Donnell TF Jr, Shepard AD. Chronic venous insufficiency. In Jarrett F, Hirsch SA, eds.* Vascular Surgery of the Lower Extremity. *St Louis: CV Mosby, 1985)*

clamped proximally and distally. The recipient vein is clamped proximally and distally with rubber-shod vascular clamps. The superficial femoral vein is divided high at its junction with the profunda femoris vein and ligated with continuous 5-0 prolene suture. Care is taken to avoid encroachment on the profunda femoris orifice with this closure. The previously mobilized superficial femoral vein is then anastomosed either end to side to the profunda femoris or end to end to its first branch. We prefer to use interrupted 7-0 monofilament sutures for this portion of the procedure, but the Carrel triangulation technique can be employed. Once the anastomosis is completed, competence of the transposed segment is retested by the 'strip' test. Intraoperative continuous wave (CW) Doppler duplex as assessment can also be employed. The wound is then carefully closed in layers, and drains are employed if it appears wet.

Vein valve transplantation

BACKGROUND

Although the topic of experimental venous autografts has been discussed extensively in the literature for some time, Taheri and colleagues deserve the credit for introducing and popularizing the use of vein valve transplantation clinically (Fig. 34.2).[19] They utilized a donor valve-containing segment of brachial vein. This 2–3 cm segment of brachial vein is inserted as an interposition graft into the superficial femoral vein approximately 4 cm below the junction of the profunda femoris vein with the superficial vein. In their initial series, Taheri and associates observed excellent clinical results in 85% of limbs, and healing of venous ulcer in over 50%.[19] Raju and associates modified the technique of vein valve transplantation by utilizing the axillary vein as the transplanted vein segment.[20] They felt that the axillary vein should provide a better size match with the diameter of the superficial femoral vein than the smaller caliber brachial vein. In addition, they enclosed the donor segment in either an 8 or 10 mm Dacron sleeve in order to minimize late vein graft dilation.

PROCEDURE

The exposure of the common femoral, superficial femoral, and profunda femoris veins is similar to that used for venous segment transposition. A longer segment of the superficial femoral vein is exposed so that at least 12–15 cm of the superficial femoral vein must be mobilized freely. A segment of the brachial vein 4–6 cm below the axilla is harvested by a second team through a longitudinal incision paralleling the vessel. Care should be taken to assure that a competent vein valve is present in the brachial or axillary vein, which should be corroborated intraoperatively by the 'strip test'. After heparin is administered and vascular occluding clamps are placed, a 2–4 cm segment of brachial vein is resected. No attempts are made to reconstruct the brachial vein, and it is merely ligated. Following application of rubber-shod vascular clamps, a small segment of superficial femoral vein is resected. The brachial vein segment is then inserted as an interposition graft into the superficial femoral vein approximately 4–5 cm below its junction with the profunda femoris vein. The distal anastomosis is performed first utilizing 7-0 monofilament sutures, which are triangulated around the valve-containing segment at 120° intervals. The anastomosis is then completed using a continuous everting suture technique.

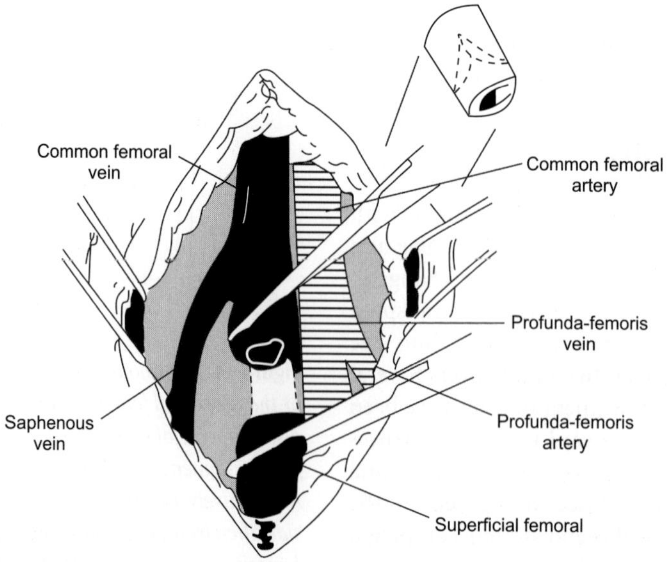

Figure 34.2 *The technique of brachial valve transplantation to the superficial femoral vein. See text for details. (Reproduced with permission from O'Donnell TF Jr, Shepard AD. Chronic venous insufficiency. In Jarrett F, Hirsch SA, eds.* Vascular Surgery of the Lower Extremity. *St Louis: CV Mosby, 1985)*

The same technique is repeated for the proximal anastomosis. In Raju's modification of the procedure, the axillary vein is employed as a donor valve-containing segment.[20] He correctly points out that this vein segment should be scrupulously checked for valve function before removal because of a 30–40% incidence of incompetent valves in the axillary vein segment. This incompetence can be repaired by valve 'reefing' with externally placed 6-0 monofilament sutures.

Popliteal vein valve transplantation

Although transplanting a valve-containing segment from the brachial to the superficial femoral vein appeared to achieve good clinical results initially, Taheri and associates observed eventual dilatation of the transplanted brachial vein segment.[21] Valvular incompetence subsequent to dilatation of the transplanted segment, as was observed with venous segment transposition, is a theoretical disadvantage of the smaller caliber brachial vein in the larger caliber superficial femoral vein circuit. Despite using a large-diameter axillary vein segment, however, Raju and Fredericks encountered progressive dilatation and deterioration of valvular function.[20] To avoid this problem, the transplanted segment was surrounded in a Dacron graft.

Approximately 15 years ago, we initiated a clinical series of vein valve transplantation that differed from other approaches.[8] This procedure employed the larger caliber axillary vein, which was transplanted to the above-knee popliteal vein (Fig. 34.3). The rationale for this approach was twofold:

- to provide a better size match of the transplanted axillary vein segment to the host popliteal vein, which might prevent late dilatation of the transplanted segment with subsequent valvular dysfunction encountered with the superficial femoral vein segment; and
- to restore a functioning valve to the popliteal vein, which would play the critical 'gatekeeper' role above the calf muscle venous pump. The rationale for the gatekeeper role of the popliteal vein valve has been discussed in detail previously.[7]

PROCEDURE

The involved lower extremity and usually the contralateral upper extremity are prepped and draped, which allows for a two-team approach. The axillary vein is exposed through a longitudinal or a transverse incision made parallel to the neurovascular bundle. Care is taken during this dissection to avoid injury to the brachial plexus or other surrounding nerve structures. A segment of axillary vein is tested for patency and valve function intraoperatively using a bidirectional Doppler probe. Usually, a segment of axillary vein measuring 6–8 cm which contains one valve is

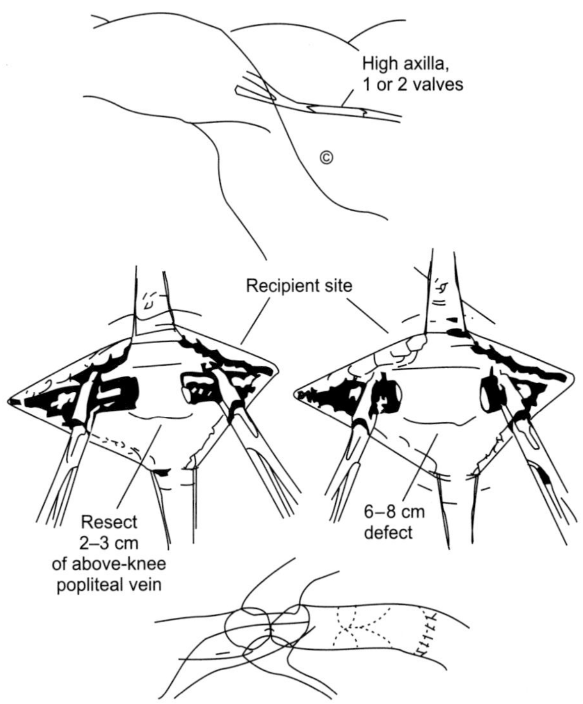

Figure 34.3 *Axillary vein-to-popliteal vein transplantation. The surgical steps involved in axillary vein-to-popliteal vein transplantation are schematically shown. (Reproduced with permission from O'Donnell TF, Mackey WC, Shepard AD, Callow AD. Clinical, hemodynamic and anatomic follow-up of direct venous reconstruction.* Arch Surg *1987;* ***122****: 474–82)*

removed. At the same time, the popliteal vein is exposed through a standard above-knee approach commonly used in arterial reconstruction for femoral above-knee popliteal bypass. The lower portion of this vein, however, is the usual site of transplantation. Alternatively the below the knee segment may be selected. The vein is dissected free from concomitant arterial structures. Usually, this dissection can be somewhat tedious if the vein has the characteristic post-thrombotic changes. After an approximately 8 cm segment of vein had been isolated, it is encircled with vessel loops. Five thousand units of heparin is administered, and the vein is clamped with soft, rubber-shod, non-crushing vascular clamps.

A 3–4 cm segment of vein is removed to receive the transplanted axillary vein valve-bearing segment. The distal anastomosis of the interposition graft is usually done first with interrupted 7-0 monofilament suture. Once the four quadrant interrupted sutures were placed, the transplanted vein segment was 'parachuted' down into the position. The remaining sutures are then placed. In placing the sutures for both anastomoses, care must be taken to avoid entrapping the valvular mechanism. The proximal anastomosis was then performed in a similar manner. The vein segment was flushed before completion of the last portion of the proximal anastomosis. The operative site then underwent intraoperative evaluation. The patient is maintained on intravenous heparin perioperatively for 3 to 5 days or low weight molecular Heparin while converted to warfarin. To increase venous flow through the transplanted segment postoperatively, the patient is maintained on intermittent pneumatic compression (50–60 mmHg) until fully ambulatory. The patient is usually up into a chair on the fourth or fifth day and ambulatory on day 6.

RESULTS

Vein valve transplant

Fifteen series were reviewed between the years 1982 through 2000 in which vein valve transplantation was performed on a total of 420 limbs (Table 34.2). A critical review of these series shows severe limitations in the reporting standards for most. Important preoperative demographic data and postoperative outcomes were noticeably absent in many, whilst several authors appeared to repeat their series periodically by adding several new limbs. In the later situation, it was difficult to determine which limbs were new.

PREOPERATIVE DEMOGRAPHIC DATA

The number of limbs reported in the series range from a low of two in the Straub clinic series which reviewed their experience with valvuloplasty and other DVRs [5] to a high of 83 limbs in Raju's series reported in 1999[27] (Table 34.2). The average number of limbs per series was 28. Only two series reported the incidence of a history of DVT, while over one-half the series described the mean age and gender ratio. The overall mean age for the 15 series was 47 years and the male-to-female ratio was 1.27. In a retrospective analysis, which applied the CEAP classification to these series, only 10 of 15 series provided sufficient information to determine 'C', the clinical status of the limb. Information regarding the etiology, anatomy and physiology were also absent in 5 of the 15 series on average. Vein valve transplantation was performed for the indication of ulcer, either C5 or C6, in 259/420 (62%) limbs. Ascending and descending phlebography was performed as a preoperative diagnostic modality in all 15 series, but not all authors presented the results of their preoperative findings. Where described, approximately 50% of the limbs demonstrated severe post-thrombotic changes on ascending phlebography. The most interesting manuscript was that of Raju in which he differentiated trabeculated from non-trabeculated recipient vein sites in the lower extremity and correlated this pathologic finding with outcome.[27] In those series that detailed results of descending phlebography, all patients were in at least the Kistner III category with the majority being in Kistner grade IV. Like preoperative ascending/descending phlebography, hemodynamic measurements were routine in the preoperative evaluation of these patients. In the early series, venous pressure was the most common technique used, while in the latter series air plethysmography was employed (e.g. Bry,[26] Raju[27] and Perrin[28]) to assess reflux and calf muscle pump function. Eight of 15 series described some type of superficial venous surgery prior to deep venous reconstruction. On average, 85% of these limbs had undergone a superficial venous operation; either ligation and stripping and/or interruption of incompetent perforating veins.

OPERATIVE PROCEDURE

Eight of the series used the axillary vein as the donor site for the valve containing segment and this site was more common in the later series. Four series employed the brachial vein as the donor site and one series used either

Table 34.2 *Results of 15 vein valve transplantation series (420 limbs 1982–2000)**

	Preoperative characteristics						
	CEAP classification	Ulcers C5/C6	Age (years)	Gender ratio M:F	Phlebography Asc/Desc	Hemodynamic studies	Superficial venous surgery
Number of series reporting	10/15	15/15	8/15	8/15	9/15	7/15	8/15
Mean OR proportion	–	62%	47	1.27	–	–	85%

	Postoperative outcome measures					
	Ulcer healing	Ulcer recurrence	Follow-up length (mean)	Phlebography Asc vs Dec	Hemodynamics	Complications
Number of series reporting	11/15 (157 limbs)	6/15 (53 limbs)	8/15	13/15 vs 11/15	12/15	6/15
Mean OR proportion	79%	28%	3 series, 5 years	5.6% occluded vs 25% reflux	27% improved over preop	1 death, 5% hematoma

*References 3, 4, 5, 19–28.

site. The recipient site for the vein transplant was at the femoral level in ten series, popliteal level in three series, and a mixture of the femoral and popliteal level in two series.

POSTOPERATIVE OUTCOME MEASURES

Twelve series provided objective evidence of a clinical outcome such as ulcer healing. In three series, it was difficult to separate the results for vein valve transplantation from that of the other DVR procedures reported. The early series mixed initial ulcer healing with ulcer recurrence, so that it was impossible to determine what was the absolute ulcer recurrence rate. Seven series described the absolute ulcer recurrence rate following vein valve transplantation, whereas three series calculated by the life-table method an ulcer-free survival rate (Bry,[26] Raju[27] and Perrin[28]). In Masuda's report, the results of vein valve transplantation were co-mingled with other DVR procedures.[5] Of the 157 limbs where ulcer healing was recorded, 124 (79%) initially healed their ulcer. The absolute ulcer recurrence rate in 53 limbs was 28% where this number was reported solely. The ulcer-free interval at 6 years in the three series where this factor was reported specifically for vein valve transplant was comparable at 6 years: 65% in our series,[26] 60% in Raju's series[27] and 50% in Perrin's series.[28] Fourteen of 15 series reported the results of the postoperative evaluation of graft patency by ascending phlebography. With the exception of the recent series of Perrin where a 37.5% occlusion rate in 32 vein valve transplants was described,[28] a low 5.6% overall mean rate of occlusion was observed in the 250 limbs which underwent ascending phlebography. Of the 215 limbs that underwent postoperative descending phlebography, 53 (25%) demonstrated significant reflux. Hemodynamic results following vein valve transplant were more variable. In the 11 series where some form of functional measurement was carried out, 46 of 168 (27%) limbs showed an improved venous pressure pattern. Postoperative results as assessed by air plethysmography were conflicting. In our series, venous filling index (VFI), a measurement of reflux, failed to show an improvement, but assessment of VFI versus ejection fraction placed the limbs in a sector where less than a 30% chance of developing an ulcer would be observed.[26] In Raju's series, however, VFI reduced postoperatively from 6 mm/s to 4 mm/s.[27]

LENGTH OF FOLLOW-UP

Only six of the 15 series provided data on length of follow-up. The series of Bry,[26] Raju[27] and Perrin[28] had follow-up data for beyond 5 years. Unfortunately, the other two series had extremely short follow-up.

MORBIDITY AND MORTALITY

There was only one death recorded in the 15 series, which occurred in Rai's report where an elderly individual died of a myocardial infarction following valve transplant.[25] Hematoma formation, however, appeared to be the most common postoperative complication and averaged approximately 5%. This is most likely related to the perioperative anticoagulation regimen.

Venous segment transfer

A review of the literature from 1975 through 2000 reveals six series reporting venous segment transfer (VST) operations (Table 34.3). Two additional reviews were discarded because they obviously contain patients reported in a publication one year earlier by the same author. Only two manuscripts focused on VST alone,[29,30] whereas the remaining four reported the results of VST along with valvuloplasty for primary valvular incompetence or vein valve transplant for post-thrombotic syndrome. Five of the six series provided data sufficient enough to classify patients retrospectively by the CEAP

Table 34.3 *Results of six venous segment transposition series (83 limbs 1980–2000)**

	Preoperative characteristics						
	CEAP classification	Age (years)	Gender ratio	Ulcers C5/C6	Phlebography Asc vs Desc	Hemodynamics	Superficial venous surgery
Number of series reporting	5/6	3/6	3/6	5/6	6/6 vs 6/6	6/6	4/6
Mean OR proportion	–	47	2:1	71%	Post-thrombotic 86%	–	78%

	Postoperative outcome measures					
	Ulcer healing	Ulcer recurrence	Phlebography Asc vs Desc	Hemodynamics	Follow-up	Complications
Number of series reporting	1/6	5/6	5/5 vs 5/5	4/5	1/5	1/5
Mean OR proportion	35%	36%	22% reflux 9.6% occluded	35% improved		0 deaths, 3.4% hematoma

*References 5, 18, 24, 28–30.

classification. The mean age and gender ratio were available only in three series and averaged 47 years and the gender ratio 2 to 1. Five of the six series described the incidence of preoperative ulcer, whilst two of the later series described whether ulcers healed (C6) or remained open C5/6. There was a 71% incidence of ulcer (C5 or C6) preoperatively, which was comparable to this finding in the vein valve transplant series. Three series differentiated post-thrombotic syndrome from PVI in regards to etiology. VST was performed for post-thrombotic syndrome in 86% of the limbs. All limbs underwent ascending and descending phlebography. The former helped to identify the disease process, whereas the later showed the level of reflux. The majority of limbs had Kistner 4+ reflux. With the exception of the series by Querel[29] and the subsequent long-term follow-up of that series by Johnson,[30] all other series reported either previous or associated treatment of superficial venous incompetence.

POSTOPERATIVE OUTCOMES

It was difficult to determine the ulcer healing rate in the VST series, but ulcer recurrence was well detailed. The crude ulcer recurrence rate in 40 limbs was 35%. Only Perrin's series reported cumulative ulcer-free interval by the life-table method, which was 75% at 5 years.[28] In Masuda and Kistner's recent report, VST was combined with other DVR procedures such as vein valve transplant.[5] The ulcer-free interval for VST was less than with primary valvuloplasty. Ascending and descending phlebographic data was available in five of the six series. Eight of 83 limbs (9.6%) showed surgical site thrombosis on postoperative ascending phlebography. The highest incidence was in Perrin's series – 27.8%.[28] Of the 63 limbs that underwent late descending phlebography, 14 (22%) demonstrated major reflux or failure of the VST. Only one series detailed postoperative complications specific to VST. Perrin demonstrated a 1.3% incidence of bleeding complications requiring surgery and a 3.4% incidence of wound hematoma.[28]

CONCLUSIONS

As we enter the new millennium, there are several outstanding questions regarding the surgical treatment of venous disease that have not been answered:

- Do patients with advanced chronic venous insufficiency and tissue injury-class C5 or C6, benefit to a greater degree from external compression and wound care than from surgery?
- If surgery is chosen, what are the effects of superficial venous surgery alone in patients with C5/C6 disease and with deep venous incompetence?
- Finally, what is the role of deep venous reconstruction in the management of C5/C6 disease?

To answer these questions, the most powerful evidence will come from large randomized controlled trials (RCT). Currently, there is a proposal before NIH which compares compression and wound care to superficial venous surgery. The later cohort – superficial surgery – has been subdivided further into saphenectomy alone or treatment of ICVPs alone. Obviously, for most surgeons patients who are offered deep venous reconstruction are a distillate of those who have failed superficial venous surgery and, in most instances, a preceding course of elastic compression and wound care. To properly answer whether DVR is helpful to patients with C5/C6 disease an additional large RCT would be required.

As has been detailed previously in this paper, the results of DVR on 420 limbs have been published during the 18-year period from 1982 through 2000 for an average of 23 cases per year. Therefore, to set up a RCT, multiple sites would be required to attain the appropriate numbers for statistical validity. Such a trial would take at least 10 years to assess the long-term results, because short-term results in any vascular procedure can be misleading, e.g. early results of polytetrafluoroethylene (PTFE) versus autogenous vein graft in lower extremity reconstruction. In the end, surgeons will be left to an analysis of data from less powerful trials or clinical series to guide them in their present management of advanced chronic venous insufficiency. Unfortunately, those data are quite weak.

There are large gaps in information which characterize the preoperative status of patients undergoing either vein valve transplant or venous segment transposition. Over one-third of the series on vein valve transplants lack descriptive data by which patients can be classified by CEAP criteria. Postoperative outcome measures were weak, particularly in venous segment transposition. Ulcer healing was co-mingled with recurrent ulcer so no meaningful interpretation of the results could be obtained in several series. Only three series provided ulcer recurrence rate in life-table analysis form and an additional series co-mingled the results of vein valve transplant and venous segment transposition together so the effect of one procedure could not be sorted out from the other.

What do we do now?

Vein valve transplantation and venous segment transposition were performed for the preoperative indication of ulcer in over half the limbs for vein valve transplantation and nearly three-quarters of the limbs undergoing venous segment transfer. We feel that this procedure should be restricted to C5/C6 patients. The axillary vein site appears to be the preferred donor site for vein valve transplantation.[7] While Sottiurai's prospective but nonrandomized series suggests that a distal (popliteal) recipient site has better results,[24] 10 of the 15 series reviewed had vein valve transplants performed at the femoral level. Over 60% of patients undergoing vein valve transplantation will be ulcer free for 6 years by life-table format. The surgical site thrombosis rate is relatively low (5.6%) for this procedure if anticoagulation is utilized. Competence of the transplanted valve may be observed in over three-quarters of the limbs. There is a paradox, however, between clinical and hemodynamic results. Only a quarter of patients undergoing vein valve transplantation demonstrated improvements in venous pressure. Moreover, there appears to be a difference between venous refill time, which appears to improve postoperatively, and the percentage drop in venous pressure, which usually does not change following surgery. Finally, deep venous reconstructive surgery is a relatively safe procedure with only one death reported in more than 400 procedures. Besides graft site occlusion, hematoma formation related to perioperative anticoagulation is the most common complication and is quite low (around 5%). Following venous segment transfer the surgical site thrombosis rate appears to be higher than that for vein valve transplant (9.6%). Few data are available on ulcer recurrence rate by the life-table method for VST other than that of Perrin's study where 25% of patients had recurrence at 5 years. One would conclude, at present, that axillary vein valve transplant appears to be the preferred procedure for deep venous reconstruction in the post-thrombotic limb.

Patient algorithm

In the absence of a large RCT which would dictate an optimal method of treatment, our approach has been as follows for the patient with C5 or C6 disease. Patients in C5/C6 classification who have failed to respond to elastic compression and wound care or develop ulcer recurrence, undergo treatment of superficial venous incompetence as demonstrated by duplex scanning.[2] Data from the North American SEPS Trial shows that approximately 50% of patients with post-thrombotic deep venous involvement will have maintenance of an ulcer-free state in excess of 3 years. If an ulcer recurs, then axillary vein valve transplantation is utilized.

REFERENCES

1. Rodrigues AA, O'Donnell TF. Reconstructions for valvular incompetence of the deep veins. In Gloviczki P, Yao JST, eds. *Handbook of Venous Disorders*. London: Chapman & Hall Medical, 1996: 434–445.
2. O'Donnell TF. Lessons from the past guide the future: is history truly circular? *J Vasc Surg* 1999; **30**: 776–86.
3. Raju S, Fredericks RK, Neglen PN, *et al.* Durability of venous valve reconstruction techniques for 'primary' and postthrombotic reflux. *J Vasc Surg* 1996; **23**: 357–67.
4. Raju S. Venous insufficiency of the lower limb and status ulceration. *Ann Surg* 1983; **197**(6): 688–97.
5. Masuda EM, Kistner RL. Long-term results of venous valve reconstruction: a four- to twenty-one-year follow-up. *J Vasc Surg* 1994; **19**: 391–403.
6. Raju S. Venous reconstruction for treatment of post-phlebitic syndrome. In Haimovici H, ed. *Vascular Surgery: Principals and Techniques.* Cambridge: Blackwell Science, 1996.
7. O'Donnell TF. The Surgical management of deep venous valvular incompetence. In Rutherford RB, ed. *Vascular Surgery.* Philadelphia: WB Saunders, 1989: Chapter 14.
8. O'Donnell TF, Mackey WC, Shepard AD, Callow AD. Clinical, hemodynamic, and anatomic follow-up of direct venous reconstruction. *Arch Surg* 1987; **122**: 474–82.
9. Raju S, Frederick R. Venous obstruction and analysis of one hundred and thirty-seven cases with hemodynamic, venographic and clinical correlation. *J Vasc Surg* 1991; **14**: 305–13.
10. Pierik EGJM, van Urk H, Hop WCJ, Wittens CHA. Endoscopic versus open subfascial division of incompetent perforating veins in the treatment of venous leg ulceration: a randomized trial. *J Vasc Surg* 1997; **26**: 1049–54.
11. Iafrati M, O'Donnell TF. Subfascial dissection and perforating vein ablation. In Gloviczki P, Bergan JJ, eds. *Atlas of Endoscopic Perforator Vein Surgery.* London: Springer-Verlag, 1998: Chapter 14.
12. Akesson H, Brudin L, Cwikiel W, Ohlin P, Plate G: Does the correction of insufficient superficial and perforating veins improve venous function in patients with deep venous insufficiency? *Phlebology* 1990; **5**: 113–23.
13. Gloviczki P, Bergan JJ, Rhodes JM, *et al.* Mid-term results of endoscopic perforator vein interruption for chronic venous insufficiency: lessons learned from the North American Subfascial Endoscopic Perforator Surgery Registry. *J Vasc Surg* 1999; **29**: 489–502.
14. Porter JM, Moneta GL, Kistner RL, *et al.* An international consensus committee on chronic venous disease: reporting standards in venous disease, an update. *J Vasc Surg* 1995; **21**: 635–45.
15. van Bemmelen PS, Bedford G, Beach K, *et al.* Quantitative segmental evaluation of venous valvular reflux with ultrasonic duplex scanning. *J Vasc Surg* 1989; **10**: 425–31.
16. Welch HJ, Faliakou EC, Mclaughlin RL, *et al.* Comparison of descending phlebography with quantitative photo plethysmography, air plethysmography and duplex quantitative valve closure time in assessing deep venous reflux. *J Vasc Surg* 1992; **16**: 913–20.
17. O'Donnell TF, Burnand KG, Clemenson G, *et al.* A prospective study to compare Doppler examination with clinical and phlebographic detection of the location of incompetent perforating veins. *Arch Surg* 1977; **112**: 31–9.
18. Kistner RL, Sparkuhl MD. Surgery in acute and chronic venous disease. *Surgery* 1979; **85**: 31–43.

19. Taheri SA, Lazar L, Elias S. Status of vein valve transplant after 12 months. *Arch Surg* 1982; **117**: 1313–17.
20. Raju S, Fredericks R. Valve reconstruction procedures for nonobstructive venous insufficiency: rationale, techniques, and results in 107 procedures with two- to eight-year follow-up. *J Vasc Surg* 1988; **7**: 301–10.
21. Taheri SA, Pendergast DR, Lazar E. Vein valve transplantation. *Am J Surg* 1985; **150**: 201–2.
22. Eriksson I, Almgren B. Surgical reconstruction of incompetent deep vein valves. *Uppsala J Med Sci* 1988; **93**: 139–43.
23. Nash T. Long-term results of vein valve transplants placed in the popliteal vein for intractable post-phlebitic venous ulcers and pre-ulcer skin changes. *J Cardiovasc Surg* 1988; **29**: 712–16.
24. Sottiurai VS. Surgical correction of recurrent venous ulcer. *J Cardiovasc Surg* 1991; **32**: 104–9.
25. Rai DB, Lerner R. Chronic venous insufficiency disease: its etiology. A new technique for vein valve transplantation. *Int Surg* 1991; **76**(3): 174–8.
26. Bry JD, Muto PA, O'Donnell TF, Isaacson LA. The clinical and hemodynamic results after axillary-to-popliteal vein valve transplantation. *J Vasc Surg* 1995; **21**: 110–19.
27. Raju S, Neglen P, Doolittle J, Meydrech EF. Axillary vein transfer in trabeculated postthrombotic veins. *J Vasc Surg* 1999; **29**: 1050–64.
28. Perrin M. Reconstructive surgery for deep venous reflux: a report on 144 cases. *J Cardiovasc Surg* 2000; **8**(4): 246–55.
29. Queral LA, Whitehouse WM, Flinn WR, *et al.* Surgical correction of chronic deep venous insufficiency by valvular transposition. *Surgery* 1980; **87**(6): 688–95.
30. Johnson HD, Queral LA, Finn WR, *et al.* Late objective assessment of venous valve surgery. *Arch Surg* 1981; **116**: 1461–6.

35

Endovascular reconstruction for chronic iliac vein and inferior vena cava obstruction

PATRICIA E THORPE, FRANCISCO J OSSE AND HAI P DANG

Endovascular therapy for venous occlusion has derived largely from experience with thrombolysis and stents in the arterial system.[1–3] Relative success with venous thrombolysis was reported as early as 1968,[4] but subsequent complication rates using systemic infusions of streptokinase proved to be a deterrent to widespread application of the therapy.[5] Eventually, peripheral vascular interventionists treating acute vascular thrombosis adopted multi-sidehole infusion wires and catheters, and preferred the proven safety margin of urokinase to streptokinase.[6] These tools served to broaden the use of thrombolysis. During the same period, we saw the evolution of adjunctive therapies including stenting and mechanical thrombectomy.[7,8] These techniques were extended to venous thrombosis in the late 1980s and early 1990s.[9–11] Differences in application have evolved, depending on the site, e.g. upper extremity, dialysis fistula, lower extremity, but the principles of percutaneous over-the-wire intervention have been widely used to treat both acute and chronic venous occlusion. Sequential or synchronous application of these interventional techniques, using percutaneous access, requires familiarity with various catheters and wires to safely secure 'purchase' of the residual lumen. Since the lumen is frequently not detectable with magnetic resonance venography (MRV) or duplex, progressive intraluminal advancement of wires and catheters through organized thrombus and synechiae can be tedious. It must be done without rushing and with patience.

Interest in treating venous insufficiency led to development of standards for evaluation and classification of patients.[12,13] The CEAP classification is used to assess patient status and monitor outcome. Appropriate patient selection for intervention depends on clinical assessment, noninvasive studies and, occasionally, phlebography. Patient histories can be vague and, often, do not correlate with observed venous pathology. Patients with a history of immobilization, due to trauma or surgery, may have had unsuspected DVT. Even occlusive thrombus in the deep system can be clinically occult, especially when a patient is at bed rest or not ambulatory. Discovery of large venous collaterals during surgery can indicate a prior episode of thrombosis. Occult chronic common iliac vein disease can be present in patients undergoing surgery (Fig. 35.1). Chronic iliac vein thrombosis can result in confusing and misleading duplex data. Left iliac vein compression or occlusion (May–Thurner syndrome) can be missed when brisk flow in the external iliac is diverted to the hypogastric system. Normal flow will be seen in the common femoral segment. This, combined with poor visualization in the upper pelvis, can make the examination appear unremarkable, even when the common iliac is occluded. Chronic pelvic vein obstruction can also produce misleading air plethysmography data. The outflow fraction can be normal, due to collaterals, and the degree of valvular reflux can be obscured by a low flow state. Hemodynamic testing can identify and separate superficial and deep vein reflux, which must be distinguished from obstruction.[14,15]

After reviewing clinical and noninvasive data, if there is incongruity between physical examination, history, or noninvasive studies, symptomatic patients undergo phlebography. Observation of contrast flow, from a pedal injection, reveals venous flow patterns. Then, a

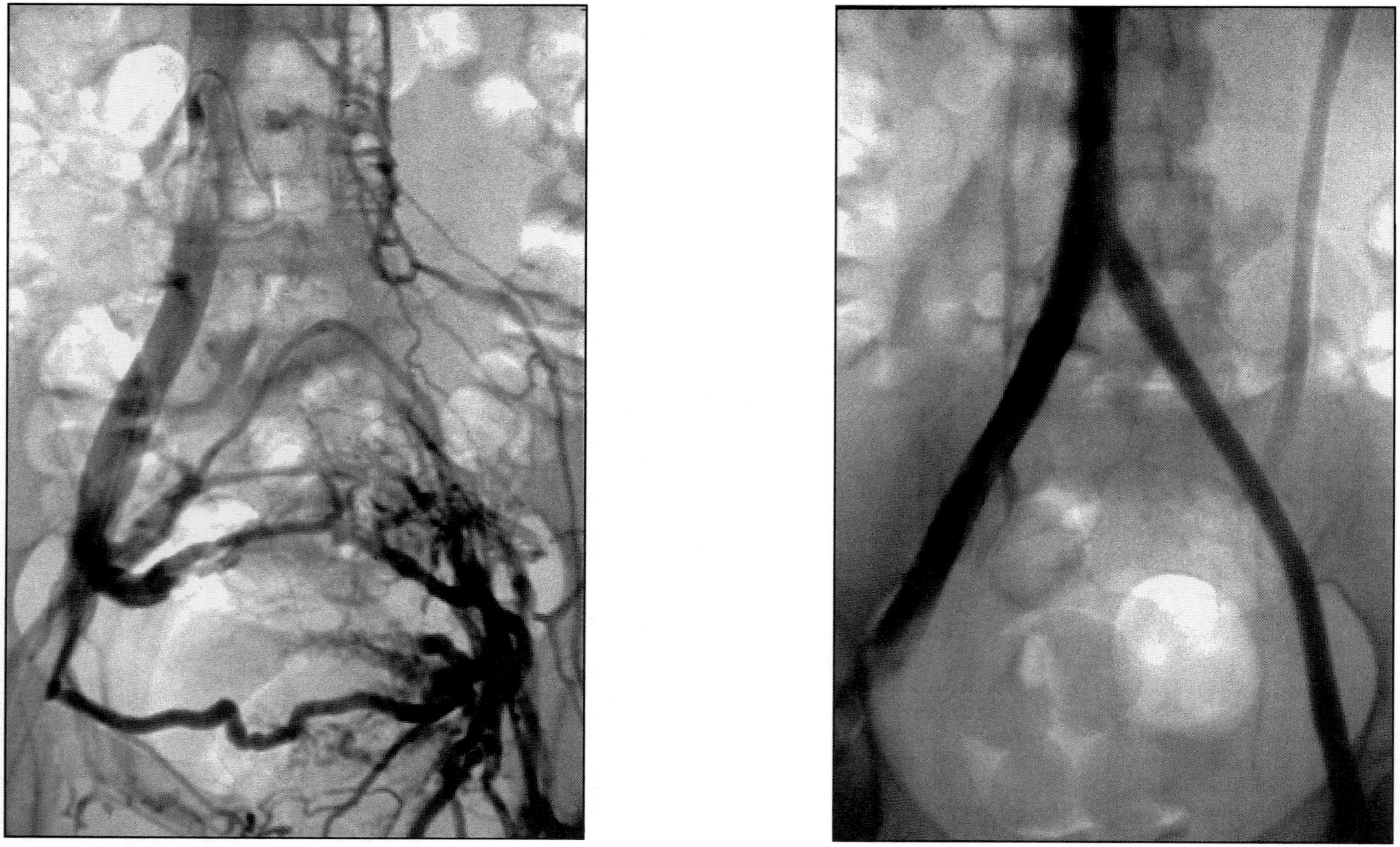

(a) (b)

Figure 35.1 *May–Thurner syndrome. (a) A 46-year-old female, with 12-month history of debilitating pain and edema after DVT. (b) Following urokinase and three Wallstents 10×94, 10×68, 10×42, patent at 29 months.*

decision can be made whether or not a suboptimal pattern might be improved with endovascular therapy. Each procedure is tailored to correct the flow abnormalities identified by dynamic phlebography. It is important for the interventionist to perform the contrast injection, with and without tourniquets, to observe the flow patterns. This critical information cannot be obtained by looking at static images. In chronic disease, comparing video sequences is much more informative than looking at cut films.

To a patient, the most important gauge of therapeutic success is improved daily existence. The amount of time spent with the leg(s) elevated decreases when therapy reduces the obstructive component contributing to venous pressure. Increasing venous outflow can diminish pain and edema, even though the issue of valvular reflux is not addressed. In fact, re-establishing flow often unmasks reflux that was unapparent in a low-flow state. Thus, as in arterial interventions, treatment of chronic venous conditions is palliative. By addressing the obstructive component of venous hypertension we hope to give patients a better quality of life.

RATIONALE OF THROMBOLYSIS FOR CHRONIC VENOUS THROMBOSIS

The main principle in thrombolytic therapy is effective and efficient delivery of an agent to the thrombosed vascular segment(s). In larger axial veins, this is best achieved with catheter delivery utilizing multi-sidehole infusion catheters and wires. When there is thrombus in deep calf veins and the popliteal, simultaneous flow-directed infusion, utilizing tourniquets, serves to improve flow in these areas. It is most important to optimize venous flow in the distal deep system. Persistent diversion of distal flow into the superficial system will place the newly opened and stented proximal segments at greater risk for re-thrombosis. Optimizing resting flow velocities, by re-establishing continuity of flow from the foot to the cava, has proven to give the best hemodynamic and clinical results.

Between 1980 and 1999, peripheral vascular thrombolysis was largely performed with urokinase (Abbokinase, Abbott Laboratories, Chicago, IL, USA). This agent was preferred over streptokinase for the safety margin relative to bleeding complications. Problems centered on manufacturing protocols led to a shortage of urokinase and indefinite withdrawal of this agent from the US market. Alternative lytic agents such as alteplase (Activase, Genentech Inc., South San Francisco, CA, USA) and reteplase (Retavase, Centocor Inc., Malvern, PA, USA) are now being used in peripheral interventions.[16,17] Early in our experience with alternative lytic agents, there has been an increase in bleeding complications, compared with urokinase. This has required dose adjustments for concomitant heparin as well as the lytic infusions. Nevertheless, the value of thrombolysis appears well accepted by the interventional community, and, therefore, remains an important tool in therapy.

It is not immediately obvious nor well understood how thrombolytic therapy functions in the case of chronic venous occlusion. It does, however, make a difference. Physicians attempting to recanalize chronic thrombus frequently fail to advance the wire or stay intraluminal if they do not infuse a thrombolytic agent prior to and during the wire recanalization phase. Only short, subtotal occlusions can be readily treated without lytic therapy. In treating chronic occlusions, we share, with Semba and Dake,[11] the impression that a thrombolytic infusion can 'soften' more organized thrombus and, thereby, facilitate passage of wires and catheters. Although catheter-directed thrombolytic therapy has been shown to be most successful in removing acute thrombus,[18] in chronic conditions, clinical improvement observed after thrombolytic infusion is often greater than the image would suggest. That is because improvement of venous flow, particularly in the calf, depends on the cumulative effect of many unnamed veins remaining patent. Restoring flow in these small conduits can make a significant clinical difference. Analysis of National Venous Registry (NVR) data suggested thrombolysis of chronic thrombus was unsuccessful. In truth, images of distal veins often look as abnormal after lytic infusion as they do before. Whereas comparison images show dramatic difference when lysing acute DVT, the phlebographic appearance of chronic venous obstruction changes less, even though the venous flow can improve significantly. Interpretation of static contrast images fails to explain the clinical improvement in patients after thrombolytic infusion for chronic obstruction. Reducing venous resistance, by augmenting small and medium-size venous channels, does not dramatically alter the post-infusion images, but it is an important adjunct to stenting larger veins. Video/digital phlebography, as mentioned above, can demonstrate a clear difference in rate of flow/contrast clearance after thrombolytic infusion. Vascular physiology and fluid dynamics studies show how flow in a tubular conduit is proportional to r^4, where r represents the radius.[19] If we apply this concept to venous flow, we see that augmenting multiple-occluded or tiny lumens from <1 mm to >2–3 mm significantly increases venous flow despite minimal change on radiographic images. According to this principle, Poiseuille's law, delivery of thrombolytic agents to the extremity via catheter or flow-directed techniques, can promote flow by enlarging the residual lumen. Although not restored to original caliber, lysing acute and subacute thrombus, superimposed upon chronic organized thrombus, increases the luminal diameter. This may not produce a dramatic change on x-ray images, but the increase in flow can be documented with duplex and correlated with post-treatment clinical improvement. Ambulatory venous pressure, as indirectly measured with air plethysmography, should decrease as resistance to flow decreases. However, in our examinations, the numbers often do not reflect the degree of clinical improvement. Reasons for this are complex and most likely involve the effects of long-standing obstruction on valves and the calf muscle pump.

TECHNIQUES OF ENDOVENOUS RECONSTRUCTIONS

Access sites and venous cannulation

When treating an iliac or caval obstruction, the popliteal approach is generally selected. If necessary, a bilateral approach is used simultaneously. Occasionally, resistance from old thrombus will require use of the 'pull-through' technique, to provide sufficient force to advance a catheter through the tight residual lumen.[20] This requires access from the contralateral or jugular approach. This technique allows one to keep the wire from buckling or pushing back, as the catheter is advanced. Although the baseline phlebogram is performed with the patient supine, the endovascular procedure requires use of a Foley catheter and placement of the patient in a prone position. Initial deep venous access is acquired using a combination of contrast infusion from a pedal vein and ultrasound guidance of a 21 gauge needle from a Micropuncture Set (Cook Inc., Bloomington, IN, USA) into the back wall of the popliteal vein or a superficial tributary. Successful entry into a patent distal vein, in continuity with occluded proximal deep venous segment(s), permits placement of a working sheath for catheter exchange and contrast injection. Spasm and missed passes are significantly less with the combination 3–5.5F, coaxial, micropuncture dilators and 0.018 inch nitinol wire than with standard intravenous catheters. An angled 4–5F hydrophilic catheter, in combination with a 0.035 inch Glidewire™ (Boston Scientific, Na, MA, USA) or 0.035 inch Roadrunner™ (Cook Inc.), is carefully advanced from the popliteal level, through the superficial femoral vein to the common femoral level.

Thrombolysis and balloon angioplasty

During the initial 24–48 hours, the goal is to place a multi-sidehole catheter along the length of the abnormal segments traversed by the wire. An overnight infusion of thrombolytic agent will decrease the intraluminal resistance and set the stage for subsequent catheter advancement, balloon dilatation and stent placement. Following passage of a wire into the normal cava, an exchange is made to position a stiffer exchange length wire that is maintained as the working wire during stent deployment. Sequential predilatation in the cava and iliac vein is conducted, from proximal to distal, using 8–14 mm balloons (4 cm length). Balloon selection depends on the estimated size of the native vessel and the observed resistance to balloon expansion (Fig. 35.2). Overdilatation is avoided. Some vessels are very tenacious

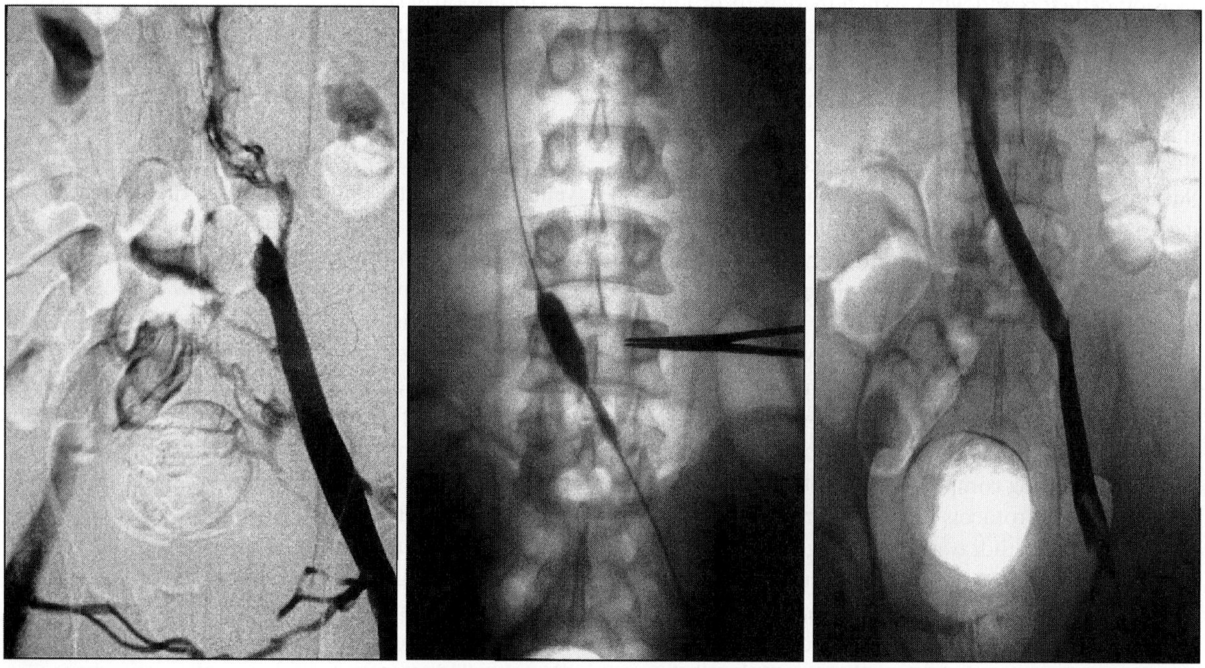

(a) (b) (c)

Figure 35.2 *Endovascular treatment of May–Thurner occlusion. (a) Left iliac occlusion. (b) Balloon dilatation 12×4 cm. (c) 12×60 mm Wallstent.*

whereas others dilate with relative ease. Great care is taken to 'feel' the balloon as one slowly proceeds to expand the residual lumen.

Metallic stents

The interventionist must have a working knowledge of stent properties and be familiar with a wide variety of commercially available products. The number of stents now on the market has grown significantly over the past decade and currently there are more than 40 different stents available for coronary use and more than 20 for use in the periphery.[21] Significant improvement in patency rates has been observed in iliac lesions treated with stents in addition to angioplasty. In the NVR, at 1 year, 74% of limbs treated with stents remained patent compared with 53% of limbs not receiving stents (P <0.001).[18]

No stent possesses all the qualities of an ideal stent, e.g. good radio-opacity, ease of positioning, flexibility, tractability, fidelity of shape and low restenosis rate. Evaluation of the characteristics of the properties of metallic stents is gained with experience as new stents are introduced and compared with those in use. Clinical use of stents in the iliac vein was first reported by Zollikofer *et al.* in 1988.[22] Prior to that, others had reported use of stents in the inferior and superior vena cava.[23] Migration and intimal hyperplasia were documented with early use of the Gianturco Z stent.[24] Modifications were made to prevent slippage; modular stent units were connected with nylon suture and small hooks were added. Migration has been a rare event with all stent designs.[25] When this does occur, misplaced or migrated Palmaz and Wallstents can be effectively retrieved using endovascular techniques.[26]

All stents have been shown to become endothelialized and/or covered with neointima.[22] Sawada reported this in all Z stents observed at autopsy.[24] The neointima appears rapidly and the endothelialization process occurs within 2–6 weeks. The amount of intimal thickening has been correlated to design. More rigid stents, exerting greater axial force on the vessel wall, seem to accelerate intimal hyperplasia.[27,28] In these animal studies, and our experience, the Wallstent is less likely to induce compromising intimal hyperplasia due to the small wire size, pliability and longitudinal flexibility.[7] Zollikofer noted two important observations in animal studies:

- regression of intimal hyperplasia occurred with time; and
- restenosis is more common at a site of high-pressure flow, e.g.arteriovenous fistula.[22]

This appears true for stented and non-stented vein segments. Intravascular ultrasound (IVUS) has allowed us to examine symptomatic patients and document restenosis caused by intimal hyperplasia.

The majority of interventionists use the Wallstent for venous stenting (Table 35.1). In the common iliac location, with extrinsic pressure a factor in causing compression, flexibility and self-expansion may give the Wallstent an advantage. A study comparing long-term patency of self-expanding versus balloon expandable stents, placed in the common iliac vein, has not been done. The choice of lengths and diameters make this design suitable for 1–2 cm vein diameters. The newer nitinol stents have less foreshortening than the Wallstent, but they are somewhat less visible under fluoroscopy, especially in large patients. Currently available stents are used 'off label', as the 8–16 mm diameter stents are only FDA approved for biliary and iliac artery use. Covered stents, suitable for repair of venous tears, are still unavailable in the USA, although different designs are now used in Europe and elsewhere. Another stent limitation is length. Many of the venous occlusions are long, and reconstruction requires tandem stent deployment. The fully expanded stent length ranges from 4.0 to 10.0 cm. Stents remain correspondingly longer if full expansion is not achieved. As in the arterial system, crossing the origin of branch vessels does not appear to be associated with problems. We have closely followed, with duplex imaging, iliac vein Wallstents in place for more than 7 years. There is no indication of strut fracture or failure. Stents with larger interstices have a tendency to look more deformed when deployed in veins damaged with chronic mural thrombus. These vessels are not smooth tubular structures, like normal veins or arteries. The Wallstent most consistently excludes the irregular endothelial surface and creates a smooth, sufficiently widened diameter.

ENDOVENOUS TREATMENT OF CHRONIC ILIAC VEIN THROMBOSIS

When Zollikofer *et al.*[22] first placed a stent in the iliac system, the indication was treatment of intimal hyperplasia, at the proximal anastomosis of a common femoral-to-common iliac bypass graft. Since then, stents have been shown to be an effective adjunct to surgery and balloon dilatation, particularly in the left common iliac segment.[29,30] As in arterial disease, 'culprit' lesions are frequently discovered after removal of acute thrombus. Verhaeghe *et al.* reported discovery of an underlying anatomical anomaly or lesion in 13/19 (68%) of limbs treated with catheter-directed rt-PA for iliofemoral thrombosis.[31] Ten of the venous lesions (77%) were unknown before lysis and eight (62%) were treated with stent therapy. For the most part, the condition is diagnosed in association with thrombosis, and as Cockett observed, early on, in acute cases, 'mere removal of the clot does little good in these cases as it does not deal with the real cause of venous obstruction (i.e. the stricture)'.[32]

Table 35.1 *Venous stent types implanted in 600 patients*

Year	First author	Stent type					
		Wallstent	Palma	Gianturco	Nitinol	Other	
1988	Zollikofer[22]	3					
1992	Zollikofer[41]	7					
1992	Freidrich	7					
1992	Sawada[24]			4			
1993	Grenier[42]	1					
1993	Mickley[52]	6					
1994	Semba[11]	4	41				
1995	Berger[43]		2				
1996	Nazarian[29]	Yes	Yes	Yes			
1996	Buelens[53]	6					
1996	Vorwerk[44]	7					
1996	Rilinger[45]		6				
1997	LaHei[46]						
1997	Akesson[48]	3	2	11			
1997	Bjarnason[54]	75					
1997	Verhaeghe[31]	9					
1998	Henderson[49]	5					
1998	Heniford[50]	2					
1998	Fearon[47]		1				
1998	Binkert[51]	11				1 Cragg	
1998	Mickley[30]	4	3		1		
1999	Blattler[55]	12					
1999	Mewissen[18]	Yes	Yes		Yes		
1999	Thorpe[56]	159	1		3		
2000	Neglen[40]	203					
	TOTAL	524	56	15	4	1	600
	PERCENT	87	9	3	1	<1	

Although the majority of large vein thromboses recanalize sufficiently, a certain percentage of iliofemoral DVT patients do not recover satisfactorily. Following standard therapy of heparin, bed rest and oral anticoagulation, they remain symptomatic with pain and/or edema. Some develop ulcers. Unfortunately, it is not possible to predict which patients will develop a severe post-thrombotic syndrome. Cockett and Thomas identified the relative lack of iliac recanalization and associated post-inflammatory perivenous scarring as the main etiologies of serious post-thrombotic sequelae. The degree of uncompensated residual obstruction causes venous claudication, and the cutaneous changes associated with persistent venous hypertension. Patients in this category were among those first considered for surgical bypass.[33,34]

The May–Thurner syndrome

The evolution and application of endovascular techniques for treatment of acute iliofemoral thrombosis led to an increased awareness of the left common iliac compression syndrome initially described in 1906.[35,36] Opinions regarding whether or not the abnormality represents an acquired venous lesion or residual congenital anomaly seem to be influenced by observations during surgery versus postmortem analysis, as done originally by May and Thurner in 1957.[37–39] Between 1906 and 1963, four studies (960 cadaver dissections) were conducted to look at venous anatomy. Compression of the left common iliac vein was documented in 22%.[36–39] Based on these investigations, the frequency of occurrence cited in adults was between 20 and 34%, with an incidence of 4–17% in newborns up to 10 months and 10–26% in children between 1 and 8 years of age.[38]

Left iliac compression (LIC) explains why deep vein thrombosis predominantly affects the left leg. Many persons with occult left iliac compression or occlusion are, in fact, asymptomatic. Prethrombotic venous hypertension may be present, but remains largely undiagnosed. Subtle asymmetry in leg or foot size may be noticed, but is mostly ignored. Iliac compression patients frequently present with associated femoral thrombosis. In fact, the condition should be suspected in anyone with acute left extremity DVT and/or symptoms of venous insufficiency. The youngest patient in whom we have seen venous claudication and edema, with a normal saphenous vein and phlebographic confirmation of left iliac compression, was a 12-year-old girl. In addition, we have treated three young women, aged between 17 and 24, with iliac stents to alleviate symptoms caused by May–Thurner compression not yet complicated by thrombosis. In their study of 94 patients with suspected iliac vein obstruction, Neglen and Raju have reported on primary stenting of May–Thurner compression.[40] Forty-three symptomatic limbs, with no history or phlebographic evidence of prior DVT, showed better long-term results than patients presenting with iliac compression complicated by thrombosis (personal communication).

Results of endovenous treatment for iliac vein thrombosis

Most published reports of endovascular therapy for iliac and iliofemoral thrombosis involve single case reports or small series of patients treated for acute DVT. A review of the English literature dealing with endovascular treatment of thrombotic iliac occlusion or May–Thurner syndrome reveals numerous accounts of limited experience with short follow-up There are 12 reports of one to three patients,[22,24,41–50], and 12 publications with more than six patients (Table 35.2).[17,18,29–31,40,51–56] Early on, Mickley and colleagues documented use of stents after thrombectomy. Self-expanding stents were used to correct 10 severely stenosed venous segments in 8/30 patients operated on for iliofemoral thromboses.[52] Stenoses occurred within 3–6 months after thrombectomy and arteriovenous fistula surgery. The lesions were treated with percutaneous Wallstent placement. Median follow-up at 17 months (range 3–23 months) showed 100% primary patency. In 1998, Mickley *et al.* reported experience stenting left iliac spurs discovered after thrombectomy.[30] Comparing results of stented versus unstented iliac spurs revealed re-thrombosis of 16/22 in 73% of untreated spurs, despite adequate anticoagulation, whereas only 1/8 (13%) of stented spurs reoccluded ($P = 0.01$).

THE STANFORD EXPERIENCE

In 1994, the Stanford group reported their initial study.[11] They treated 27 limbs in 21 patients (20 acute, 7 chronic) with catheter-directed thrombolysis. The average dose of urokinase was 4.9 million IU (range 1.4–16 million IU) infused over an average of 30 hours (range 15–74 hours). Sixteen limbs had underlying stenoses that were treated with angioplasty (2) or angioplasty and stent (14). Two chronically occluded iliac veins could not be traversed with a guidewire. Although primary patency at 3 months was reported as 11/12 (92%), longer-term group follow-up was not included.

THE UNIVERSITY OF MINNESOTA EXPERIENCE

Nazarian and colleagues, at Minnesota, discussed on the role of metallic stents after failure of balloon angioplasty or surgery.[29] Over a 65-month period, 55 patients received stents in the subclavian veins (9), innominate veins (3), superior vena cava (4), inferior vena cava (3), iliac veins (29), femoral veins (5) and portal veins (6). The series included patients treated for malignant stenoses and benign, chronic iliac occlusions. They noted no significant difference of 1-year patency between patients with and without a history of DVT, or relative to the type of stent used (i.e. Gianturco, Palmaz or Wallstent). Stenotic lesions had a 1-year primary assisted patency of 74% compared with 57% for veins with prestent occlusions ($P = 0.15$). Among the iliac veins, 13 were initially occluded. Primary-assisted patency for iliac veins was 66% compared with 37% when femoral thrombosis accompanied iliac DVT ($P = 0.06$). Two-year patency rates were significantly lower in patients with known malignancy. Technical problems were associated with single-module Z stents that persistently slipped above or below the stenosis. One external iliac Z stent fracture was identified at 5 months with no adverse outcome.

In 1997, Bjarnason *et al.* reported on treatment of 77 patients.[54] The majority of the patients, mean age 47 years (range 14–78 years) presented with acute DVT symptoms of <14 days' duration (69/86,78%) while 9 (10%) had subacute thrombus (14–28 days) and 9 (10%) had thrombus older than 28 days. The mean length of symptoms prior to thrombolysis was 15 days (range 0–256 days). The average dose of urokinase was 10.5 million IU (range 0.4–24 million IU) and the average infusion time was 75 hours (range 8–247 hours). They reported greater technical success in treating iliac veins (79%) versus femoral veins (63%). We have also seen this pattern. It reflects the fact that subclinical thrombosis is present prior to clinical presentation with acute iliofemoral DVT. Even though the initial technical success was similar between patients undergoing stent placement versus those who did not, it was less for patients with thrombus older than 4 weeks than those with more acute conditions. Thrombosed superficial femoral veins are often poorly recanalized and respond poorly to thrombolysis alone. Eighty-six stents were placed in 38 (44%) of the 87 limbs treated for iliofemoral thrombosis. Seventy-five Wallstents were placed in 36 limbs and 11 Gianturco stents were placed in two limbs. Interestingly, they found a lower 6-month primary patency rate between stented (60%) and non-stented (75%) iliac veins and 54% versus 75% at one year ($P = 0.011$). At 1 year, the secondary patency rate was 76% for stented and 82% for non-stented vessels ($P = 0.46$). They hypothesized that patients requiring stents presented with more severe chronic venous disease, accounting for the poorer long-term results. Stented patients were not

Table 35.2 *Results of 707 venous stents*

														Adjuvant treatment		
Year	First author	Reference	No. patients	Limbs	No. Stents	Site Iliac	Site Fem	Site IVC	Technical success Success	F/U Range	F/U Mean	Primary patency	Assisted patency	Last F/U with imaging	Warfarin	Aspirin
1988	Zollikofer	22	2	2	6	3	3		100%	4–12 m	NR	75%	NR			
1992	Zollikofer	41	2	2	6	1	5		100%	1–54 m	NR	100%		4 y		
1992	Sawada	24	2	2	3	3			100%	7–13 m	10 m	50%	100%	6 m		
1993	Grenier	42	1	1	1	1			100%	8 m		100%		8 m		
1993	Mickley	51	8	8	6	6			100%	3–23 m	17 m	100%		17 m		
1994	Semba	17	21	25	14	14	0		85%	1–46 m	NR	85%		3 m	8–12 wk	yes
1995	Berger	43	1	1	1	1			100%	6 m		100%		6 m		
1996	Nazarian	29	55	NA	34	29	5		76%	6–65 m	24 m	59%	63%	1 & 4 y	3–6 mo	no
1996	Buelens	52	6	6	6	6			100%	NR		NA				
1996	Vorwerk	44	1	2	7	4	3		100%	1 m		0%				
1996	Rilinger	45	3	3	6	6			100%	3–10 m	6 m	59%	63%	6 m	12 mo	
1997	LaHei	46	1	1	1	1			100%	6 m		0%			6 m	
1997	Akesson	48	3	3	7	6			100%	13–20 m	18 m	100%		18 m		
1997	Bjarnason	54	77	87	86	60	18	8	79%	6–72 m	NR	63%	78%	1 y		
1997	Verhaeghe	31	24	24	9	9			79%	6 m	NR	75%	NA			
1998	Henderson	49	3	3	5	5			100%	8–12 m	8 mo	66%	100%	6 m	6 mo	no
1998	Heniford	50	1	1	2	2			100%	24 m	NR	100%		2 y		
1998	Fearon	47	1	1	1	1			100%	NR		NA				
1998	Binkert	53	8	8	8	8			87%	10–121 m	36 m	100%		3 y		
1998	Mickley	30	8	8	12	12			88%	4–30 m	NR	73%	82%	2 y		
1999	Blattler	55	14	12	12	12			86%	1–43 m	15 m	92%	92%	1 y		
1999	Mewissen*	18	287	303	105	99	5		97%	12–36 m	NR	74%**		1 y	6 mo or >	no
1999	Thorpe	56	84	93	162	100	44	18	95%	6–20 m	38 m	77%	91%	3 y	indefinite	no
2000	Neglen	40	94	102	118	118	0		95%	1–21 m	12 m	82%	91%	1 y	no	yes
	TOTAL		707	698	618	507	83	26								
	PERCENTAGE					82	14	4								

*483 patients entered in NVR but only 287 had adequate 1-year follow-up data.

uniformly maintained on warfarin longer that 6 months.

THE NATIONAL VENOUS REGISTRY

An important report in the literature regards the National Venous Registry (1994–97).[55] This was a multicenter registry that collected data on 473 iliofemoral DVT patients treated with endovascular techniques. The study included 287 patients with adequate follow-up. The majority had acute presentation of iliofemoral thrombosis (70%). The average dose of urokinase was 7.8 million IU and nearly 50% required placement of an iliac stent. Technical success, including placement of 104 stents, was 97%. Results were reported in terms of lysis grade. Complete lysis was achieved in 60% of patients presenting with acute thrombus (<10 days). Among this group, 90% remained patent at 12 months compared with 70% of those with less than complete lysis. Patients were maintained on warfarin for 4–6 months. The study revealed greater 1-year patency in limbs with iliac stenosis treated with angioplasty plus stent (74%) versus angioplasty alone (53%). A remarkably lower patency rate (20% at 2 months) was observed in the five stents placed in femoral segments. In our experience, stenting lower segments requires careful assessment of flow patterns and intimal hyperplasia. The study was based on analysis of pre- and postphlebograms and duplex ultrasound with minimal follow-up of 12 months.

THE CREIGHTON UNIVERSITY EXPERIENCE

Between 1988 and 1999, 116 patients received urokinase for lower extremity DVT at Creighton. Eighty-four underwent endovascular therapy for chronic lower extremity thrombosis. The mean age was 47.5 years (range 12–90 years). Patients received a mean dose 8.7 million IU (range 2–27 million IU with a minimum 24-hour infusion of urokinase (range 24–120 hours). Persistent venous stenoses, after thrombolysis, required stent placement in 53% (62 patients and 71 limbs). Among these patients, thirty-two (51% of those stented and 28% of the total) had stents placed in the common femoral and/or superficial femoral veins. Sixteen patients had a single iliac stent placed for focal common iliac compression associated with acute thrombosis (L/15, R/1). In this subgroup, there is 100% primary patency with median follow-up of 24 months (range 8–50 months). Three patients have developed intimal hyperplasia within the stented segment, causing increase in edema and discomfort compared to post-stenting. This occurred between 6 and 12 months and all were treated with balloon dilatation resulting in resolution of symptoms. All patients treated for chronic iliofemoral and iliocaval occlusion were examined before and after lysis/stenting with ultrasound. In 16 patients, peak velocities in diseased and non-affected iliac and femoral veins were suitable for analysis. We found the median common iliac velocity in the normal limb to be 44 cm/s ($n = 16$). Comparison of pre-stent mean (7.25 cm/s) and post-stent mean (41.3 cm/s), common iliac vein velocity demonstrated a significant difference ($P < 0.0001$) whereas the mean stented left iliac vein velocity (41.3 cm/s) was not significantly different from the untreated right iliac vein mean velocity (47 cm/s) ($P = 0.4569$).[57] Bjarnason *et al.* also reported that velocities of less than 25 cm/s in the stented iliac segment correlated with poor patency.[54] Further analysis of stented patients showed 19 required two iliac stents, 20 received three stents and three large patients (>250 pounds) had more than three stents placed in the left iliac vein. Overall, 1-year primary patency of patients with iliac stents, including those with femoral stents, is 80% (57/71). Re-thrombosis occurred within 30 days in 8/71 (11%). Six of these patients were retreated with thrombolysis and additional stents to improve inflow. This group included the three large patients with more than three stents in their long iliac veins. Symptomatic restenosis was documented and dilated in 6/71 (9%) limbs. In all, the restenosis became clinically apparent between 6 and 12 months. One-year secondary patency is 94% (67/71).

All patients are discharged in class II compression hosiery and/or the Velcro CircAid™ legging (CircAid, San Diego, CA, USA) Patients are seen at follow-up at 3, 6 and 12 months and yearly thereafter. In addition to the pertinent physical examination, duplex imaging and hemodynamic testing (APG) are repeated at these intervals or if clinical decline occurs. Warfarin is usually continued indefinitely except in patients with a single iliac stent placed after successful lysis of acute thrombus. Normal distal veins provide sufficient confluence of deep venous flow to favor patency. Low molecular weight heparin (LMWH; 1 mg/kg every 12 hours or 1.5 mg/kg every 24 hours) has been used, in place of unfractionated heparin, without complication. Patients remain at bed rest for at least 24 hours after sheath removal, to prevent hematoma. Oral anticoagulation (PT/INR) is maintained at <2.0 or >4.5 seconds. Low levels can be supplemented with LMWH. Elevated levels are often associated with antibiotics requiring temporary adjustments of warfarin dose. Patients undergoing surgery or dental work are given a schedule for LMWH coverage while discontinuing warfarin.

VENOUS STENTING WITHOUT THROMBOLYSIS

Neglen and Raju are the only authors to report on a large endovascular series in which thrombolysis was not used in treating chronic venous obstruction. They treated a highly selected group of patients suspected of having iliac vein occlusion.[40] They placed 118 Wallstents in 77 iliac veins, 43 of which were diagnosed with non-thrombotic iliac occlusion or stenosis. In the remaining limbs, there was evidence of prior DVT. As in the other large patient series, technical success was high (97%). Eighty-seven limbs were treated with a 1-year primary patency of 82% and assisted and secondary patency of 91% and 92%, respectively. Their data support the Creighton finding that focal iliac vein stenoses or occlusions can be opened effectively and safely stented with good 1-year patency rates.[57,58] Clinical improvement usually parallels technical success. However, in severe chronic DVT, involving multiple venous segments, relief of large vein obstruction can produce clinical improvement even when chronic venous insufficiency remains.

COMPLICATIONS OF ILIAC VEIN THROMBOLYSIS AND STENTING

Bleeding complications can occur with prolonged thrombolytic infusions, but they are relatively uncommon in the post-thrombotic patient population compared with cardiac patients. In reviewing the complications reported in the literature, clearly the most common problem is minor bleeding at the sheath site (Table 35.3). Major bleeding, requiring transfusion, has been reported in 1–25% of patients. This is more likely to occur in obese patients; the use of ultrasound guidance for initial puncture is strongly recommended. Pulmonary embolus occurred one time in our series, and continued thrombolysis resolved all symptoms. It has been reported in <1% of all reported cases. Therefore, IVC filters are not routinely recommended. Among nearly 1000 iliofemoral venous thrombolysis patients reported in the literature, death has occurred in <1% due to pulmonary embolism (1),[18] sepsis (1),[29] retroperitoneal hematoma (1),[56] and intracranial hemorrhage (2)[18,56] and MI (1).[54] Re-thrombosis <30 days is generally due to poor outflow or inflow and/or subtherapeutic anticoagulation. When this occurs, re-treatment with thrombolysis and additional stents is effective. Intimal hyperplasia, causing symptomatic restenosis occurred in approximately 10% of stented veins, and can be effectively treated with angioplasty.[40,56]

ENDOVENOUS TREATMENT OF INFERIOR VENA CAVAL OCCLUSION

Among the most symptomatic post-thrombotic patients are individuals with a combination of iliac vein and inferior vena cava (IVC) obstruction. Not infrequently, bilateral iliac vein thrombosis is associated with infra-renal IVC occlusion. The severity of symptoms implies inadequate collateral outflow in the face of multisegmental obstruction that is poorly recanalized. While not as common as isolated iliofemoral thrombosis, patients with iliocaval involvement are represented between 1 and 10% in the larger reported series.

Etiology and presentation

Although relatively uncommon, the causes of IVC obstruction are varied. In addition to primary caval malignancy, which is rare, causes of caval thrombosis include renal cell carcinoma, retroperitoneal fibrosis, radiation therapy, aortic aneurysm, ascites, trauma, surgery and filter placement. Regardless of etiology, affected persons generally develop significant retroperitoneal and abdominal collaterals to compensate for occlusion of the infra-renal IVC. The condition may remain occult when collaterals are adequate, and only become clinically evident upon a subsequent thrombotic episode.

Patients with IVC obstruction often complain that elevation does little to relieve extremity edema. Poorly compensated iliocaval obstruction can cause unrelenting elevation of venous pressure, resulting in a constant sensation of fullness in the groin area, severe leg discomfort, and stasis ulceration. More severe hemodynamic dysfunction, per clinical class of disease, can be identified in patients with chronic deep vein obstruction.[59] Clearly, quality of life can be significantly diminished. Ultimately, some patients disabled by iliocaval occlusion have been considered for bypass surgery. Patency results of long bypass grafts for large vein obstruction are inconsistent, at best.[60] Believed to require assistance from an arteriovenous fistula to maintain patency, some go on to fail due to intimal hyperplasia at the anastomosis. Ironically, intimal hyperplasia may be accelerated by arterial pressures.[22]

Techniques of endovenous IVC reconstructions

Endovascular reconstruction of chronic iliocaval occlusion is feasible (Fig. 35.3). Whilst technically more challenging, it is an attractive therapeutic option for carefully selected patients. The first endovenous stent was placed in the IVC in 1986 by Zollikofer and collegues.[22] Since then, the literature contains reports of 89 patients receiving stents to treat benign (67%) and malignant (33%) IVC obstructions. The Stanford group has reported on a series of 17 consecutive patients, with chronic IVC occlusion, treated over a 6-year period.[61] The mean duration of symptoms was 32 months. Thrombolysis and/or stents were used with technical success in 15 (88%) patients. After mean follow-up of 19 months, primary patency rate was 80% and the primary assisted rate was 87% (13/15). There were no procedure-related complications, although four patients died during the follow-up period due to underlying disease.

THE CREIGHTON UNIVERSITY EXPERIENCE WITH IVC RECONSTRUCTION

Seven patients, six males, one female, ranging in age from 16 to 72 years (mean 45), underwent endovascular

Table 35.3 *Complications of 935 endovascular reconstructions for venous thrombosis*

Year	First author	No patients	None reported	<30 d death	Intracranial hemorrhage	PE	Stent migration	Acute <30 d thrombosis	Major hematoma	Minor hematoma	Retroperitoneal hematoma	GI bleeding	Sepsis/ infection
1988	Zollikofer[22]	2	0										
1992	Zollikofer[41]	2	0										
1992	Sawada[24]	2	0										
1993	Grenier[42]	1	0										
1993	Mickley[52]	8	0										
1994	Semba[11]	21	0										
1995	Berger[43]	1	0										
1996	Nazarian[29]	55		1	0	0	8	0	1	.3	.0	1	1
1996	Buelens[53]	6						1					
1996	Vorwerk[44]	1						1					
1996	Rilinger[45]	3	0										
1997	LaHei[46]	1						1					
1997	Akesson[48]	3	0										
1997	Bjarnason[54]	77		1		1	1		3	11	.1	1	
1997	Verhaeghe[31]	24						4	6				
1998	Henderson[49]	3						1					
1998	Heniford[50]	1	0										
1998	Fearon[47]	1	0										
1998	Binkert[51]	8	0										
1998	Mickley[30]	8						1					
1999	Blattler[55]	14						1					
1999	Mewissen[18]	483		2	1	6	0	75	54	77	.7		
1999	Thorpe[56]	116		2	1(SDH)	0	0	3	3	.8	.1	1	2
2000	Neglen[40]	94		0	0	0	0	5	1	.0	.1	0	0
	TOTAL	935		6	2	7	9	93	68	99	10	3	3
	PERCENTAGE			<1	<0.5	<1	1	10.00	7.27	11	.1	<0.5	<0.5

*483 patients enrolled in NVR after receiving thrombolysis for DVT; 287 analyzed with 1-year follow-up.

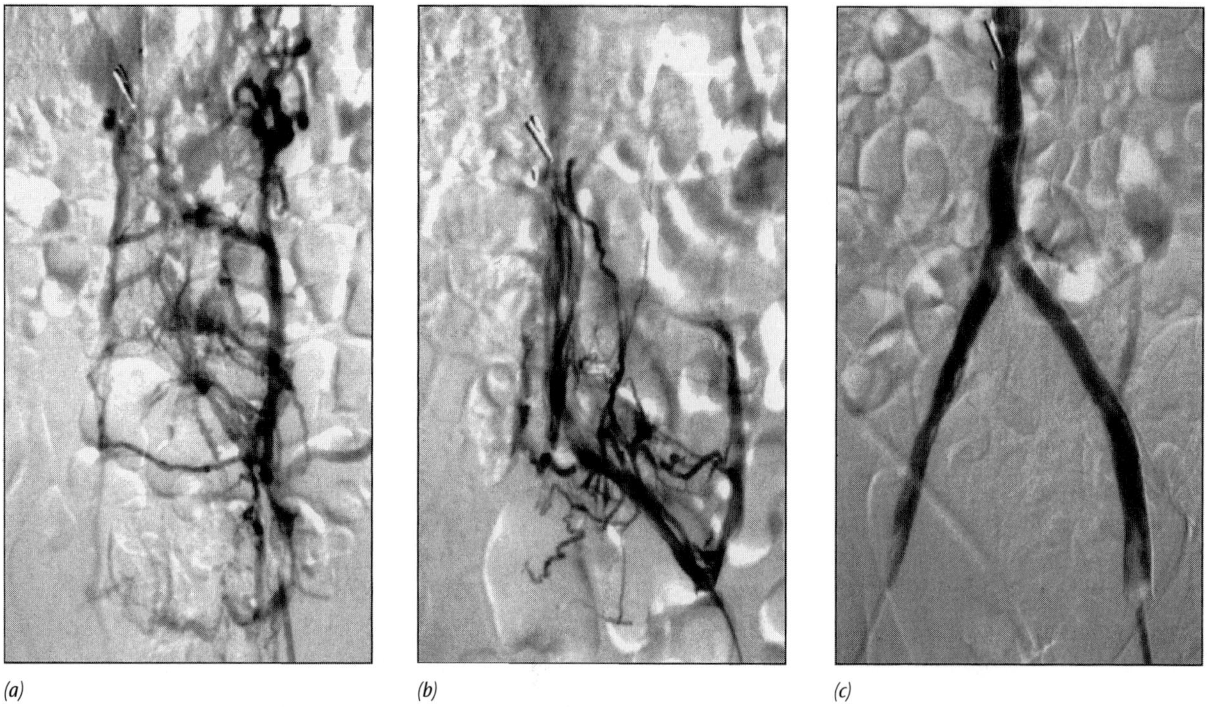

Figure 35.3 *Iliocaval occlusion. (a) Bilateral iliac and caval occlusion in 38-year-old male with history of trauma and ATIII deficiency. (b) Caval plication performed 17 years before intervention. (c) Bilateral popliteal access for thrombolytic infusion of 3.4 million IU urokinase and placement of six 10 mm self-expanding stents.*

therapy for symptomatic chronic IVC and iliac vein occlusion. CEAP classification included C4 (3), C5 (2) and C6 (2). Prior to intervention, the mean clinical score was 10.25 and the average and median disability score was 3. All patients wore compression hosiery and were on warfarin. Three had a history of pulmonary embolus (PE) treated with a filter (1), a DeWeese caval plication (1) and caval ligation (1). One patient had a prophylactic filter placed prior to back surgery. One patient had popliteal transposition valvuloplasty, another underwent a Palma bypass previously. The etiology of IVC occlusion was post-thrombotic in all patients. All had bilateral iliac obstructions, with femoral obstruction in 10 limbs. One presented with acute left DVT extending from the calf to the iliac. Chronic changes were noted in the calf and popliteal regions in 5/7 (71%) patients. Reflux was documented in 11 limbs. Two patients had prior below-the-knee amputation due to stasis ulcers, and presented with nonhealing ulcers on the surviving limb.

Endovascular reconstruction of the occluded iliac and IVC segments was accomplished in all patients. The median length of stay was 8 days (range 6–15 days). Urokinase was used in six patients and a combination of urokinase and rt-PA was used in one. The average dose was 8.8 million IU infused over 48–96 hours (range 36–120 hours). The average number of stents placed was 2.8 (range 2–4). In three patients, stents extended the entire length of the IVC.

Complications related to thrombolysis included access site infection, urinary tract infection, transient hematuria and retroperitoneal and groin hematoma, in one patient each. The retroperitoneal hematoma occurred in the patient receiving rt-PA and was associated with wire perforation at the site of caval ligation. Clinical follow-up with physical examination, duplex and hemodynamic testing has been conducted for all patients for an average of 29 months (range 6–52 months). Clinical improvement was noted rapidly in all patients. The disability decreased in every patient, from 3 to 2, and in one young patient to 1 (this patient is asymptomatic and has normal venous filling index on plethysmography). The mean clinical score decreased to 3.8 following therapy (P = 0.0001). In two patients, ulcer healing occurred in <30 days, but recurred at 18 months in one, due to poor compliance with warfarin and a recurrent popliteal DVT.

Patients previously unable to work resumed gainful employment. Most of all, other meaningful activities abandoned due to exertional pain and swelling could once again be enjoyed. Long-term follow-up shows mean primary patency at 19 months and mean assisted patency at 27.3 months. Three patients have undergone re-intervention for restenosis in the left common iliac stent. In two of these, no further treatment has been necessary at 1 and at 2 years. One patient, noncompliant with warfarin, experienced recurrent popliteal DVT; decreased flow in the stents was documented after this event.

DISCUSSION

Endovenous therapy for iliac vein or IVC thrombosis is feasible yet it is in a state of evolution. In limbs with acute thrombosis, with or without short segment iliac stenosis/occlusion, catheter-directed thrombolysis can effectively remove thrombus and thereby restore flow and limit valve injury. Stenting appears to effectively treat iliac compression and venous stenosis much better than angioplasty alone. In patients with little or no residual obstruction, flow is generally adequate to promote long-term iliac stent patency, even without warfarin.[40,49]

Chronic venous occlusive disease is technically more challenging to treat. It takes longer to complete the procedure and attention must be focused on creating continuity of flow within the limb to optimize venous drainage. Just as success in arterial revascularization procedures often depends on the state of distal runoff, so the fate of iliac vein revascularization relies upon inflow. Neglect of distal inflow status, i.e. tibial and popliteal veins, can result in compromised deep venous flow, which jeopardizes stent patency. As Bjarnason *et al.* acknowledged,[54] failure to adequately restore flow in the superficial femoral vein poses a threat to iliac patency. However, we share their impression that superficial femoral vein lysis is most successful when performed with acute thrombus during the first episode of DVT. Chronic SFV occlusion is more difficult to correct than chronic iliac obstruction. Again, the status of the tibial and popliteal veins is not insignificant in any of these patients, as demonstrated by those who remain very symptomatic with distal disease only despite normal appearing proximal venous segments.

The higher long-term patency rates in the Creighton series, despite the extensive disease in many patients, can be explained in two ways. First is initial attention to distal inflow. A pedal phlebogram is performed in all patients to assess the flow pattern in the entire leg. Re-established flow in the thigh and pelvis can fail if tibio-popliteal veins remain occluded. Distal thrombotic obstruction is simultaneously treated with flow-directed thrombolysis during all catheter-directed procedures. Also, femoral stenoses are treated with angioplasty and/or stent if they are hemodynamically significant. Stasis and persistence of dominant collaterals indicate this. If there is a pullback pressure differential of >5 mmHg, above and below a stenosis, we may consider placement of an additional stent.

Second, patients are maintained on long-term warfarin diligently monitored by the endovascular service. Patients are encouraged to be involved and to understand anti-coagulation. Most of the Creighton patients have extensive evidence of distal post-thrombotic change. When patients have no prior history or evidence of DVT, iliac stents appear to remain patent without long-term oral anticoagulation. Neglen and Raju, for example, maintain their patients on aspirin, not warfarin.[40] At Creighton, since placement of the first iliac stents in 1993, more complications (re-thrombosis) have occurred due to subtherapeutic anticoagulation than due to excessive anticoagulation. One bleeding complication occurred in a 40-year-old patient taking Zyban (Catalytica Pharmaceutical, Greenville, NC, USA) an anti-smoking medication. This spontaneous elbow hemarthrosis resolved without sequelae.

CONCLUSION

Endovascular therapy for chronic iliac vein or IVC thrombosis is focused on restoring patency by thrombus removal, angioplasty or stent placement, to treat the obstructive component of venous hypertension. Several successful series have been reported but standard reporting guidelines are still sorely absent in the literature. However, the evolution of endovascular therapy has engendered respect for the complexity of venous disease. Treatment of chronic obstructive disease makes us keenly aware of how much this condition adversely affects a patient's quality of life. Not surprisingly, those who have undergone successful revascularization, with the tools and techniques discussed in this chapter, are the strongest advocates for endovascular therapy.

REFERENCES

1. Gardiner G, Koltin W, Kandarpa K, *et al.* Thrombolysis of occluded femoropopliteal grafts. *Am J Roentgenol* 1986; **147**: 621–6.
2. Durham J, Geller S, Abbott W, *et al.* Regional infusion of urokinase into occluded lower extremity bypass grafts: long-term clinical results. *Radiology* 1989; **172**: 83–7.
3. Ouriel K, Shortell C, DeWeese J, *et al.* A comparison of thrombolytic therapy with operative revascularization in the initial treatment of acute peripheral arterial ischemia. *J Vasc Surg* 1995; **21**: 26–34.
4. Browse NL, Thomas ML, Pim HP. Streptokinase and deep vein thrombosis. *Br Med J* 1968; **3**: 717–20.
5. Meissner AJ, Misiak A, Ziemski JM, *et al.* Hazards of thrombolytic therapy in deep vein thrombosis. *Br J Surg* 1987; **74**: 991–3.
6. McNamara TO, Goodwin SC, Kandarpa K. Complications of thrombolysis. *Semin Interv Radiol* 1994; **11**: 134–44.
7. Sigwart U, Puel J, Mirkovitch V, *et al.* Intravascular stents to prevent occlusion and restenosis after angioplasty. *N Engl J Med* 1987; **316**: 701–6.
8. Sharafuddin MJA, Hicks ME. Current status of percutaneous mechanical thrombectomy. *J Vasc Interv Radiol* 1997; **8**: 911–21.

9. Okrent D, Messersmith R, Buckman J. Transcatheter fibrinolytic therapy and angioplasty for left iliofemoral thrombosis. *J Vasc Interv Radiol* 1991; **2**: 195–200.
10. Molina JE, Hunter DW, Yedlicka JW. Thrombolytic therapy for iliofemoral venous thrombosis. *Vasc Surg* 1992; **26**: 630–7.
11. Semba CP, Dake MD. Iliofemoral deep venous thrombosis: aggressive therapy with catheter-directed thrombolysis. *Radiology* 1994; **191**: 487–94.
12. Porter JM, Moneta GL. International consensus committee on chronic venous disease. Reporting standards in venous disease: an update. *J Vasc Surg* 1995; **21**: 635–45.
13. Kistner RL. Definitive diagnosis and definitive treatment in chronic venous disease: a concept whose time has come. *J Vasc Surg* 1996; **24**: 703–10.
14. Raju S. New approaches to the diagnosis and treatment of venous obstruction. *J Vasc Surg* 1986; **4**: 42–54.
15. Illig KA, Oriel K, DeWeese JA, *et al.* Increasing the sensitivity of the diagnosis of chronic venous obstruction. *J Vasc Surg* 1996; **24**: 176–8.
16. McNamara TO, Chen JL, Temmins CJ, *et al.* Complications associated with use of rt-PA vs Retavase during thrombolysis of peripheral arteries and veins (abstract). *J Vasc Interv Radiol* 2000; **11**(2): 301.
17. Semba CP, Bakal CW, Karim AC, *et al.* Alteplase as an alternative to urokinase. *J Vasc Interv Radiol* 2000; **11**: 279–87.
18. Mewissen MW, Seabrooke GR, Meissner MH, *et al.* Catheter-directed thrombolysis for lower extremity deep vein thrombosis: report of a multi-center registry. *Radiology* 1999; **211**: 39–49.
19. Mohrman DE, Heller LJ. Homeostasis and cardiovascular transport. In Hefta J, Melvin S, eds. *Cardiovascular Physiology*, 4th edn. New York: McGraw-Hill, 1997: 1–8.
20. Ginsburg R, Thorpe P, Bowles CR, Wright AM, Wexler L. Total iliac occlusions: pull-through technique for establishing access for balloon angioplasty. *Radiology* 1989; **172**: 111.
21. Dyet JF, Watts WJ, Ettles DF, *et al.* Mechanical properties of metallic stents: how do these properties influence the choice of stent for specific lesions? *Cardiovasc Interv Radiol* 2000; **23**: 47–54.
22. Zollikofer C, Largiader I, Bruhlmann WF. Endovascular stenting of veins and grafts: preliminary clinical experience. *Radiology* 1988; **167**: 707–12.
23. Charnsangavej C, Carrasco CH, Wallace S, *et al.* Stenosis of the vena cava: preliminary assessment of treatment with expandable metallic stents. *Radiology* 1986; **161**: 295–8.
24. Sawada S, Fujiwara Y, Koyama T, *et al.* Application of expandable metallic stents to the venous system. *Acta Radiol* 1992; **33**: 156–9.
25. El Feghaly M, Soula P, Rousseau H, *et al.* Endovascular retrieval of two migrated venous stents by means of balloon catheters. *J Vasc Surg* 1998; **28**: 541–56.
26. Slonim SM, Dake MD, Rasavi MK, *et al.* Management of misplaced or migrated endovascular stents. *J Vasc Interv Radiol* 1999; **10**: 851–9.
27. Duprat G, Wright KC, Charnsangavej C, *et al.* Self-expanding metallic stents for small vessels: an experimental evaluation. *Radiology* 1987; **162**: 469–72.
28. Duprat G, Wright KC, Charnsangavej C, *et al.* Flexible balloon-expanded stent for small vessels. *Radiology* 1987; **162**: 276–8.
29. Nazarian GK, Austin WT, Wegryn AS. Venous recanalization by metallic stents after failure of balloon angioplasty or surgery: four-year experience. *Cardiovasc Interv Radiol* 1996; **19**: 227–33.
30. Mickley V, Schwagierek R, Rilinger N. Left iliac venous thrombosis caused by venous spur: treatment with thrombectomy and stent implantation. *J Vasc Surg* 1998; **28**: 942–97.
31. Verhaeghe R, Stockx L, Lacroix H, Vermylen J, Baert AL. Catheter-directed lysis of iliofemoral vein thrombosis with use of rt-PA. *Eur Radiol* 1997; **7**: 996–1001.
32. Cockett FB, Thomas ML. The iliac compression syndrome. *Br J Surg* 1965; **52**: 816–21.
33. Jaszczak P, Mathiesen FR. The iliac compression syndrome. *Acta Chir Scand* 1978; **144**: 133–6.
34. Moller JW, Eickhoff JH, Buchhardt Hansen HJ, *et al.* The iliac compression syndrome. *Acta Chir Scand* 1989; **502**: 141–5.
35. McMurrich JP. The valves of the iliac vein. *Br Med J* 1906; **2**: 1699–700.
36. McMurrich JP. The occurrence of congenital adhesions in the common iliac veins, and their relation to thrombosis of the femoral and iliac veins. *Am J Med Sci* 1908; **135**: 342–6.
37. Ehrich WE, Krumbhaar EB. A frequent obstructive anomaly of the mouth of the left common iliac vein. *Am Heart J* 1943; **26**: 737–50.
38. May R, Thurner J. The cause of the predominantly sinistral occurrence of thrombosis of the pelvic veins. *Angiology* 1957; **8**: 419–27.
39. Negus D, Fletcher EW, Cockett FB, Thomas ML. Compression and band formation at the mouth of the left common iliac vein. *Br J Surg* 1968; **55**(5): 369–74.
40. Neglen P, Raju S. Balloon dilatation and stenting of chronic iliac vein obstruction: technical aspects and early clinical outcome. *J Endovasc Ther* 2000; **7**: 79–91.
41. Zollikofer CL, Antonucci F, Stuckmann G, *et al.* Use of the Wallstent in the venous system including hemodialysis-related stenoses. *Cardiovasc Interv Radiol* 1992; **15**: 334–41.
42. Grenier H, Roussear H, Douws C, *et al.* External iliac vein stenosis after segmental pancreatic transplantation: treatment by percutaneous endoprosthesis. *Cardiovasc Interv Radiol* 1993; **16**(3): 186–8.
43. Berger A, Jaffe JW, York TNN. Iliac compression syndrome treated with stent placement. *J Vasc Surg* 1995; **21**: 510–14.
44. Vorwerk D, Guenther RW, Wendt G, *et al.* Iliocaval stenosis and iliac venous thrombosis in retroperitoneal fibrosis: percutaneous treatment by use of hydrodynamic thrombectomy and stenting. *Cardiovasc Interv Radiol* 1996; **19**: 40–2.

45. Rilinger N, Gorisch J, Mickley V, *et al.* Endovascular stenting in patients with iliac compression syndrome: experience in three cases. *Invest Radiol* 1996; **31**: 729–33.
46. LaHei ER, Appleberg M, Roche J. Surgical thrombectomy and stent placement for iliac compression syndrome. *Australas Radiol* 1997; **41**(3): 243–6.
47. Fearon WF, Semba CP. Iliofemoral venous thrombosis treated by catheter-directed thrombolysis, angioplasty and endoluminal stenting. *West J Med* 1998; **168**: 277–9.
48. Akesson H, Lindh M, Ivancev K, *et al.* Venous stents in chronic iliac vein occlusions. *Eur J Vasc Endovasc Surg* 1997; **13**(3): 334–6.
49. Henderson AM, McIntyre KE, Hunter G, *et al.* May–Thurner syndrome: three patients treated with catheter-directed thrombolysis and stent placement. *Vasc Surg* 1998; **32**(5): 439–46.
50. Heniford TB, Senleer SO, Olsoffka JM, *et al.* May–Thurner syndrome: management with endovascular surgical techniques. *Ann Vasc Surg* 1998; **12**: 482–6.
51. Binkert CA, Schoch E, Stuckmann G, *et al.* Treatment of pelvic spur (May–Thurner syndrome) with self-expanding metallic endoprostheses. *Cardiovasc Interv Radiol* 1998; **21**: 22–6.
52. Mickley V, Friedrich JM, Huttschenreiter S, *et al.* Long-term results of percutaneous transluminal angioplasty and stent implantation in venous stenoses following transfemoral thrombectomy. *Vasa* 1993; **2**(1): 44–52.
53. Buelens C, Vandenbosch G, Stockx L, *et al.* Cockett's syndrome: initial results with percutaneous treatment in 6 patients. *J Belg Radiol* 1996; **79**: 132–5.
54. Bjarnason H, Kruse JR, Asinger DA, *et al.* Iliofemoral deep venous thrombosis: safety and efficacy outcome during 5 years of catheter-directed thrombolytic therapy. *J Vasc Interv Radiol* 1997; **8**: 405–18.
55. Blattler W, Blattler IK. Relief of obstructive pelvic venous symptoms with endoluminal stenting. *J Vasc Surg* 1999; **29**(3): 484–8.
56. Thorpe PE. Endovascular therapy for chronic venous obstruction. In Ballard JL, Began JJ, eds. *Chronic Venous Insufficiency.* New York: Springer, 1999: 179–219.
57. Thorpe PE. Endovascular therapy for chronic venous occlusion. *J Endovasc Surg* 1999; **6**: 118–19.
58. Thorpe PE, Osse FJ, Dang HP. Evaluating and treating chronic lower extremity venous obstruction: endovascular tools and techniques. In press.
59. Welkie JF, Comerota AJ, Katz ML, *et al.* Hemodynamic deterioration in chronic venous disease. *J Vasc Surg* 1992; **16**: 733–40.
60. Gloviczki P, Pairolero PC, Toomey BJ, *et al.* Reconstruction of large veins for non-malignant venous occlusive disease. *J Vasc Surg* 1992; **16**: 750–61.
61. Razavi MK, Hansch EC, Kee ST, *et al.* Chronically occluded inferior venae cavae: endovascular treatment. *Radiology* 2000; **214**: 133–8.

36

Autogenous venous bypass grafts for chronic iliac or infrainguinal venous occlusive disease

STEPHEN G LALKA

In appropriately selected patients, estimated to be one-third of those having deep venous insufficiency with a predominantly obstructive component documented by venography and a hemodynamically significant pressure gradient, reconstructive surgery alone or in combination with standard ablative surgical (i.e. perforator ligation) and non-surgical (i.e. compression therapy) modalities may provide dramatic symptomatic relief.[1]

ETIOLOGY

Of patients with chronic venous disease, only 10–30% have predominantly chronic venous obstruction. The vast majority of these cases result from absent or incomplete recanalization after deep vein thrombosis. Post-traumatic occlusion can also affect any segment of the venous system. Non-thrombotic proximal outflow obstruction at the iliofemoral level can be due to iatrogenic operative injury, pelvic tumor ingrowth or extrinsic compression, irradiation sequelae, retroperitoneal fibrosis, or left common iliac vein compression from the overlying right common iliac artery with or without associated intraluminal adhesions.

PATHOLOGIC ANATOMY AND PHYSIOLOGY

If chronic occlusion is the end point of venous thrombosis, collateral veins develop around the area of occlusion (Fig. 36.1). The extent of collateral venous circulation decreases as the site of venous obstruction becomes more cephalad. Even if well-developed collaterals are present, these vessels have a higher resistance to flow than the native veins and rarely contain competent valves.[2] Venographically documented anatomic obstruction does not correlate with functional obstruction to venous outflow: resting venous hypertension, exacerbated by increased venous flow with exercise, can exist with obstruction, whereas normal pressures may be obtained in other patients with similarly obstructed venous outflow. Therefore, hemodynamically significant, symptomatic venous outflow obstruction is the result of inadequate quantity and/or quality of collateral formation.

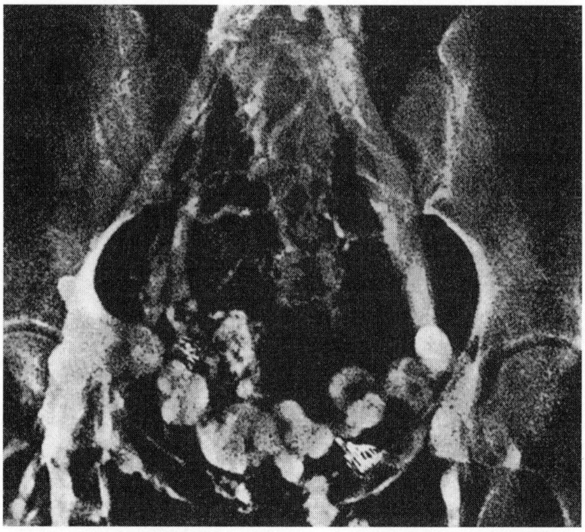

Figure 36.1 *Chronic right iliofemoral occlusion with cross-pelvic venous collaterals.*

Non-thrombotic chronic obstructive venous disease occurs less frequently than post-thrombotic occlusion. Trauma or iatrogenic surgical injury can cause short-segment venous occlusion. If there are sufficient collaterals around the obstruction, symptoms will be minimal. Irradiation, malignant disease, and retroperitoneal fibrosis often involve long segments and tend to obliterate potential collaterals. In these cases, obstructive symptoms may be severe. However, some large retroperitoneal tumors with extensive compression of the iliac veins and the inferior vena cava (IVC) may be asymptomatic due to their relatively slow growth allowing time for development of a profuse collateral circuit.[3]

Another mechanism of chronic lower extremity venous obstruction is the iliac compression syndrome (May–Thurner syndrome). The 3:1 predominance of left-sided iliofemoral thrombosis is explained by the peculiar anatomic relationship of the left iliac vein to the overlying right common iliac artery in its course along the pelvic brim. In addition to the extraluminal compression of the vein, fibrous adhesions or 'webs' may develop within the lumen at the site of compression and produce intraluminal obstruction by binding the anterior and posterior walls of the vessel together.[4]

Three rare, non-thrombotic forms of chronic lower extremity venous obstructive symptoms caused by extravascular anatomic abnormalities are compression of the femoral vein (Gullmo syndrome), popliteal vascular entrapment, and the soleal arch syndrome described by Servelle.[5] However, these may be of more venographic than physiological significance. If they are found to be physiologically relevant, surgical therapy involves simple correction of the extravascular pathology.

The underlying pathophysiology in all forms of chronic lower extremity venous obstruction is chronic venous hypertension. With significant deep venous obstruction as a component of chronic venous disease, the normal fall in ambulatory venous pressure is compromised. Indeed, with the most severe form of proximal venous obstruction associated with poorly developed collaterals, venous pressure may actually increase during exercise as outflow is impeded (Fig. 36.2).

DIAGNOSIS

The two most common signs and symptoms of segmental venous occlusive disease of the lower extremity are edema and pain on ambulation. The edema resulting from proximal venous obstruction involves the entire lower extremity and is usually greater than that in patients with valvular incompetence alone. Those who experience severe swelling within 2–4 hours of standing are distinguished as having a much more serious degree of venous insufficiency than those with lesser amounts of swelling noticed only at the end of the day. An occasional patient with only partial proximal obstruction may have episodic edema.

Comparison between patients with valvular incompetence and those with outflow obstruction has shown that swelling of the affected limb in the latter group is usually less important to the patient than the exercise-induced calf pain. The pain pattern of chronic obstructive venous disease is characteristic, described by the patient as a 'bursting, stretching ache' with forceful

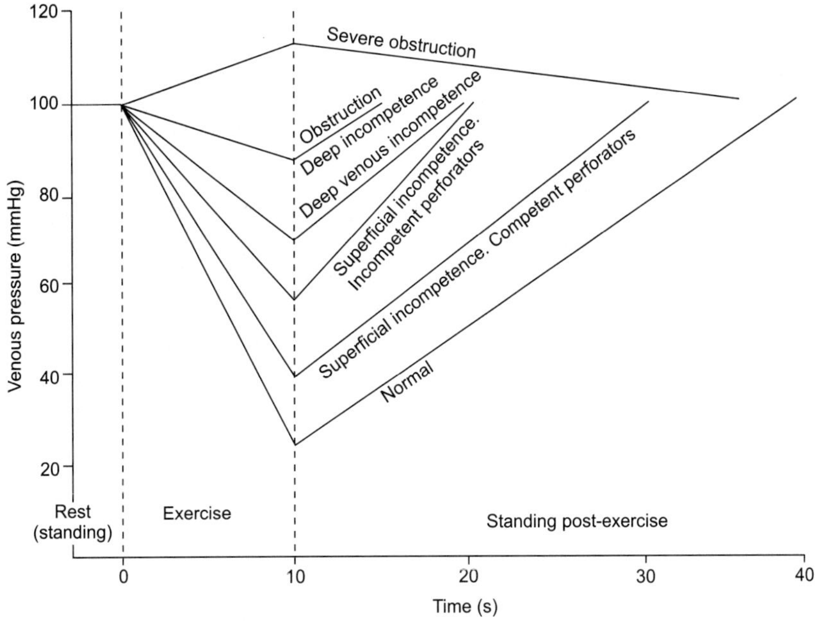

Figure 36.2 *Ambulatory venous pressure measurements in normal and diseased states.*

exertion. Patients with valvular incompetence alone often complain of 'aching' or 'heaviness' in the thigh or calf but not of pain sufficient to limit activity. Because this bursting pain develops after exercise and requires the patient to be off his or her feet to obtain relief, it has been termed 'venous claudication'. The claudication is less severe than with arterial disease, with patients having a usual walking limit of 514 ± 225 m; it may occur sooner after climbing or running. In addition, venous claudication may be accompanied by the appearance of cyanosis, a sensation of further swelling, and increased prominence of the superficial veins of the thigh. The pain in venous claudication is caused by increased intramuscular pressure as blood is propelled cephalad by the calf muscle pump against an outflow obstruction.[6]

The various noninvasive diagnostic tests used to evaluate patients with symptomatic chronic venous disease are discussed in detail in preceding chapters. If the noninvasive tests indicate significant obstructive venous disease, venous pressure studies and venography are mandatory before reconstructive surgical intervention. Ascending venography through the foot is designed to visualize the venous system distal to the inguinal ligament. Ascending and descending femoral venography (via ipsilateral, contralateral, or brachial approaches) is then performed to assess the entire iliocaval system for patency and to identify extraluminal compression or intraluminal webs (Fig. 36.3). Under fluoroscopy in the 65° erect position, the valvular competence of the infrainguinal veins in the affected limb is also assessed.

Cannulation of the common femoral vein allows measurement of iliac and femoral venous pressures.[7] By measurement of pressure gradients across intraluminal defects, partial obstruction of hemodynamic significance can be identified (Fig. 36.4). With simultaneous bilateral supine femoral pressure measurements, the hemodynamic significance of an iliofemoral obstruction is better delineated. A significant obstruction exists with a vertical gradient of greater than 2 mmHg at rest or if the horizontal gradient (compared with contralateral femoral pressure) exceeds 2 mmHg. Exercise pressures can be measured with a pedal ergometer or during postpneumatic tourniquet hyperemia while the patient remains supine to detect subcritical partial obstruction that is magnified by the increase in venous flow. With this method, an exercise venous pressure increase (from resting level) of greater than 3 mmHg indicates a significant proximal obstructive lesion. To reiterate, venographic venous obstruction is not necessarily associated with functional venous obstruction, as can be shown by these pressure studies.

Raju[8] has greatly refined the use of venous pressure measurements in the diagnosis of chronic obstructive venous disease. With the patient in the supine position, venous pressure is simultaneously measured in the dorsum of the foot and hand, and a resting arm–foot

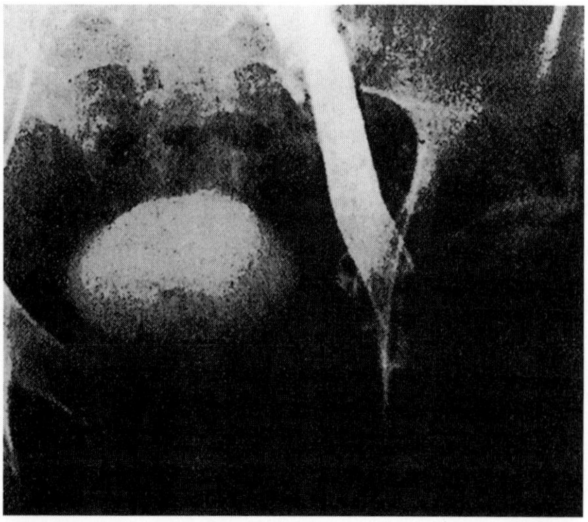

Figure 36.3 *Retrograde cannulation of the left common iliac vein from the right. Injection of contrast agent is coupled with a Valsalva maneuver to demonstrate intraluminal obstruction of the left common femoral vein. The arrow points to the rounded clot within the lumen.*

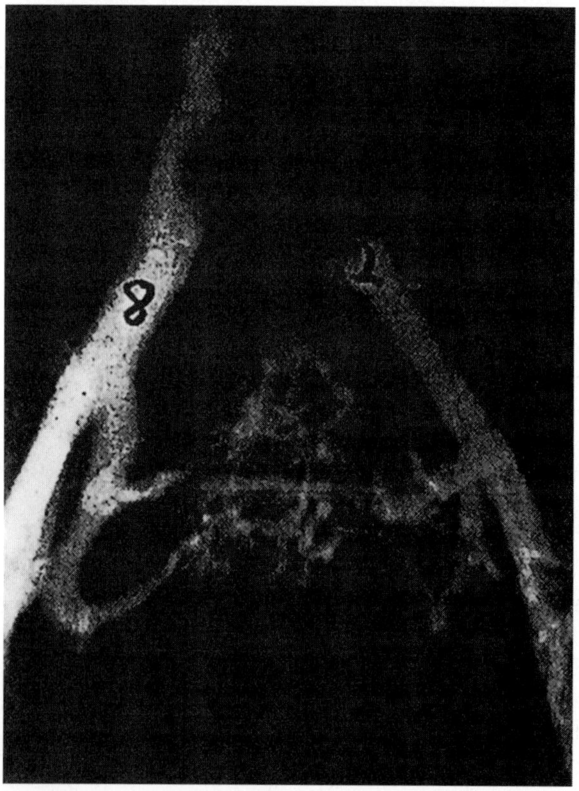

Figure 36.4 *Phlebogram of a young woman with long-standing edema of the left lower extremity. Near-total obstruction by the right iliac artery and development of numerous collateral channels through the presacral plexus are evident. The superimposed numbers represent the manometric determinations at supine rest, indicating a horizontal gradient of 5 cmH_2O.*

venous pressure differential is obtained. Next, a thigh cuff is inflated to 300 mmHg for 3 minutes and then released. This causes a foot venous pressure elevation due to the increased venous flow stimulated by reactive hyperemia. An arm–foot differential of greater than 4 mmHg and a foot venous pressure elevation of greater than 6 mmHg were found to be abnormal.[8] Raju described grades of pressure measurements that determine physiologic significance of the extent of collateralization seen on the venogram:

- grade I (fully compensated): normal arm–foot venous pressure differential without significant increase in foot pressure with stress (in this group, hemodynamic function was normal despite venographically documented obstruction, due to hemodynamically adequate collaterals);
- grade II (partially compensated): normal arm–foot differential with abnormal response to reactive hyperemia (indicating that the collaterals were adequate at rest but insufficient during increased flow);
- grade III (partially decompensated): abnormal arm–foot differential and abnormal response to hyperemia;
- grade IV (totally decompensated): abnormally elevated arm–foot differential and absent reactive hyperemia-induced venous pressure increase (due to severely inadequate collaterals even at rest; with maximum venous filling of the limb due to the venous outflow obstruction, elevated pressure at the venular and capillary level prevents further inflow at the arteriolar level during exercise).

Raju concluded that large profuse collaterals on venograms can be hemodynamically inadequate owing to the presence of stenosis or other high-resistance areas not readily identified venographically.[8] Such precise venous pressure studies are necessary to identify which patients will benefit from venous reconstructive surgery. Postoperatively, such pressure studies are required to assess the efficacy of various therapeutic modalities.

Without documentation of hemodynamically significant venous obstruction, reconstructive surgery should not be undertaken because it is doomed to failure. The lack of a sufficient pressure differential between the diseased inflow segment and the normal outflow segment of a proposed bypass graft will result in inadequate flow through the bypass conduit, resulting in graft thrombosis after closure of the adjunctive arteriovenous fistula (AVF). The minimum values of physiologic significance mentioned previously (2–3 mmHg) are not sufficient to subject a patient to reconstructive surgery. A review of the available data suggests that venous reconstructive surgery has an excellent chance of success with a preoperative pressure differential >10 mmHg, a good chance of success with a differential of 4–10 mmHg, and a poor success rate if the measured gradient is <4 mmHg. Similarly, reconstructive surgery would be indicated, with a good chance of success, if the exercise/hyperemia-induced change in pressure in the diseased limb exceeded 6 mmHg.[9]

SURGICAL MANAGEMENT

In the management of chronic venous disease, the goals are to treat the presenting symptoms and to prevent the adverse effects of continued venous hypertension on the skin and subcutaneous tissues by restoring the venous physiology of the limb to as normal a state as possible. Conservative treatment with elastic compression stockings and elevation of the legs remains the first line of management and will be adequate for the overwhelming majority of patients with chronic venous disease. When obstructive venous insufficiency is documented, venous reconstructive surgery must be preceded or supplemented by standard ablative surgery, such as ligation of incompetent perforating veins with ulcer excision and skin grafting, as venous bypass surgery alone cannot adequately palliate a patient with multiple mechanisms/sites of venous pathology.

Based on the CEAP classification,[10] for patients with class 4–6 chronic venous disease or class 3 disease (edema without skin pathology) with livelihood-/lifestyle-limiting venous claudication, who have failed aggressive treatment with compression stockings, elevation, and standard ablative therapy, venous reconstructive surgery should be considered and the diagnostic plan as outlined previously should be instituted.[1,11] The number of patients with chronic venous insufficiency who are suitable candidates for deep venous reconstruction for obstructive pathology range from 1% to 3%.[1,12,13]

Cross-femoral venous bypass

Segmental venous obstruction of the iliofemoral system can be bypassed by a crossover femoral vein–femoral vein graft. This is the most frequently performed reconstruction procedure for chronic obstructive venous disease.

PATIENT SELECTION

The most suitable cases for a cross-femoral venous bypass involve persistent isolated unilateral iliac or common femoral vein occlusions in young and middle-aged patients with class 3–6 (as above) chronic deep venous insufficiency unresponsive to conservative measures. The venous outflow obstruction should be venographically and hemodynamically stable or worsening and of at least 1 year's duration, suggesting that no further resolution is likely to occur by recanalization and collateralization.

Prerequisites for success of cross-femoral grafts include:[14,15]

- patent contralateral iliofemoral and caval runoff;
- the presence of a supine resting pressure gradient in excess of 4 mmHg between the femoral veins in the involved and contralateral limbs;
- an adequate distal venous system (i.e. a patent profunda femoris vein, preferably with an open or a partially recanalized superficial femoral vein);
- a patent, competent greater saphenous vein on the recipient (runoff) side with a minimal diameter of 4.5 mm and no varicosities.

Venous pressure measurements are essential to assess the functional efficacy of a reconstructive procedure; one cannot rely solely on venography, which only provides evidence of technical operability. Of patients with a post-thrombotic syndrome, 10% are operable according to venography, whereas only one-third of these patients should have reconstruction based on physiologic significance. The main technical obstacle to cross-femoral venous reconstruction is a destroyed femoral vein with multiple septa resulting from recanalization in combination with poor outflow.[1]

A second, less frequent type of candidate for cross-femoral venous bypass is a patient with the subacute onset of progressive severe leg swelling secondary to extrinsic disease affecting one iliac vein. If diagnostic studies reveal that the cause of vein compression is lymphoma, subsequent irradiation or chemotherapy may dramatically improve the extrinsic compression. If cervical, colonic, ovarian, prostatic, or bladder carcinoma is found, cross-femoral bypass should be considered after surgical management of the cancer, if survival is estimated to be at least 6 months. A bypass should also be performed if the extrinsic compression is found to be due to periadventitial scarring from prior surgery, irradiation, or retroperitoneal fibrosis. The recommendation of waiting 1 year with symptoms of venous disease before reconstruction (see above) does not apply in these subacute cases since the nature of their disease process and treatment limits the likelihood of collateral formation.

One other indication for cross-femoral bypass is in the acute limb-threatening situation of phlegmasia for which venous thrombectomy has failed to relieve the iliofemoral obstruction. The rationale behind this approach is to perform reconstruction before the patency of the thrombectomized femoral vein and the competence of its delicate valves have been irreparably damaged by post-thrombotic changes.[16]

OPERATIVE TECHNIQUE

General or spinal anesthesia can be used. Low-molecular-weight dextran (LMD) infusion (1 ml/kg over the first hour and then 25 ml/h thereafter) is begun at the start of the case.

The first step with autogenous conduit is exposure of the donor greater saphenous vein from the groin to the knee in the leg contralateral to the iliofemoral obstruction (Fig. 36.5). This vein can be rotated at the saphenofemoral junction and used as the cross-femoral conduit (classic Palma technique); if this rotation causes kinking at the saphenofemoral junction, the vein should be excised and translocated with an additional anastomosis to the 'outflow' (nondiseased) femoral vein. A vertical groin incision is then made in the affected limb for exposure of the common femoral, proximal superficial femoral, and profunda femoral veins, and the saphenofemoral junction. To avoid difficult dissection and to preserve every possible collateral, one needs to dissect only the anterior 180° of the vein in the affected limb and use a U-shaped vascular clamp to perform the anastomosis without complete dissection of the posterior aspect. In post-thrombotic proximal obstruction, the common femoral and superficial femoral veins should be dissected caudally until a patent segment is found.[17]

A subcutaneous tunnel is dissected suprapubically between the vertical groin incisions. The patient is then heparinized with a bolus of 100 units/kg (heparin monitoring with activated clotting time is advisable). An anteromedial longitudinal venotomy is made that is three times the diameter of the saphenous vein. A 2–3 mm ellipse of vein wall is removed. The femoral vein at the site of anastomosis may have intraluminal webs, resulting from recanalization, which should be excised in the area of the anastomosis. A saphenous vein is anastomosed to the affected common femoral vein either side to side (if a 'skip fistula'[1] is to be constructed) or end to side with standard vascular surgery techniques. The creation of an adjunctive arteriovenous fistula is recommended (see below).

Intraoperative and then early postoperative/predischarge venography, femoral venous pressure measurements, and duplex studies should be obtained. The heparin should not be reversed with protamine. All wounds should be closed in layers, with the placement of closed suction drains that remain for a maximum of 48 hours. Systemic LMD is continued for 72 hours. Locally delivered heparin is continued through a thin catheter introduced via a branch of the superficial femoral vein or profunda femoris, or even a tributary of the AVF, with the catheter end placed opposite the inflow anastomosis (this catheter may be used for intraoperative and postoperative (pre-discharge) venography[18]). This local heparin irrigation is begun at 400 units/h and slowly increased until the PTT exceeds 1.5 normal at 48 hours. The LMD can be discontinued the next day when the heparin has been increased to achieve a PTT of 2–2.5 times normal. Sodium warfarin is begun when the patient is adequately anticoagulated with heparin and is continued as long as the graft is patent. Heparin is stopped after 4 days of concomitant heparin and

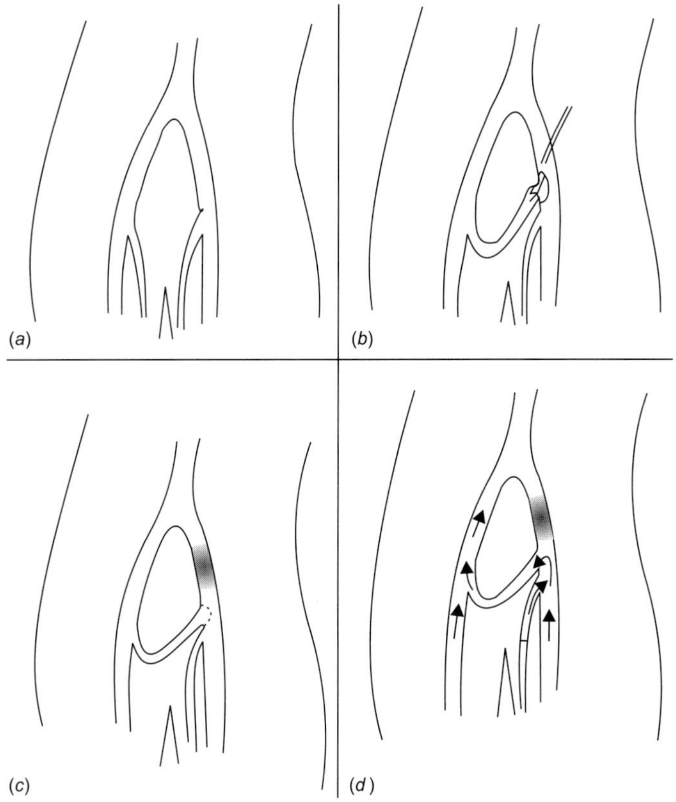

Figure 36.5 *Technique of crossover saphenous vein graft. (a) The left iliofemoral segment is obstructed. (b) The contralateral competent saphenous vein has been passed subcutaneously across the pubis to the left groin. (c) An end-to-side anastomosis has been completed. (d) Venous flow from the left leg crosses through the graft to the right iliac system.*

warfarin therapy if the international normalized ratio exceeds 2.5. An intermittent pneumatic compression device is used to increase lower extremity venous flow during the entire perioperative period. After 72 hours at bed rest, the patient ambulates wearing graded elastic compression stockings which are worn daily until the AVF is closed.[1]

For acute iliofemoral venous thrombosis, Eklof[16] obtains a cannula venogram the day after iliofemoral thrombectomy (with arteriovenous fistula). If this shows complete obstruction of the iliac vein with poor collateral capacity and the leg is severely swollen, the obstructed leg is revascularized acutely with femoro-femoral crossover bypass grafting with flow augmented by the previously constructed arteriovenous fistula. Anticoagulation is continued as long as the graft is patent. The arteriovenous fistula is maintained for a much longer time than after thrombectomy (as long as 26 months in one case in which the graft remained patent at the 36-month follow-up visit).[16]

RESULTS

After discharge, graft patency can be assessed by duplex scanning at 1 month and then every 3 months for the first year. If there is some question of patency by duplex, magnetic resonance venography or radionuclide venography can be obtained during this time. After 1 year, conventional contrast venograms can be obtained with a low risk of graft thrombosis; this can be correlated with duplex scanning and the patient should then be followed noninvasively every 6 months for life, with a low threshold for venography if there is a suspicion of a failing graft on duplex. To evaluate venous graft patency while an adjunctive temporary arteriovenous fistula remains open, magnetic resonance venography is useful for determining patency but cannot delineate areas of stenosis. For conventional venography in such cases, simple foot venipuncture, temporary lower extremity venous occlusion with a thigh cuff during injection of contrast, and digital subtraction angiography during and after release of the cuff are used to opacify the graft with a rapid bolus of contrast. Venography appears to be a more reliable method of postoperative follow-up of cross-femoral grafts than duplex scanning because of the difficulty in distinguishing between a patent graft and the normal flow produced by a well-developed venous collateral circuit when using noninvasive imaging.[16,19]

In a thoroughly evaluated clinical series, involving 47 patients who underwent cross-femoral venous bypass, Halliday and associates[19] found that 89% of the grafts were clinically patent at 5 years, compared with a 75% cumulative venographic patency. The patients whose grafts were incorrectly thought to be patent clinically were shown to have either large venous collaterals or recanalized iliac veins on venography. The authors proposed that although recanalization of the iliac venous segment was uncommon, a slowly occluding cross-femoral graft may allow sufficient time for recanalization to occur silently or for collaterals to develop, so that the improvement gained with the bypass graft was not completely lost. In this series, most patients with disabling venous claudication had relief of their symptoms, but return of their complaints suggested a stenosing graft, which was confirmed by venography. Those patients with minimal post-thrombotic changes in the calf but with disabling symptoms during exercise had the best clinical response to surgery. Resolution of venous ulceration was correlated with graft patency. Twenty-four patients with moderate-to-severe symptoms without ulceration did not require further surgical treatment to control their venous disease. There were no wound infections or hematomas, 6% had recurrent venous thrombosis, and there was a 2% incidence of post-bypass pulmonary embolism. There was no documented recanalization of an occluded graft in their series. They documented dilation of the autogenous bypass conduit over time, suggesting that the valves in the transposed saphenous vein segment could become incompetent secondary to the dilation.

Danza and associates[20] reported on 27 symptomatic patients with iliac vein thrombosis who underwent the standard Palma procedure (8 patients) or a modified Palma technique using a free femorofemoral saphenous vein graft (19 patients). Their modified technique avoids the torsion that may occur when the proximal saphenous vein is left attached to the femoral vein. With this modified technique, 12 patients (63%) had excellent results, four patients (21%) had good results, and three patients (16%) had no improvement. This is in contrast to the patients undergoing the standard Palma procedure, of whom only three (37.5%) had excellent results, three (37.5%) had good results, and two (25%) had poor results. Table 36.1 presents selected clinical reports that provide long-term follow-up information, including hemodynamic and anatomic evaluation of efficacy.[21–25]

Saphenopopliteal bypass

Venous reconstructive surgery to transpose the saphenous vein into the popliteal vein in order to bypass isolated occlusion of the femoropopliteal segment is based on the principle that the calf muscle pump acts almost exclusively on the deep venous system to empty the leg. Thus, a new outflow connecting the deep system distally and proximally should provide relief from obstructive venous hypertension.

PATIENT SELECTION

Saphenopopliteal bypass is performed rarely and only if the following six conditions are met:

- there is isolated occlusion of the superficial femoral vein, the popliteal vein, or both in the presence of tibial veins (inflow) patent at least to the level of major popliteal tributaries;
- the common femoral and iliocaval systems (outflow) must be patent;
- the patient has a patent non-varicosed saphenous vein with competent valves unaffected by previous phlebitis (this is the most significant factor that precludes this reconstructive option); if the ipsilateral saphenous is unsuitable, the contralateral saphenous may be used as the bypass conduit;
- femoral phlebitis has been inactive for at least one year;
- elevated ambulatory venous pressure exists (see above); for example, after exercise (10 tiptoes or 10 knee bends), venous pressure on the occluded side should not drop by more than one third of the erect resting pressure on the contralateral side;
- compression and ablative surgery have failed to relieve severe symptoms of deep venous insufficiency.

The diagnostic evaluation should be the same as for a cross-femoral bypass, including noninvasive testing as well as venography and venous pressure studies.[1] Because of the stringent inclusion/exclusion criteria, saphenopopliteal bypass is performed much less frequently than cross-femoral bypass.

OPERATIVE TECHNIQUE

With the patient under either general or spinal anesthesia and with LMD begun at the start of the case, a medial incision is made in the proximal calf posterior to the medial border of the tibia, and the saphenous vein is carefully exposed without creation of a flap (Fig. 36.6). Intraoperative exposure of the saphenous vein is made

Table 36.1 *Results of autogenous cross-femoral venous bypass*

Author	Year	No. patients	Follow-up (mo.)	% Clinical success	% Patency
Husni[21]	1978	78	7–144	74	73
Hutschenreiter[22]	1979	20	6–78	69	44
O'Donnell[23]	1987	6	24	100	100
AbuRahma[24]	1991	24	66	88	75

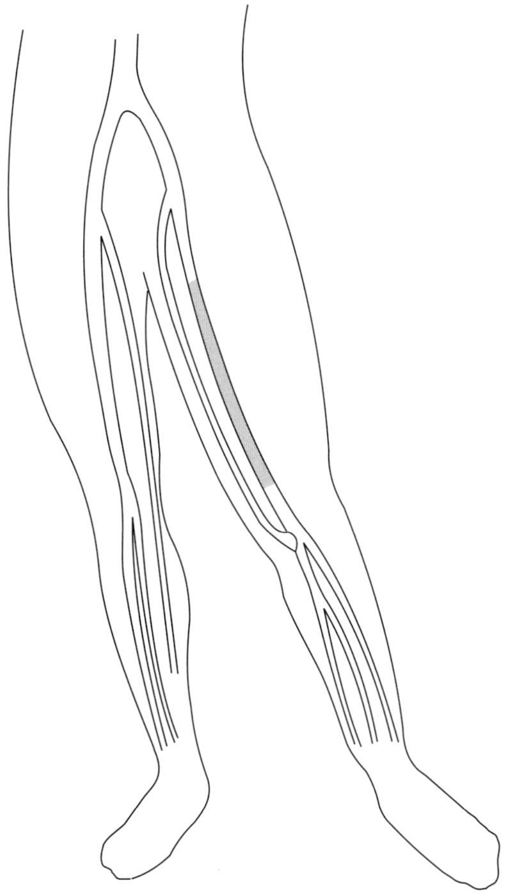

Figure 36.6 *Completed* in situ *saphenopopliteal anastomosis for superficial venous obstruction.*

easier by preoperative marking with indelible ink (using duplex imaging). The saphenous vein is mobilized over a distance of approximately 10 cm to provide enough length to allow it to lie in a gentle curve in its course to the popliteal anastomosis. Occasionally, a confluence of tibial veins just caudad to the popliteal vein is the most cephalad uninvolved segment, and the dissection must expose it as well as the popliteal vein and tibial veins. After heparin anticoagulation (as above) and control of the inflow and outflow vessels, a longitudinal venotomy three times the diameter of the saphenous vein is made in the anteromedial popliteal segment, and a 1–2 mm ellipse of vein is excised. The saphenous vein is transected only after determining the exact length required (with the knee in the extended position). The saphenous vein is carefully brought down to the recipient vein (without twisting or kinking) and anastomosed end to side to the popliteal vein. A generous window of gastrocnemius-soleus fascia is excised to avoid compression of the transposed saphenous vein conduit. An adjunctive AVF can be created using the saphenous conduit in a 'skip fistula' configuration (i.e. side-to-side anastomosis of saphenous conduit to popliteal vein then caudad end of saphenous to posterior tibial artery anastomosis). Alternatively, a separate distal leg incision can be made for a side-to-side posterior tibial AVF. Intraoperative and postoperative anticoagulation and serial graft surveillance techniques are the same as for cross-femoral bypass discussed previously. Both Bergan and coworkers[12] and Dale[17] described a side-to-side saphenopopliteal anastomosis; however, that technique is made possible only when the saphenous vein is elongated, as in the postphlebitic leg, allowing a side-to-side anastomosis without tension. Annous and Queral[26] reported 18-month patency in a case of mid-thigh superficial femoral vein occlusion for which a distal superficial femoral–greater saphenous bypass with an end-to-side anastomosis was performed. The authors believed that such a configuration had an advantage over the typical saphenopopliteal bypass because the saphenous outflow collateral pathway was not interrupted and there was redirection of the total drainage of the popliteal vein into the saphenous vein.

RESULTS

Gruss[27] reported on 14 operations (five without and nine with peripheral adjunctive arteriovenous fistulae). Of the 14 patients with standard saphenopopliteal bypass, three developed postoperative thrombosis and continued to suffer severe venous hypertension symptoms. Four patients with patent bypasses exhibited worsening of their venous pressure and volumetric curves, which reverted to preoperative levels. Seven patients with patent grafts showed lasting improvement of function 10–15 years postoperatively despite varicose degeneration in two of these grafts. Gruss emphasized two important points:

- the transposed saphenous vein can develop varicose degeneration without decreased function;
- deterioration of function can occur despite having a venographically patent bypass graft.

Table 36.2 summarizes reported clinical trials with autogenous saphenopopliteal bypass.[21,24,28] In a case report, Schanzer and Skladany[29] describe the successful combination of autogenous saphenopopliteal and cross-femoral bypasses with a distal posterior tibial–saphenous AVF, for occlusion of an external iliac vein and superficial femoral vein with preserved common femoral vein.

It should be noted that clinical success of both saphenopopliteal and cross-femoral bypass procedures is limited if patients also have severe infrainguinal valvular reflux.[24]

Raju perforator bypass

This very selectively performed bypass is intended to correct venous hypertension in cases of severe post-thrombotic syndrome causing occlusion of the popliteal vein extending into the cephalad segments of the tibial

Table 36.2 *Results of saphenopopliteal bypass*

Author	Year	No. patients	Follow-up (mo.)	% Clinical success	% Patency
Frileux[28]	1972	23	12–36	31	67
Husni[21]	1978	26	6–120	69	63
AbuRahma[24]	1991	19	66	58	56

veins. Although multiple incompetent perforating veins drain blood from the deep veins toward the greater and lesser saphenous veins, they are functionally inadequate.[8,18]

PATIENT SELECTION

The inadequate collateral function of the perforators is documented by venous pressure measurement; values >6 mmHg after reactive hyperemia are considered a functional indication for the Raju perforator bypass.[8] The saphenous vein must be patent and competent.

OPERATIVE TECHNIQUE

The greater saphenous vein in the calf is mobilized. Through the same incision, the posterior tibial vein is dissected distal to the occluded segment and below the incompetent perforators. The caudad greater saphenous is anastomosed end to side to the posterior tibial vein. Raju initially employed a distal adjunctive AVF but these had a high rate of spontaneous fistula closure.[8,18]

RESULTS

In a series of six cases, Raju[8] reported 100% long-term patency even though some grafts thrombosed in the immediate postoperative period only to recanalize later. This striking observation may be related to the high rate of spontaneous thrombolysis known to occur in the calf.[18]

Technical adjuncts to venous bypass grafting

Grafts in the venous system, either autogenous or prosthetic, do not perform as well as their counterparts in the arterial system because of several unique characteristics of the venous environment:

- a capacity for recanalization of native vessels with frequent formation of intraluminal webs;
- low intraluminal pressure;
- slow flow against a hydrostatic pressure gradient;
- low oxygen tension;
- irregular flow as a result of the phasic component and turbulence around valves;
- thin, fragile vessel walls;
- a propensity for formation of large, profuse collateral pathways that can compete with and diminish flow in an implanted graft.[1]

Consistent problems unique to autogenous grafts in the venous system are marked anastomotic stricturing as a result of the organization of excessive fibrin and platelets at the suture lines and narrowing of the entire graft due to intense perigraft fibrosis; synthetic grafts in the venous system are subject to the same anastomotic failures. Because of the thin, nonrigid, highly elastic vein walls, suture lines are under greater tension than in the arterial system; this adds to the tendency for anastomotic stricture. To prevent excessive tension, it has been necessary to interpose a graft longer than the excised vein segment.

There is unanimous agreement that the most non-thrombogenic conduit in the venous system is autogenous vein. However, controversy exists as to the preferential use of autogenous saphenous vein versus polytetrafluoroethylene (PTFE) for cross-femoral venous bypass. Saphenous vein grafts often provide inadequate symptomatic relief of venous hypertension because of the high resistance of the small saphenous vein conduit. The author and his associates developed a clinically based mathematical model of unilateral iliac vein obstruction to establish a theoretical basis for selecting saphenous vein or a larger-diameter prosthetic conduit for cross-femoral bypass.[30] Saphenous vein less than 4.5 mm diameter should not be used as a bypass conduit for cross-femoral venous revascularization due to the inability of such a small graft to relieve a hemodynamically significant iliac obstruction. Based on their data, the author and his associates believe that with such an inadequate saphenous vein, a 10 mm PTFE graft with an adjunctive AVF would be the appropriate conduit for cross-femoral venous revascularization of a unilateral iliac vein occlusion.[30]

Arteriovenous fistulae

Adjunctive arteriovenous fistulae for venous reconstructive surgery, whether used with autogenous or prosthetic conduits, improve long-term graft patency. The minimal shunt flow required to keep both the adjunctive arteriovenous fistula and the bypass graft patent appears to be at least 100 ml/min if technical errors are excluded. Fistula flows of 0.3–4.7 l/min have been reported with no adverse sequelae.[1] Various configurations of adjunctive arteriovenous fistulae have been used with venous reconstructions (Fig. 36.7).

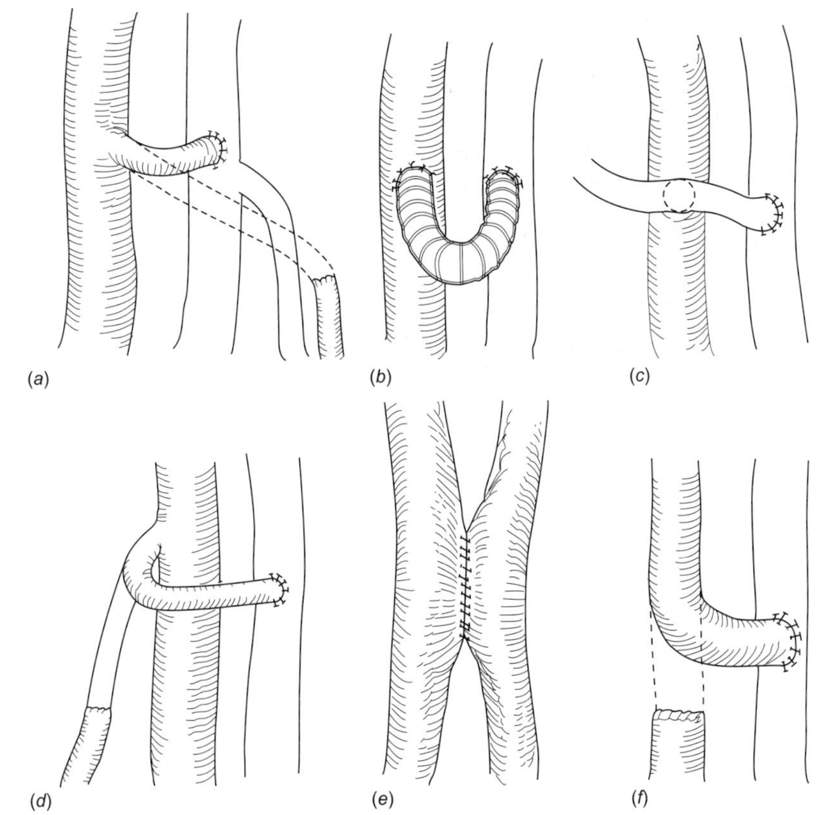

Figure 36.7 *Configurations of adjunctive arteriovenous fistulas for venous reconstruction. (a) Superficial femoral vein (SFV) tributary end to side to superficial femoral artery (SFA). (b) PTFE interposition graft between SFA and SFV. (c) Sequential or 'skip' fistula: venous bypass graft side to side to SFV and end to side to SFA. (d) Saphenous vein branch end to side to SFA ('bucket handle' configuration). (e) Side-to-side SFA to SFV fistula. (f) Distal saphenous end to side to posterior tibial artery, which is used with saphenopopliteal bypass.*

Closure of an adjunctive arteriovenous fistula has been found to be technically difficult owing to the often severe desmoplastic reaction that occurs in the vicinity of venous reconstruction. A simple technique to facilitate ligation of an arteriovenous fistula is to doubly wrap a heavy 0/0 nonabsorbable monofilament suture loosely around the body of the fistula. The two ends of suture are passed on a needle through the fascia to a subcutaneous position, where they are threaded through a button and loosely tied. The button is buried under the skin 2–3 cm medial to the vertical incision. At the time of fistula ligation, local anesthesia is used for a small skin incision over the button. The suture is untied, the button is removed, and the suture is then tied down snugly over the fascia to ligate the fistula. Wire loops have similarly been used to occlude the AVF. A percutaneous method for closure of temporary arteriovenous fistulae involves entry of the contralateral femoral artery for placement of a detachable balloon in the fistula under direct radiographic control. Before inflation and detachment of the balloon, an arteriovenogram is obtained to evaluate the patency of the venous bypass graft. After release of the balloon, a repeated angiogram documents complete obliteration of the fistula.

The timing of closure of an adjunctive arteriovenous fistula remains unsettled. The benefits of the fistula are maintenance of an increased venous pressure, prevention of the collapse of the anastomotic suture line, and elevated flow velocity, which may wash away procoagulant substances and loosely adherent platelets. Because these two thrombogenic factors should not continue to be a problem after anastomotic healing is complete, ligation of the arteriovenous fistula at 3–6 months after venous reconstruction should be appropriate. Chronic effects of late ligation include vein graft dilation (with secondary valve incompetence) and stimulation of native venous collaterals. The latter effect argues for ligation at an even later date. Arguments against prolonged maintenance of the fistula are that distal venous hypertension is created, causing peripheral edema and potentially causing caudad venous valvular incompetence or even thrombosis. In addition, cardiac output is increased, there is a continuing threat of subacute bacterial endoarteritis, and arterial ischemia may be exacerbated. These facts argue for early closure of the arteriovenous fistulae at 6 weeks.

Primary arteriovenous fistulae have been created between the femoral artery and vein and the posterior tibial and saphenous vein in patients not considered candidates for the venous bypass grafts just described.[31] This technique results in enlarged, hemodynamically significant venous collaterals which, after closure of the fistula, can alleviate venous hypertension. Therefore, in selected patients, creation of an arteriovenous fistula without venous reconstruction can occasionally be considered. One possible theoretical mechanism for the sustained effect of a temporary arteriovenous fistula is that it may take more venous pressure and flow to open or to dilate existing venous collaterals than to sustain them.

ACKNOWLEDGMENT

I am grateful to the WB Saunders Company of Philadelphia for permission to reproduce the illustrations in this chapter from Lalka (1995).[1]

REFERENCES

1. Lalka SG. Management of chronic obstructive venous disease of the lower extremity. In Rutherford R, ed. *Vascular Surgery*, 4th edn. Philadelphia: WB Saunders, 1995: 1862–82.
2. Kiliewich LA, Strandness DE Jr. The natural history of deep venous thrombosis. In Bergan JJ, Yao JST, eds. *Surgery of the Veins.* Orlando, FL: Grune & Stratton, 1985: 123–39.
3. Beck SDW, Lalka SG, Donohue JP. Long-term results after inferior vena cava resection during retroperitoneal lymphadenectomy for metastatic germ cell cancer. *J Vasc Surg* 1998; **28**: 808–14.
4. Cockett FB. Iliac vein compression – its relation to iliofemoral thrombosis and the post-thrombotic syndrome. *Br Med J* 1967; **2**: 14–19.
5. Eklof B, Juhan C. Venous compression syndromes caused by anatomical anomalies. In Eklof B, Gjores JE, Thulesias O, *et al.*, eds. *Controversies in the Management of Venous Disorders.* London: Butterworths, 1989: 291–307.
6. Qvarfordt P, Eklof B, Ohlin P, *et al.* Intramuscular pressure, blood flow, and skeletal muscle metabolism in patients with venous claudication. *Surgery* 1984; **95**: 191–5.
7. Negus D, Cockett FB. Femoral vein pressures in post-phlebitic iliac vein obstruction. *Br J Surg* 1967; **54**: 522–5.
8. Raju S. New approaches to the diagnosis and treatment of venous obstruction. *J Vasc Surg* 1986; **4**: 42–54.
9. Lalka SG, Malone JM. Surgical management of chronic obstructive venous disease of the lower extremity. *Semin Vasc Surg* 1998; **1**: 113–23.
10. Porter JM, Moneta GL, International Consensus Committee on Chronic Venous Disease. Reporting standards in venous disease: an update. *J Vasc Surg* 1995; **21**: 635–45.
11. O'Donnell TF Jr. Chronic venous insufficiency: an overview of epidemiology, classification, and anatomic consideration. *Semin Vasc Surg* 1988; **1**: 60–5.
12. Bergan JJ, Yao JST, Flinn WR, McCarthy WJ. Surgical treatment of venous obstruction and insufficiency. *J Vasc Surg* 1986; **3**: 174–81.
13. Gloviczki P, Pairolero PC. Venous reconstruction for obstruction and valvular incompetence. *Perspect Vasc Surg* 1988; **1**: 75–93.
14. Vollmar J. Reconstruction of the iliac veins and inferior vena cava. In Jobbs JT, ed. *The Treatment of Venous Disorders.* London: MTP Press, 1977: 320.
15. Lalka SG, Lash JM, Unthank JL, *et al.* Inadequacy of saphenous vein grafts for cross-femoral venous bypass. *J Vasc Surg* 1991; **13**: 622–30.
16. Eklof B. Temporary arteriovenous fistula in reconstruction of iliac vein obstruction using PTFE grafts. In Eklof B, Gjores JE, Thulesius O, *et al.*, eds. *Controversies in the Management of Venous Disorders.* London: Butterworths, 1989: 280–90.
17. Dale WA. Reconstructive venous surgery. *Arch Surg* 1979; **114**: 1312–18.
18. Gruss JD, Hiemer W. Bypass procedures for venous obstruction: Palma and May–Husni bypasses, Raju perforator bypass, prosthetic bypasses, and primary and adjunctive arteriovenous fistulae. In Raju S, Villavicencco JL, eds. *Surgical Management of Venous Disease.* Baltimore, MD: Williams & Wilkins, 1997: 289–305.
19. Halliday P, Harris J, May J. Femoro-femoral crossover grafts (Palma operation): a long-term follow-up study. In Bergan KK, Yao JST, eds. *Surgery of the Veins.* Orlando, FL: Grune & Stratton, 1985: 241–54.
20. Danza R, Navarro T, Baldizan J. Reconstructive surgery in chronic venous obstruction of the lower limbs. *J Cardiovasc Surg* 1991; **32**: 98–103.
21. Husni EA. Clinical experience with femoropopliteal venous reconstruction. In Bergan JJ, Yao, JST, eds. *Venous Problems.* Chicago: Yearbook Medical Publishers, 1978: 485–91.
22. Hutschenreiter S, Vollmar J, Leoprecht H, *et al.* Rekonstructive Eingriffe am Venensystem; Spatergebnisse unter Kritischer Bewertung funktioneller und gefassmorphologischer Kriterien. *Chirurgie* 1979; **50**: 555–63.
23. O'Donnell TF Jr, Mackey WC, Shepard AD, Callow AD. Clinical, hemodynamic and anatomic follow-up of direct venous reconstruction. *Arch Surg* 1987; **122**: 474–82.
24. AbuRahma AF, Robinson PA, Boland JP. Clinical hemodynamic and anatomic predictors of long-term outcome of lower extremity venovenous bypasses. *J Vasc Surg* 1991; **19**: 635–44.
25. Eklof BG, Kistner RL, Masuda EM. Venous bypass and valve reconstruction: long-term efficacy. *Vasc Med* 1998; **3**: 157–64.
26. Annous MO, Queral LA. Venous claudication successfully treated by distal superficial femoral-to-greater saphenous venous bypass. *J Vasc Surg* 1985; **2**: 870.

27. Gruss JD. The saphenopopliteal bypass for chronic venous insufficiency (May–Husni operation). In Bergan JJ, Yao JST, eds. *Surgery of the Veins.* Orlando, FL: Grune & Stratton, 1985: 255–65.
28. Frileux C, Pillot-Bienayme P, Gillot C. Bypass of segmental obliteration of ilio-femoral venous axis by transposition of saphenous vein. *J Cardiovasc Surg* 1972; **13**: 409–14.
29. Schanzer H, Skladany M. Complex venous reconstruction for chronic ilio-femoral vein obstruction. *Cardiovasc Surg* 1996; **4**: 837–40.
30. Lalka SG, Lash JM, Unthank JL, *et al.* Inadequacy of saphenous vein grafts for cross-femoral venous bypass. *J Vasc Surg* 1991; **13**: 622–30.
31. Edwards WS. Femoral AV fistula as a complementary or primary procedure for iliac venous occlusion. In Bergan JJ, Yao JST, eds. *Surgery of the Veins.* Orlando, FL: Grune & Stratton, 1985: 267–71.

37

Prosthetic bypasses for non-malignant occlusion of the inferior vena cava or iliac veins

JAE-SUNG CHO AND PETER GLOVICZKI

Reconstructions of iliac veins and inferior vena cava (IVC) with prosthetic grafts have been performed more frequently since early 1980s, when experimental studies suggested good results with expanded polytetrafluoroethylene (ePTFE) grafts.[1–4] Early results of case reports and small series of venous reconstructions have been encouraging, but long-term follow-up and objective documentation of patency have been scant. Progress in endovascular technology will undoubtedly affect indications for surgical reconstruction, which likely will be reserved for those patients who present with symptomatic, long segment occlusion of large veins and for those who failed or were not candidates for venous stenting.

There are several reasons why patency of grafts implanted in the venous system is inferior to those used for arterial replacement. These include low pressure and low flow in the venous system, competitive collateral flow around the graft, external compression of the graft in tightly confined spaces, such as the area under the inguinal ligament and the retrohepatic space.[1,5] Distal venous obstruction and valvular incompetence further decrease inflow to the graft.[5,6] The thrombogenic potential of the prosthetic grafts and hypercoagulability of many patients with deep venous thrombosis also account for increased risk of graft failure. Nevertheless, results of venous reconstructions have been better because of improved preoperative evaluation and accurate patient selection, refinement of surgical technique and due to the availability of large-diameter externally supported ePTFE grafts with relatively low thrombogenicity. In addition, the use of adjuncts such as an arteriovenous fistula (AVF) and perioperative anticoagulation, combined with aggressive postoperative graft surveillance have contributed to improved patency and clinical outcome.

Chapter 36 describes in detail the etiology, clinical presentation, preoperative evaluation of patients with chronic venous outflow obstruction and presents technique and results of autologous venous reconstructions. This chapter focuses on indications and patient selection for prosthetic reconstructions and discusses the technique and results of prosthetic bypass grafts, implanted for non-malignant occlusion of the inferior vena cava (IVC) and iliac veins. Chapter 43 discusses venous reconstruction in patients with malignant tumors.

PATIENT SELECTION

Symptomatic, good-risk patients with post-thrombotic obstruction of the iliac vein and the IVC are most frequently the candidates for surgical reconstruction. Venous occlusion may also develop due to trauma or irradiation, or as a result of external compression of deep veins by retroperitoneal fibrosis,[7] tumors,[8–10] cysts, aneurysms, abnormally inserted muscles, fibrous bands or ligaments.[11,12] Compression of the left common iliac vein by the overlying right common iliac artery (May–Thurner Syndrome) is a frequently overlooked cause of left iliofemoral venous thrombosis.[13–16] Congenital anomalies, such as membranous occlusion of the suprahepatic IVC, with or without associated thrombosis of hepatic veins (Budd–Chiari syndrome),[17] or hypoplasia of the iliofemoral veins, as in

Klippel–Trenaunay syndrome,[18,19] can also cause chronic venous insufficiency.

The Mayo Clinic experience with 44 large vein reconstructions, performed in 42 patients for benign iliocaval or femoral venous thrombosis, was recently reported.[20] The etiology of venous obstruction was congenital in 2 and secondary to other causes in 40: of these, deep vein thrombosis was the etiology in 25, trauma in 5, retroperitoneal fibrosis in 4, caval occlusion devices in 4, and others in 2. Thirty-six patients had limb swelling or venous claudication, and 38 had pain. Fourteen patients had healed or active ulcers (classes 5 and 6).

PREOPERATIVE EVALUATION

Preoperative evaluation of patients with venous occlusive disease is discussed in detail in Chapter 36 by Lalka. It is important to emphasize that evaluation must reveal the etiology and functional significance of deep venous obstruction, and the extent and severity of associated venous incompetence. Of note, in at least two-thirds of the patients with venous outflow obstruction, distal reflux due to incompetent valves will contribute to development of chronic venous insufficiency (CVI).[6]

Noninvasive venous evaluation of deep venous obstruction

Duplex scanning and strain-gauge or air plethysmography are used to confirm occlusion and also to determine the extent of distal valvular incompetence and calf muscle pump failure. It is important to exclude any abdominal or pelvic pathology (tumor, cyst, retroperitoneal fibrosis) with computed tomography (CT) or magnetic resonance imaging (MRI). Outflow plethysmography is useful to confirm functional venous outflow obstruction, and to document improvement following treatment.

Contrast and magnetic resonance venography

In our practice, patients considered for reconstruction undergo detailed contrast venography. Both ascending and descending venography are performed to evaluate obstruction and the severity of valvular incompetence.[5,20,21] Iliocavography and abdominal cavography through a brachial approach may also be necessary in some patients to visualize the IVC proximal to the occlusion. The femoral access is useful not only for descending venography and iliocavography, but also for measuring femoral venous pressures. In recent years magnetic resonance venography has been used with increasing frequency, but this technology has not yet replaced contrast studies in our experience.

Venous pressure measurement

Femoral venous pressure measurements are performed during venography. As discussed in more detail in Chapter 17, resting pressure in the common femoral vein should be higher on the affected side than the contralateral, unaffected side. Normal pressure at that level is 4 mmHg, whilst it should be at least 6 mmHg or more on the affected side.[22] However, in the presence of well-developed collateralization, venous pressure may be normal at rest and manifest hemodynamic significance only under the conditions of exercise. For the purpose of testing, exercise consists of 10 dorsiflexions of the ankle or 20 isometric contractions of the calf muscle which should increase the pressure by twofold in the setting of significant obstruction.[22] In potential candidates for proximal venous reconstruction, femoral and central venous pressure measurements are also helpful. In supine patients, a pressure difference of at least 5 mmHg between the femoral and the central pressures, or a twofold increase in femoral vein pressure after exercise indicates hemodynamic significance of a lesion.[5,20–24]

Venous pressure measurement following reactive hyperemia is another means of assessing hemodynamic significance. With the transducer in the dorsum of the foot, a thigh cuff is inflated to 300 mmHg for 2 minutes and the pressure measured 5 seconds after cuff deflation. The increase in pressure up to 30 mmHg indicates the functional significance.[22] However, in cases of severe post-thrombotic syndrome, the increase in pressure either does not take place or is only very small; this is termed paradoxical reaction, the mechanism of which remains to be defined.

INDICATIONS FOR PROSTHETIC GRAFTS

Anatomic in-line iliac, iliocaval or femorocaval reconstruction can be performed for unilateral disease when autologous conduit for suprapubic graft is not available, or for bilateral iliac, iliocaval or IVC occlusion. Extensive venous thrombosis, not infrequently following previous placement of an IVC clip, tumors or retroperitoneal fibrosis recalcitrant to non-operative therapy, are other potential indications. Failure of previous endovascular attempts and occlusion following placement of multiple stents have also been indications for venous bypass grafting.

As discussed in detail in Chapter 35, recent literature has advocated angioplasty with stent placement for the treatment of short segmental venous stenosis such as in the proximal common iliac vein.[25–27] In our experience, however, long, chronic occlusions in the venous system seldom have had lasting results from endovascular intervention. In such cases, bypass is a better alternative in low surgical risk patients. Indications and results of following venous reconstructions for malignant tumors are reviewed in Chapter 43.

ADJUNCTS TO IMPROVE GRAFT PATENCY

Arteriovenous fistula

Multiple experiments confirmed that a distal AVF, first suggested by Kunlin in 1953,[28] improves patency of grafts placed in the venous system.[2,3,29,30] In Chapter 36, Lalka discusses in detail the indications and techniques of AVFs. Prosthetic grafts have significantly higher thrombotic threshold velocity than autologous grafts and require higher flow to maintain patency. Experimental work in our laboratory revealed that to avoid venous hypertension, the optimal ratio between the diameters of the fistula and the graft should not exceed 0.3.[31] Elevated intraoperative pressure in the femoral vein after placement of a fistula is a warning sign and fistula diameter should be decreased by banding the conduit. Disadvantages of an AVF include an increased operating time and the inconvenience of a second procedure to ligate the fistula at a later date. A potential side-effect is a high cardiac output caused by high fistula flow. If the femoral pressure rises with the AVF placement, increasing venous outflow obstruction may defeat the purpose of the operation.

If the prosthetic graft is anastomosed to the femoral artery, we prefer placement of the venous end of the AVF right onto the hood of the graft at the distal anastomosis, using either the side branch of the greater saphenous vein or a 4-mm prosthetic graft. The arterial anastomosis is usually made to the superficial femoral artery. A small Silastic sheet about 1 cm in length is placed around the fistula to avoid any dilation and a 2-0 Prolene suture is loosely tied around the fistula. The ends of the prolene are positioned in the subcutaneous tissue, close to the incision, to help find the fistula during a second procedure. In patients with iliocaval graft, the fistula is done at the groin, with the saphenous vein or one of its large

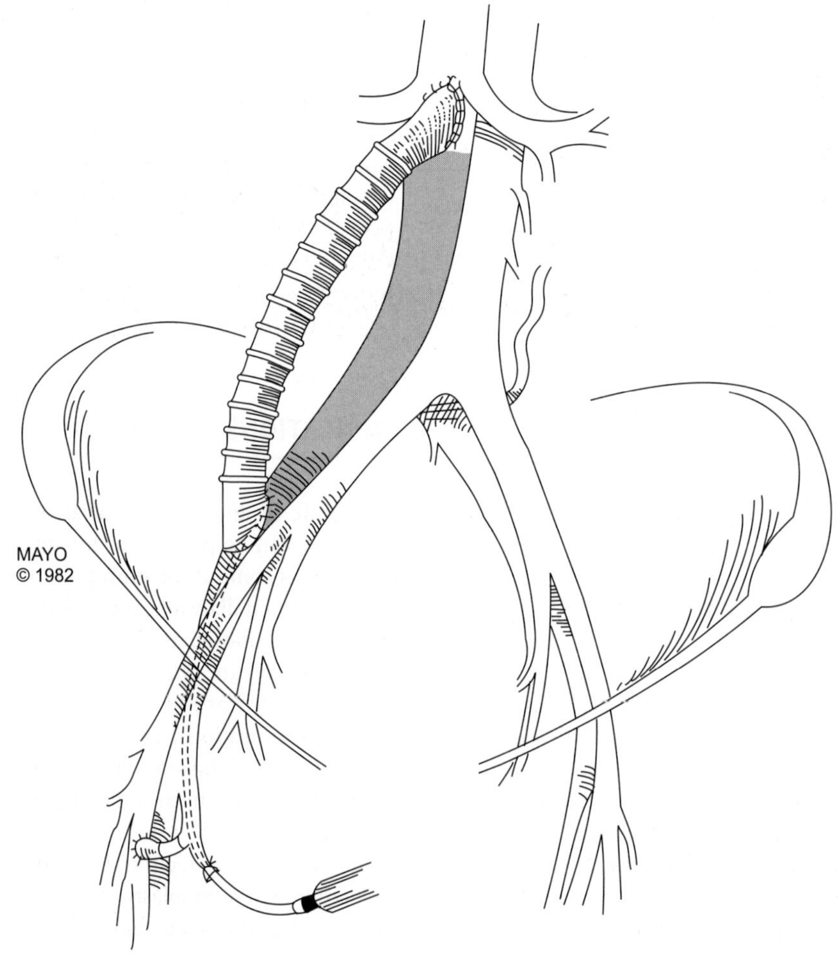

Figure 37.1 *Illustration of a right iliac vein IVC externally supported ePTFE graft. Note the arteriovenous fistula at the right groin and a 20 gauge catheter which is introduced through a tributary of the saphenous vein for perioperative heparin infusion. (Reproduced with permission from Gloviczki P, Pairolero PC, Toomey BJ,* et al. *Reconstruction of large veins for nonmalignant venous occlusive disease.* J Vasc Surg *1992;* ***16****: 750–61)*

tributaries (Fig.37.1). Intraoperative duplex scanning may be used to facilitate the identification of the fistula. Percutaneous closure of the fistula with transcatheter embolization is also an option but we prefer surgical closure.

At present we use an AVF for all prosthetic grafts anastomosed to the femoral vein and for all longer (>10 cm) iliocaval grafts. The fistula is kept open for at least 6 months postoperatively, but in patients without any side-effects, it is kept open for as long as possible to help maintain patency.

Thrombosis prophylaxis

Intravenous heparin (5000 units) is given before cross-clamping and anticoagulation is maintained during and after the procedure in most patients. Low-dose heparin (500–800 units/h), administered locally through a small polyethylene catheter (Fig. 37.1), is continued until complete systemic heparinization is achieved by increasing the dose and adjusting partial thromboplastin time to twice normal by 48 postoperative hours. The catheter is then removed and the patient converted to oral anticoagulation. Intermittent pneumatic compression pump, leg elevation, elastic bandages and early ambulation are also encouraged.[32] The patients are fitted with 30–40 mmHg compression stockings before discharge. Unfractionated heparin can be replaced by low molecular weight heparin to facilitate early dismissal from the hospital. Warfarin is continued indefinitely.

SURGICAL PROCEDURES

Cross-pubic venous bypass

For unilateral iliac or femoral venous occlusion, cross-pubic venous bypass with ePTFE may be an alternative in the absence of or small (<4 mm diameter) greater saphenous vein (GSV).[32–34] Optimal results may be achieved with normal inflow when the ipsilateral infrainguinal deep veins are not afflicted with either valvular incompetence or obstruction.

TECHNIQUE

Bilateral femoral veins are exposed through a groin incision. Excision of synechiae within the vein lumen may be necessary. An 8-mm ePTFE graft is tunneled through the suprapubic space to the contralateral femoral vein. The anastomosis between the graft and femoral vein is performed end to side with a running 5-0 nonabsorbable suture. The AVF is constructed before restoration of flow through the graft. A small polyethylene catheter is placed to the level of the distal anastomosis for postoperative infusion of low-dose heparin and for venography. An alternative approach is to place the graft in the suprapubic position under the rectus sheet and anastomose it to the contralateral external or common iliac artery that is exposed through a small flank incision (Fig. 37.2).

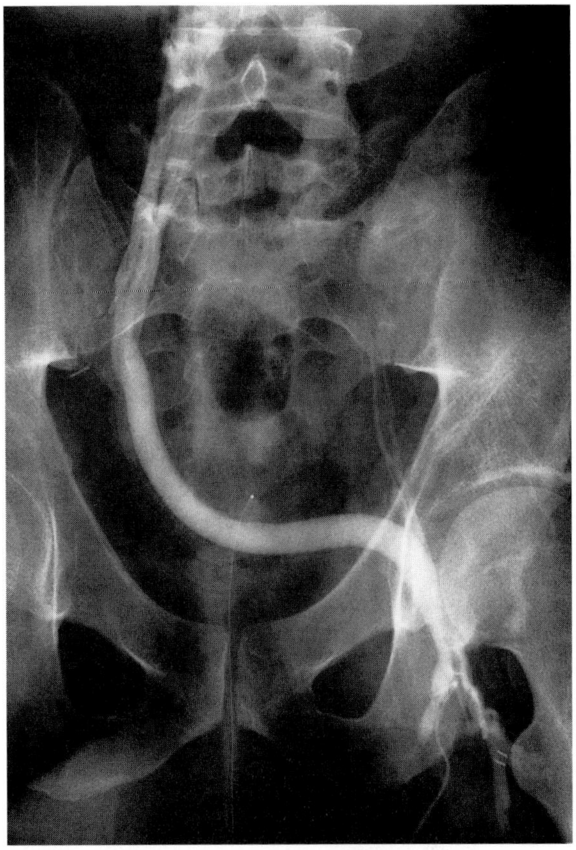

Figure 37.2 *Postoperative venogram of a patent left femoral–right iliac crossover polytetrafluoroethylene (PTFE) graft with external support.*

RESULTS

Eklof and colleagues[35,36] reported results on seven femoral crossover grafts with non-externally supported ePTFE and temporary AVF for the treatment of acute DVT (Table 37.1). Although all six surviving patients reported only minimal leg swelling, five grafts had thrombosed within 31 months, and one graft was patent at 36 months. Comerota *et al.*[37] reported use of cross-pubic venous bypass with ePTFE for residual iliofemoral thrombosis following thrombectomy, thrombolysis or both; two of three grafts were patent at 40 and 63 months. We have not favored this technique and after three failures we changed to in-line femorocaval bypass.

Sottiurai and associates observed 100% patency (26/26) at a follow-up ranging from 11 to 139 months with ulcer healing in 11 of 14 patients.[38] Gruss *et al.* have the largest experience with ePTFE; they reported an 85% (27/32) patency rate in a long-term follow-up.[22,39] Based

Table 37.1 *Results of femorofemoral bypass grafting with prosthesis*

First author	Year	No. limbs	Follow-up (months)	Postoperative imaging (%)	Patency (%)	Clinical improvement (%)
Eklof[45]	1985	7	2–31	86	17	86
Yamamoto[46]	1986	5	1–18	100	60	60
Comerota[37]	1994	3	40–60	100	67	67
Gruss[22]	1997	32	N/A	N/A	85	N/A

on his results and those of others,[40] Gruss now recommends using externally supported ePTFE grafts with AVF for all cross-pubic venous bypasses.

Femoro-ilio-caval bypass

Anatomic in-line reconstruction can be performed for unilateral disease when autologous conduit for suprapubic graft is not available, or for bilateral iliac, iliocaval or IVC occlusion. Extensive venous thrombosis, not infrequently following previous placement of an IVC clip, tumors or retroperitoneal fibrosis, resistant to non-operative therapy, are potential indications. Failure of previous endovascular attempts and occlusion following placement of multiple stents have also been indications for bypass. Even if occlusion is bilateral, unilateral iliocaval graft may offer significant improvement in collateral drainage of the opposite side as well (Fig. 37.3).

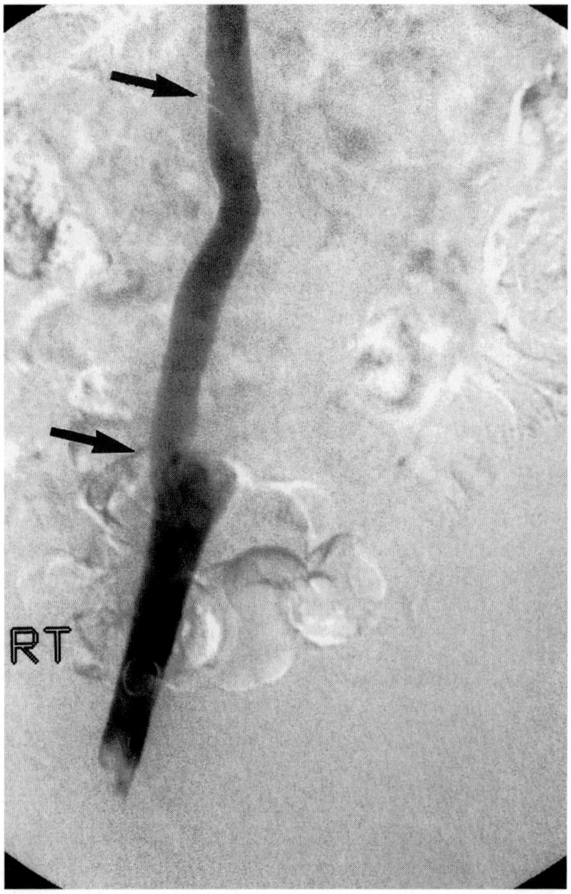

Figure 37.3 *Patent right iliocaval PTFE graft 4.5 years after placement for iliocaval occlusion caused by retroperitoneal fibrosis (arrows indicate anastomosis).*

TECHNIQUE

The femoral vessels are exposed at the groin through a vertical incision. The iliac vein or the distal segment of the IVC is exposed through the retroperitoneal approach utilizing an oblique flank incision. The IVC at the level of the renal veins is best exposed through a midline or a right subcostal incision. The infrarenal IVC is reconstructed with a 16–20 mm graft, the iliocaval segment usually with a 14 mm graft and the femorocaval segment with a 10 or 12 mm ePTFE graft. The AVF is constructed first in patients who undergo a long iliocaval bypass (Figs 37.1, 37.3).

Short iliocaval bypass with significant pressure gradient or reconstruction of the IVC with a straight ePTFE graft, in the presence of good inflow, can be performed without an AVF (Fig. 37.4).

RESULTS

Experience with femorocaval or iliocaval bypass is limited to several series with small numbers and difficult to interpret due to poor reporting standards (Table 37.2). Ijima and colleagues[40] in 1985 reported three of five femoral crossover ePTFE grafts with temporary AVF to be patent at a 22–36 months follow-up. In Eklof's series,[35] only one of three grafts were patent at 108 months. Okadome[41] reported that all four iliofemoral ePTFE grafts were patent at last follow-up ranging from 1.5 to 4 years as compared with two of four thrombo-endovenectomized segments being patent. They noted that the flow rate through AVF of 100 ml/min was necessary to help maintain graft patency, supporting the earlier findings of Ijima *et al.*[40]

We reported earlier on 11 patients with a follow-up extending up to 5 years.[5] Seven grafts were patent at a median follow-up of 9 months (range, 2 weeks to 5 years); six of the seven patients remained free of symptoms while the remaining patient experienced symptomatic relief. It should be noted that all five grafts originating from the iliac vein or the IVC were patent at last follow-up, whereas only two of six grafts originating

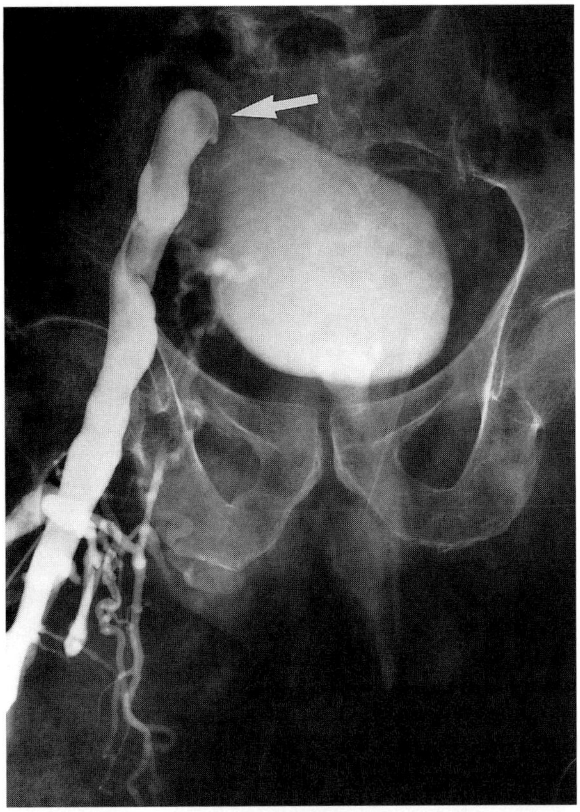

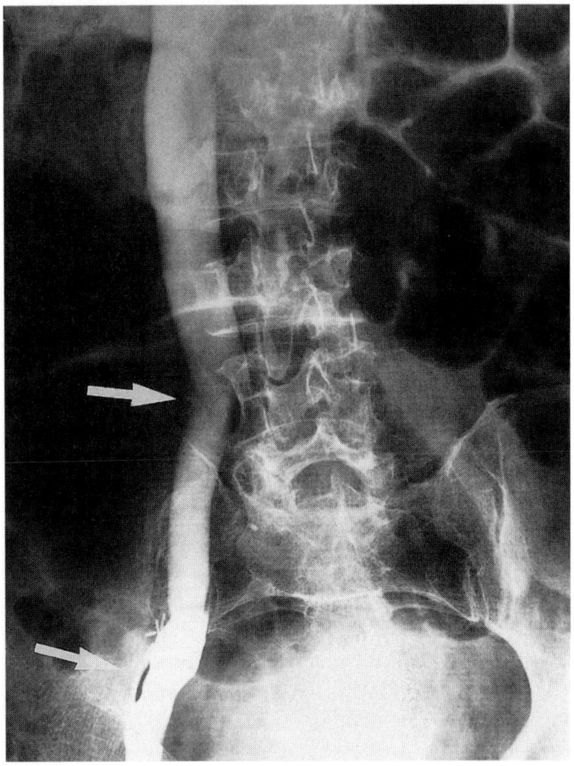

(a) (b)

Figure 37.4 *(a) Right iliocaval occlusion (arrow) with a remarkable lack of collateral circulation. (b) Patent iliocaval PTFE graft 3 months later. The patient had patent graft and excellent clinical result 5 years later (arrows indicate proximal and distal anastomosis) (Courtesy of the Mayo Foundation)*

from common femoral vein were patent. Preoperative valvular incompetence was associated with poor clinical outcome.

Alimi and colleagues[42] reported results of eight iliac vein reconstructions with femorocaval or iliocaval bypass grafting for both acute and chronic obstructions, four patients each. In an average follow-up of 20 months (range 10–45 months) seven of eight grafts were patent; early graft failure occurred in one patient operated for chronic occlusion. Sottiurai *et al.* noted long-term patency in 16 of 19 ePTFE grafts at last follow-up ranging from 80 to 113 months following femoro-femoro-caval (5), femoro-iliac (6) and femoro-caval (8) bypass grafting with an aid of AVF.[38] Ulcer healing was noted in 10 of 13 (77 %) patients and improvement of limb edema in 16 of 19 patients. Gruss and Hiemer[22] have the largest experience; they observed an 85% graft patency rate in 32 patients with ePTFE bypass grafts and temporary AVF, although routine venography was not employed.

Results of the Mayo Clinic series of 44 large vein reconstructions in 42 patients were recently updated; all

Table 37.2 *Results of femorocaval/iliocaval prosthetic bypass grafting*

First author	Year	No. limbs	Follow-up (months)	Patency (%)	Clinical improvement (%)
Husfeldt[47]	1981	4	4–30	100	100
Dale[48]	1984	3	1–30	100	100
Ijima[40]	1985	5	22–36	60	60
Eklof[45]	1985	7	2–31	29	86
Plate[49]	1985	3	1–11	33	67
Okadome[41]	1989	4	17–48	100	100
Gloviczki[5]	1992	12	1–60	58	67
Alimi[42]	1997	8	10–45	88	88
Jost[20]	2001	13	1–150	54	49
Sottiurai[38]	In press	19	80–113	84	84

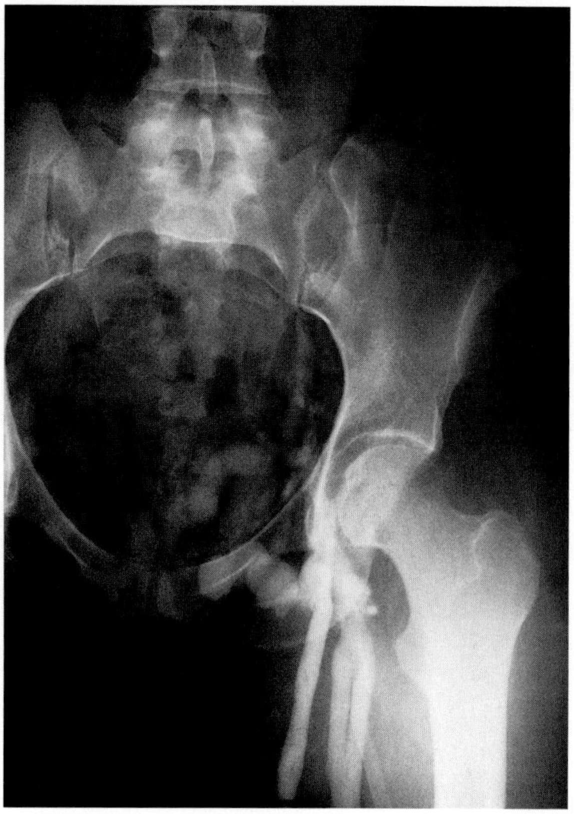

(a)

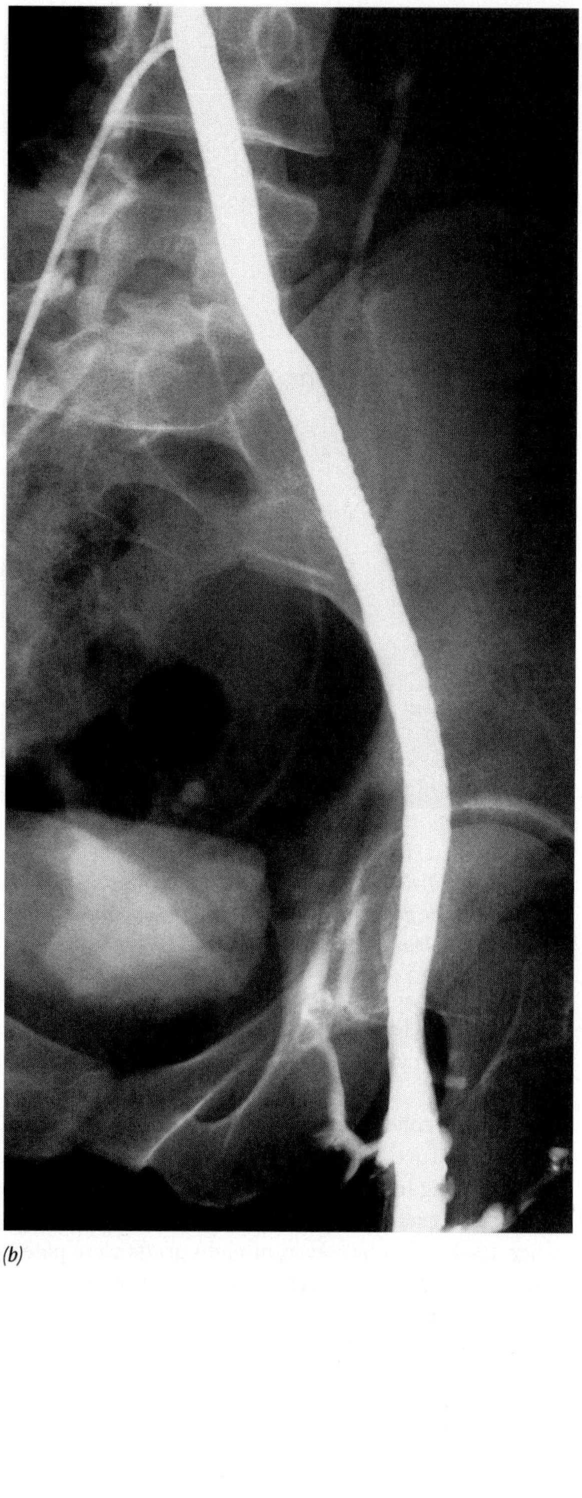

(b)

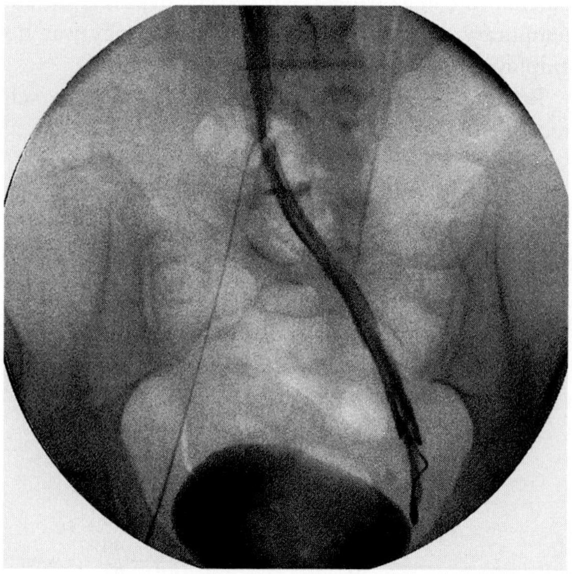

(c)

Figure 37.5 *(a) Venogram of a 36-year-old female confirms left iliac vein thrombosis. (b) Venogram 1.6 years after implantation confirms widely patent left femorocaval ePTFE graft. (c) Venogram at 11.7 years after graft placement. The patient has excellent clinical result. (Courtesy of the Mayo Foundation)* underwent surgical treatment for benign iliocaval or femoral venous thrombosis.[20] Seventeen patients had ePTFE grafts placed (femorocaval, 8; iliocaval, 5; cross-femoral, 3; cavoatrial, 1); 6 had spiral vein grafts (5 iliofemoral and 1 cavoatrial) and one femoral vein patch angioplasty was performed. Clinical follow-up averaged 3.5 years (median 2.5), and graft follow-up with imaging studies averaged 2.6 years (median 1.6). Secondary 3-year patency rate of ilio/femorocaval ePTFE bypasses at 2 years was 54% (Figs 37.5, 37.6). Secondary patency was lower in patients with an arteriovenous fistula (P = 0.023), although these data probably reflected the more extensive disease in those requiring a fistula to maintain patency. Femoro-femoral saphenous vein grafts (Palma procedure) had a patency of 83% (P = NS).

Early patency of caval reconstruction performed in patients together with excision of primary or secondary malignant disease is excellent and is discussed in detail in Chapter 43.

Suprarenal inferior vena cava reconstruction

The most common reason to reconstruct the suprarenal IVC for benign disease is membranous occlusion of the IVC, which is frequently associated with occlusion of the hepatic veins (Budd–Chiari syndrome) and consequent portal hypertension and liver failure. Occlusion of the suprahepatic IVC usually does not cause significant congestion of lower extremity veins, although leg edema and venous claudication may still develop in affected patients.

Most surgeons would agree that externally supported ePTFE graft is superior to either spiral vein graft or superficial femoral vein for vena caval or cavoatrial bypass. If percutaneous balloon angioplasty, stenting or transatrial dilatation of the membranous occlusion fails and portosystemic shunting is not required, cavoatrial bypass is an effective technique to decompress the IVC.

TECHNIQUE

The retrohepatic segment of the vena cava and the right atrium are exposed through a right anterolateral thoracotomy, extending the incision across the costal arch such that the peritoneal cavity is entered through the diaphragm. The suprarenal segment of the IVC is controlled with a partial occlusion clamp above the renal vein, and a 16- or 18-mm externally supported ePTFE graft is sutured end to side using a running either 5-0 or 6-0 Prolene suture. The graft is then passed parallel to the IVC up to the right atrium or to the suprahepatic IVC. Before completion of the anastomosis, the graft is de-aired to prevent air embolization.

An anterior approach was suggested by Kieffer, who replaced a short segment of the suprahepatic IVC with a ringed ePTFE graft.[43] Tunneling of a long cavoatrial graft in front of the liver or under the left lobe was also reported.

RESULTS

Wong and associates reported on 12 patients who underwent cavoatrial bypass grafting for Budd–Chiari syndrome.[17] Clinical improvement with patent graft was noted in 10 patients at a median follow-up of 1.5 years

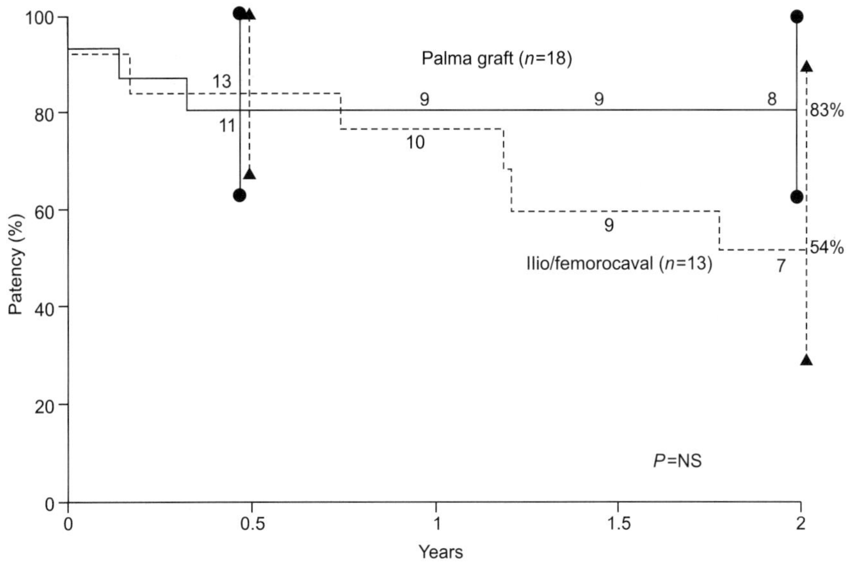

Figure 37.6 *Cumulative secondary patency rates of ePTFE ilio/femorocaval bypasses and saphenous vein crossover bypass grafts (Palma procedure). (Reproduced with permission from Jost CJ, Gloviczki P, Cherry KJ,* et al. *Surgical reconstruction of iliofemoral veins and the inferior vena cava for nonmalignant occlusive disease.* J Vasc Surg *2001;* ***33****: 320–8)*

after surgery. Kieffer's group[43] reported on long-term patency in five of six grafts placed for membranous occlusion of the vena cava. In another series, Victor *et al.* reported patent grafts at 21 months to 6 years after the operation in five patients.[44]

Three cavoatrial grafts placed for non-malignant disease were reported by our group: the patient with ePTFE graft was asymptomatic at 10 years, the long Dacron graft failed at 3 years and the spiral vein graft occluded within 1 year.[5]

GRAFT SURVEILLANCE

Direct pressure measurements are done before closure in every patient with and without graft flow to document hemodynamic benefit. In vein or polyester conduits, fistula flow can be measured and calibrated using an electromagnetic flow meter. If flow exceeds 300 ml/min, banding of the fistula should be considered. On the first postoperative day, contrast venography is obtained through the catheter which is positioned at the distal anastomosis of the graft (Fig. 37.1). Postoperatively duplex surveillance imaging is obtained at 3 and at 6 months and twice yearly thereafter. Outflow plethysmography is also performed to objectively document hemodynamic changes following the bypass procedure.

REFERENCES

1. Gloviczki P, Cho JS. Surgical treatment of chronic deep venous obstruction. In Rutherford RB, ed. *Vascular Surgery.* Philadelphia: Saunders, 1999: 2049–66.
2. Plate G, Hollier LH, Gloviczki P, Dewanjee MK, Kaye MP. Overcoming failure of venous vascular prostheses. *Surgery* 1984; **96**: 503–10.
3. Gloviczki P, Hollier LH, Dewanjee MK, Trastek VF, Hoffman EA, Kaye MP. Experimental replacement of the inferior vena cava: factors affecting patency. *Surgery* 1984; **95**: 657–66.
4. Chan EL, Bardin JA, Bernstein EF. Inferior vena cava bypass: experimental evaluation of externally supported grafts and initial clinical application. *J Vasc Surg* 1984; **95**: 657–66.
5. Gloviczki P, Pairolero PC, Toomey BJ, *et al.* Reconstruction of large veins for nonmalignant venous occlusive disease. *J Vasc Surg* 1992; **16**: 750–61.
6. Schanzer H, Skladany M. Complex venous reconstruction for chronic iliofemoral vein obstruction. *Cardiovasc Surg* 1996; **4**: 837–40.
7. Rhee RY, Golviczki P, Luthra HS, Stanson AW, Bower TC, Cherry KJ Jr. Iliocaval complications of retroperitoneal fibrosis. *Am J Surg* 1994; **168**: 179–83.
8. Dzsinich C, Gloviczki P, van Heerden JA, *et al.* Primary venous leiomyosarcoma: a rare but lethal disease. *J Vasc Surg* 1992; **15**: 595–603.
9. Bower TC. Primary and secondary tumors or the inferior vena cava. In Gloviczki P, Yao JST, eds. *Handbook of Venous Disorders: Guidelines of the American Venous Forum.* London: Chapman & Hall, 1996: 529–50.
10. Bower TC, Nagorney DM, Toomey BJ, *et al.* Vena cava replacement for malignant disease: is there a role? *Ann Vasc Surg* 1993; **7**: 51–62.
11. Rich NM, Hughes CW. Popliteal artery and vein entrapment. *Am J Surg* 1967; **113**: 696–8.
12. Gullmo A. The strain obstruction syndrome of the femoral vein. *Acta Radiol* 1957; **47**: 119–37.
13. May R, Thurner J. Ein gefasporn in der Vena iliaca communis sinistra als Ursache der ubegend linksseitigen Beckenvenenthrombosen. *Z Kreislaufforsch* 1956; **45**: 912.
14. Cockett FB, Thomas ML, Negus D. Iliac vein compression – its relation to iliofemoral thrombosis and the postthrombotic syndrome. *Br Med J* 1967; **2**: 14–19.
15. David M, Striffling V, Brenot R, Barault JF, Trigalou D. Syndrome de Cockett acquis: a propos de trois cas operes dont deux fores inhabituelles. *Ann Chir* 1981; **35**: 93–8.
16. Steinberg JB, Jacocks MA. May–Thurner syndrome: a previously unreported variant. *Ann Vasc Surg* 1993; **7**: 577–81.
17. Wang ZG, Zhu Y, Wang SH, *et al.* Recognition and management of Budd–Chiari syndrome: report of one hundred cases. *J Vasc Surg* 1989; **10**: 149–56.
18. Gloviczki P, Stanson AW, Stickler GB, *et al.* Klippel–Trenaunay syndrome: the risks and benefits of vascular interventions. *Surgery* 1991; **110**: 469–79.
19. Jacob AG, Driscoll DJ, Shaughnessy WJ, Stanson AW, Clay RP, Gloviczki P. Klippel–Trenaunay syndrome: spectrum and management. *Mayo Clin Proc* 1998; **73**: 28–36.
20. Jost CJ, Gloviczki P, Cherry KJ, *et al.* Surgical reconstruction of iliofemoral veins and the inferior vena cava for nonmalignant occlusive disease. *J Vasc Surg* 2001; **33**: 320–8.
21. Gloviczki P, Pairolero PC, Cherry KJ Jr, Hallett JW Jr. Reconstruction of the vena cava and of its primary tributaries: a preliminary report. *J Vasc Surg* 1990; **11**: 373–81.
22. Gruss JD, Hiemer W. Bypass procedures for venous obstruction: Palma and May–Husmi bypasses, Raju perforator bypass, prosthetic bypasses, and primary and adjunctive arteriovenous fistulae. In Raju S, Villavicencio JL, eds. *Surgical Management of Venous Disease.* Baltimore: Williams & Wilkins, 1997: 289–305.
23. Negus D, Cockett FB. Femoral vein pressures in post-phlebitic iliac vein obstruction. *Br J Surg* 1967; **54**: 522–5.
24. May R. The Palma operation with Gottlob's endothelium preserving suture. In May R, Weber J, eds. *Pelvic and Abdominal Veins: Progress in Diagnostics and Therapy.* Amsterdam: Excerpta Medica International Congress Series 550, 1981: 192–7.
25. Rilinger N, Gorisch J, Mickley V, *et al.* Endovascular stenting in patients with iliac compression syndrome: experience in three cases. *Invest Radiol* 1996; **31**: 729–33.

26. Binkert CA, Schoch E, Stuckmann G, *et al.* Treatment of pelvic spur (May–Thurner syndrome) with self-expanding metallic endoprostheses. *Cardiovasc Interv Radiol* 1998; **21**: 22–6.
27. Akesson H. Venous stents in chronic iliac vein occlusions. *Eur J Vasc Endovasc Surg* 1997; **13**: 334–6.
28. Kunlin K, Kunlin A. Experimental venous surgery. In May R, ed. *Major Problems in Clinical Surgery, Volume 23, Surgery of the Veins of the Leg and Pelvis.* Philadelphia: WB Saunders, 1979: 37–75.
29. Yamaguchi A, Eguchi S, Iwasaki T, Asano K. The influence of arteriovenous fistulae on the patency of synthetic inferior vena caval grafts. *J Cardiovasc Surg* 1968; **9**: 99–103.
30. Wilson SE, Jabour A, Stone RT, Stanley TM. Patency of biologic and prosthetic inferior vena cava grafts with distal limb fistula. *Arch Surg* 1978; **113**: 1174–9.
31. Menawat SS, *et al.* Effect of a femoral arteriovenous fistula on lower extremity venous hemodynamics after femorocaval reconstruction. *J Vasc Surg* 1996; **24**: 793–9.
32. Hobson RW, Lee BC, Lynch TG, *et al.* Use of intermittent pneumatic compression of the calf in femoral venous reconstruction. *Surg Gynecol Obstet* 1984; **159**: 284.
33. Lalka SG, Lash JM, Unthank JL, *et al.* Inadequacy of saphenous vein grafts for cross-femoral venous bypass. *J Vasc Surg* 1991; **13**: 622–30.
34. Halliday P, Harris J, May J. Femoro-femoral crossover grafts (Palma operation): a long-term follow-up study. In Bergan JJ, Yao JST, eds. *Surgery of the Veins.* Orlando, FL: Grune & Stratton, 1985: 241–54.
35. Eklof B. Temporary arteriovenous fistula in reconstruction of iliac vein obstruction using PTFE grafts. In Eklof B, Gjores JE, Thulesius O, Berqvist D, eds. *Controversies in the Management of Venous Disorders.* London: Butterworths, 1989: 280–90.
36. Eklof BG, Kistner RL, Masuda EM. Venous bypass and valve reconstruction: long-term efficacy. *Vasc Med* 1998; **3**: 157–64.
37. Comerota AJ, Aldridge SC, Cohen G, Ball DS, Pliskin M, White JV. A strategy of aggressive regional therapy for acute iliofemoral venous thrombosis with contemporary venous thrombectomy or catheter-directed thrombolysis. *J Vasc Surg* 1994; **20**: 244–54.
38. Sottiurai VS, Gonzales J, Cooper M, Lyon R, Hatter D, Ross C. A new concept of arteriovenous fistula in venous bypass requiring no fistula interruption: surgical technique and long-term results. Submitted to *Cardiovascular Surgery.*
39. Gruss JD. Venous bypass for chronic venous insufficiency. In Bergan JJ, Yao JST, eds. *Venous Disorders.* Philadelphia: WB Saunders, 1991: 316–30.
40. Ijima H, Kidama M, Hori M. Temporary arteriovenous fistula for venous reconstruction using synthetic graft: a clinical and experimental investigation. *J Cardiovasc Surg* 1985; **26**: 131–6.
41. Okadome K. Venous reconstruction for iliofemoral venous occlusion facilitated by temporary arteriovenous shunt. Long-term results in nine patients. *Arch Surg* 1989; **124**: 957–60.
42. Alimi YS, DiMauro P, Fabre D, Juhan C. Iliac vein reconstructions to treat acute and chronic venous occlusive disease. *J Vasc Surg* 1997; **25**: 673–81.
43. Haswell DM, Berrigan TJ Jr. Anomalous inferior vena cava with accessory hemiazygos continuation. *Radiology* 1976; **119**: 51–4.
44. Victor S, Jayanthi V, Kandasamy I, *et al.* Retrohepatic cavoatrial bypass for coarctation of inferior vena cava with a polytetrafluoroethylene graft. *J Thorac Cardiovasc Surg* 1986; **91**: 99–105.
45. Eklof B. The temporary arteriovenous fistula in venous reconstructive surgery. *Int Angiol* 1985; **4**: 455–62.
46. Yamamoto N, *et al.* Reconstruction with insertion of expanded polytetrafluoroethylene (ePTFE) for iliac venous obstruction. *J Cardiovasc Surg* 1986; **27**: 697–702.
47. Husfeldt KJ. Venous replacement with Gore-Tex prosthesis: experimental and first clinical results. In May R, Weber J, eds. *Pelvic and Abdominal Veins: Progress in Diagnostics and Therapy.* Amsterdam: Excerpta Medica. International Congress Series 550, 1981: 249–58.
48. Dale WA, Harris J, Terry RB. Polytetrafluoroethylene reconstruction of the inferior vena cava. *Surgery* 1984; **95**: 625–30.
49. Plate G, Einarsson E, Eklof B, Jensen R, Ohlin P. Iliac vein obstruction associated with acute iliofemoral venous thrombosis. Results of early reconstruction using polytetrafluoroethylene grafts. *Acta Chir Scand* 1985; **151**: 607–11.

38

Management of incompetent perforators: conventional techniques

RALPH G DEPALMA

Stasis dermatitis, liposclerosis, and ulceration are end results of transmission of elevated venous pressures to the microcirculation of the skin and subcutaneous tissues of the lower leg. Linton's classic 1938 paper[1] described the anatomy of the lower leg veins, emphasizing interruption of incompetent communicating or perforating veins to mitigate the effects of venous hypertension. These principles for perforator control set standards of general agreement conforming to current concepts of perforator interruption. With time and a better understanding of patterns of chronic venous insufficiency (CVI), many technical variations have evolved.

While the principles cited by Linton remain valid, the variable anatomy and physiology of CVI gives rise to complex flow patterns in areas of skin involvement. These individual patterns are now better understood and require different operative interventions.

Later approaches included both subfascial[2] and extrafascial[3] perforator interruptions applicable to particular types and extent of venous or lower leg cutaneous involvement. In choosing a procedure for perforator interruption, important principles include avoiding incisions in densely liposclerotic skin and quantifying the contributions of obstruction or valvular reflux. Both obstruction and valvular reflux, alone or in combination, can cause ulceration.

Another concept long recognized,[3] but more recently acknowledged,[4,5] is that incompetent greater and lesser saphenous veins are of themselves important 'perforators', transmitting venous hypertension proximally and distally, contributing to cause skin breakdown.

ANATOMY

As discussed in more detail in Chapter 2, 90–150 veins connecting the superficial and deep systems[6,7] traverse the deep fascia. These veins are called the perforating or communicating veins. Direct perforators connect with the major veins of the deep system; indirect perforators connect with the muscular venous sinusoids. Lower limb incompetent perforating veins are capable of transmitting exceedingly high pressures to the skin surrounding the ankle during standing, but particularly so during calf and foot muscular contractions. While not as well appreciated, numerous submalleolar and foot veins draining into the distal saphenous veins also contribute to venous hypertension in certain cases.[5]

Classically, three relatively constant and important perforating veins drain the medial lower leg communicating with the posterior or deep tibial veins. Cockett[8] recognized the importance of these perforators, which are named in his honor. Cockett's perforating veins lie in an axis along the posterior venous arcade (Fig. 38.1). The upper perforator, said to be the most constant, pierces the fascia at the junction of the lower and upper half of the leg at the posterior tibial margin. This vein communicates either directly or indirectly with the long saphenous vein. The middle Cockett perforator is consistently located 'one hand's breadth above the tip of the medial malleolus',[3] or 18.5 cm above the sole of the foot.[6] The lower perforator, described by Cockett,[3] lies just behind and below the medial malleolus. Other authors[6,7] depict this perforator above the malleolus, 13.5 cm from the sole of the foot.

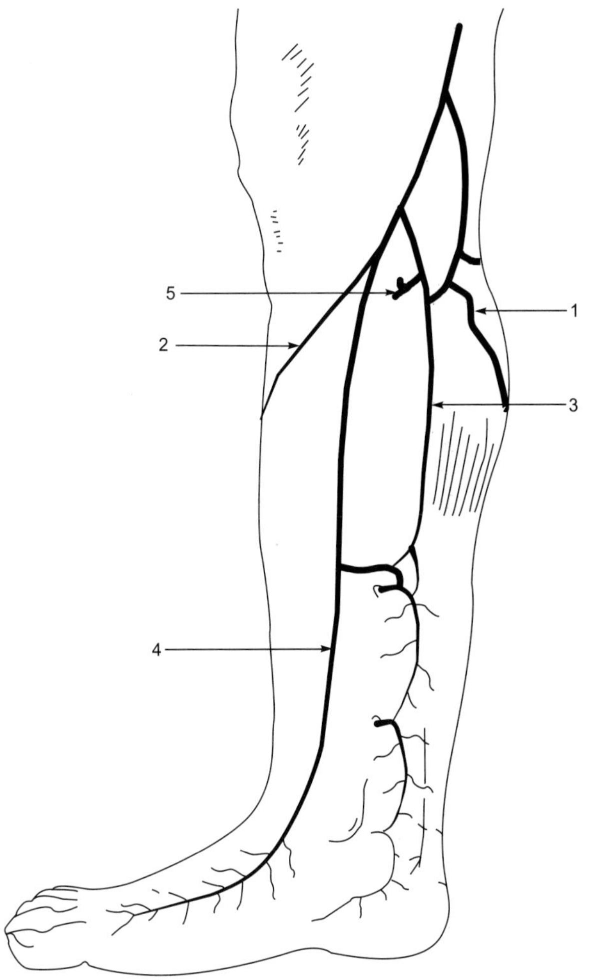

Figure 38.1 *Diagram of medial veins and perforators of the leg from Cockett's original descriptions:[3] 1, connection with short saphenous vein; 2, anterior leg tributary; 3, posterior arcade tributary linking the three internal ankle perforating veins; 4, greater saphenous vein; 5, direct communicator from deep system (Boyd's perforator). (Reproduced with permission from Dodd H, Cockett FB.* The Pathology and Surgery of the Veins of the Lower Limb. *Edinburgh, London and New York: Churchill Livingstone, 1976)*

Boyd's perforators are upper leg veins situated in the calf just below the knee. These veins are usually large and direct, usually divided into two groups, upper and lower, and sometimes intermediate. These occur with a peak frequency of 9 cm from the femorotibial line. The upper Boyd perforator is usually quite large. A large medial leg perforator situated just midway up the tibia is named in honor of Sherman. It links with the soleus and gastrocnemius veins and can become a potent source of reflux. In the lower third of the thigh, femoral perforators occur in Hunter's canal (Hunterian perforators), and in the middle and upper third of the canal, lateral perforators occur. A spectacular anatomic atlas by Claude Gillot[9] details venous anatomy drawn from 123 injected lower limbs; this valuable surgical resource outlines variations in venous anatomy which have an impact on surgical treatment.

Laterally (Fig. 38.2), one large constant external perforating vein connects with the lesser saphenous vein, along with a midcalf perforating vein, and drains into the soleus muscle sinusoids. Actually, considerable variation in perforator size and location exits, particularly in the location of lower medial perforators. An Achillean tributary is a branch of the short saphenous vein in the leg which appears along the medial side of the Achilles tendon.[9] This vein has often been identified in association with ulceration in the author's experience; it is frequently associated with important retromalleolar perforators. For more anatomic information the reader is also referred to the chapter on anatomy included in this volume (Chapter 2).

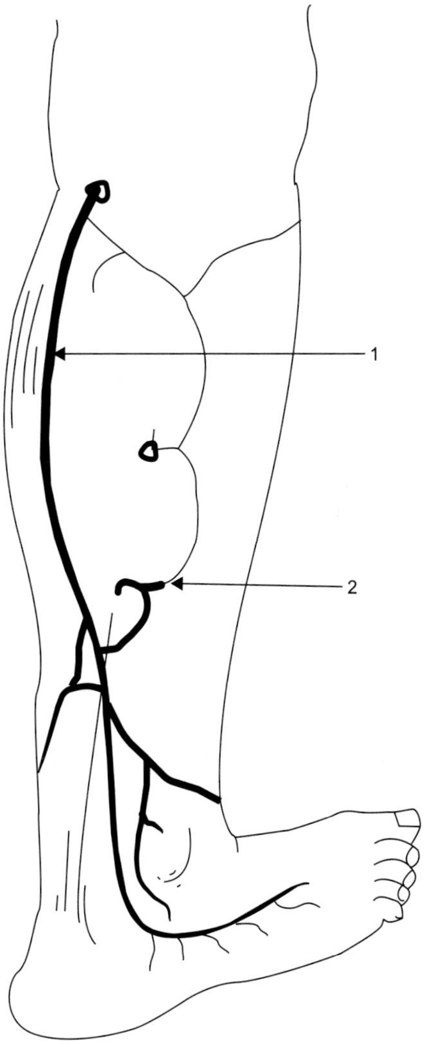

Figure 38.2 *External leg and ankle perforating veins from Cockett's original description:[3] 1, lesser saphenous vein; 2, large constant perforator connecting with lesser saphenous vein. (Reproduced with permission from Dodd H, Cockett FB.* The Pathology and Surgery of the Veins of the Lower Limb. *Edinburgh, London and New York: Churchill Livingstone, 1976)*

DIAGNOSIS

The underlying pattern and physiology of chronic venous insufficiency (CVI) should be determined before perforator interruption. This may require anatomic and physiologic studies to determine whether obstruction, valvular insufficiency, superficial deep, or both are contributing factors. In uncomplicated cases color-flow duplex scanning is an important aid for this purpose.[10] After duplex scanning, for class 4–6 disease, both ascending and descending phlebography[11] are recommended to assist in planning operations, as other interventions in the deep system such as valve repair or correction of iliac occlusion may be needed. With superficial reflux alone, contributions of the long or short saphenous veins or deep veins can usually be evaluated solely by duplex scanning. The saphenous veins, either through axial incompetence or along with secondary perforator involvement, are known to contribute to skin pathology[3,5,12] more frequently than previously thought. Detection of abnormal directional flow patterns in calf perforating veins using duplex scanning is difficult, particularly when lipodermatosclerosis is severe. When edema is controlled, fascial defects at the sites of the Cockett and Sherman perforators can sometimes be palpated along with bulging veins. With proximal obstruction, perforator 'blow out' often dominates the pattern of CVI. This abnormality should be corrected without interfering with a competent long saphenous vein. When the long saphenous is incompetent, particularly in CVI without obstruction, this vein should be considered as another 'perforator' and accordingly removed.

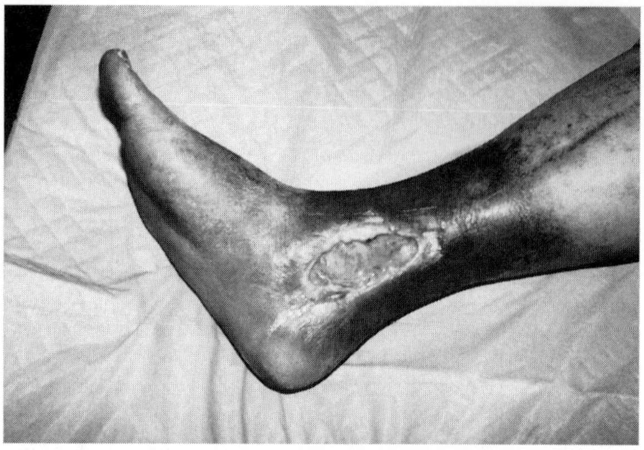

(a)

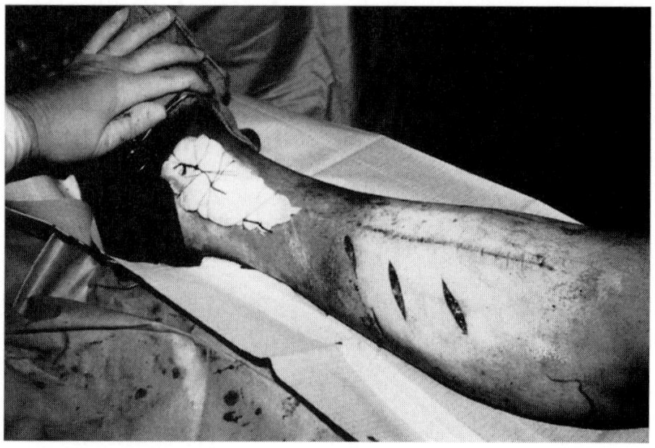

(b)

Figure 38.3 *(a) Failure of a classic subfascial perforator ligation performed elsewhere 1 year previously. Note longitudinal incision and recurrent ulcer. This patient had occlusion of the vena cava. (b) Extrafascial division of perforating veins and elevation of skin using skin line parallel incisions followed by deep ulcer excision and grafting. The posterior venous arcade and perforators were found to be patent and extensive.*

CHOICE OF PROCEDURES

The classic operative approach[1] used subfascial perforator ligation via a long vertical incision directly into the fascia. All perforating veins between the posterior tibial border and the midline posteriorly were divided and ligated. This incision extended below the malleolus to include the lowest of the three medial perforators. Prior to this extensive dissection, ulcer healing using bed rest, elevation and hospitalization for extended periods was required. The disadvantages of the classic procedure included poor healing of the longitudinal incision (Fig. 38.3) and the detection of fewer veins[2,5] in the deep compartment than one might expect.

Alternative approaches for subfascial perforator interrupter used a vertical posterior 'stocking seam' incision[13] for access to either medial or lateral perforating veins. Browse *et al.*[7] pointed out that the incidence of skin necrosis with this incision was a problem in their hands; I have not used this approach. Since the operation is performed in a prone position, access cannot be achieved to the greater saphenous vein. An interesting but temporary technical evolution was subfascial perforator shearing using a blunt phlebotome.[14] This approach offered incision through normal skin; the blind approach, subfascial hematoma, and possible injury to the posterior tibial artery or other structures in the deep compartment have rendered this approach obsolete.

EXTRAFASCIAL AND COMBINED DISSECTIONS

Cockett[3] used the extrafascial approach when the subcutaneous tissues were not severely effaced: 'an accurate incision of the line of perforating veins' was recommended. Cockett cautioned that the longitudinal incision was not to be carried below the medial malleolus. Apart from the disadvantage of the long incision, an advantage of this extrafascial approach was considered to be 'removal of . . . the enlarged . . . tortuous veins in the area . . . is really as important as tying the perforating veins from which they arise'.

Beginning in 1970, the author modified intra- and extrafascial dissections to interrupt perforating veins.[12,15] The original procedure had as its goal complete interruption of the perforating veins (either extra or intrafascial), removal of incompetent long saphenous and collateral veins, and excision with grafting of skin ulcers during one operation (Fig. 38.4). The incision for perforator interruption differed from the traditional approach in that, rather than creating a longitudinal flap, a series of bipedicled flaps in the natural skin lines were fashioned. Inframalleolar and foot perforators were also ligated through the skin line incisions. The ulcer was dissected subfascially; perforators passing into the ulcer bed from the posterior tibial veins were ligated under direct vision, and a split-thickness skin graft applied.

The procedure using a phlebotome was further developed as described in 1990.[16,17] Access to the perforators was obtained by an incision in normal skin in the proximal leg medially over Boyd's perforator which was also ligated. An extrafascial shearing operation using the phlebotome[11,14] was then employed to interrupt perforators. In early cases with superficial or small ulcers, the instrument was passed below the lesion severing underlying perforating veins (Fig. 38.5). This extrafascial shearing procedure has proved to be quite safe. With deep ulcers, formal excision and perforator

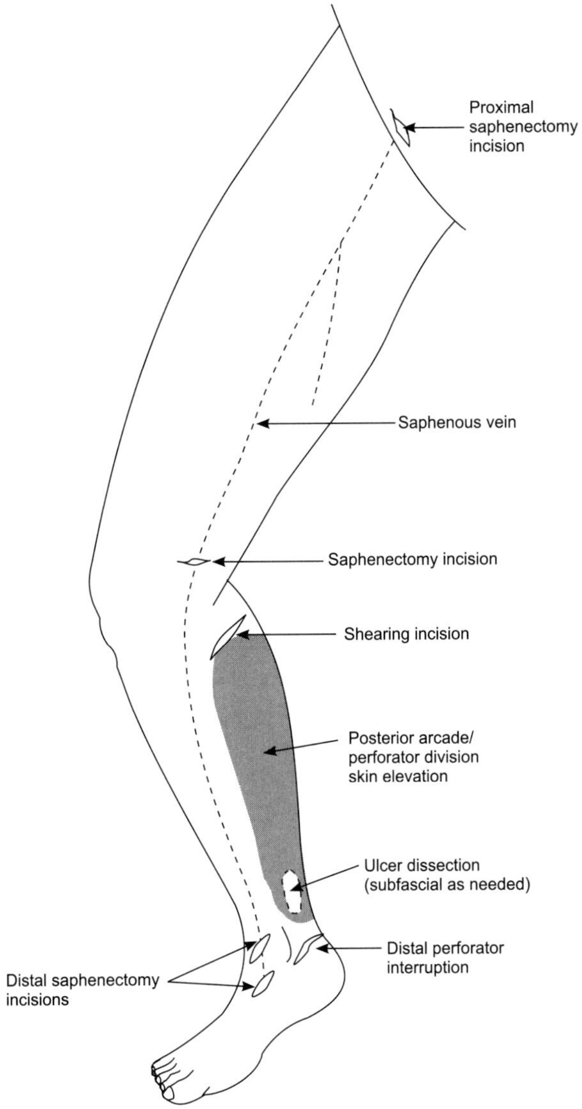

Figure 38.4 *Operation for stasis ulceration and reflux: medial perforator and long saphenous incompetence. Note area dissected to ensure complete perforator interruption as well as submalleolar skin line incisions. (Reproduced with permission from DePalma RG. Evolving surgical approaches for venous ulceration. In Negus D, Janet G, Coleridge-Smith PD, eds.* Phlebology '95. *London: Springer, 1995: Suppl 1, 980–2)*

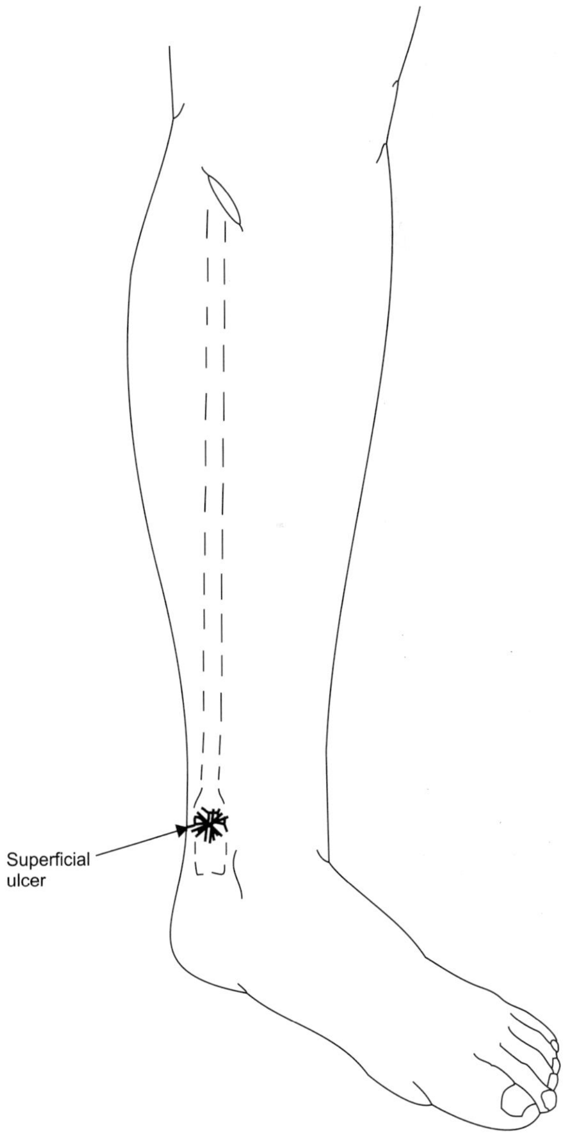

Figure 38.5 *Passage of phlebotome below superficial ulcer in shearing operation. (Reproduced with permission from DePalma RG. Surgical treatment of venous ulceration. In Bergan JJ, Yao JST, eds.* Venous Disorders. *Philadelphia: WB Saunders, 1990: 396–406)*

ligation was done subfascially through the ulcer bed as previously described.[12] The instrument was then passed extrafascially as shown in Fig. 38.6. The axis of phlebotome passage is shown in Fig. 38.7; this line encompasses the posterior venous arcade and Cockett's perforators, avoiding the skin over the tibia as well as the saphenous vein and nerve. A completed operation is shown in Fig. 38.8 and 10-year results of a similar operation are shown in Fig. 38.9.

COMMENTS

Results of conventional perforator interruption vary depending upon the etiology of CVI. These procedures are most effective when venous reflux into the skin and subcutaneous tissues can be minimized. While not within the scope of this discussion, the author has combined perforator interruption with the Palma cross-femoral bypass for iliac vein obstruction and valvuloplasty of the superficial vein in combination with perforator interruption. These combined approaches are indicated in obstruction or with severe, deep reflux. In many cases, however, conventional perforator interruption yields gratifying results. Recurrence rates in three series ranged from 9 to 10% in 168 limbs amongst 141 patients with observations ranging from 5 to 10 years.[15,18,19] Combined deep procedures were done in about 10% of these cases. Recurrences related mainly to uncorrected obstruction. Specifically, severe venous hypertension due to caval or iliac occlusion appeared to preclude success. Recently, our more liberal use of phlebography has uncovered undiagnosed iliac or caval pathology amongst 4 of 29 patients with class 5–7 disease.

The introduction of the shearing extrafascial modification greatly reduced hospital time to 3–4 days for ulcers less than 3 cm in diameter, where skin grafts are not usually needed. With skin grafting for large ulcers, bed rest, leg elevation, heparin prophylaxis, and hospital care are needed for at least 7–8 days.

Postoperatively and long term, all patients with venous ulceration require graded elastic support. However, lightweight below-knee support of 20–30 mmHg may become adequate in many cases postoperatively. Perforator interruption often allows a change to lightweight, more comfortable support and actually enhances patient compliance. These modifications of perforator interruption conform to traditional models of pioneering surgical interventions for venous ulceration. Shearing procedures are one step into the evolution of modern minimally invasive techniques. These approaches can be easily combined with direct visualization using laparo-

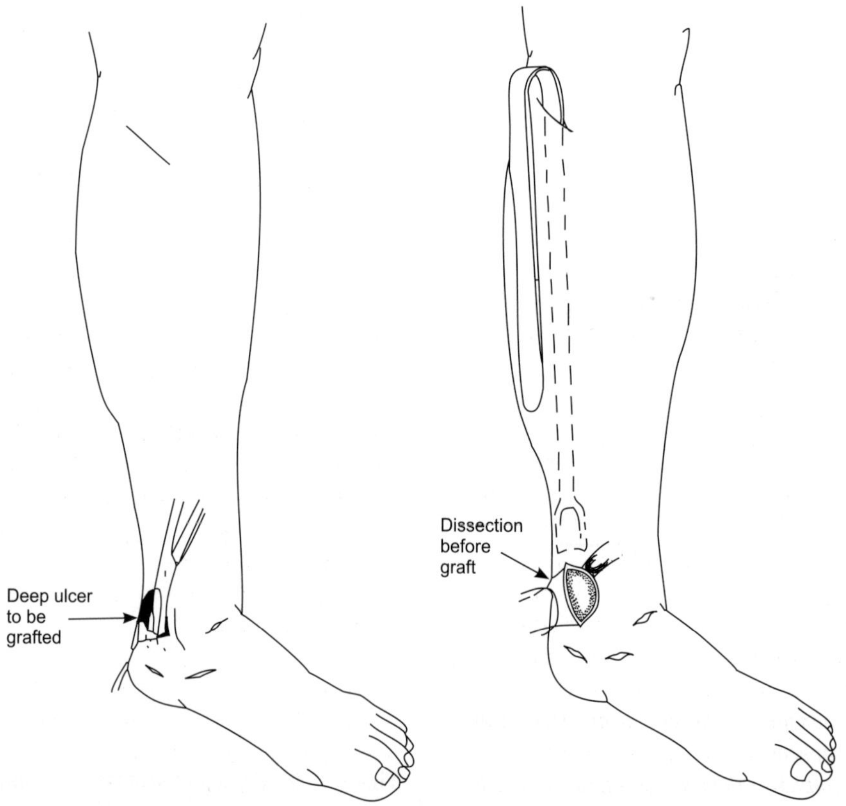

Figure 38.6 *Excision and dissection of a deep ulcer prior to extrafascial shearing operation. (Reproduced with permission from DePalma RG. Surgical treatment of venous ulceration. In Bergan JJ, Yao JST, eds.* Venous Disorders. *Philadelphia: WB Saunders, 1990: 396–406)*

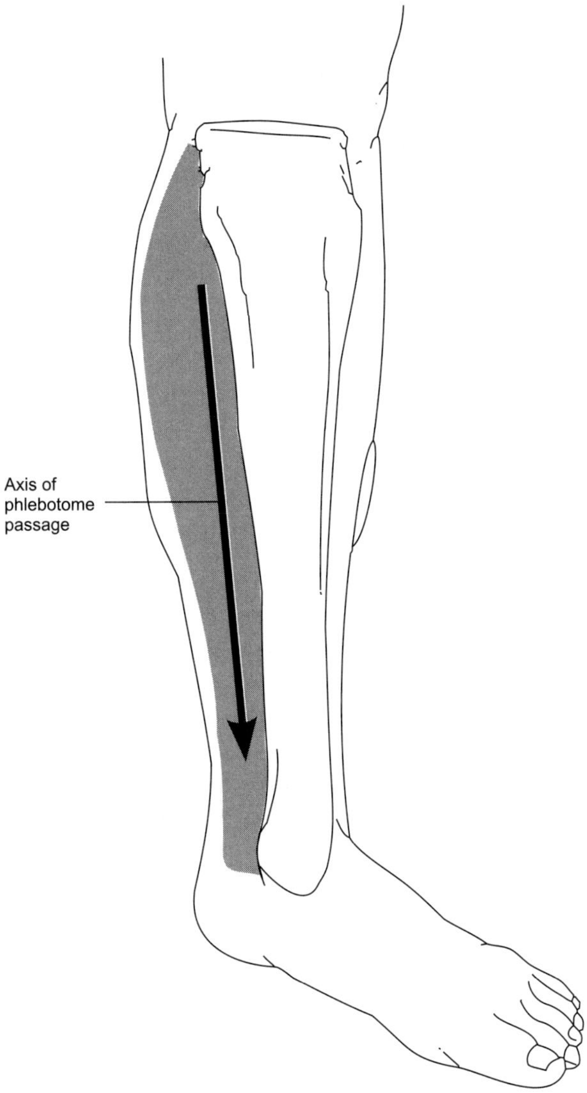

Figure 38.7 *Axis of phlebotome passage to interrupt posterior arcade Cockett's perforators. (Reproduced with permission from DePalma RG. Surgical treatment of venous ulceration. In Bergan JJ, Yao JST, eds.* Venous Disorders. *Philadelphia: WB Saunders, 1990: 396–406)*

scopic equipment for subfascial endoscopic surgical procedures (SEPS).

The 'conventional' procedures might be considered to require comparison to alternatives such as venous bypass, valve repair alone, valve transplantation, and SEPS. Given the variable anatomy and physiology leading to venous ulceration, it appears likely that combinations of interventions are needed in certain cases. A 22% ulcer recurrence rate at 30 months with SEPS[20] suggests a need to re-evaluate indications and the techniques of this procedure. For class 5–6 disease with dominant inframalleolar and foot perforators, and also when skin grafting is required, the author now uses extrafascial perforator interruption in the lower leg and

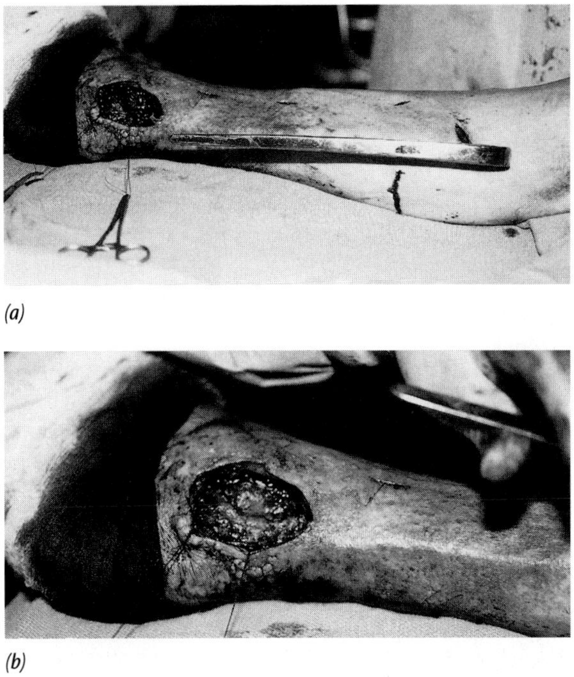

Figure 38.8 *(a) Operative photograph of shearing procedure to interrupt posterior arcade; ulcer recurrence 2 years after SEPS. (b) Note ligatures of perforators from posterior-tibial vein at posterior rim of ulcer excision.*

foot along with SEPS to deal with upper perforators. The retromalleolar space and inframalleolar perforators are not accessible with SEPS as this space is quite tight.

To assess results, we compared preoperative non-operative treatment for 3 years in compliant patients with postoperative results.[21] Perforator interruption was mainly used along with other procedures. Data included number of occurrences of ulceration amongst 10 individuals (range 3–8 per individual) with average time of 13 weeks to heal. Nine of ten patients remained healed postoperatively up to 5 years at present; one recurrence was treated with a second extrafascial procedure; this individual remains healed. Clinical severity score was reduced from 12 (9–17) preoperatively, to a mean of 3.5. Using carefully characterized cohorts methods of quantification such as these can be used to quantify results pre and postoperatively. Since additional procedures along with perforator interruption might be required, prospective randomization of a single method of perforator interruption would appear to be a daunting task.

As this chapter is written, progress is still being made. With each case of venous disease we learn something new and we write at the same time as we search for answers. The vexing problems of lipodermatosclerosis and ulceration are identical end results of differing and chaotic patterns of venous disease. It appears unlikely that one answer will emerge from linear analyses of fractal data or from a single surgical procedure.

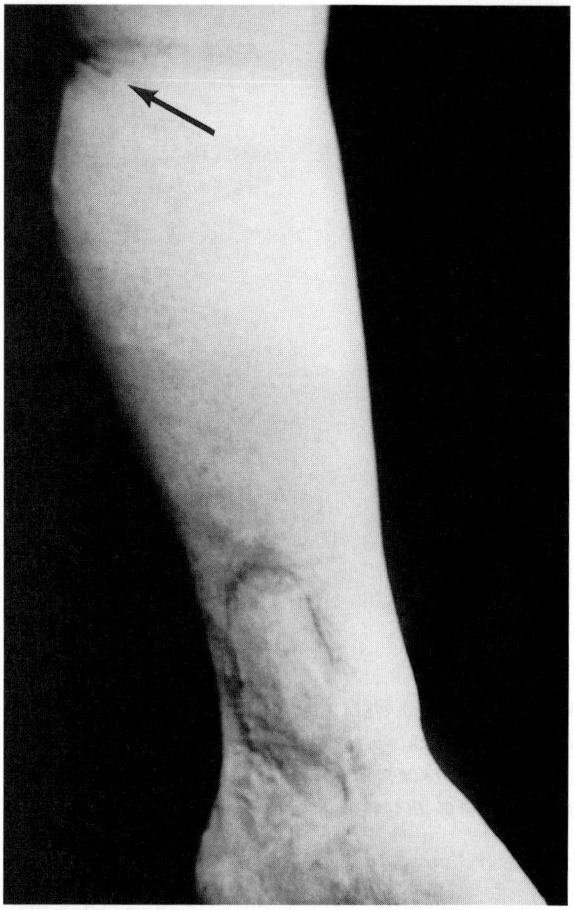

Figure 38.9 *Ten-year result of shearing procedure and skin graft performed upon a 50-year-old woman with thrombosis of superficial femoral vein. Arrow indicates shearing access incision. Patient continues to wear a 30 mmHg graded support stocking.*

Generally, the principle of perforator interruption which prevents transmission of venous hypertension to vulnerable skin areas, benefits many patients.

REFERENCES

1. Linton RR. The communicating veins of the lower leg and the operative techniques for their ligation. *Ann Surg* 1938; **107**: 582.
2. Linton RR. The post thrombotic ulceration of the lower extremity: its etiology and surgical treatment. *Ann Surg* 1953; **138**: 415.
3. Dodd H, Cockett FR. The management of venous ulcers. In *The Pathology and Surgery of the Veins of the Lower Limbs.* Edinburgh, London and New York: Churchill Livingstone, 1976: 269–96.
4. Walsh TC, Bergan JJ, Beewan S, Mouton SL. Proximal venous reflux adversely effects distal venous function. *Surgery* 1994; **8**: 566.
5. Negus D. The distal long saphenous vein in recurrent venous ulceration In Raymond-Martimbeau P, Prescott R, Zummo M, eds. *Phlebologie '92.* Paris: John Libbey Eurotext, 1992: 1291.
6. Haeger K. Anatomy of the veins of the leg. In Hobbs JT, ed. *The Treatment of Venous Disorders.* Philadelphia: JB Lippincott, 1977: 18–33.
7. Browse NL, Burnand KG, Thomas ML. The natural history and treatment of varicose veins. In *Diseases of the Veins. Pathology, Diagnosis and Treatment.* London: Arnold, 1988: 201–51.
8. Cockett FB, Elgan-Jones DE. The ankle blow out syndrome *Lancet* 1953; **1**: 17.
9. Guillot C. In Henreit JP, ed. *Anatomical Atlas of the Superficial Venous Network of the Lower Limbs.* Cabourg-France, Corlet Imprimeur SA, 1998.
10. Bergan JJ. New developments in surgery of the venous system. *Cardiovasc Surg* 1993; **1**: 624–31.
11. Kamida CB, Kistner RL. Descending phlebography, the Staub technique. In Bergan JJ, Kistner RL, eds. *Atlas of Venous Surgery.* Philadelphia: WB Saunders, 1992: 105–10.
12. DePalma RG. Surgical therapy for venous stasis. *Surgery* 1974; **76**: 910.
13. Dodd H. The diagnosis and ligation of incompetent ankle perforating veins. *Ann R Coll Surg Engl* 1964; **34**: 186–96.
14. Edwards JM. Shearing operation for incompetent perforating veins. *Br J Surg* 1976; **63**: 885–6.
15. DePalma RG. Surgical therapy for venous stasis: results of a modified Linton operation. *Am J Surg* 1979; **137**: 810–13.
16. DePalma RG. Surgical treatment of chronic venous ulceration. In Bergan JJ, Yao JST, eds. *Venous Disorders.* Philadelphia: WB Saunders, 1990: 396–406.
17. Simpson CJ, Smellie GD. The phlebotome in the management of incompetent perforating veins and venous ulceration. *J Cardiovasc Surg (Torino)* 1987; **78**: 279–81.
18. DePalma RG. Surgical treatment of chronic venous ulceration. In Raymond-Martimbeau P, Prescott, R, Zummo PM, eds. *Phlebologie '92.* Paris: John Libbey Eurotext, 1992: 1235–7.
19. DePalma RG. Evolving surgical approaches for venous ulceration. In Negus D, Jantet G, Coleridge Smith PD, eds. *Phlebology '95.* London: Springer, 1995: Suppl I, 980–2.
20. Gloviczki P, Bergan JJ, Rhodes JM, Canton LG, Harmsen S, Ilstrup DM. Mid-term results of endoscopic perforator vein interruption for chronic venous insufficiency: lessons learned from the North American subfascial endoscopic perforator surgery registry. The North American Study Group. *J Vasc Surg* 1999; **29**: 489–502.
21. DePalma RG, Kowallek DL. Venous ulceration: a cross-over study from nonoperative to operative treatment. *J Vasc Surg* 1996; **24**: 788–92.

39

Subfascial endoscopic perforating vein surgery

JEFFREY M RHODES, PETER GLOVICZKI, MANJU KALRA AND AUDRA A NOEL

Incompetent perforating veins have been linked to chronic venous insufficiency and its most severe manifestation, venous ulceration, for over a century.[1] The hallmark of treatment of chronic venous insufficiency has been compression therapy.[2] Over the past two decades, however, the emergence of minimally invasive surgical techniques has led to increasing interest and much debate about appropriate surgical therapy for the treatment of severe chronic venous insufficiency and venous ulcers.

The classic operation, as suggested by Linton in 1938 to ligate perforating veins to treat venous ulcers, has been abandoned because of an estimated 24% major wound complication rate.[3,4] Although several authors have made modifications to Linton's original technique to decrease wound complications, a major change in practice did not occur until the development of subfascial endoscopic perforator surgery (SEPS). In 1985, Hauer reported his technique of perforator vein division using an endoscope inserted at a site distant from the ulceration.[5–7] In contrast to the Linton procedure, wound complication rate with SEPS, including minor wound problems, is of the order of only 5%.[4] SEPS has become the surgical technique of choice for perforator ablation. However, the efficacy of perforator ablation, regardless of which technique is used, remains intensely debated.

This chapter discusses indications and preoperative evaluation for SEPS, presents the currently used endoscopic techniques and discusses the available hemodynamic and clinical results following SEPS.

SURGICAL ANATOMY OF PERFORATING VEINS

Chapter 2 in this volume presents important details on the anatomy of the perforating veins. To emphasize key points, a few observations need to be mentioned here. Perforating veins are those that connect the superficial venous system to the deep veins. Valves within the calf and thigh perforators prevent blood from refluxing into superficial from the deep system, although in some normal limbs reversal of flow in the perforators can be demonstrated.[8,9] The Cockett perforators are the most important clinically and they originate from the posterior arch vein (Leonardo's vein) and connect to the paired posterior tibial veins. Although the posterior arch vein does connect to the greater saphenous vein just below the knee, if saphenous stripping alone is performed, incompetent Cockett perforators will frequently be left intact. In addition to the Cockett perforators, the more proximal paratibial perforators are also believed to be of clinical significance. These connect either the posterior arch vein or the greater saphenous vein and its tributaries to the posterior tibial and popliteal veins.

One must be aware of variations in the perforator system that would limit their accessibility with the endoscope. Anatomic dissections by Mozes *et al.* demonstrated that only 63% of the medial perforators can be identified in the posterior superficial compartment alone.[10] The remaining Cockett II, III and some of the paratibial perforators lie within the intermuscular septum dividing the deep and superficial compartments or within the posterior deep compartment itself. Therefore, one must perform a paratibial fasciotomy (incise the fascia of the deep posterior compartment, distal to edge of the soleus muscle). The incision in the fascia is made close to the tibia, to avoid injury to the posterior tibial vessels and tibial nerve. Exploration of the deep compartment is now done routinely during SEPS in order to identify and interrupt all clinically relevant perforating veins.

INDICATIONS FOR PERFORATOR INTERRUPTION

Many patients with advanced chronic venous insufficiency have incompetent perforators. Although isolated perforator incompetence is seen in only 5% of patients with venous ulceration, it occurs in conjunction with superficial reflux (without deep reflux) in 32% of patients (Table 39.1). Incompetent calf perforators in conjunction with either superficial or deep reflux have been reported in 73% of limbs with venous ulceration. The presence of incompetent perforators in patients with advanced CVI (clinical classes 4–6, i.e. lipodermatosclerosis, healed or active ulceration[11]) and low operative risk constitute indications for surgical intervention. An open ulcer is not a contraindication for SEPS. Contraindications include associated arterial occlusive disease, infected ulcer, a nonambulatory or a medically high-risk patient. Diabetes, renal failure, liver failure, morbid obesity or ulcers in patients with rheumatoid arthritis or scleroderma are relative contraindications. Presence of deep venous obstruction at the level of the popliteal vein or higher on preoperative imaging is also a relative contraindication. Patients with extensive skin changes, circumferential large ulcers, recent deep venous thrombosis, severe lymphedema or large legs may not be suitable candidates. SEPS has been performed for recurrent disease after previous perforator interruption, however it is technically more demanding in this situation. Limbs with lateral ulcerations should be managed by open interruption of lateral or posterior perforators where appropriate.

PREOPERATIVE EVALUATION

Preoperative evaluation includes imaging studies to document superficial, deep and/or perforator incompetence and to guide the operative intervention. The preferred test is duplex scanning. Ascending and descending phlebography are reserved for patients with underlying occlusive disease or recurrent ulceration after perforator division in whom deep venous reconstruction is being considered. Preoperative duplex mapping assists the surgeon in identifying all incompetent perforators at the time of operation. Duplex scanning is performed with the patient on a tilted examining table with the affected extremity in a near upright non-weight-bearing position. Perforator incompetence is defined by retrograde (outward) flow lasting greater than 0.3 seconds or longer than antegrade flow during the relaxation phase after release of manual compression.[12] Duplex scanning has 100% specificity and the highest sensitivity of all diagnostic tests to predict the sites of incompetent perforating veins.[13,14] In addition to duplex scanning, a functional study such as strain-gauge or air plethysmography is performed before and after surgery to quantify the degree of incompetence, identify abnormalities in calf muscle pump function, aid in the exclusion of outflow obstruction and assess hemodynamic results of surgical intervention.[15,16]

Table 39.1 *Distribution of valvular incompetence in patients with advanced chronic venous disease*

Author, Year	No. limbs	Sup no. (%)	Perf no. (%)	Deep no.(%)	Sup + Perf no. (%)	Sup + Perf + Deep no. (%)
Schanzer,[34] 1982	52	3 (6)	20 (38)	4 (8)	11 (21)	14 (27)
Negus,[32] 1983	77	0 (0)	0 (0)	0 (0)	35 (46)	42 (54)
Sethia,[45] 1984	60	0 (0)	5 (8)	20 (33)	17 (28)	18 (30)
Hanrahan,[46] 1991	91	16 (17)	8 (8)	2 (2)	18 (19)	47 (49)
van Bemmelen,[47] 1991	25	0 (0)	0 (0)	2 (8)	3 (12)	20 (80)
Darke,[48] 1992	213	0 (0)	8 (4)	47 (22)	83 (39)	75 (35)
Lees,[49] 1993	25	3 (12)	0 (0)	3 (12)	10 (40)	9 (36)
Shami,[50] 1993	59	0 (0)	0 (0)	19 (32)	31 (53)	9 (15)
van Rij,[64] 1994	120	48 (40)	6 (5)	10 (8)	31 (26)	25 (21)
Myers,[51] 1995	96	15 (16)	2 (2)	7 (8)	25 (26)	47 (49)
Labropoulos,[52] 1996	120	26 (22)	1 (1)	5 (4)	23 (19)	65 (54)
Gloviczki,[25] 1999	146	0 (0)	7 (5)	0 (0)	66 (45)	73 (50)
Total	1084	111 (10)	57 (5)	119 (11)	353 (32)	444 (41)

Sup, superficial incompetence; Perf, perforator incompetence; Deep, deep vein incompetence.

SURGICAL TECHNIQUE

Hauer's initial description of SEPS was of a single port approach to gain access to the subfascial space.[7] This has since been refined with the advent of an endoscope that is designed specifically for SEPS. This device has two channels that allow for both viewing and instrumentation through a single port (Fig. 39.1). To provide a bloodless operative field, the limb is first exsanguinated with an Esmarque bandage and a pneumatic tourniquet placed on the proximal thigh is then inflated to 300 mmHg. A skin and fascial incision is then made in the mid-calf 4 cm posterior to the medial tibial border. The endoscope is inserted to the level of the medial malleolus and the subfascial space is bluntly dissected and explored as the endoscope is withdrawn. All perforating veins that are encountered are clipped and divided. Some of the single port endoscopic equipment now allows for CO_2 insufflation that aids in visualization of the subfascial space.

Our preferred technique for perforator ablation is the two-port technique. This utilizes standard laparoscopic instrumentation and two ports, one for the camera and another for dissection. O'Donnell[17] initially described this approach, which was then simultaneously developed by our group at the Mayo Clinic[18–20] and by Conrad in Australia.[21] We use a thigh tourniquet and limb exsanguination to provide a bloodless field. Two 10 mm diameter endoscopic ports are placed in the medial aspect of the calf 10 cm distal to the tibial tuberosity and about 10–12 cm apart, proximal to the diseased skin (Fig. 39.2). More recently, we have changed to a 5 mm distal port, since the availability of 5 mm harmonic scalpel and excellent 5 mm instruments (scissors, dissecting instruments). The distal port is now placed halfway between the first port and the ankle, for easier dissection. The camera through the 10 mm port reaches all the way to the medial malleolus. Too proximal a placement will make distal visualization more difficult. We are now routinely using balloon dissection to widen the subfascial space and facilitate access after port placement.[22] We use a 10 mm video camera, since they withstand the torque better than the smaller, 5 or 2 mm scopes. Carbon dioxide is insufflated into the subfascial space and pressure is maintained around 30 mmHg to improve visualization and access to the perforators. Using laparoscopic scissors inserted through the second port, the remaining loose connective tissue between the calf muscles and the superficial fascia is sharply divided.

The subfascial space is widely explored from the medial border of the tibia to the posterior midline and down to the level of the ankle. All perforators encountered are divided either with the harmonic scalpel, electrocautery or sharply between clips (Fig. 39.3a). A paratibial fasciotomy is next made by incising the fascia of the posterior deep compartment (Fig. 39.3b). The Cockett II and Cockett III perforators are located frequently within an intermuscular septum, and this has to be incised before identification and division of the perforators can be accomplished. The medial insertion of the soleus muscle on the tibia may also have to be exposed to visualize proximal paratibial perforators. By rotating the ports cephalad and continuing the dissection up to the level of the knee the more proximal perforators can also be divided. Whilst

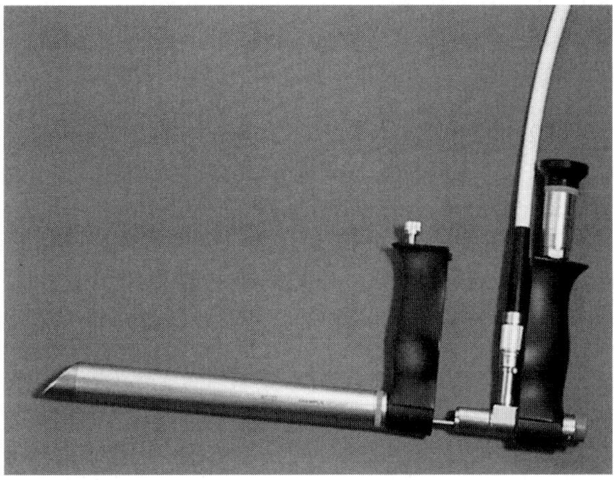

Figure 39.1 *Olympus endoscope for the subfascial perforating vein interruption. The scope can be used with or without CO_2 insufflation. It has an 85° field of view and the outer sheath is either 16 or 22 mm in diameter. The working channel is 6 × 8.5 mm, with a working length of 20 cm. (Reproduced with permission from Bergan JJ, Ballard JL, Sparks S. Subfascial endoscopic perforator vein surgery: the open technique. In Gloviczki P, Bergan JJ, eds.* Atlas of Endoscopic Perforator Vein Surgery. *London: Springer-Verlag, 1998: 141–9)*

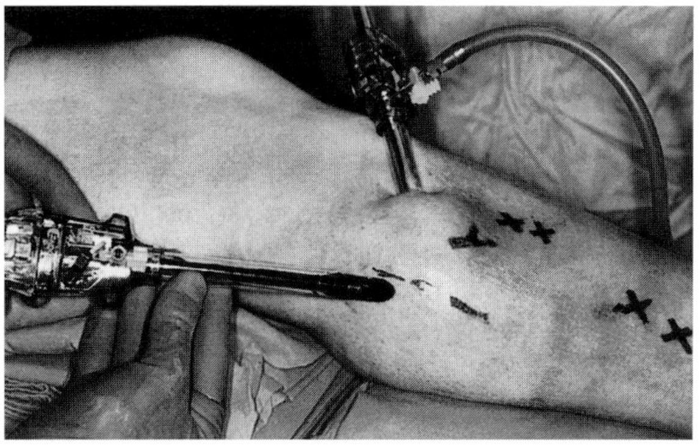

Figure 39.2 *Two-port technique for SEPS. Carbon dioxide is insufflated through first port, that is used for the video camera. Placement of a second 10 mm port is performed under video control. Note that incompetent perforators were marked with an X preoperatively using duplex scanning. (Reproduced with permission from Gloviczki P, Cambria RA, Rhee RY, Canton LG, McKusick MA. Surgical technique and preliminary results with endoscopic subfascial division of perforating veins.* J Vasc Surg *1996;* ***23****: 517–23)*

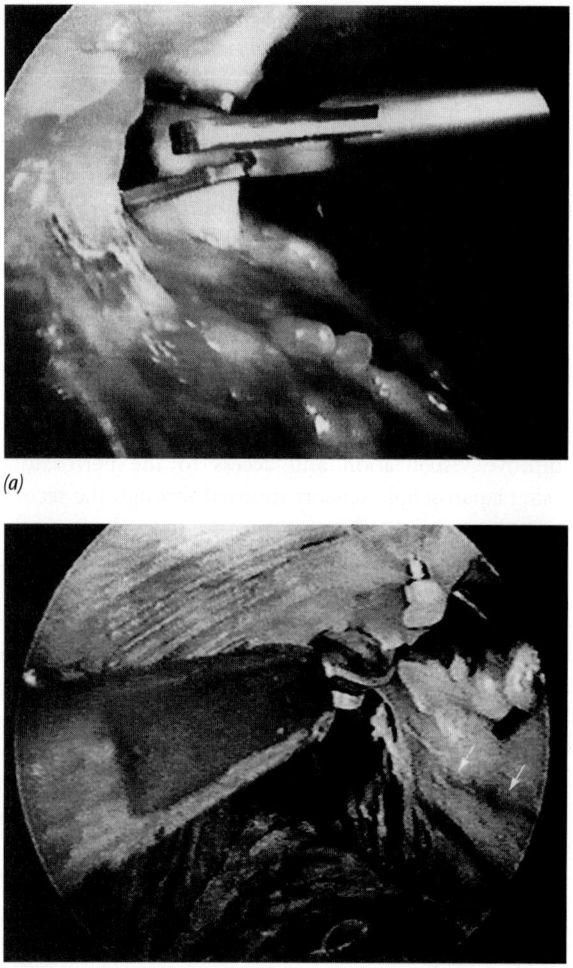

(a)

(b)

Figure 39.3 *(a) Division of the perforator (left leg) with endoscopic scissors after placement of vascular clips. (Reproduced with permission from Gloviczki P, Cambria RA, Rhee RY, Canton LG, McKusick MA. Surgical technique and preliminary results with endoscopic subfascial division of perforating veins.* J Vasc Surg *1996;* ***23****: 517–23) (b) Paratibial fasciotomy of the right leg performed with endoscopic scissors. The posterior tibial vessels (arrow) can often be seen through the fascia separating the superficial and deep compartments. (Reproduced with permission from Gloviczki P, Canton LG, Cambria RA, Rhee RY. Subfascial endoscopic perforator vein surgery with gas insufflation. In Gloviczki P, Bergan JJ, eds.* Atlas of Endoscopic Perforator Vein Surgery. *London: Springer-Verlag, 1998: 125–38)*

the paratibial fasciotomy can aid in distal exposure, reaching retromalleolar Cockett I perforator endoscopically is usually not possible, and if incompetent, may require a separate small incision over it to gain direct exposure.

After completion of the endoscopic portion of the procedure, the instruments and ports are removed, the CO_2 is manually expressed from the limb and the tourniquet is deflated. Bupivacaine hydrochloride (Marcaine), 20 ml 0.5% solution is instilled into the subfascial space for postoperative pain control. Stab avulsion of varicosities in addition to high ligation and stripping of the greater and/or lesser saphenous vein, if incompetent, is performed. The wounds are closed and the limb is elevated and wrapped with an elastic bandage. Elevation is maintained at 30° postoperatively for 3 hours after which ambulation is permitted. Unlike the in-hospital stay after an open Linton procedure, this is an outpatient procedure and patients are discharged the same day or next morning following overnight observation. Restrictions are the same as with greater saphenous stripping. Patients are allowed to return to work after 10 days to 2 weeks.

RESULTS OF SURGICAL TREATMENT

Clinical results

To provide level 1 evidence on the efficacy of perforator interruption in the treatment of advanced chronic venous disease, prospective, randomized, multicenter trials will be needed.[23] Presently such trials are being designed and initiated both in Europe and North America. Until such data are available, one must analyze the results of retrospective and prospective studies from single institutions or benefit from the recently presented data of the North American (NASEPS) registry.[24,25] Comparison of the reported data on medical and surgical treatment of chronic venous disease is not without its flaws, however. There are several important clinical variables that make the comparison difficult. First, many series have not adequately documented the pathophysiology of venous disease and only the most recent publications use the CEAP classification scheme proposed by the International Consensus Committee on Chronic Venous Disease.[11] Second, the larger series on nonoperative management have divided their patients into compliant and noncompliant groups.[2,26] While such studies demonstrate the importance of patient compliance in achieving clinical success, it is difficult to compare results with surgical series, when such separation of patients following surgical treatment was not reported. Third, since concomitant ablation of superficial reflux is often performed at the same time as SEPS, clinical benefit attributed directly to perforator interruption has been difficult to assess. Fourth, in many studies, extended follow-up with large numbers of patients was insufficient to accurately predict ulcer recurrence. Despite these limitations, valuable insight can be gained from the growing body of literature.

The classic papers of Linton[3,27] and Cockett[28,29] reported significant clinical benefit from open perforator ligation. This has been supported by subsequent data from several other investigators.[6,30–36] By combining data from the larger series, it is estimated that the crude ulcer recurrence rate was approximately 22% (range 0–55%) and the wound complication rate was significant, averaging 24% (range 12–53%) (Table 39.2).[4] Combined with the concern over the high wound complication rate, the open Linton procedure was dealt a critical blow with the 1976 *Lancet* publication authored by Burnand *et al.*[37] They reported a 55% overall ulcer recurrence rate, with 100% recurrence in a subset of 23 patients with post-thrombotic syndrome.[37] These data are often cited by those who argue against perforating vein ablation; however, a point often overlooked is that ulcer recurrence in the other subset of patients, those without post-thrombotic damage of the deep veins, was only 6%. This distinction between post-thrombotic limbs and those with primary valvular incompetence is critical. As evidenced in Burnand's paper, excellent outcome after surgical intervention is possible with proper patient selection.

Only a few small prospective randomized studies have been reported on treatment of chronic venous disease, mostly with medical management. In a non-controlled trial that compared 37 SEPS procedures with 30 antedated open perforator ligations, SEPS resulted in lower calf wound morbidity, shorter hospital stay and comparable short-term ulcer healing.[38] A single prospective randomized trial, conducted by Pierik *et al.*, compared the incidence of wound complications in 39 patients following open perforator ligation or SEPS.[39] Wound complications occurred in 53% in the open group versus 0% in the SEPS group with no ulcer recurrence in either group at a mean follow-up of 21 months. These studies indicate that SEPS is as effective as open perforator ablation during early follow-up, with the additional benefit of significantly fewer wound complications, thereby establishing it as the procedure of choice for perforator vein surgery, when indicated.

Experience with SEPS continues to grow and the midterm results from single centers as well as the North American registry are now available (Tables 39.3 and 39.4). The Mayo Clinic series included 57 consecutive

Table 39.2 *Clinical results of open perforator interruption for the treatment of advanced chronic venous disease*

Author, Year	No. limbs treated	No. limbs with ulcer	Wound complications no. (%)	Ulcer healing no. (%)	Ulcer recurrence* no. (%)	Mean follow-up (years)
Silver,[35] 1971	31	19	4 (14)	–	– (10)	1–15
Thurston,[36] 1973	102	0	12 (12)	†	11 (13)	3.3
Bowen,[53] 1975	71	8	31 (44)	–	24 (34)	4.5
Burnand,[37] 1976	41	0	–	†	24 (55)	–
Negus,[32] 1983	108	108	24 (22)	91 (84)	16 (15)	3.7
Wilkinson,[54] 1986	108	0	26 (24)	†	3 (7)	6
Cikrit,[31] 1988	32	30	6 (19)	30 (100)	5 (19)	4
Bradbury,[15] 1993	53	0	–	†	14 (26)	5
Pierik,[39] 1997	19	19	10 (53)	17 (90)	0 (0)	1.8
Total	565 (100)	184 (33)	113/468 (24)	138/157 (88)	97/443 (22)	–

*Recurrence calculated where data available and percentage accounts for patients lost to follow-up.
†Only class 5 (healed ulcer) patients admitted in study.

Table 39.3 *Clinical results of SEPS for the treatment of advanced chronic venous disease*

Author, Year	No. limbs treated	No limbs with ulcer*	Concomitant saphenous ablation no. (%)	Wound complications no. (%)	Ulcer healing no. (%)	Ulcer recurrence† no. (%)	Mean follow-up (months)
Jugenheimer,[55] 1992	103	17	97 (94)	3 (3)	16 (94)	0 (0)	27
Pierek,[56] 1995	40	16	4 (10)	3 (8)	16 (100)	1 (2.5)	46
Bergan,[57] 1996	31	15	31 (100)	3 (10)	15 (100)	(0)	–
Wolters,[58] 1996	27	27	0 (0)	2 (7)	26 (96)	2 (8)	12–24
Padberg,[41] 1996	11	0	11 (100)	–	‡	0 (0)	16
Pierek,[59] 1997	20	20	14 (70)	0 (0)	17 (85)	0 (0)	21
Rhodes,[16] 1998	57	22	41 (72)	3 (5)	22 (100)	5 (12)	17
Gloviczki,[25] 1999	146	101	86 (59)	9 (6)	85 (84)	26 (21)	24
Illig,[60] 1999	30	19	–	–	17 (89)	4 (15)	9
Total: no. limbs (%)	465 (100)	237 (51)	284/435 (65)	23/424 (5)	214/237 (90)	38/329 (12)	–

*Only class 6 (active ulcer) patients are included.
†Recurrence calculated for class 5 and 6 limbs only, where data available and percentage accounts for patients lost to follow-up.
‡Only class 5 (healed ulcer) patients were admitted in this study.

Table 39.4 *Clinical results of SEPS (perforator ligation) alone for the treatment of advanced chronic venous disease*

Author, Year	No. limbs	Recurrence no. (%)
Jugenheimer,[55] 1992	16	0 (0)
Pierik,[56] 1995	34	1 (3)
Wolters,[58] 1996	26	2 (8)
DePalma,[61] 1996	3	1 (33)
Pierik,[59] 1997	2	0 (0)
Sparks,[62] 1997	7	0 (0)
Pierik,[39] 1997	3	0 (0)
Rhodes,[16] 1998	4	1 (25)
Gloviczki,[25] 1999	38	11 (29)
Murray,[63] 1999	18	2 (11)
Total	151	18 (12)

SEPS procedures in 48 patients.[40] Correction of superficial reflux, when present, is a critical step in the surgical management of venous disease and consequently 41 limbs had concomitant ablation of saphenous reflux. The minor wound complication rate was 5% and one patient developed an early recurrent deep venous thrombosis. All 22 limbs with active ulcers demonstrated healing within a median of 36 days after surgery. New or recurrent ulcers developed in 9% of all patients and in 12% of those with preoperative class 5 and class 6 disease during follow-up that extended to 52 months and averaged 17 months. Post-thrombotic deep vein obstruction was associated with both delayed healing and ulcer recurrence while patients with primary valvular incompetence had no ulcer recurrences.

The relative safety of SEPS was also confirmed in the early report of North American (NASEPS) registry, with a 6% wound complication rate and one deep venous thrombosis at 2 months after surgery.[26] The midterm (24 months) results in 146 patients followed up in the registry demonstrated an 88% cumulative ulcer healing rate at 1 year.[25] The median time to ulcer healing was 54 days (Fig. 39.4). Using life-table methods, a significant rate of ulcer recurrence (1 year, 16% and 2 year, 28%) following SEPS was predicted (Fig. 39.5a). Similar to the Mayo Clinic series, post-thrombotic limbs had a higher 2-year cumulative recurrence rate (46%) than those with primary valvular incompetence (20%) ($P < 0.05$) (Fig. 39.5b). The nine post-thrombotic limbs with a component of deep vein obstruction fared particularly poorly, with failure to heal ulcers in four limbs and ulcer recurrence in the remaining five. Twenty-eight (23%) of the 122 patients who had an active or healed ulcer (class 5 or 6) before surgery, had an active ulcer at last follow-up. Despite experiencing an ulcer recurrence, these patients still demonstrated improvement over their preoperative state based on scoring of the clinical signs and symptoms. Pain was less, the ulcer was smaller, easier to manage and it was single more often than multiple. So while the observed recurrence rates in the Registry were high, they still compare favorably to results of nonoperative management.

Hemodynamic results

Given the chronicity of venous disease and the extended follow-up required to fully assess the results of interventions, many authors have focused on measuring parameters of venous hemodynamics, both to quantify the results of therapy and to follow patients over time. These hemodynamic studies should be considered analogous to the noninvasive studies that many surgeons use to follow their arterial reconstructions. Whilst most studies, including the NASEPS Registry, lacked sufficient hemodynamic data to support the clinical results,

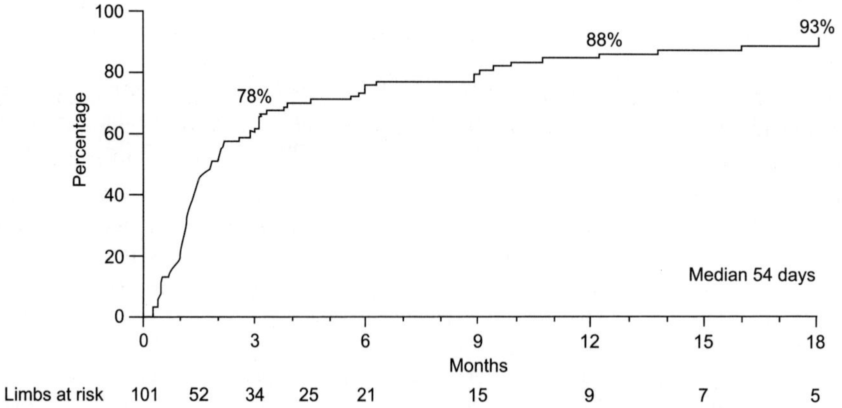

Figure 39.4 *Cumulative ulcer healing in 101 patients following SEPS. The 90-day, 1- and 1.5-year healing rates are indicated. The standard error is less than 10% at all time points. (Reproduced with permission from Gloviczki P, Bergan JJ, Rhodes JM, Canton LG, Harmsen S, Ilstrup DM and the North American Study Group. Mid-term results of endoscopic perforator vein interruption for chronic venous insufficiency: lessons learned from the North American Subfascial Endoscopic Perforator Surgery (NASEPS) registry.* J Vasc Surg *1999;* ***29****: 489–502)*

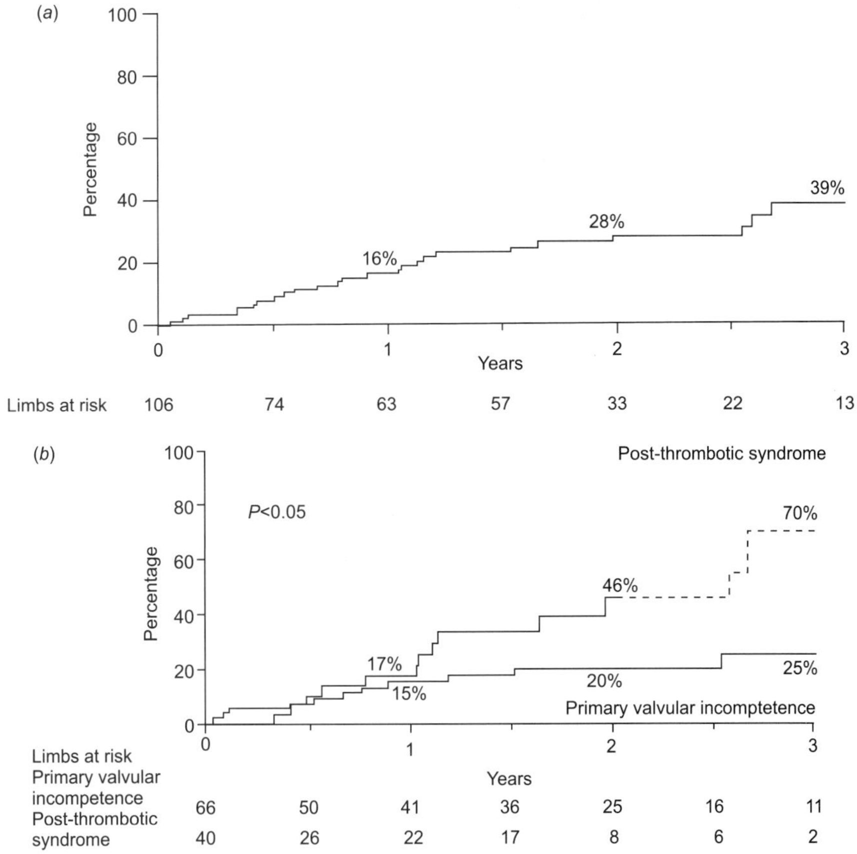

Figure 39.5 *(a) Cumulative ulcer recurrence in 106 patients following SEPS. The 1-, 2- and 3-year recurrence rates are indicated. All class 5 limbs at the time of SEPS and class 6 limbs that subsequently healed were included. The start point (day 0) for time to recurrence in class 6 patients was the date of initial ulcer healing. The standard error is less than 10% at all time points. (b) Ulcer recurrence based on etiology of chronic venous insufficiency. Limbs were separated into primary valvular incompetence (*n *= 66) and post-thrombotic syndrome (*n *= 40). The 1-, 2- and 3-year recurrence rates are indicated. The dashed line represents a standard error of greater than 10% (*P *<0.05). (Reproduced with permission from Gloviczki P, Bergan JJ, Rhodes JM, Canton LG, Harmsen S, Ilstrup DM and the North American Study Group. Mid-term results of endoscopic perforator vein interruption for chronic venous insufficiency: Lessons learned from the North American Subfascial Endoscopic Perforator Surgery (NASEPS) registry.* J Vasc Surg *1999;* ***29****: 489–502)*

functional improvement after perforator interruption has been reported. Bradbury *et al.* used foot volumetry and duplex scanning to assess hemodynamic improvement after saphenous and perforator ligation in 43 patients with recurrent ulcers.[15] Expulsion fraction and half-refilling time (T50) improved significantly after surgery in the 34 patients with no ulcer recurrence at 66 months. Recent air plethysmographic studies by Padberg *et al.* have documented persistent hemodynamic improvement up to 2 years following perforator ligation with concomitant correction of superficial reflux.[41] We have studied hemodynamic consequences of incompetent perforator vein interruption, using strain-gauge plethysmography to assess calf muscle pump function, venous incompetence and outflow obstruction before and within 6 months following endoscopic perforator vein surgery.[16] Both calf muscle pump function and the degree of venous incompetence improved significantly following SEPS (Figs 39.6 and 39.7). The improvement in venous incompetence (measured by refill rate) correlated strongly with the clinical improvement of our patients (Fig. 39.8). In the subset of patients that underwent SEPS alone ($n = 7$), without concomitant superficial reflux ablation, a significant improvement in hemodynamic status could not be demonstrated. This was most likely due to both the small numbers in this group and the relative predominance of post-thrombotic limbs. It is also logical to assume that perforator interruption alone would result in a lesser hemodynamic improvement than perforator interruption with concomitant superficial reflux ablation.

Hemodynamic improvement was significantly better in patients with primary valvular incompetence compared to post-thrombotic limbs.[16] Proebstle *et al.* using light reflection rheography before and 8 weeks following SEPS had very similar results to the Mayo Clinic series, showing significant improvement in limbs with primary valvular incompetence.[42] Similar to findings of Burnand

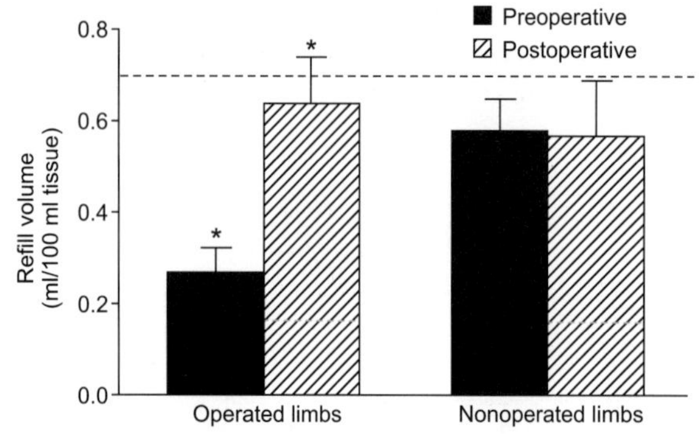

Figure 39.6 *Calf muscle pump function as measured by refill volume both pre- and postoperatively in the operated* (n = 28) *and nonoperated contralateral limbs* (n = 18). *P *<0.01; dashed line indicates normal refill volume (0.7 ml/100 ml tissue. (Adapted from Rhodes JM, Gloviczki P, Canton LG, Heaser TV, Rooke T. Endoscopic perforator vein division with ablation of superficial reflux improves venous hemodynamics.* J Vasc Surg *1998;* ***28****: 839–47)*

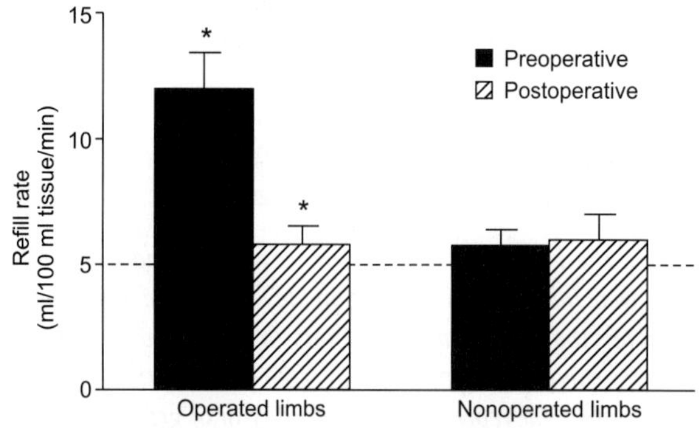

Figure 39.7 *Venous incompetence as assessed by refill rate after passive drainage both pre- and postoperatively in the operated* (n = 30) *and nonoperated contralateral limbs* (n = 20). *P *<0.001; dashed line indicates normal refill rate <5.0 ml/100 ml tissue/min. (Adapted from Rhodes JM, Gloviczki P, Canton LG, Heaser TV, Rooke T. Endoscopic perforator vein division with ablation of superficial reflux improves venous hemodynamics.* J Vasc Surg *1998;* ***28****: 839–47)*

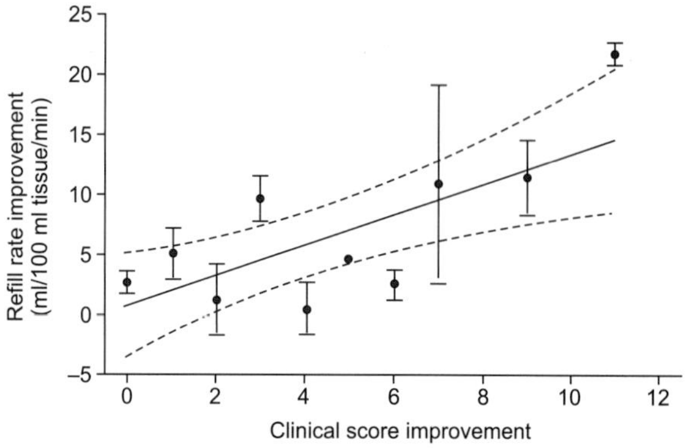

Figure 39.8 *Correlation between clinical and hemodynamic improvement measured by refill rate after SEPS with or without ablation of superficial reflux* (n = 29). *The mean values ± SEM and the results of linear regression analysis are depicted with 95% confidence intervals* (r = *0.77,* P *<0.01). (Adapted from Rhodes JM, Gloviczki P, Canton LG, Heaser TV, Rooke T. Endoscopic perforator vein division with ablation of superficial reflux improves venous hemodynamics.* J Vasc Surg *1998;* ***28****: 839–47)*

et al.[43] and Stacey *et al.*,[44] neither we nor the University of Ulm group were able to show significant hemodynamic improvement in post-thrombotic patients. It is important to note, however, that the number of patients studied in this subgroup has been low, less than 15 in all reported studies.[42,44] The benefits in these patients are clearly not of the same magnitude as in those with primary valvular incompetence.

CONCLUSION

Perforator incompetence, caused by primary valvular incompetence or by previous deep venous thrombosis, contributes to ambulatory venous hypertension and the development of chronic venous disease. Although the exact role and contribution of perforators in the development of venous ulcers is under debate, poor results of nonoperative management to prevent ulcer recurrence justify surgical attempts at perforator ligation, in addition to ablation of superficial reflux. The endoscopic technique of perforator interruption has significantly fewer wound complications than the open technique and is the preferred method for ablation of medial perforating veins. Interruption of incompetent perforators with ablation of superficial reflux, if present, is effective and durable in decreasing symptoms of CVI and rapidly healing ulcers. Ulcer recurrence following correction of perforator and superficial reflux in patients with post-thrombotic syndrome is much higher than in patients with primary valvular incompetence. A prospective randomized trial is needed and the NAVUS (North American Venous Ulcer Surgery) Trial is currently under peer review. If funded, this study will define the long-term benefit of surgical treatment of venous ulcers over medical management and it will also define the role of SEPS in the treatment of patients with advanced chronic venous disease.

REFERENCES

1. Gay J. Lettsonian Lectures 1867. *Varicose Disease of the Lower Extremities.* London: Churchill, 1868.
2. Mayberry JC, Moneta GL, Taylor LMJ, Porter JM. Fifteen-year results of ambulatory compression therapy for chronic venous ulcers. *Surgery* 1991; **109**: 575–81.

3. Linton RR. The operative treatment of varicose veins and ulcers, based upon a classification of these lesions. *Ann Surg* 1938; **107**: 582–93.
4. Gloviczki P, Rhodes JM. The management of perforating vein incompetence. In Rutherford RB, ed. *Vascular Surgery*, 5th edn. Philadelphia: WB Saunders, 2000.
5. Edwards JM. Shearing operation for incompetent perforating veins. *Br J Surg* 1976; **63**: 885–6.
6. DePalma RG. Surgical therapy for venous stasis: results of a modified Linton operation. *Am J Surg* 1979; **137**: 810–13.
7. Hauer G. [Endoscopic subfascial discussion of perforating veins – preliminary report]. [German]. *Vasa* 1985; **14**: 59–61.
8. Sarin S, Scurr JH, Smith PD. Medial calf perforators in venous disease: the significance of outward flow. *J Vasc Surg* 1992; **16**: 40–6.
9. Lofgren EP, Myers TT, Lofgren KA, Kuster G. The venous valves of the foot and ankle. *Surg Gynecol Obstet* 1968; **127**: 289–90.
10. Mozes G, Gloviczki P, Menawat SS, Fisher DR, Carmichael SW, Kadar A. Surgical anatomy for endoscopic subfascial division of perforating veins. *J Vasc Surg* 1996; **24**: 800–8.
11. Porter JM, Moneta GL. Reporting standards in venous disease: an update. International Consensus Committee on Chronic Venous Disease [see comments]. *J Vasc Surg* 1995; **21**: 635–45.
12. Gloviczki P, Lewis BD, Lindsey JR, McKusick MA. Preoperative evaluation of chronic venous insufficiency with duplex scanning and venography. In Gloviczki P, Bergan JJ, eds. *Atlas of Endoscopic Perforator Vein Surgery.* London: Springer-Verlag, 1998: 81–91.
13. Pierik EG, Toonder IM, van Urk H, Wittens CH. Validation of duplex ultrasonography in detecting competent and incompetent perforating veins in patients with venous ulceration of the lower leg. *J Vasc Surg* 1997; **26**: 49–52.
14. O'Donnell TFJ, Burnand KG, Clemenson G, Thomas ML, Browse NL. Doppler examination vs clinical and phlebographic detection of the location of incompetent perforating veins: a prospective study. *Arch Surg* 1977; **112**: 31–5.
15. Bradbury AW, Stonebridge PA, Callam MJ, Ruckley CV, Allan PL. Foot volumetry and duplex ultrasonography after saphenous and subfascial perforating vein ligation for recurrent venous ulceration. *Br J Surg* 1993; **80**: 845–8.
16. Rhodes JM, Gloviczki P, Canton LG, Heaser TV, Rooke T. Endoscopic perforator vein division with ablation of superficial reflux improves venous hemodynamics. *J Vasc Surg* 1998; **28**: 839–47.
17. O'Donnell TF. Surgical treatment of incompetent communicating veins. *Atlas of Venous Surgery.* Philadelphia: WB Saunders, 2000: 111–24.
18. Gloviczki P, Cambria RA, Rhee RY, Canton LG, McKusick MA. Surgical technique and preliminary results of endoscopic subfascial division of perforating veins. *J Vasc Surg* 1996; **23**: 517–23.
19. Rhodes JM, Gloviczki P, Canton LG, Rooke T, Lewis BD, Lindsey JR. Factors affecting clinical outcome following endoscopic perforator vein ablation. *Am J Surg* 1998; **176**: 162–7.
20. Gloviczki P, Canton LG, Cambria RA, Rhee RY. Subfascial endoscopic perforator vein surgery with gas insufflation. In Gloviczki P, Bergan JJ, eds. *Atlas of Endoscopic Perforator Vein Surgery.* London: Springer-Verlag, 1998: 125–38.
21. Conrad P. Endoscopic exploration of the subfascial space of the lower leg with perforator interruption using laparoscopic equipment: a preliminary report. *Phlebology* 1994; **9**: 154–7.
22. Allen RC, Tawes RL, Wetter A, Fogarty TJ. Endoscopic perforator vein surgery: creation of a subfascial space. In Gloviczki P, Bergan JJ, eds. *Atlas of Endoscopic Perforator Vein Surgery.* London: Springer-Verlag, 1998: 153–62.
23. Sackett DL. Rules of evidence and clinical recommendations on the use of antithrombotic agents. *Chest* 1989; **95**: 2S–4S.
24. Gloviczki P, Bergan JJ, Menawat SS, *et al.* Safety, feasibility, and early efficacy of subfascial endoscopic perforator surgery: a preliminary report from the North American registry. *J Vasc Surg* 1997; **25**: 94–105.
25. Gloviczki P, Bergan JJ, Rhodes JM, Canton LG, Harmsen S, Ilstrup DM. Mid-term results of endoscopic perforator vein interruption for chronic venous insufficiency: lessons learned from the North American subfascial endoscopic perforator surgery registry. The North American Study Group. *J Vasc Surg* 1999; **29**: 489–502.
26. Erickson CA. Healing of venous ulcers in an ambulatory care program: the role of chronic venous insufficiency and patient compliance. *J Vasc Surg* 1995; **22**: 629–36.
27. Linton RR. The post-thrombotic ulceration of the lower extremity: its etiology and surgical treatment. *Ann Surg* 1953; **138**: 415–32.
28. Cockett FB, Jones BD. The ankle blow-out syndrome: a new approach to the varicose ulcer problem. *Lancet* 1953; **1**: 17–23.
29. Cockett FB. The pathology and treatment of venous ulcers of the leg. *Br J Surg* 1956; **44**: 260–78.
30. Anning ST. Leg ulcers: the results of treatment. *Angiology* 1956; **7**: 505–16.
31. Cikrit DF, Nichols WK, Silver D. Surgical management of refractory venous stasis ulceration. *J Vasc Surg* 1988; **7**: 473–8.
32. Negus D, Friedgood A. The effective management of venous ulceration. *Br J Surg* 1983; **70**: 623–7.
33. Dodd H, Cockett FR. The management of venous ulcers. In *The Pathology and Surgery of the Vein of the Lower Limbs.* New York: Churchill-Livingstone, 1976: 269–96.
34. Schanzer H, Peirce EC. A rational approach to surgery of the chronic venous statis syndrome. *Ann Surg* 1982; **195**: 25–9.
35. Silver D, Gleysteen JJ, Rhodes GR, Georgiade NG, Anlyan WG. Surgical treatment of the refractory postphlebitic ulcer. *Arch Surg* 1971; **103**: 554–60.

36. Thurston OG, Williams HT. Chronic venous insufficiency of the lower extremity. Pathogenesis and surgical treatment. *Arch Surg* 1973; **106**: 537–9.
37. Burnand K, Thomas ML, O'Donnell T, Browse NL. Relation between postphlebitic changes in the deep veins and results of surgical treatment of venous ulcers. *Lancet* 1976; **1**: 936–8.
38. Stuart WP, Adam DJ, Bradbury AW, Ruckley CV. Subfascial endoscopic perforator surgery is associated with significantly less morbidity and shorter hospital stay than open operation (Linton's procedure) [see comments]. *Br J Surg* 1997; **84**: 1364–5.
39. Pierik EG, van Urk H, Hop WC, Wittens CH. Endoscopic versus open subfascial division of incompetent perforating veins in the treatment of venous leg ulceration: a randomized trial. *J Vasc Surg* 1997; **26**: 1049–54.
40. Rhodes JM, Gloviczki P, Canton LG, Rooke T, Lewis BD, Lindsey JR. Factors affecting clinical outcome following endoscopic perforator vein ablation. *J Vasc Surg* 1998; **176**: 162–7.
41. Padberg FTJ, Pappas PJ, Araki CT, Back TL, Hobson RW. Hemodynamic and clinical improvement after superficial vein ablation in primary combined venous insufficiency with ulceration [see comments]. *J Vasc Surg* 1996; **24**: 711–18.
42. Proebstle TM, Weisel G, Paepcke U, Gass S, Weber L. Light reflection rheography and clinical course of patients with advanced venous disease before and after endoscopic subfascial division of perforating veins. *Dermatol Surg* 1998; **24**: 771–6.
43. Burnand KG, O'Donnell TFJ, Thomas ML, Browse NL. The relative importance of incompetent communicating veins in the production of varicose veins and venous ulcers. *Surgery* 1977; **82**: 9–14.
44. Stacey MC, Burnand KG, Layer GT, Pattison M. Calf pump function in patients with healed venous ulcers is not improved by surgery to the communicating veins or by elastic stockings. *Br J Surg* 1988; **75**: 436–9.
45. Sethia KK, Darke SG. Long saphenous incompetence as a cause of venous ulceration. *Br J Surg* 1984; **71**: 754–5.
46. Hanrahan LM, Araki CT, Rodriguez AA, Kechejian GJ, LaMorte WW, Menzoian JO. Distribution of valvular incompetence in patients with venous stasis ulceration. *J Vasc Surg* 1991; **13**: 805–12.
47. van Bemmelen PS, Bedford G, Beach K, Strandness DE Jr. Status of the valves in the superficial and deep venous system in chronic venous disease. *Surgery* 1991; **109**: 730–4.
48. Darke SG, Penfold C. Venous ulceration and saphenous ligation. *Eur J Vasc Surg* 1992; **6**: 4–9.
49. Lees TA, Lambert D. Patterns of venous reflux in limbs with skin changes associated with chronic venous insufficiency. *Br J Surg* 1993; **80**: 725–8.
50. Shami SK, Sarin S, Cheatle TR, Scurr JH, Smith PD. Venous ulcers and the superficial venous system [see comments]. *J Vasc Surg* 1993; **17**: 487–90.
51. Myers KA, Ziegenbein RW, Zeng GH, Matthews PG. Duplex ultrasonography scanning for chronic venous disease: patterns of venous reflux. *J Vasc Surg* 1995; **21**: 605–12.
52. Labropoulos N, Delis K, Nicolaides AN, Leon M, Ramaswami G. The role of the distribution and anatomic extent of reflux in the development of signs and symptoms in chronic venous insufficiency. *J Vasc Surg* 1996; **23**: 504–10.
53. Bowen FH. Subfascial ligation (Linton operation) of the perforating leg veins to treat post-thrombophlebitic syndrome. *Am Surg* 1975; **41**: 148–51.
54. Wilkinson GEJ, Maclaren IF. Long term review of procedures for venous perforator insufficiency. *Surg Gynecol Obstet* 1986; **163**: 117–20.
55. Jugenheimer M, Junginger T. Endoscopic subfascial sectioning of incompetent perforating veins in treatment of primary varicosis. *World J Surg* 1992; **16**: 971–5.
56. Pierik EGJM, Wittens CHA, van Urk H. Subfascial endoscopic ligation in the treatment of incompetent perforator veins. *Eur J Vasc Endovasc Surg* 1995; **5**: 38–41.
57. Bergan JJ, Murray J, Greason K. Subfascial endoscopic perforator vein surgery: a preliminary report. *Ann Vasc Surg* 1996; **10**: 211–19.
58. Wolters U, Schmit-Rixen T, Erasmi H, Lynch J. Endoscopic dissection of incompetent perforating veins in the treatment of chronic venous leg ulcers. *Vasc Surg* 1996; **30**: 481–7.
59. Pierik EG, van Urk H, Wittens CH. Efficacy of subfascial endoscopy in eradicating perforating veins of the lower leg and its relation with venous ulcer healing. *J Vasc Surg* 1997; **26**: 255–9.
60. Illig KA, Shortell CK, Ouriel K, Greenberg RK, Waldman D, Green RM. Photoplethysmography and calf muscle pump function after subfascial endoscopic perforator ligation. *J Vasc Surg* 1999; **30**: 1067–76.
61. DePalma RG, Kowallek DL. Venous ulceration: a cross-over study from nonoperative to operative treatment. *J Vasc Surg* 1996; **24**: 788–92.
62. Sparks SR, Ballard JL, Bergan JJ, Killeen JD. Early benefits of subfascial endoscopic perforator surgery (SEPS) in healing venous ulcers. *Ann Vasc Surg* 1997; **11**: 367–73.
63. Murray JD, Bergan JJ, Riffenburgh RH. Development of open-scope subfascial perforating vein surgery: lessons learned from the first 67 patients. *Ann Vasc Surg* 1999; **13**: 372–7.
64. Van Rij AM, Soloman C, Christie R. Anatomic and physiologic characteristics of venous ulceration. *J Vasc Surg* 1994; **20**: 759–64.

40

Superior vena cava syndrome: endovascular therapy

ROBERT L VOGELZANG AND NANCY SCHINDLER

Superior vena cava (SVC) syndrome was first described in 1757 in a patient with a syphilitic thoracic aortic aneurysm. In that era, inflammatory/infectious entities were the most common cause of caval obstruction but in modern times, most is due to mediastinal or pulmonary malignancy with far fewer being inflammatory or infectious in nature.

Obstruction of the SVC affects about 15 000 people per year. The vena cava is a thin-walled, low-pressure vessel in close contact with lymph nodes, lung and major vascular structures. It is thus particularly prone to mechanical obstruction by any number of intrathoracic processes.

As stated above, by far the most common cause of SVC syndrome is malignancy (85–97% of cases) with lung cancer representing 80% of all cases. Indeed, 3–5% of patients with lung cancer will develop SVC syndrome during the course of their illness. Metastatic cancers and lymphomas cause another 10–15% of these cases.[1–9]

Benign causes for SVC syndrome include, most importantly, central venous catheters. Other benign etiologies that have caused the syndrome are inflammatory processes (mediastinitis, tuberculosis, actinomycosis, histoplasmosis), teratoma, cysts, goiter, thymoma, vascular diseases (aneurysms) and penetrating or blunt trauma.

SVC syndrome secondary to central venous catheters and/or pacemakers is now a widely reported problem. Caval obstruction has been a well-recognized complication of pacemakers but any catheter placed for chemotherapy, dialysis access, or hyperalimentation can cause the problem as well. As the number of patients with chronic central venous catheters increases, we fully expect a marked increase in the incidence of this problem.

CLINICAL PRESENTATION

The clinical manifestations of SVC syndrome include venous congestion, upper body (including face) edema, severe continuous headache, visual disturbances, cyanosis, hoarseness, dyspnea on exertion and shortness of breath.[10] Patients with SVC syndrome can present gradually or acutely with the severity of the condition depending mainly on the presence and/or development of collaterals such as the azygos that is the most important pathway for central venous decompression in the face of obstruction. Severe cases can present with syncope, seizures, or coma. In our experience, most patients have symptoms that range in duration from several weeks to months with a gradual rather than abrupt onset.

DIAGNOSIS

The diagnosis of SVC syndrome is quite readily made clinically but modern imaging tests are almost always necessary for confirmation. Chest x-ray may show a mass and duplex scan generally reveals the presence of venous obstruction and collaterals but neither ever images the cause or the precise point of obstruction.[6] For these obvious reasons, CT or MRI is almost now universally performed, except in those who are being treated (Fig. 40.1). In those individuals, venography is

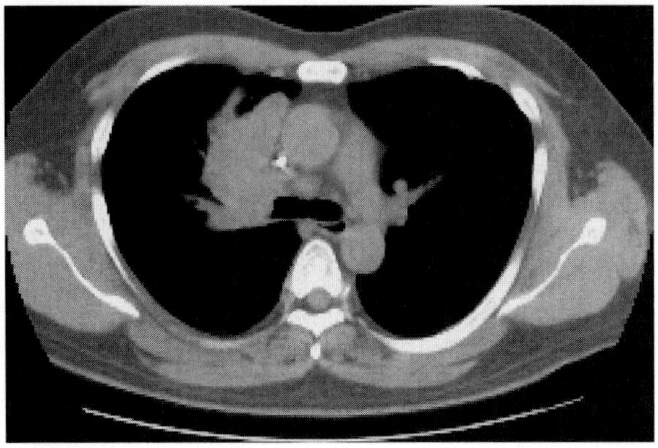

Figure 40.1 *CT of SVC obstruction.*

used to guide therapeutic decision making such as biopsy, stent placement or bypass. A tissue diagnosis can usually be obtained by sputum cytology, bronchoscopy, percutaneous fine needle aspiration, mediastinoscopy, or rarely, thoracotomy.

TREATMENT

In the past, the major treatment options for malignant SVC obstruction were conservative: anticoagulation and radiation with or without chemotherapy. For the most part, however, anticoagulation and other medical regimens including steroids and diuretics have not been effective. Radiation therapy, until recently, was considered the first-line therapy for many cases of SVC syndrome but the results in malignancy are quite poor with complete responses of only 15–60% as well as a significant recurrence rate of up to 33%. Furthermore, additional treatments for recurrence are usually not possible and complications such as esophagitis, weight loss, skin irritation, and initial worsening of symptoms secondary to edema can be seen.[11–13] Radiation is, however, most appropriate as a single therapy for non-small-cell lung cancers, and may be used alone or as part of combination therapy in the treatment of small-cell cancer or lymphoma, but it plays no role in the treatment of benign SVC syndrome. Chemotherapy is very useful in treating other sites of malignancy but it is not truly effective for relief of this problem, except in certain lesions like small-cell cancer and lymphoma. Even in these tumors, response and relief of symptoms is usually only partial (reported to be about 60% at best) and may not occur for several weeks.

Recent innovations in endovascular therapy have effected a major change in the treatment of this problem so that for almost all patients with symptomatic malignant SVC obstruction, endovascular techniques such as thrombolysis, angioplasty and stenting now represent the best method to relieve the disabling symptoms.

The first percutaneous management of SVC syndrome was reported in a child in 1982; the first successful adult caval angioplasty was performed by Sherry who dilated a lesion caused by a pacemaker wire.[14,15] Since that time the treatment of SVC syndrome with percutaneous techniques has advanced considerably so that the vast majority of lesions can be treated with a high degree of safety and effectiveness. Currently, the two major endovascular treatment modalities that are used are thrombolysis and stenting.

Thrombolysis is an important part of endovascular management of SVC obstruction when thrombosis of the cava or central veins occurs. In these cases clot removal helps relieve or reduce symptoms, uncover the morphology of the lesion and permit stenting or angioplasty to take place.[16,17] Most of the time, lysis must be accompanied by treatment of the high-grade stenosis that caused the thrombosis except in the case of benign catheter-related clotting where an underlying lesion is not present and angioplasty or stenting is not necessary. For example, Grey described 16 patients with central line-related SVC syndrome who were treated with thrombolysis only with an overall success rate of 56%.[18]

Angioplasty of SVC stenotic lesions can occasionally be useful but for the most part balloon dilatation without stent placement results in rapid recurrence or outright failure due to the fibrous, elastic nature of many venous lesions. Recognition of the limitations of angioplasty has led to the near-universal adoption of stenting of malignant SVC lesions.[19] To date, there are more than 300 reports of SVC stent therapy with the majority of reported experiences with three stents: the Gianturco Z stent, the Palmaz stent and the Wallstent. Other new stent designs have also been used.

Gianturco Z stents are self-expanding stainless steel stents with anchoring hooks that prevent migration. It is the only device available with diameters up to 40 mm; its principal advantages are size, rigidity, ease of placement and lack of shortening. The open construction of the stent itself could theoretically make this device more prone to tumor ingrowth than other stents although we have not seen this problem occur (Fig. 40.2).

Palmaz stents are balloon-expandable stents whose major advantage is accurate positioning, and the increased radial force of the balloon, which may be helpful in expanding obstructions due to tumor or fibrosis. The chief disadvantage of Palmaz stents is their relatively short length and lack of flexibility (Fig. 40.3).

The Wallstent is a self-expanding stainless steel device that is by far the most commonly used stent for venous applications, principally because the stent is flexible and available in multiple lengths. It is an effective stent for SVC applications (Fig. 40.4).

Charnsangavej first reported stenting of malignant SVC occlusion with a Gianturco Z stent that relieved the patient's symptoms until her death 3 weeks later. An

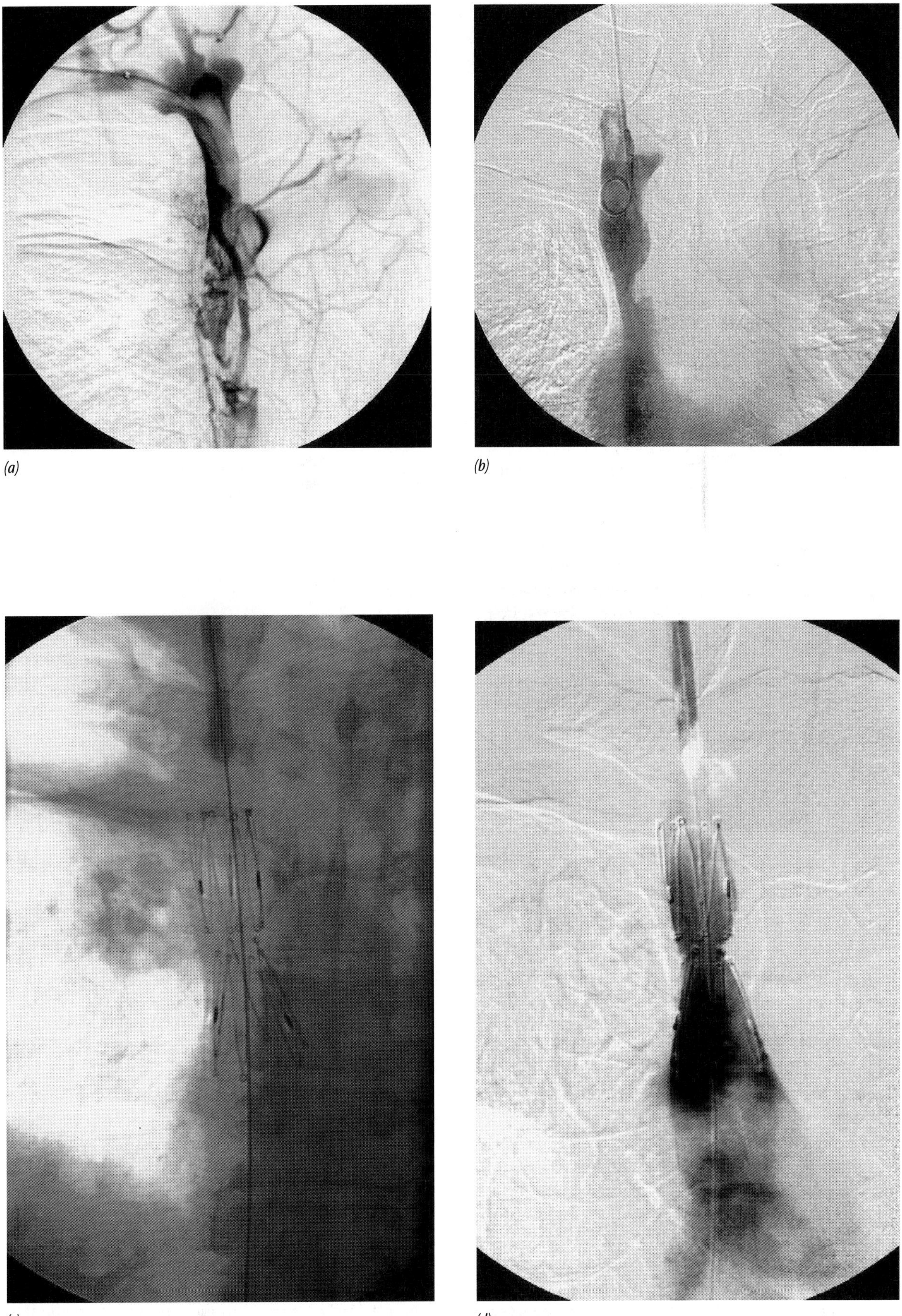

Figure 40.2 *(a–d) Treatment of SVC obstruction with thrombolysis and Gianturco stents.*

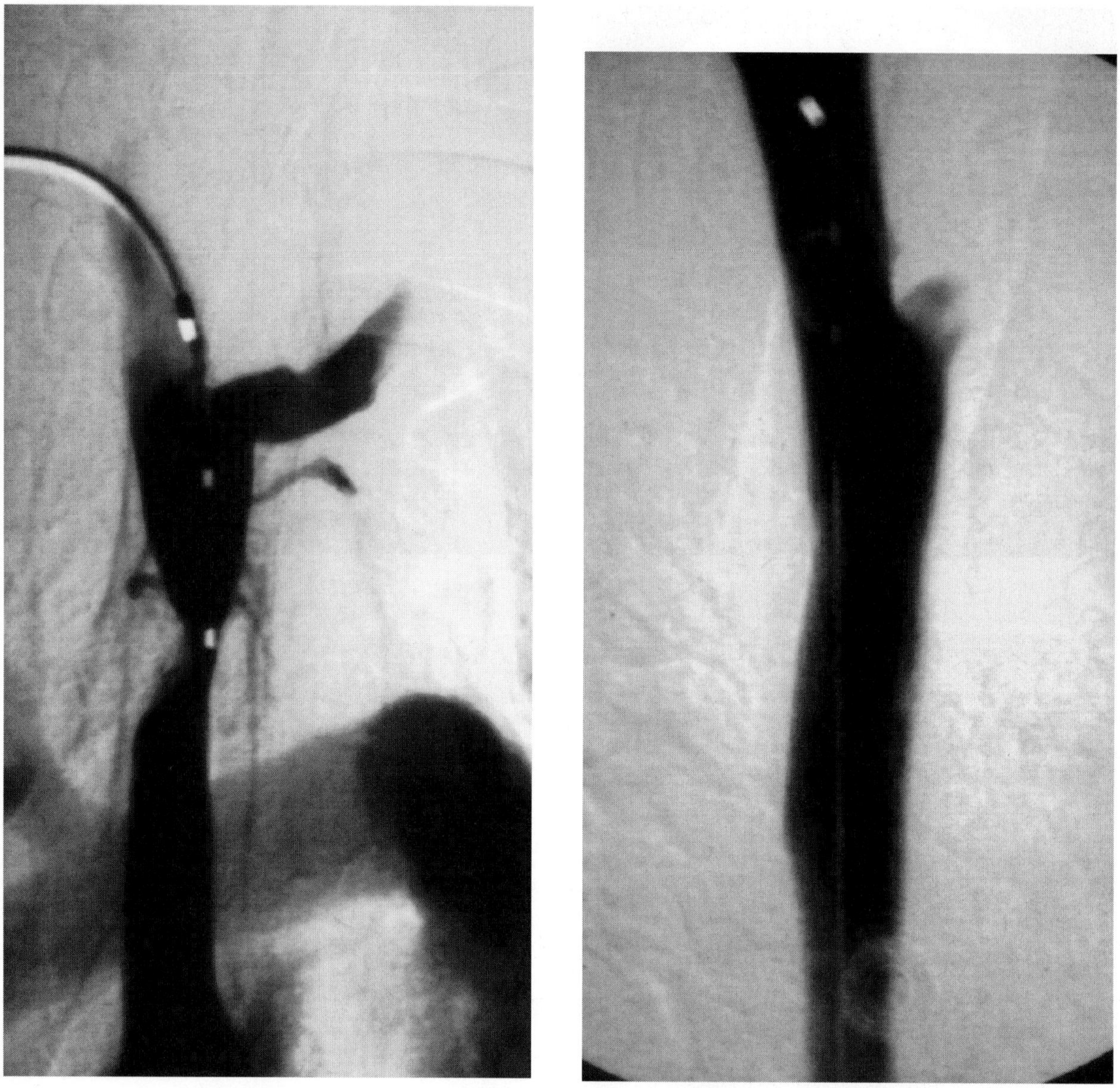

(a) *(b)*

Figure 40.3 *(a, b) Use of Palmaz stent in SVC obstruction.*

autopsy revealed a patent stent.[20] Shortly thereafter, Rosch reported two patients with radiation-resistant SVC obstruction also treated with Gianturco stents. Both patients had rapid resolution of symptoms, and remained asymptomatic for 6 months.[21]

Since the initial reports, there have been larger series with more substantial follow-up. Solomon reported the first use of Palmaz stents for SVC syndrome was in 1991; in 1992 Zollikofer published the use of Wallstents in this condition.[22,23] Thus far, unfortunately, the SVC stent literature has been somewhat spotty with very few papers attempting to compare stents. It should be noted that prospective, randomized data comparing stent types does not exist. One exception was Oudkerk *et al.* who reported their experience with Gianturco and Wallstents; they found Wallstents to be more prone to reocclusion and postulated that this was related to the increased surface area of exposed wire.[24]

Most reports have emphasized the use of combination therapy with use of thrombolysis, angioplasty and stenting all used in a variety of combinations. With these newer methods, technical success can be achieved in almost 100% of cases and primary patency of SVC stents for malignant obstruction has ranged from 50 to 100%. Secondary procedures such as repeat stenting and angioplasty of course improve these results considerably.

Total occlusion of the superior vena cava does not appear to be a contraindication to stent therapy. For example, Crowe reported a technical success rate of 84.6% in patients who had a total occlusion of the SVC

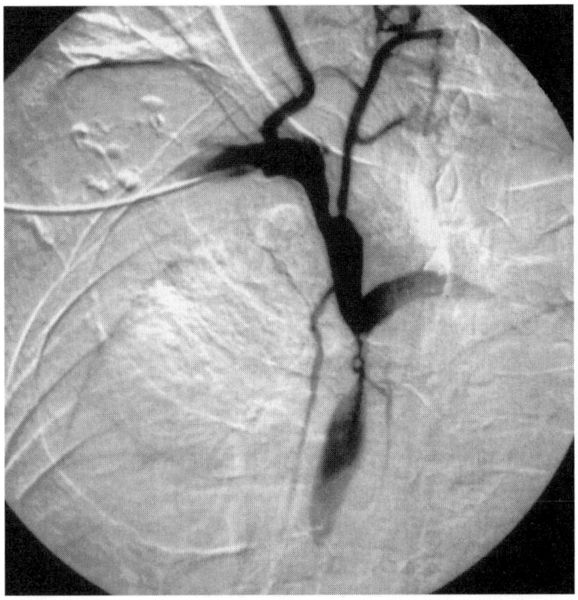

(a)

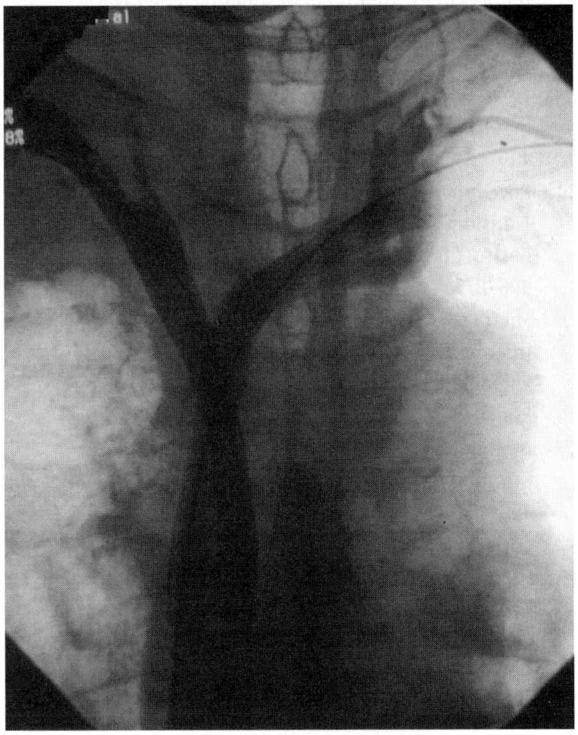

(b)

Figure 40.4 *(a, b) Use of Wallstents in SVC obstruction.*

with a strategy including thrombolysis and percutaneous transluminal angioplasty (PTA) prior to stenting.[25]

The largest published report of SVC syndrome stenting is in 75 patients with malignant obstruction treated with Wallstents.[13] All (100%) patients had improvement of symptoms within 48 hours of the procedure, and 90.2% remained free of symptoms until they died. Interestingly, this study also compared stent therapy results with radiation; it found that only 12% of the radiation-treated patients had durable symptomatic relief.

The major complication rates for stent therapy are low and include bleeding complications of thrombolysis and anticoagulation, stent migration, stent occlusion, and pulmonary embolus; however, most complications can be successfully treated with percutaneous methods. For example, shortening of Wallstents after deployment can cause the stent to migrate or embolize. Migration or shortening can be easily treated with restenting, but we have learned that balloon dilatation of the stenosis before stent placement generally avoids this problem. Stent migration into the atrium or pulmonary artery has been described, but even these can often be treated with endovascular procedures. For example, Bartorelli described a case in which a Palmaz stent that embolized to the right atrium was managed by retrieval with a balloon catheter and deployment of the stent in the iliac vein.[26]

Stent obstruction secondary to tumor ingrowth between stent struts or elements or by compression has been described in all stent types. At least one case of the use of a covered stent graft to repair this problem has been described.[27]

Many issues in SVC stenting are unresolved, due in no small part to the small volume of cases any one institution sees. For example, the question of whether anticoagulation is necessary post-stenting is not fully answered. Some authors report anecdotal experiences with patients who acutely thrombose their stents after cessation of anticoagulation therapy. Others who do not use systemic anticoagulation report excellent results comparable to those who use anticoagulation and another group believe in temporary anticoagulation for a period of weeks to months until the stent is presumably covered with a pseudointima and is therefore less thrombogenic.[28,29]

The above discussion points out again that the SVC stent therapy literature lacks any prospective randomized data and therefore, many questions remain unanswered. The role of stents in benign caval obstruction is quite controversial. It is obvious that SVC stenting is a highly effective palliative remedy for malignant SVC syndrome because long-term results are not really important in patients with a short life expectancy. In those with benign disease, however, the answers to questions become even more important, yet the data on which to base clinical decision-making are deficient.

Even though the first cases of central venous angioplasty were reported for benign disease, there are no large studies of endovascular treatment of 'benign' SVC syndrome available. This fact partly reflects the low percentage of all patients with a benign cause of SVC syndrome. The largest series of patients with SVC syndrome secondary to benign causes was submitted by Kee, who included 16 patients treated for disease such as catheter-related, fibrous mediastinitis and other causes which were treated with thrombolysis, PTA and stents.[30]

Of the 13 with follow-up (mean 17.1 months), the primary patency was 77% and secondary patency was 85%. The largest reported series of patients with endovascular treatment of SVC syndrome related to catheter complications alone was published by Rosenblum and included six patients with central line-related SVC syndrome.[31] They reported excellent results with patency up to 2 years and no recurrences. Three of their patients were able to have central lines placed across the stented lesion. Larger series of venous stenting for hemodialysis patients involving veins other than the SVC have not had as good results, but found that larger veins tended to have the best patency when stented. It is important to consider that whilst life expectancy in patients with malignant SVC syndrome is frequently less than 1 year, the same is not true of patients with benign disease. They may survive many years, and therefore long-term patency is critical. The gold standard upon which to compare endovascular treatment in these patients is obviously surgical bypass since recent series of selected patients with surgical bypass for SVC syndrome have shown 5-year patency of up to 86%.[32–36] On the other hand, advances in stent technology including medical therapy for restenosis may reduce or eliminate the problem of chronic stent occlusion and make surgical bypass an even less frequently used procedure.

CONCLUSION

SVC syndrome is a serious complication that can disable patients and threaten their lives. We anticipate that the incidence of both benign and malignant forms of this disease will increase in frequency due to more effective cancer therapy and the widespread use of central venous catheters. Traditional treatments for malignant SVC obstruction such as anticoagulation and radiation are generally ineffective; most physicians believe that endovascular techniques in general (and stenting in particular) are the best palliative methods now available. Benign occlusions, however, are far more problematic and to date, the results of stenting are mixed with no true long-term data available.

REFERENCES

1. Hunter, W. *Medical Observations and Inquiries*, 1757.
2. Perez CA, Van Amburg AL 3d. Management of superior vena cava syndrome. *Semin Oncol* 1978; **5**(2): 123–34.
3. Parish JM, Marschke PF Jr, Dines DE, Lee RE. Etiologic considerations in superior vena cava syndrome. *Mayo Clin Proc* 1981; **56**: 407–13.
4. Stanford W, Doty DB. The role of venography and surgery in the management of patients with superior vena cava syndrome. *Ann Thorac Surg* 1986; **41**: 158–63.
5. Tayade, BO, Salvi SS, Agarwal IR. Study of superior vena cava syndrome: aetiopathology, diagnosis and management. *J Assoc Physicians India* 1994; **42**(8):609–11.
6. Armstrong BA, Perez CA, Simpson JR, Hederman MA. Role of irradiation in the management of superior vena cava syndrome. *Int J Radiat Oncol Biol Phys* 1987; **13**: 531–9.
7. Fincher RM. Superior vena cava syndrome: experience in a teaching hospital. *South Med J* 1987; **80**: 1243–5.
8. Ostler PJ, Clarke DP, Watkinson AF, Gaze MN. Superior vena cava obstruction: a modern management strategy. *Clin Oncol* 1997; **9**: 83–9.
9. Escalante CP. Causes and management of superior vena cava syndrome. *Oncology* 1993; **7**(6): 61–8.
10. Shimm DS, Logue DL, Rigsby LC. Evaluating the superior vena cava syndrome. *J Am Med Assoc* 1981; **245**: 951–3.
11. Rodrigues CI, Njo KH, Karim AB. Hypofractionated radiation therapy in the treatment of superior vena cava syndrome. *Lung Cancer* 1993; **10**: 221–8.
12. Davenport D, Ferree C, Blake D, Raben M. Radiation therapy in the treatment of superior vena caval obstruction. *Cancer* 1978; **42**: 2600–3.
13. Nicholson AA, Ettles DF, Arnold A, Greenstone M, Dyet JF. Treatment of malignant superior vena cava obstruction: metal stents or radiation therapy. *J Vasc Interv Radiol* 1997; **8**: 781–8.
14. Rocchini AP, Cho KJ, Byrum C, Heidelberger K. Transluminal angioplasty of superior vena cava obstruction in a 15-month-old child. *Chest* 1982; **82**: 506–8.
15. Sherry CS, Diamond NG, Meyers TP, Martin RL. Successful treatment of superior vena cava syndrome by venous angioplasty. *AJR Am J Roentgenol* 1986; **147**: 834–5.
16. Rantis PC Jr, Littooy FN. Successful treatment of prolonged superior vena cava syndrome with thrombolytic therapy: a case report. *J Vasc Surg* 1994; **20**: 108–13.
17. Enders GC, Sodums MT. Local thrombolytic therapy in superior vena cava syndrome secondary to malignant thymoma: a case report and literature review. *Cathet Cardiovasc Diagn* 1994; **31**: 215–18.
18. Gray RJ, Horton KM, Dolmatch BL, *et al.* Use of Wallstents for hemodialysis access-related venous stenoses and occlusions untreatable with balloon angioplasty. *Radiology* 1995; **195**: 479–84.
19. Hemphill DJ, Sniderman KW, Allard JP. Management of total parenteral nutrition-related superior vena cava obstruction with expandable metal stents. *J Parenter Enteral Nutr* 1996; **20**(3): 222–7.
20. Charnsangavej C, Carrasco CH, Wallace S, *et al.* Stenosis of the vena cava: preliminary assessment of treatment with expandable metallic stents. *Radiology* 1986; **161**: 295–8.
21. Rosch J, Bedell JE, Putnam J, Antonovic R, Uchida B. Gianturco expandable wire stents in the treatment of superior vena cava syndrome recurring after maximum-tolerance radiation. *Cancer* 1987; **60**: 1243–6.

22. Solomon N, Wholey MH, Jarmolowski CR. Intravascular stents in the management of superior vena cava syndrome. *Cathet Cardiovasc Diagn* 1991; **23**: 245–52.
23. Zollikofer C, Antonucci F, Stuckmann G, Mattias P, Bruhlmann WF, Salmonowitz EK. Use of the Wallstent in the venous system including hemodialysis-related stenoses. *Cardiovasc Interv Radiol* 1992; **15**: 334–41.
24. Oudkerk M, Kuijpers TJ, Schmitz PI, Loosveld O, de Wit R.. Self-expanding metal stents for palliative treatment of superior vena caval syndrome. *Cardiovasc Interv Radiol* 1996; **19**: 146–51.
25. Crowe MT, Davies CH, Gaines PA. Percutaneous management of superior vena cava occlusions. *Cardiovasc Interv Radiol* 1995; **18**: 367–72.
26. Bartorelli A., Fabbiocchi F, Montorsi P, Loaldi A, Tamborini G, Sganzerla P. Successful transcatheter management of Palmaz stent embolization after superior vena cava stenting. *Cathet Cardiovasc Diagn* 1995; **34**: 162–6.
27. Chin D, Peterson BD, Timmermans H, Rosch J. Stent-graft in the management of superior vena cava syndrome. *Cardiovasc Interv Radiol* 1996; **19**: 302–4.
28. Rosch J, Uchida BT, Hall LD, *et al.* Gianturco-Rosch expandable Z-stents in the treatment of superior vena cava syndrome. *Cardiovasc Interv Radiol* 1992; **15**: 319–27.
29. Irving JD, Dondelinger RF, Reidy JF, *et al.* Gianturco self-expanding stents: clinical experience in the vena cava and large veins. *Cardiovasc Interv Radiol* 1992; **15**: 328–33.
30. Kee ST, Kinoshita L, Razavi MK, Myman UR, Semba CP, Dake MD. Superior vena cava syndrome: treatment with catheter-directed thrombolysis and endovascular stent placement. *Radiology* 1998; **206**: 187–93.
31. Rosenblum J, Leef J, Messersmith R, Tomiak M, Beck F. Intravascular stents in the management of acute superior vena cava obstruction of benign etiology. *J Parenter Enteral Nutr* 1994; **18**: 362–6.
32. Doty DB. Bypass of superior vena cava: six years' experience with spiral vein graft for obstruction of superior vena cava due to benign and malignant disease. *J Thorac Cardiovasc Surg* 1982; **83**: 326–38.
33. Magnan PE, Thomas P, Giudicelli R, Fuentes P, Branchereau A. Surgical reconstruction of the superior vena cava. *Cardiovasc Surg* 1994; **2**: 598–603.
34. Gloviczki P, Pairolero PC, Cherry KJ, Hallett JW Jr. Reconstruction of the vena cava and its primary tributaries: a preliminary report. *J Vasc Surg* 1990; **11**: 373–81.
35. Dartevelle PG, Chapelier AR, Pastorino U, *et al.* Long-term follow-up after prosthetic replacement of the superior vena cava combined with resection of mediastinal-pulmonary malignant tumors. *J Thorac Cardiovasc Surg* 1991; **102**: 259–65.
36. Moore WM Jr, Hollier LH, Pickett TK. Superior vena cava and central venous reconstruction. *Surgery* 1991; **110**: 35–41.

41

Surgical treatment of superior vena cava syndrome

PETER GLOVICZKI, PETER PAIROLERO, MICHAEL MCKUSICK, THOMAS C BOWER, LINDA C CANTON AND KENNETH J CHERRY

Obstruction of the superior vena cava (SVC) or innominate veins occurs most frequently in patients with metastatic malignant disease. Nonmalignant causes are, however, increasing due to the more frequent use of central venous lines and catheters and the widespread use of pacemakers. Signs and symptoms of venous congestion of the head, neck and upper extremities are determined by the duration, progression and extent of the venous occlusive disease, and by the amount of collateral venous circulation that develops. Mortality is high in patients with metastatic malignant disease, and usually occurs at 6–12 months after the onset of symptoms.

This chapter reviews the etiology of SVC syndrome and discusses clinical presentation, preoperative evaluation and surgical treatment of these patients. Endovascular treatments with thrombolysis, angioplasty and stents are discussed in detail in Chapters 15, 21 and 40.

ETIOLOGY

Obstruction of the SVC caused by a syphilitic aortic aneurysm was first described in 1757 by William Hunter.[1] The most frequent etiology of SVC syndrome today is metastatic malignant disease. In a review of multiple large series, 85% of 1986 patients with SVC syndrome had metastatic pulmonary or mediastinal malignancy.[2] The most frequent tumor was metastatic adenocarcinoma of the lung. Benign disease causing SVC syndrome is less frequent. Severe venous congestion of the head and neck can be caused by fibrosing mediastinitis or granulomatous fungal diseases such as histoplasmosis. Previous radiation treatment to the mediastinum or retrosternal goiter are additional etiologies. Central venous lines and catheters used for either hemodynamic monitoring, parenteral alimentation, or drug administration have become more frequent causes of SVC, innominate veins or subclavian vein thrombosis.[3,4] Because of the large number of pacemaker implantations, some of these patients also develop severe symptoms, usually after multiple line placements using bilateral access sites. Superior vena cava thrombosis can also be associated with thrombophilia, caused by deficiencies in circulating natural anticoagulants (antithrombin III, protein S, protein C) or by factor V Leiden mutation.

Figure 41.1 (opposite) *(a) A 69-year-old man with severe symptomatic superior vena cava syndrome. (b) Bilateral upper extremity venogram confirms thrombosis of the superior vena cava and both innominate veins following bilateral pacemaker line placement. (c) Postoperative venogram confirms patency of a right internal jugular vein–right atrial appendage spiral saphenous vein graft. Arrow indicates jugular anastomosis. (Reproduced with permission from Gloviczki P, Pairolero PC, Toomey BJ* et al. *Reconstruction of large veins for nonmalignant venous occlusive disease.* J Vasc Surg *1992;* **16***: 750–61) (d) Photograph 5 days after spiral vein graft placement. The patient has excellent clinical result 5 years after the operation.*

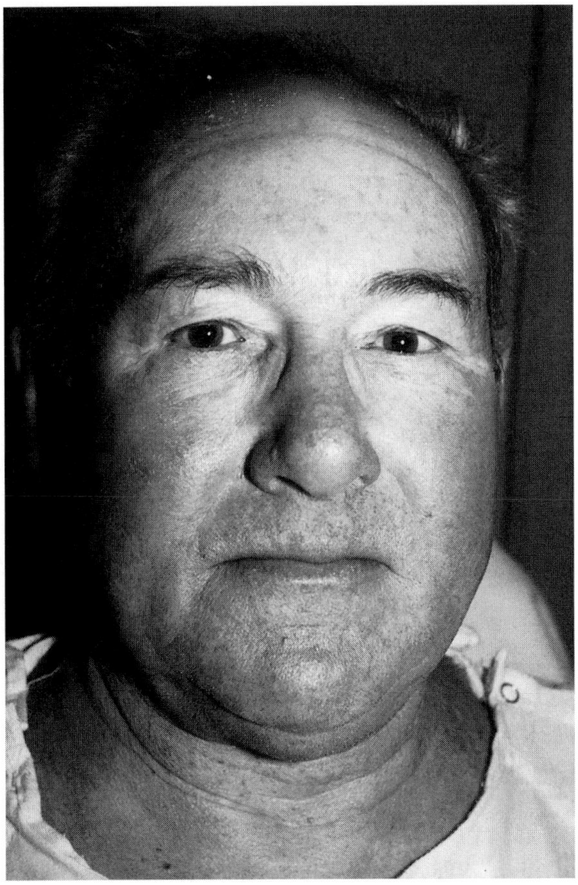

(a)

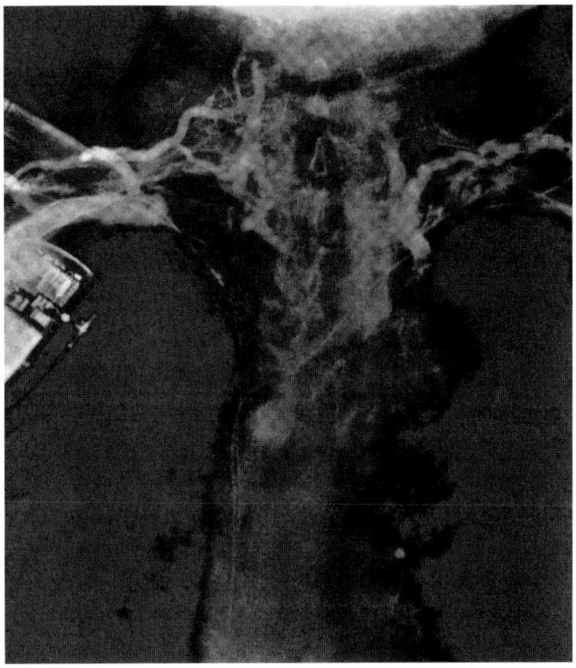

(b)

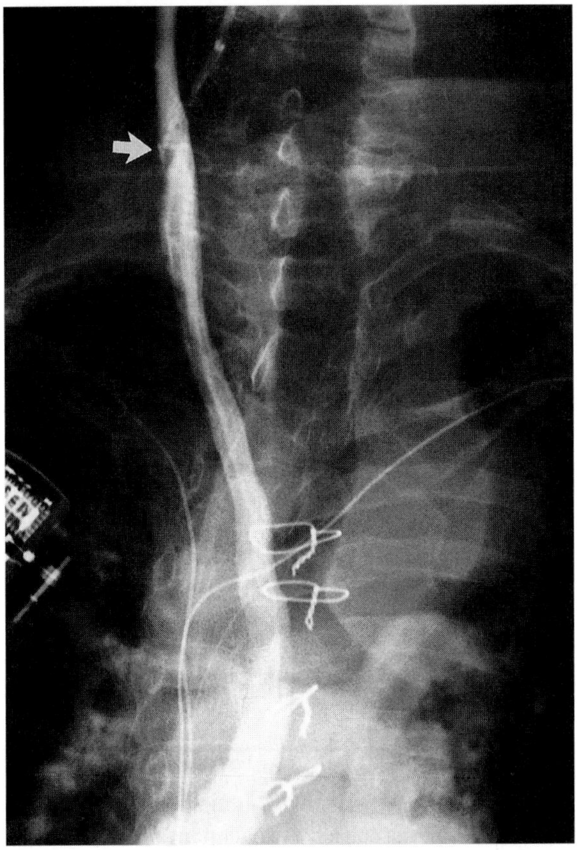

(c)

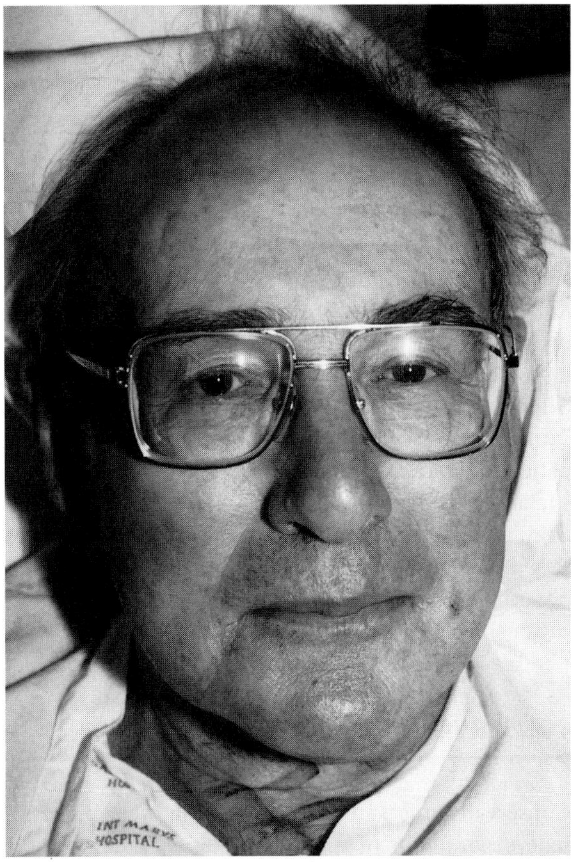

(d)

CLINICAL PRESENTATION

The most frequent symptom of SVC syndrome is the feeling of fullness in the head and neck, that is more severe when the patient bends over or lies flat in bed. These patients can only sleep by elevating the head on multiple pillows. Headache, dizziness, visual symptoms or occasional blackout spells may result from cerebral venous hypertension. Additional symptoms may include mental confusion, dyspnea, orthopnea or cough. Swelling of the face and eyelids is evident and the patient notes the need for larger size shirts because of enlargement of the neck (Fig. 41.1). Ecchymosis, and dilated jugular veins accompany cyanosis of the upper body. Extensive venous collaterals of the chest will frequently develops. Mild-to-moderate upper extremity swelling may occur, but the primary symptoms in these patients are localized to the head and neck.

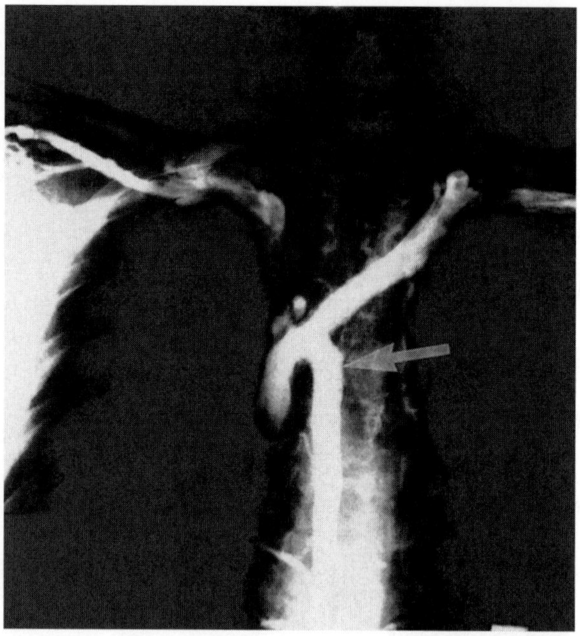

Figure 41.2 *Obstruction of the superior vena cava. There is retrograde flow in the azygos vein (arrow) that drains venous blood from the upper half of the body through lumbar collaterals into the inferior vena cava.*

DIAGNOSTIC EVALUATION

A detailed clinical history with physical examination can usually establish the diagnosis of SVC syndrome. Routine laboratory tests, chest roentgenogram and computed tomography of the chest are performed in all patients to exclude underlying malignant disease. Fast computed tomography (Imatron scan) provides more details of the mediastinal structures, and we prefer this to the conventional computed tomography if mediastinal tumor or fibrotic process is suspected (see Chapter 16). Magnetic resonance venography (MRV) is also suitable to define anatomy, although patients with pacemakers are not candidates for these tests. Patency of at least one internal jugular vein should be confirmed with duplex scanning in those patients who are candidates for surgical reconstruction.

Evaluation of patients considered for endovascular or open surgical treatment is continued with bilateral upper extremity venography (Fig. 41.2). Based on the extent of venous occlusion, as defined by bilateral upper extremity venography, Stanford and Doty[5] classified patients with SVC syndrome into four types (Fig. 41.3a–d). Bronchoscopy, mediastinoscopy, thoracoscopy, thoracotomy or median sternotomy may be necessary in some patients to provide tissue diagnosis or occasionally to attempt resection of a localized tumor causing superior vena cava occlusion.

CONSERVATIVE THERAPY

Conservative measures are used first in every patient to relieve symptoms of venous congestion. These include elevation of the head during the night on pillows, modifications of daily activities by avoiding bending over, and avoidance of wearing constricting garments or tight collar. Patients frequently need diuretics to decrease venous edema and anticoagulation with heparin and warfarin are used to protect the venous collateral circulation. Thrombolytic treatment should be considered in most patients with benign acute superior vena cava syndrome. Patients in the end stage of metastatic malignant disease are frequently not candidates for thrombolysis. Since external compression by the tumor is the usual pathomechanism of caval occlusion in these patients, endovascular treatment, as discussed later, using stents is the best technique to alleviate symptoms.

Symptoms of SVC syndrome associated with metastatic malignant disease frequently improve following irradiation or chemotherapy. Chen *et al.* treated 42 patients with malignant superior vena cava syndrome using external beam radiotherapy and/or chemotherapy.[6] Symptoms of superior vena cava syndrome resolved in 80% of the patients who underwent radiotherapy, with a mean interval of 4 weeks. A similar benefit of radiation or chemotherapy was noted by others as well.[7]

ENDOVASCULAR TREATMENT WITH CAVAL STENTS

In symptomatic patients with significant stenosis of the superior vena cava caused by malignant disease, expandable intravascular wire stents can provide rapid sympto-

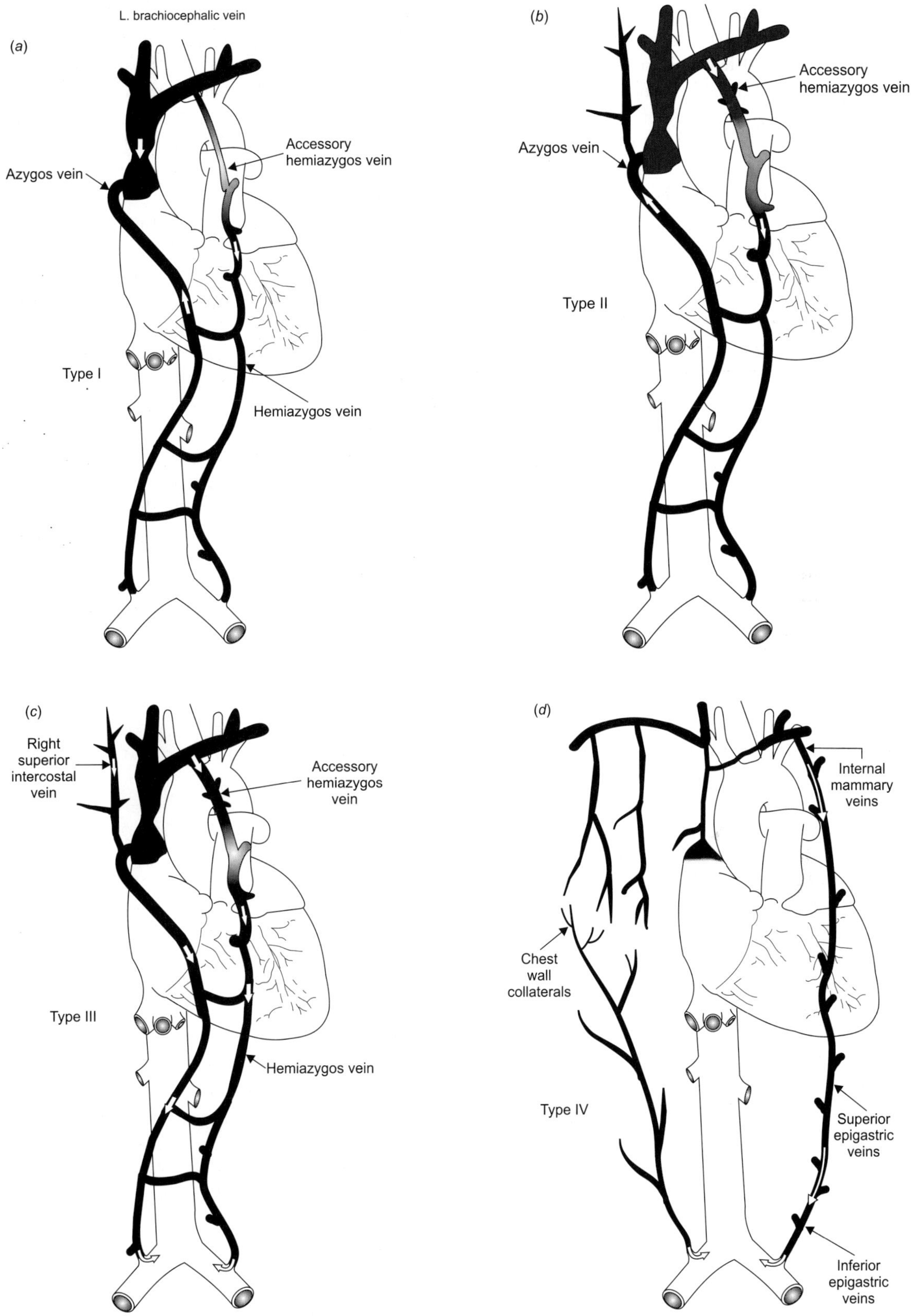

Figure 41.3 *Venographic classification of superior vena cava syndrome. (a) Type I: high-grade superior vena cava stenosis but still normal direction of blood flow through superior vena cava and azygos veins. Increased collateral circulation through hemiazygos and accessory hemiazygos veins. (b) Type II: greater than 90% stenosis or occlusion of superior vena cava with normal direction of blood flow through the azygos vein. (c) Type III: occlusion of superior vena cava with retrograde flow in both azygos and hemiazygos veins. (d) Type IV: extensive occlusion of superior vena cava, innominate and azygos with chest wall and epigastric venous collaterals.*

matic relief. Long-term results of stents placed in young patients for benign lesions are not well known, and rethrombosis or intimal hyperplasia can be significant. For patients with benign disease there is no generally accepted policy because of lack of long-term results. However, our current practice is to offer endovascular treatment first to all suitable patients, including those with mediastinal fibrosis, once biopsy excluded malignancy.

Techniques and results of endovascular treatment are discussed in detail in Chapter 40.

SURGICAL TREATMENT

Indication

The best indication for superior vena caval replacement is persistent, symptomatic superior vena cava syndrome caused by benign disease.[4] Causes for venous thrombosis in 19 operated patients in our recent series included mediastinal fibrosis (n = 12), indwelling foreign bodies (n = 4), idiopathic thrombosis (n = 2) and antithrombin III deficiency (n = 1).[8] Surgical reconstruction of the SVC has been performed also in patients with end stage malignancy,[9] although we rarely operate in these patients. We believe that patients with malignant tumor should undergo reconstruction only if their life expectancy is greater than one year. This group of patients may include those with lymphoma, thymoma or metastatic medullary carcinoma of the thyroid gland.[8,10] Indications and results of surgical treatment for malignant caval obstruction are discussed in detail by Bower in Chapter 43. Dartavelle *et al.* reported on a group of patients who had successful caval resection and reconstruction with resection of pulmonary and mediastinal malignant tumors.[11]

Selection of graft

For replacement of the superior vena cava or the innominate vein in patients with benign disease, autogenous spiral saphenous vein graft is our first choice. This graft was described in experiments by Chiu in 1974[12] and Doty used it first in patients.[13] Our technique of preparing and implanting the spiral graft was described previously in detail.[4,10,14] The saphenous vein is harvested, it is opened longitudinally, valves are excised and the vein is wrapped around a 32 or 36 French polyethylene chest tube. The edges of the vein are then approximated with running 6-0 monofilament polypropylene sutures (Figs 41.4 and 41.5). More recently, we have used non-penetrating vascular clips (US Surgical, Inc.) for this purpose, with good result (Fig. 41.4d). The vein is continuously irrigated during the phase of preparation with heparinized papaverine solution to preserve integrity of endothelial cells and to prevent desiccation. Spiral saphenous vein graft is a relatively non-thrombogenic autologous tissue. Disadvantages include the additional incision and the time (60–90 min) needed to prepare the graft and that the length of the graft is limited by the availability of the saphenous vein. Placement of clips rather than suturing reduces this time considerably.

Of the available autologous graft materials, greater saphenous vein, panel vein graft, autologous pericardium and superficial femoral vein have been used to reconstruct the superior vena cava in a limited number of patients.[15–20] Iliocaval allograft can also be considered in those patients, who receive immunosuppressive treatment for protection of another transplanted organ, kidney or liver.[21] Cryopreserved femoral vein grafts are also potential alternatives.

The advantages of externally supported polytetraflouroethylene (ePTFE) grafts are the easy availability in different length and sizes and the blow surface thrombogenicity among all prosthetic materials. Short, large-diameter grafts have excellent long-term patency, since flow through the grafts usually amounts to several hundred ml/min. If the peripheral anastomosis is

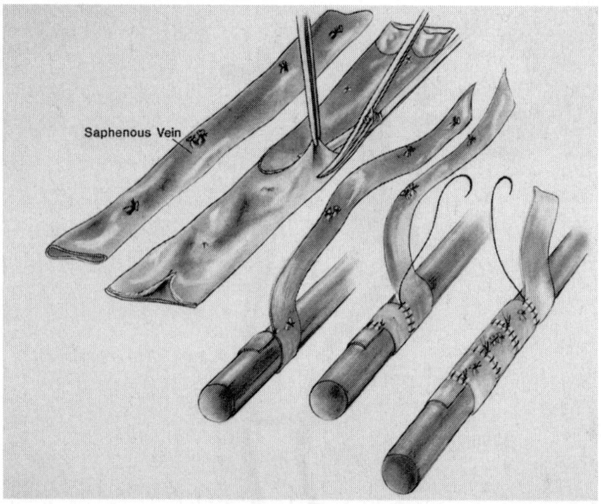

(a)

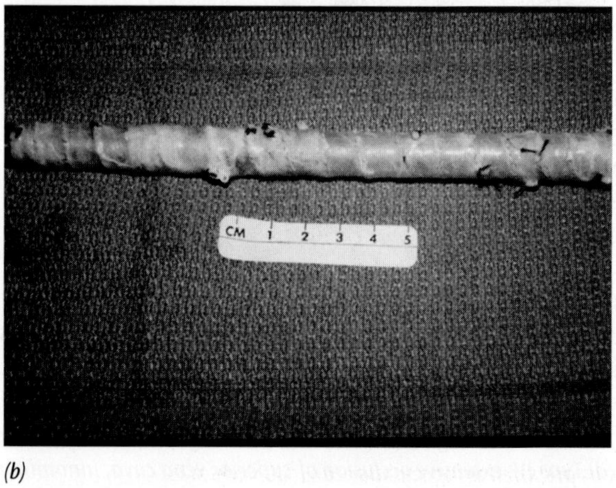

(b)

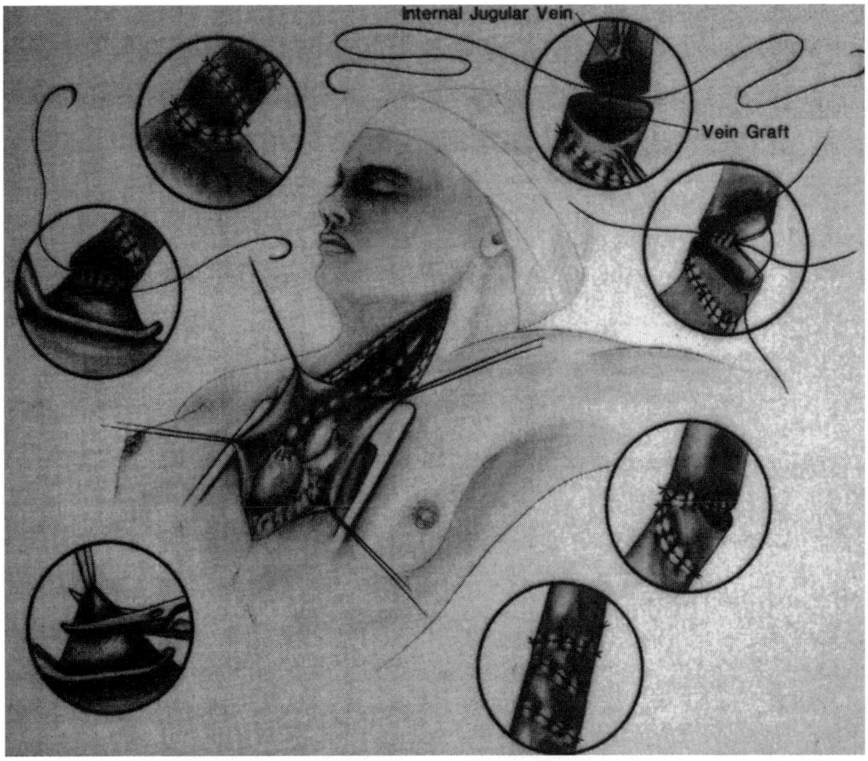

(c)

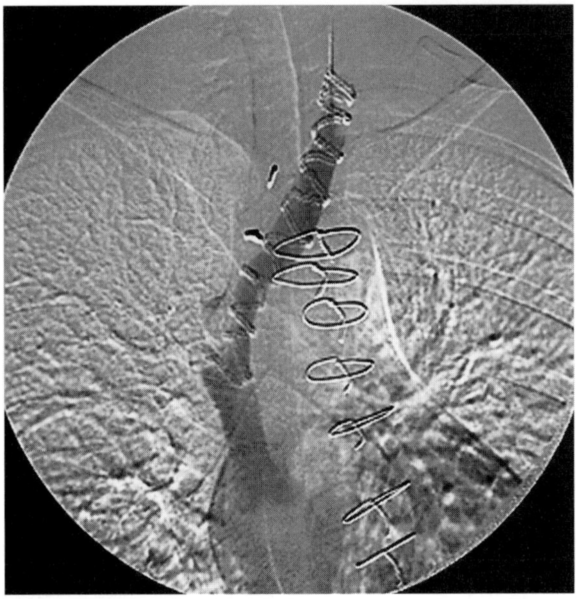

(d)

Figure 41.4 *(a) Technique to prepare a spiral saphenous vein graft. Note that the saphenous vein is opened longitudinally, valves are excised, the vein is wrapped around an Argyle chest tube, and the vein edges are approximated with sutures. (b) A 15 cm long spiral saphenous vein graft ready for implantation (c) Technique of left internal jugular–right atrial spiral vein graft implantation. (Reproduced with permission from Gloviczki P, Pairolero PC. Venous reconstruction for obstruction and valvular incompetence. In Goldstone J, ed.* Perspectives in Vascular Surgery. *St Louis, MO: Quality Medical Publishing, 1988: 75–93) (d) Left internal jugular, right atrial spiral vein graft. The graft was prepared using vascular clips (US Surgical).*

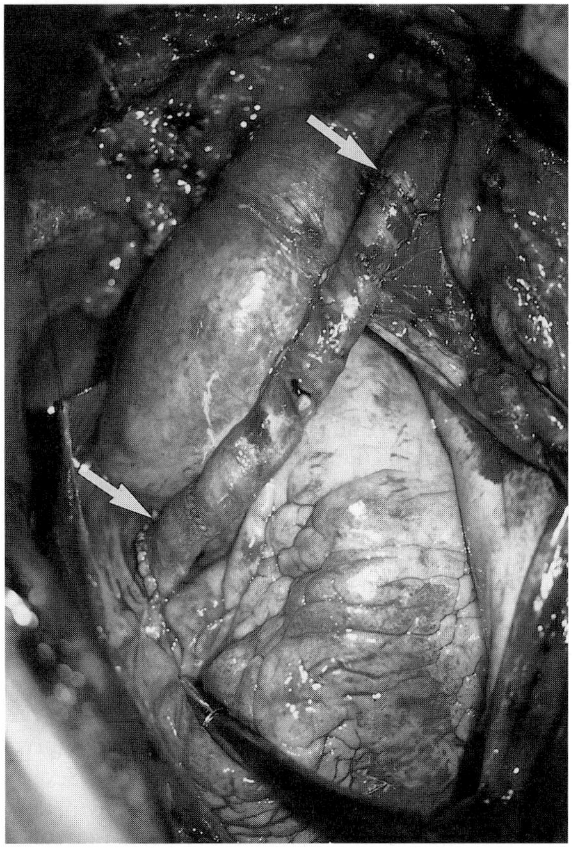

Figure 41.5 *Left innominate vein–right atrial spiral saphenous vein graft. Arrows indicate anastomoses.*

performed with the subclavian vein, the addition of an arteriovenous fistula is needed in the arm to assure long-term patency. In patients who need internal jugular–atrial appendage bypass, we prefer to use spiral saphenous vein graft. Prosthetic graft is our choice in patients with a tight mediastinum, or with persistent malignancy, since increasing external compression of the vein graft following closure of the sternum in such patients is most likely.

Surgical technique

Median sternotomy is required to explore the mediastinum and replace the obstructed innominate vein or superior vena cava. If the internal jugular vein is used for inflow, the midline skin incision is extended using an n oblique neck incision anterior to the sternocleidomastoid muscle of the appropriate side (Fig 41.4c). The mediastinum is exposed and biopsy, or, if possible, resection of the tumor is performed before caval reconstruction. The pericardiac sac is opened, since the graft in most patients is attached to the right atrial appendage. In some, the patent portion of the superior vena cava can be used for this purpose. The peripheral anastomosis of the graft can be performed to the internal jugular vein or to tone of the innominate veins, in an end-to-side or, preferably, an end-to-end fashion.

Postoperative anticoagulation is started 36–48 hours later with heparin and the patient is dismissed on oral anticoagulation. Patients with spiral vein graft who have no underlying coagulation abnormality are maintained on warfarin sodium for 3 months only. Those with underlying coagulation disorders, or those with ePTFE grafts, usually benefit from lifelong anticoagulation.

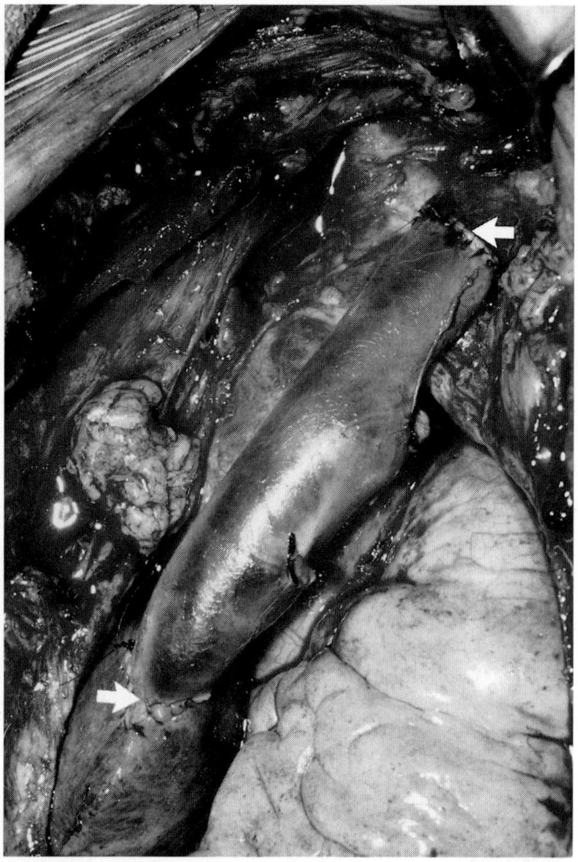

Figure 41.6 *Left innominate vein-right atrial appendage bypass using a cadaver iliocaval allograft. Arrows indicate the anastomoses. (From Rhee RY, Gloviczki P, Steers JL, Krom RAF, Kitabayashi K, Wiesner RH. Superior vena cava reconstruction using an iliocaval allograft.* Vasc Surg *1996;* ***30****: 77–83)*

Results of surgical treatment

Reconstruction of the occluded superior vena cava or innominate vein gives the most gratifying result of venous bypasses (Fig. 41.6). Patency rate is very good, since the mean flow through the graft is usually high (mean 1440 ml/mm, range 750–2000 ml/mm).[9] Shorter grafts placed entirely within the mediastinum have a better chance of long-term patency than those with an anastomosis in the neck.

Doty *et al.* reported on long-term results in nine patients who underwent spiral vein grafting for superior vena cava syndrome, caused by benign disease.[22] Seven of nine grafts remained patent during follow-up that extended from 1 to 15 years and all but one of the patients became asymptomatic.

We reported earlier our results in 12 patients who underwent superior vena cava reconstruction for benign disease.[4] More recently, Alimi *et al.* updated our experience at the Mayo Clinic that included 19 patients, who underwent underwent SVC (Table 41.1) reconstruction for symptomatic nonmalignant disease.[8] Spiral saphenous vein graft (n = 14), polytetrafluoroethylene (PTFE; n = 4), or human allograft (n = 1) was implanted. No early death or pulmonary embolism occurred. Four early graft stenoses or thromboses (spiral saphenous vein graft, n = 2; PTFE, n = 2) required thrombectomy, with success in three. Four of 19 grafts occluded during follow-up (two PTFE, two spiral saphenous vein graft). The primary, primary-assisted and secondary patency rates were 53%, 70%, and 74% at 5 years, respectively (Fig. 41.7). Straight SSVGs had a 70% primary patency rate and a 90% secondary patency rate at 5 years (Fig. 41.8). Most secondary interventions included endovascular therapy, angioplasty or stenting.

Results with expanded PTFE (ePTFE) grafts implanted into the mediastinum in several reported series showed excellent patency.[11,22–29] Dartevelle *et al.* observed continued patency in 20 of 22 ePTFE grafts, with a mean follow-up of 23 months.[11] Moore and Hollier observed no graft occlusion at a mean follow-up

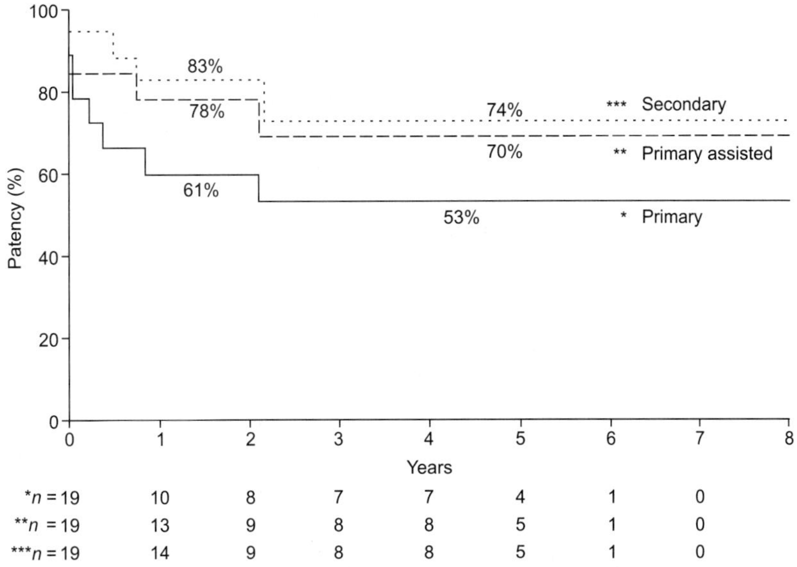

Figure 41.7 *Cumulative patency rates of 19 bypass grafts used for superior vena cava reconstruction.*

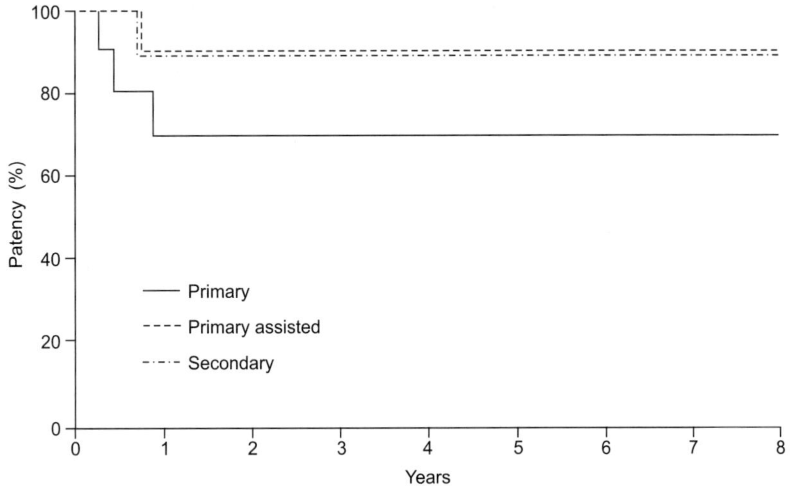

Figure 41.8 *Cumulative patency rates of 12 straight spiral saphenous vein grafts used for superior vena cava reconstruction.*

of 30 months among 10 patients who underwent large central vein reconstruction.[29] In 8 of these 10 patients an additional arteriovenous fistula at the arm was used to increase flow and maintain patency. Reviewing other series from the literature, we found that patency of ePTFE grafts at 2 years was approximately 70%.[9,20, 21,23–26] In our experience some thrombus formation occurs even in patent ePTFE grafts. Thrombosis occurs much less in patients in whom the distal anastomosis is performed with the internal jugular or the subclavian veins, and results appear much better in patients with innominate or SVC interposition grafts. Although spiral vein graft continues to be our first choice for superior vena cava replacement, short, large-diameter ePTFE is an excellent alternative for SVC replacement.

However, increasing success with superficial femoral vein as an arterial conduit has resurrected this autologous graft for large vein reconstructions as well. Autologous femoropopliteal vein shows promise for replacement of large central veins.[18] Still, the morbidity of harvesting a deep vein in patients with thrombotic potentials and venous thrombosis elsewhere in the body is not well known. We warn our patients that harvesting of the superficial femoral vein may result in persistent limb swelling and venous claudication.

MRV is the best technique to follow intrathoracic grafts, although patients with pacemakers are not candidates for this imaging study and these undergo contrast venography. Postoperative imaging is performed before discharge, and once at 3–6 months after surgery. In our experience, most graft stenosis presents within 1 year after implantation. Endovascular therapy is most useful as an adjunctive measure to correct graft stenosis and improve long-term graft patency (Figs 41.7, 41.8).[8]

Table 41.1 *Signs and symptoms of SVC syndrome in 19 patients with benign disease**

	No. patients	%
Signs		
Head and neck swelling	19	100
Large chest wall venous collaterals	17	89
Arm swelling	11	58
Facial cyanosis	8	42
Symptoms		
Feeling of fullness in head or neck	14	74
Dyspnea on exertion or orthopnea	12	63
Headaches	7	37
Visual problems, painful eyes	5	26
Cough	6	32

*Adapted from Alimi YS, Gloviczki P, Vrtiska TJ *et al.* Reconstruction of the superior vena cava: benefits of postoperative surveillance and secondary endovascular interventions. *J Vasc Surg* 1998; **27**: 287–301.

CONCLUSIONS

Surgical treatment of SVC syndrome with spiral vein graft or prosthetic grafts is effective and provides predictable long-term relief. As experience with endovascular techniques increases, it is likely that surgical treatment will be reserved for those who fail thrombolysis, angioplasty or stenting or for those who are not candidates for endovascular management. Endovascular techniques are also helpful adjuncts to prolong patency of grafts used for SVC replacement.

REFERENCES

1. Hunter W. The history of an aneurysm of the aorta with some remarks on aneurysms in general. *Med Obstet Soc Phys Lond* 1757; **1**: 323 to end.
2. Ahmann FR. A reassessment of the clinical implications of the superior vena cava syndrome. *J Clin Oncol* 1984; **4**: 961–9.
3. Sculier JP, Feld R. Superior vena cava obstruction syndrome: recommendations for management. *Cancer Treatment Rev* 1985; **12**: 209–18.
4. Gloviczki P, Pairolero PC, Toomey BJ, *et al.* Reconstruction of large veins for nonmalignant venous occlusive disease. *J Vasc Surg* 1992; **16**: 750–61.
5. Stanford W, Doty DB. The role of venography and surgery in the management of patients with superior vena cava obstruction. *Ann Thorac Surg* 1986; **41**: 158–63.
6. Chen JC, Bongard F, Klein SR. A contemporary perspective on superior vena cava syndrome. *Am J Surg* 1990; **160**: 207–11.
7. Yellin A, Rosen A, Reichert N, Lieberman Y. Superior vena cava syndrome. The myth – the facts. *Am Rev Respir Dis* 1990; **141**: 1114–18.
8. Alimi YS, Gloviczki P, Vrtiska, TJ, *et al.* Reconstruction of the superior vena cava: benefits of postoperative surveillance and secondary endovascular interventions. *J Vasc Surg* 1998; **27**: 287–301.
9. Doty DB. Bypass of superior vena cava: six years' experience with spiral vein graft for obstruction of superior vena cava due to benign and malignant disease. *J Thorac Cardiovasc Surg* 1982; **83**: 326–38.
10. Gloviczki P, Pairolero PC, Cherry KJ Jr, Hallett JW Jr. Reconstruction of the vena cava and of its primary tributaries: a preliminary report. *J Vasc Surg* 1990; **11**: 373–81.
11. Dartevelle PG, Chapelier AR, Pastorino U, *et al.* Long-term follow-up after prosthetic replacement of the superior vena cava combined with resection of mediastinal-pulmonary malignant tumors. *J Thorac Cardiovasc Surg* 1991; **102**: 259–65.
12. Chiu CJ, Terzis J, Mac Rae ML. Replacement of superior vena cava with the spiral composite vein graft. *Ann Thorac Surg* 1974; **17**: 555–60.
13. Doty DB, Baker WH. Bypass of superior vena cava with spiral vein graft. *Ann Thorac Surg* 1976; **22**: 490–3.
14. Gloviczki P, Pairolero PC. Venous reconstruction for obstruction and valvular incompetence. In: Goldstone J, ed. *Perspectives in Vascular Surgery.* St Louis, MO: Quality Medical Publishing, 1988: 75–93.
15. Benvenuto R, Rodman FSB, Gilmour J, Phillips AF, Callaghan JC. Composite venous graft for replacement of the superior vena cava. *Arch Surg* 1962; **84**: 570–3.
16. Bass J Jr, Pan HC, Gottesman L. Superior vena cava syndrome: report of a new operative technique. *J Int Med Assoc* 1980; **72**: 1105–9.
17. Gladstone DJ, Pillai R, Paneth M, Lincoln JCR. Relief of superior vena caval syndrome with autologous femoral vein used as a bypass graft. *J Thorac Cardiovasc Surg* 1985; **89**: 750–2.
18. Marshall WG Jr, Kouchoukos NT. Management of recurrent superior vena caval syndrome with an externally supported femoral vein bypass graft. *Ann Thorac Surg* 1988; **46**: 239–41.
19. Zembala M, Kustrzycki A, Ostapczuk S, Dutkiewicz R, Hirnle T. Pericardial tube for obstruction of superior vena cava by malignant teratoma. *J Thorac Cardiovasc Surg* 1986; **91**: 469–71.
20. Hagino RT, Bengtson TD, Fosdick DA, Valentine RJ, Clagett GP. Venous reconstructions using the superficial femoral-popliteal vein. *J Vasc Surg* 1997; **26**: 829–37.
21. Rhee RY, Gloviczki P, Steers JL, Krom RAF, Kitabayashi K, Wiesner RH. Superior vena cava reconstruction using an iliocaval allograft. *Vasc Surg* 1996; **30**: 77–83.
22. Doty DB, Doty JR, Jones KW. Bypass of superior vena cava. Fifteen years' experience with spiral vein graft for obstruction of superior vena cava caused by benign disease. *J Thorac Cardiovasc Surg* 1990; **99**: 889–95.
23. Bergeron P, Reggi M, Jausseran J, *et al.* Our experience in superior vena cava surgery (in French). *Ann Chir: Chir Thorac Cardiovasc* 1985; **39**: 485–91.

24. Herreros J, Glock Y, Fuente A, *et al.* The superior vena cava compression syndrome. Our experience of twenty six cases (in French). *Ann Chir: Chir Thorac Cardiovasc* 1985; **39**: 495–500.
25. Masuda H, Ogata T, Kikuche K, Takagi K, Tanaka S. Total replacement of superior vena cava because of invasive thymoma: seven years' survival. *J Thorac Cardiovasc Surg* 1988; **95**: 1083–5.
26. Ricci C, Benedetti VF, Colini GF, Gossetti B, Mineo TC. Reconstruction of the superior vena cava: 15 years' experience using various types of prosthetic material. *Ann Chir* 1985; **39**: 492–5.
27. Bardi K, Bouziri S, Jaafoura H, *et al.* Venous involvement in Takayasu's disease: does it exist? *Ann Vasc Surg* 1988; **2**: 231–4.
28. Gloviczki P, Pairolero PC. Prosthetic replacement of large veins. In Bergan JJ, Kistner RL, eds. *Atlas of Venous Surgery.* Philadelphia: WB Saunders, 1992: 191–214.
29. Moore WM Jr, Hollier LH. Reconstruction of the superior vena cava and central veins. In Bergan JJ, Yao JST, eds. *Venous Disorders.* Philadelphia: WB Saunders, 1991; 517–27.

PART 5

Special venous problems

42

Venous trauma in the lower extremity

ROBERT W HOBSON II, NORMAN M RICH, DAVID L GILLESPIE AND PETER J PAPPAS

Management of venous trauma continues to be a challenging and controversial topic for clinical investigation. Historically, the principles and techniques for surgical repair of injured major veins were well established in practice during the late nineteenth and early twentieth centuries by surgeons including Murphy, Dorfler, Carrel and Guthrie.[1,2] Successful direct venous reconstruction remains a significant surgical challenge, whether for repair of an injured vein or the elective reconstruction of the venous system compromised by thrombus or tumor. In contrast to the wide application and success of arterial reconstruction, success in venous reconstruction has been more limited. Early recommendations in favor of venous repair were modified based on clinical observations made during World War I by Makins,[3] who reported improved limb survival after arterial occlusion or ligation by the performance of concomitant venous ligation. These data also were interpreted inappropriately as an indication for ligation of isolated venous injuries. As clinical reports from World War II were analyzed, however, the concepts of improved results after venous ligation and preferential venous ligation over repair were dismissed.[4] Subsequent clinical reports of acute lower extremity edema and in some cases venous gangrene after ligation of major venous injuries, even in the presence of patent arterial repairs, resulted in a more aggressive recommendation for venous repair.[5,6] Furthermore, some patients developed chronic venous insufficiency when ligation of major injured veins was practiced, particularly at the level of the popliteal or common femoral veins in the lower extremity.[7,8] The purpose of this chapter is to review current recommendations for the management of venous trauma in the lower extremity including iliac and caval injuries and to outline technically important considerations and adjunctive methods to improve the patency of venous repairs.

PATHOPHYSIOLOGY: RATIONALE FOR VENOUS REPAIR

Stimulated by clinical reports from the Korean War[5,6] and the Vietnam Vascular Registry,[7,9] laboratory investigations were directed toward elucidating the pathophysiology of acute venous occlusion and repair. Several authors[10,11] documented the physiologic effects of acute and chronic femoral venous occlusion on femoral arterial blood flow, femoral venous pressure, and femoral vascular resistance (Fig. 42.1). The gradual improvement in femoral arterial blood flow associated with a reduction in venous pressure and peripheral vascular resistance 48 hours after ligation resulted from an improvement in venous outflow through collateral veins in the canine hindlimb.[11] Consequently, the first 24–72 hours were described as the important period of patency for venous repairs. These data supported the recommendation for direct venous repair of major injured veins in an attempt to avoid these adverse hemodynamic consequences, particularly when the venous injury occurred at the common femoral or popliteal levels or was associated with a concomitant arterial injury. However, it was recognized that the presence of venous hypertension in the extremity constituted an important hemodynamic indication for venous repair. In the absence of acute venous hypertension, repair of the injured vein would appear to have a lesser influence on limb survival and subsequent incidence of chronic venous insufficiency.

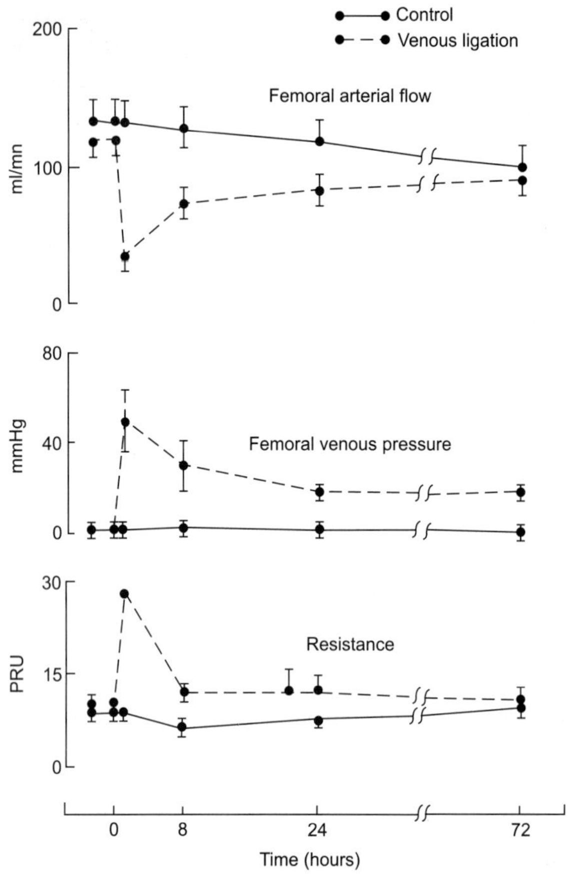

Figure 42.1 *Changes in femoral arterial blood flow, venous pressure, and resistance (mean ± standard error) after femoral venous ligation in the canine hindlimb. (Adapted from Hobson RW, Howard EW, Wright CB,* et al. *Hemodynamics of canine femoral venous ligation: significance in combined arterial and venous injuries.* Surgery *1973;* ***74****: 824)*

Based on these clinical reports and laboratory information, the earlier recommendation for universal repair of major injured veins in the lower extremity has been modified by knowledge of the hemodynamic significance of these injuries and the clinical necessity for performance of venous ligation in some cases, particularly when the patient is a multiple trauma victim. Although ligation of upper extremity venous injuries has been well tolerated, routine repair of common femoral and popliteal venous injuries has been recommended. However, management of these cases has been tempered during recent years by clinical reports that suggest a lack of major complications when venous injuries are ligated rather than repaired. Mullins and colleagues[12] reported on the results of venous ligation in the lower extremity after venous trauma. No early amputations were required and no cases of massive edema or ulceration were reported. Timberlake and associates[13] reported venous injuries managed by ligation that were unassociated with major long-term complications. This series of cases included ligation of 21 of 31 popliteal venous injuries. However, these authors emphasized the importance of elevation of the extremity pending complete resolution of edema and recommended four-compartment fasciotomy based on clinical findings or documentation of elevated compartmental pressures. Although the mean clinical follow-up was confined to less than 3 years in these reports, no clinical sequelae were reported during this limited period. However, as emphasized during the Vietnam Vascular Registry,[14] further follow-up was recommended on patients undergoing venous reconstruction to define the incidence of chronic venous insufficiency which may not be apparent until 5–10 years after venous ligation or occlusion of repairs. Although the reported incidence of edema after ligation or occlusion of primary femoral venous injuries was 75% in the author's experience,[15] recommendations for universal venous repair should be modified by the realization that all venous injuries in the lower extremity are not associated with adverse hemodynamic consequences. More recently, Sharma and colleagues[16] reported on an analysis of 191 major venous injuries in 163 patients. Fifty-two of the injuries occurred in the femoral or popliteal regions. These authors documented the incidence of measured venous hypertension before repair and emphasized the importance of correcting adverse hemodynamics by venous reconstruction. They also emphasized the importance of precise clinical repair using meticulous suture technique and intraoperative venography.[17] Aitken and associates[18] devised a functional grading system for lower vein ligation or various repair options. Although not specifically related to the type of repair, 'poor' results were observed in two-thirds of patients treated by ligation as compared with only one-third treated by repair. Functional outcome among 26 patients with lower extremity venous trauma was reported, 60–66 months after ligation or venous repair. Edema was present in five of six patients initially treated with ligation and nine of 20 who underwent repair. Venograms demonstrated venous occlusion in 11 of the 17 patients. Nine of the 11 patients with occlusion had edema, including all patients treated with ligation, whereas five of six patients with patent repairs were doing well without reported incidence of edema. A recent study by Zamir *et al.* examined the functionality of 46 patients who underwent simple or complex venous repairs for traumatic injuries. This study found that 81% of patients regained full function of their extremity following these repairs. In this study the incidence of perioperative edema was 2/46 (4%) and postoperative venous occlusion in 4/46 (9%).[19]

These experimental and clinical data suggest the importance of adverse hemodynamics and the emphasis for repair in the common femoral and popliteal veins of the lower extremity. One would anticipate a lower incidence of complications if ligation were performed in patients without venous hypertension.

COMPLICATIONS OF VENOUS RECONSTRUCTION

Thrombosis of direct venous repairs or interposition grafts within the venous system constitutes a major complication. However, several considerations are important in minimizing this complication. Meticulous surgical technique in experimental and clinical venous repairs is a major factor and requires some additional emphasis.[2,16] Use of interposition grafting, which has not been recommended by all authors,[20] constitutes one of the more controversial issues in venous reconstruction. Myer *et al.*[20] reported a 59% failure rate with venous grafting and commented that use of similar techniques in the arterial system had resulted in much higher rates of success. Unfortunately, hemodynamic measurements were not reported and operative venography was not performed to evaluate the technical adequacy of these venous reconstructions. With regard to the technical aspects of the venous repair (Fig. 42.2), the margin for error in completion of the venovenous anastomosis is less than that for the arterial anastomosis. Ideally, sutures must be placed loosely to avoid undue tension on the suture line; such tension would result inevitably in narrowing of the anastomosis and occlusion. These lessons have been emphasized in laboratory experience and subsequent clinical reports. Venography is recommended to confirm a successful repair; technically inadequate repairs will result in an early venous occlusion. Occlusion of the venous repair in the presence of combined arterial and venous trauma, particularly at the level of the popliteal artery and vein, may be associated with adverse clinical results. Rich *et al.*[8] reported that patency of repaired popliteal veins was an important factor resulting in the high amputation rate for combined popliteal arterial and venous trauma. Reports on the patency of femoral venous reconstruction in both the research laboratory and the clinical setting have been highly variable. This obviously relates to the choice of surgical technique and the use of various methods (Fig. 42.2) for repair of major injured veins.[21] Although the lengthy venous reconstruction should not be performed in the multiple trauma victim, use of interposition grafting can be associated with clinically acceptable results provided certain technical requirements are fulfilled rigorously and adjunctive measurements are used. Cases from our clinical experience[15] have confirmed that ligation can be associated with subsequent requirements for remedial reconstruction. That series has been expanded to more than 75 patients with femoral venous injuries and patency has continued to be in the 75–80% range (RW Hobson, unpublished data, 1995). Symptomatic pulmonary embolus has not occurred in this series, but approximately 10% of patients have demonstrated tibial venous thrombi on venography. All of these patients were maintained on anticoagulant therapy and edema resolved after 1 week, again without symptomatic pulmonary emboli. Schramek and colleagues[22] reported similarly successful results in managing 15 femoral and popliteal venous injuries in a group of 82 vascular injury cases. Interposition grafting was used in four femoral venous injuries supplemented with distal arteriovenous fistulas.[23] Follow-up venograms in these cases demonstrated patent grafts prompting the investigators to recommend use of interposition grafting for venous repair as necessary.

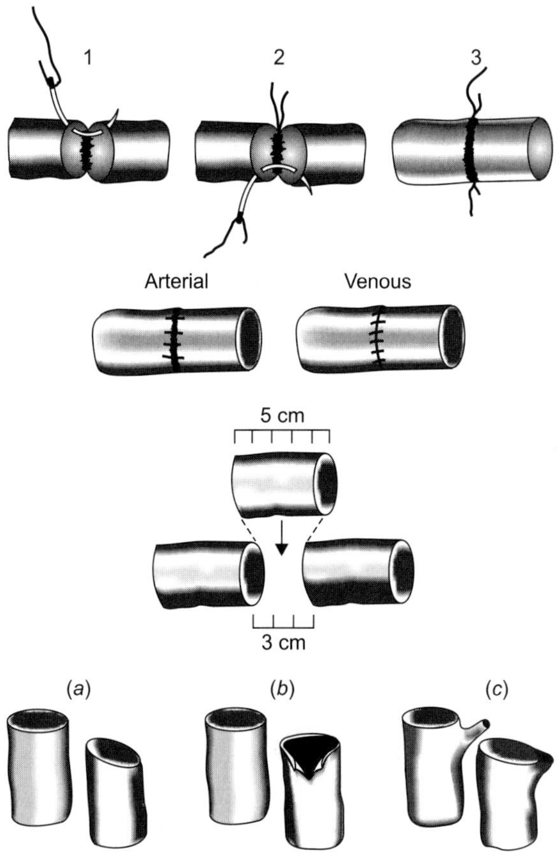

Figure 42.2 *Drawings demonstrating basic principles in performing venous anastomoses. Continuous sutures must be placed loosely in contrast to the usual technique for arterial anastomosis. Grafts in the venous system should be somewhat longer than the defect and of similar diameter. Diagonal cuts (a), 'fishmouthing' (b), and use of adjacent branches (c) may help prevent stenosis at suture lines. (Adapted from Rich NM, Hobson RW, Wright CB,* et al. *Techniques of venous repair. In Swan KG, ed.* Venous Surgery in the Lower Extremity. *St Louis, MO: Warren H. Green, 1974)*

Rich and colleagues[24] reported on 51 autogenous venous interposition grafts for repair of major injured veins; 36 involved the superficial femoral vein, eight the popliteal vein, and seven the common femoral vein. They reported a 2% incidence of thrombophlebitis, no pulmonary emboli, and an 11.8% incidence of residual edema in the lower extremities. Recent reports on vascular trauma have also emphasized the value of femoral and popliteal venous repair.[16–18,25,26] Although some investigators have reported an increased incidence of thrombosis with interposition venous grafting, the addition of adjunctive techniques to their clinical protocol may have improved the reported poor results.[2] Techniques designed to improve patency of direct venous repair include the following:

- administration of pharmacologic agents such as intraoperative heparin and postoperative low molecular weight dextran;
- intermittent pneumatic compression after popliteal and femoral venous injuries;
- creation of distal arterial venous fistulas.

In addition, certain technical features at the level of the common femoral vein requiring use of paneled or spiral vein grafts, if not used would certainly result in heightened thrombosis rate.

Ultimately, the clinical recommendation for venous repair should be selective and related to presence of venous hypertension or venographic evidence of absence of venous collateralization in the limb. This is particularly true of the superficial femoral vein but perhaps less so in cases of common femoral and popliteal venous injuries, which have been acknowledged as preferentially treated by repair when feasible. The only major exception to this recommendation is the multiple trauma victim, who might be jeopardized by the additional operative time required for venous repair.

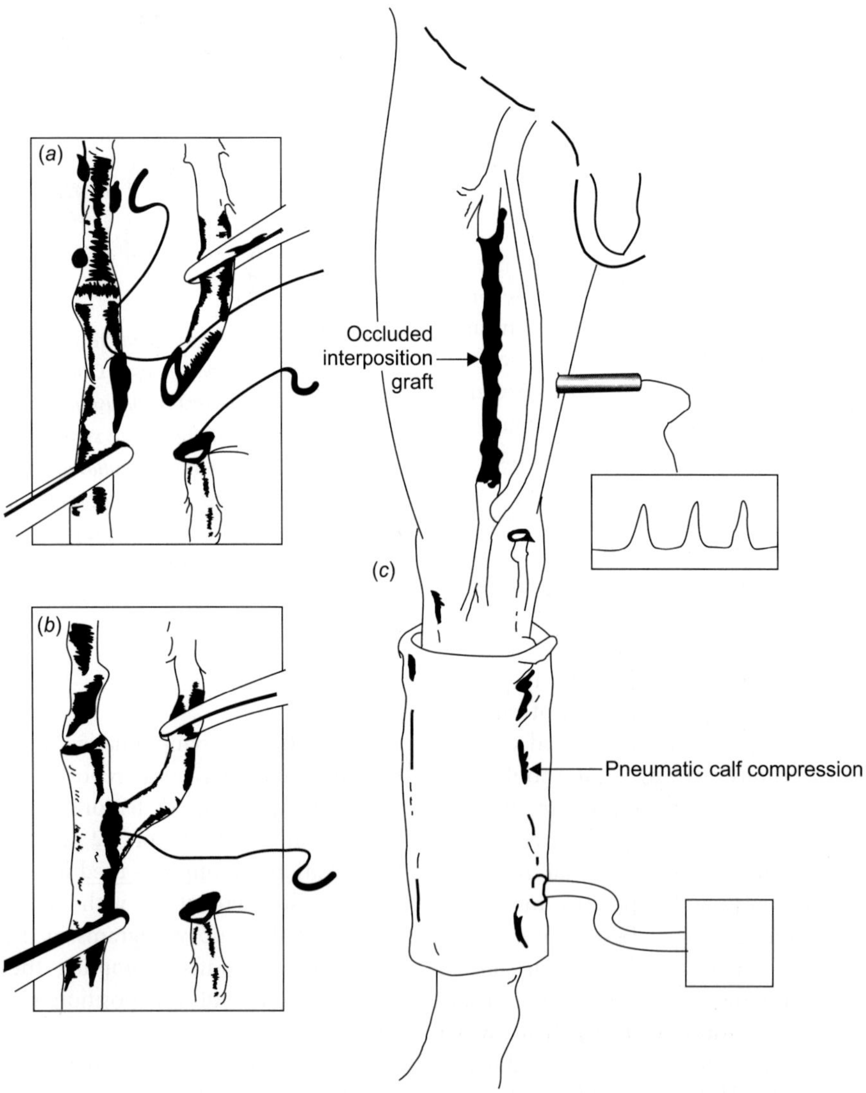

Figure 42.3 *Application of pneumatic calf compression is considered a valuable adjunct in achieving acceptable patency after repair of popliteal and femoral venous injuries. In this case a saphenopopliteal bypass (a–c) was performed after occlusion of a contralateral interposition saphenous vein graft in the superficial femoral vein. Augmentation of venous flow (c) was confirmed by use of continuous-wave Doppler. (Adapted from Hobson RW, Lee BC, Lynch TG,* et al. *Use of intermittent pneumatic compression of the calf in femoral veins reconstruct.* Surg Gynecol Obstet *1984;* **159***: 284)*

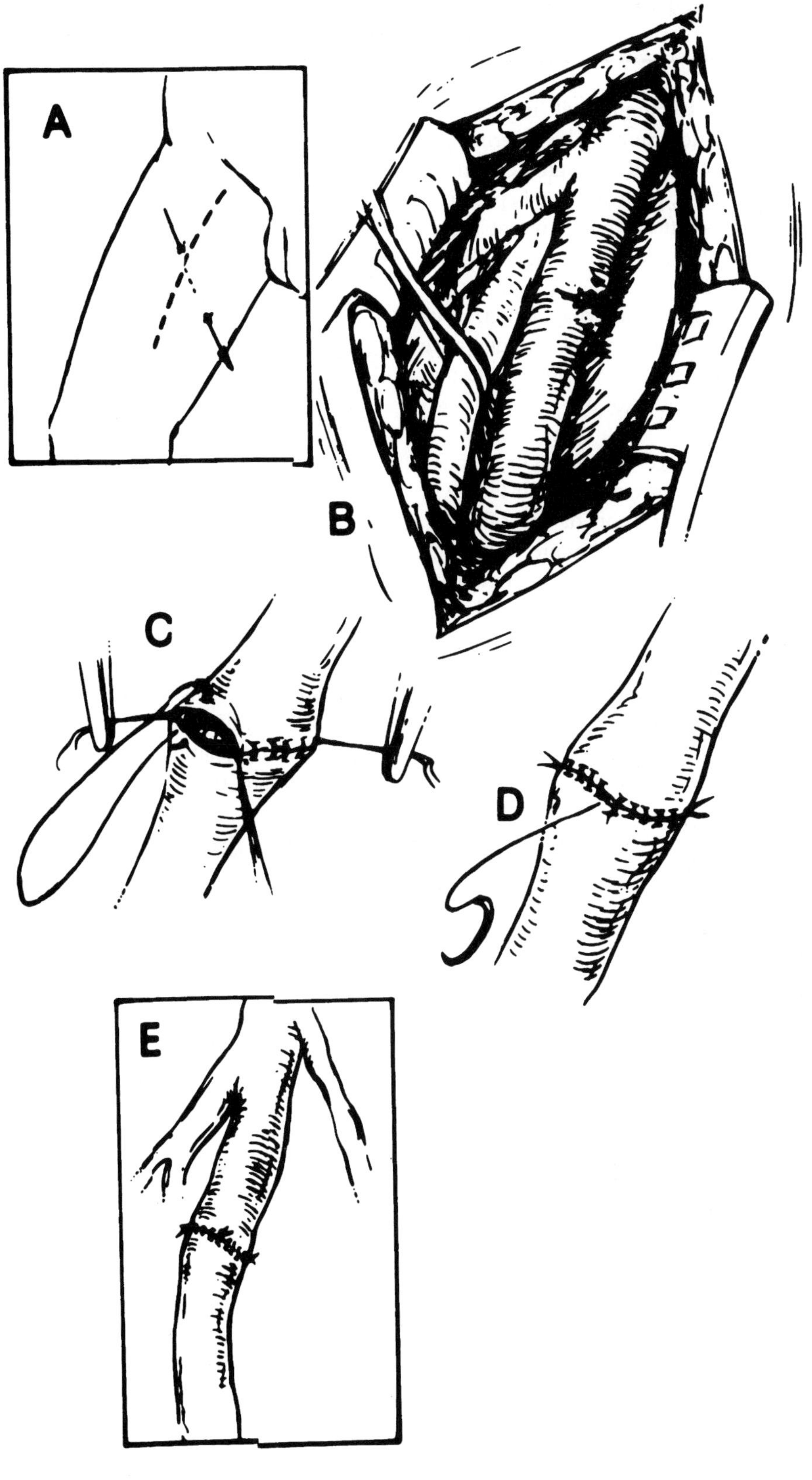

Figure 42.4 *The technique of end-to-end anastomosis is demonstrated in this superficial femoral venous injury (a,b). Although two-point fixation may be suitable for some injuries, three-point Carrel fixation (c, d) is recommended for lower extremity venous injuries. Any narrowing at the anastomosis indicates revision. (Adapted from Bergan JJ, Kistner RL, eds.* Atlas of Venous Surgery. *Philadelphia: WB Saunders, 1992)*

ADJUNCTIVE TECHNIQUES TO IMPROVE VENOUS PATENCY

Application of adjunctive techniques will improve the patency of venous repair after trauma. The experimental rationale for the use of low molecular weight dextran has been reported.[27] Interestingly, postoperative heparinization did not appear to be efficacious. A recent report from Smith *et al.* found a 6-week patency rate of 88% in the management of simple and complex venous repairs without the use of any long-term anticoagulation.[28] Our current recommendation includes use of intraoperative heparinization and administration of low molecular weight dextran that is continued for 48–72 hours postoperatively.[15]

Mechanical methods designed to increase the velocity of blood flow through the deep venous repair by use of intermittent pneumatic compression of the calf (Fig. 42.3) has been a useful adjunctive technique.[29] Although the increase in velocity of blood flow is intermittent with compression boots, this technique has been used by us[15] routinely to achieve a reported patency of 74% with femoral venous reconstructions, including use of interposition grafts.

Finally, the experimental value of distal arteriovenous fistulas has been established by several investigators.[30–32] The increased velocity of blood flow and arterialization of the venous repair should contribute to improved patency. Whether the fistula should be placed immediately adjacent to the venous repair is controversial since a secondary operation might then be required for its repair. However, recent techniques involving the construction of smaller fistulas, which can be ligated percutaneously or occluded by use of radiographic intervention, offer innovative clinical options. A more distal placement of the fistula also would allow its ligation or repair without disruption of the venous anastomosis. Although these fistulas have been reported as being an attractive alternatives for experimental reasons, clinical application, particularly after trauma, has been limited.[22] However, their use after elective venous reconstruction has been suggested and recommended by others after venous thrombectomy.

TECHNICAL CONSIDERATIONS

Venous reconstruction should be performed with special attention to surgical technique. Sutures must be placed loosely in the performance of end-to-end anastomoses to avoid undue tension, which results in narrowing of the anastomosis and the requirement for operative revision. Triangulation methods as originally described by Carrel are recommended (Fig. 42.4). Interrupted

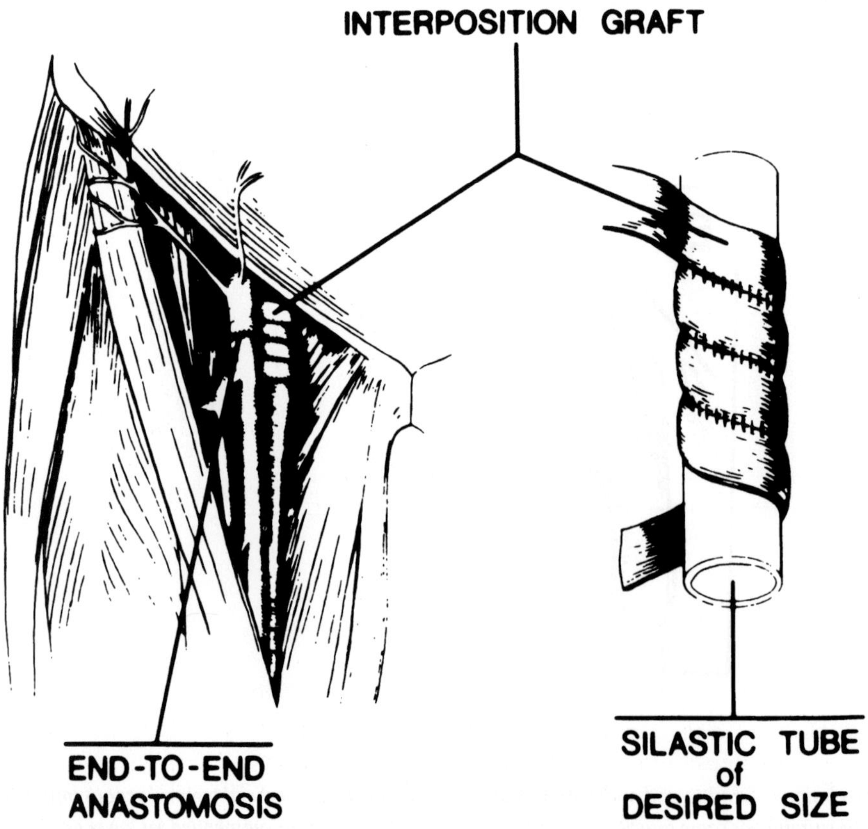

Figure 42.5 *Spiral vein interposition graft for femoral venous reconstruction. (Adapted from Hobson RW, Yeager RA, Lynch TG,* et al. *Femoral venous trauma: techniques for surgical management and early results.* Am J Surg *1983;* ***146****: 220)*

sutures are recommended for injury to smaller veins including the popliteal vein. Occlusion of the venous repair in the presence of combined arterial and venous trauma, particularly at the level of the popliteal artery and vein, may be associated with adverse clinical results.

Adequately sized interposition grafts may also require specialized techniques including paneled or spiral[15] vein grafts (Fig 42.5) for the common femoral vein. Several authors have reported patency of over 70% of these reconstructions; however, use of adjunctive methods is particularly important if high patency is to be achieved. Iliac and vena caval injuries are encountered as part of the operative management of penetrating abdominal trauma and require additional considerations in a discussion of lower extremity venous trauma. Although 5–10% of these injuries may occur as a result of blunt trauma, most are due to civilian or military reports of penetrating trauma. General principles of maintaining a patent airway, crystalloid fluid resuscitation followed by type-specific blood transfusions, and early operative intervention, apply. The midline incision is preferred and control of retroperitoneal bleeding is accomplished after mobilization of the right colon. Application of pressure by use of sponge sticks proximally and distally allows control of bleeding after which appropriate repair by lateral venorrhaphy or patch angioplasty can be accomplished. Rarely, interposition grafting can be considered. In the multiple trauma victim with intra-

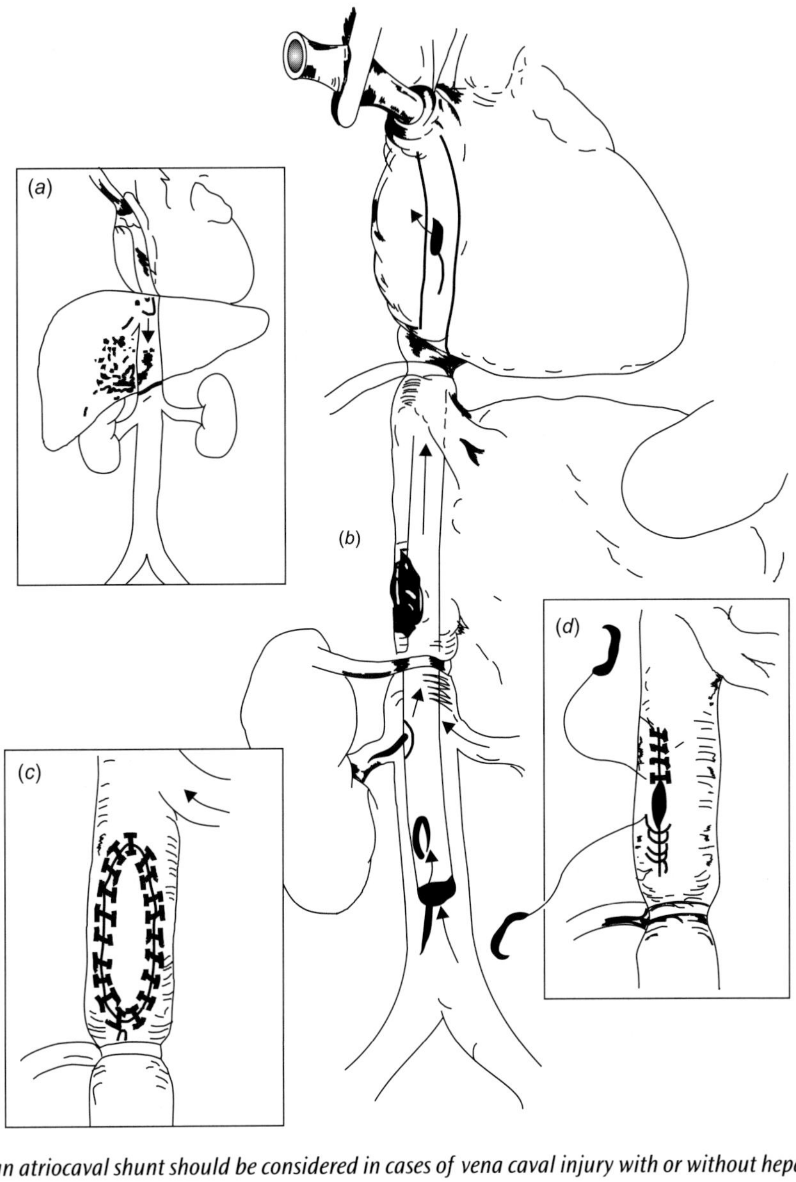

Figure 42.6 *Use of an atriocaval shunt should be considered in cases of vena caval injury with or without hepatic venous injury associated with major retrohepatic hematomas. (a) Placement of the shunt is recommended before mobilization of the right lobe of the liver. (b) Although a modified shunt may also be introduced through the infrarenal portion of the inferior vena cava, insertion of the shunt through the right atrial appendage, as demonstrated, is the preferred method. Repair by patch angioplasty (c) or lateral venorrhaphy (d) can then be accomplished (Adapted from Bergan JJ, Kistner RL, eds.* Atlas of Venous Surgery. *Philadelphia: WB Saunders, 1992)*

abdominal iliac or caval injuries, however, associated injuries to adjacent arteries, bowel, and other intra-abdominal structures frequently dictate ligation of the venous injuries in an effort to salvage the patient's life. As emphasized in several reports, the mortality of the iliac or caval venous injuries ranges from 20% to 40% and is often related to other multiple associated injuries.[33,34]

Injuries to the retrohepatic vena cava and hepatic veins are unusual (Fig. 42.6). When retrohepatic venous injuries are suspected by the presence of a significant retroperitoneal hematoma, several authors have recommended the use of atriocaval shunts.[35,36] These injuries are associated with high mortality. Use of appropriate shunts has been reported to improve survival in 30–50% of cases. Burch and associates reported survival in six of 18 patients after use of the atriocaval shunt.[35] Rovito also reported use of a no. 8 or no. 9 endotracheal tube as a modified atriocaval shunt.[36] The endotracheal tube was passed through the right atrial appendage and the balloon inflated in the suprarenal cava below the area of the injury. A vascular tourniquet was also placed at the level of the suprahepatic vena cava. Four of eight patients survived after use of this technique.

CONCLUSIONS

Most data favor the repair of injured common femoral and popliteal veins, whilst repair of injuries to the superficial femoral vein are more controversial. Repair by lateral venorrhaphy, end-to-end anastomosis, patch angioplasty, or interposition grafting is recommended for common femoral and popliteal venous injuries and for those superficial femoral venous injuries associated with venous hypertension. Follow-up and functional data suggest superiority for venous repair.

REFERENCES

1. Bergan JJ, Yao JST. *Venous Problems.* Chicago: Year Book Medical Publishers, 1978.
2. Hobson RW, Rich NM, Wright CB. *Venous Trauma: Pathophysiology, Diagnosis, and Surgical Management.* Mt Kisco, NY: Futura Publishing, 1983.
3. Makins GH. *Gunshot Injuries to the Blood Vessels.* Bristol: John Wright & Sons, 1919.
4. DeBakey ME, Simeone EA. Battle injuries of the arteries in World War II. *Ann Surg* 1946; **123**: 534.
5. Hughes CW. Acute vascular trauma in Korean War casualties. *Surg Gynecol Obstet* 1954; **99**: 91.
6. Spencer FC, Grewe RV. The management of arterial injuries in battle casualties. *Ann Surg* 1955; **141**: 304.
7. Rich NM, Hughes CW. Vietnam Vascular Registry: a preliminary report. *Surgery* 1969; **65**: 218–26.
8. Rich NM, Jarstfer BS, Geer TM. Popliteal arterial repair failure: Causes and possible prevention. *J Cardiovasc Surg* 1974; **15**: 34–51.
9. Rich NM, Hughes CW, Baugh JH. Management of venous injuries. *Ann Surg* 1970; **171**: 724–30.
10. Barcia PJ, Nelson TJ, Whelan TG. Importance of venous occlusion in arterial repair failure: an experimental study. *Ann Surg* 1972; **175**: 223–7.
11. Hobson RW, Howard EW, Wright CB, *et al.* Hemodynamics of canine femoral venous ligation: significance in combined arterial and venous injuries. *Surgery* 1973; **74**: 824–9.
12. Mullins RJ, Lacas CE, Ledgerwood AM. The natural history following venous ligation for civilian injuries. *J Trauma* 1980; **20**: 737–43.
13. Timberlake GA, O'Connell RC, Kerstein MD. Venous injury: to repair or ligate, the dilemma. *J Vasc Surg* 1986; **4**: 553–8.
14. Rich NM, Gomez ER, Coffoy JA, *et al.* Long-term follow-up of venous reconstruction following trauma. In Bergan JJ, Yao JST, eds. *Venous Disorders.* Philadelphia: WB Saunders, 1991: 471–81.
15. Hobson RW, Yeager RA, Lynch TG, *et al.* Femoral venous trauma: techniques for surgical management and early results. *Am J Surg* 1983; **146**: 22–4.
16. Sharma PVP, Shah PM, Vinzons AT, *et al.* Meticulously restored lumina of injured veins remain patent. *Surgery* 1992; **112**: 928–32.
17. Sharma PVP, Ivatory RR, Simon RJ, Vinzons AT. Central and regional hemodynamics determine optimal management of major venous injuries. *J Vasc Surg* 1992; **16**: 887–94.
18. Aitken RJ, Matley PJ, Immelman EJ. Lower limb vein trauma: a long-term clinical and physiological assessment. *Br J Surg* 1989; **76**: 585–8.
19. Zamir G, Berlatzky Y, Rivkind A, Haim A, Wolf YG. Results of reconstruction in major pelvic and extremity venous injuries. *J Vasc Surg* 1998; **28**(5): 901–8.
20. Meyer J, Walsh J, Schuler J, *et al.* The early fate of venous repair after civilian vascular trauma. *Ann Surg* 1987; **206**: 458–64.
21. Rich NM, Hobson RW, Wright CB, *et al.* Techniques of venous repair. In Swan KG, ed. *Venous Surgery in the Lower Extremity.* St Louis, MO: Warren H. Green, 1974: 22–4.
22. Schramek A, Hashmonai M, Farbstein J, *et al.* Reconstructive surgery in major vein injuries in the extremities. *J Trauma* 1975; **15**: 816–22.
23. Schramek A, Hashmonai M. Distal arteriovenous fistula for prevention of occlusion of venous interposition grafts to veins. *J Cardiovasc Surg (Torino)* 1974; **15**: 39–45.
24. Rich NM, Collins GJ, Andersen CA, *et al.* Autogenous venous interposition grafts in repair of major venous injuries. *J Trauma* 1977; **17**: 512–20.
25. Sayoyan RM, Kerstein MD. Role of concomitant venous repair in the management of extremity arterial injuries. In Ernst CB, Stanley JC, eds. *Current Techniques in Vascular Surgery*, Vol. 2. Philadelphia: BC Decker, 1991.

26. Ellenby MI, Schuler JJ. Repair or ligation in extremity venous injuries. In Bergan JJ, Yao JST, eds. *Venous Disorders.* Philadelphia: WB Saunders, 1991: 451–70.
27. Hobson RW, Croom RD, Rich NM. Influence of heparin and low molecular weight dextran on the patency of autogenous vein grafts in the venous system. *Ann Surg* 1973; **178**: 773.
28. Smith LM, Block EF, Buetcher KJ, Draughn DC, Watson D, Hedden W. The natural history of extremity venous repair performed for trauma. *Am Surg* 1999; **65**(2): 116–20.
29. Hobson RW, Lee BC, Lynch TG, *et al.* Use of intermittent pneumatic compression of the calf in femoral venous reconstruction. *Surg Gynecol Obstet* 1984; **159**: 284–6.
30. Levin PM, Rich NM, Hutton JE, *et al.* Role of arteriovenous shunts in venous reconstruction. *Am J Surg* 1971; **122**: 183–91.
31. Hobson RW, Croom RD, Swan KG. Hemodynamics of the distal arteriovenous fistula in venous reconstruction. *J Surg Res* 1973; **14**: 483–9.
32. Hobson RW, Wright CB. Peripheral side-to-side arteriovenous fistula: hemodynamics and application to venous reconstruction. *Am J Surg* 1973; **126**: 411–14.
33. Mattox KL, Rea J, Ennix CL, *et al.* Penetrating injuries to the iliac arteries. *Am J Surg* 1978; **136**: 663–7.
34. Millikan IS, Moore EE, Van Way CW III, *et al.* Vascular trauma in the groin: contrast between iliac and femoral injuries. *Am J Surg* 1981; **142**: 695–8.
35. Burch IM, Feliciano DV, Mattox KL. The atriocaval shunt: facts and fiction. *Ann Surg* 1988; **207**: 555–68.
36. Rovito PF. Atrial caval shunting in blunt hepatic vascular injury. *Ann Surg* 1987; **205**: 318–21.

43

Primary and secondary tumors of the vena cava

THOMAS C BOWER

Tumors which involve the vena cava are rare and often malignant.[1] Most patients with these tumors either have metastases or are too debilitated to tolerate operation. For these individuals, there are very few treatment alternatives.

At present, surgical resection remains the only hope for cure or palliation of symptoms from caval malignancies because chemotherapy and radiation therapy alone have had no proven benefit. Surgeons have long been aggressive in the treatment of selected individuals with renal cell carcinoma and intracaval tumor thrombus.[2–13] In most of these cases, the tumor thrombus can be removed without the need for caval replacement. More recently, a number of surgeons have reported successful resection and graft replacement of the vena cava in patients with other primary or secondary tumors.[1,14–20] Discussion is limited to tumors that affect the inferior vena cava (IVC) in this chapter. For reference, the IVC from the confluence of the common iliac veins to the renal veins is the infrarenal segment, from the renal veins to the hepatic veins is the suprarenal portion, and from the hepatic veins to the right atrium is the suprahepatic segment. The suprarenal IVC is further divided into an infrahepatic and retrohepatic segment.

TUMOR TYPES

Vena cava tumors originate primarily from the smooth muscle cell of the vein wall or secondarily from endothelial or mesothelial cells of abdominal or retroperitoneal organs.[21] Local growth or regional extension of these tumors occurs by either extraluminal or intraluminal growth or by a combination of these mechanisms.[22] Distant metastases occur either by lymphatic or hematogenous routes, depending on the type of malignancy. Renal cell or adrenocortical carcinoma, pheochromocytoma, some germ cell tumors, and sarcomas of uterine origin may grow as tumor thrombus within the vena cava.[1–13,23] The various types of primary and secondary tumors of the IVC tumors are shown in Table 43.1.

Table 43.1 *Tumors of the inferior vena cava*

Primary
IVC leiomyosarcoma
Secondary
Retroperitoneal soft tissue tumors
Liposarcoma
Leiomyosarcoma
Malignant fibrous histiocytoma
Hepatic tumors
Cholangiocarcinoma
Hepatocellular carcinoma
Metastatic (e.g. colorectal)
Pancreaticoduodenal cancers
Secondary tumors which may have tumor thrombus
Renal cell carcinoma
Pheochromocytoma
Adrenocortical carcinoma
Sarcomas of uterine origin
Leiomyomatosis
Endometerial stromal cell
Germ cell tumors
Embryonal
Teratocarcinoma

IVC, inferior vena cava.

The most common primary tumor of the venous system is leiomyosarcoma. Venous leiomyosarcomas are extremely rare but are more common than their arterial counterparts.[24] Primary venous leiomyosarcoma arises in the inferior vena cava in 50–60% of patients and the IVC is a more common site of origin than the other central or peripheral veins.[17,25] Primary caval tumors may arise from any segment of the vena cava. In a review of 144 cases by Mingoli *et al.*,[26] the suprarenal IVC was involved in three-fourths of patients, the infrarenal segment in one-third, and the suprahepatic segment in one-fourth.

Primary venous leiomyosarcoma of the IVC is more prevalent in women than in men.[17,26] In the report by Mingoli and colleagues, over 80% were women and the mean age was 54.4 years. However, these tumors do occur in patients over a wide age range.[26]

Pathologically, these tumors are usually polypoid or nodular in appearance and firmly attached to the vessel wall of origin.[22,24,26,27] They represent approximately 6% of all types of retroperitoneal sarcomas but typically exhibit less intra-tumor hemorrhage and necrosis than the other sarcomas.[22,24] Although intraluminal growth occurs most commonly, these tumors may invade through the caval wall and become adherent to or invade adjacent structures. When this latter growth pattern occurs, these tumors are difficult to differentiate from other retroperitoneal sarcomas.[1,21] Metastases occur early in the course of disease and are present in almost one-half of patients at the time of diagnosis. Lung, liver, kidney, bone, pleura, or chest wall are the most common sites for metastatic spread.[17,24,27] If surgical resection is not possible, survival of these patients is measured in months. Mingoli *et al.* reported a mean survival of only 3 months for untreated patients in one of their series.[26]

Secondary IVC tumors include primary cancers of the solid or hollow organs within the abdomen; cancers or germ cell tumors metastatic to the pericaval lymph nodes; retroperitoneal sarcomas such as leiomyosarcoma, liposarcoma, or malignant fibrous histiocytoma; or malignancies which develop tumor thrombus.[1,21] These tumors are most often noted in patients in their fifth, sixth or seventh decades of life.[1,16,18–21]

Abdominal cancers invade or obstruct the segment of IVC in anatomic proximity to their site of origin. Hepatocellular carcinoma, cholangiocarcinoma, mixed liver tumors, and metastatic lesions to the liver involve the retrohepatic segments, and pancreatic, duodenal, and large renal or adrenal malignancies involve the suprarenal IVC. All of these cancers typically compress or invade the IVC.[1]

Retroperitoneal sarcomas can involve any segment of the IVC. These tumors usually have a pseudocapsule and often displace but do not invade adjacent organs. In two-thirds of cases, the sarcomas grow extrinsic to the major arteries and veins.[22,28] However, in the other third, the tumors invade the IVC and develop a component of intraluminal growth which makes them indistinguishable pathologically from primary caval tumors.[1,21] Retroperitoneal sarcomas are the most common cause of malignant obstruction of the infrarenal IVC segment.[1]

The most common malignancy which affects the vena cava is renal cell carcinoma.[1–13,29] Tumor thrombus is found in the IVC in 4–15% of patients[1,11,13,29] and is associated more commonly with large (greater than 4.5 cm diameter) renal cell carcinomas and right-sided tumors.[1,4,11,13,29,30] The extent of tumor thrombus within the IVC can be classified in a number of ways, depending on whether the thrombus extends above or below the level of the diaphragm, and whether it involves the retrohepatic or infrahepatic IVC.[1] Nearly one-half of patients have thrombus extending to the renal vein confluence with the IVC, 40% of patients have thrombus in the infrahepatic or retrohepatic segments, and only 10% have extension of tumor thrombus into the right heart.[1,4,13,29]

In general, secondary malignancies of the IVC carry a poor prognosis with survival less than 1 year without treatment.[1,20,21] The exception is patients with renal cell carcinoma and tumor thrombus who may live several years or more with aggressive surgical management (see section on outcomes).

CLINICAL PRESENTATION

Patients with caval malignancies present with symptoms and signs related to the primary tumor or to metastatic disease. Rarely, the clinical presentation is related to obstruction of the vena cava alone.[1] In a few cases, the tumors are detected at any early stage as an incidental finding during evaluation of other nonspecific symptoms such as abdominal or back pain. In a recent report from the Mayo Clinic of 29 patients who had IVC replacement for malignant disease, over two-thirds of the patients presented with one or more symptoms.[20] Pain was the most common symptom and occurred in 58.6% of patients; weight loss, fatigue or nausea occurred in 24.1%, and lower extremity edema in 10.3%. Only one patient presented with a lower extremity deep vein thrombosis. Nine patients (31%) were asymptomatic but had a mass discovered either by physical examination or incidentally with an imaging study.[20] By contrast, only four of 144 patients with primary venous leiomyosarcomas of the IVC, reported by Mingoli and colleagues, were asymptomatic at the time of diagnosis.[26] All other patients in this series had multiple symptoms or signs when first seen. Abdominal pain occurred in 95 patients (66.0%) and an abdominal mass was noted in 69 (47.9%). Lower limb edema occurred in 56 (38.9%), weight loss in 44 (30.6%), and Budd–Chiari syndrome in 32 (22.2%).[26] Nonspecific symptoms such as fever, anorexia, nausea, vomiting, weakness, nocturnal sweating, and dyspnea were seen in less than 15% of patients.[26]

Consumption coagulopathy and red blood cell abnormalities have also been noted in patients with primary caval tumors.[24]

Obstruction of the IVC may result in a variety of symptoms or signs.[1,21] The segment of IVC involved by the tumor and the degree of venous outflow obstruction of the adjacent organs determines the clinical presentation. Obstruction to blood flow in the right heart may cause cardiac arrhythmias, syncope, pulmonary hypertension or embolism, and even right heart failure. Hepatic vein outflow obstruction results in Budd–Chiari syndrome with hepatomegaly, massive ascites, jaundice, and in late stages liver failure. Occlusion of the suprarenal IVC may lead to renal or lower extremity deep venous insufficiency. Cancers which invade the retrohepatic IVC cause back or right upper quadrant abdominal pain, biliary tract symptoms, nausea, vomiting, or tenderness on abdominal examination. Obstruction of the IVC at the renal vein confluence may result in renal insufficiency or nephrotic syndrome but dialysis-dependent renal failure is unusual because of venous decompression of the left kidney by gonadal, adrenal, or lumborenal vein branches.[1,21] Tumor thrombus which obstructs renal venous blood flow may cause hematuria, flank pain, or a varicocele. The most common symptoms or signs of tumors involving the infrarenal segment include abdominal or back pain, or a palpable mass.[1,20,21] Lower extremity pain, dysesthesias, or weakness occur from tumor involvement of the lumbosacral plexus, the nerve roots, or the psoas muscle. Lower extremity edema occurs with acute caval occlusion but is rare in patients who have chronic IVC obstruction.[31–33] The initial venous hypertension in the latter case is gradually decompressed through pelvic, paravertebral, or abdominal wall collateral veins. Deep vein thrombosis is very unusual and is more typically seen in patients with primary venous leiomyosarcoma of the iliac or peripheral veins.[1,4,16–22,24,26,34]

EVALUATION

A multidisciplinary approach to the evaluation and treatment of patients with IVC tumors is important.[1,20,21] Specialists in medical and surgical oncology, vascular, general, hepatobiliary, urologic or cardiothoracic surgery are needed to help direct the work-up and choose the type of imaging studies which will best determine resectability of the cancer.

The goals of evaluation are to determine the type of tumor, to define the local extent of the malignancy, to exclude the presence of metastatic disease, and to assess the degree of caval obstruction and the status of venous collaterals.[1,20,21]

Much of the patient evaluation and the decision to treat is based on radiologic studies. Chest roentgenography is useful to exclude metastatic lung lesions and hilar or mediastinal adenopathy. Abdominal roentgenograms are rarely diagnostic but may show calcification within a retroperitoneal mass suggestive of sarcoma.[17] Excretory urography in patients with renal malignancies may show distortion, displacement, or a filling defect of the kidney, the ureter, or the renal calices.[1,21,22]

The four most useful modalities to image the vena cava and the cancer are computed tomography (CT), magnetic resonance imaging (MRI), vena cavography, and ultrasonography.[1,4,21,29,30] Often, a combination of tests is used to determine surgical resectability, and plan vena cava reconstruction.

Computed tomography and magnetic resonance imaging are the two studies used most often.[1,21,35] CT and MRI scans of the chest and abdomen define the local extent of the cancer, the level of venous involvement, the presence of regional or distant metastases, and the studies allow good imaging of the IVC at all levels (Fig. 43.1). MRI is a very versatile technique because the tumor and the IVC can be imaged in axial, coronal and sagittal planes (Fig. 43.2).[30,35] A combination of axial and sagittal T1-weighted and SE pulse sequences with axial single breath-hold gradient echo images may be the optimal method for detection of IVC tumor thrombus related to renal cell carcinoma.[30] False-positive studies with MRI are usually caused by flow artifacts.[30] Whether the use of gadolinium contrast will further improve the accuracy of this technique is yet to be determined. Additionally, both scans can be used for postoperative cancer surveillance and to monitor graft patency if venous reconstruction has been performed.[20]

The entire IVC can be imaged by ultrasonography as well, but the image may be distorted by the tumor or by overlying bowel gas. However, in selected individuals, ultrasonography is as sensitive as MRI and vena cavography in defining patency of the IVC and the presence and extent of intraluminal tumor thrombus.[30]

Vena cavography has long been the gold standard test for evaluation of patients with suspected peripheral or central venous obstruction. This study provides detailed information about the location and extent of caval involvement by the cancer. Both antegrade and retrograde approaches may be necessary to define the anatomy.[16] Vena cavography was used routinely in our early experience but at the present time we only use this study if the venous anatomy is not well-shown by other imaging tests.[20]

Once resectability has been determined, the next step in evaluation is medical risk assessment for operation. A thorough cardiopulmonary evaluation is essential as most of the postoperative mortality and morbidity is related to heart or lung problems.[1,4,13,20,21] Additionally, assessment of the patient's physical condition preoperatively is important. We use the performance status scale outlined by Zubrod *et al.*,[36] which has been a useful predictor of the anticipated functional quality of life for

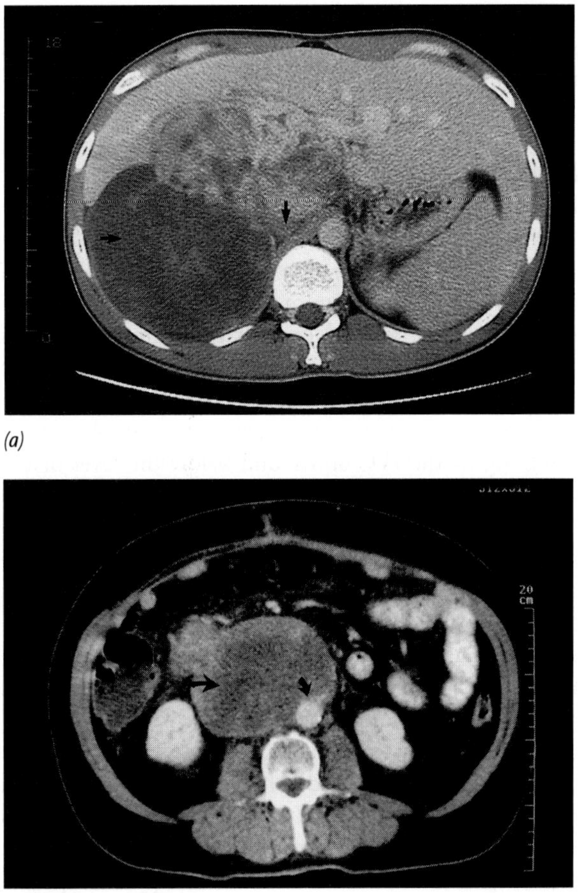

(a)

(b)

Figure 43.1 *Computed tomographic scan (CT) of a patient with a large leiomyosarcoma (a) involving the right lobe of the liver, right kidney, and retroperitoneum (white arrows). The retrohepatic segment of the suprarenal inferior vena cava was invaded by the tumor (black arrow). The patient underwent tumor and liver resection with IVC replacement. CT scan of a patient with a retroperitoneal leiomyosarcoma surrounding the infrarenal IVC (b). The tumor is shown by the large black arrow. This patient also required resection of the infrarenal aorta shown by the smaller black arrow. [(b) Reproduced with permission from Bower TC, Stanson AW. Evaluation and management of malignant tumors of the inferior vena cava. In Rutherford RB, ed.* Vascular Surgery, *5th edn. Orlando, FL: WB Saunders, 2000]*

cancer patients postoperatively. A score of 0 indicates that the patient is fully active with no limitations while a score of 4 indicates that the patient is bedridden and unable to perform self-care. Patients with performance status scores of 0–1 have a low operative risk. Although we have operated on patients with performance status scores of 2, these few patients have had prolonged hospital recoveries and have not shown improvement in their physical well-being during follow-up.[20] Patients with scores of 3 or 4 should not be operated.

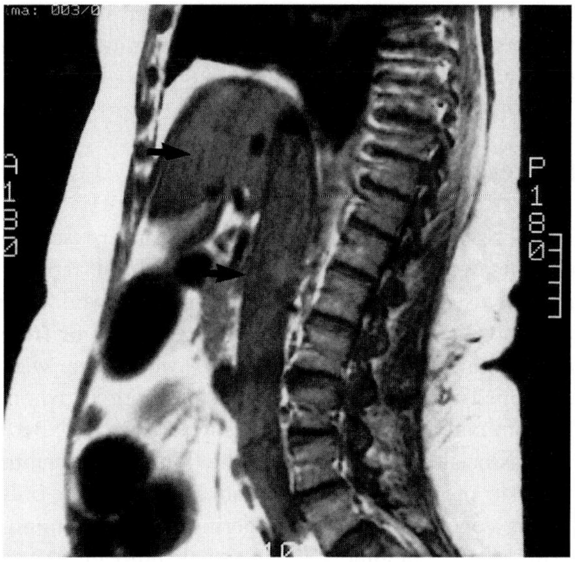

Figure 43.2 *Magnetic resonance imaging scan showing intracaval tumor thrombus extending into the right heart chambers secondary to an endometrial stromal cell sarcoma.*

TREATMENT

Most patients with cancers involving the IVC have advanced disease, are debilitated, or have metastases – all of which exclude them for consideration of operation.[20] Most primary or secondary caval tumors are not amenable to chemotherapy or radiation and thus, surgical resection of the tumor is the mainstay of therapy.[1,21] This may require resection or replacement of the vena cava. Patients with localized tumors, few medical co-morbidities, and a good performance status should be considered candidates for operation.[1,20,21]

Surgical approach

Operative treatment depends on the type and extent of the malignancy, the segment of vena cava involved by the tumor, the degree of caval obstruction, and the status of the collateral veins. Exposure of the tumor and the vena cava can be achieved through several different incisions depending on the patient's body habitus, the segment of IVC to be reconstructed, the possible need for cardiopulmonary or venovenous bypass, and the need for concomitant major liver resection.[1,16,19–21] A midline abdominal incision is useful for tumors involving the IVC up to the confluence of the renal veins. A bilateral subcostal or a midline incision may be used to replace the infrahepatic segment of the IVC.[1,11,16,18–21] We prefer a right thoracoabdominal approach through the eight or ninth interspace for patients who require retrohepatic IVC replacement in conjunction with major liver resection.[18,20] For patients who require cardiopulmonary bypass to remove intracaval tumor thrombus, a median sternotomy together with a midline or subcostal abdominal incision usually affords excellent exposure.[1,11,21]

IVC resection without replacement

The decision to replace the IVC during cancer resection is controversial.[16,18–20,33] IVC resection without replacement is usually well tolerated in patients in whom the vena cava is occluded or scarred from tumor or from prior adjuvant therapy, for those who have well-developed venous collaterals, and for those in whom concomitant intestinal resection is necessary.[19,20,33,34] Beck and associates have reported the long-term venous sequelae of 24 patients who had IVC resection only during operations for retroperitoneal, nonseminomatous germ cell tumors.[33] Acute renal failure developed in four patients postoperatively, lower extremity edema in four, and chylous ascites in three. Interestingly, these authors were unable to predict late venous sequelae on the basis of a patient's preoperative venous symptoms, signs, or imaging results.[33] A clinical course of slow, progressive occlusion of the infrarenal IVC by tumor suggests IVC resection alone should result in few complications. However, if the IVC occlusion occurs rapidly, postoperative edema may occur in 36–70% of patients and long-term edema or venous problems may affect over one-third.[31,32]

Resection of the suprarenal segment of the vena cava without venous replacement has been reported but carries more risk of renal dysfunction and lower extremity edema than resection of the infrarenal segment.[19,37] With suprarenal IVC occlusion, venous blood flow is rerouted through collateral lumbar, epigastric, renal, adrenal, gonadal, and paravertebral pathways which may adequately relieve venous hypertension of the kidneys and the lower extremities.[19,38] However, the ability to predict preoperatively which patients will tolerate suprarenal IVC ligation or resection alone without postoperative complications is difficult.[1,19,20] Renal insufficiency is more likely to occur in patients who have had, or will need, right nephrectomy, in whom the left renal vein requires ligation at operation to remove the tumor.[19] Transient or permanent renal insufficiency has been reported in as many as one-half of patients who require left renal vein ligation in these situations.[39] In a report of six patients who had suprarenal IVC resection, with or without replacement, one patient with chronic caval occlusion preoperatively tolerated the resection without sequelae.[19] Another patient with rapid IVC occlusion developed renal failure, and a third patient required reimplantation of the left renal vein onto a caval graft to reverse intraoperative anuria.[19] These authors now recommend renal vein reconstruction if the suprarenal IVC requires resection and the patient develops anuria or has a reduction in urine output during the period of renal vein cross-clamping.[19] This principle applies whether the right or left renal vein requires reimplantation.[20]

Renal cell carcinoma with IVC tumor thrombus

The most common operation performed on the IVC is removal of intracaval tumor thrombus in patients with renal cell carcinoma.[1–13,29] Patients with tumor thrombus confined to the IVC at the renal vein confluence or the infrahepatic segment tolerate removal of thrombus with little hemodynamic consequence by simple cross-clamping of the IVC above and below the level of the thrombus.

Patients with thrombus extending into the retrohepatic segment up to the hepatic veins require complete mobilization of the liver to allow access to the suprahepatic IVC.[13] Intraoperative transesophageal echocardiography is a useful adjunct in these cases to define the proximal extent of the thrombus and to determine the need for cardiopulmonary bypass.[1,13] If only a small tongue of tumor thrombus extends to the caval–atrial junction, then the supradiaphragmatic extrapericardial portion of the IVC should be isolated. Some surgeons prefer to gently manipulate the tumor back into the suprahepatic IVC so that a vascular clamp can be placed below the caval–atrial junction which avoids the need for cardiopulmonary bypass.[5,13] However, this maneuver must be carefully performed to prevent tumor embolization. Hepatic vascular exclusion with cross-clamping of the suprahepatic and infrarenal IVC as well as the arterial and venous inflow to the liver isolates the retrohepatic vena cava and facilitates tumor removal at this level with little blood loss.[1,20,40] The cavotomy may need to be extended into the infrahepatic caval segment to be certain that all the thrombus has been removed. The cavotomy can then be closed to a point where the suprahepatic clamp can be released and moved to the infrahepatic segment to minimize liver ischemia. Resection of large renal cell cancers with tumor thrombus in the retrohepatic IVC is difficult, especially for right-sided ones that extend behind the liver to the diaphragm. Nesbitt *et al.*[13] suggest performing nephrectomy first in these situations with ligation and amputation of the renal vein rather than complete *en bloc* tumor resection. They believe this maneuver facilitates access to and exposure of the suprarenal IVC.[13] Preoperative renal artery embolization for large cancers may reduce vascularity and contract the tumor thrombus, but the technique is not performed universally.[13,41]

Tumor thrombus in the right heart should be removed with cardiopulmonary bypass, with or without circulatory arrest or concomitant deep hypothermia.[13] The use of deep hypothermia or circulatory arrest is advantageous in selected individuals but is probably not necessary in every case. The risk of coagulopathy and organ dysfunction during circulatory arrest or with cooling must be weighed against the advantage these techniques provide for tumor removal.[1,4–10,13,23,29]

In most cases, the vena cavotomy can be closed primarily. If primary closure narrows the IVC or if a cuff of vena cava is removed in the course of tumor resection, the cavotomy should be closed with a synthetic or venous patch.[1,21] Partial resection of the IVC wall with patch angioplasty is a useful technique to reconstruct the vena cava at all levels and is preferable to graft replacement of the IVC because patch closure is simpler and safer.[16]

IVC replacement

Vena cava replacement should be considered at all levels for patients in whom the IVC is not obstructed but requires resection for tumor clearance, in individuals without well-developed venous collaterals, for those in whom collateral veins are ligated or resected during tumor removal, and for patients who require IVC replacement at or above the level of the renal vein confluence.[20] Externally supported expanded polytetrafluorethylene (PTFE) grafts are used most often to replace the IVC.[1,14–20,42] These grafts are advantageous because they are readily available, easily size-matched to the diameter of the vena cava, and theoretically resistant to compression by the abdominal viscera.[16,18–20] They are preferable, in our opinion, to the use of spiral saphenous vein or superficial femoral vein in this location.[1,20,42]

In general, the need to add an arteriovenous fistula either at the femoral level or centrally for IVC reconstructions is controversial.[16–20] In the Mayo Clinic series, only three of 29 patients had an arteriovenous fistula. An arteriovenous fistula is not necessary with suprarenal caval grafts because of the large blood flow volume at this level.[16,19,20] Although experience with IVC prosthetic grafts for malignancy is limited, the experience with caval grafts for benign disease suggests that addition of an arteriovenous fistula is useful for patients who require reconstruction of more than one caval segment and for those with small diameter (< 14 mm) grafts.[20,42]

Lower extremity pneumatic compression devices are used postoperatively in all patients with IVC grafts. Subcutaneous heparin and aspirin suppositories are administered the first 2–3 days after operation, and all patients with IVC replacement are dismissed from the hospital on warfarin.[20]

Replacement of the suprarenal IVC in conjunction with major liver resection

Successful resection of primary and secondary tumors of the suprarenal IVC in conjunction with major liver resection has been reported by a number of authors.[14–16,18–20] Careful patient selection is critical to a good outcome. A number of operative principles can minimize the mortality and morbidity in these cases.[18–20] Intra-abdominal exploration is important to exclude metastatic disease. Intraoperative ultrasonography is used to clarify the intrahepatic extent of tumor and to confirm hepatic venous outflow and portal vein and hepatic artery inflow to the anticipated hepatic remnant. If the tumor is deemed resectable, the IVC is isolated above and below the level of the tumor before resection is begun. Early ligation of the appropriate afferent and efferent lobar vasculature before parenchymal division, the use of hepatic vascular exclusion to complete tumor resection and perform the IVC reconstruction, and the selected use of venovenous bypass to maintain patient hemodynamics are important adjuncts to minimize blood loss and lower operative risk.[1,20] Our surgical technique has been previously described and is illustrated schematically in Fig. 43.3.[18,20] We have performed major liver resection and retrohepatic IVC replacement in 13 patients. Liver ischemia was less than 30 minutes in most of them and was under 1 hour in all but one patient,[20] well within the tolerable limits of liver ischemia reported by others.[40] Transient elevation in liver function tests are common postoperatively, usually peak within the first 2–3 days after operation, and then return to normal.[20] These patients remain auto-anticoagulated for 24–48 hours. Otherwise, these patients are cared for as outlined previously.

OUTCOMES AND SURVIVAL

Selected patients with graft replacement of the IVC for malignant disease appear to do well though the experience at any one center remains limited.[16,19,20] Kieffer and associates had two deaths among 18 patients surgically-treated for caval tumors.[16] Huguet *et al.*[19] reported one death among four patients with suprarenal IVC graft replacement. The mortality rate was 6.9% in the recent Mayo Clinic report.[20] Major morbidity in this series included cardiopulmonary problems in five patients, bleeding in five, chylous ascites or large pleural effusions in two, and bile leak, lower extremity edema with tibial vein thrombosis, and wound infection in one patient each.[20] Renal failure or graft infection have been reported but the overall incidence of these problems is low.[16,19,20]

Mortality rates for patients undergoing radical nephrectomy and IVC tumor thrombectomy range from 2.7 to 13%.[4,5,7,8,10,12,13] The mortality rate does not appear to be influenced by the addition of cardiopulmonary bypass or hypothermic circulatory arrest.[6,7,9,10] Major morbidity occurs in 10–31% of patients with cardiopulmonary problems occurring most often.[4,12,13] However, postoperative bleeding, lower extremity edema, renal or venous insufficiency, and ascites may occur.[1] Some authors report pulmonary emboli as a major postoperative problem and recommend IVC clipping or

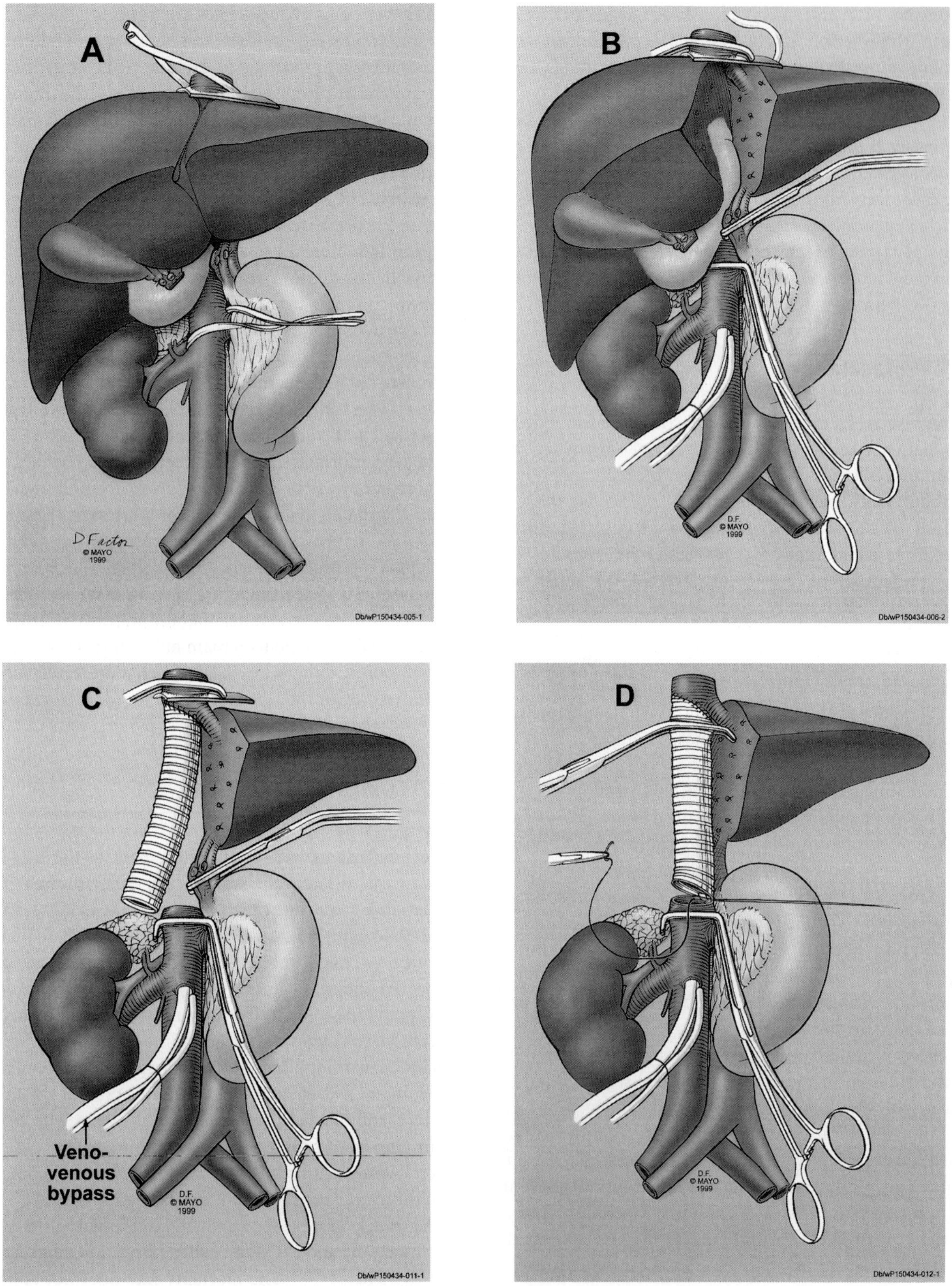

Figure 43.3 *Key steps in performance of retrohepatic inferior vena cava replacement and liver resection. (a) Early isolation of the suprahepatic and infrahepatic IVC. (b) Vascular isolation of the liver just prior to completion of tumor and IVC resection. (c) Upper caval anastomosis performed with vascular isolation of the liver. Some patients require venovenous bypass to maintain stable hemodynamics. (d) Blood flow is reestablished through the liver and the lower caval anastomosis is completed. [(a, c, d) Adapted from Bower TC, Stanson AW. Evaluation and management of malignant tumors of the inferior vena cava. In Rutherford RB, ed.* Vascular Surgery, *5th edn. Orlando, FL: WB Saunders, 2000. (b) Adapted from Bower TC, Nagorney DM, Toomey BJ,* et al. *Vena cava replacement for malignant disease: is there a role?* Ann Surg *1993;* **7**: *51–62]* (continued)

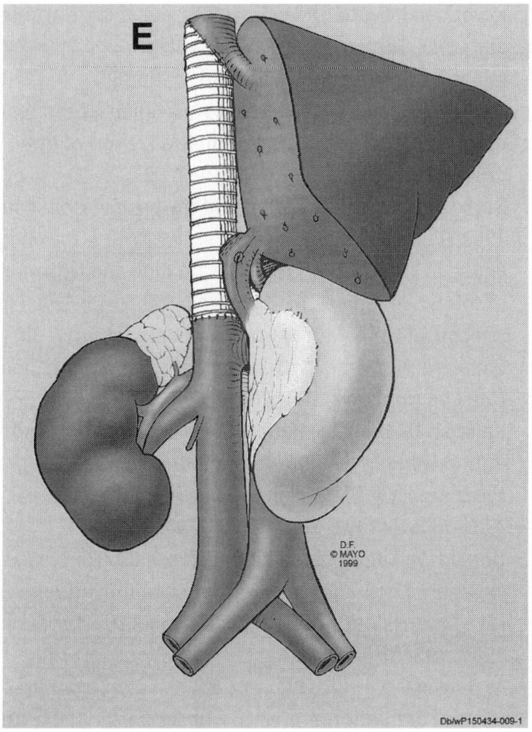

Figure 43.3 (continued) *Key steps in performance of retrohepatic inferior vena cava replacement and liver resection. (e) Completed graft reconstruction with reattachment of the ligaments of the liver to avoid torsion of the hepatic venous outflow.*

filter placement for patients with residual bland thrombus in the infrarenal IVC.[4,13,29]

The patency of short, large diameter prosthetic grafts used for caval replacement for either benign or malignant disease is good.[1,16,19,20,42] No graft occlusions occurred among three survivors with suprarenal IVC replacement in one report[19] and only three of 29 grafts occluded (10.7%) at a median follow-up of 2.9 years in the Mayo Clinic report.[20] The longest patent graft documented in the latter report was 6.3 years.[20]

The most important outcome measures are the impact of operation on survival, tumor recurrence, and quality of life of the patient. Survival of patients with primary IVC leiomyosarcomas reported by Mingoli *et al.*[26] averaged 3 months in patients not subjected to operation, 21 months in those with palliative resection, and 36.8 months in those treated with radical resection. Among 120 operated patients in their current registry,[34] neither the pattern of growth or tumor size, patency or the segment of the IVC involved by tumor, the use of adjuvant therapy, nor the extent of caval resection and replacement affected long-term survival or disease recurrence by multivariate analysis. However, almost 60% of patients who had radical tumor resection developed local or distant recurrent disease at a mean of 32 months postoperatively.[34]

Survival after operation in patients with secondary caval malignancies is difficult to determine because of the limited number of patients operated and the diverse etiology of the cancers.[16,18–20] The majority of operations performed in the Mayo Clinic series were for secondary tumors.[20] The 1-year patient survival was 89.3%, 2-year survival was 80.3%, and 3-year survival was 75%.[20] The mean survival was 3.14 years in the group with infrarenal IVC replacement, 2.88 years in the group who had the infrarenal and suprarenal segments replaced, and 2.26 years in the group with suprarenal caval replacement. The longest survivor in that series lived 6.33 years.[20] Local tumor control was good and most deaths occurred from regional or distant metastases. Although there was a trend toward improvement in survival in operated patients, the authors were unable to make any conclusions regarding the impact of these operations on survival for the reasons mentioned above.[20]

The greatest chance for survival is in patients with renal cell carcinoma and caval tumor thrombus who have no evidence of distant disease. Aggressive surgical treatment in this group has resulted in 5-year survival rates of 50% or more.[4,13,29] The primary determinants of survival for these patient are completeness of tumor resection and the presence of regional nodal or distant metastases.[4,5,8–10,13] Tumor thrombus, as an independent factor, probably does not affect long-term survival.[3,5,7,9,13]

Postoperative quality of life is an important but difficult issue to assess objectively and few clinical reports have addressed this. With careful patient selection, most patients who have an excellent performance status preoperatively tolerate the operation with minimal restriction in their physical activity postoperatively. In our initial review, almost 82% of operated patients had a good or excellent performance status and this trend has persisted.[18,20] Nonetheless, the beneficial role of aggressive tumor resection and caval replacement is still unknown and will require more experience with longer patient follow-up.

REFERENCES

1. Bower TC, Stanson AW. Diagnosis and management of tumors of the inferior vena cava. In Rutherford RB, ed. *Vascular Surgery*, 5th edn, vol 1. Orlando, FL: WB Saunders, 2000: 2077–92.
2. Clayman RV, Gonzalez R, Fraley EE. Renal cell cancer invading the inferior vena cava: clinical review and anatomic approach. *J Urol* 1980; **123**: 157–63.
3. Cherrie RJ, Goldman DG, Lindner A, *et al.* Prognostic implications of vena caval extension of renal cell carcinoma. *J Urol* 1982; **128**: 910–12.
4. Neves RJ, Zincke H. Surgical treatment of renal cancer with vena cava extension. *Br J Urol* 1987; **59**: 390–5.
5. Skinner DG, Pritchett TR, Lieskovsky G, *et al.* Vena caval involvement by renal cell carcinoma. *Ann Surg* 1989; **210**: 387–94.
6. Shahain DM, Libertino JA, Zinman LN, *et al.* Resection of cavoatrial renal cell carcinoma employing total circulatory arrest. *Arch Surg* 1990; **125**: 727–32.

7. Novick AC, Kaye MC, Cosgrove DM, *et al.* Experience with cardiopulmonary bypass and deep hypothermic circulatory arrest in the management of retroperitoneal tumors with large vena caval thrombi. *Ann Surg* 1990; **212**: 472–7.
8. Libertino JA, Burke WE, Zinman L. Long-term results of 71 patients with renal cell carcinoma with venous, vena caval, and atrial extension. *J Urol* 1990; **143**: 294A.
9. Hatcher PA, Anderson EE, Paulson DF, *et al.* Surgical management and prognosis of renal cell carcinoma invading the vena cava. *J Urol* 1991; **145**: 20–4.
10. Montie JE, El Ammar R, Pontes JE, *et al.* Renal cell carcinoma with inferior vena cava tumor thrombi. *Surg Gynecol Obstet* 1991; **173**: 107–15.
11. Stewart JA, Carey JA, McDougal WS, *et al.* Cavoatrial tumor thrombectomy using cardiopulmonary bypass without circulatory arrest. *Ann Thorac Surg* 1991; **51**: 717–22.
12. Suggs WD, Smith RB, Dodson TF, *et al.* Renal cell carcinoma with inferior vena caval involvement. *J Vasc Surg* 1991; **14**: 43–8.
13. Nesbitt JC, Soltero ER, Dinney CPN, *et al.* Surgical management of renal cell carcinoma with inferior vena cava tumor thrombus. *Ann Thorac Surg* 1997; **63**: 1592–600.
14. Kumada K, Shimahara Y, Fujui K, *et al.* Extended right hepatic lobectomy: combined resection of inferior vena cava and its reconstruction by ePTFE graft. *Acta Chir Scand* 1988; **154**: 481–3.
15. Iwatsuki S, Todo S, Starzl TE. Right trisegmentectomy with a synthetic vena cava graft. *Arch Surg* 1988: **123**: 1021–2.
16. Kieffer E, Bahnini A, Koskas F. Nonthrombotic disease of the inferior vena cava: surgical management of 24 patients. In Bergan JJ, Yao JST, eds. *Venous Disorders.* Philadelphia: WB Saunders, 1991: 501–16.
17. Dzsinich C, Gloviczki P, van Heerden JA, *et al.* Primary venous leiomyosarcoma: a rare but lethal disease. *J Vasc Surg* 1992; **15**: 595–603.
18. Bower TC, Nagorney DM, Toomey BJ, *et al.* Vena cava replacement for malignant disease: is there a role? *Ann Vasc Surg* 1993; **7**: 51–62.
19. Huguet C, Ferri M, Gavelli A. Resection of the suprarenal inferior vena cava: the role of prosthetic replacement. *Arch Surg* 1995; **130**: 793–7.
20. Bower TC, Nagorney DM, Cherry KJ, *et al.* Replacement of the inferior vena cava for malignancy: an update. *J Vasc Surg* 2000; **31**: 270–81.
21. Bower TC. Primary and secondary tumors of the inferior vena cava. In Gloviczki P, Yao JST, eds. *Handbook of Venous Disorders.* London: Chapman & Hall, 1996: 529–50.
22. Hartman DS, Hayes WS, Choyke PL, Tibbetts GP. Leiomyosarcoma of the retroperitoneum and inferior vena cava: radiologic–pathologic correlation. *Radiographics* 1992; **12**: 1203–20.
23. Concepcion RS, Koch MO, McDougal WS, *et al.* Management of primary nonrenal parenchymal malignancies with vena caval thrombus. *J Urol* 1991; **145**: 243–7.
24. Enzinger FM, Weiss SW. Soft tissue tumors. In Gay SM, ed. *Soft Tissue Tumors*, 3rd edn. St Louis, MO: Mosby Year Book, 1995: 505–10.
25. Kevorkian J, Cento DP. Leiomyosarcoma of large arteries and veins. *Surgery* 1973; **73**: 390–400.
26. Mingoli A, Feldhaus RG, Cavallaro A, Stipa S. Leiomyosarcoma of the inferior vena: analysis and search of world literature on 141 patients and report of three new cases. *J Vasc Surg* 1991; **14**: 688–99.
27. Burke AP, Virmani R. Sarcomas of the great vessels. *Cancer* 1993; **71**: 761–73.
28. Chang AE, Sondak VK. Clinical evaluation and treatment of soft tissue tumors. In Gay SM, ed. *Soft Tissue Tumors*, 3rd edn. St Louis, MO: Mosby Year Book, 1995: 17–38.
29. Couillard DR, White RWD. Surgery of renal cell carcinoma. *Urol Clin North Am* 1993; **20**: 263–75.
30. Kallman DA, King BF, Hattery RR, *et al.* Renal vein and inferior vena cava tumor thrombus in renal cell carcinoma: CT, US, MRI and venacavography. *J Comput Assist Tomogr* 1992; **16**: 240–7.
31. Donaldson MC, Wirthlen LS, Donaldson GA. Thirty-year experience with surgical interruption of the inferior vena cava for prevention of pulmonary embolism. *Ann Surg* 1980; **191**: 367–72.
32. Agrifoglio G, Edwards EA. Venous stasis after ligation of femoral or inferior vena cava. *J Am Med Assoc* 1961; **178**: 1–7.
33. Beck SDW, Lalka SG, Donohue JP. Long-term results after inferior vena caval resection during retroperitoneal lymphadenectomy for metastatic germ cell cancer. *J Vasc Surg* 1998; **28**: 808–14.
34. Mingoli A, Sapeinza P, Cavallaro A, *et al.* The effect of extent of caval resection in the treatment of inferior vena cava leiomyosarcoma. *Anticancer Res* 1997; **17**: 3877–82.
35. Stanson AW, Breen JF. Computed tomography and magnetic resonance imaging. In Gloviczki P, Yao JST, eds. *Handbook of Venous Disorders: Guidelines of the American Venous Forum.* London: Chapman & Hall, 1996: 529–50.
36. Zubrod CG, Schneiderman M, Frei E III, *et al.* Appraisal of methods for the study of chemotherapy of cancer in man: comparative therapeutic trial of nitrogen mustard and triethylene thiophosphoramide. *J Chron Dis* 1960; **11**: 7–33.
37. Duckett JW, Lifland JH, Peters PC. Resection of the inferior vena cava for adjacent malignant diseases. *Surg Gynecol Obstet* 1973; **136**: 711–16.
38. Perhoniemi V, Salmenkivi K, Vorne M. Venous haemodynamics in the legs after ligation of the inferior vena cava. *Acta Chir Scand* 1986; **152**: 23–7.
39. McCullough, DL, Gittes, RF. Ligation of the renal vein in the solitary kidney: effects on renal function. *J Urol* 1975; **113**: 295–8.
40. Huguet C, Gavelli A, Addario Chieco P, *et al.* Liver ischemia for hepatic resection: where is the limit? *Surgery* 1992; **111**: 251–9.
41. Swanson DA, Wallace S, Johnson DE. The role of embolization and nephrectomy in the treatment of metastatic renal carcinoma. *J Urol Surg* 1980; **7**: 719–30.
42. Gloviczki P, Pairolero PC, Toomey BJ, *et al.* Reconstruction of large veins for nonmalignant venous occlusive disease. *J Vasc Surg* 1992; **16**: 750–61.

44

Venous malformations and aneurysms: evaluation and treatment

ELIZABETH RACHEL AND WILLIAM H PEARCE

Congenital vascular malformations (CVM) are rare complex lesions of malformed vessels that occur as a result of maturational arrest during embryogenesis (weeks 4–10). CVMs may produce a variety of clinical manifestations ranging from port-wine stains to more complex lesions involving large, arteriovenous fistula. These large, high-flow malformations may produce skeletal abnormalities, hemodynamic changes with cardiac decompensation to disfiguring cutaneous lesions. Whilst these lesions are present at birth, they may not be discovered until early childhood or adolescence. When found, CVMs present a difficult diagnostic problem for the clinician. It is important to first understand the abnormal development of the circulatory system and how each part of the circulatory system may be involved in these lesions. From the clinician's point of view, the initial step is to describe the predominant abnormality, whether it is venous, arterial, lymphatic or a combination. Therefore, multiple imaging modalities are often required to define the anatomic distribution and the predominant component of the vascular malformation. Once defined, appropriate therapy for the CVM can be tailored to the patient's needs. Unfortunately, in many of the more complex lesions, both surgery and percutaneous interventions have a high recurrence rate and such lesions are best treated conservatively. This chapter deals with the embryology, diagnosis and management of the wide variety of congenital vascular malformations and venous aneurysms.

ETIOLOGY

Congenital vascular malformations develop as a result of the abnormal development of the vascular system. Embryologic development of the vascular system was described by Woollard as occurring in three stages:[1]

- The first stage consists of a syncytial network of undifferentiated capillary blood spaces (Fig. 44.1).
- During the second stage the retiform plexus develops as the capillary network becomes organized into central channels. Some of these channels will ultimately coalesce and differentiate further into named extremity vessels. Some primitive structures will normally regress.
- Finally, the development of the axial vessels in the limb bud occurs during the last maturational stage.

Remodeling of vessels is influenced by blood flow and pressure, mechanical tension, hormones and metabolic demands of the recipient tissues. High-flow areas develop thick-walled, large-caliber vessels and formation of capillaries occurs in areas with increased blood pressure. Conversely, in areas of reduced pressure, capillary density is decreased. Tension on vessels in the developing limb bud result in increased vessel length.

Developmental arrest can occur at any time during development and can give rise to specific disorders. Port-wine stain and cutaneous vascular nevi represent abnormalities at the earliest stage, the undifferentiated capillary syncytial network. Cavernous hemangiomas

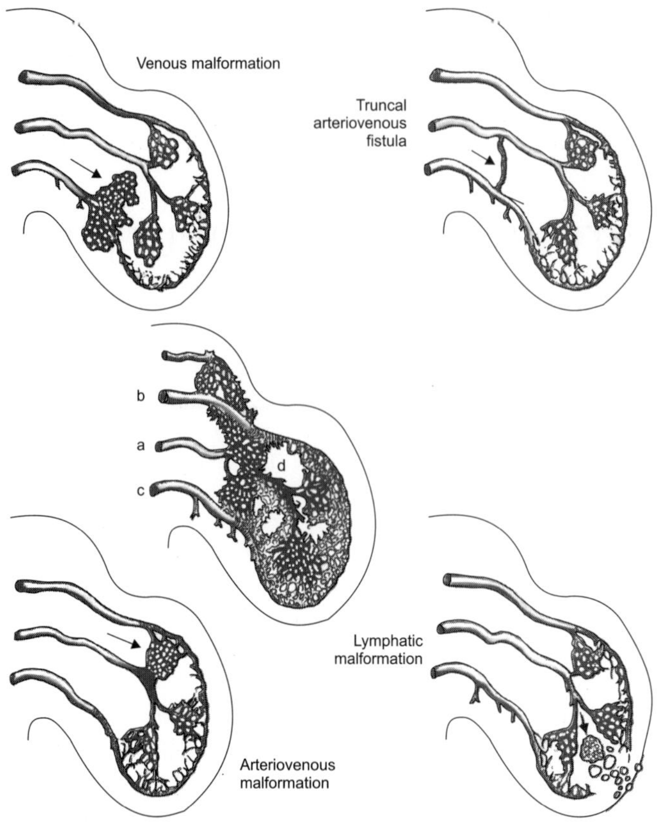

Figure 44.1 *Early development of blood vessels in the anterior appendage bud of a 12 mm long pig embryo. a, Persistent axial artery (retiform); b, cephalic vein; c, basilic vein; d, resorption of primitive capillary network. (Reproduced with permission from Mulliken JB, Young AE, eds.* Vascular Birthmarks: Hemangiomas and Malformations. *Philadelphia: WB Saunders, 1988)*

and venous lakes represent arrest at retiform stage as do many arteriovenous malformations with various degrees of shunting. Developmental abnormalities of the final stage of maturational results in absence or hypoplasia of mature arteries and veins and the persistence of immature, primitive elements.

Only recently has the biology of arteriovenous fistulas been studied extensively. Folkman found that cells derived from congenital hemangiomas displayed abnormal division and tube formation.[2] More recent studies suggest that such elemental cells continue to produce vascular derived endothelial growth factor (VEGF), which may be responsible for the remarkable neovascularity produced by these lesions.[3] Recently, several laboratories have identified specific genetic abnormalities in families with CVMs. Using linkage analysis Boon *et al.*[4,5] reported a specific mutation of chromosome 21 that acted in consort with TIE-2. It appeared that this gene was inherited as an autosomal dominant in five families. It was also linked to a new locus on 1p21-p22 called 'VMGLOM.'[6] Other venous malformations have been located to specific mutation, at position 849 in the kinase domain of receptor tyrosine kinase TIE-2. This mutation, which is also inherited as autosomal dominant, was discovered occurring in distinct families with CVMs. And finally, Bielenberg *et al.* studied cutaneous hemangiomas and found an imbalance in angiogenic factors in the dermis surrounding these neoplasms.[7] This, along with the observation by Wautier, suggests these lesions have an uncontrolled growth rate with autocrine cytokine input from angiogenic factors.[8] Anti-angiogenic treatment may be an option for aggressive hemangiomas and CVMs.

CLASSIFICATION

Historically, vascular malformations were identified by descriptive terms such as hemangioma simplex, cavernous hemangioma or port-wine stain. Various classification systems have been proposed based on anatomic, clinical and embryologic criteria and no real consensus exists regarding nomenclature. Several well-recognized syndromes are still routinely identified by their eponyms, such as Klippel–Trenaunay syndrome (KTS) and Parkes–Weber syndrome (PWS). Mulliken divided lesions based on biology as either hemangiomas or CVMs[9] (Table 44.1). Criteria suggested by Belov[10] in the Hamburg system in 1988 is anatomic and divides lesions into primarily arterial, venous and mixed arteriovenous lesions with or without lymphatic involvement. These are further subdivided into truncal versus extra-truncal lesions. Truncal lesions are identified by congenital absence, hypoplasia, or dilata-

Table 44.1 *Characteristics of vascular birthmarks**

	Hemangioma	Malformation
Clinical	Usually nothing seen at birth; 30% present as red macule	All present at birth; may not be evident
Clinical	Rapid postnatal proliferation and slow involution	Commensurate growth; may expand as a result of trauma, sepsis, hormonal modulation
Clinical	Female-to-male ratio 3:1	Female-to-male ratio 1:1
Cellular	Plump endothelium, increased turnover	Flat endothelium, slow turnover
Cellular	Increased mast cells	Normal mast cell count
Cellular	Multilaminated basement membrane	Normal thin basement membrane
Cellular	Capillary tubule formation *in vitro*	Poor endothelial growth *in vitro*
Hematologic	Primary platelet trapping: thrombocytopenia (Kasabach–Merritt syndrome)	Primary stasis (venous); localized consumptive coagulopathy
Radiologic	Angiographic findings: well circumscribed, intense lobular-parenchymal staining with equatorial vessels	Angiographic findings: diffuse, no parenchyma
Radiologic		Low flow: phleboliths, ectatic channels
Radiologic		High flow: enlarged, tortuous arteries with arteriovenous shunting
Skeletal	Infrequent 'mass effect' on adjacent bone; hypertrophy rare	Low flow: distortion, hypertrophy or hypoplasia
Skeletal		High flow: destruction, distortion or hypertrophy

Reproduced with permission from Mulliken JB. Classification of vascular birthmarks. In Mulliken JB, Young AE, eds. *Vascular Birthmarks: Hemangiomas and Malformations.* Philadelphia: WB Saunders Company, 1988: 35.

tion of differentiated vascular trunks. Truncal defects are more localized than diffuse lesions and often are hemodynamically significant. They frequently involve the upper extremity. KTS is an example of a truncal defect where there is congenital absence or hypoplasia of the deep venous system of the lower extremity in association with a cutaneous vascular stain (capillary malformation) and limb hypertrophy. Alternative venous drainage of the extremity is maintained through compensatory hypertrophy of the superficial system and persistence of the primitive lateral leg vein. Extra-truncal forms are subdivided into limited versus infiltrating lesions and include those defects resulting from persistent immature fetal venous lakes. These lesions may be limited and discrete and of little clinical consequence, especially with microfistulous connections. More typically they are diffuse with infiltration into multiple tissue planes including skin, muscle, bone and soft tissue and may involve the lymphatic system. Extensive lesions, especially with macrofistulous connections, can lead to limb length discrepancy and hypertrophy, massive edema, vascular steal and even hyperdynamic high-output cardiac failure. The latter is more common in infants with diffuse, infiltrating visceral lesions.

Mulliken suggested that vascular malformations be categorized according to flow characteristics, either high flow or low flow, with further subdivision into anatomic subgroups designated by the predominant element, i.e. arterial, venous, capillary or lymphatic.[11] In this scheme, venous, lymphatic and capillary malformations are all low-flow lesions. Pure arterial malformations, including aneurysms and ectasia, arteriovenous malformations and arteriovenous fistulae are considered high-flow lesions. The predominant element is identified first by an A, then a V, C, or L for arterial, venous, capillary and lymphatic malformations, respectively. This is followed with M for malformation. An arteriovenous malformation is a high-flow lesion identified as an AVM and a pure venous malformation is a low-flow lesion identified simply as a VM. Complex and mixed malformations such as Klippel–Trenaunay syndrome and Parkes–Weber syndrome are characterized as regional defects. KTS has capillary, lymphatic and venous anomalies and is designated as CLVM. Parkes–Weber is similar to KTS with capillary, lymphatic and venous malformations, but in addition has associated high-flow arteriovenous fistulae, AVF. Syndromes with extravascular systemic abnormalities, such as Maffucci's syndrome (lymphovenous malformations, LVM, venous ectasia and deep system anomalies in association with endochondromas) are categorized as diffuse malformations. This rare disorder, which usually presents in adolescence with clusters of venous malformations of the extremities, has a 50% malignant transformation rate to sarcoma.

Primary venous aneurysms are very rare and few case reports exist in the literature. Historically they were called cavernous malformations. They generally are not associated with shunting and symptoms are due to venous distension, reflux, ulceration and thrombosis, especially of the lower extremities. Venous aneurysms have been reported in the jugular system, the vena cava, the axillary-subclavian veins, the common femoral vein, the popliteal vein and the saphenous systems. The superior vena cava and popliteal veins are most common. Like other vascular malformations, there does not appear to be a gender bias.

The etiology of pure venous aneurysms is unclear (Fig. 44.2). They may be secondary to congenital defects, degenerative or inflammatory changes and perhaps to

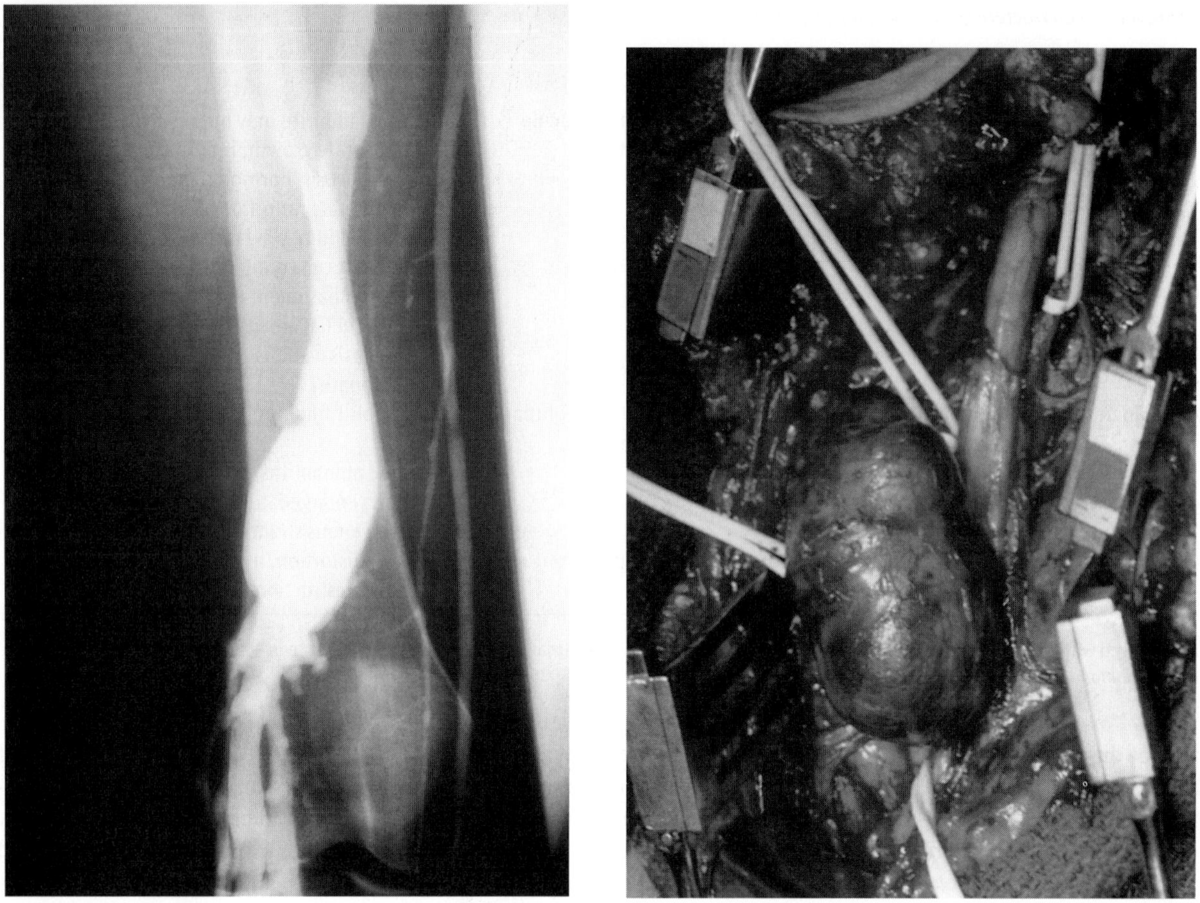

(a) (b)

Figure 44.2 *A 19-year-old boy presented with a compressible mass behind the right knee. (a) Ascending venography demonstrated a popliteal venous aneurysm. (b) Intraoperative photograph demonstrating the popliteal aneurysm and the closely adherent sciatic nerve.*

chronic local trauma from adjacent arteries. The histologic characteristics of the vessel wall differ depending on the site of the venous aneurysm, etiology and perhaps with the age of the lesion. There is thinning of the wall and smooth muscle cell attenuation in some lesions and fibrous tissue deposition in others.[12,13]

It is important to differentiate true congenital vascular malformations from hemangiomas, as the clinical course and long-term consequences are distinctly different (Table 44.1). Congenital vascular malformations are present at birth, exhibit normal endothelial cell structure, function and turnover. They grow proportionately with the child and do not regress over time. Hemangiomas, commonly called 'strawberry marks' are the most common benign tumor of infancy. They are well-circumscribed lesions and are not usually present at birth. Hemangiomas generally manifest during the first several weeks of life, grow rapidly, with disproportionate growth relative to the child, then slowly involute over a period of years.[9] Although highly vascular during the early proliferative phase, hemangiomas are not considered true vascular malformations. More than half these lesions are present on the head and neck, and approximately 20–25% are located on the extremities. Hemangiomas are more common in female infants. They are usually isolated lesions, but can have visceral, i.e. hepatic, cardiac and pulmonary, involvement. Observation, patience, watchful waiting and serial photography to document lesion regression are warranted along with parental education and reassurance. Most patients will have entered the involution phase by the second half of their first year of life with the great majority having complete resolution by school age.[11] Craniofacial hemangiomas, especially lesions involving periorbital tissues and oropharyngeal lesions, deserve special consideration and a more aggressive approach is taken with these lesions. Untreated eyelid lesions can result in permanent refractive errors, strabismus and the failure to develop normal binocular vision. Oropharyngeal lesions can result in an abnormal suck response, neonatal feeding problems and even airway obstruction. Steroids and laser therapy are potentially useful during the proliferative phase for patients with complicated hemangiomas. Systemic steroids should be dosed at 2–3 mg/kg/day and then weaned over a period of 4–6 weeks.[9] Systemic steroid therapy in the neonate should be approached with caution and if no clinical improvement is noted after the first 7–10 days steroid therapy should be stopped. Limited surgical excision remains an option.

Patients with hemangioma and visceral involvement have a high mortality secondary to congestive heart failure and should be treated with systemic steroids; regression should be followed with serial CT scan. Cutaneous and mucosal hemangiomas may ulcerate and bleed during the proliferative phase.

These complications may require surgical excision if they fail local wound care. Patients with hemangioma can develop thrombocytopenia and coagulopathy due to platelet trapping, known as Kasabach–Merritt syndrome.[9] These patients develop petechiae, persistent bleeding or a tense, rapidly enlarging hemangioma due to an intralesional bleed. Supportive care is indicated with transfusion of packed cells as necessary and occasionally systemic steroids. Platelet transfusion is generally not helpful due to continued sequestration. Embolization with gel, coils, methacrylate glues, polyvinyl alcohol and detachable balloons has been used alone and in combination with surgical excision for complicated lesions. Plasmapheresis and chemotherapeutic agents have also been used for life-threatening complications.

PHYSIOLOGY

Evaluation and treatment of CVM depends on accurate and full understanding of the anatomic and hemodynamic consequences (Fig. 44.3). Total body blood volume, heart rate and stroke volumes are increased in patients with CVM with compensatory cardiac hypertrophy. There is increased flow through the lesion itself

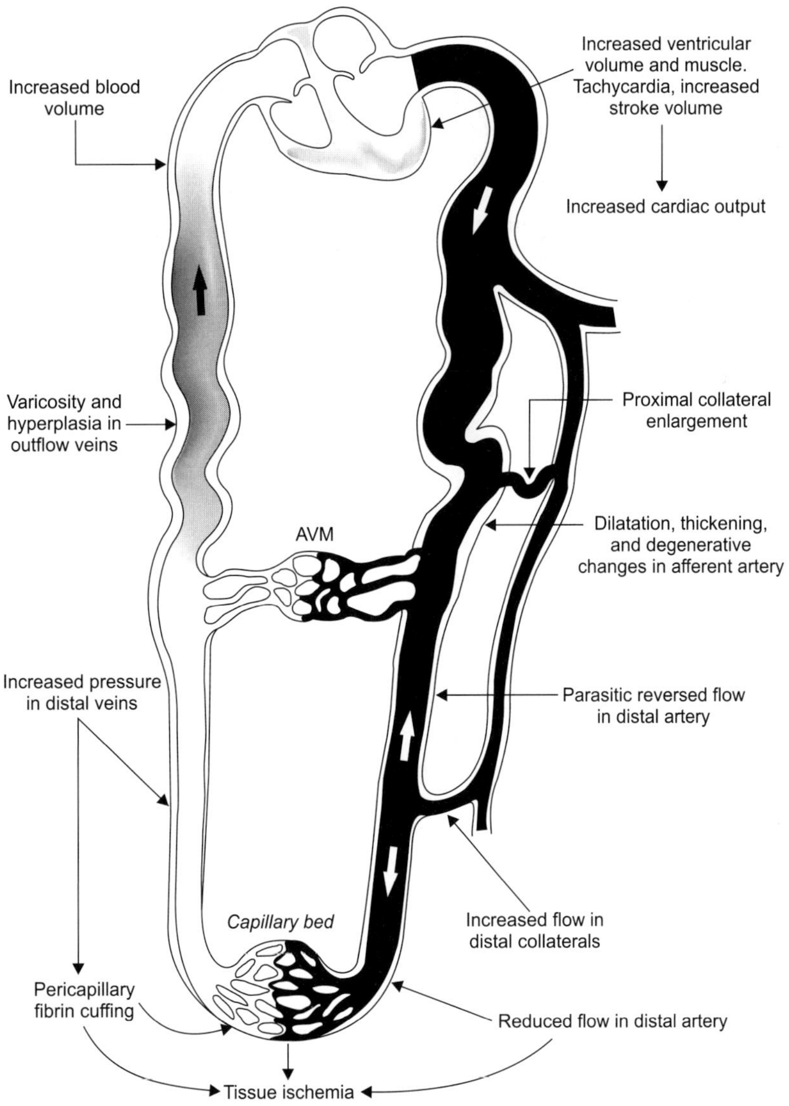

Figure 44.3 *Hemodynamic response to abnormal arteriovenous communication. (Reproduced with permission from Mulliken JB, Young AE, eds.* Vascular Birthmarks: Hemangiomas and Malformations. *Philadelphia: WB Saunders, 1988: 234)*

secondary to decreased peripheral resistance with increased venous return. Feeding arteries proximal to the malformation dilate and hypertrophy, including collaterals. Histologically, the dilated arteries have disrupted elastic lamina and loss of medial smooth muscle. Arteries distal to AVF exhibit reversed flow and the distal capillary bed may be ischemic as flow is preferentially shunted through the low-resistance malformation. Draining veins dilate, thicken and are arterialized under pressure in patients with AVF. Varicose veins and venous hypertension can develop with eventual chronic stasis changes.

Compression of the feeding artery and AVF itself results in reflex bradycardia and a decrease in the cardiac output, known as the Nicoladoni–Branham sign.

Total blood flow through the lesion can be estimated using Doppler-derived data. Shunting can also be evaluated by measuring the oxygen saturation of the draining veins. More accurate quantitative evaluation of flow through the malformation uses radiolabeled microspheres to evaluate the shunt fraction. Labeled microspheres of known dimension are injected intra-arterially proximal to a CVM. Spheres are trapped in normal capillary beds but traverse dilated abnormal arteriovenous connections, and are trapped in the pulmonary vascular bed. A lung scan follows. The ratio of trapped signal to total dose given provides an estimate of the shunt fraction.

CLINICAL PRESENTATION

Clinical presentation of congenital vascular malformations depends largely on the dominant feature, i.e. venous, arterial, capillary or lymphatic, location of the lesion, and duration of symptoms. Some lesions remain quiescent for many years, presenting only after some minor trauma, with pregnancy or with the onset of menses. It seems likely that antecedent trauma can disturb a previously stable collateral system and unmask a CVM. The relationship to hormones remains unclear. The reported incidence is less than 2% of the population and, unlike hemangiomas, there is no gender predilection for CVM.[14] The most common lesions, approximately half, are venous in origin and nearly two-thirds affect the extremities.[15] Pure arterial defects are rare, accounting for less than 1.0% of all malformations. Mixed lesions with arterial and venous defects are not uncommon, affecting 15–30% of individuals.

Patients most often seek medical attention for a cosmetic deformity such as cutaneous vascular stain, palpable mass, limb edema, varicosities, thrombophlebitis or other complications of venous hypertension (Table 44.2). When palpable, the mass is firm, may be pulsatile and usually incompressible. A continuous mechanical bruit may be audible over arteriovenous fistulae and a thrill may be palpable. An involved limb may be warmer than the uninvolved limb and patients complain of increased girth and heaviness from increased venous volume. Young adolescents may develop scoliosis and limb length discrepancies. The finding of lateral leg varicosities, vascular stains, unilateral limb hypertrophy or other venous abnormalities in a young person should alert the examiner to the possibility of an underlying CVM. Patients with extremity lesions and significant shunting of blood from the distal arterial bed can present with ischemic rest pain or ulceration. Pelvic malformations are complex and can produce rectal pain, sexual dysfunction, massive uterine bleeding and ureteral outlet obstruction with hydronephrosis. Central, high-flow lesions in the pelvis and abdomen can produce high-output cardiac failure. Although physical examination alone is often sufficient to make a diagnosis of a vascular malformation, it often will not define the extent of the lesion and further evaluation is indicated prior to any planned intervention.

Table 44.2 *Incidence of physical changes in 82 affected extremities**

Changes	No.	%
Color changes	57	69.5
Erythema	(33)	
Cyanosis	(24)	
Venous varices	49	59.7
Edema	46	56.0
Increased length	20	24.3
Deformity	9	11.0
Ulceration	8	9.8
Pulse deficit	3	3.6
Bleeding	3	3.6

*Reproduced with permission from Szilagyi DE, Smith RF, Elliott JP, Hageman JH. Congenital arteriovenous anomalies of the limbs. *Arch Surg* 1976; **111**: 423–9.

Presentation of pure venous aneurysms depends mostly on location. Jugular and superficial venous aneurysms present usually as soft, compressible, nonpulsatile masses that distend with Valsalva. There is no thrill. Vena caval aneurysms are usually asymptomatic and are found on chest x-ray or CT scan performed for some other reason. Popliteal venous aneurysms are associated with thrombosis and pulmonary embolus. This diagnosis should be considered in patients with recurrent pulmonary emboli in the absence of other risk factors. Rupture of venous aneurysms is rare.

DIAGNOSIS AND EVALUATION

Plain radiographs, computed tomography (CT), angiography, venography, duplex ultrasonography and

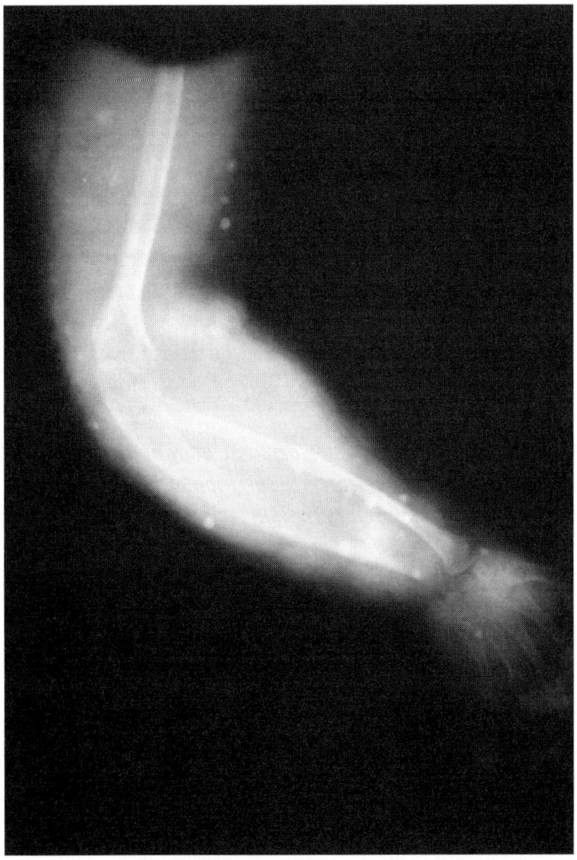

(a)

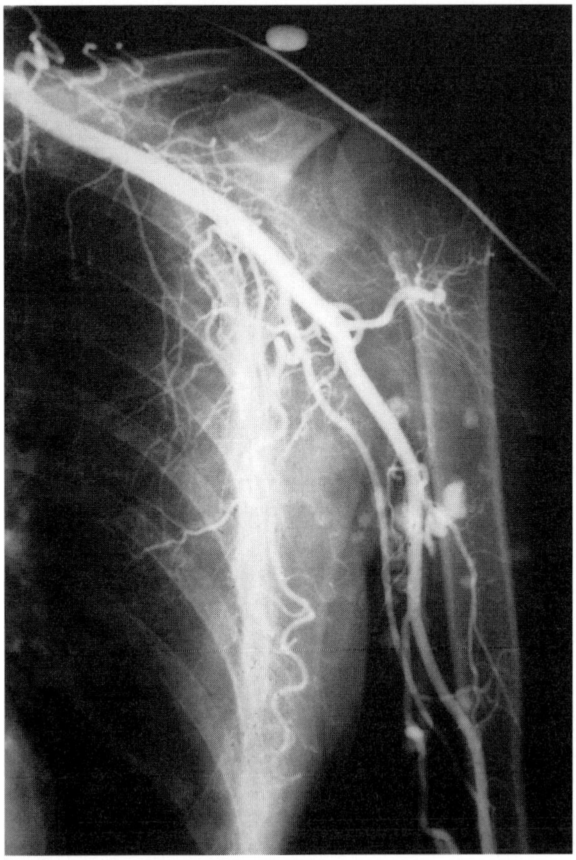

(b)

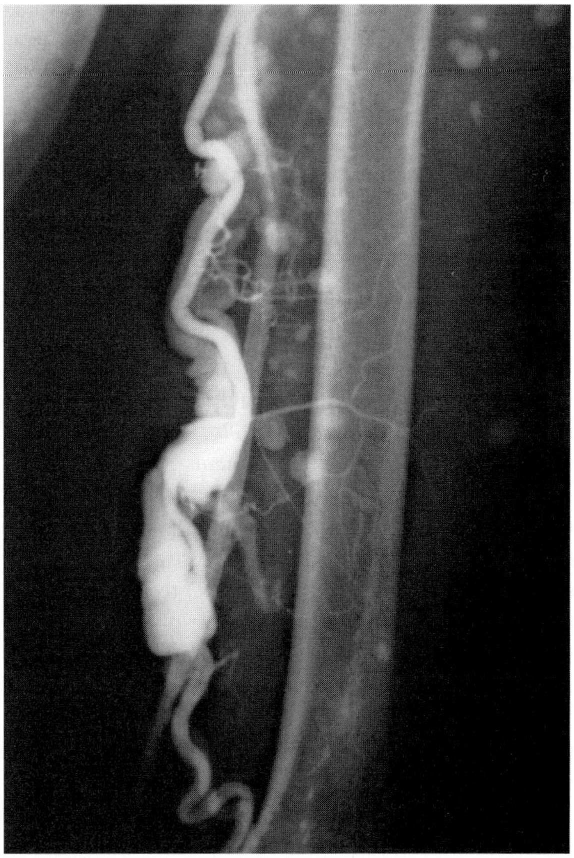

(c)

Figure 44.4 *A 19-year-old female presenting with swollen left arm with extensive bluish cutaneous lesions and loud bruit. (a) Plain radiograph demonstrating numerous calcified phleboliths. (b) Arteriogram of the left arm demonstrating normal axillary subclavian arteries. (c) Extensive tortuosity aneurysm formation of both artery and vein demonstrating a high-flow fistula.*

magnetic resonance imaging (MRI) are techniques currently used in evaluation of vascular malformations. Plain films can demonstrate soft tissue and bony hypertrophy, limb length discrepancy and phleboliths (Fig. 44.4). Contrast-enhanced computed tomography can identify the location of the CVM, bony involvement, vessel ectasia and aneurysm formation. True extent of the lesion into soft tissue, however, is underestimated as only contrast-enhanced vessels opacify. Selective arteriography identifies multiple anomalous feeding arteries and early filling of draining veins. Although essential prior to any intervention, it too, underestimates the true extent of these lesions. Ill-advised early surgical treatment including isolated ligation of major feeding vessels is not curative and prevents further endovascular therapy. Recruitment of nondominant collaterals re-establishes flow to the nidus of the lesion and recurrence. Also, direct puncture phlebography may be necessary to fully demonstrate venous anomalies including venous lakes, ectasia and venous aneurysm. Superselective arteriography is useful as both a diagnostic and therapeutic method, and can be used in combination with surgical resection.

Duplex ultrasonography is a portable, noninvasive imaging technique that provides both functional and anatomic data in the evaluation of CVM.[16] Continuous-wave Doppler of the proximal arteries demonstrates increased flow velocity above baseline and absence of the reversed diastolic flow component consistent with a low resistance circuit. Distal to the fistula, arterial flow is reversed and digital pressures may be decreased. Interrogation of the venous outflow demonstrates increased flow velocity and turbulence. Venous outflow may be continuous or pulsatile. Segmental arterial studies are useful to evaluate ischemia distal to a CVM with significant shunting. The systolic occlusion pressure is reduced distal to the fistula and increases with compression of the lesion and restoration of antegrade arterial flow distally.[16] Pulse-volume recording amplitudes are increased over CVM reflecting increased flow volume through that segment. PVRs may be reduced distal to a CVM with significant shunting.

MRI is the diagnostic imaging modality of choice in patients with vascular malformations.[17] It allows imaging in both axial and sagittal planes and more importantly can identify extension into soft tissue and bone (Figs 44.5, 44.6). Using routine spin-echo technique, vascular channels appear as black holes or flow voids. Exposure of tissue to a static magnetic field causes proton alignment in the direction of the field. In high-flow lesions that signal is lost as the blood leaves the imaging slice and the flow void appears black. Time of flight MRI uses pulsed waves to suppress soft tissue signals and allows flow-related enhancement of vessels supplying and draining the lesion.

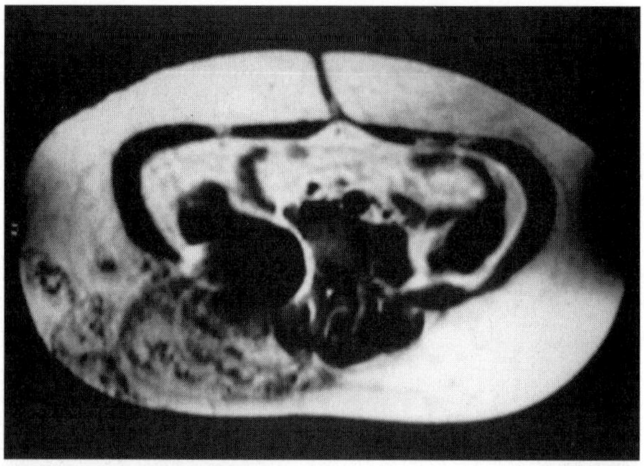

Figure 44.6 *Left flank lesion demonstrating numerous flow voids. Note the involvement of the peri-spinal muscles and anatomic detail provided by the MRI.*

MANAGEMENT

Vascular malformations often involve more tissue than is clinically apparent. Intervention depends on the type of lesion, location, extent and patient symptoms (Fig. 44.7). Minimally symptomatic patients and patients with asymptomatic lesions should be fully evaluated to ensure an accurate diagnosis and reassurance that vascular malformations are not neoplastic. Venous anomalies should be treated conservatively with external support where appropriate (Fig. 44.8). Jugular aneurysms are usually benign, but large lesions may be ligated without a problem for cosmetic reasons. Caval malformations present special problems for aortic surgery, in terms of

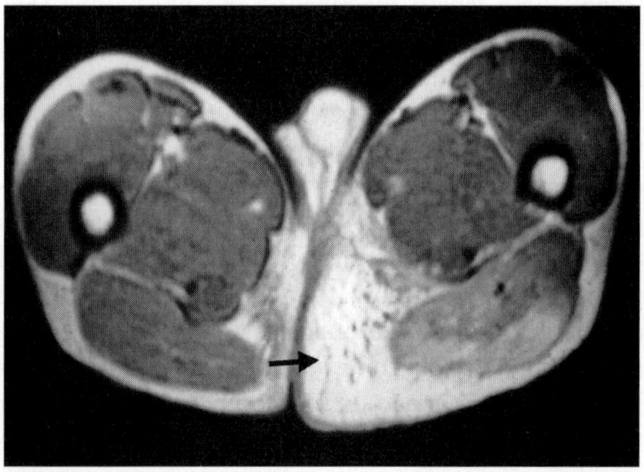

Figure 44.5 *Cross-sectional MRI demonstrating enhancing lesion in the medial aspect of the left thigh. Note multiple flow voids (arrow).*

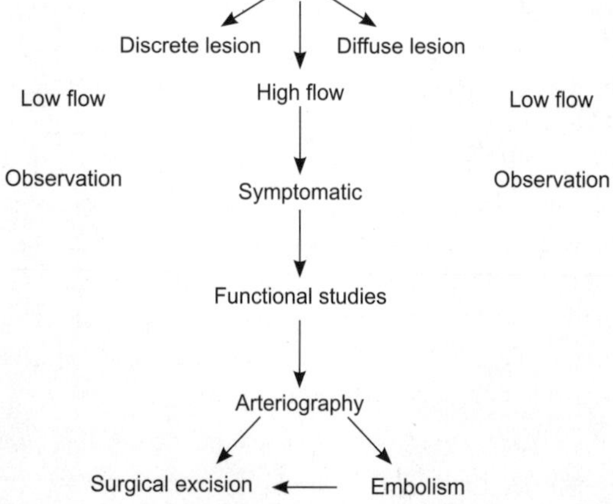

Figure 44.7 *Algorithm for diagnostic evaluation of patients with peripheral congenital vascular malformation. (Reproduced with permission from Pearce WH, Rutherford RB, Whitehill TA, Davis K. Nuclear magnetic resonance imaging: its diagnostic value in patients with congenital vascular malformations of the limbs.* J Vasc Surg *1988;* **8***: 64–70)*

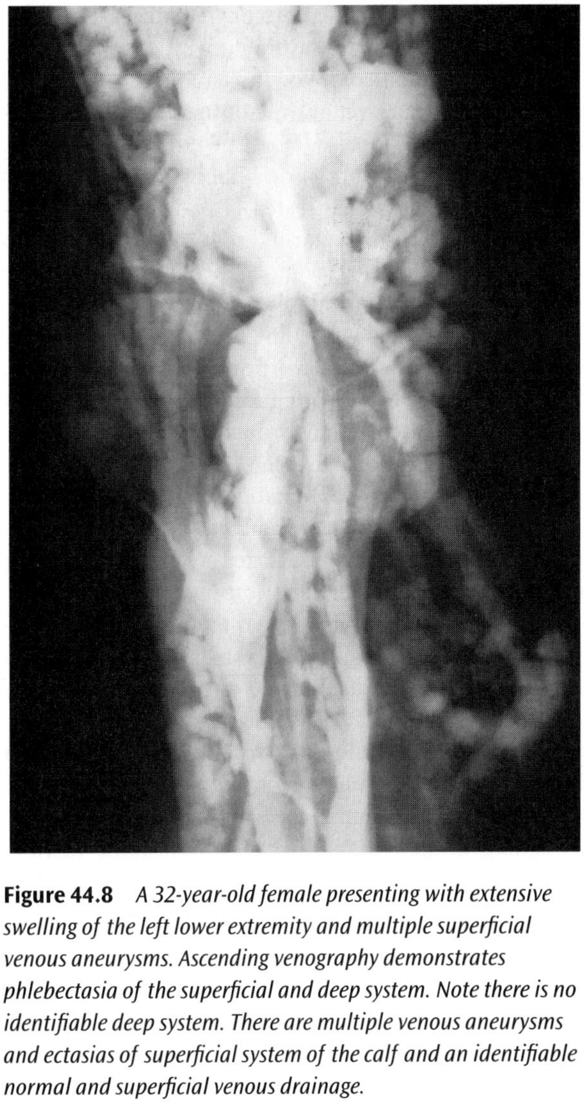

Figure 44.8 *A 32-year-old female presenting with extensive swelling of the left lower extremity and multiple superficial venous aneurysms. Ascending venography demonstrates phlebectasia of the superficial and deep system. Note there is no identifiable deep system. There are multiple venous aneurysms and ectasias of superficial system of the calf and an identifiable normal and superficial venous drainage.*

access, but caval aneurysms do not need specific treatment once diagnosis is confirmed. Saccular aneurysms of the vena cava may be ligated at the base and excised.[18] It is particularly important that patients with venous malformations have accurate assessment of their deep system. Surgical resection of dilated superficial varicosities in a patient with an absent or hypoplastic deep venous system is disastrous. The remaining venous collateral system is not adequate to drain the limb and massive lower-extremity swelling and ulceration develop. Patients undergoing surgery for popliteal venous aneurysm are at high risk for perioperative and postoperative deep venous thrombosis and consideration should be give to short-term anticoagulation.[18,19] Patients with venous malformations should be placed in compressive stockings and sleeves early on to offset long-term complications of venous stasis.

Evaluation with a plan toward intervention, in patients with vascular malformations, is best done by a multidisciplinary team including vascular surgeons, interventional radiologists, plastic and orthopedic surgeons. Patients, their families and the entire team must be committed to long-term treatment, multiple re-interventions and control of the lesion rather than cure in the majority of cases. Indications for treatment of vascular malformations using interventional techniques and/or surgical excision include congestive heart failure, ischemia, bleeding and ulceration. Functional impairment and severe cosmetic deformity are also considerations. Treatment options include multiple, staged transcatheter embolizations, surgical excision. Although arterial embolization can decrease symptoms from inflow, the venous changes, i.e. dilatation, varicosities, insufficiency and thrombosis, do not respond. The vast majority of patients require lifelong compressive therapy.

Definitive cure is possible in patients with limited, superficial lesions that are amenable to complete surgical excision. In reviewing the literature, only 20–30% of patients with vascular malformations are candidates for complete excision.[20] No single author has a significant surgical experience. The largest surgical series were published in 1976, 1983, 1990 and 1992 comprising fewer than 100 patients.[20–22] Szilagyi reported on 18 patients with vascular malformations treated surgically. Fifty-five percent of patients reported improvement in their symptoms following excision, 11% were unchanged and fully a third were worse after surgery than before.[21] In 1992, Pearce reported the Northwestern experience in 15 patients with vascular malformations treated surgically.[20] Five patients were lost to follow-up. Assuming those patients did well and did not seek further intervention, two-thirds of those undergoing excision improved. Thirteen percent were unchanged and 20% were worse after surgical excision. Ford reported that more than 85% patients were improved following embolic therapy for vascular malformation, although not cured, and that surgical excision was associated with a 50% complication rate.[23]

If complete excision of the malformation is not possible, some authors suggest isolation of the lesion as an alternative. Skeletonization of lesions by ligation of all vessels feeding and draining the lesion is conceptually appealing, but more difficult in practice. Even minor collateral inflow can compensate over time and result in recurrence. Proximal ligation or embolization of major feeding vessels results in temporary improvement of symptoms. Recurrence of the lesion occurs as collaterals restore inflow to the vascular mass. Occlusion of the main feeding trunk surgically or through endovascular means precludes further interventional approaches and should be avoided.

By contrast, superselective catheterization and embolization of secondary feeders and the nidus of the lesion are appropriate therapy either alone or in combination with surgical excision to decrease operative blood loss (Fig. 44.9). Materials used for embolic therapy should be permanent and include stainless steel coils,

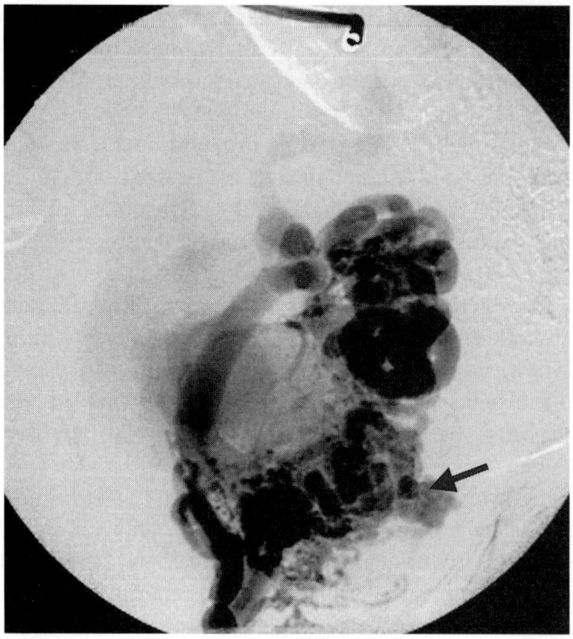

(a)

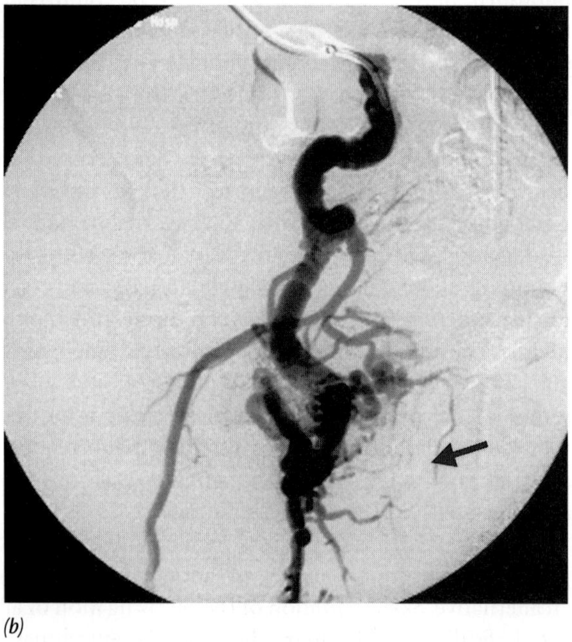

(b)

Figure 44.9 *A 42-year-old woman with right internal iliac arteriovenous malformation with pre- (a) and post- (b) alcohol embolization of a large superior feeder. A small venous AVM is seen inferiorly following embolization (arrow).*

alcohol foam (Ivalon), detachable balloons and cyanoacrylate glues that polymerize at body temperature.[24] Synthetic adhesives delivered at the nidus of the lesion forms a cast of the malformation and decreases recurrence. Temporary agents such as gel foam are not used because recanalization of embolized vessels results in recurrence. These are complicated, long procedures requiring multiple injections that can be painful and general anesthesia is appropriate.

The results of embolization for treatment of vascular malformations compare favorably with surgical series. Yakes *et al.* obtained follow-up studies in 19 of 20 patients with arteriovenous malformations treated with ethanol embolization.[25] All patients showed persistent occlusion of the malformation radiographically at up to 24 months. Widlus *et al.* treated 11 patients with cyanoacrylate embolization. During a 40-month follow-up period, 82% reported complete resolution of their symptoms and the remaining patients improvement.[26] No patients reported worsening of their symptoms with superselective embolization in these two series. Rosen, Riles and Berenstein reported follow-up on 108 of 120 patients with vascular malformations treated by interventional means.[15] Fifty-five percent were asymptomatic at 3 years, 21% were symptomatic, but improved. Twenty percent had had no significant change in symptoms post-procedure and 4% reported worsening of their symptoms following embolization.

Complications of endovascular therapies occur in less than 6% of patients with vascular malformations.[24] They include swelling, ischemia and distal tissue necrosis, contrast nephrotoxicity, allergic reactions, and rarely, inadvertent embolization of particulate matter through large fistulae and subsequent pulmonary emboli or stroke. Distal ischemia can range from superficial sloughing of skin to compartment syndrome to limb ischemia requiring amputation. Nevertheless, Ford and others from the Los Angeles Children's Hospital concluded that superselective angiography and embolization should be primary therapy for symptomatic peripheral arteriovenous malformations in children, reserving surgery for complicated residual disease.[23] When embolization is used as an adjunct to surgical excision, it should be performed as close to the time of surgery as possible to decrease the time available for collateral recruitment.

COMMENT

Arteriovenous malformations are a difficult clinical problem. The lesions that are present at birth are often not found until early childhood or adolescence. Multiple imaging modalities are often required to identify the predominant component of the malformation (arteriovenous, lymphatic, or capillary). Once the predominant component is identified, treatment is considered based on the patient's symptoms. In general, most extremity arteriovenous malformations are best treated with observation. With limb growth abnormalities, congestive heart failure, bleeding or other complications, intervention may be required. Destruction of the nidus in arteriovenous malformations is essential for cure. Absolute alcohol appears to be the treatment of choice for obliterating the nidus. For more superficial venous malformations, surgery or sclerotherapy has been successful. For venous aneurysms, treatment is usually not necessary except for instances of repeat embolization or for cosmetic reasons. Reconstruction of deep veins is essential to prevent chronic edema.

REFERENCES

1. Woollard HH. The development of the principle arterial stems in the forelimb of the pig. *Cont Embryol* 1922; **14**: 139.
2. Mulliken JB, Zetter BR, Folkman J. In vitro characteristics of endothelium from hemangiomas and vascular malformations. *Surgery* 1982; **92**: 348.
3. Chang J, Most D, Bresnick S, Reinisch J, Longaker MT, Turk AE. Gene expression of basic fibroblast growth factor and vascular endothelial growth factor is upregulated in proliferating hemangiomas: a possible mechanism of angiogenesis. *Surg Forum* 1997; **48**: 686-8.
4. Boon LM, Brouillard P, Irrthum A, *et al.* A gene for inherited cutaneous venous anomalies (glomangiomas) localizes to chromosome 1. *Am J Human Genet* 1999; **6**(1): 125–33.
5. Vikkula M. Boon LM, Carraway KL, *et al.* Vascular dysmorphogenesis caused by an activating mutation in the receptor tyrosine kinase TIE2. *Cell* 1996; **87**(7): 1181–90.
6. Boon LM, Brouillard P, Irrthum A, *et al.* A gene for inherited cutaneous venous anomalies ('glomangiomas') localizes to chromosome 1p21-22. *Am J Human Genet* 1999; **65**(1): 125–33.
7. Bielenberg DR, Bucana CD, Sanchez R, Mulliken JB, Folkman J, Fidler IJ. Progressive growth of infantile cutaneous hemangiomas is directly correlated with hyperplasia and angiogenesis of adjacent epidermis and inversely correlated with expression of the endogenous angiogenesis inhibitor, IFN-beta. *Int J Oncol* 1999; **14**(3): 401–8.
8. Wautier MP, Boval B, Chappey O, *et al.* Cultured endothelial cells from human arteriovenous malformations have defective growth regulation. *Blood* 1999; **94**(6): 2020–8.
9. Mulliken JB, Young AE, eds. *Vascular Birthmarks: Hemangiomas and Malformations.* Philadelphia: WB Saunders, 1988.
10. Belov S. Classification of congenital vascular defects. *Int Angiol* 1990; **9**(3): 141–6.
11. Mulliken JB, Glowacki GA. Hemangiomas and vascular malformations in infants and children: a classification based on endothelial characteristics. *Plast Reconstr Surg* 1982; **69**: 412–20.
12. Winchester D, Pearce WH, McCarthy WJ, McGee GS, Yao JST. Popliteal venous aneurysms. *Surgery* 1993; **114**: 600–7.
13. Gillespie DL, Villavicencio JL, Gallagher C, *et al.* Presentation and management of venous aneurysms. *J Vasc Surg* 1997; **26**(5): 845–52.
14. Tasnadi G. Epidemiology and etiology of congenital vascular malformations. *Semin Vasc Surg* 1993; **6**(4): 200–3.
15. Rosen RJ, Riles TS, Berenstein A. Congenital vascular malformations. In Rutherford RB, ed. *Vascular Surgery*, 4th edn. Philadelphia: WB Saunders, 1995: 1218–32.
16. Rutherford RB. Noninvasive testing in the diagnosis and assessment of arteriovenous fistula. In Berenstein EF, ed. *Noninvasive Diagnostic Techniques in Vascular Disease.* St Louis, MO: CV Mosby, 1985: 666–79.
17. Pearce WH, Rutherford RB, Whitehall TA, *et al.* Nuclear magnetic resonance imaging: its diagnostic value in patients with congenital vascular malformations. *J Vasc Surg* 1988; **8**: 64–70.
18. Freidman SG, Krishnasastry KV, Doscher W, Deckoff SL. Primary venous aneurysms. *Surgery* 1990; **108**(1): 92–5.
19. Ross GJ, Violi L, Barber LW, Vujic I. Popliteal venous aneurysm. *Radiology* 1988; **168**(3): 721–2.
20. Scott EE, Pearce WH, McCarthy WJ, Flinn WR, Yao JST. Arteriovenous malformation: long-term follow-up. In Yao JST, Pearce WH, eds. *Long-term Results in Vascular Surgery.* Norwalk, CT: Appleton & Lange, 1993: 401–10.
21. Szilagyi DE, Smith RF, Elliot JP, *et al.* Congenital arteriovenous anomalies of the limbs. *Arch Surg* 1976; **111**: 423–9.
22. Flye WW, Jordan BP, Schwartz MZ. Management of congenital arteriovenous malformations. *Surgery* 1983; **94**(5): 740–7.
23. Ford EG, Stanley P, Tolo V, *et al.* Peripheral arteriovenous fistulae: observe, operate obturate? *J Pediatr Surg* 1992; **27**(6): 714.
24. Rosen RJ. Embolization in the treatment of arteriovenous malformations. In Goldberg HI, Higgins CB, Ring EJ, eds. *Contemporary Imaging.* San Francisco, CA: University of California Press, 1985: 153.
25. Yakes WF, Luethke JM, Parker SH, *et al.* Ethanol embolizations of vascular malformations. *Radiographics* 1990; **10**(5): 787–96.
26. Widlus DM, Murray RR, White RI, *et al.* Congenital arteriovenous malformations: tailored embolotherapy. *Radiology* 1988; **2**: 511–16.

PART **6**

Lymphedema

45

Lymphedema: pathophysiology, classification and clinical evaluation

JOHN J BERGAN

Lymphedema is frustrating to physician and patient alike. This is true because it is incurable and, despite intensive investigations, its cause is poorly understood.

Lymphedema is the accumulation of tissue fluid in interstitial spaces, principally in subcutaneous tissues (Fig. 45.1). This fluid sequestration is caused by a variety of defects in lymphatic transport. Lymphedema is the result of a functional overload of the lymphatic system in which lymph volume exceeds transport.[1]

The prime function of the lymphatic system is to clear the interstitial spaces of excess water, large molecules and particulate matter. These are transported from the tissues back into the intravascular circulation by way of the venous system. A large proportion of plasma proteins pass through the capillary wall daily and not all of these return directly to the circulation. The lymphatic system absorbs those protein molecules that fail to return to the circulation by way of veins. As much as a third of the proteins escaping from the blood are cleared by the lymphatics. Failure of any part of the lymphatic system will result in accumulation of plasma proteins in interstitial fluid. This increases interstitial fluid colloid osmotic pressure and directs more movement of water toward the interstitial space.

The most common clinical presentation of primary lymphedema occurs in 80% of cases. This is a mild swelling of the feet, ankles, and lower legs in women, beginning at puberty. The swelling progresses slowly but may become quite disfiguring. First, there is no limitation of activity. Later, there may be increasing disability from size and weight of the limb (Fig. 45.2). There may be a family history, and though the swelling is unilateral

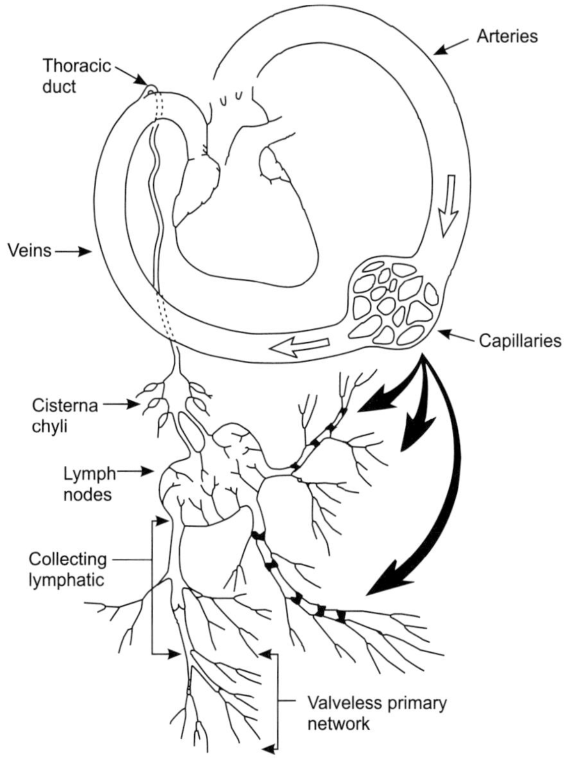

Figure 45.1 *This simplified diagram shows the valveless primary connecting network of lymphatics and the valve containing collecting lymphatics as they progress to the lymph node. From the lymph node, lymph passes to main lymph ducts within the body cavities and eventually returns to the circulation by way of major veins. The lymph is derived from tissue fluid exuding from the capillaries, and nourishes peripheral tissues.*

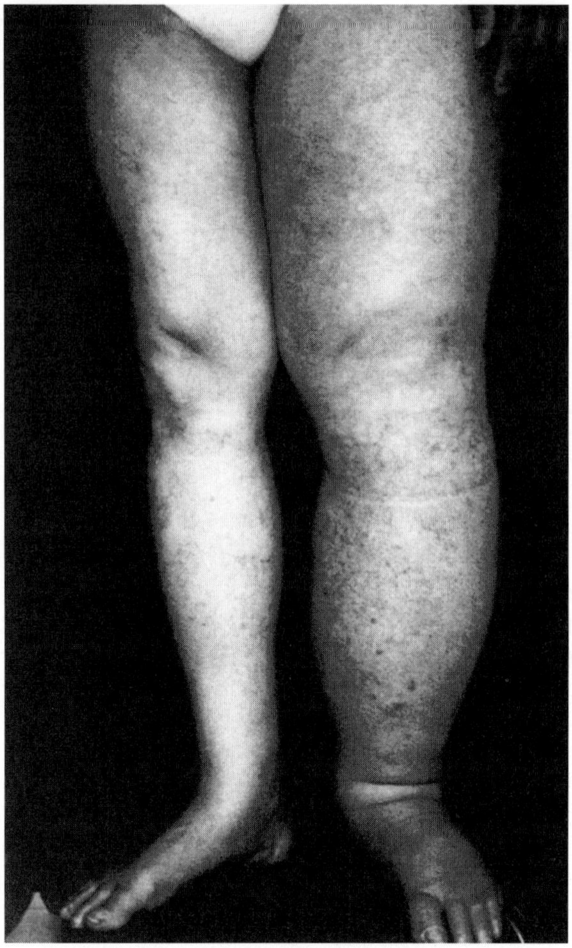

Figure 45.2 *Progressive lymphedema as shown in this photograph is not only disfiguring but disabling as well. The sheer size and weight of the limb interfere with daily mobility.*

on presentation, it is common to find a trace of edema in the opposite extremity.

The second most common presentation of lymphedema occurs in 10% of patients, both men and women. This involves the entire limb, develops quickly within 6–8 weeks, and may be related to a minor event such as an ankle sprain, insect bite, episode of infection, or blunt trauma. Occasionally, it follows a groin operation.

The last and least common mode of presentation is true congenital edema, affecting one or several limbs, present at birth or at an early age, and associated with lymph vesicles of the skin. These three clinical forms of lymphedema are referred to as primary (Table 45.1; Fig. 45.3).

Table 45.1 *Classification of lymphedema*

I	Congenital	Appearing at birth or early age
II	Lymphedema praecox	Presenting under age 35
III	Lymphedema tarda	Presenting over age 35
IV	Secondary	Presenting after surgery and/or radiation or developing as a result of parasitic infection or other identifiable cause (Fig. 45.3)

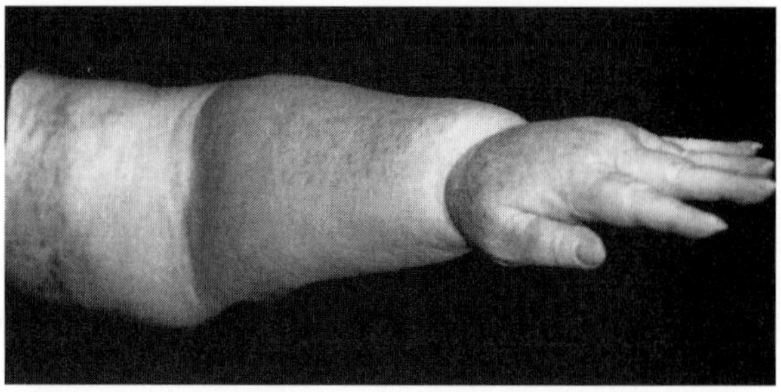

Figure 45.3 *This photograph of the lymphedematous arm following radical mastectomy. Proximal radiation is typical of a common form of lymphedema encountered in clinical practice.*

CLASSIFICATION

Rudolph Matas[2] in New Orleans produced a wordy definition of lymphedema, calling attention to high protein concentration within the tissues. Arthur Allen[3] in the 1930s said that primary lymphedema was caused by a congenital underdevelopment of lymph vessels. He coined the term 'lymphedema praecox' to separate lymphedema presenting in early life from the congenital variety. However, it was Kinmonth who provided the most useful and practical classification of lymphedema. He suggested the terms primary and secondary without indicating the cause of the primary variety.[4] Kinmonth's most famous contribution was the development of lymphangiography. This has fallen into disuse and has been replaced by less invasive, less traumatic methods of visualizing lymphatics.[5]

FUNDAMENTAL CAUSES OF LYMPHEDEMA

As is true of most conditions in which the actual cause has not been established with certainty, there are several theories which attempt to explain the reason that fluids and proteins accumulate in interstitial tissue.[6] Some, but not all, are supported by scientific evidence.

Perhaps the most common cause of lymphedema is a simple overload of the fluid transport system. This occurs in trauma, heat, irradiation, and infections. All of these increase capillary permeability and fluid egress into interstitium. If lymphatic pathways are normal, the edema is eventually cleared.

As there is strong evidence that interstitial tissue pressure is usually negative, it is difficult to understand why fluids and proteins pass into the positive pressure lymphatic system.[7] Perhaps the passage of fluid and macromolecules into the lymphatics is an active mechanical process.[8] Clearly, small molecules such as water enter the terminal segments of lymphatics and move proximally when lymphatics respond to adjacent arterial pulsations, contract, or are compressed. Thus, the distal fluid content becomes concentrated and osmotic pressure assists movement of water into the vessels during the next spell of lymphatic relaxation.[9] As all lymphatics except the terminal segments contain smooth muscle cells and spontaneous contraction of lymphatics has been noticed in animals, it may be that the transport of fluid and macromolecules is aided by such spontaneous contractile movement. Confirmation of this hypothesis has been difficult,[10,11] but it is highly likely that a derangement of this pump system leads to inefficient transport of lymph.

Because of Arthur Allen's influence in America and his early work in investigation of vascular diseases, most clinicians believe that lymphedema is caused by insufficient lymphatics. It was Allen who suggested that primary lymphedema was caused by underdevelopment of lymphatic vessels.[3] Lymphangiography confirmed that fact but has left unexplained whether this is a congenital or an acquired defect. Nevertheless, this explanation is intuitive, logical, and understandable.

Lymph node abnormalities, either acquired by surgical removal and/or radiation destruction or developed in response to inflammatory processes, are another acknowledged cause of lymphedema.[12] John Wolfe, working with Kinmonth,[13] showed that some patients with unilateral whole limb lymphedema had small and shrunken lymph nodes with an increased amount of fibrous tissue in the hilum. The radiologic description suggested that hilar fibrosis caused obstruction to lymph flow. Wolfe had the advantage of working in a clinic with extensive lymphangiographic experience, and noted that patent, distended peripheral lymphatics, and reduced number of proximal vessels was seen in situations of proximal obstruction. When small fibrotic nodes are not seen with distal vessel distension and a reduced number of distal lymphatics, it does not refute this theory but simply indicates that a wide spectrum of peripheral appearances may occur with proximal obstruction.

Finally, just as obstruction may occur in limb lymphatics, defects in central, abdominal, or thoracic collecting trunks may cause either lymphedema in the limbs or chylous reflux in the body cavities. The latter phenomenon is described as chylous ascites in the peritoneum, chylothorax affecting pleura, chyluria when renal lymphatics are involved, and chylometrorrhagia if the uterus is afflicted.[6] In such situations, lymphangiography has shown dilated, incompetent, megalymphatics in the abdomen and limbs.[14] Such defects are often associated with cutaneous angiomata and appear at an early age, which suggests an embryonic maldevelopmental origin of the lymphatic system.

All forms of lymphedema caused by conditions not originating in the lymphatics, lymph nodes, or other conducting elements may be referred to as secondary lymphedema. Obvious causes would be surgical *en bloc* removal of lymph nodes, lymphatic trunks, or radiation to these tissues before or after surgery for malignancy. Filariasis is also an important secondary cause of lymphedema.[14]

DIFFERENTIAL DIAGNOSIS

Increased peripheral venous pressure is the most common cause of lower extremity edema. Various conditions may precipitate this, the most common being chronic venous insufficiency. This, in turn, may be due to primary cause such as intrinsic valve failure or weakness of vein walls which allows venous dilation, elongation, and tortuosity. A secondary cause is the sequelae of deep venous thrombosis.[15]

Increased peripheral venous pressure and resultant edema may be cardiac in origin as in biventricular or right heart failure, pulmonary hypertension, or valvular heart disease. An indication of this as a cause of peripheral edema may come from other symptoms such as dyspnea, orthopnea, or paroxysmal nocturnal dyspnea. In such situations, the patient must be quizzed for insomnia, and physical examination should emphasize presence or absence of rales, ventricular gallop, distended neck veins, or cardiomegaly.

Edema may be present in Graves' disease. This may appear as a dermopathy occurring over the dorsum of the feet and legs. This is commonly referred to as localized or pretibial myxedema. The orange-peel appearance of the skin associated with pruritus and hyperpigmentation is characteristic but may be confused with venous obstructive edema.[16]

Hypothyroidism is another cause of localized edema. In this condition, hyaluronic acid-rich protein is deposited within the dermis of the skin. These deposits draw additional fluid into the skin, reducing elasticity and disrupting structural integrity.

Lipedema is another condition that can be confused with lymphedema. Lipedema is the abnormal accumulation of subcutaneous fat in the thighs and legs, sparing the feet. It is different from usual lymphedema in that it is symmetric, often painful, associated with easy bruising, and spares the feet and toes (absent Stemmer sign). Further confusion about this condition arises from the fact that it may progress into frank, florid lymphedema as the patient grows older.[17]

Just as treatment of malignancy can produce lymphedema, recurrence of malignancy can initiate lymphedema. This is because malignant cells may obstruct lymphatics and tumor growth can cause obstruction by extrinsic pressure. This condition is characterized by rapid onset, relentless progression, pain, and a more central distribution. The tissue is more firm and less soft.[18]

CLINICAL COURSE

As indicated above, the presentation of lymphedema may be at birth, sudden, or slowly developing. Early edema is painless, begins on the dorsum of the foot and ankle, and progresses proximally. Early, it subsides during recumbency and worsens towards the end of the waking day. The swelling becomes permanent secondary to fibrosis of skin and subcutaneous tissue. Early, as the edema involves the dorsum of the feet, the toes may be swollen also. This may be termed Stemmer sign, thickening of the skin on the dorsum of the second toe (Fig. 45.4). In later stages, the affected skin becomes thickened, darkened, and develops multiple warty projections (Fig. 45.5). This is referred to as lymphostatic verrucosis.[19]

Investigation of this condition by isotope lymphography and indirect or interstitial lymphography has revealed lymphostasis, cutaneous reflux or dermal backflow, as well as lymph cysts. Lymph collectors and subcutaneous fat in this condition are rarefied, tortuous, or ectatic.[20]

The physical findings described above have led to a system of grading of lymphedema. In grade I, the lymphedema pits on pressure, is reduced by limb elevation, and no fibrosis is present. In grade II, the lymphedema does not pit on pressure, does not reduce on elevation, and moderate fibrosis is present. In grade III, the lymphedema is irreversible and there is skin and subcutaneous fibrosis as well as sclerosis.

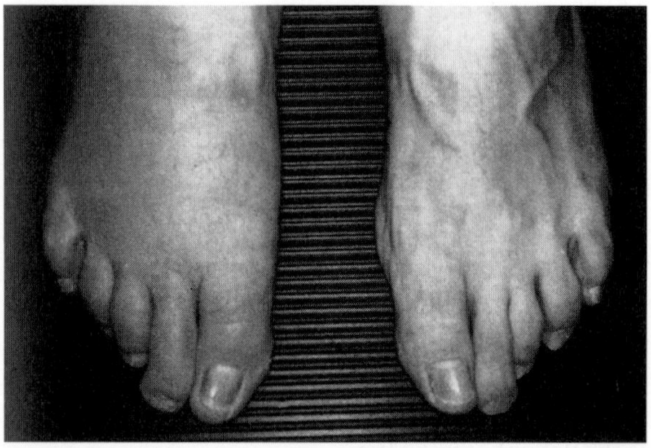

Figure 45.4 *This photograph shows the subtle early changes of lymphedema. Note the smooth swelling of the dorsum of the foot and the swelling that involves the toes. This, in comparison to the normal contralateral left foot, presents a striking and unforgettable clinical picture that allows easy early diagnosis.*

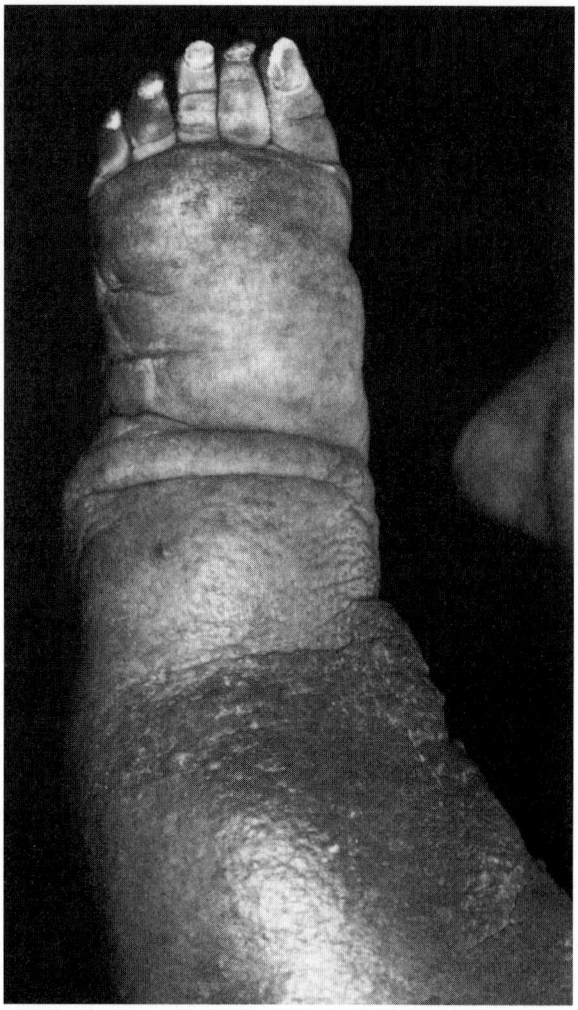

Figure 45.5 *Late, poorly treated lymphedema causes severe cutaneous changes as shown in this photograph. The epidermal, warty excrescences allow repeated attacks of recurrent cellulitis. Prevention of these chronic changes can be achieved by meticulous attention to principles of care that has as its object the reduction of edema and maintenance of a relatively edema-free limb.*

DIAGNOSTIC AIDS

Although lymphedema is a clinical diagnosis, objective verification is often desirable. As indicated above, direct lymphangiography, developed by Kinmonth, has been largely replaced by more modern techniques. This includes lymphoscintigraphy using a variety of radiocolloids.[21] Lymphoscintigraphy describes the anatomy of the lymph vessels and the dynamics of lymph flow. It is discussed in detail in Chapter 46.

Lymphoscintigraphy is largely descriptive. It does not influence choice of therapy. Findings in secondary lymphedema, for example, are quite characteristic but simple history taking and physical examination reveal the cause of the condition in every case. In primary lymphedema, lymphoscintigraphy shows obstructive lymphatics or deficient number of lymphatic vessels. However, prompt extravasation of the tracer cephalad to the injection site and subsequent slow transport often causes a poor definition of lymphatic trunks. Conventional lymphangiography delineates nodal abnormalities but lymphoscintigraphy does not. Thus, neither primary nor metastatic malignancy is detectable with lymphoscintigraphy.[22] Nevertheless, the technique is minimally invasive, patient acceptable, and may find its greatest utility in establishing the diagnosis in rare or difficult cases.[23,24] When the cause of lymphedema is obvious, there is certainly no need for lymphangiography or lymphoscintigraphy.

Imaging techniques have their place in differential diagnosis and perhaps in quantitation of results of treatment. The simplest imaging technique is duplex imaging of the venous system to assessment venous insufficiency, if present. However, the most rewarding is computed tomography (CT). A single axial slice through the mid-calf will establish the diagnosis.[25] This is a quick, noninvasive study. It displays abnormalities that are present in the most common forms of limb swelling. Venous obstruction is seen as an increased cross-sectional area of the muscle compartment, but not the subcutaneous fat layer. The latter is homogeneous. Subfascial fluid between muscles may be present. In obesity (lipedema), the subcutaneous fat layer is also increased and homogeneous but muscles are unaffected and no fluid is present in either the subcutaneous or the subfascial spaces. By contrast, in lymphedema, fluid collects in the subcutaneous interstitial tissues as seen in the CT image. There is no subfascial fluid. A honeycomb pattern is often present which is a result of increased cystic interstitial fluid collections and subsequent fibrosis. Other common causes of limb swelling such as popliteal cysts and hematomas are easily differentiated by CT. It has been natural to apply magnetic resonance imaging (MRI) to study lymphedema simply because this technique reflects water content of various tissues. In lymphatic edema, trabecular structures suggesting dilated collateral lymphatic vessels are observed in the swollen subcutaneous tissue (Fig. 45.6). In venous edema, fat intensity is found in the subfascia.[26] MRI examinations have confirmed those of CT which describe diffuse dermal and subcutaneous abnormalities and non-edematous but occasionally hypertrophied, skeletal muscle. Laking or honeycombing consistent with dermal collateral lymphangiectasis and sequestered lymph as well as increased subcutaneous fat is visualized by MRI.

Lymphoscintigraphy has been compared with MRI. Scintigraphy has shown dermal diffuse, crossover and retrograde tracer backflow. Delayed tracer transport and poorly defined lymph trunks with delayed or nonvisualization of regional lymph nodes has been demonstrated.[27] By contrast, MRI has visualized the lymph trunks, nodes and soft tissues proximal to the sites of lymphatic obstruction but not in a similar fashion. Combined techniques of lymphoscintigraphy and MRI should probably be used in the most difficult cases to document more completely which lymphatic abnormalities are present.

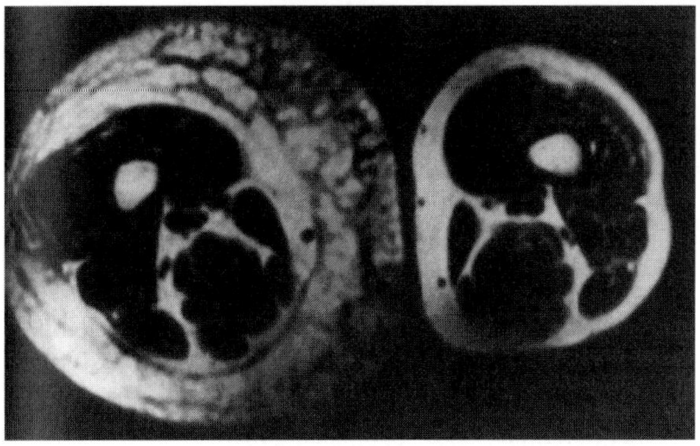

Figure 45.6 *This magnetic resonance photograph shows the characteristic picture of lymphedema in the thigh. Trabecular structures suggesting dilated collateral lymphatic vessels are observed. The honeycomb collections of fluid are consistent with dermal collateral lymphangiectasis and sequestered lymph.*

Duplex imaging of the lymphedematous limb is the most inexpensive and noninvasive technique. The lymphedematous limb and the dilated lymph channels may be visualized. However, the greatest utility of duplex ultrasound is to provide a way of detecting and estimating venous physiology and pathophysiology, if present. Severe chronic venous insufficiency may be found in the lymphedematous limb as an inciting or accompanying cause for the abnormalities that are seen.[28] When patients with clear venous abnormalities are studied, their lymphatics do show various abnormalities. Lymphatic abnormalities have been found to be present in nearly all patients with severe chronic venous insufficiency. Extravasation of fluid in the area of the ulcer, dermal backflow, tortuosity and irregularity of the lymph channels, as well as retention of the contrast agent for more than 24 hours has been seen on lymphangiography in venous disease. This is not lymphedema *per se* but is lymphatic damage secondary to the inflammatory processes that accompany severe chronic venous insufficiency.[29]

REFERENCES

1. Mortimer PS. The pathophysiology of lymphedema. *Cancer* 1998; **83**: 2798–803.
2. Matas R. The surgical treatment of elephantiasis and elephantoid states dependent upon chronic obstruction of the lymphatic and venous channels. *Am J Trop Dis* 1913; **1**: 60–85.

3. Allen EV. Lymphoedema of the extremities. Classification, etiology, and differential diagnosis: a study of 300 cases. *Arch Intern Med* 1934; **54**: 606–24.
4. Kinmonth JB. Lymphangiography in man. *Clin Sci* 1952; **II**: 13.
5. Kinmonth JB, Kemp Harper RA, Taylor GW. Lymphangiography. A technique for its clinical use in the lower limb. *Br Med J* 1955; **1**: 940–2.
6. Browse NL, Stewart G. Lymphoedema: pathophysiology and classification. *J Cardiovasc Surg* 1985; **26**: 91–106.
7. Guyton AC, Armstrong GE, Crowell JW. Negative pressure in interstitial spaces. *Physiologist* 1960; **3**: 70.
8. Guyton AC, Granger HJ, Taylor AE. Interstitial fluid pressure. *Physiol Rev* 1971; **51**: 527–63.
9. Casley-Smith JR. The fine structure and functioning of tissue channels and lymphatics. *Lymphology* 1980; **12**: 177–83.
10. Olszewski W, Engeset A. Intrinsic contractility of leg lymphatics in man. Preliminary communication. *Lymphology* 1979; **12**: 81–4.
11. Olszewski W, Engeset A. Intrinsic contractility of prenodal lymph vessels and lymph flow in human leg. *Am J Physiol* 1980; **239**: H775–83.
12. Gough MH. Primary lymphoedema: clinical and lymphographic studies. *Br J Surg* 1966; **53**: 917–25.
13. Kinmonth JB, Wolfe JH. Fibrosis in the lymph nodes in primary lymphoedema. *Ann R Coll Surg (Eng)* 1980; **62**: 344–54.
14. Manson P. In Manson-Bahr PH, ed. *Manson's Tropical Disease*, 16th edn. London: Cassell, 1966. Originally published 1898.
15. Bergan JJ, Yao JST, Flinn WR, McCarthy WJ. Surgical treatment of venous obstruction and insufficiency. *J Vasc Surg* 1986; **3**: 174–81.
16. Bull RH, Cobum PR, Mortimer PS. Pretibial myxedema: a manifestation of lymphedema? *Lancet* 1993; **341**: 403–4.
17. Ryan TJ, Curri SB. Hypertrophy and atrophy of the fat. *Clin Dermatol* 1989; **7**: 93–106.
18. Scanlon EF. James Ewing Lecture. The process of metastases. *Cancer* 1985; **55**: 1163–6.
19. Browse NL. The diagnosis and management of primary lymphedema. *J Vasc Surg* 1986; **3**: 181–5.
20. Schultz-Ehrenburg U, Niederauer HH, Tiedjen KU. Stasis papillomatosis: clinical features, etiopathogenesis, and radiological findings. *J Dermatol Surg Oncol* 1993; **19**: 440–6.
21. Richards TB, McBiles M, Collins PS. An easy method for diagnosis of lymphedema. *Ann Vasc Surg* 1990; **4**: 255–9.
22. McNeill GC, Witte MH, Witte CL, *et al.* Whole-body lymphangioscintigraphy: preferred method for initial assessment of the peripheral lymphatic system. *Radiology* 1989; **172**: 495–502.
23. Vaqueiro M, Gloviczki P, Fisher J, Hollier LH, Schirger A, Wahner HW. Lymphoscintigraphy in lymphedema: an aid to microsurgery. *J Nucl Med* 1986; **27**: 1125–30.
24. Nawaz MK, Hamad MM, Abdel-Dayem HM, Sadek S, Eklof BGH. Lymphoscintigraphy in lymphedema of the lower limbs using ^{99m}Tc HSA. *Angiology* 1992; **43**: 147–54.
25. Vaughan BF. CT of swollen legs. *Clin Radiol* 1990; **41**: 24–30.
26. Fujii K. MR imaging of edematous limbs in lymphatic and non-lymphatic edema. *Acta Radiol* 1994; **3**: 262–9.
27. Case TC, Witte CL, Witte MH, Unger EC, Williams WH. Magnetic resonance imaging in human lymphedema: comparison with lymphangioscintigraphy. *Magn Reson Imaging* 1992; **10**: 549–58.
28. Drinan KJ, Wolfson PM, Steinitz D, Mocco P, Cherney D. Duplex imaging in lymphedema. *J Vasc Technol* 1993; **17**(1): 23–6.
29. Meade JW, Mueller CB. Lymphatic and venous examination of the ulcerated leg: a preliminary report. *Surgery* 1992; **112**: 872–5.

46

Lymphoscintigraphy and lymphangiography

ROBERT A CAMBRIA, MARY F HAUSER, CLAIRE E BENDER AND PETER GLOVICZKI

LYMPHOSCINTIGRAPHY

Kinmonth, who described the technique of direct cannulation and injection of radio-opaque contrast material into pedal lymphatic vessels, revolutionized imaging of the lymphatic system during the decade of the 1950s.[1] His systematic review and classification of contrast lymphangiograms obtained using this technique provided the basis of our understanding of lymphatic anatomy in patients with lymphedema.[2] However, with the development of less invasive techniques for the imaging of the lymphatic system, and with limited potential for direct reconstruction of lymphatic vessels, contrast lymphography is rarely required. There remain several situations where contrast lymphography has distinct advantages, and where required, the anatomic resolution of this technique is unparalleled. The current indications for and technique of lymphangiography are discussed later in this chapter.

Lymphoscintigraphy, broadly described as an assessment of the lymphatic clearance of injected radioactive particles, was also pioneered in the 1950s. Because it is less invasive, easier to perform, and associated with fewer complications, lymphoscintigraphy has largely replaced contrast lymphangiography in the evaluation of lymphatic function. With newer imaging equipment and modern radiolabeled tracers, normal and pathologic lymphatic function can be accurately determined, and a great deal of anatomic information can also be obtained. Recently, lymphoscintigraphic techniques have been most commonly employed for the delineation of lymphatic drainage and potential nodal metastasis from a variety of neoplastic lesions. Magnetic resonance lymphangiography is a new, promising imaging modality of the lymphatic system.

History of lymphoscintigraphy

Sherman *et al.* first reported the transport of radioactive colloids by the lymphatic system in 1953.[3] He utilized colloidal gold (^{198}Au) in rabbit experiments, hoping to deliver tumoricidal doses of beta irradiation to regional lymph nodes as a treatment for metastatic cancer. Sherman performed autoradiographs of the regional lymph nodes, demonstrating the potential of this technique for lymphatic imaging. In the same year, Jepson *et al.* demonstrated the feasibility of using plasma protein radiolabeled with ^{131}I in the evaluation of lymphatic transport.[4] He demonstrated the slower clearance of interstitial protein via the lymphatic system as compared to crystalloid ^{131}I via the capillary network. In 1957, Taylor *et al.* demonstrated a delay in the transport of radiolabeled protein from the subcutaneous injection site in patients with lymphedema, as compared to normal subjects.[5] Although many lessons regarding the physical properties and rate of lymphatic transport of colloidal materials were gleaned from these early studies, it became evident that high-energy irradiation emitters are not appropriate for use in diagnostic imaging. The development of ^{99m}Tc-labelled radiocolloids and macromolecules, however, has made lymphoscintigraphy a safe and practical technique.

Technique of lymphoscintigraphy

The first consideration in the performance of lymphoscintigraphic imaging and evaluation of lymphatic function is the selection of an appropriate radiolabeled macromolecule or colloidal material. Characteristics such as particle size and surface charge affect the biokinetic behavior of subcutaneously injected materials.

Particles greater than 10 nm in diameter are transported by the lymphatics, whilst smaller particles are transported via the capillary network. Lymphatic transport time is directly related to particle size, and particles over 100 nm in size are transported very slowly. Optimal size for the delineation of lymphatic vessels and nodes in extremity lymphoscintigraphy is between 10 and 40 nm.[6] Most of our experience has been with ^{99m}Tc-antimony trisulfide colloid, but more recently this compound has not been available in the USA. ^{99m}Tc-human serum albumin (Tc-HSA) is available for lymphoscintigraphy in the USA, and we have had good results with this macromolecule as well. Both of these compounds are of appropriate size for extremity lymphoscintigraphy.

Exercise is known to influence the rate of lymphatic transport, and therefore must be standardized during the performance of lymphoscintigraphy.[7] Patients are comfortably positioned supine on the imaging table. For studies of the lower extremities, the feet are attached to a foot ergometer, and the patient is instructed on its use. For upper extremity studies, the patients are given a squeezable ball, which they compress during the study.

For studies of a lymphedematous extremity, subcutaneous injection of the radiolabeled tracer utilizing a tuberculin syringe and 27 gauge needle is performed into the web space between the second and third digits of the hand or foot. The volume of the injection is kept between 0.1 and 0.2 ml, which is associated with a brief period of discomfort at the injection site, but is otherwise tolerated extremely well. We have used 11 MBq (350–450 μCi) of ^{99m}Tc-antimony trisulfide colloid or 37 MBq (1 mCi) of Tc-HSA. Over 3 hours, 30–40% of the injected activity is transported from the injection site using these compounds.

A gamma camera with a large field of view is positioned immediately following injection of the tracer

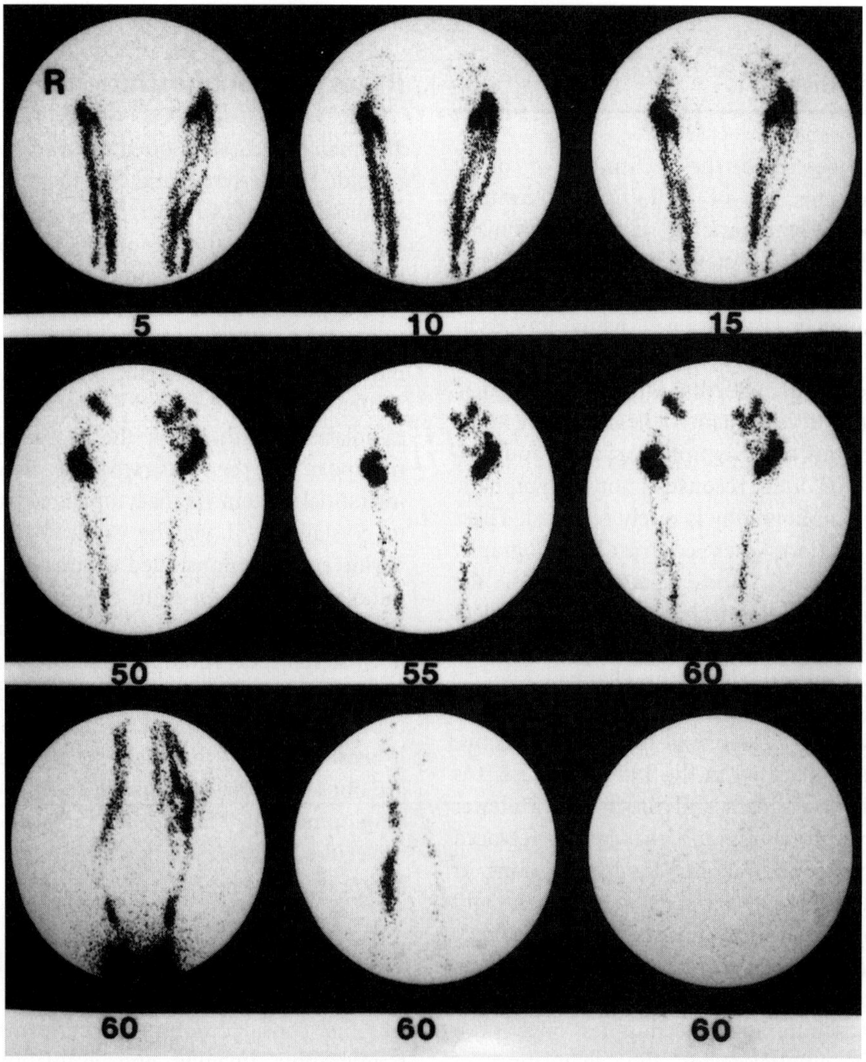

Figure 46.1 *Dynamic anterior images obtained every 5 minutes for 60 minutes following tracer injection. This 64-year-old man with long-standing bilateral leg swelling had rapid lymphatic transport, with activity appearing in the groin nodes on the first image. (Reproduced with permission from Cambria RA, Gloviczki P, Naessens JM, Wahner H. Noninvasive evaluation of the lymphatic system with lymphoscintigraphy: a prospective, semiquantitative analysis in 386 extremities.* J Vasc Surg *1993;* **18***: 775)*

to include the groin region in the upper field of view. An all-purpose collimator is used, and a 20% window is placed symmetrically around the 140 keV photopeak of the ^{99m}Tc isotope. Dynamic anterior images are obtained every 5 minutes during the first hour (Fig. 46.1). Exercise using the foot ergometer or plastic ball is begun immediately following injection of the tracer compound. The patient is requested to exercise for 5 minutes initially and then for 1 minute out of every five for the remainder of the first hour while dynamic images are being obtained.

Total body images over 20 minutes are obtained after 1 and 3 hours following the injection (Fig. 46.2). Patients are encouraged to ambulate between these images, although the degree of exercise is no longer standardized at this point in the study. In selected patients with delayed lymphatic transport, total body images may also be obtained at 6 and 24 hours to further delineate the degree of lymphatic obstruction.

Mapping of lymphatic drainage in neoplastic disease

The primary focus of this chapter is on the evaluation of the extremity with lymphedema. However, injection of radiolabeled particles to detect nodal drainage from the area of a tumor has become a more common use of lymphoscintigraphic techniques, and deserves mention. As noted above, the potential for detection and treatment of lymph nodes draining a neoplasm was appreciated in the earliest days of lymphoscintigraphy, and later confirmed in the 1970s.[8,9] However, clinical application of these techniques and analysis of their utility in the management of malignant neoplasia has only become popular in the last decade.[10] Initially employed in the treatment of melanoma, lymphatic mapping is being utilized in a growing number of cancers, including those affecting the breast, vulva and penis.

A distinguishing feature of lymphoscintigraphy for the delineation of sentinel lymph nodes is the choice of radioactive tracer and particle size. Since the primary aim is to identify the first lymph node draining a particular region, rather than depict the entire lymphatic system, a larger particle size is selected. ^{99m}Tc-sulfur colloid, with particle sizes ranging from 100 to 1000 nm is frequently employed. A hand-held gamma probe is then used intraoperatively to identify the lymph nodes where radioactivity has accumulated. Tracer injections in the dermis, subcutaneous tissue and peritumor locations have all been used with reasonable results. Most reports have agreed that a combination of radioactive tracer with a visible dye (isosulfan blue) has yielded the best results.[11]

The utility and long-term impact of sentinel node mapping and examination in the management of

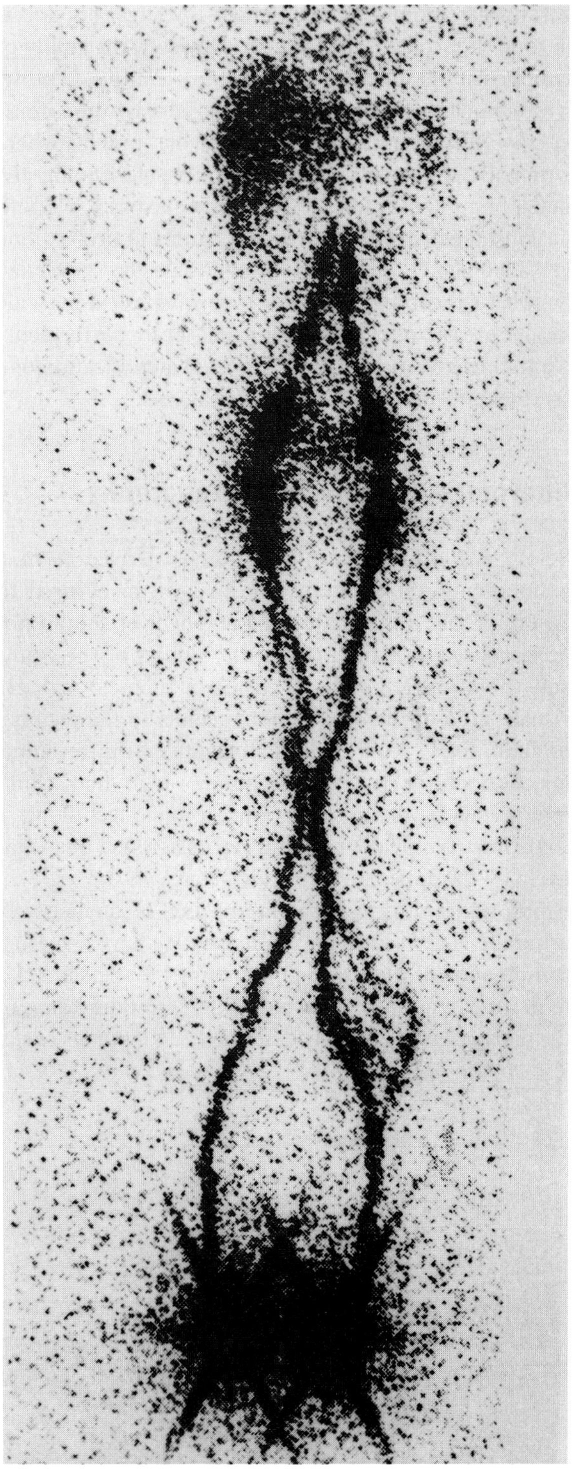

Figure 46.2 *Total body lymphoscintigram 1 hour after injection of tracer. This 38-year-old woman was admitted with a 15-year history of bilateral lower extremity swelling. Lymph vessels, nodes, and transport kinetics appear normal. There are several collateral lymph channels at left popliteal region. (Reproduced with permission from Cambria RA, Gloviczki P, Naessens JM, Wahner H. Noninvasive evaluation of the lymphatic system with lymphoscintigraphy: a prospective, semiquantitative analysis in 386 extremities.* J Vasc Surg *1993;* ***18****: 776)*

various carcinomas remains under investigation, and is beyond the scope of this chapter. However, the ability of lymphoscintigraphic techniques to identify sentinel lymph nodes is indisputable. Preoperative lymphoscintigraphy with gamma camera is valuable in areas where lymphatic drainage is ambiguous in determining the nodal basin(s) of interest. When only one basin needs to be considered, exploration with a handheld probe alone is adequate.[12] Although somewhat controversial, lymphatic mapping is accurate even when previous wide local excision of a skin lesion has been performed.[13] Numerous investigators have reported identification of a sentinel node in well over 90% of patients.[14]

Interpretation of lymphoscintigraphy

Before any diagnostic information is derived from a lymphoscintigraphic study, the images can be used to ensure proper injection technique. The liver should not be visualized over the first 10–15 minutes of the study, and should only be faintly visible after 1 hour. Early visualization of the liver without activity in the regional or abdominal lymph nodes is suggestive of intravenous injection of the tracer compound, which may cloud interpretation of the study. Once proper technique is confirmed, lymphatic function can be assessed quantitatively by the appearance of radioactivity in the regional lymph nodes during dynamic imaging, or qualitatively using the visual scintigraphic images. We have favored a combination of these techniques, using the visual images to derive a lymphatic transport index, a modification of the scoring system initially described by Kleinhans *et al.*[15]

The transport index is a scoring system for the lymphoscintigraphic images that can range from near 0 in normal scans to a maximum of 45 in scans demonstrating the absence of lymphatic transport. The components of the score and criteria for scoring the studies are depicted in Fig. 46.3. By examining the images, information on the appearance tracer in the regional nodes, location and number of lymphatic channels and nodes, and distribution pattern of tracer can be scored and tabulated. This semiquantitative score can then be used for comparison of serial scans in an individual patient, or comparison of lymphatic function between patients.

We have reported on the prospective evaluation of 386 extremities using the transport index.[16] Asymptomatic extremities (n = 79) had an average transport index of 2.6, while lymphedematous extremities (n = 124) had a mean index of 23.8. In our series, a transport index of greater than 5 was highly suggestive of lymphedema (sensitivity 80%, specificity 94%). Unfortunately, the transport index was unable to distinguish those extremities with primary lymphedema from those with secondary lymphedema, which is not surprising since the lymphatic anatomy in the end stages of these disorders can be quite similar. However, lymphoscintigraphy allowed us to exclude lymphatic pathology as a cause for extremity swelling in one-third of our patients.

Several reports have noted the accuracy of lymphoscintigraphy using a variety of tracer compounds and interpretation methods. Stewart *et al.* reported very high sensitivity and specificity rates using visual interpretation of lymphoscintigraphic images alone[17] and these findings are supported by others.[18,19] However, some authors have recommended the use of time–activity

Patient's Initials ____________________

Clinic Number ____________________ Date __________

LYMPHOSCINTIGRAPHY

DATE EVALUATION

______ Arms ______ Legs

	1 hr		3 hr		6 hr		24 hr	
Image	R	L	R	L	R	L	R	L
Lymph transport kinetics: 0 = no delay, 1 = rapid, 3 = low grade delay, 5 = extreme delay, 9 = no transport								
Distribution pattern: 0 = normal, 2 = focal abnormal tracer, 3 = partial dermal, 5 = diffuse dermal, 9 = no transport								
Lymph node appearance time: Minutes								
Assessment of lymph nodes: 0 = clearly seen, 3 = faint, 5 = hardly seen, 9 = no visualization								
Assessment of lymph vessels: 0 = clearly seen, 3 = faint, 5 = hardly seen, 9 = no visualization								
Abnormal sites of tracer accumulation (describe)								

Figure 46.3 *Evaluation form for calculation of lymphatic transport index.*

curves obtained with dynamic imaging over the regional lymph nodes for the analysis of lymphatic function.[20–22] Weissleder *et al.* reported an improvement in sensitivity of the examination when quantitative clearance data were used.[7] Our previous experience with quantitative analysis of regional lymph node tracer accumulation has demonstrated a great deal of variability in normal extremities, making interpretation of these data difficult.[23] Therefore, we have come to rely heavily on the visual interpretation of the lymphoscintigraphic images for a given study, and use the semiquantitative transport index as described above to compare serial exams or studies in different patients.

Lymphoscintigraphic patterns in normal and swollen extremities

In the normal lymphoscintigram, the areas of highest tracer activity usually remain at the injection site. As mentioned previously, only 30–40% of the injected activity is normally transported from the injection site over the period of the study. In the case of the lower extremity, this intense area of activity overshadows any anatomic detail in the area of the foot. Gradual ascent of the tracer from the foot occurs, and with normal transit, activity is detected in the inguinal lymph nodes on the dynamic images between 15 and 60 minutes from the time of

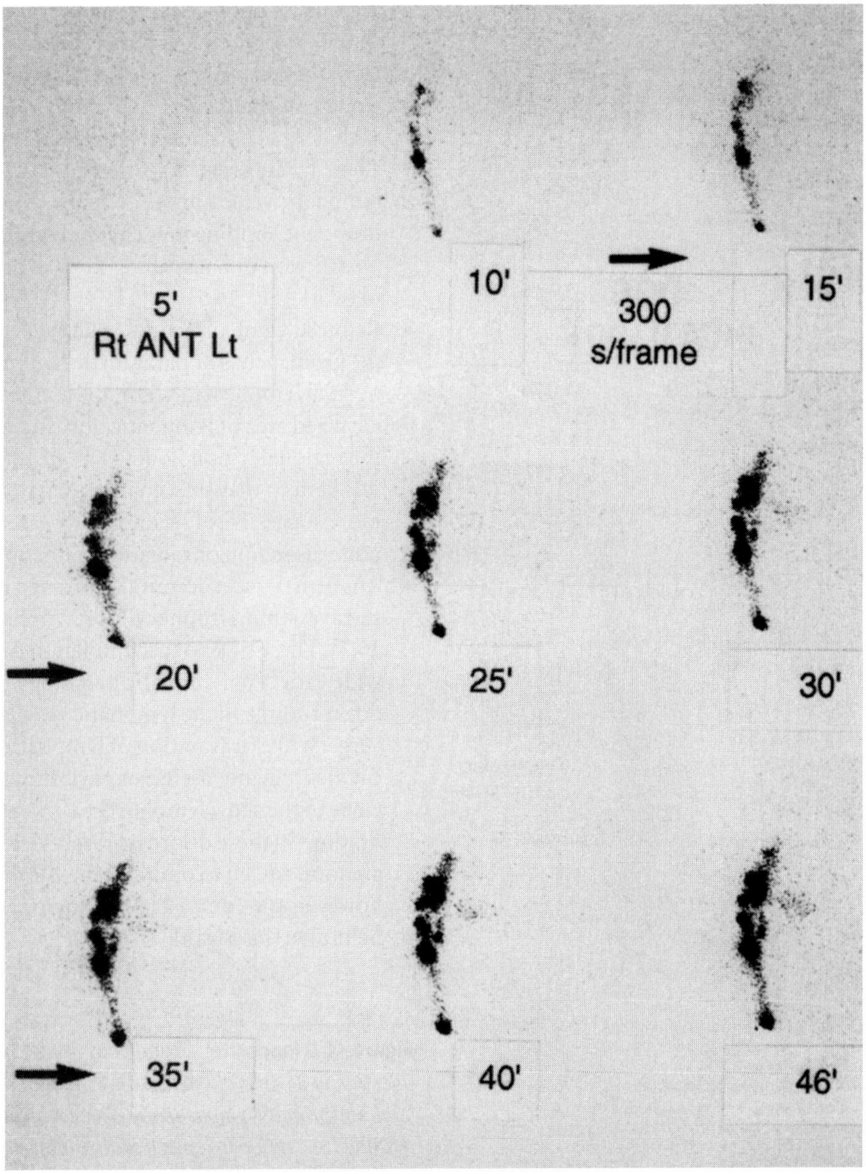

Figure 46.4 *Lymphoscintigraphic images of the groin taken every 5 minutes after injection of the colloid into both feet. There is normal lymphatic transport and image pattern of the inguinal nodes on the right, and no visualization of the lymphatics of the left. This 30-year-old woman had primary lymphedema of the left leg. (Reproduced with permission from Gloviczki P, Wahner HW. Clinical diagnosis and evaluation of lymphedema. In Rutherford RB, ed.* Vascular Surgery, *4th edn. Philadelphia: WB Saunders, 1995: 1906)*

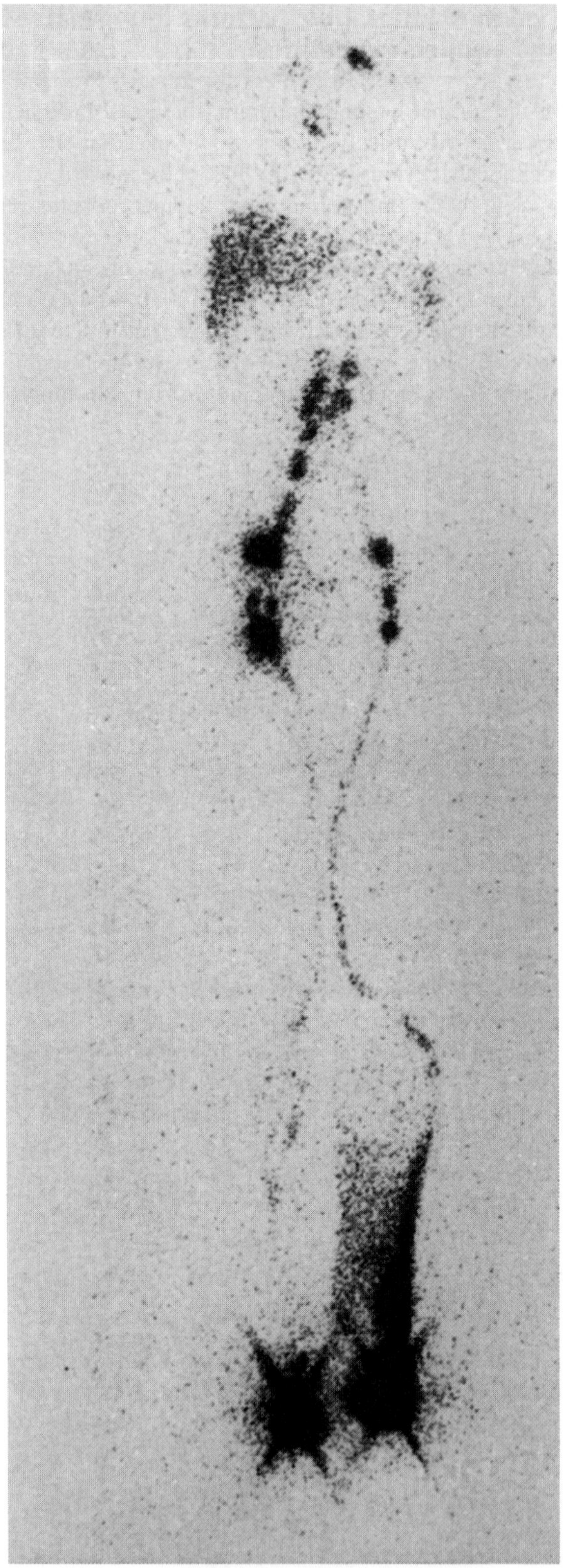

injection. Appearance of significant activity in the groin in less than 15 minutes indicates rapid transport, and absence of activity after 1 hour is suggestive of delayed lymphatic transport (Fig. 46.4). On the total body images, several lymphatic channels may be seen in the area of the calf, but in the thigh the lymphatics run close together on the medial aspect, and separate activity in each of the channels is seldom seen. With normal transit times, the inguinal nodes should be clearly visualized 1 hour following injection, and faint visualization of the para-aortic nodes, liver and bladder may be seen (Fig. 46.2). On the 3-hour image, the uptake in the pelvic and abdominal nodes and liver should be intense (Fig. 46.5), and occasionally the area of the distal thoracic duct in the left supraclavicular fossa will be visible.

In lymphedematous extremities, several lymphoscintigraphic patterns may be observed either alone or in combination.[24] These can be broadly classified as follows:

- Delay or absence of lymphatic transport from the injection site. Little or no activity is detected in the regional lymph nodes by 1 hour following injection. In the extreme circumstance, no transport of activity from the foot can be detected (Fig. 46.6).
- Collateral channels or a cutaneous pattern consistent with dermal backflow may be seen in the extremity. These findings are suggestive of obstruction of lymphatic vessels in the extremity, with lymphatic flow either finding new channels around the obstruction or back-filling the rich dermal lymphatic network (Fig. 46.5).
- Reduced, faint, or no uptake in the lymph nodes of the groin, pelvis or para-aortic regions, with relatively normal lymph channels in the extremity, indicating a localized area of lymphatic obstruction at the level of the regional lymph nodes (Fig. 46.10(a)). Although this pattern may be seen in primary lymphedema, it is more suggestive of secondary disease following lymph node dissection or radiation for neoplastic disease.
- Abnormal tracer accumulation suggestive of extravasation, lymphocele, or lymphangiectasia (Fig. 46.7). These types of accumulation can be seen in a wide variety of lymphatic pathology ranging from direct trauma to the lymphatic vessels following surgery, to extravasation of lymphatic fluid into body cavities (chylous ascites or chylothorax) or reflux of chyle to the skin (lymphorrhea). Scintigraphic findings in these disorders rarely yield enough anatomic detail to pinpoint the site of lymphatic leak, however, and contrast lymphangiography may be helpful in this regard.

Figure 46.5 (opposite) *Total body image 3 hours after injection in 34-year-old man with 18-month history of left leg swelling (primary lymphedema). There is localized area of dermal distribution in left calf with diminished number of lymph nodes in left inguinal region. (Reproduced with permission from Cambria RA, Gloviczki P, Naessens JM, Wahner H. Noninvasive evaluation of the lymphatic system with lymphoscintigraphy: a prospective, semiquantitative analysis in 386 extremities.* J Vasc Surg *1993;* ***18****: 777)*

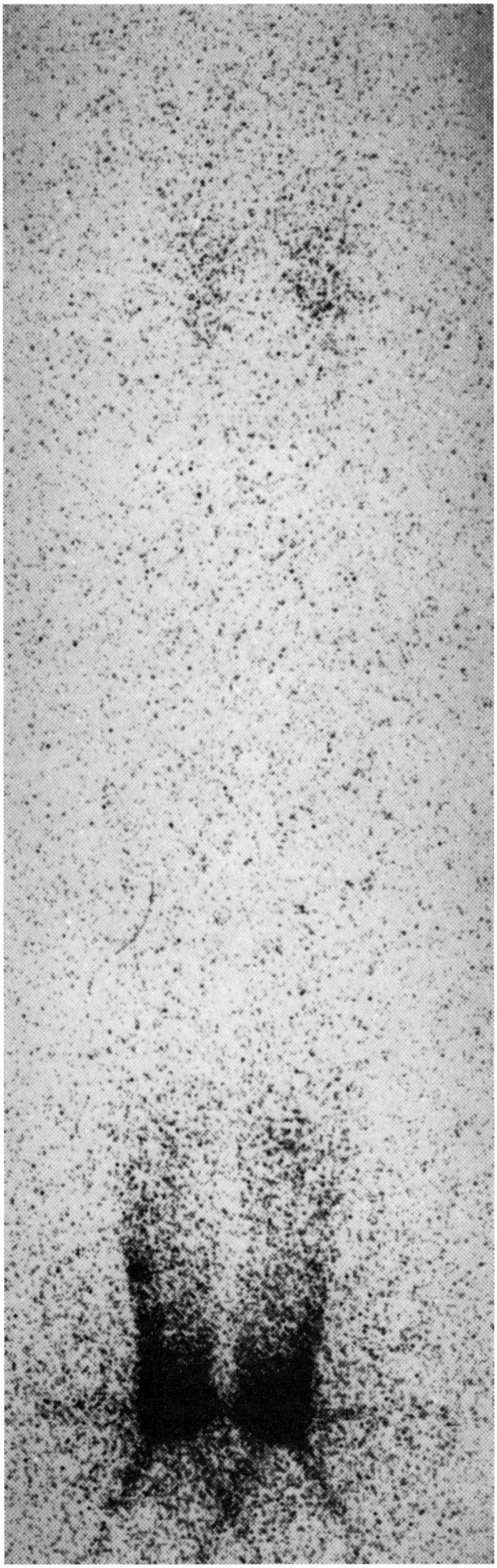

Lymphoscintigraphy can be used to monitor the effects of therapeutic intervention or the progression of lymphedema over time. In one study, over 80% of extremities demonstrated an improvement in lymphoscintigraphic findings following a regimen of complex physical therapy and compression.[25] Similarly, alterations in lymph flow with the application of either hot or cold compresses can be measured with lymphoscintigraphy.[26] In our study, the transport index correlated well with degree of symptoms on repeated examination in several patients.[16]

Lymphoscintigraphy has become quite useful in the evaluation of patients considered for direct lymphatic reconstruction. In the ideal patient (secondary lymphedema due to obstruction at the groin or axillary level), lymphoscintigraphy can identify dilated lymphatics in the involved extremity with sufficient accuracy to proceed with surgical exploration on the basis of these findings.[23] In addition, this study is suitable to follow the effectiveness of some lymphatic reconstructions. While patency of lymphovenous anastomoses cannot be directly demonstrated,[27] the study can image patent suprapubic or axillary lymphatic grafts placed for unilateral lymphatic obstruction[15] (Fig. 46.8).

Lymphoscintigraphic findings in extremities with venous disease vary depending on the duration and extent of venous pathology. Early in the course of venous disease, before extensive edema formation or the development of lipodermatosclerosis, the lymphatic system is normal and lymphoscintigraphic appearance will reflect this. An increase in lymphatic transport (rapid transit) develops as capillary filtration and edema in the extremity increases. This was noted in early studies of lymphatic flow with ^{131}I-labeled albumin[28] and has been confirmed in both animal models[29] and humans.[17] The increase in lymphatic transport occurs as a homeostatic mechanism where the lymphatic system attempts to reduce the increased tissue fluid. Others have demonstrated a decrease in lymphatic transport associated with venous pathology.[7,22,30] Lymphatic vessels are damaged in areas of extensive lipodermatosclerosis that accompanies advanced venous disease, leading to delayed lymphatic transport and exacerbation of edema in the extremity. In our series, 31 patients had evidence of deep venous insufficiency; 4 of these (13%) had rapid transport, 9 (29%) had normal lymphatic transport, and 18 (58%) had delayed transport.[16]

Figure 46.6 (opposite) *Lymphoscintigram of a 25-year-old woman with congenital familial lymphedema of both lower extremities. Note absence of lymph vessels and lymph nodes at 6 hours, with only minimal dermal backflow visible in the distal calves. (Reproduced with permission from Gloviczki P, Wahner HW. Clinical diagnosis and evaluation of lymphedema. In Rutherford RB, ed.* Vascular Surgery, *4th edn. Philadelphia: WB Saunders, 1995: 1908)*

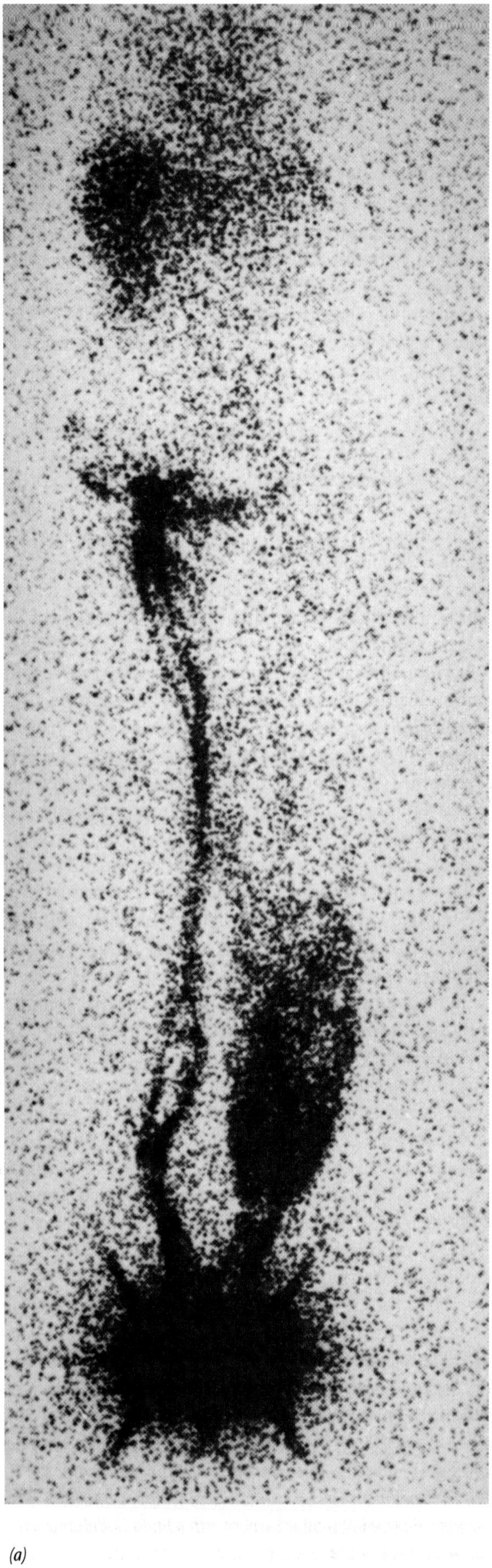

(a)

Summary

Lymphoscintigraphy has become the test of choice in patients with suspected lymphedema. Unlike contrast lymphangiography, it is noninvasive, well tolerated, and associated with very few complications. When necessary, it can be repeated serially to follow the clinical course of lymphatic function. Although initially developed as a functional study, newer imaging techniques and equipment can yield a great deal of anatomic information,

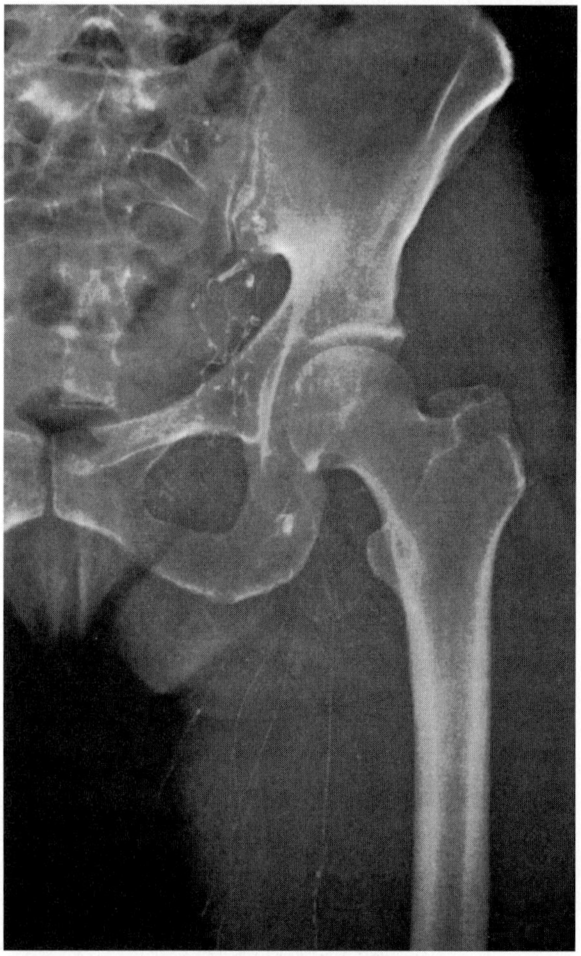

(b)

Figure 46.7 *(a) Lymphoscintigram of a 43-year-old woman with left lower extremity lymphedema following hysterectomy and bilateral iliac node dissection for cervical cancer. Dermal pattern is seen on left with no visualization of the inguinal nodes. Transport was mildly delayed in the clinically asymptomatic right limb. Note lack of visualization of iliac nodes bilaterally. (b) Contrast lymphangiography in the same patient confirms the lymphoscintigraphic findings. Few small lymph vessels and two small nodes are seen only in the thigh. (Reproduced with permission from Gloviczki P, Wahner HW. Clinical diagnosis and evaluation of lymphedema. In Rutherford RB, ed.* Vascular Surgery, *4th edn. Philadelphia: WB Saunders, 1995: 1909)*

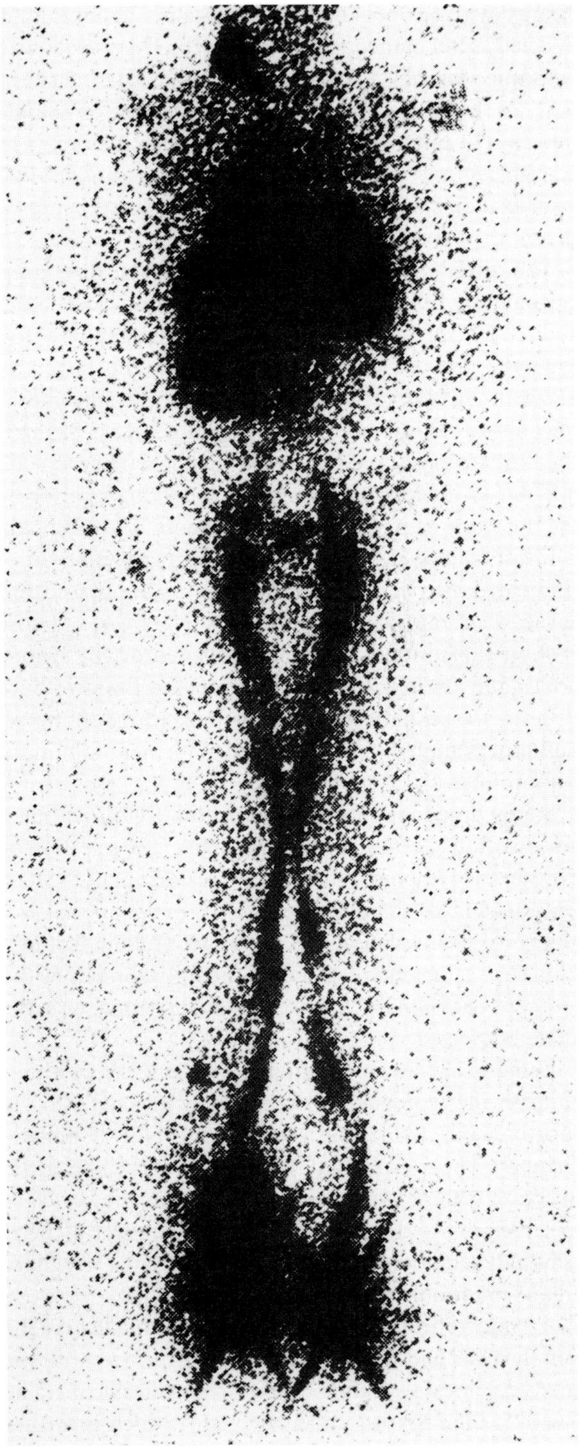

(a)

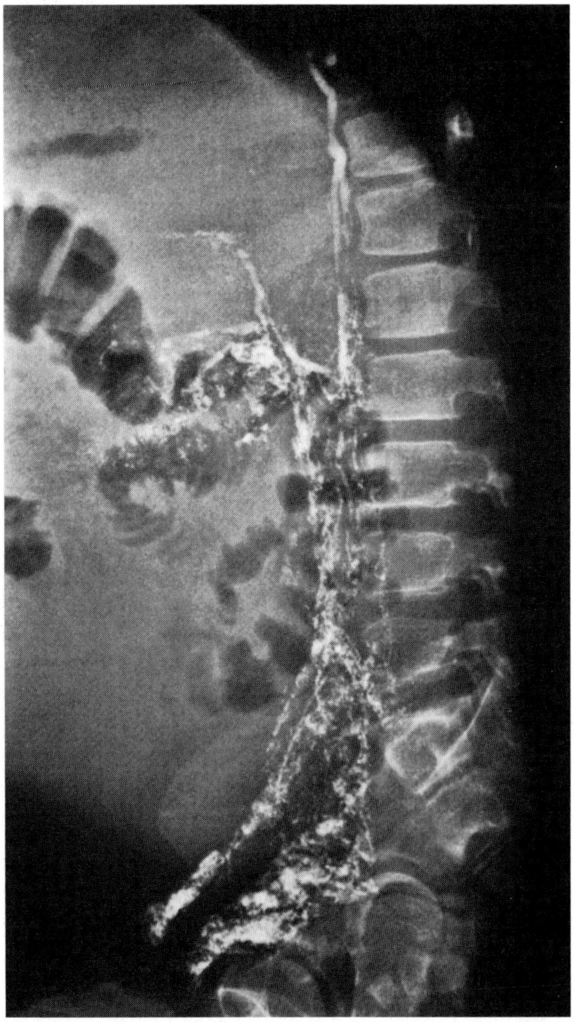

(b)

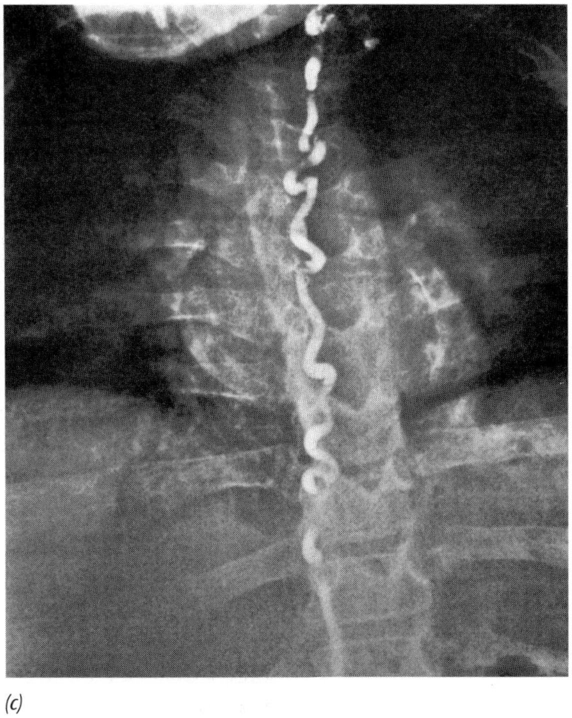

(c)

Figure 46.8 *(a) Lymphoscintigram of an 18-year-old man with lymphangiectasia, protein-losing enteropathy, and chylous ascites. Note large leg lymphatics and reflux of colloid into the mesenteric lymph vessels, filling almost the entire abdominal cavity. (b) Lymphangiogram of the same patient reveals reflux of dye into the dilated mesenteric lymphatics. (c) Note extremely dilated and tortuous but patent thoracic duct. (Reproduced with permission from Gloviczki P, Wahner HW. Clinical diagnosis and evaluation of lymphedema. In Rutherford RB, ed.* Vascular Surgery, *4th edn. Philadelphia: WB Saunders, 1995: 1910)* which in certain cases may be sufficient for direct surgical intervention on the lymphatic system. While diagnostic accuracy utilizing several methods of interpretation has been reported, we have come to rely largely on visual interpretation of scintigraphic images. Where necessary, a simple scoring system can be applied to derive a lymphatic transport index, which can then be used to compare individual scintigraphic studies to one another. Most recently, these techniques are being employed with increasing frequency for the mapping of lymphatic drainage from a variety of neoplastic lesions, and for the biopsy of sentinel lymph nodes.

LYMPHANGIOGRAPHY

In 1943, Servelle performed the first contrast lymphangiogram. Nearly a decade later, Kinmonth described the basic technique of the subcutaneous injection of a vital dye for identification of superficial dorsal foot lymphatics for cannulation and direct injection of contrast material.[1] Almost 50 years later, there have been only modifications in the injected contrast agents and the radiographic filming of the examination.

The continued development and refinement of cross-sectional imaging techniques (computed tomography, magnetic resonance imaging, ultrasonography) and isotope lymphoscintigraphy have seen a reduced need for diagnostic lymphangiography.

Although lymphangiography is a time-consuming, technically challenging interventional radiologic procedure, it provides a highly detailed examination of both the lymphatic vessels and nodes.

Technique of lymphangiography

Lymphangiography is performed as an outpatient procedure. The patient is instructed not to eat or drink 8 hours prior to the examination. Medications and clear liquids are permitted. Conscious sedation may be given if the patient is anxious or unable to remain quiet for 30–60 minutes. The patient is placed supine on a padded radiographic fluoroscopic table.

A variety of blue dyes have been used for opacification of lymphatic channels, including methylene blue, patent blue violet and isosulfan blue (Lymphazurin 1%, Hirsch Industries, Cherry Hill, NJ, USA). Ninety percent of isosulfan blue is excreted via the bilary tract and the remaining 10% is excreted in the urine. The urine can be discolored for a few days.

In patients with allergy to blue dye, lymph vessels are identified as thin-walled in contrast to the thicker walls of nearby veins. Fluorescein can be used to localize the lymph vessels, but is less intense than the traditional blue dyes.

In the initial phase, the skin between each toe is cleaned with alcohol and 0.5 ml lidocaine (lignocaine) is injected intracutaneously in each web. This is followed with injection of 0.5 ml of isosulfan blue (Lymphazurin 1%). Some authors have mixed the solutions for a single injection in each web.[31] The patient is then instructed to actively flex and extend the toes and ankles until optimal visualization has occurred. The hair on the dorsum of the foot is shaved if necessary.

The sites for blue dye injection to visualize deep lymphatics of the leg are the sole of the foot, close to the abductor hallucis muscle. For lymphangiography of the arm, the dorsum of the hand, between the fingers is injected, and for cervical lymphangiography the site of injection is behind the ears. Striking blue streaks through the skin are visualized lymphatic channels. They may be difficult to identify by color-blind individuals performing the study or in dark-skinned patients. The iodinated contrast material used for lymphangiography is Ethiodol (iodinated ethyl esters of fatty acids of poppyseed oil, Savage Laboratories, Missouri City, TX, USA). Almost 90% of the contrast material is retained by the lymph nodes and the remainder flows into the thoracic duct entering the pulmonary bed. In patients with diminished pulmonary function, this may lead to further pulmonary compromise.

Sterile drapes are placed around both feet providing a large working surface for the examiners. The selection of the optimal lymphatic channel on the dorsum of the foot includes a large channel oriented in a direction that will accept easy cannulation and subsequent tubing fixation. This channel is often located on the mid-dorsum of the foot, but occasionally, a more proximal channel near the ankle is selected.

Using a cut-down technique, lidocaine 1% without epinephrine (adrenaline) is generously injected into the subcutaneous tissues surrounding the blue lymphatic channel. The purpose of this liberal local anesthetic injection is to obtain a pain-free environment as well as to facilitate the delicate procedure of removal of perilymphatic adipose and other tissue. Lidocaine may have an antispasmodic effect on the small channel.

A 2 cm vertical or transverse incision is made over the lymph vessel and blunt dissection is performed until the channel is located. A thin 3 cm × 1 cm malleable metallic wedge is then slipped under the vessel, which is further cleaned of any adjacent fat or fibrous tissue. At both the proximal and distal ends of the exposed vessel, a 5-0 silk tie is gently positioned for further use. Next the proximal tie (toward the ankle) is taped with a Steri-strip. This tie is put under slight tension in order to distend the lymph vessel. The more distal tie can be used as a repair for leaks, but the needle must pass through the tie.

We use either a 27 or 30 gauge lymphangiography needle based on the diameter of the visualized lymphatic vessel. The needle tip is held nearly parallel to the lymphatic channel for cannulation. The needle can be gently test injected with sterile saline to check position.

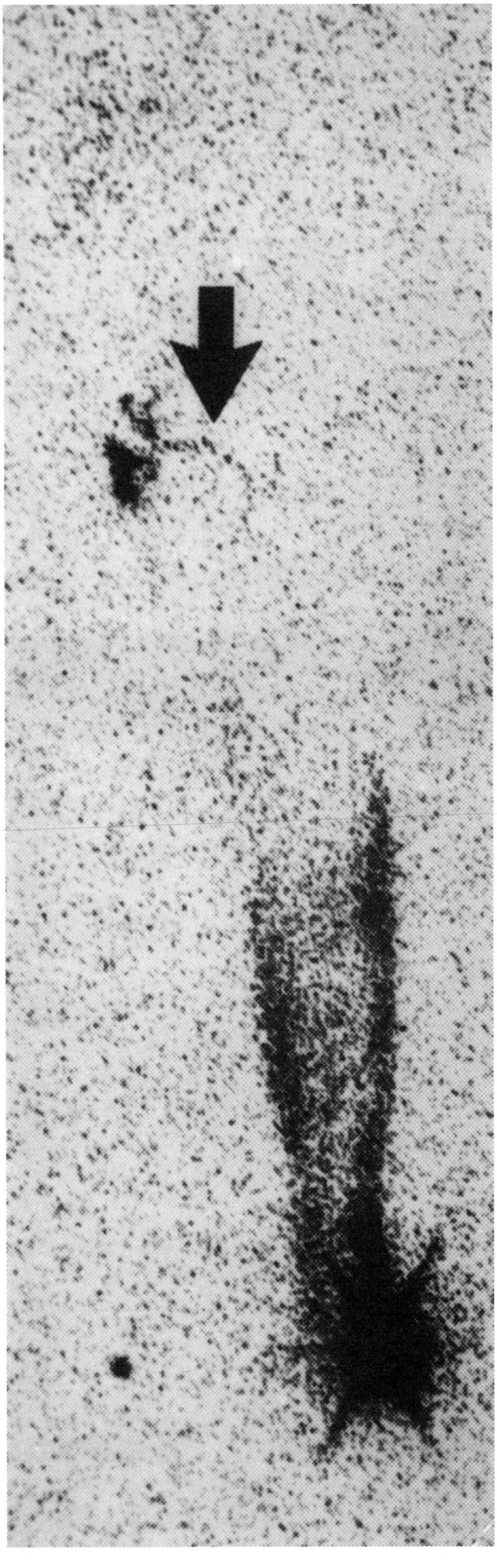

Once in position, a Steri-Strip is used to secure the needle or the dorsum of the foot. The proximal tie is then relcased to allow flow; it can be moved just proximal to the bevel of the needle and tightened for a better seal. The tubing of the needle can be draped between the appropriate toes and then taped to the skin.

A Harvard infusion pump apparatus (Bard Medsystems, North Reading, MA, USA) is used to inject the heated contrast material at 0.10–0.15 ml/min for a total of 5–7 ml per leg without leakage. If unsuccessful on one side, overfilling of the infused side using 10–12 ml can cross-fill at the bilateral para-aortic lymph node level. After 1–2 ml of injection, brief fluoroscopy or a radiograph is taken to confirm lymphatic filling. Patients can experience leg cramping as contrast material ascends in the lower leg. After the injection, both incisions are washed with sterile saline. Single or double vertical mattress prolene sutures are used to close the incision. Antimicrobial ointment and a small dressing are applied. Sutures should be removed after 10 days.

The standard series of radiographs are obtained immediately after the procedure (for vessel evaluation) and at 24 hours (for node architecture and location) include:

- pelvic: AP, both obliques, lateral;
- lumbosacral spine: AP, lateral, both obliques;
- chest: PA, lateral.

Radiographic spot films are useful to identify sites of extravasation in the trunk, chest or limbs. Early, frequent fluoroscopic observation can assist in localization of leaks. Extremity films are taken in addition if the test is being performed for lymphedema.

Interpretation of lymphangiography

Complete evaluation of the lymphangiogram includes interpretation of the channel (immediate) and nodal (24 hours) phases of the study as well as any spot films taken (Fig. 46.9). The lymphatic channels are evaluated for size, number, obstruction, or metastatic involvement. The lymph nodes are individually evaluated for size, number, contour and internal architecture.

Ethiodol usually clears from the lymphatic vessels within 3–4 hours. Delayed emptying occurs in proximal obstruction. Extravasation into the perilymphatic tissues can occur in lymphatic obstruction or too rapid infusion rates.

Figure 46.9 (opposite) *A 52-year-old man with secondary lymphedema of the left lower extremity who underwent suprapubic lymphatic grafting 5 years ago. Arrow indicates patent lymphatic graft. Note that injection of the colloid was made into the left foot and that the suprapubic graft fills the right inguinal lymph nodes.*

The appearance of the lymph nodes depends on:

- the degree of opacification, and
- histology.

Contrast material is located within the sinuses. A normal lymph node appears as a sharply defined round or oval density with a fine, homogeneous and granular appearance. From the hilus of the node, efferent lymphatic channels emanate centrally.

Complications of lymphangiography

The contrast lymphangiogram is a tedious, time-consuming invasive radiological procedure. Lymphangiography is relatively safe as long as patients are carefully selected and standard precautions are taken.[32] Complications are classified as follows:

- idiosyncratic reactions to blue dyes and Ethiodol
- pulmonary complications
- central nervous system embolization of oily contrast
- local wound complications
- accidental intravenous injection of Ethiodol
- post-lymphography pyrexia
- progression of lymphedema.

Mild or anaphylactic reactions to either the blue dyes or Ethiodol are rare (less than 1%). Life-support measures must be available in the procedure room. Delayed reactions within a few hours can also occur. Weg and Harkleroad[33] have detected modest decreases in total lung diffusion and capillary volume after lymphangiography in patients without pre-existing lung disease. Severity of pulmonary complications is related to pre-existing pulmonary disease and larger volumes (>20 ml) of Ethiodol. Extremely rare cases of hemoptysis, pulmonary infarction and respiratory distress syndrome have been reported.[34,35]

Pulmonary embolization of Ethiodol has been reported by Bron[36] in 55% of patients. Clinically significant pulmonary complications were observed by Hessel *et al.*[37] in only 0.4% of patients. Pulmonary complications are more likely to occur in patients with lymphatic obstruction or in patients infused with large (>20 ml) volumes of Ethiodol. If lymphangiography must be performed in patients with pulmonary disease, a single extremity study using 4–5 ml Ethiodol can be offered. The overall mortality rate reported by Hessel is 0.01%.[37]

Clouse *et al.*[38] have described mild-to-moderate fevers in 5% of patients in their series of 108 procedures. Worsening of the chronic obstructive lymphedema after contrast lymphangiography has also been reported.[24]

Indications for lymphangiography

The current uses of lymphangiography are small in number. Lymphoscintigraphy is our examination of choice for routine evaluation of lymphedema. Contrast lymphangiography is rarely and selectively used for the diagnosis of lymphedema (Fig. 46.10).[24] It can be useful in those patients who are candidates for microvascular lymphatic reconstruction. It is very helpful, however, in the evaluation of patients with lymphangiectasia and reflux of chyle. The details of extent and location of the dilated ducts are much better delineated with contrast

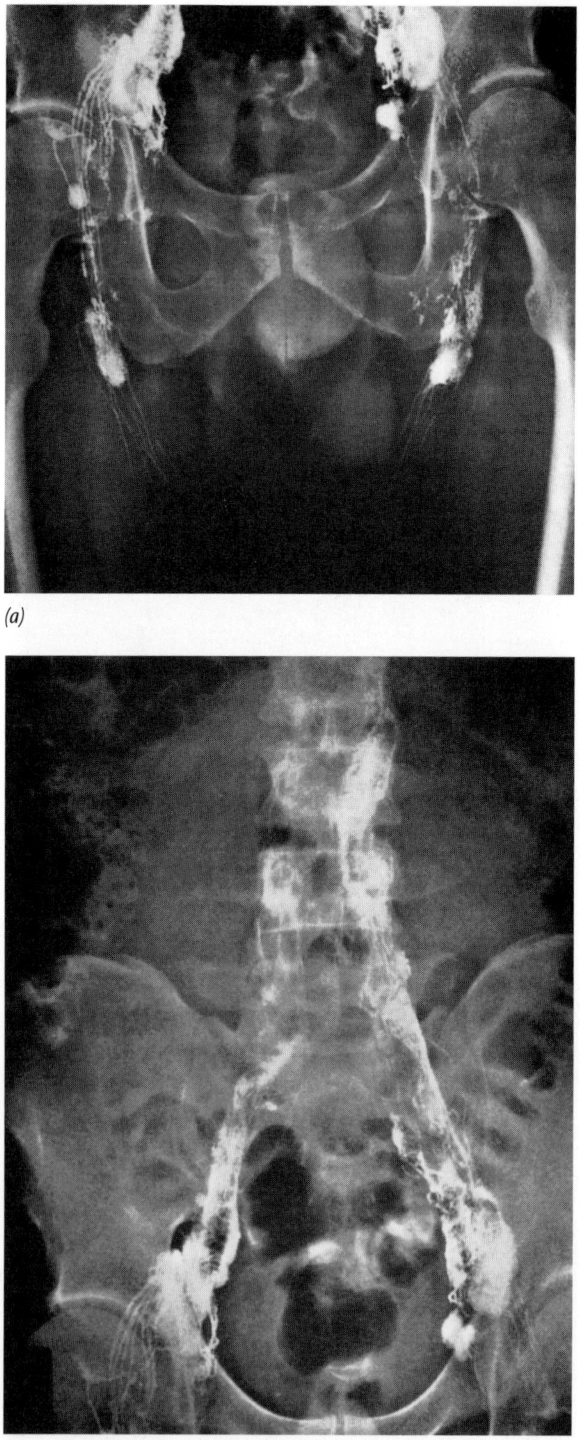

(a)

(b)

Figure 46.10 *(a, b) Normal lymphatic anatomy demonstrated by bipedal contrast lymphangiography.*

lymphangiography than with lymphoscintigraphy (Fig. 46.7). Obstruction of the thoracic duct and localization of pelvic, abdominal or thoracic lymphatic fistulae is best studied by lymphangiography.

Lymphangiography now plays a very limited role in the evaluation of patients with early stages of Hodgkin's lymphoma and seminoma.

Contraindications for lymphangiography

Careful selection of patients and routine precautions are the keys to the success of this invasive procedure. Patients with prior history of significant contrast reactions, pulmonary disease, or intracardiac or intrapulmonary shunts should be excluded. Lymphangiography should not be performed in patients undergoing pulmonary radiation therapy. It should not be performed in patients with possible extensive lymphatic obstruction (e.g. bulky pelvic or retroperitoneal adenopathy).

CONCLUSIONS

Lymphoscintigraphy has become the test choice in patients with suspected lymphedema. Unlike contrast lymphangiography, it is noninvasive, well tolerated, and associated with very few complications. When necessary, it can be repeated serially to follow the clinical course of lymphatic function. Although initially developed as a functional study, newer imaging techniques and equipment can yield a great deal of anatomic information, which in certain cases may be sufficient for direct surgical intervention on the lymphatic system. Although diagnostic accuracy utilizing several methods of interpretation has been reported, we have come to rely largely on visual interpretation of scintigraphic images. In addition, a simple scoring system can be applied to derive a lymphatic transport index, which can then be used to compare individual scintigraphic studies to one another.

Contrast lymphangiography should be used very selectively in patients with lymphedema. It provides useful information, however, in the evaluation of patients with lymphangiectasia, with abdominal or thoracic lymphatic fistulae, or in patients with anomalies of the thoracic duct.

Recently magnetic resonance lymphangiography has been introduced as a noninvasive technique to better evaluate the thoracic duct and superficial and deep lymphatic channels in patients with focal or diffuse vascular diseases or swelling of extremities. Using a heavily T2-weighted fast spin-echo sequence and a maximum-intensity projection algorithm, this modality can obtain further information about various vascular anomalies, which may be useful in current and future therapeutic considerations. Both axial and off-axial evaluation of lymphatic channels in conjunction with magnetic resonance venography can help differentiate lymphatics from veins.[39]

REFERENCES

1. Kinmonth JB. Lymphangiography in man; a method of outlining lymphatic trunks at operation. *Clin Sci* 1952; **11**: 13–20.
2. Kinmonth JB, Taylor GW, Tracy GD, Marsh JD. Primary lymphedema. Clinical and lymphangiographic studies of a series of 107 patients in which the lower limbs were affected. *Br J Surg* 1957; **45**: 1–10.
3. Sherman AI, Ter-Pogossian M. Lymph node concentration of radioactive colloidal gold following interstitial injection. *Cancer* 1953; **6**: 1238–40.
4. Jepson RP, Simeone FA, Dobyns BM. Removal from skin of plasma protein labelled with radioactive plasma protein. *Am J Physiol* 1953; **175**: 443–8.
5. Taylor GW, Kinmonth JB, Rollinson E, Rotblat J, Francis GE. Lymphatic circulation studied with radioactive plasma protein. *Br Med J* 1957; **1**: 133–7.
6. Bergqvist L, Strand SE, Persson BRR. Particle sizing and biokinetics of interstitial lymphoscintigraphic agents. *Semin Nucl Med* 1983; **13**: 9–19.
7. Weissleder H, Weissleder R. Lymphedema: Evaluation of qualitative and quantitative lymphoscintigraphy in 238 patients. *Radiology* 1988; **167**: 729–35.
8. Fee HJ, Robinson DS, Sample WF, Graham LS, Holmes EC, Morton DL. The determination of lymph shed by colloidal gold scanning in patients with malignant melanoma: a preliminary study. *Surgery* 1978; **84**: 626–32.
9. Meyer CM, Lecklitner ML, Logic JR, *et al.* Technetium-99m sulfur colloid cutaneous lymphoscintigraphy in the management of truncal melanoma. *Radiology* 1979; **131**: 205–9.
10. Morton DL, Wen DR, Cochran AJ. Management of early-stage melanoma by intraoperative lymphatic mapping and selective lymphadenectomy: an alternative to routine elective lymphadenectomy or 'watch and wait'. *Surg Oncol Clin North Am* 1992; **1**: 247–59.
11. Cox CE, Pendas S, Cox JM, *et al.* Guidelines for sentinel node biopsy and lymphatic mapping of patients with breast cancer. *Ann Surg* 1998; **227**: 645–53.
12. Burak WE, Walker MJ, Yee LD, *et al.* Routine preoperative lymphoscintigraphy is not necessary prior to sentinel node biopsy for breast cancer. *Am J Surg* 1999; **177**: 445–9.
13. Kelemen PR, Essner R, Foshag LJ, Morton DL. Lymphatic mapping and sentinel lymphadenectomy after wide local excision of primary melanoma. *J Am Coll Surg* 1999; **189**: 247–52.
14. Krag D, Weaver D, Ashikaga T, *et al.* The sentinel mode in breast cancer: a multicenter validation study. *N Engl J Med* 1998; **339**: 941–6.

15. Kleinhans E, Baumeister RGH, Hahn D, Siuda S, Bull U, Moser E. Evaluation of transport kinetics in lymphoscintigraphy: Follow-up study in patients with transplanted lymphatic vessels. *Eur J Nucl Med* 1985; **10**: 349–52.
16. Cambria RA, Gloviczki P, Naessens JM, Wahner HW. Noninvasive evaluation of the swollen extremity with lymphoscintigraphy: a prospective semiquantitative analysis in 386 extremities. *J Vasc Surg* 1993; **18**: 773–82.
17. Stewart G, Gaunt JI, Croft DN, Browse NL. Isotope lymphography: a new method of investigating the role of the lymphatics in chronic limb oedema. *Br J Surg* 1985; **72**: 906–9.
18. Golueke PJ, Montgomery RA, Petronis JD, Minken SL, Perler BA, Williams GM. Lymphoscintigraphy to confirm the clinical diagnosis of lymphedema. *J Vasc Surg* 1989; **10**: 306–12.
19. Richards TB, McBiles M, Collins PS. An easy method for the diagnosis of lymphedema. *Ann Vasc Surg* 1990; **4**: 255–9.
20. Ohtake E, Matsui K. Lymphoscintigraphy in patients with lymphedema. *Clin Nucl Med* 1986; **11**: 474–8.
21. Carena M, Campini R, Zelaschi G, Rossi G, Aprile C, Paroni G. Quantitative lymphoscintigraphy. *Eur J Nucl Med* 1988; **14**: 88–92.
22. Rijke AM, Croft BY, Johnson RA, de Jongste AB, Camps JAJ. Lymphoscintigraphy and lymphedema of the lower extremities. *J Nucl Med* 1990; **31**: 990–8.
23. Vaqueiro M, Gloviczki P, Fisher J Hollier LH, Schirger A, Wahner HW. Lymphoscintigraphy in lymphedema: an aid to microsurgery. *J Nucl Med* 1986; **27**: 1125–30.
24. Gloviczki P, Wahner HW. Clinical diagnosis and evaluation of lymphedema. In Rutherford RB, ed. *Vascular Surgery.* Philadelphia: WB Saunders, 1995: 1899–920.
25. Hwang JH, Kwon JY, Lee KW, *et al.* Changes in lymphatic function after complex physical therapy. *Lymphology* 1999; **32**: 15–21.
26. Meeusen R, van der Veen P, Joos E, Roeykens J, Bossuyt A, De Meirleir K. The influence of cold and compression on lymph flow at the ankle. *Clin J Sport Med* 1998; **8**: 266–71.
27. Gloviczki P, Fisher J, Hollier LH, Pairolero PC, Schirger A, Wahner HW. Microsurgical lymphovenous anastomosis for treatment of lymphedema: a critical review. *J Vasc Surg* 1988; **7**: 647–52.
28. Hollander W, Reilley P, Burrows BA. Lymphatic flow in human subjects as indicated by the disappearance of I^{131}-labelled albumin from the subcutaneous tissue. *J Clin Invest* 1961; **40**: 222–33.
29. Szabo G, Magyar Z, Papp M. Correlation between capillary filtration and lymph flow in venous congestion. *Acta Med Hung* 1963; **19**: 185–9.
30. Larcos G, Wahner HW. Lymphoscintigraphic abnormalities in venous thrombosis. *J Nucl Med* 1991; **32**: 2144–8.
31. Kadir S. The lymphatic system. In Kadir S, ed. *Diagnostic Angiography.* Philadelphia: WB Saunders, 1986: 617–41.
32. Lossef SV. Complication of lymphangiography. *Semin Interv Radiol* 1994; **11**: 107–12.
33. Weg JG, Harkleroad LE. Aberrations in pulmonary function due to lymphangiography. *Dis Chest* 1986; **53**: 534–40.
34. Koehler PR. Complications of lymphography. *Lymphology* 1986; **1**: 116–20.
35. Silvestri RC, Huseby JS, Rughani I, *et al.* Respiratory distress syndrome from lymphangiography contrast medium. *Am Rev Respir Dis* 1980; **122**: 543–9.
36. Bron KM, Baum S, Abrams HL. Oil embolism in lymphangiography: incidence, manifestations, and mechanisms. *Radiology* 1963; **80**: 194–202.
37. Hessel SJ, Adams DF, Abrams HL. Complications of angiography. *Radiology* 1981; **138**: 273–81.
38. Clouse ME, Hallgrimsson J, Wenlund DE. Complications following lymphography with particular reference to pulmonary oil embolization. *Am J Roentgenol Rad Ther Nucl Med* 1966; **96**: 972–8.
39. Laor T, Hoffer FA, Burrows PE, Kozakewich HP. MR lymphangiography in infants, children and young adults. *Am J Roentgenol* 1998; **171**: 1111–17.

47

Lymphedema: medical and physical therapy

THOM W ROOKE AND CINDY L FELTY

Lymphedema is a frustrating condition to treat. Most patients cannot be helped by surgery and are subsequently managed with elastic compression, physical therapy, drugs, proper hygiene, education, and other noncurative 'conservative' measures.[1,2] Unfortunately, many health professionals render suboptimal care because they do not fully understand the theoretical and practical aspects of nonsurgical therapy for lymphedema. It is essential that those who choose to treat patients with lymphedema not only recognize and properly use the therapeutic modalities available in their own communities, but also familiarize themselves with options available elsewhere so that difficult patients can be referred to specialized centers when appropriate.

WHY TREAT LYMPHEDEMA?

There are four major reasons for treating lymphedema.

Pain

Lymphedema is usually a painless condition, but patients will occasionally complain of significant discomfort associated with limb swelling. In rare instances, pain in the extremities is the major symptom for which the patient seeks treatment.

Impaired function

Many patients have problems with limb strength and/or mobility because of lymphedema. Severely swollen limbs (especially those with 'elephantiasis') may be so heavy that the patient cannot lift them, and when this occurs a normal lifestyle is obviously impossible. Lesser degrees of swelling can also produce significant disability. Jobs requiring fine motor skill, heavy lifting, unusual posturing, or repetitive movements may be difficult to perform when the upper extremity is swollen, especially if the dominant arm is involved. Lower limb edema can likewise limit the ability to perform activities in which prolonged standing, bending, or climbing is necessary.

Even when the edema is relatively minor, limbs that become chronically indurated and 'woody' may suffer from movement limitations which are out of proportion to the amount of swelling present in them. In some cases the inability to wear shoes, gloves, or other articles of clothing can be functionally disabling.

Cosmesis

The biggest problem caused by lymphedema is often cosmetic disfigurement. A surprisingly small amount of edema may, in the eyes of certain patients, be perceived as a major cosmetic catastrophe.

Prevention of future problems

This is probably the most common reason for treating lymphedema. Left unmanaged, there may be a tendency for limb swelling to worsen over time, or for relatively minor annoyances caused by pain, functional impairment, cosmetic disfigurement, etc., to evolve into major problems. Whether (and to what extent) aggressive therapy will prevent these problems remains uncertain. The treatment of lymphedema may reduce the chance of cellulitis in limbs with a history of recurrent infections, but the impact of this effect has not been well quantified. The ability to prevent progressive limb enlargement, fibrosis, or lymphedema-associated malignancy (Stewart–Treves syndrome) also remains uncertain.

THE TREATMENT OF LYMPHEDEMA

Step 1: make a diagnosis

Although the work-up of patients with suspected lymphedema has been discussed elsewhere, the importance of accurately diagnosing the cause of the swelling deserves re-emphasis. The diagnosis of lymphedema can usually be made from the history and physical examination. Most patients with primary lymphedema will give a 'typical' history in which swelling develops spontaneously; this often occurs at birth or in association with puberty, childbirth, or a minor injury. A familial history of limb swelling may also be present. Patients with secondary lymphedema can usually describe the precipitating event such as surgery, radiation therapy, infection, etc. The physical examination generally reveals limb swelling of a type and distribution consistent with lymphedema. If necessary, a confirmatory study such as a lymphoscintigram can be performed to confirm or document lymphatic obstruction.[3]

Conditions which may mimic lymphedema include congestive heart failure, venous disease, infective cellulitis, drug-induced swelling, reflex sympathetic dystrophy, tumor, lipedema, and a host of others. These entities can usually be differentiated from lymphedema on purely clinical grounds, but occasionally the presentation is atypical enough to warrant specific testing.

It is surprisingly common to find two or more co-morbid processes occurring simultaneously in a swollen limb. For example, patients with true lymphedema may have additional swelling caused by one or more of the conditions mentioned above (such as congestive heart failure, venous disease, drugs, etc.). The need to identify and treat these non-lymphedematous components of limb swelling is obvious but often overlooked.

Once a diagnosis of lymphedema has been confirmed with reasonable certainty, and the co-morbid causes of swelling (if any) have been identified and treated, the underlying etiology of the lymphedema should be re-addressed. Specifically, one needs to determine whether 'something else' can be done to improve the lymph flow. For example, are the lymphatic vessels obstructed by an infection or neoplastic process, which might respond to antibiotics or chemotherapy? Are antiparasitic drugs indicated? Can lymphatic reconstructive surgery be performed? Unfortunately, while the decision to proceed with 'conservative' therapy must be made in conjunction with the decision to treat the underlying cause of the lymphedema, most types of lymphedema do not have etiologies that are curable by definitive medical therapy.

Step 2: make the decision to treat

The next step in lymphedema therapy is to decide who should be treated and how aggressive the treatment should be. Numerous issues need to be considered. For example, does every patient with edema need to be treated? Is the goal of treatment to completely eliminate all traces of limb swelling? How much consideration should be given to the patient's desires and expectations with regard to therapy? As in most cases in which options exist, the correct approach is generally one that balances the benefits of treatment against the problems associated with therapy.

The benefits of treatment may be divided into those that are real and obvious (such as relief of pain, improved limb function, or significant cosmetic improvement) and those that are theoretical and/or uncertain (such as the possible prevention of complications like cellulitis, fibrosis, or malignancy). The drawbacks of treatment can likewise be subdivided into various categories. For example, there may be significant financial expense associated with the purchase of stockings, pumps, or massage services. A certain amount of physical discomfort and time commitment is inherent in the religious use of stockings, pumps, or other forms of treatment. Finally, the decision to treat creates a potential for emotional stress because it forces the patient to concede that he/she has a 'disease' that cannot be 'cured' and for which the patient must be 'treated'.

Treatment decisions must therefore be individualized for every patient based upon the potential for benefit versus the likelihood that the patient will experience difficulties tolerating or complying with treatment. In some cases the practitioner must try to convince a reluctant patient that edema therapy should be instituted; in others, the patient will demand from the practitioner extraordinary, time-consuming, or uncomfortable therapies for seemly minor degrees of edema. The art of therapy lies in matching the intensity of treatment with the severity of disease in a way that meets the needs and expectations of both the practitioner and the patient, and in doing so assures that the patient will comply with recommendations.

Step 3: assess the patient's overall prognosis and establish short/long-term goals

This is really an extension of the 'whether or not to treat' and 'how aggressively to treat' issues. Once a decision has been reached to initiate therapy, the ultimate goal of treatment should be defined. For example, treatment strategies in a poor-prognosis patient with lymphedema secondary to metastatic cancer (or another life-threatening disease) may emphasize short-term goals like pain relief, moderate control of swelling with elastic wraps or garments, treatment or prevention of cellulitis, and other measures directed largely at maintaining comfort. Extremely aggressive therapeutic measures that require expensive pumps, prolonged and costly massage treatments, rigorous dietary and exercise programs, or fanatical compliance may not be in the patient's best interests. By contrast, patients with lymphedema and a 'good prognosis' (such as those with primary lymphedema) need to think in terms of lifelong management strategies. Expensive, aggressive, time-consuming therapies make more sense for these patients; the commitments made early to accept the cost, discomfort, and discipline of therapy will usually be justified by the expected long-term benefits.

Step 4: get the swelling down

The most important aspect of lymphedema therapy is to maximally reduce the limb swelling prior to instituting maintenance therapy, and failure to do this is the most common reason for treatment failures. It is much easier to maintain the size of a fully reduced limb (using elastic compression, pumps, etc.) than it is to control edema in a partially reduced limb in which significant residual swelling remains. Patients with lymphedema who are fitted with graduated elastic compression stockings prior to achieving maximal limb reduction are almost always doomed to a future of poor swelling control.

A lymphedematous limb can be reduced using a number of methods, alone or in combination.

BED REST/LEG ELEVATION

Although it is one of the best methods available for decreasing limb swelling, the aggressive use of strict bed rest and leg elevation usually requires hospitalization to be maximally effective. Not surprisingly, this approach has fallen out of favor in recent years; the rising cost of hospital stays and the reluctance of third party payers to cover such 'non-essential' hospitalizations has made this form of therapy relatively uncommon. Nonetheless, it is a method of 'last resort' for patients with severe lymphedema, especially when the swelling is resistant to less aggressive forms of outpatient therapy, and it is a treatment that clearly deserves further study to determine its cost-efficiency relative to other forms of reduction therapy.

Leg elevation utilizes gravity to drain fluid from the edematous limb, and the higher the limb can be elevated, the greater the theoretical benefit. Simply elevating the foot of the bed, or propping the limb up on pillows is a reasonable option between periods when other forms of treatment are being used. Special foam 'wedges' can be purchased and placed on the end of the bed to elevate the legs more efficiently and comfortably than can be achieved with pillows alone. However, truly aggressive elevation therapy requires the use of special slings to hoist the arm or leg as high as the patient can tolerate (Fig. 47.1). Several days of aggressive treatment with these slings will usually reduce all but the most resistant cases of lymphedema.

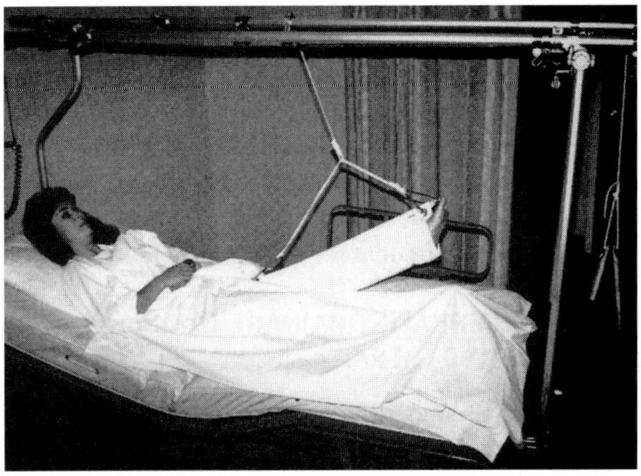

Figure 47.1 *Lymphedema sling. The sling enables the patient to keep his/her leg elevated while in bed, typically to 45° or more.*

PUMPS

In most US practices, pneumatic pumping has become the mainstay of reduction therapy. Patients are typically pumped for one to three sessions per day, with each session lasting 30–60 minutes. The pumps are often located in a hospital or outpatient setting; if this is the case, patients must therefore come to the facility for treatment. Between sessions the limb is wrapped with elastic to prevent re-accumulation of edema. Some types of pumps can be left on for prolonged periods while the patient is in bed; treatment sessions lasting 6 hours or more are possible with this approach. Pumping is generally pursued until no further reduction in limb size can be achieved, at which time maintenance therapy is instituted.

Several types of pump are currently available for patients with lymphedema. These include:

- single chamber. These pumps have an inflatable single chamber sleeve that encases the limb. During the inflation period the limb is cyclically compressed at a predetermined pressure (usually 60–100 mmHg) for a fixed length of time (usually 20–40 seconds). The uniform pressure forces fluid out of the limb through the veins and remaining lymphatics. Experience shows that many edematous limbs can be adequately reduced with single chamber pumps.
- multichamber pumps. Pneumatic pumps utilizing multi-chambered sleeves are popular devices for treating lymphedema. By sequentially inflating the chambers in the sleeve, fluid can be 'milked' out of the swollen limb. Although these pumps appear to be more effective than single chamber units, they are also more expensive.
- cardiac-gaited pumps. Some pumps use single chamber sleeves which inflate in a cardiosynchronous fashion (i.e. they inflate during a specific portion of the cardiac cycle, usually to a pressure of

approximately 60 mmHg, then deflate during the remainder of the cardiac cycle).

Although these pumps can be used to reduce or treat lymphedema, they are expensive to purchase (US$10 000 or more) and usually require trained assistance to operate. It is uncertain whether these pumps offer any benefit over conventional single or multi-chamber units.

MANUAL LYMPHATIC DRAINAGE/COMPLEX DECONGESTIVE THERAPY

Massage has been used for centuries to force fluid from swollen limbs, but the modern form of massage-based therapies for lymphedema known as manual lymphatic drainage (MLD) and complex decongestive therapy (CDT) have largely emerged over the last hundred years.[4] MLD refers to the actual massage technique used to push edema from swollen limbs; it was developed in the early 1930s by Dr Emil Vodder and has evolved into one of the most accepted methods for massaging swollen limbs. CDT combines the use of massage to reduce the limb with a well-defined program of exercise, elastic compression, hygiene, and bandaging to control the swelling once reduction is achieved. These techniques enjoy considerable popularity in Europe and Australia, and are now becoming widely available in the USA and Canada. Clinics specializing in this approach are currently accessible to many North American patients with lymphedema.

MLD massage is typically performed by a therapist who has been properly trained in the technique (training programs are now conducted in the USA and Canada as well as in Europe). Treatment is usually initiated by massaging the chest or abdomen in order to empty the central lymphatic vessels and prepare them to receive peripheral lymph fluid from the limbs (Fig. 47.2). The therapist then massages distally along the affected limb (Figs 47.3, 47.4). Light massage is generally favored to stimulate lymphatic flow and gently push fluid through the obstructed vessels. Two or three massage sessions may be conducted per day; between each session, the limb is tightly wrapped with bandages to prevent fluid re-accumulation. The massage sessions, which can require 2 weeks or more to maximally reduce a limb, are generally performed in conjunction with regular educational sessions stressing hygiene, specific exercise, diet, elastic compression, and other aspects of edema management.

At this time there are only limited data comparing the edema-reducing efficacy (or cost/benefit ratio) of massage-oriented techniques to other modalities such as bed rest with limb elevation or pneumatic pump therapy.

Compression bandaging can be a primary therapy for lymphedema, or may be used in conjunction with other reduction measures such as pumping or massage. Bandaging forces fluid from the limb and prevents its return when the limb is dependent. Compression bandaging also compensates for the loss of tissue elasticity and helps restore limb shape.

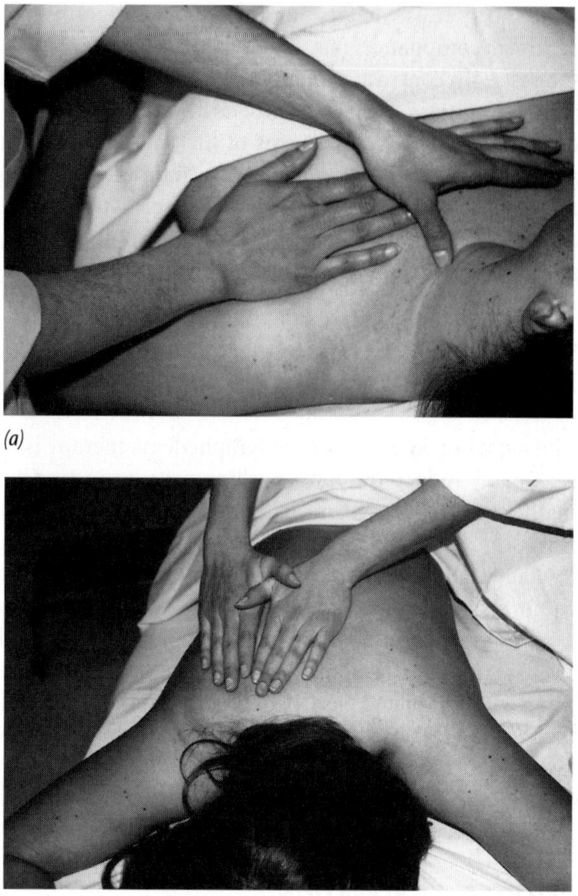

(a)

(b)

Figure 47.2 *Manual lymphatic drainage – chest massage. Massage therapy for an edematous arm begins with the thorax. Gentle massage is performed over both the anterior (a) and posterior (b) portions of the chest to stimulate thoracic lymph flow and empty the central lymphatic vessels. The region of the chest contralateral to the affected limb is massaged first, followed by the ipsilateral region of the chest.*

OTHER TECHNIQUES

Numerous adjuvant techniques for reducing lymphedema have been touted as useful. These include oddities such as high-compression pumps which utilize mercury-filled bladders to compress the limbs,[5] the use of microwave diathermy or ovens to heat the swollen limb prior to bandaging,[6] and simply puncturing the skin so that the edema fluid leaks out. In general, the safety, effectiveness, and proper role (if any) of these methods remains uncertain or dubious.

Step 5: maintaining limb reduction

After the edema in the limb is maximally reduced, the re-accumulation of fluid must be prevented. This is

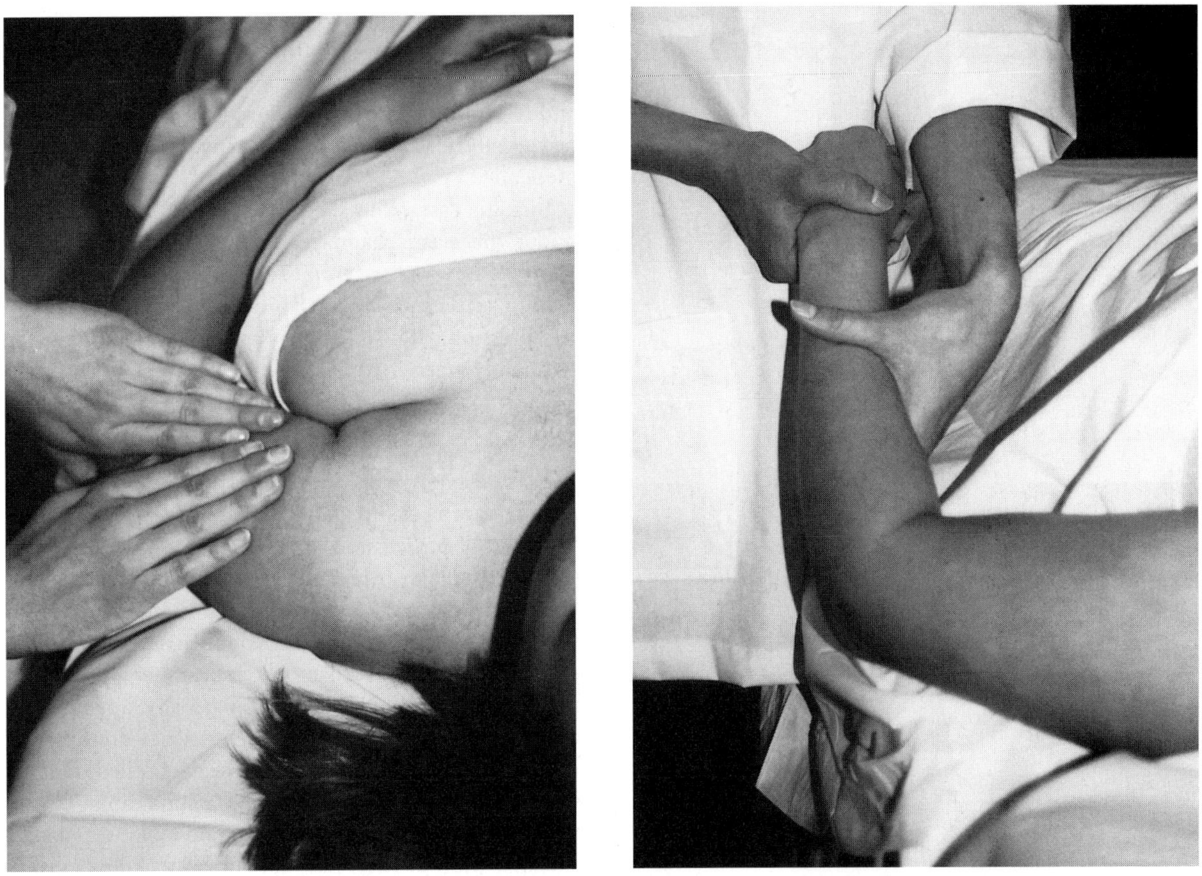

(a) (b)

Figure 47.3 *Manual lymphatic drainage – arm massage. After the thoracic lymphatic vessels have been emptied, the arm is massaged. Using gentle, often circular motions, the therapist stimulates the lymphatics and pushes fluid along the arm toward the thorax. Massage proceeds slowly in a proximal (a) to distal (b) direction.*

accomplished by using either elastic or non-elastic compression, sometimes in conjunction with various adjunctive therapies when necessary.[7]

The most important aspect of maintenance therapy is to correctly match the intensity of the treatment to the severity of the patient's disease. Maintenance therapy is a lifelong process; if the program is too aggressive, then rigorous compliance may be difficult to achieve, and if it is inadequate the swelling will return. The key to success is therefore in developing a maintenance program which is so simple, comfortable, and easy to comply with, that the patient will follow it religiously, yet still intensive enough to control the swelling. Unfortunately, practitioners often forget that therapies that are not complied with (because they are too expensive, uncomfortable, or difficult to use) will fail as surely as those which are intrinsically inadequate.

ELASTIC COMPRESSION

Compression is the mainstay of most maintenance programs, and it is generally applied in the form of elastic wraps or graduated elastic compression stockings.

Elastic wraps

Elastic bandages come in a variety of types, widths, thicknesses, and materials. The most important distinction is between long- and short-stretch types. Long-stretch wraps, including brands such as ACE®, CoNCo®, DuPey®, and Setopress®, are relatively compliant and tend to 'give' more when applied around the limb (these wraps typically stretch to 100% or more of their original length). By contrast, short-stretch wraps, including brands such as Komprex® and Durelast®, are 'stiffer' and may provide better control of swelling (these typically stretch to 70% or less of their original length). Short-stretch bandages tend to be more expensive and (in some cases) less comfortable to wear than the long-stretch variety. An extreme example of a short-stretch wrap is the Esmark® bandage, which is basically a long piece of rubber that can be wound around the leg to provide exceptional compression. By exploring different wraps, a suitable match can usually be found for any given limb.

There are several methods for applying wraps, including the spiral and figure-of-eight techniques (Fig. 47.5). Using either method, the 'tightness' can be controlled by

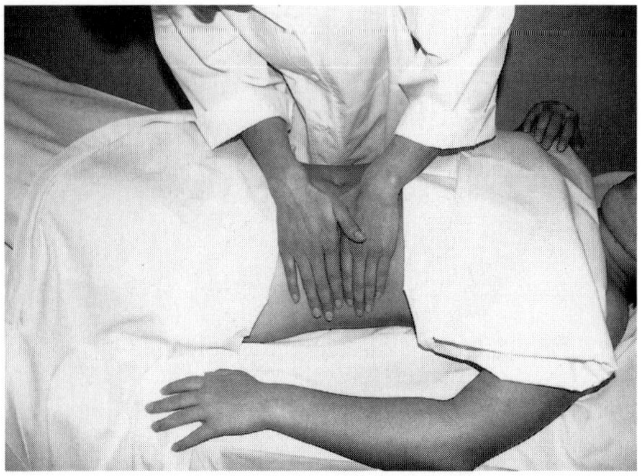

(a)

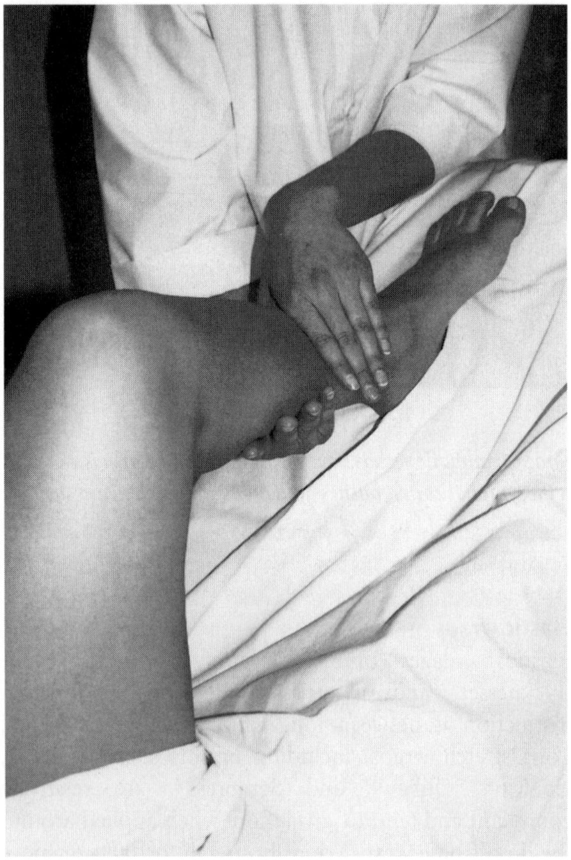

(b)

Figure 47.4 *Manual lymphatic drainage – lower extremities. Lower extremity edema reduction begins with massage of the trunk (a) including regions both contralateral and ipsilateral to the swollen limb. Massage then proceeds distally along the leg (b).*

manually determining the degree to which the wrap is stretched during the application, and the 'stiffness' can be altered by varying the amount of overlap that occurs each time the limb is encircled (the usual overlap is approximately 2.5–5 cm at the ankle). Wraps must be applied proximally enough on the limb to directly compress the regions in which the control of swelling is desired (for example, thigh swelling can not be controlled if the wrap is applied exclusively to the calf), and re-wrapping needs to be performed every 3–6 hours because the elastic tends to loosen over time and become ineffective.

In some cases, thin sheets of foam rubber are applied under the elastic bandages to add extra stiffness and compression to the wrap. This foam can also protect delicate areas such as bony prominences from excessive compression. Re-wrapping may be required less frequently when foam is used.

Graduated elastic compression stockings

Stockings, like bandages, come in a variety of materials, styles, and types (Fig. 47.6). Custom-fit and ready-made products are available, and the most popular brands come from the USA, Germany and Switzerland. Stockings have several advantages over bandages, including their ability to be worn all day without need for significant readjustment (unlike wraps, which must be reapplied several times per day) and improved cosmetic appearance. Drawbacks include cost (which may be US$100 per stocking or more) and the difficulties some people experience donning and doffing them. Patients with joint disease, limited mobility, weakness, poor eyesight, general debilitation, or any significant disability may find it impossible to put on a stocking without help. Like bandages, stockings must be worn religiously to control swelling.

Important factors to assess when prescribing a stocking including:

- fit: stocking measurements must be made by a fitting expert after the limb has been maximally reduced. If a ready-made garment of proper size is not available, or if a custom-made stocking is needed, the reduction in limb size must be maintained with elastic bandages or other devices until the desired stocking arrives. The accuracy of the fit must be reassessed once the stocking is worn.
- material and brand: these factors affect the cost, comfort, and longevity of a stocking. As long as an accurate fit and proper compression is provided, the material and brand are largely a matter of patient preference. The life span of a typical stocking (worn daily) is usually 3–4 months, although specific guarantees on workmanship, compression, etc., may vary among brands.
- length: stockings should reach proximally enough on the limb to cover the swollen areas, and steps must be taken to ensure that the stockings stay up; these steps may include the use of skin glue, garter belts, or pantyhose. In some patients (especially men) compliance with the recommendation to use stockings will be much better with a shorter garment, and the use of shorter stockings should occasionally be considered even if the edema in the proximal leg is not well controlled.

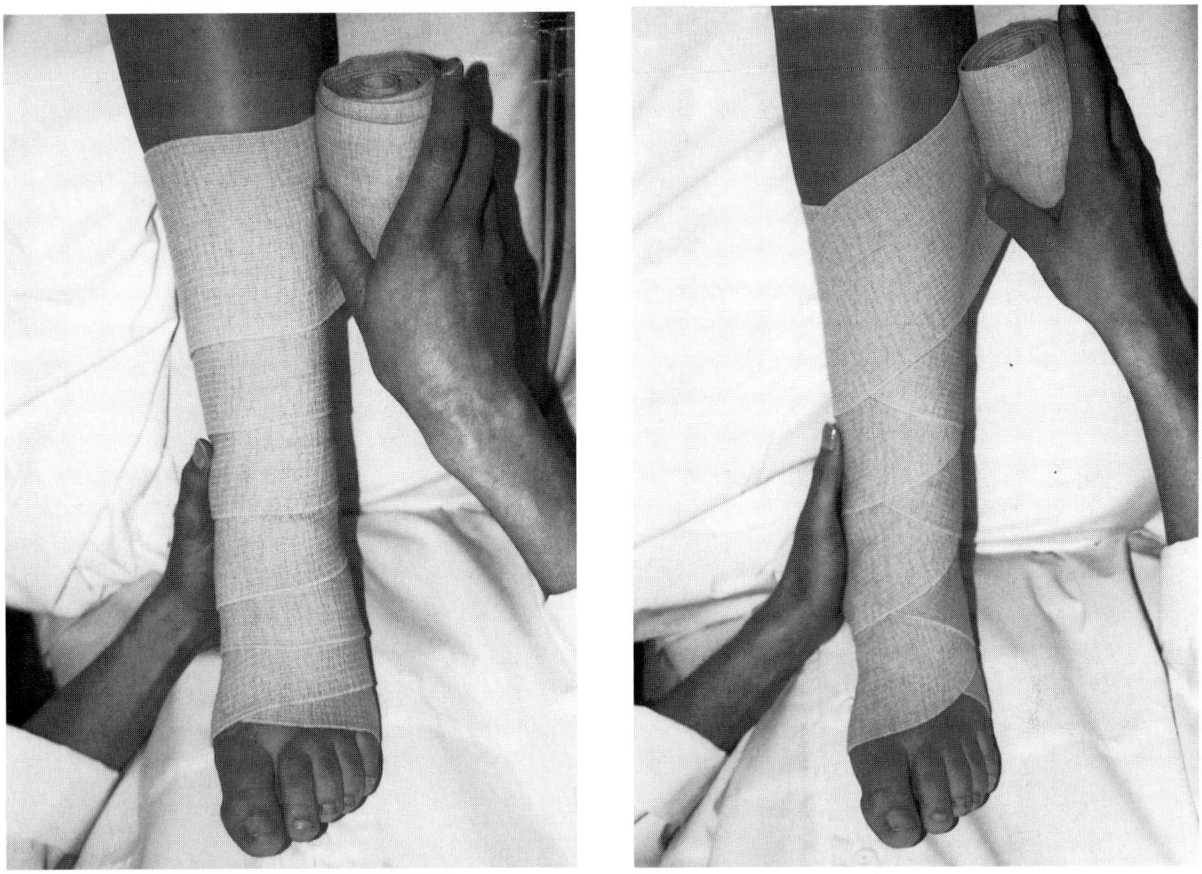

Figure 47.5 *Techniques for applying elastic wrap. (a) Spiral: beginning at the foot, the wrap is applied up the leg in a spiral fashion. The overlap should be greatest at the foot and ankle (2.5–5 cm) and progressively less as the wrap ascends the leg. This technique is easier for the patient to use than most others, but the wrap tends to loosen and slip during the day. (b) Figure-of-eight: the extra overlap inherent in this technique tends to provide more compression and less 'slipping' than the spiral approach.*

- compression: a pressure of 40–50 mmHg (at the ankle) is usually needed to control lymphedema, but pressures of 50–60 mmHg or greater may sometimes be required. The difficulty associated with donning and wearing a stocking increases as the amount of compression arises.

NON-ELASTIC COMPRESSION

Non-elastic wraps can be used to compress limbs and prevent the swelling of lymphedema. One such non-elastic system is the CircAid®. The device is a series of non-stretch, adjustable compression bands, which are applied over the ankle and calf. The adjustable compression bands are closed with Velcro and can be tightened as limb reduction occurs.

SUPPLEMENTARY USE OF 'REDUCTION' MEASURES TO HELP MAINTAIN LIMB SIZE

Elevation

Many of the measures described previously for reducing limb swelling can also be used on an intermittent or as-needed basis to help maintain a limb in the reduced state. The simplest of these is elevation. Patients should always be encouraged to elevate their affected limb as high and as often as possible each day, allowing gravity to periodically help drain the fluid from their limbs.

Pumps

The use of pumps is more controversial. Many patients can purchase or rent a pump for use at home; typical therapeutic approaches with these units range from use on an as-needed basis to religious overnight and daily sessions. Single-chamber pumps may be purchased for less than US$1000, while top-of-the-line sequential models can approach US$10 000. Although the multi-chamber sequential pumps may be more effective at maintaining reduction, it is clear that some patients can be adequately treated with less expensive single-chamber models. If pump therapy is to be used for long-term maintenance treatment, it makes financial sense to acquire the least expensive type that will 'do the job'. Not surprisingly, some manufacturers have campaigned aggressively to persuade physicians and patients to invest early in expensive multi-chamber sequential pumps –

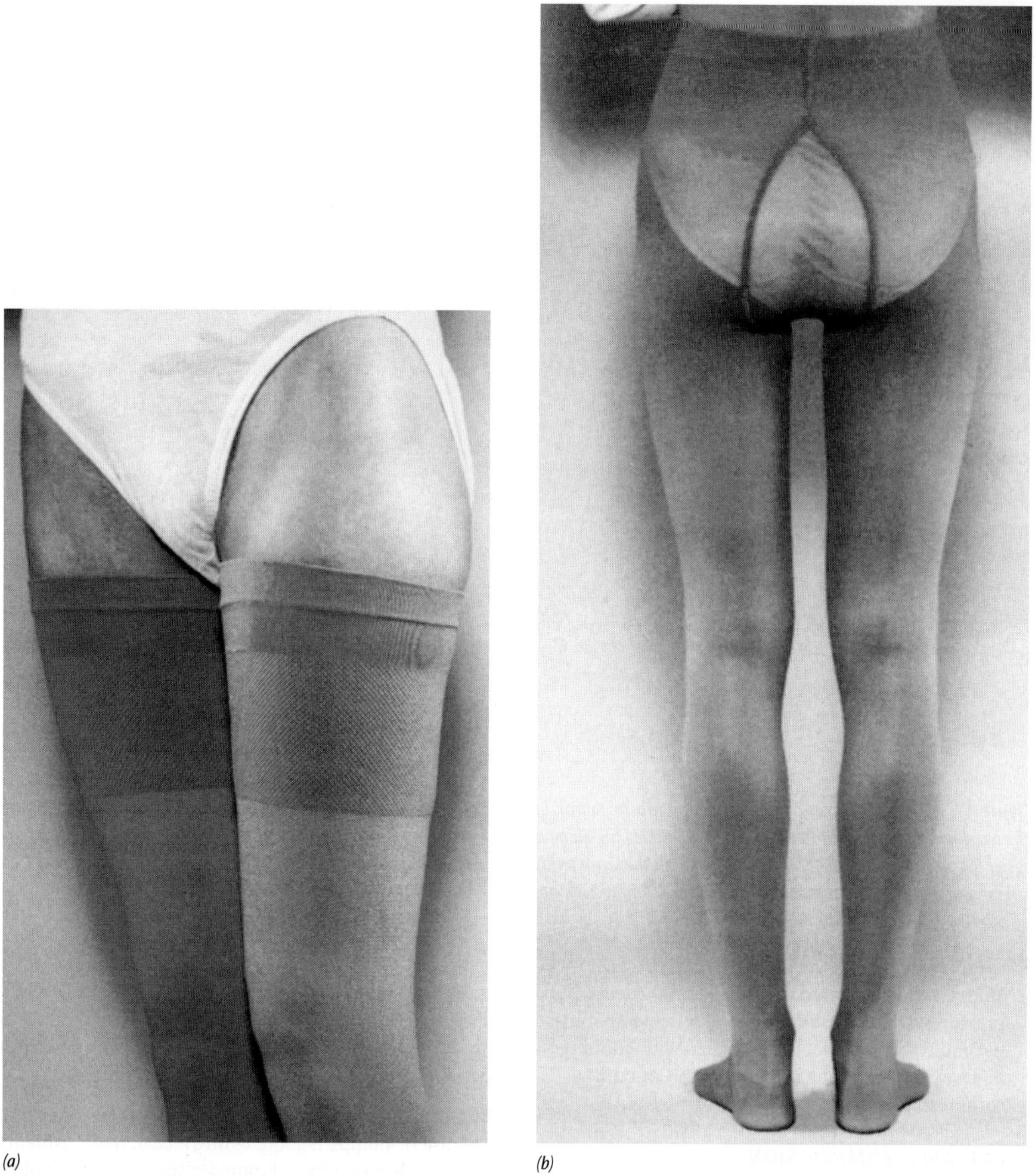

(a) (b)

Figure 47.6 *Graduated elastic compression stockings. Compression stockings come in various lengths including calf, thigh-high (a), and pantyhose (b). The compression must be adequate to control the swelling (typically 40–50 mmHg or more) and the length must be sufficient to cover the affected regions of the leg.*

even when the lymphedema may be minor – on the pretext that all lymphedema patients deserve 'the best' pump available to treat and prevent swelling. This knee-jerk approach should be discouraged; it clearly fails to recognize that low-cost alternatives may be sufficient for a particular patient.

Whenever possible, pumps should be rented rather than purchased until a decision can be made about a particular model's comfort and performance, or whether a different model should be tried. The ability to get a pump repaired or serviced locally should influence a decision about 'what brand to buy'.

Massage

Manual lymphatic drainage can be performed on either a regular or as-needed basis to help maintain limb reduction. There may be financial, social, or practical problems in visiting a massage therapist regularly for the rest of a patient's life, but in selected situations the benefits of a rigorous long-term maintenance massage program might outweigh the risks and costs.

It is obvious that not every patient with lymphedema will need an aggressive long-term massage program, just as not every patient requires an expensive pump. More research is needed to identify ways to determine which patient should be treated with pumps versus massage versus other adjunct measures. It would also be valuable to objectively explore whether pumps and massage can be used in a complementary fashion; at this time most clinicians offering massage therapy advise strongly against the use of pumps, arguing that pumping can damage tissue and is a poor method for removing lymph fluid.[8,9]

Exercise

In many patients, specific exercises (frequently performed with the limbs wrapped and/or elevated) constitute the major component of maintenance therapy. The exercises usually emphasize gentle motions that not only activate the muscle pumps to move lymph fluid, but also help to keep the affected limb toned and flexible.

Step 6: additional considerations

DIET

Although specific dietary measures have been advocated to treat lymphedema,[10] the most important dietary considerations are to avoid:

- unnecessary salt intake, and
- excessive weight gain.

Too much salt can lead to an increase in total body fluid, which in turn may aggravate lymphedema. Obesity also tends to worsen lymphedema. Fatty limbs are not only larger and more difficult to compress than lean limbs, but the excess adipose tissue seems to make the limb more susceptible to lymphedema formation. Generalized obesity may also contribute to swelling by impairing venous return, or by interfering with exercise, pneumatic pump therapy, limb elevation, and other edema-reducing activities that are dependent upon limb mobility.

DIURETICS

Diuretics are probably most important during the initial phase of aggressive lymphedema therapy when rapid reduction is occurring and large quantities of fluid are moving from the tissue space into the systemic circulation. In some cases, diuretics may play a minor role in maintaining the reduction in lymphedema, but they are certainly not curative. Just as chronic, excessive salt intake may aggravate lymphedema, the daily removal of salt by dietary measures and/or diuretics may improve it. Unfortunately, diuretics cannot remove the excess protein that has become trapped in the interstitial space; this protein is the major cause of lymphedema. If used, diuretics should be taken sparingly and only in conjunction with other measures aimed at controlling the edema.

AVOIDANCE OF DRUGS THAT EXACERBATE EDEMA

Many drugs cause fluid retention and aggravate lymphedema; their use should be avoided whenever possible. Some of the worst offenders include non-steroidal anti-inflammatory drugs, calcium blockers and steroids. Estrogens may cause edema to worsen in some individuals, and whenever they are used their benefits as contraceptives or replacement agents should be carefully weighed against their potential to cause additional swelling.

ANTIBIOTICS

All patients with significant lymphedema are at risk for cellulitis and lymphangitis. These infections may develop spontaneously, but they usually result from an identifiable episode of trauma, or occur in conjunction with an obvious portal of entry through the skin (such as a foreign body, cutaneous fungal infection, ingrown hair, etc.). The causative agent is typically *Streptococcus*, and recurrent episodes are common.

Each attack of cellulitis or lymphangitis tends to destroy some of the remaining lymphatic vessels, which in turn may cause the edema to worsen. For this reason infections should be treated promptly when they develop, and prophylactic antibiotic therapy should be instituted without hesitation if repeated episodes occur. The drug of choice is penicillin (usually 500 mg orally three or four times a day for cellulitis, and less for prophylaxis) although occasionally drugs with broader spectrums are used (especially in penicillin-allergic patients). Patients with lymphedema who have a history of cellulitis or lymphangitis should be given a prescription for antibiotics which can be filled and kept at home; therapy should be initiated at the first sign of infection and maintained for 7–10 days once it is started. Small doses of antibiotics may be taken daily for prophylaxis, although a popular alternative regimen is to treat with therapeutic doses for 1 week out of each month.

MALIGNANCY SCREENING

Patients with long-standing lymphedema, either primary or secondary, are at a small but definite risk of developing malignancies such as angiosarcoma in the affected limb. This phenomenon (the Stewart–Treves syndrome) may affect up to 1% of those with chronic lymphedema, and regular monitoring for unusual masses or skin changes is therefore indicated.[11] Patients need to be educated about the problem and taught to check their limbs carefully for abnormalities; physicians must likewise inspect and palpate for tumors at every follow-up visit. Any suspicious lesion should be biopsied or removed promptly.

BENZOPYRONES

This class of drugs is not currently approved by the FDA for use in the USA, but they are widely available elsewhere in the world.[12] These agents are thought to exert a beneficial effect by, in part, stimulating macrophages to increase the breakdown of proteins trapped in the interstitial space. This theoretically reduces both swelling and fibrosis, making the limb easier to reduce in size. One of the most popular benzopyrones for treating lymphedema is coumarin; this drug does not have anticoagulant properties and should not be confused with Coumadin (warfarin). The standard dose of coumarin is 400–800 mg/day, given in a single or divided dose. Once instituted, coumarin takes months or even years to exert a maximal effect on limb reduction.

Recent evidence suggests that coumarin may not be as effective as originally thought, and that the incidence of side-effects, including serious liver toxicity, is significant.[13] For these reasons the use of coumarin cannot be endorsed for routine practice.

GENETIC COUNSELING

Certain forms of primary lymphedema are heritable including Milroy's disease (in which the swelling is present at or near birth) and Meige's disease (which is familial lymphedema praecox).[14] Genetic counseling to discuss the risk of having affected offspring should be provided for all patients with familial lymphedema.

PSYCHOLOGICAL COUNSELING

Most patients adapt well to the limitations and adversities associated with lymphedema. Some do not. When necessary, counseling may be a valuable addition to physical and medical therapy. This is especially true for the adolescent with new onset disease in whom body image, physical appearance, and self-esteem may be tightly linked.[15] Rarely, patients may receive significant, often unrecognized secondary gains from their lymphedema. In a few cases the edema may be factitial (Secretan's syndrome or *oedème bleu*).[16,17] Not surprisingly, factitial edema can be extremely resistant to any form of therapy, including psychiatric.

REFERENCES

1. Kobayashi M, Miller T. Lymphedema. *Clin Plast Surg* 1987; **14**(2): 303–13.
2. Cooke J, Rooke T. Lymphedema. In Loscalzo J, Creager M, Dzau V, eds. *Vascular Medicine*, 1st edn. Waltham, MA: Little, Brown, and Company, 1992: 1099–113.
3. Cambria R, Gloviczki P, Naessens J, *et al.* Noninvasive evaluation of the lymphatic system with lymphoscintigraphy: a prospective, semiquantitative analysis in 386 extremities. *J Vasc Surg* 1993; **18**: 773–82.
4. Földi E, Földi M, Clodius L. The lymphedema chaos: a lancet. *Ann Plast Surg* 1989; **22**(6): 505–15.
5. Palmer A, Macchiaverna J, Braun A, *et al.* Compression therapy of limb edema using hydrostatic pressure of mercury. *Angiology* 1991; **42**(7): 533–42.
6. Liu N, Olszewski W. The influence of local hyperthermia on lymphedema and lymphedematous skin of the human leg. *Lymphology* 1993; **26**: 28–37.
7. Pappas C, O'Donnell T. Long-term results of compression treatment for lymphedema. *J Vasc Surg* 1992; **16**: 555–64.
8. Eliska O, Eliskova M. Are peripheral lymphatics damaged by high pressure manual massage? *Lymphology* 1995; **28**: 21–30.
9. Eliska O, Eliskova M. Massage and damage to lymphatics (editorial). *Lymphology* 1995; **28**: 1–3.
10. Soria P, Cuesta A, Romero H, *et al.* Dietary treatment of lymphedema by restriction of long-chain triglycerides (abstract). *Angiology* 1994; **45**(8): 703.
11. Schmitz-Rixen T, Horsch S, Arnold G. Angiosarcoma in primary lymphedema of the lower extremity – Stewart–Treves syndrome. *Lymphology* 1984; **17**: 50–3.
12. Casley-Smith J, Morgan R, Piller N. Treatment of lymphedema of the arms and legs with 5,6-benzo-[α]-pyrone. *N Engl J Med* 1993; **329**(16): 1158–63.
13. Loprinzi CL, Kugler JW, Sloan JA, *et al.* Lack of effect of coumarin in women with lymphedema after treatment for breast cancer. *N Engl J Med* 1999; **340**(5): 346–50.
14. Wheeler E, Chan V, Wassman R, *et al.* Familial lymphedema praecox: Miege's disease. *Plast Reconstr Surg* 1981; **67**(3): 362–4.
15. Smeltzer D, Stickler G, Schirger A. Primary lymphedema in children and adolescents: a follow-up study and review. *Pediatrics* 1985; **76**(2): 206–18.
16. Brunning J, Gibson A, Perry M. Oedème bleu: a reappraisal. *Lancet* 1980; **1**: 810–12.
17. Jørgensen J, Gammeltoft M, Schmidt H. Factitious lymphoedema, Secretan's syndrome. *Acta Derm Venereol (Stockh)* 1983; **63**(3): 271–3.

48

Principles of surgical treatment of chronic lymphedema

PETER GLOVICZKI

Congenital or acquired obstruction of lymph vessels or lymph-conducting elements of lymph nodes result in impaired lymphatic transport. Primary or secondary valvular incompetence also decreases normal lymphatic transport capacity. Protein-rich extracellular fluid accumulates and chronic lymphedema develops when the collateral lymphatic circulation becomes insufficient and when all compensatory mechanisms, including the tissue macrophage activity or drainage through spontaneous lymphovenous anastomoses have been exhausted. Since the transport of excess tissue fluid containing lymphocytes, different plasma proteins, immunoglobulins and cytokines is impaired, chronic inflammatory changes in the subcutaneous tissue and skin also occurs.

A variety of surgical techniques have been attempted to treat patients with chronic lymphedema. The large number of individual techniques of physiologic and excisional operations that are practiced today worldwide is testimony to our frustration to deal with this difficult problem.

The principles of excisional operations have been to remove the excess tissue to decrease the volume of the extremity.[1,2] Physiologic operations (Fig. 48.1) have been aimed at restoring lymphatic transport capacity with lymphovenous anastomoses, lymphatic grafting, enteromesenteric bridge operation or free transfer of normal lymphatic tissue.[3–12] Lymphatic valvular incompetence has been treated by ligation and excision of retroperitoneal lymphatics, with or without lymphovenous anastomoses.

PREOPERATIVE DIAGNOSTIC EVALUATION

Imaging studies are used selectively, depending on the age of the patient, the presentation of the disease and whether surgical treatment is planned or not. Computed tomography is important to exclude underlying malignancy and magnetic resonance imaging is used in patients with suspected congenital vascular malformation. Duplex scanning of deep veins excludes venous occlusion or valvular incompetence. Lymphoscintigraphy is used now most frequently as the main diagnostic tool to evaluate the lymphatic system. The study involves interstitial injections of small amounts of radiolabeled antimony trisulfide colloid (technetium-99m-labeled Sb_2S_3colloid) into the interdigital space and subsequently imaging the extremity with dual-headed gamma counter. Details of this text are discussed in Chapter 46. The semiquantitative transport index of Kleinhans and Baumeister has been used in our experience to document the severity of the edema.[9] In our institution, the sensitivity of the semiquantitative interpretation is excellent (92%) with a specificity of close to 100% for the diagnosis of lymphedema. It remains the test of choice in differentiating lymphedema from edemas of other origin.

Contrast lymphangiography in our experience is reserved for patients with chylous reflux, abdominal or thoracic chylous fistulas or for evaluation of the thoracic duct. We have used contrast lymphangiogram occasionally, however, for preoperative assessment of chronic lymphedema before lymphatic microsurgery.

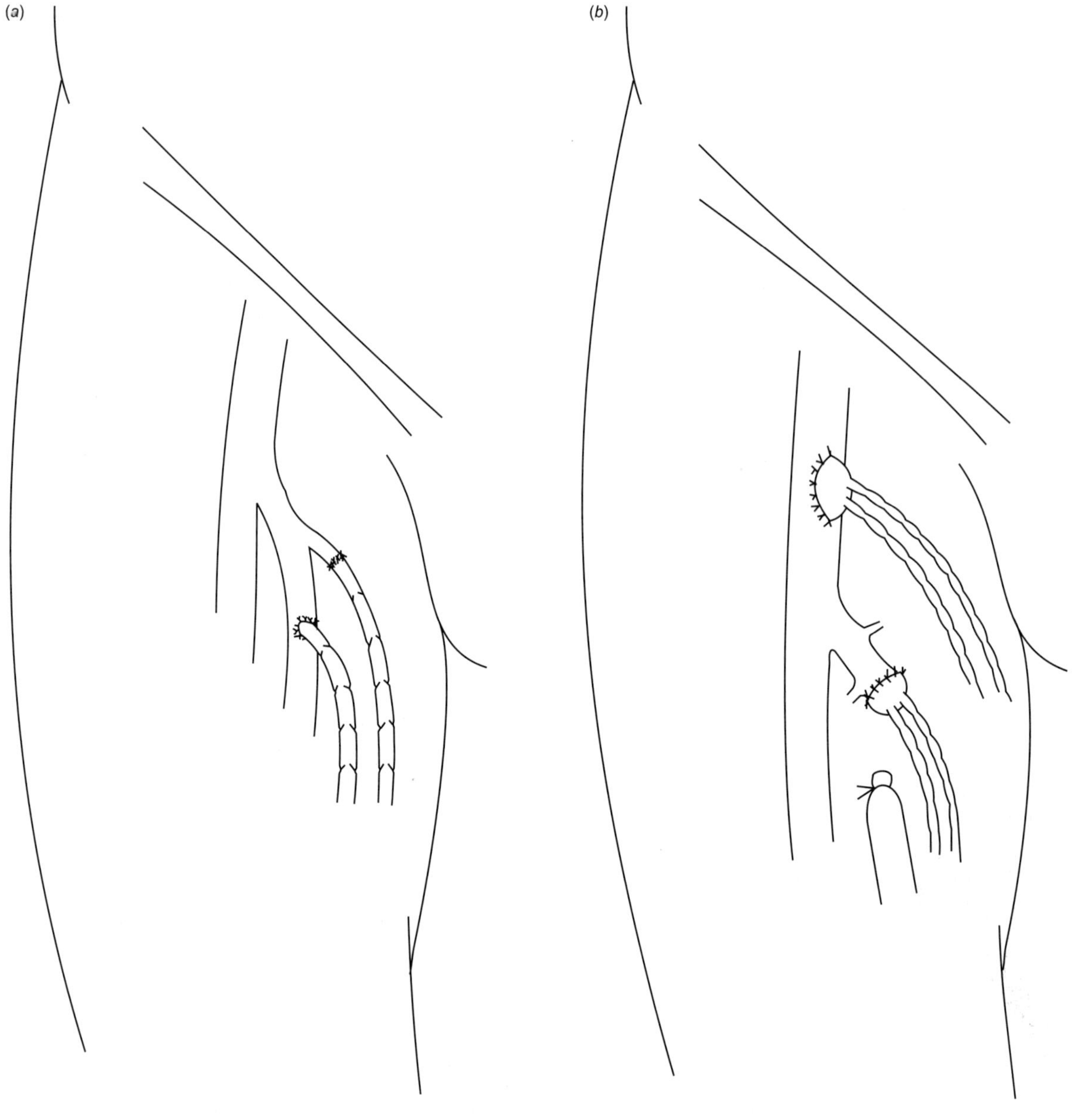

Figure 48.1 *Reconstruction for lymphatic obstruction in secondary lymphedema. (a) End-to-end and end-to-side lymph node–vein anastomosis. (b) End-to-end and end-to-side lymph vessel–vein anastomosis.*

SURGICAL TREATMENT

Potential indications for surgical intervention are:

- impaired function and movement of the involved extremity due to its large size and weight in patients, not responding to medical management;
- recurrent episodes of cellulitis and lymphangitis;
- intractable pain;
- lymphangiosarcoma; and
- cosmesis (patient unwilling to undergo more conservative treatment and willing to proceed even with experimental operations).

Operations for lymphedema are divided into two major groups: excisional and lymphatic reconstruction.

Excisional operations

Excisional procedures usually include staged removal of the lymphedematous subcutaneous tissue of the leg. If the skin is diseased and has to be resected, coverage with skin grafting is necessary. The most radical excisional operation, the Charles procedure, includes total skin and subcutaneous tissue excision of the lower extremity from the tibial tuberosity to the malleoli. It is seldom performed today. The skin grafts are unfortunately difficult to manage with frequent localized sloughing (especially in areas of recurrent cellulitis), excessive scarring, hyperkeratosis and dermatitis.

The modified Homans operations (Servelle's excisional operation, Miller's staged subcutaneous

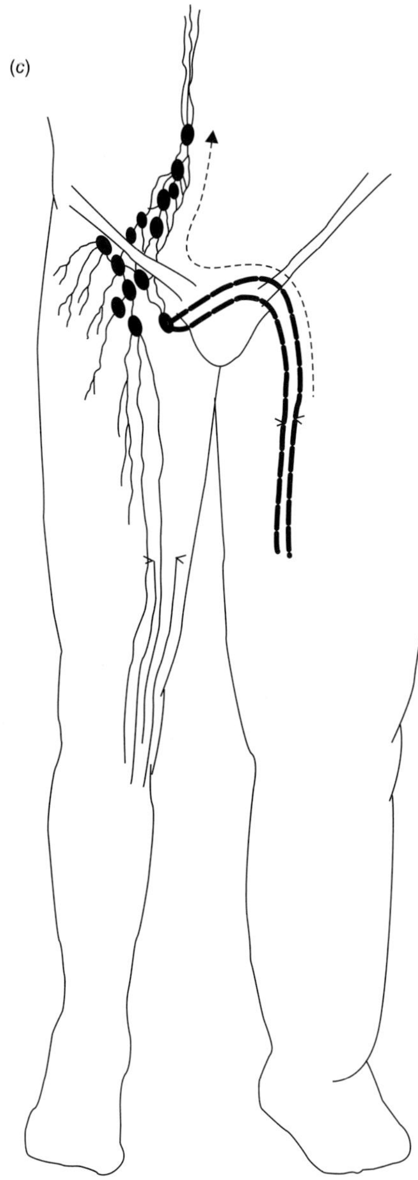

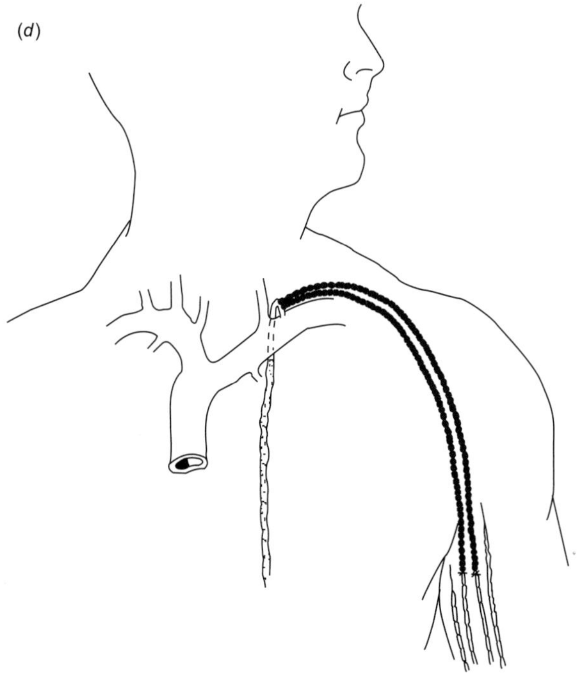

Figure 48.1 *(c) Cross-femoral lymph vessel transposition for secondary lymphedema of the left lower extremity. (d) Treatment of postmastectomy lymphedema with transplantation of two lymph channels from the lower to the upper extremity.*

excision, Pflug's staged excisional operations) involve localized excision of the fibrosed edematous subcutaneous tissue. Moderately thick flaps (1–1.5 cm) are elevated anteriorly and posteriorly to the mid-sagittal plane in the calf and/or thigh. The redundant skin is excised and the wound is closed usually in one layer only. Since not all edematous tissue is excised, most of these are palliative procedures and the results are directly related to the amount of subcutaneous tissue excised. The patients are susceptible to recurrences and should continue to wear elastic compression stockings. The results of most of these procedures are good as far as volume reduction is concerned. However, prolonged hospitalization, poor wound healing, long surgical scars, sensory nerve loss, residual edema of the foot and ankle can be problems and prevent offering such procedures short of disabling lymphedema, not responding to medical measures. Results reported by the UCLA group have been most satisfactory.[1]

Lymphatic reconstructions

Developments in microvascular techniques have allowed surgical attempts at direct lymphatic reconstructions, performance of lymphovenous anastomoses or lymphatic grafting.[3–12] Although some of these operations have been performed for several decades, the long-term patency of such reconstructions has not been sufficiently proven and their use continues to be controversial. Such reconstructions would potentially be indicated in only a subset of patients who have proximal obstruction at the root of the involved extremity, with preserved lymphatics distally. Unfortunately, patients with primary lymphedema usually have diffuse disease and are not considered candidates for reconstruction. Efforts to increase lymph transport by implanting a piece of omentum or a segment of ileum (mesenteric bridge operations) to the affected areas in order to promote neolympho-lymphatic communication have had reported success in small groups of patients, but very few surgeons have personal experience with such procedures.

LYMPHOVENOUS ANASTOMOSES

Direct lymphovenous anastomoses have had varying degrees of reported success. The rationale for the operation is based on the observation that in patients with chronic lymphedema, spontaneous lymphovenous anastomosis could occasionally be demonstrated by lymphangiography. Ideally, direct reconstructions on the lymphatic system must be initiated early in the course of the lymphedema, prior to the development of subcutaneous fibrosis and lymphatic vessel sclerosis.

Potential indications for lymphovenous anastomoses are limited. The patients must have had recent onset secondary to lymphedema without previous episodes of cellulitis or lymphangitis. They must also have undergone a trial of conservative, nonoperative treatment prior to being considered for surgery. Venous hypertension is also a contraindication to this type of reconstruction. An ideal candidate is a patient with a proximal pelvic lymphatic obstruction with dilated infrainguinal lymph vessels. Anastomoses in the leg are performed usually between the superficial medial lymphatic bundle and tributaries of the saphenous or deep femoral vein (Fig. 48.2). We have used lymphovenous anastomoses in patients with chylous reflux to divert chyle into the venous system, in addition to distal ligation of the dilated incompetent lymph vessels. Thoracic duct–azygos vein anastomosis can also be successful in patients with thoracic duct occlusion, to prevent recurrent chylothorax.

Technically, lymphovenous anastomosis can be performed after significant practice, using good microsurgical technique and high-power magnification. In experiments, the author had objective evidence of late patency. Anastomoses using normal femoral lymph vessels and a tributary of the femoral vein in dogs yielded a patency rate of 50% at 3–8 months after surgery by cinelymphangiography.[10] The effectiveness of this operation is difficult to prove in humans. In 14 patients who underwent lymphovenous anastomoses at the Mayo Clinic, only five limbs maintained the initial improvement at an average of 46 months after surgery.[7] This improvement occurred in four of the seven patients with secondary lymphedema and in only one of the seven patients with primary lymphedema. Lymphoscintigraphy can provide only indirect evidence of improved lymph transport but cannot document patency of the anastomoses. Postoperative lymphangiography would be the only way to confirm anastomosis patency, but it is not practical, invasive, unacceptable for the patient and progression of lymphedema after such studies have also been reported.

Experience from Italy, Holland, China and Australia indicates that clinical improvement in a large number of operated patients can be achieved.[3–6,8] In O'Brien's series from Australia, 73% of the patients had subjective improvement and 42% experienced long-term improvement.[8] This technique is claimed to be of value in a select group of patients with secondary lymphedema. However, direct confirmation of long-term patency and lymphovenous anastomoses according to the author's knowledge is not available.

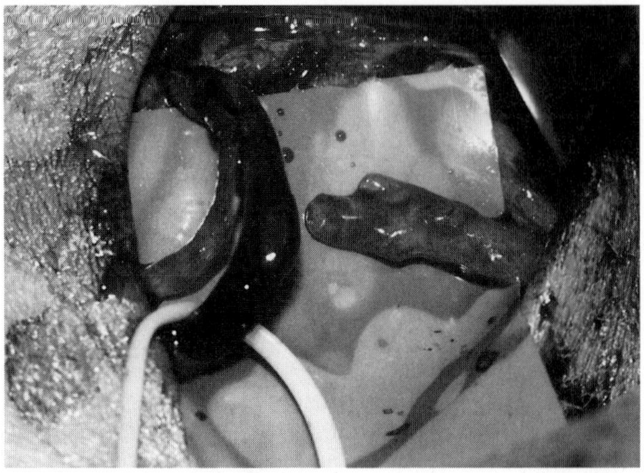

(a)

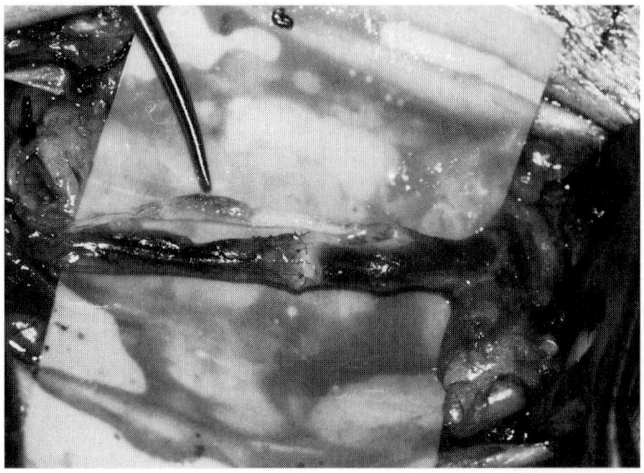

(b)

Figure 48.2 *Microsurgical lymphovenous anastomosis performed at the right groin. (a) Two dissected lymph vessels and a tributary of the saphenous vein (arrow) with a side branch prepared for anastomosis. (b) Patent end-to-end lymphovenous anastomoses.*

LYMPHATIC GRAFTING

The concept of lymphatic grafting is attractive in that the problems inherent in lymphovenous anastomoses (such as venous hypertension causing reversal of flow into the lymphatic circuit) can be avoided. Also, patency of lymph–lymphatic anastomoses should in theory be better than patency of blood-filled system. This technique, pioneered by Baumeister, has been offered to patients with unilateral secondary lymphedema of the lower extremities or to patients with postmastectomy lymphedema of the arm.[9,11,12] It is important to document normal lymphatics in the donor leg with lymphoscintigraphy before considering surgery.

In postmastectomy lymphedema, autotransplantation of two or three lymph vessels from the major lymphatic bundle from the medial aspect of the thigh to the arm is done. The distal anastomosis is performed on the proximal arm with epifascial and subfascial lymph vessels in an end-to-end fashion. The proximal anastomosis is best performed in the neck to one of the larger cervical descending lymphatic vessels. The procedure for lower extremity reconstruction is a transposition of two or three normal lymphatic trunks in the thigh to the diseased limb with a lympholymphatic anastomoses in the groin (cross-femoral grafting). In a report of 55 patients undergoing such procedures, 80% of the patients were noted by Baumeister to have improvement (volume reduction) after a mean follow-up of three years.[12] Objective documentation of flow through the lymphatic graft can be obtained with lymphoscintigraphy (Fig. 48.3). In our limited experience with this operation, we observed long-term patency of suprapubic lymphatic graft, although graft patency in this patient was not followed by late clinical improvement. Lymphatic grafting is a promising operation but it requires true microsurgical expertise and commitment to treat this frequently frustrating and difficult disease. Long-term patency rates associated with documented clinical improvement have to be reported in a larger number of patients, operated on in more than one center before this operation can be recommended for routine treatment as an alternative to conservative measures.

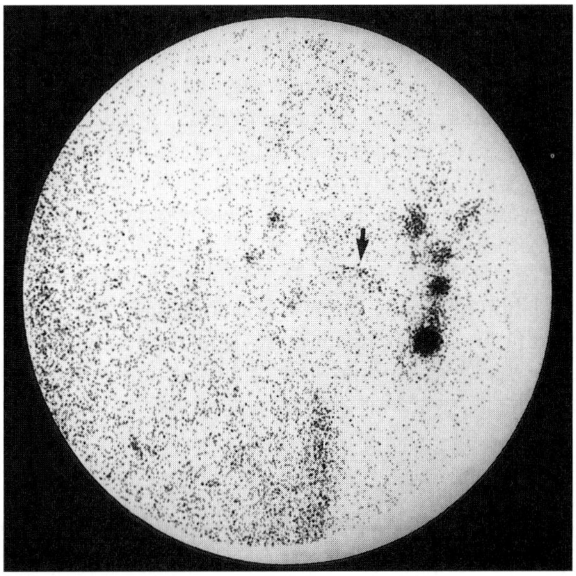

Figure 48.3 *Lymphoscintigraphy three months after cross-femoral lymphatic transposition. Note visualization of the left inguinal nodes following injection of isotope into the right edematous foot. There was no uptake prior to operation.*

REFERENCES*

1. Miller TA, Wyatt LE, Rudkin GH. Staged skin and subcutaneous excision for lymphedema: a favorable report of long-term results. *Plast Reconstr Surg* 1998; **102**: 1486.
2. Puckett CL, Silver D. Staged skin and subcutaneous excision for lymphedema: a favorable report of long-term results (Discussion). *Plast Reconstr Surg* 1998; **102**: 1499.
3. O'Brien BMcC, Shafiroff BB. Microlymphaticovenous and resectional surgery in obstructive lymphedema. *World J Surg* 1979; **3**: 3–15.
4. Huang GK, Ru-Qi H, Zong-Zhao L, Yao-Liang S, Tie De L, Gong-Ping P. Microlymphaticovenous anastomosis for treating lymphedema of the extremities and external genitalia. *J Microsurg* 1981; **3**: 32–9.
5. Gong-Kang H, Ru-Ai H, Zong-Zhao L, Yao-Liang S, Tie De L, Gong-Ping P. Microlymphaticovenous anastomosis in the treatment of lower limb obstructive lymphedema: analysis of 91 cases. *Plast Reconstr Surg* 1985; **76**: 671–85.
6. Campisi C, Tosatti E, Casaccia M, *et al.* Lymphatic microsurgery (in Italian). *Minerva Chir* 1986; **41**: 469–81.
7. Gloviczki P, Fisher J, Hollier LH, Pairolero PC, Schirger A, Wahner HW. Microsurgical lymphovenous anastomosis for treatment of lymphedema: a critical review. *J Vasc Surg* 1988; **7**: 647–52.
8. O'Brien BMcC, Mellow CG, Khazanchi RK, Dvir E, Kumar V, Pederson WC. Long-term results after microlymphatico-venous anastomoses for the treatment of obstructive lymphedema. *Plast Reconstr Surg* 1990; **85**: 562–72.
9. Kleinhaus E, Baumeister RGH, Hahn D, *et al.* Evaluation of transport kinetics in lymphoscintigraphy: follow-up study in patients with transplanted lymphatic vessels. *Eur J Nucl Med* 1985; **10**: 349–62.
10. Gloviczki P, Hollier LH, Nora FE, Kaye MP. The natural history of microsurgical lymphovenous anastomoses: an experimental study. *J Vasc Surg* 1986; **4**: 148–56.
11. Baumeister RG, Siuda S, Bohmert H, Moser E. A microsurgical method for reconstruction of interrupted lymphatic pathways: autologous lymph-vessel transplantation for treatment of lymphedemas. *Scand J Plast Reconstr Surg* 1986; **20**: 141–6.
12. Baumeister RG, Siuda S. Treatment of lymphedemas by microsurgical lymphatic grafting: what is proved? *Plast Reconstr Surg* 1990; **85**: 64–74.

*A complete list of references is available in Gloviczki P. The management of lymphatic disorders (Section XVIII). In Rutherford RB, ed. *Vascular Surgery*, 5th edn. Philadelphia: WB Saunders, 1995: 1883–949.

49

The management of chylous disorders

AUDRA A NOEL AND PETER GLOVICZKI

Chylous disorders develop due to abnormal circulation of chyle, the lipid- and protein-rich lymph fluid collected by the mesenteric lymphatic system. Primary developmental abnormalities of the lymph vessels (lymphangiectasia, obstruction)[1,2] or secondary causes (tumor, trauma)[3,4] lead to accumulation of the chyle in abnormal areas of the body. Disruption of the lymphatics causes chylous fistulae or effusions such as chylothorax or chylous ascites. Chylous reflux is the term used to describe retrograde flow in the incompetent lymphatic system due to lymphangiectasia and loss of lymphatic valve function. This chapter focuses on the most frequent primary chylous disorder, lymphangiectasia, associated with reflux of chyle to the limbs and genitalia, and discusses the management of chylous ascites and chylothorax. Many of the principles used for the treatment of primary chylous disorders can also be applied to those patients who develop chylous effusions due to iatrogenic or penetrating trauma or due to malignant tumors, most frequently due to lymphoma.

ETIOLOGY AND PRESENTATION

Primary chylous disorders are fortunately rare and they are usually caused by congenital lymphangiectasia.[1,2,3,5] Lymphatic dilatation (megalymphatics) may develop without proximal occlusion, although associated agenesis or obstruction of the thoracic duct has also been documented.[6,7]

Patients may present with lymphedema of one or both lower limbs or with swelling of the scrotum or the labia. The typical sign of lymphangiectasia and chylous reflux is, however, leakage of milky fluid due to disruption of the dilated lymphatics. Rupture of the distended lymph vessels or lymphatic cysts may manifest in protein losing enteropathy (malabsorption associated with chyle leaking into the lumen of the bowel),[5,6] chylous ascites,[8] chylothorax,[3,9] chyloptysis (chyle in the sputum, due to reflux into the lungs and tracheobronchial tree),[10] chyluria, chylometrorrhagia or chylocutaneous fistula, with or without lymphedema of the limbs or genitalia.[1,2,11,12]

Symptoms develop at a young age, since the underlying abnormality is congenital. Most patients are in their early teens at the onset of severe symptoms, although occasionally older patients may also present with chylous effusions, without underlying malignancy or the history of trauma. The mean age of 35 patients, 15 men and 20 women, treated for primary chylous disorders at the Mayo Clinic was 29 years and ranged from 1 day to 81 years.[13] The patients presented with lower limb edema (54%), dyspnea (49%), scrotal or labial edema (43%) and abdominal distension (37%). The etiology was primary lymphangiectasia in 66%, yellow nail syndrome in 11%, lymphangioleiomyomatosis in 9% and other in 18%.

Loss of chyle results in malnourishment due to depletion in lipids, protein, calcium and cholesterol. Significant loss of lymphocytes and immunoglobulins will cause severe compromise of the immune system and these patients are susceptible to infections.

EVALUATION

History and physical examination are most important and will frequently reveal the diagnosis. Chest x-ray shows effusion; paracentesis or thoracentesis reveals milky fluid, rich in albumin and lipids. Computed tomography (CT) is performed to confirm effusion and exclude malignancy.

The dilated lymphatics (megalymphatics, lymphangiomyomatosis) are better seen with magnetic resonance imaging (MRI). The benefits of lymphoscintigraphy are discussed in detail in Chapter 46. The radioactive colloid will reflux to the affected limb from the pelvis (Fig. 49.1a). Although lymphoscintigraphy is our initial diagnostic test, pedal lymphangiography performed with lipid-soluble contrast will confirm the diagnosis, localize the dilated retroperitoneal lymphatics and frequently confirm the sites of lymphatic leak.

NONSURGICAL MANAGEMENT

Patients with lymphedema of the limbs are treated with external compression, using elastic or non-elastic bandaging, elastic stockings or garments. Patients with advanced lymphedema benefit from the use of intermittent pneumatic compression pumps or manual lymphatic drainage. Since lymphatic occlusion is rare, leg elevation with conservative measures are usually more effective than in patients with congenital lymphedema caused by lymphatic hypoplasia or obstruction. Return of the swelling with the erect position, however, is more instantaneous and the amount of chylous leak from ruptured cutaneous blisters is directly dependent on the lipid content of the ingested food.

Meticulous skin care in the areas of chylous leak is important since the open blisters are potential sites for infection. Chyle production should be decreased by instituting a medium-chain triglyceride diet and sometimes parenteral nutrition is required to achieve improvement. Diuretics are needed frequently to

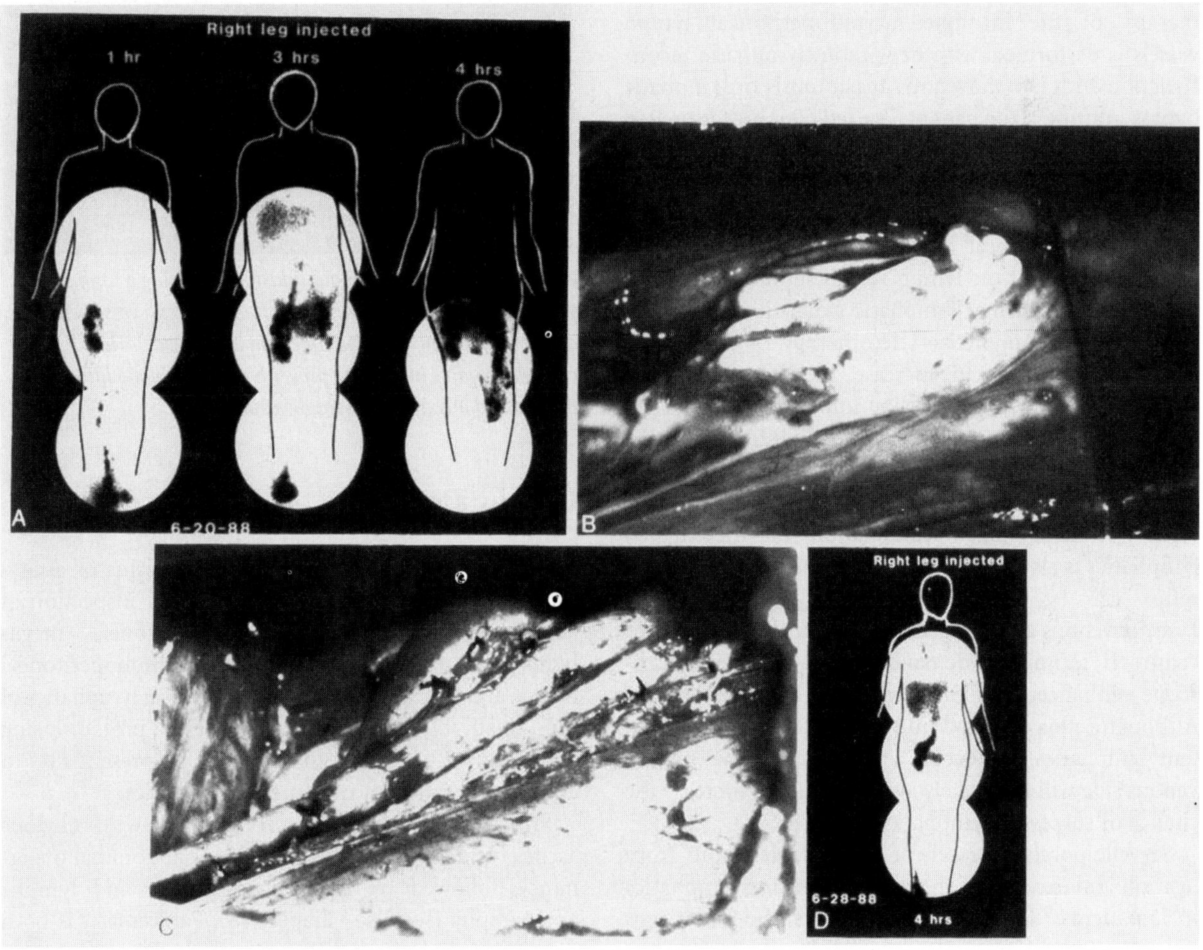

Figure 49.1 *(a) Right lower extremity lymphoscintigraphy in a 16-year-old female with lymphangiectasia and severe reflux into the genitalia and left lower extremity. Injection of the isotope into the right foot reveals reflux into the pelvis at 3 hours and into the left lower extremity at 4 hours. (b) Intraoperative photograph reveals dilated incompetent retroperitoneal lymphatics in the left iliac fossa containing chyle. (c) Radical excision and ligation of the lymph vessels were performed. In addition, two lymphovenous anastomoses were also performed between two dilated lymphatics and two lumbar veins. (d) Postoperative lymphoscintigram performed in a similar fashion reveals no evidence of reflux at 4 hours. The patient has no significant reflux 4 years after surgery. (a–d Reproduced with permission from Gloviczki P, Calcagno D, Schirger A,* et al. *Noninvasive evaluation of the swollen extremity: experiences with 190 lymphoscintigraphic examinations.* J Vasc Surg *1989;* **9**: *683–9)*

decrease chyle production, and furosemide and spironolactone (Aldactone) are used in high doses in severe cases.[8]

Nutritional management is used in conjunction with diuresis and paracentesis or thoracentesis in order to control symptomatic ascites or pleural effusions. Although these are only palliative measures, many patients may be controlled adequately. If not, surgical intervention is considered to provide long-term improvement.

SURGICAL TREATMENT

Chylous reflux

In patients with lymphedema and reflux of chyle to the genitalia and the limbs, excision, ligation and sclerotherapy of the incompetent retroperitoneal lymph vessels is performed, with or without lymphatic reconstruction with lymphovenous anastomosis or lymphatic bypass grafting.[7] The patients are fed 60 g butter melted in milk or cream 4 hours before the procedure. The retroperitoneal lymphatics are approached through a flank incision. The fatty meal allows ready visualization of the retroperitoneal lymphatics during exploration. Careful ligation of the lymph vessels should be done in order to avoid further lymphatic avulsion and leaking (Fig. 49.1a–d). Adjunctive sclerotherapy of the dilated lymphatics is done to increase the efficacy of the operation. We inject tetracycline solution, 500–1000 mg diluted in 20 ml normal saline directly into the dilated retroperitoneal lymph vessels to provoke obstructive lymphangitis. Percutaneous computed tomography (CT-) or MRI-guided cannulation of the dilated lymphatics is also possible and sclerotherapy to decrease reflux can be performed repeatedly, if necessary.[14] Lymphovenous anastomoses can also be done. This procedure is technically demanding and requires microscope enhancement to complete the anastomosis. Although reflux of blood into the dilated and incompetent lymphatics can occur, a competent valve on the venous side will completely avoid reflux and increase the chance of successful lymphatic drainage.[13]

Servelle published excellent and durable results from ligation and excision of the dilated refluxing lymphatics in 55 patients.[11] In a series of 19 patients who underwent ligation of the retroperitoneal lymphatics for chylous reflux to the limbs and genitalia (antireflux procedure) by Kinmonth, permanent cure was achieved in five patients and alleviation of symptoms, frequently after several operations, in 12 patients.[2] No improvement or failure was noted in only two cases.

We recently reviewed the results of 35 patients with primary chylous disorders treated over a 24-year period.[13] Twenty-one (60%) patients underwent 26 surgical procedures. Eighteen procedures were performed for chylous ascites or reflux, 10 of these patients (53%) underwent resection of retroperitoneal lymphatics ± sclerotherapy of lymphatics, 3 (17%) had lymphovenous anastomosis or saphenous vein interposition grafts (Fig. 49.2), 4 (21%) had peritoneovenous shunts, and one (5%) patient had a hysterectomy for periuterine lymphangiectasia. All patients improved initially, but 29% had recurrence of symptoms at a mean of 25 months (range 1–43). Three patients had postoperative lymphoscintigraphy confirming improved lymphatic transport and diminished reflux.

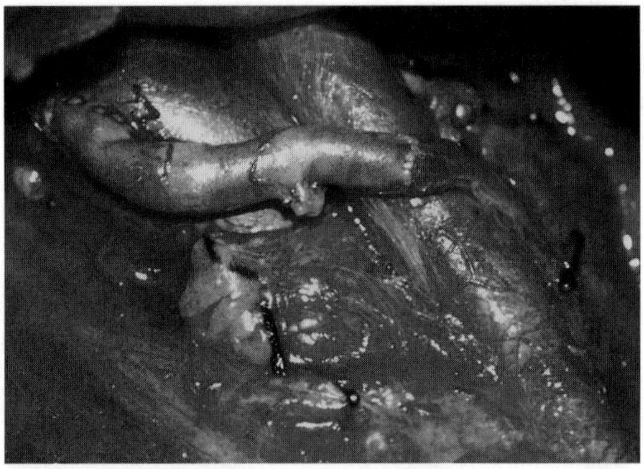

Figure 49.2 *Lymphovenous anastomosis using a saphenous vein graft between a large retroperitoneal lymph vessel (end to end) and the right common iliac vein (end to side). The competent valve in the vein prevents reflux of blood into the dilated and incompetent lymph vessel.*

Chylous ascites

Browse identified two principal mechanisms of ascites formation, using lymphangiography and inspection at laparotomy: leakage from retroperitoneal megalymphatics, usually through a visible lymphoperitoneal fistula, and leakage from dilated subserosal lymphatics of the small intestine, associated with protein-losing enteropathy.[8] Chylous cysts can also be present due to extreme dilatation of mesenteric lymphatics.

Preoperative evaluation of patients with chylous ascites includes CT or MRI to exclude abdominal malignancy, followed by lymphoscintigraphy and lymphangiography (see also Chapter 46). Paracentesis is both diagnostic and therapeutic. If conservative measures, including nutritional regulation and serial paracentesis, fail, surgical intervention should be considered.

Preparation of the patient for surgery is the same as used for retroperitoneal lymphatic ligation. Four hours after a fatty meal is ingested, abdominal exploration will confirm dilated and ruptured lymphatics, which can be oversewn, ligated or clipped (Fig. 49.3). Chylous cysts, when found, should be excised. The most involved

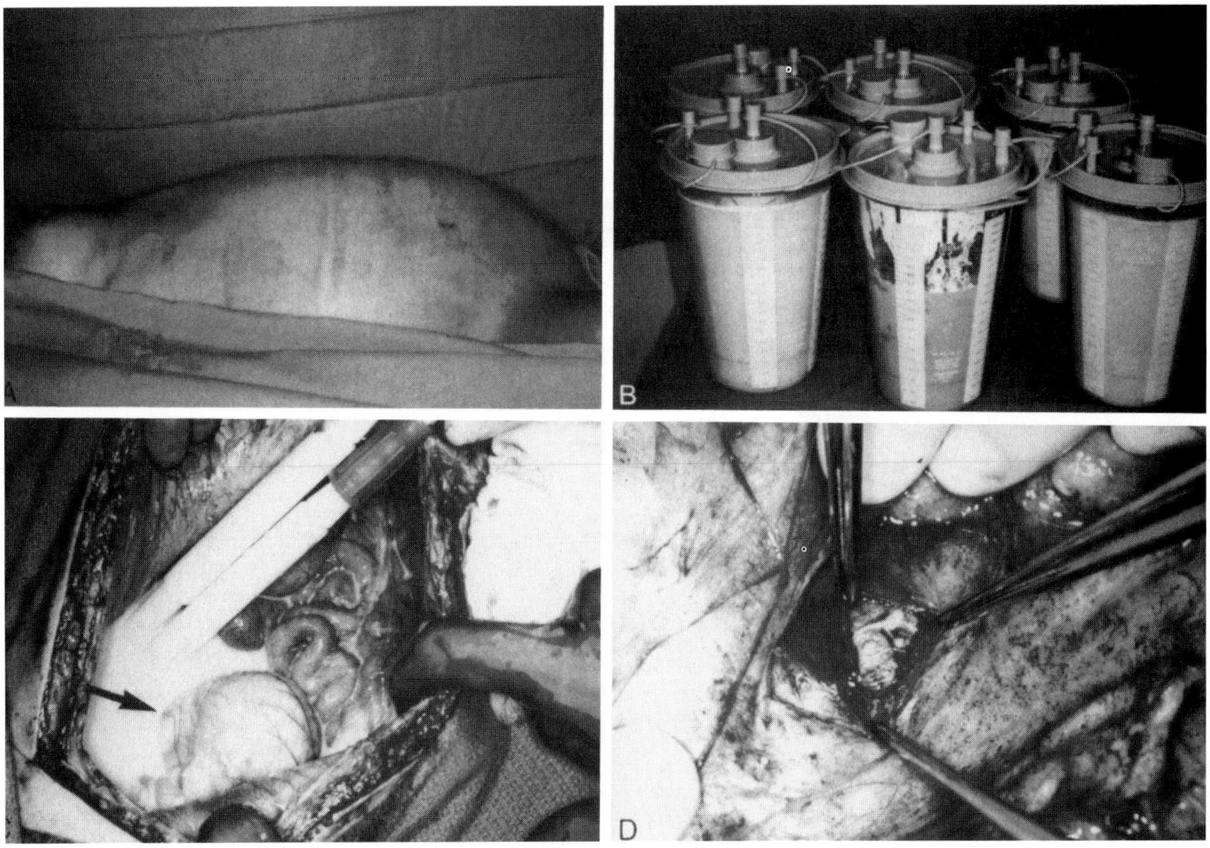

Figure 49.3 *(a) Photograph of an 18-year-old female with lymphangiectasia and recurrent chylous ascites. (b) During the operation, 12 liters of chyle were aspirated from the abdomen. (c) The chylous ascites was caused by ruptured lymphatic and leaking large mesenteric lymphatic cysts (arrow). (d) The dilated retroperitoneal lymphatics containing chyle were ligated and excised. The patient maintains an excellent clinical result 8 months after the operation. (Reproduced with permission from Gloviczki P, Noel A.A. Lymphatic reconstructions. In Rutherford RB, ed.* Vascular surgery, *5th edn. Philadelphia: WB Saunders, 2000: 2159–74)*

segments of the short bowel can be resected in patients who have severe protein-losing enteropathy. Success of the exploration is improved if a well-defined abdominal fistula is identified. However, if the mesenteric lymphatic trunks are fibrosed, aplastic, or hypoplastic, and exudation of the chyle is the main source of the ascites, the prognosis is poor, and recurrence is frequent. In these patients, ascites may be controlled with a peritoneal–venous shunt.

Browse *et al.* reported on a series of 45 patients with chylous ascites.[8] The age at presentation ranged from 1 to 80 (median 12) years; 23 patients were aged ≤15 years. Thirty-five patients had an abnormality of the lymphatics (primary chylous ascites); in the remaining ten, the ascites was secondary to other conditions, principally non-Hodgkin's lymphoma (six patients). Associated lymphatic abnormalities were present in 36 patients, lymphedema of the leg being the commonest (26 patients). All patients were initially treated conservatively with dietary manipulation with best results in patients with leaking small bowel lymphatics. Surgery (fistula closure, bowel resection or insertion of a peritoneovenous shunt) was performed in 30 patients. Closure of a retroperitoneal or mesenteric fistula, when present, was the most successful operation, curing seven of the 12 patients treated by Browse and colleagues.[8] In those patients who develop chylous ascites due to iatrogenic trauma, frequently after aortic reconstructions, a short period of conservative management is justified. If chylous ascites re-accumulates, reoperation with ligation of the fistula is the most effective treatment.[4]

Results with peritoneal–venous shunts have been mixed, patency is usually judged by recurrence of ascites. In Browse's experience with nine peritoneal–venous shunt placements, all occluded within 3–6 months after insertion.[3] We have use the Le Veen shunt with good results, although one of four patients developed symptomatic superior vena cava syndrome due to thrombosis around the shunt.[13]

Chylothorax

Chylothorax may result from lymphangiectasia with or without thoracic duct obstruction (Fig. 49.4), or from

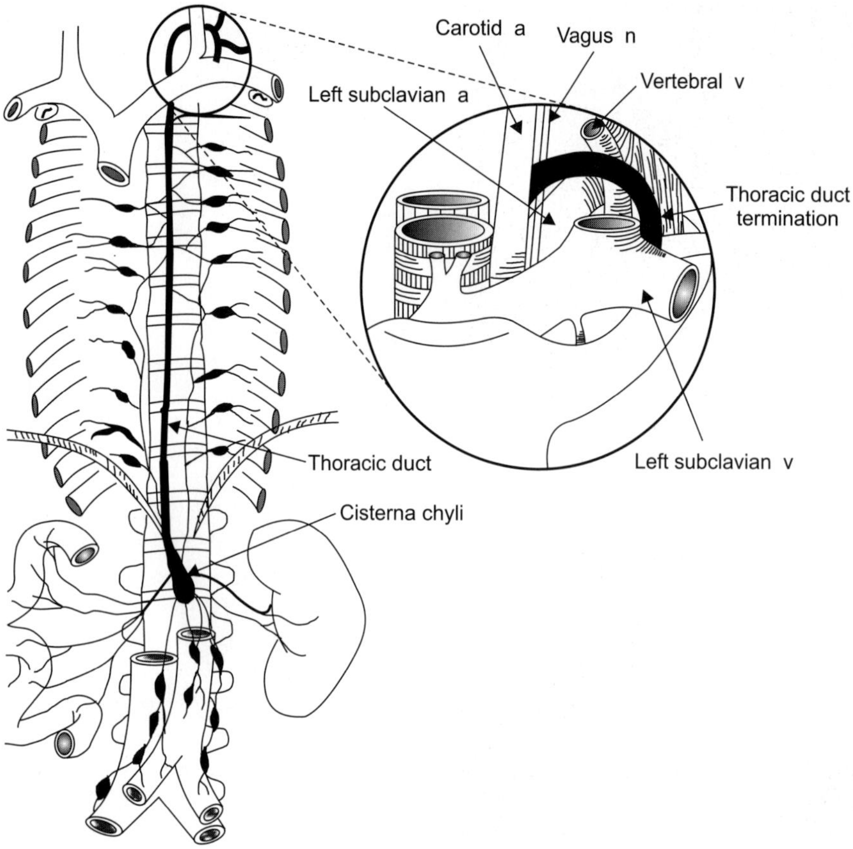

Figure 49.4 *Cervical and thoracoabdominal anatomy of the thoracic duct. (Reproduced with permission from Gloviczki P, Noel A.A. Lymphatic reconstructions. In Rutherford RB, ed.* Vascular surgery, *5th edn. Philadelphia: WB Saunders, 2000: 2159–74)*

chylous ascites passing through the diaphragm. In the latter group of patients, the chylothorax improves when the chylous ascites is controlled. Preoperative lymphangiography may localize the site of the chylous fistula or document occlusion of the thoracic duct. Thoracentesis is diagnostic but rarely therapeutic, as chyle from the thoracic duct or large intercostal, mediastinal, or diaphragmatic collaterals will re-accumulate. Although percutaneous or tube pleurodesis may be effective in other forms of nonmalignant chylothorax, it is less effective for primary chylothorax. Surgical pleurodesis, either with video-assisted thoracoscopy (VATS) or open thoracotomy, with excision of the parietal pleura is the optimal treatment.[8,9] After a fatty meal, thoracotomy or VATS is performed and lymphatics oversewn or clipped, followed by pleurodesis. In the Mayo Clinic series, eight procedures for chylothorax included thoracotomy with decortication and pleurodesis (two patients, four procedures), ligation of thoracic duct (three patients) and resection of thoracic duct cyst (one patient), with excellent early results in all patients.[13] In two patients, reported earlier, thoracic duct azygos vein anastomosis was performed, with good result.[7]

A recent prospective study from Cope described 11 patients with primary and secondary chylothorax treated with percutaneous catheterization and embolization of the thoracic duct with a 45% technical success rate, suggesting a role for percutaneous intervention.[15] Silk *et al.*,[16] and more recently Engum and colleagues[17] reported on using pleuroperitoneal shunts in children with good results.

If the upper thoracic duct is occluded, resulting in reflux of chyle into the pleural or peritoneal cavity, thoracic duct–azygos vein anastomosis can be attempted to reconstruct the duct and improve lymphatic transport. Preoperative imaging of the duct with contrast pedal lymphangiography in these patients is important because occlusion of the entire duct precludes anastomoses. Through a right posterolateral thoracotomy, an anastomosis between the lower thoracic duct and the azygos vein is performed in an end-to-end fashion, with 8-0 or 10-0 nonabsorbable interrupted sutures and magnification using loupes or the operating microscope (Fig. 49.5a–c). Kinmonth, who performed this operation in several patients, suggested that the anastomosis alone is not effective for decompressing the thoracic duct; ligation of the abnormal mediastinal lymphatics and oversewing of the sites of the lymphatic leak are also necessary.[2] Browse reported on three patients, who underwent thoracic duct–azygos vein anastomosis, but all shunts occluded by 1 year after intervention.[8] In the series of Browse a total of 20

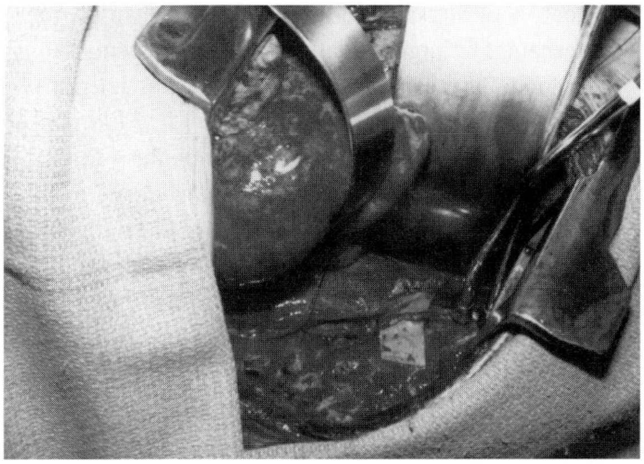

(a)

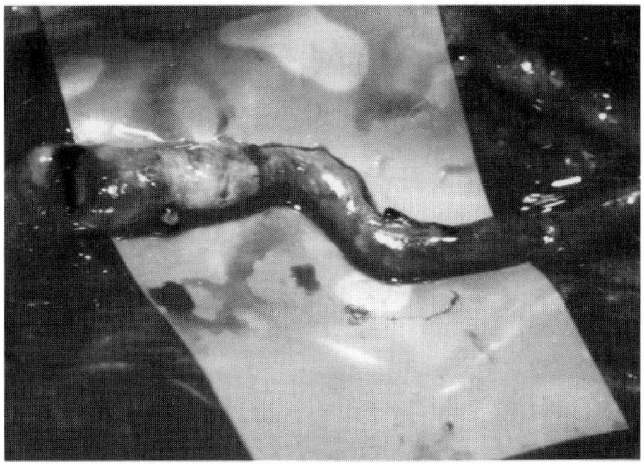

(b)

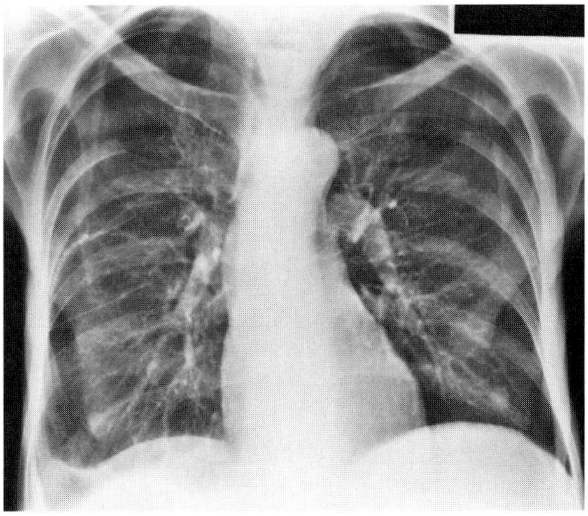

(c)

Figure 49.5 *(a, b) Thoracic duct–azygos vein anastomosis performed through a right posterolateral thoracotomy in an end-to-end fashion with interrupted 8-0 Prolene sutures. (c) Chest roentgenogram 2 years later confirms absence of chylothorax. (Reproduced with permission from Gloviczki P, Noel A.A. Lymphatic reconstructions. In Rutherford RB, ed.* Vascular surgery, *5th edn. Philadelphia: WB Saunders, 2000: 2159–74)*

patients were treated for primary or secondary chylothorax.[3] They suggest initial conservative treatment, but it should be abandoned if the fluid loss exceeds 1.5 l/day for more than 5–7 days in an adult or more than 100 ml/day in a child. Open pleurectomy was the most successful treatment in preventing re-accumulation of the effusion. Twelve of 20 patients were alive and free from an effusion 3–22 years after treatment.

CONCLUSIONS

Chylous disorders are fortunately rare. The underlying abnormality of primary chylous disorders is congenital lymphangiectasia, with or without occlusion or atresia of the thoracic duct. Secondary chylous effusions develop due to tumor, most frequently lymphoma or iatrogenic or penetrating trauma. Although medical management with diet, paracentesis or thoracentesis may control symptoms temporarily, surgical treatment is frequently the only permanent solution. Ligation of the incompetent retroperitoneal lymphatics and oversewing the sites of rupture can produce long-term improvement in many patients with lymphangiectasia and lymphatic reflux. Chylous ascites can effectively be treated with ligation of the mesenteric or retroperitoneal lymphatic fistula, if it can be identified. The role of peritoneovenous shunts remains controversial. Chylothorax requires surgical intervention in most patients and pleurodesis and ligation of the leaking lymphatics or the thoracic duct is frequently effective. In selected patients with chylothorax a thoracic duct–azygos vein anastomosis or pleuroperitoneal shunt may be considered as surgical options.

REFERENCES

1. Servelle M, Nogues, C. *The Chyliferous Vessels.* Paris: Expansion Scientifique Francaise, 1981: 40–59.
2. Kinmonth JB. Chylous diseases and syndromes, including references to tropical elephantiasis. In *The Lymphatics: Surgery, Lymphography and Diseases of the Chyle and Lymph Systems*, 2nd edn. London: Edward Arnold, 1982: 221–68.
3. Browse NL, Allen DR, Wilson NM. Management of chylothorax. *Br J Surg* 1997; **84**: 1711–16.
4. Gloviczki P, Lowell RC. Lymphatic complications of vascular surgery. In Rutherford RB, ed. *Vascular surgery*, 5th edn. Philadelphia: WB Saunders, 2000: 781–9.
5. Servelle M. Congenital malformation of the lymphatics of the small intestine. *J Cardiovasc Surg* 1991; **32**: 159–65.
6. Kinmonth JB, Cox SJ. Protein-losing enteropathy in lymphoedema. Surgical investigation and treatment. *J Cardiovasc Surg* 1975; **16**: 111–14.

7. Gloviczki P, Noel AA. Lymphatic reconstructions. In Rutherford RB, ed. *Vascular Surgery*, 5th edn. Philadelphia: WB Saunders, 2000: 2159–74.
8. Browse NL, Wilson NM, Russo F, al-Hassan H, Allen DR. Aetiology and treatment of chylous ascites. *Br J Surg* 1992; **79**: 1145–50.
9. Peillon C, D'Hont C, Melki J, *et al.* Usefulness of video thoracoscopy in the management of spontaneous and postoperation chylothorax. *Surg Endosc* 1999; **13**: 1106–9.
10. Sanders JS, Rosenow EC, Piehler JM, Gloviczki P, Brown LR. Chyloptysis (chylous sputum) due to thoracic lymphangiectasis with successful surgical correction. *Arch Intern Med* 1988; **148**: 1465–6.
11. Servelle M. Surgical treatment of lymphedema: a report on 652 cases. *Surgery* 1987; **101**: 485–95.
12. Gloviczki P, Calcagno D, Schirger A, *et al.* Noninvasive evaluation of the swollen extremity: experiences with 190 lymphoscintigraphic examinations. *J Vasc Surg* 1989; **9**: 683–9.
13. Noel AA, Gloviczki P, Bender CE, Whitley D, Stanson AW, Dechamps C. Surgical treatment for lymphedema and chylous effusions caused by lymphangiectasia. *J Vasc Surg* (Submitted 2001).
14. Molitch HI, Unger EC, Witte CL, vanSonnenberg E. Percutaneous sclerotherapy of lymphangiomas. *Radiology* 1995; **194**(2): 343–7.
15. Cope C, Salem R, Kaiser LR. Management of chylothorax by percutaneous catheterization and embolization of the thoracic duct: prospective trial. *J Vasc Interv Radiol* 1999; **10**(9): 1248–54.
16. Silk YN, Goumas WM, Douglass HOJr, Huben RP. Chylous ascites and lymphocyst management by peritoneovenous shunt. *Surgery* 1991; **110**: 561–5.
17. Engum SA, Rescorla FJ, West KW, Scherer LR3, Grosfeld JL. The use of pleuroperitoneal shunts in the management of persistent chylothorax in infants. *J Pediatr Surg* 1999; **34**: 286–90.

PART 7

Issues in venous disease

50

Venous outcomes assessment

ROBERT B RUTHERFORD, FRANK T PADBERG JR, ANTHONY J COMEROTA, ROBERT L KISTNER, MARK H MEISSNER AND GREGORY L MONETA*

Clinical papers from earlier decades in the last half century most often characterized treatment groups with chronic venous disease (CVD) in simple terms, such as the percentage with 'stasis dermatitis' or with 'stasis ulcers', the latter sometimes being separated into healed or active groups. After a variable 'mean follow-up period' after treatment, the percentage of ulcers healed, or staying healed, or, if patients with stasis dermatitis were included, the percentage without a new ulcer, were commonly reported as evidence of improvement. Pain and swelling were also mentioned, and sometimes graded, in an attempt to show the symptomatic relief provided by treatment. Even individual components of 'stasis dermatitis' (cutaneous pigmentation, inflammation, induration, subcutaneous fibrosis) were graded in a few reports. However, none of the above characteristics of CVD was assessed in a universally accepted, standardized fashion. As the use of life-table methods became popular among vascular surgeons, primarily as a way of reporting patency rates, it was occasionally used in preference to the mean follow-up period, in characterizing the 'ulcer-free interval'. Finally, in most evaluations of surgical treatments, the impact on outcome of background differences in the use of compressive therapy or in adjunctive procedures were commonly ignored. Such was the state of the art before reporting standards were developed.

The first version of the SVS/ISCVS reporting standards in venous disease, published in 1988,[1] did much to improve this. In addition to a number of other specific suggestions [e.g. a multifactorial factor grading system for assessing the risk of deep venous thrombosis (DVT), and proposed standards for reports on pulmonary embolism, DVT prophylaxis and appropriate diagnostic studies], it proposed a three-level classification for CVD, suggested that the segmental anatomy and etiology of the venous disease be described, and recommended using functional means of objective assessment before and after treatment [e.g. ambulatory venous pressures (AVP) or one of the then current noninvasive tests (NITs) for assessing obstruction or reflux]. It also recommended a +3 to −3 scale for gauging change in status after treatment, much like that proposed for lower extremity arterial disease,[2] in which change in clinical class plus a significant change in a physiologic test value were required in order to claim significant improvement (or worsening). Although some of the flawed reporting practices mentioned above were not addressed, it was a major step in the right direction.

Subsequently, a consensus meeting of an *ad hoc* international committee of the American Venous Forum (AVF) was held in Hawaii in 1994 at which the CEAP system of classification of venous disease was conceived and developed.[3] The CEAP system categorizes the basic

*From the American Venous Forum's Ad Hoc Committee on Venous Outcomes Assessment.

elements of the venous condition at a given point in time. It separately categorizes the clinical condition of the extremity ('C'), the etiology ('E'), the anatomic location of the problem ('A') and the underlying pathophysiology ('P'). The major value of this classification is to standardize the key elements in a way that patients or groups of patients with venous disease can either be distinguished from each other, or grouped in common classes and compared in a standard manner in reports from different practice groups or institutions. This system was recommended and outlined as the main feature of a revision in the venous reporting standards published in 1995.[4] It has also been promulgated in the previous *Venous Handbook*[5] and is again presented in this edition. The importance of the uniform classification framework provided by CEAP is acknowledged and seen in its increasing use, in scores of publications world wide. It has been translated into at least six languages and promulgated in Europe, Asia and South America as well as in North America. However, the executive committee of the AVF, who own its copyright, while not wishing to change the basic system, recognized it as a dynamic document that would need to be augmented or changed with time. Almost 3 years ago it appointed an Ad Hoc Committee on Venous Outcomes to consider additional methods for assessing the results of treatment of chronic venous disease (CVD) and particularly venous severity scoring.

This chapter represents an update on the deliberations of this *ad hoc* committee, the additional needs for venous outcomes assessment it has identified, and what it has done to date to try to fill those needs. They include:

- the need for a venous severity scoring system;
- the need for standard practices in dealing with differences in the background of conservative therapy and in controlling for the concomitant use of adjunctive methods or procedures when evaluating an interventional treatment or procedure;
- the need to modify the current venous disability score;
- the need to assess current instruments for the patient-based assessment of the impact of venous disease and its treatment on their quality of life, and to either endorse one of them or incorporate the best of them into an improved version;
- the need for an updated comparison of venous diagnostic tests and their ability to assess venous dysfunction; and
- the need to identify and grade those risk factors that significantly affect outcome after DVT (as opposed to risk factors which predict the risk of developing DVT).

Although this latter need does not directly relate to assessing the treatment of CVD, it is important in comparing methods of treating DVT when judged in terms of its late sequelae, and thus is included here. The need for proper cost-benefit studies is an additional need that is recognized by the committee, but it was felt that proper methodology for this was already available and simply needed to be applied in comparing treatment methods. The remainder of this chapter will separately discuss these six additional approaches to venous outcomes assessment and the current status of the committee's deliberations on them.

VENOUS SEVERITY SCORING

Methods of outcomes assessment need to be able to gauge change in status following treatment in a meaningful and objective way and, for purposes of analysis and comparison, should usually be quantitative rather than qualitative. They should result in a practical assessment of the success of a given treatment over time, whether applied to groups of patients of varying levels of severity or patients grouped into similar levels of severity. Both, but particularly the former, require a quantitative method of gauging the severity of disease. Properly comparing the outcomes of two or more treatments in the same institution, or the reported results of the same treatment from different institutions, or the results of the same treatment using different adjunctive measures, is not possible unless the relative severities of the underlying disease in the treatment groups are known.[6] However, if the severity of the disease is uniformly quantified and the score changes significantly with treatment, a disease severity score can not only serve as a background against which to view other outcome criteria, in comparing treatment groups, but also can itself reflect the degree of change in disease severity associated with treatment. As such, disease severity scores can be very useful in outcomes assessment. The widespread use of a properly designed disease severity scoring scheme should allow patient groups of similar degrees of severity to be selected for entry into clinical trials and to be compared in regard to outcome following different therapies. If generally adopted, the outcomes following a given treatment reported by different practices groups or institutions can also be compared knowing the relative severity of disease of the treated patients in each report. Thus a venous severity scoring system can become a valuable adjunct in venous outcomes assessment.

The CEAP classification system (Clinical–Etiology–Anatomic–Pathophysiologic),[2] and particularly its clinical classes, C1–C6, does represent a progressive gradation of disease severity. It gauges the severity of disease at a given point in time, but because a number of its components are relatively static and do not change significantly in response to treatment, and other components have alphabetic designations, it cannot be used for disease severity scoring in its current form. For example, the healing of an active ulcer would drop the patient from C6 to C5, but no further. Some of the elements of C4, particularly subcutaneous fibrosis and cutaneous atrophy, are unlikely to change significantly with treatment. The elimination of edema (C3) or varicose veins (C2), or reticular veins and telangiectasias (C1) for that matter, conceivably could produce an improvement in clinical class, but the results of their treatment are not usually so absolute, and significant improvements short of complete elimination of the characteristic venous state would not result in categorical improvement.

So the clinical class of CEAP does not allow a practical assessment of change in response to treatment or adverse events, but then it was not intended to do so. However, the Ad Hoc Committee on Venous Outcomes of the AVF felt that CEAP identifies most if not all the necessary components involved in comprehensive outcomes assessment and many of its elements could be individually graded to produce a venous severity scoring system. This is the approach that was selected in producing a Venous Clinical Severity Score (CVSS).

It should be noted that a 'clinical score' is included in the full CEAP document and is included in the previous *Venous Handbook* (see Table 38.3, page 656).[3] It uses a 0–2 grading of a number of symptoms and signs, which include pain and venous claudication, as well as the characteristic elements of the C3–C6 levels of CEAP, for a maximum score of 18. Varicose veins are not included in this clinical score, so a patient with successful removal of these could only be gauged by a change in pain, at the most 2 points. Although the approach used in this clinical score is conceptually sound, it is rather simplistic. Furthermore, the scores assigned can be rather arbitrary and subjective because many of the scoring levels are inadequately delineated by the descriptive terms associated with them. It has not gained widespread acceptance or use, and was not included in the current version of venous reporting standards.[4]

In developing a severity scoring system based on CEAP, it was clear, on the one hand, that a clinical severity score could be primarily based on the 'C' of CEAP, and on the other, that the 'E' or etiology is fixed and could not be incorporated. However, both the anatomic segments 'A' and the pathophysiology, 'P', of CEAP represent objective, gradable data. Since each segment (A) is or is not involved in the essential pathophysiologic processes (P) of reflux and/or obstruction, they could be combined and adapted into a grading scheme capable not only of reflecting disease severity, but in some situations even gauge change with treatment, as in a comparison of anticoagulant therapy, thrombolysis or thrombectomy for deep venous thrombosis (DVT). Importantly, it was felt that such a scheme could be scored using duplex scan findings. Therefore a Venous Segmental Disease Score (VSDS) was also developed, in addition to a CVSS. These two elements of the proposed venous severity scoring system will thus be seen to be closely allied to CEAP.

However, in developing these venous severity scores, it was considered important to avoid confusion with, or undermining, the CEAP classification system. Thus, this venous severity scoring scheme is not intended to replace or change any aspect of CEAP, but to augment it with additional compatible methods to further improve our ability to assess venous outcomes.

The Venous Clinical Severity Score (VCSS) – a modification to replace the Clinical Score of CEAP

DESIGN CONSIDERATIONS AND RATIONALE

The following rationale evolved in developing a venous clinical severity score. Whilst it was felt desirable to use the basic clinical elements of CEAP where possible, it was important not to mimic them so closely as to cause confusion with CEAP classification. For this reason simply scoring each of the six clinical classes from 0 to 3 was rejected.

We wished to take advantage of the progressive order of severity intrinsic to the clinical classes of CEAP, but also to give additional weight to the upper levels, C4–C6. This was done by separately scoring certain attributes of each of these levels.

It was necessary to avoid elements that are static and use only those with ability to reflect change over a relatively short period of time (months). Thus subcutaneous fibrosis, one of the hallmarks of C4–C6, was not considered.

Because of its success in the SVS/ISCVS reporting standards[2] and its common use by clinicians, we employed the 0–3 grading scheme and applied it to all clinical descriptors (0 = absent, 1 = mild, 2 = moderate, and 3 = severe). This allowed improvement at each level to be gauged.

In addition, it was felt important to define and describe each level and each grade in sufficient detail to minimize overlap and arbitrariness in assigning scores.

Both ascending and flat scales were considered and several were constructed. An ascending scale assigns the score to the highest level achieved. Thus if six descriptors were each scored 0–3, the score would increase from 0 to 18 for each box in ascending fashion. However, this approach did not fit with our goal to develop a severity scoring scheme which covered the full spectrum of disease with a wide spread of scores capable of significant change with treatment. One might achieve improvement in lower descriptors (e.g. remove varicosities, relieve edema and pain), but if there were little change in a higher descriptor, the score would change little (e.g. an ulcer healed but pigmentation and induration remained). In a flat scale, where points for each descriptor are added to give the total score, this same degree of improvement would be result in a greater score change. Therefore a flat scale was chosen.

CLINICAL DESCRIPTORS CONSIDERED AND CHOSEN

All six clinical class levels (C1–C6) as well as separate characteristics of C4–C6 (pigmentation, inflammation, induration, ulcer size, number, multiplicity, duration) were considered as gradable clinical descriptors. In addition, pain, disability, neuropathy, venous eczema and venous claudication were considered.

C1 (telangiectasias and reticular veins) was eliminated because it was not considered a major pathologic characteristic of the patient with CVD, the treatment of which was the focus of these outcome assessment methods.

Disability scoring was felt to be important in its own right and was retained as a separate score. A new Venous Disability Score is presented separately below.

Venous claudication was not included. It was felt to be much rarer than other features of CVD and besides, patients with this degree of venous obstruction would be represented with high scores for pain and swelling.

Neuropathy, whilst commoner than realized, was not considered common enough or easily gauged by most investigators.

Venous eczema was considered for inclusion, not separately but as a severe form of inflammatory change.

Ultimately, nine clinical descriptors were selected: pain, varicose veins, edema, pigmentation, induration, inflammation, total number of ulcers, duration of active ulceration, and size of largest current ulcer.

There was considerable sentiment for trying to compensate, in scoring, for background differences in the use of compressive therapy and limb elevation, because it was realized that, for example, advanced skin changes without ulceration in a very compliant patient may well represent more severe disease than multiple active ulcers in a noncompliant patient, or one who had never been introduced to compressive therapy and elevation. At one point, when working on a 30-point flat scale, a superimposed sliding scale of 0–3 was considered, with the score not to exceed 30. When one of the descriptors (telangiectasias and reticular veins) was dropped in the final deliberations, it was decided to simply include 0–3 points for differences in background conservative therapy, bringing the severity score back to an even 30-point scale.

The Venous Clinical Severity Score finally recommended is presented in Table 50.1. It is accompanied

Table 50.1 *Venous Clinical Severity Score*

Attribute	Absent = 0	Mild = 1	Moderate = 2	Severe = 3
Pain	None	Occasional, not restricting activity or requiring analgesics	Daily, moderate activity limitation, occasional analgesics	Daily, severely limits activities, regular use of analgesics
Varicose veins*	None	Few, scattered: branch VVs with competent GS/LS	Multiple: single segment GS/ LS reflux	Extensive: multisegment GS/ LS reflux
Venous† edema	None	Evening ankle edema only	Afternoon edema above ankle	Morning edema above ankle requiring activity change, elevation
Skin pigmentation	None or focal, low intensity (tan)	Diffuse, but limited in area and old (brown)	Diffuse over gaiter distribution (lower third) or recent pigmentation (purple)	Wider distribution (above lower third) and recent pigmentation
Inflammation	None	Mild cellulitis, limited or marginal area around ulcer	Moderate cellulitis, involves most of gaiter area	Severe cellulitis (lower third or above) or venous eczema
Induration	None	Focal, circum-areolar (<5 cm)	Medial or lateral, less than lower third	Entire lower third or more
Total no. ulcers‡	0	1	2–4	>4
Active ulceration, duration	None	<3 months	>3 months, <1 year	Not healed >1 year
Active ulcer, size	None	<2 cm diameter	2–4 cm diameter	>4 cm diameter
Compressive therapy¶	Not used or not compliant	Intermittent use of stockings	Wears elastic stockings most days	Full compliance stockings + elevation

Qualifying comments:

*To assure differentiation between C1 and C2, 'varicose' veins must be <4 mm diameter to qualify for inclusion here. Occasional or mild edema and focal pigmentation over VVs does not qualify for inclusion under the two subsequent attributes.

†Presumes venous origin by characteristics, e.g. brawny (not pitting or spongy) edema, with significant effect of standing/limb elevation and/or other clinical evidence of venous etiology, i.e. varicose veins, h/o DVT. Edema must be regular finding, e.g. daily occurrence.

‡Total number equals active and healed.

¶Sliding scale to adjust for background differences in use of compressive therapy.

by qualifying comments regarding its application. As a minimum, it is recommended that each of these nine clinical characteristics be scored, as separate items, from 0 to 3 in each patient. Their total, along with the tenth item, the degree of use of compressive therapy, can then be combined to facilitate numeric comparison. It is realized that the final version represents considerable arbitrariness and another group of 'experts' might have come up with a different scheme that might also serve well. However, after months of deliberation, the committee could not arrive at a better scheme and it was felt that future field testing, as recommended below, would provide a more objective basis for further modifying it.

The Venous Segmental Disease Score (VSDS) – a combination of the anatomic and pathophysiologic components of CEAP

DESIGN CONSIDERATIONS AND RATIONALE

The following rationale evolved in developing a venous segmental disease score. The concept behind the VSDS was to combine the pathophysiologic designation of reflux and obstruction with the venous segments of the anatomic classification. Points are assigned for the pathophysiologic findings of reflux and/or obstruction. It was intended that an objective score could weight the importance of the pathophysiology in the specific anatomic segments. VSDS is intended to complement the venous clinical severity score. Since duplex has become a commonly accepted imaging standard, the scoring scheme is intended to incorporate this as the primary source of anatomic and pathophysiologic data. Although phlebography is not required as often as in the past, these examinations are usually obtained when the duplex is inconclusive, and thus often add valuable information that may be used in scoring. It is important to emphasize that the venous segmental disease scores are solely derived from anatomic evidence of reflux and venous obstruction, and do not attempt to evaluate or score the physiologic severity of the reflux or obstruction.

ANATOMIC SEGMENTS CONSIDERED AND ASSIGNED

Although 18 venous segments are designated for the anatomic localization of disease in the CEAP classification system, we recognized that scoring all 18 would be unwieldy and unnecessarily complex. Some were easy to eliminate as playing relatively insignificant roles when incompetent or obstructed; however, the relative roles of the remainder were not considered equal. For example, superficial venous incompetence is a common and significant cause of venous insufficiency; however, thrombosis or occlusion of superficial veins is usually of minor physiologic consequence.

More proximal veins (IVC, iliac, CFV) are generally considered to play a greater role in symptomatic venous obstruction than most of the distal veins; conversely, the virtual absence of valves in these veins makes reflux a normal physiologic parameter in this location. Popliteal vein incompetence has an enhanced significance in both reflux and obstruction; this probably results from its unique situation as the outflow of the calf muscle pump. A pathologic tibial vein, as well as the popliteal vein, is more highly associated with venous insufficiency than the proximal veins.[7,8] Therefore, 2 points were assigned for the venous segments considered to play a significant role in obstruction or reflux. Whilst 1 point was assigned to most veins, the point value was reduced to 0.5 for those deemed to be of lesser significance.

In recognition of the higher morbidity associated with post-thrombotic venous insufficiency, it seemed reasonable to assign points for both obstruction and reflux scales to these limbs. This approach is consistent with the original concept of the CEAP system. Previously, long-term evaluations of outcome following prior venous thrombosis relied upon phlebography for confirmation of diagnosis in the era prior to accurate ultrasound imaging.[9,10] Recently, duplex-based studies have achieved widespread acceptance.[11] Although it could be said that any given abnormal venous segment would not be refluxing if totally obstructed – or, not obstructed if patent and refluxing – in fact, there are recanalized post-thrombotic veins that are incompetent but are also significantly narrowed.

The final version of the VSDS is presented in Table 50.2, which includes qualifying comments regarding its application. It is clear that this final VSDS is also arbitrary, albeit the product of long deliberations. The committee therefore recommends that further modifications be done after appropriate field testing, using objective correlative data.

RECOMMENDED REPORTING PRACTICES TO COMPENSATE FOR DIFFERENCES IN ADJUNCTIVE TREATMENTS WHILE ASSESSING A PRIMARY INTERVENTION

As has been pointed out, background differences in conservative therapy are often ignored when evaluating an operative procedure. The patient who has major extremity venous surgery characteristically spends more time than usual in the recumbent position, often with legs elevated, during the postoperative rehabilitation period. Frequently the legs are wrapped in Ace bandages initially and subsequently the patient may be given a prescription for new elastic stockings, and may be more likely to wear them regularly when still under closer

Table 50.2 *Venous Segmental Disease Score (based on venous segmental involvement with reflux or obstruction*)*

Reflux	Obstruction (excised/ligated)
½ Lesser saphenous	
1 Greater saphenous	1 Greater saphenous (only if from groin to below knee)
½ Perforators, thigh	
1 Perforators, calf	
2 Calf veins, multiple (PT alone = 1)	1 Calf veins, multiple
2 Popliteal vein	2 Popliteal vein
1 Superficial femoral vein	1 Superficial femoral vein
1 Profunda femoris vein	1 Profunda femoris vein
1 Common femoral vein & above†	2 Common femoral
	1 Iliac vein
	1 IVC
10 Maximum reflux score‡	10 Maximum obstruction score‡

*As determined by appropriate venous imaging (phlebography or duplex scan).
†Normally there are no valves above the common femoral vein.
‡Not all of the 11 segments listed can be involved in reflux or obstruction.
Qualifying comments:

- Reflux means that all the valves in that segment are incompetent. Obstruction means there is total occlusion at some point in the segment or >50% narrowing of at least half of the segment.
- Most segments are assigned one point but some segments have been weighted more or less to fit with their perceived significance, e.g. increasing points for common femoral or popliteal obstruction and for popliteal and multiple calf vein reflux and decreasing points for lesser saphenous or thigh perforator reflux.
- Points can be assigned for both obstruction and reflux in the same segment. This will be uncommon but can occur in some post thrombotic states, potentially giving secondary venous insufficiency higher severity scores than primary disease.

physician supervision. This may contribute to improved initial outcome, as in enhanced ulcer healing, and has been called 'the placebo effect of venous surgery'. Its impact should be recognized but, as part of proper postoperative care, it cannot be controlled.

However, background differences in conservative therapy before and after the perioperative period can and should be controlled for, not only in assessing the results of interventional treatments in individual patients, but also in group comparisons. This has been only partly addressed by points awarded in the recommended venous clinical severity score. *Therefore it is recommended, in addition, that assessments of the outcome of venous surgery use randomized or concomitant matched controls with conservative treatment alone, if the intent is to demonstrate a benefit from such intervention over and above conservative treatment. Alternatively, investigators should take adequate measures to assure that the background treatment of compressive therapy and limb elevation remains constant in the period before, and beyond the perioperative period, after surgery.*

An equally vexing reporting practice is failure to control for concomitant adjunctive procedures carried out at the time of the primary operation under assessment. The classic example of this is carrying out ligation and stripping of superficial veins and/or perforator interruption at the same time as deep venous surgery is being evaluated, and then claiming improvement. It is not possible to assign improvement to the primary procedure being assessed under such circumstances, particularly when there are numerous studies claiming to show sufficient improvement from correcting superficial and/or perforator insufficiency alone that deep venous insufficiency does not require correction. Of course the same can be said for assessing perforator interruption when saphenous stripping is also carried out in many of the patients. The excuse is made that it is unfair to the patient not to fully treat their CVD at one operation. This is true, but misleading reporting practices are also unfair to the patient. *The time has come to stop reporting retrospective outcome analyses of one's operative approach to CVD, and trying to claim benefit from one particular procedure, or combination of procedures, while sometimes performing them concomitantly with other procedures. There is nothing wrong with practicing what one feels is the most appropriate combinations of operations in a given patient, but it is wrong to expect one's colleagues to accept this as scientific proof that one approach is superior to another, or that one of several procedures used has measurable benefit.*

The recommended solution to this dilemma is to isolate the effect of the primary operation under consideration, which may be done in one of two ways:

- Do not apply the primary operation until all indicated lesser procedures have been carried out. For example, only perform deep venous valvuloplasty or valved transplant after superficial and/or perforator interruption has been carried out and the clinical status has stabilized. Since there seems to be clinical equipoise over whether or not deep venous reconstructions add sufficiently to superficial and perforator vein surgery alone to be performed at the same time, rather than being reserved for failure of the latter procedures, this approach seems quite ethical.
- Compare the outcomes of patients having the primary procedure plus the adjunctive procedure(s) to those having the adjunctive procedure(s) alone, studying patients with a similar distribution and severity of disease. This approach might work well for evaluating perforator vein interruptions.

Although the two examples given are the most common offenders, there are other operations in which the principle that a study protocol must isolate a procedure in order to assess its benefit would equally apply.

THE VENOUS DISABILITY SCORE (VDS) – A MODIFICATION OF THE ORIGINAL CEAP DISABILITY SCORE

The disability score originally developed with CEAP was featured in the previous edition of the *Venous Handbook*[3] but is not part of the revised venous reporting standards.[4] Unfortunately, in this version, disability is related (score 2) to working an 8-hour day and (score 3) to ability to work. It is felt that this should be modified in recognition of the many patients with CVD who do not ordinarily work an 8-hour day (housewives, retirees, students, etc.). That disability score also refers to ability to work with or without 'support device', which is not explained, but is presumed to mean compression and elevation. To avoid misinterpretation by others, including those in health care agencies, it was felt that 'support device' should be identified as compression therapy with or without intermittent leg elevation.

A slightly modified wording of the disability score is therefore offered to accommodate the reality that not all individuals will be expected to work an 8-hour day while retaining the original concept of compression therapy and intermittent limb elevation facilitating maintenance of reasonable or usual daily activities. 'Usual activities' is further qualified as being normal for the patient, i.e. those carried on before being disabled by venous disease. This modification, presented in Table 50.3, is intended to widen the application of this aspect of CEAP to a broader population.

Table 50.3 *Venous Disability Score*

0 = Asymptomatic
1 = Symptomatic but able to carry out usual activities* without compressive therapy
2 = Can carry out usual activities* only with compression and/or limb elevation
3 = Unable to carry out usual activities* even with compression and/or limb elevation

*Usual activities = patient's activities before onset of disability from venous disease.

PATIENT-BASED ASSESSMENTS OF THE IMPACT OF THE TREATMENT OF CVD ON THE QUALITY OF LIFE

There seems to be general agreement that proper patient based quality of life (QOL) instruments could be of significant value in evaluating the treatment of CVD. Because severity of symptoms and signs in CVD do not always closely correlate with each other, and noninvasive tests do not offer one simple parameter that correlates reasonably with severity of CVD (like the ankle or toe pressure in arterial occlusive disease) to serve as a common end point, the assessment of CVD and the outcome of its treatment is much more complex than with peripheral arterial disease. For this reason, QOL instruments might be particularly helpful in clinical investigations of CVD and its treatment. In addition, there is the need to demonstrate the value of certain treatments to health care authorities, as, for example, reimbursement for compressive therapy, for varicose vein surgery and for some aspects of venous ulcer management, all of which continue to be at issue. However, beyond this general agreement on need, there are a number of related issues that are not settled. These can be presented as a series of questions:

- Do general QOL instruments suffice for this purpose or should they be used in conjunction with disease specific (venous) questionnaires, and vice versa?
- Which general or generic QOL instrument should be used?
- Of the disease-specific questionnaires, is any one questionnaire adequate for evaluating the treatment of CVD in its broadest context, or should separate, more specific questionnaires be used (e.g. one for patients with varicose veins, another for patients with venous ulcers)?
- Depending on the answers to the above questions, should an additional venous QOL instrument be developed which is more suitable for all of CVD?

Varicose vein surgery[12,13] and long-term DVT outcome[14] have been evaluated using the Medical Outcomes Study Short Form (SF-36) health assessment questionnaire alone, but most now feel that this approach to outcome assessment would serve better if one of the generic instruments were augmented by a venous specific questionnaire. There are other generic health impairment questionnaires, like the Nottingham Health Profile and the Sickness Impact Profile, but they are quite long, and currently the SF-36, or the SF-12, seems preferred for use in conjunction with a disease-specific questionnaire.

Four disease specific instruments have been developed:

- A group of French authors have developed and validated a questionnaire for patients with venous disease.[15] It is short, consisting of only 20 questions, and has been prepared in an English version. It emphasizes four dimensions – psychological, pain, physical and social function. Internal consistency (α >0.82) and stability (r >0.82) were excellent, but external validity with the SF-36 was not measured. However, it does *not* emphasize the specific anatomic and physiologic issues of severe CVD. Rather it is limited to certain objective findings and subjective symptoms, some of which are vague. Edema, induration, skin temperature change, cyanosis/erythema were primary inclusion criteria and the symptoms included heavy legs, leg pain, nocturnal cramps, paresthesias or burning sensations. Inclusion of these vague and nonspecific end points may have been felt necessary to differentiate the potential efficacy of a venotonic flavonoid preparation under investigation. The validation was derived from a diffuse group of patients from three general practice settings who were thought to have CVD. However, the presence of lipodermatosclerosis or ulceration was not noted and objective venous testing was not performed routinely.

- The Aberdeen questionnaire[16] is well validated and has been used with the SF-36.[17] It includes 20 questions, seven of which separately detail the right and left leg. The severity of its components are weighted in a scoring system which attributes the greatest value to the anatomic distribution of varicose veins, as diagrammed by the patient, the second greatest to ulceration and the third to eczema (rash). Cosmetic considerations are juxtaposed with the severity of long-standing disease. Smith *et al.* first applied it clinically to the evaluation of varicose vein surgery[18] and further validated it against a 25-question 'patients symptoms and concerns' scale. Since varicose veins can lead to ulceration and thus run the entire CEAP spectrum, this instrument has the potential capacity for general use; however, it clearly is directed towards varicose veins primarily and there are no questions directed specifically towards deep venous disease.
- Smith and colleagues have also formulated a questionnaire specifically venous ulceration.[19] This questionnaire, which was refined from 32 down to 20 items, and the SF-36 general health measure were given to a prospective consecutive cohort of 98 patients with proven venous ulcers diagnosed on clinical and color duplex examination. The ulcer-specific questionnaire showed good reliability in regard to internal consistency (Cronbach's $\alpha = 0.93$) and test–retest analysis ($r = 0.84$). Four important health factors were identified: social function, domestic activities, cosmesis and emotional status. Validity was demonstrated by a high correlation with all eight domains of the SF-36 general health measure ($r > 0.55$, $P < 0.001$). Responsiveness was demonstrated by a significant reduction in the score of the ulcer questionnaire as ulcers healed at 6 and 11 weeks ($P < 0.05$). This questionnaire, called the Charing Cross Venous Ulcer questionnaire, has been carefully developed and validated.
- A fourth health-related quality-of-life (HR-QOL) instrument for venous disease was developed at Temple University School of Medicine and applied to the evaluation of catheter-directed thrombolytic therapy on patients with iliofemoral DVT in comparison with a group of patients treated with anticoagulant therapy alone.[20] It has been separately validated.[21] The 80-item self-administered HR-QOL questionnaire contains the Health Utilities Index, Short Form-12 and disease-targeted scales including health distress, stigma, health interference, physical functioning and symptoms (e.g. leg swelling, pain, ulcers). Psychometric testing confirmed that the questionnaire is reliable and valid. This questionnaire may be too long for general use. In addition, it has only been used for the mid-term outcome after DVT, not the treatment of CVD. However, it has many well-designed and pertinent questions.

At this point a single practical HR-QOL for evaluating the complete spectrum of CVD and its treatment has not yet been developed. The Aberdeen questionnaire, with its application to patients with varicose veins, and the Charing Cross Venous Ulcer questionnaire, for patients with venous ulcers, appear to be excellent instruments to focus on those specific manifestations of CVD. The question remains whether it would be better to take the best elements of these and the other two questionnaires and develop a universal HR-QOL for the broader spectrum of CVD. However, presuming this is feasible, the development, field testing and validation of the end product (for validity, internal consistency, stability, reliability) will take considerable time and effort. Nevertheless, such a project is under consideration by the committee.

STANDARDIZATION OF NON-INVASIVE VENOUS TESTING TO SERVE AS OBJECTIVE CRITERIA FOR REPORTING PRACTICES

The change in venous status scale featured in the current venous reporting standards to gauge the 'final outcome after surgery'[4] combines a categorical change in clinical status with a significant change in an objective functional test, in a +3 to −3 scale. It is conceptually sound, but it depends on the ability to change CEAP clinical class (see previous discussion) and accepted standards for noninvasive tests. What constitutes 'significant change' in these tests, and which tests and values are appropriate and equivalent for use as objective gauges of reflux, obstruction or overall abnormal venous function, deserves clarification and standardization.

The current venous reporting standards do not really address what test values serve to identify normal and abnormal venous function, and for evidence of 'significant change' following operation only a 10 mmHg change in ambulatory venous pressure (AVP) or a 10-second difference in venous refill time (VRT-PPG) are suggested. These recommendations are felt to be inadequate for current use and deserve updating.

The test values separating abnormal from normal venous function are somewhat better known for the more commonly used tests than what constitutes 'significant change', although the former may be specific for certain test conditions such as body or limb position, duration and method of standardizing leg muscle pump activity, release of venous occlusion. Regarding the latter, in principle, normalization of a test is clear evidence for significant change, and would qualify for +3 on the above scale. For +2, or in the absence of clinical categorical improvement, +1 designations, one basically needs to apply the least degree of change that is beyond reasonable limits of operator error. Although it might seem a simple task to determine the confidence limits of test reproducibility, these are not well established for most tests. Part of the problem is that a small change might normalize a slightly abnormal test value, and, conversely, the more abnormal the test is the greater the degree of change needed to make a significant difference. For example, for the Venous Filling Index (VFI), using air plethysmography, an abnormal value is >2.0 ml/s. Below that value, in the normal range, a change of 0.3 ml/s is said to be significant; from 2 to 10 ml/s a change of 1 ml/s is significant; and, in the very abnormal range, >10 ml/s, a change of 2 ml/s is significant (E Arkans, personal communication). In other tests, specifically those of valve reflux and venous obstruction, only normalization is accepted as significant change. Finally, the tests themselves do not correlate evenly with changes in clinical classification. It is not a simple matter.

Standardization is clearly needed, given the biases or differences of opinion and the differences in venous testing practices that still exist. The need would best be met by a multicenter study of the most widely used tests, performed together and repeatedly on the same subjects, with normal subjects and patients with different degrees of abnormality represented and CEAP staged. The committee and the Executive Council of the American Venous Forum recognize this need and support such a study.

However, accumulating and analyzing such data as the basis for solid recommendations will take some time. Meanwhile, can we propose interim guidelines? The committee attempted to do this, based on a survey of 16 recognized experts on venous testing. They were queried as to what values of which tests are acceptable to use as objective criteria to gauge 'abnormal venous function' and a 'significant change' in venous function, as well as their view of the reliability of each as either a 'stand-alone' or confirmatory test, the latter meaning acceptable in association with clinical evidence of change, as in the +3 to −3 scale. The results were viewed in the light of the Paris Consensus[22] and the following were offered as interim guidelines.

Reflux or global

- Ambulatory venous pressure: abnormal value >30 mmHg; significant change >10 mmHg.
- Photoplethysmography, venous refill time: abnormal value = VRT <20 seconds sitting, <18 seconds standing; significant change >5 seconds.
- Air plethysmography, venous filling index (venous filling time @ 90%): abnormal VFI >2 ml/s, significant change in abnormal value = improvement by >2 ml/s or normalization.
- Duplex scan valve closure time: abnormal value = VCT >0.5 seconds or >1.0 second (depending on position and technique of release of backflow). Significant change: conversion to normal.

Obstruction

- Air plethysmography, outflow fraction: abnormal value = OF <35% in 1 second, significant change >10%.
- Venous pressure gradient: resting >4 mmHg, induced hyperemia >6 mmHg. Significant change >2 mmHg and conversion to normal.
- Venous occlusion plethysmography (maximum venous outflow versus venous capacitance): abnormal value: MVO >200 ml/s or VC/VO ratio below discriminate line. Significant change conversion from abnormal to normal.

The values offered for significant change in some tests do not represent the confidence limits of reproducibility, partly because they are not well established, but also because, like the values chosen for the ankle brachial index in the arterial reporting standards,[2] it was felt that the least change that could be accepted as objective evidence of change in association with significant (e.g. categorical) clinical improvement, would better serve the intended purpose.

A number of other tests were considered but not included because they were felt to be either not widely enough used or lacking in agreement on what were the accepted values.

The tests and values listed above are based on the committee's view of current opinion, and may be subject to debate. However, they were felt to better serve the purpose of the current Venous Reporting Standards in regard to objective evidence in support of the claim of 'significant change' on its +3 to −3 scale than the present limited recommendation (10 mmHg AVP or 10 seconds VRT). These values could serve pending further definitive study as recommended above.

IDENTIFYING AND GRADING RISK FACTORS THAT SIGNIFICANTLY AFFECT LIMB OUTCOME AFTER DVT

Therapeutic anticoagulation with unfractionated or low molecular weight heparin (LMWH) followed by warfarin remains standard therapy for acute deep venous thrombosis (DVT).[23] However, different preparations and dosage schedules of LMWH are being compared, and ambulatory therapy with LMWH and compression bandages is being compared with standard inpatient therapy. In addition, new anticoagulants, catheter-directed thrombolytic therapy,[24] compression stockings[25] and surgery all might play a role in treatment in selected cases and be the focus of clinical trials. Although the incidence of recurrent venous thromboembolism, specifically PE and recurrent DVT, have been the most common end points in trials evaluating the anticoagulant treatment of acute DVT, the incidence and severity of post-thrombotic sequelae is also an important, though frequently neglected, end point of treatment. To properly compare different therapeutic regimens for acute DVT in this regard, one should knowing the determinants of long-term limb outcome and grading the treatment groups accordingly. Currently there is no scheme for doing this, so it is possible that differences in late outcome may be due to differences in the treatment groups in regard to factors that significantly affect outcome rather than differences in the treatments themselves.

To accomplish this, factors need to be identified that, when scored, would correlate with outcome, e.g. with the venous clinical severity score presented above. Ideally such a scheme should include factors that could be assessed at the time of a patient's presentation with an acute DVT. This not only would permit a precise description of populations included in clinical trials, and allow subgroups that derived the greatest benefit from any treatment to be identified, but in comparing therapeutic regimens, it would also assure comparable treatment groups. However, recognizing the current limitations, some pretreatment factors do have the potential to influence long-term outcome and they should be included in reports of any DVT treatment being evaluated in regard to the incidence of post-thrombotic syndrome. Although substantial evidence relating these factors to long-term outcome is lacking and it is not yet possible to develop on the basis of objective data a scoring scheme predictive of the severity of CVD following acute DVT, the following should be considered and included in reports comparing DVT therapies.

The extent of thrombosis

Although investigators have not been able to identify a clear relationship between the extent of thrombosis and long-term outcome,[26,27] some means of comparing the extent of thrombus among patients subjected to various therapies is necessary and currently, use of the reporting scheme proposed in the updated reporting standards in venous disease[4] is recommended.

The anatomic distribution of thrombosis

Although some investigators have found the distribution of thrombus to be unrelated to outcome,[26] others have noted a weak correlation between initial tibial and popliteal segmental scores, as defined by the reporting standards, and ultimate clinical class.[27] Furthermore, it does appear that the frequency of symptoms at 1 year is less after isolated calf vein than after proximal venous thrombosis.[28] At the very least, it would seem appropriate to specify the relative number of limbs with isolated calf vein and proximal venous thrombosis included in any clinical trial. A scoring system based on segments involved might be utilized.

Previous thrombotic events

The clinical prognosis is clearly worse after symptomatic recurrent thrombotic events, ipsilateral recurrences being associated with a sixfold increased risk of the post-thrombotic syndrome.[29] It therefore seems logical that patients with a history of previous DVT would have a worse outcome with a new episode. The relative proportion of patients with previous lower extremity thrombosis should therefore be included in reports of therapeutic clinical trials, if not specifically excluded by protocol.

Thrombotic risk factors

Irreversible thrombotic risk factors should contribute to an increased risk of recurrent thrombosis, and thus an increased risk of post-thrombotic sequelae. No individual clinical risk factors have yet been clearly related to the severity of chronic venous disease;[10] however, some assessment of overall thrombotic risk, such as the weighted scheme included in the updated venous reporting standards,[4] should be included in describing patients subjected to treatment.

In pursuing this approach, one is faced with a similar situation seen with some of the above described approaches to outcomes assessment, and the committee is at a point of choosing between one of two options:

- carrying out prospective studies of DVT patients in significant numbers to identify the relative contribution of the above risk factors and other potential determinants of long-term outcome after DVT, then use those data as the basis for a grading scheme; or
- proposing an arbitrary scheme and field test it prospectively, modifying it later on the basis of the data obtained.

Either way, this effort will likely require studies with large numbers of patients. Unfortunately, untreated patients are not available for such study for ethical reasons, so groups with standard anticoagulant therapy will have to be used instead, possibly those serving as controls for newer therapies. Meanwhile trials of new therapeutic approaches should characterize treatment groups in regard to at least the above four generally accepted risk factors.

On a separate note, it should be pointed out that there are a number of factors known to affect long-term outcome, which can only be assessed during follow-up. These include the global extent of reflux, the anatomic distribution of reflux, the rate of recanalization, and the presence of residual venous obstruction. Whilst they develop during treatment, and thus have limited utility in characterizing a population prior to treatment, they may be identified early enough to be prognostic of long-term outcome and thus be valuable in not only early identification of those needing intensive conservative management but in comparing therapies directed at mitigating the post-thrombotic syndrome. The committee feels this additional aspect might be included in the prospective longitudinal studies recommended above.

CONCLUSIONS

The additional approaches to venous outcomes assessments discussed in this chapter represent the deliberations of a single committee, at best the measured views of a few experts in the field. Much of what is recommended is admittedly arbitrary. It is clear that they would be better based on data from large multicenter studies of patients with venous disease, in whom clinical and duplex scan data were gathered and correlated with CEAP classification, other outcome criteria and tests of venous function. We enthusiastically advocate and encourage the correlative studies needed to put these efforts on a more objective basis. However, whilst 6 years of venous evaluation using CEAP have brought great improvements, there are still unmet needs in venous outcomes assessment. At the very least we hope we have identified these needs and, for some of them, have suggested additional methods or approaches that should improve venous outcomes assessment.

ACKNOWLEDGMENT

The Venous Severity Scoring System, including both the Venous Clinical Severity Score and the Venous Segmental Disease Severity Score, and the modified Venous Disability Score have been approved by the Executive Council of the American Venous Forum and have been published in the *Journal of Vascular Surgery*.[30] The tables and much of the text on those sections have been drawn from that article.

REFERENCES

1. Porter JP, Rutherford RB, Clagett GP, *et al.* Reporting standards in venous disease. *J Vasc Surg* 1988; **8**: 172–81.
2. Rutherford RB, Baker JD, Ernst C, *et al.* Recommended standards for reports dealing with lower extremity ischemia: revised version. *J Vasc Surg* 1997; **26**: 517–38.
3. Nicolaides AN, and members of the executive committee. Classification and grading of chronic venous disease in the lower limbs: a consensus statement. In Gloviczki P, Yao JST, eds. *Handbook of Venous Disorders.* London: Chapman & Hall, 1996: 652–60.
4. Porter JP, Moneta GM, and an International Consensus Committee on Chronic Venous Disease. Reporting standards in venous disease: an update. *J Vasc Surg* 1995; **21**: 635–45.
5. Porter JP, Moneta GM, and an International Consensus Committee on Chronic Venous Disease. Reporting standards in venous disease: an update. In Gloviczki P, Yao JST, eds. *Handbook of Venous Disorders.* London: Chapman & Hall, 1996: 629–51.
6. Rutherford RB. Presidential Address: Vascular surgery – comparing outcomes. *J Vasc Surg* 1996; **23**: 5–17.
7. Rosfors S, Lamke LO, Nordstroem E, Bydegman S. Severity and location of venous valvular insufficiency: the importance of distal valve function. *Acta Chir Scand* 1990; **156**: 689.
8. Gooley NA, Sumner DS. Relationship of venous reflux to the site of venous valvular incompetence: implications for venous reconstructive surgery. *J Vasc Surg* 1988; **7**: 50–9.
9. Stacey MC, Burnand KG, Thomas ML, Pattison M. Phlebographic abnormalities in the natural history of ulceration. *Br J Surg* 1991: **78**; 868–71.
10. Prandoni P, Lensing AWA, Cogo A, *et al.* The long term clinical course of acute deep venous thrombosis. *Ann Intern Med* 1996; **125**: 1–7.
11. Meissner MH, Caps MT, Zierler BK, *et al.* Determinants of chronic venous disease after acute deep venous thrombosis. *J Vasc Surg* 1998; **28**: 826–33.
12. Baker DM, Turnbull NB, Pearson JC, Makin GS. How successful is varicose vein surgery? A patient outcome study using SF-36 health assessment questionnaire. *Eur J Vasc Surg* 1995; **9**: 299–304.
13. Paisley AM, Bradbury AW. The effect of deep venous reflux on the results of superficial venous surgery. Presented at the 12th Annual Meeting of the American Venous Forum, Phoenix, AZ, Feb 5, 2000 (submitted to *J Vasc Surg*).
14. Beyth RJ, Cohen AN, Landesfeld CS. Long term outcome of DVT. *Arch Intern Med* 1995; **155**: 1031–7.
15. Launois R, Reboul-Marty J, Henry B. Construction and validation of a quality of life questionnaire in chronic lower limb venous insufficiency. *Qual Life Res* 1996; **5**: 539–54.

16. Garratt AM, MacDonald LM, Ruta DA, Russell IT, Buckingham JK, Krukowski ZH. Towards measurement of outcome for patients with varicose veins. *Qual Health Care* 1993; **3**: 5–10.
17. Garratt AM, Ruta DA, Abdalla MI, Russell IT. Responsiveness of the SF-36 and a condition specific measure of health outcome for patients with varicose veins. *Qual Life Res* 1996; **5**: 1–12.
18. Smith JJ, Garratt AM, Guest M, Greenhalgh RM, Davies AH. Evaluating and improving health related quality of life in patients with varicose veins. *J Vasc Surg* 1999; **30**: 710–19.
19. Smith JJ, Guest M, Greenhalgh RM, Davies AH. Measuring the quality of life in patients with venous ulcers. *J Vasc Surg* 2000; **31**: 642–9.
20. Comerota AJ, Throm RC, Mathias SD, Haughton S, Mewissen M. Catheter directed thrombolysis for iliofemoral deep vein thrombosis improves health related quality of life. *J Vasc Surg* 2000; **32**: 130–7.
21. Mathias SD, Preble LA, Putterman CG, Chmiel JJ, Throm RC, Comerota AJ. Health related quality of life measure in patients with deep venous thrombosis: a validation study. *Drug Inf J* 1999; **33**: 1173–87.
22. Nicolaides AN. The investigation of chronic venous insufficiency: a consensus statement. *Circulation* 2000; **102**: E126–63.
23. Hyers TM, Agnelli G, Hull RD, *et al.* Antithrombotic therapy for venous thromboembolic disease. *Chest* 1998; **114**: 561S–78S.
24. Mewissen MW, Seabrook GR, Meissner MH, Cynamon J, Labropoulos N, Haughton SH. Catheter-directed thrombolysis of lower extremity deep venous thrombosis: report of a national multicenter registry. *Radiology* 1999; **211**: 39–49.
25. Brandjes D, Buller H, Heijboer H, *et al.* Randomised trial of effect of compression stockings in patients with symptomatic proximal-vein thrombosis. *Lancet* 1997; **349**: 759–62.
26. Browse NL, Clemenson G, Thomas ML. Is the postphlebitic leg always postphlebitic? Relation between phlebographic appearances of deep-vein thrombosis and late sequelae. *Br Med J* 1980; **281**: 1167–70.
27. Meissner MH, Caps MT, Zierler BK, *et al.* Determinants of chronic venous disease after acute deep venous thrombosis. *J Vasc Surg* 1998; **28**: 826–33.
28. Meissner M, Caps M, Bergelin R, Manzo R, Strandness D. Early outcome after isolated calf vein thrombosis. *J Vasc Surg* 1997; **26**: 749–56.
29. Prandoni P, Lensing A, Cogo A, *et al.* The long term clinical course of acute deep venous thrombosis. *Ann Intern Med* 1996; **125**: 1–7.
30. Rutherford RB, Padberg FT Jr, Comerota AJ, Kistner RL, Meissner MH, Moneta GL. Venous severity scoring: an adjunct to venous outcome assessment. *J Vasc Surg* 2000; **31**: 1307–12.

51

Reporting standards in venous disease: an update

JOHN M PORTER, GREGORY L MONETA, AND AN INTERNATIONAL CONSENSUS COMMITTEE ON CHRONIC VENOUS DISEASE

ACUTE LOWER EXTREMITY VENOUS THROMBOSIS

Risk factors and predisposing conditions

The following is an attempt to quantify risk for acute lower extremity deep vein thrombosis. This quantification scheme, although unproven, may allow more precise patient characterization in reports evaluating prophylaxis and treatment of deep venous thrombosis.

PRIOR HISTORY OF DEEP VENOUS THROMBOSIS

A prior episode of lower extremity deep venous thrombosis is the greatest risk factor for a subsequent episode of deep venous thrombosis.[1] A history of an abnormal phlebogram or an abnormal objective vascular laboratory examination (phleborheography, impedance plethysmography, B-mode ultrasound imaging, or ultrasonic duplex scanning) is sufficient to establish a prior episode of proximal lower extremity deep venous thrombosis. A history of isolated calf vein thrombosis requires a previous abnormal phlebogram or a definitive duplex ultrasound examination. A patient with clinical post-thrombotic syndrome and no history of prior deep venous thrombosis should be classified as grade 1 (suspected).

Assign grade
- 0 = none
- 1 = suspected
- 2 = proven
- 3 = multiple

IMMOBILIZATION

Immobilization from illness or injury is a deep venous thrombosis risk factor.[2] Duration and cause of the immobilization influence the risk of deep venous thrombosis.

Assign grade
- 0 = none
- 1 = 1–3 days
- 2 = >3 days
- 3 = immobilization caused by acute paraplegia[3]

POSTOPERATIVE STATE

Duration of operation and type of anesthesia appear related to development of postoperative deep venous thrombosis.[4] Patients undergoing pelvic, hip and lower extremity orthopedic procedures and intercranial neurosurgical operations are at particular risk.

Assign grade
- 0 = local anesthesia
- 1 = <45 minutes, regional or general
- 2 = >45 minutes, regional or general
- 3 = extensive major (> 3 hours) and/or pelvic operation[5]

AGE

Increasing age increases the risk of deep venous thrombosis.[6]

Reprinted with permission from *Journal of Vascular Surgery* 1995; **21**: 634–45.

Assign grade

- 0 = < 40 years
- 1 = 40–70 years
- 2 = >70 years

MALIGNANCY

The presence of a malignancy and its extent may influence the development of deep venous thrombosis.[7]

Assign grade

- 0 = none
- 1 = nonrecurrence or local recurrence only
- 2 = extensive regional tumor
- 3 = metastatic

TISSUE TYPE OF MALIGNANCY

Tissue type of associated malignancy may also influence development of deep venous thrombosis.

Assign grade

- 0 = other than adenocarcinoma
- 1 = adenocarcinoma (especially mucinous adenocarcinoma), malignant glioma of the brain

CARDIAC DISEASE

Severity of cardiac disability appears to increase the risk of developing deep venous thrombosis.[8]

Assign grade

- 0 = New York Heart Association (NYHA) class 1
- 1 = NYHA class 2
- 2 = NYHA class 3
- 3 = NYHA class 4

LIMB TRAUMA

Bony and extensive soft tissue lower extremity or pelvic injury increases the likelihood of lower extremity deep venous thrombosis.[9]

Assign grade

- 0 = none
- 1 = soft tissue injury including bruise, contusion, and sprain
- 2 = fracture of tibia and/or fibula
- 3 = fracture of femur
- 4 = fracture of hip or pelvis

PRETHROMBOTIC STATE

Several coagulation abnormalities predispose to abnormal clotting, including venous thrombosis. These include but are not limited to antithrombin III deficiency; protein C or S resistance or deficiency; myeloproliferative disorders, especially thrombocytosis; plasma hyperviscosity states; lupus anticoagulant and/or anticardiolipin antibodies, factor V Leiden, prothrombin gene mutation, hyperhomocysteinemia.[10–14]

Assign grade

- 0 = none suspected
- 1 = suspected
- 2 = proven, treated
- 3 = proven, untreated

HORMONAL THERAPY

Prolonged erogenous ethinyl estradiol in a dosage in excess of 50 μg daily is associated with an increased risk of venous thrombosis.[15,16] Neither low-dose estrogen therapy nor any other hormonal therapy has such a clear relationship to deep venous thrombosis, although others are suspected.

Assign grade

- 0 = no
- 1 = yes

PREGNANCY AND POSTPARTUM STATE

Venous thrombosis is five times more likely in a pregnant or post-puerperal woman compared with a non-pregnant, non-puerperal woman not taking oral contraceptive medication.[17]

Assign grade

- 0 = absent
- 1 = present

OBESITY

Extreme obesity may be a mild independent risk factor in deep venous thrombosis.[18]

Assign grade

- 0 = normal to 175% ideal body weight
- 1 = >175% ideal body weight

SUMMARY

The factors listed represent our impression of the risk factors relevant to the development of deep venous thrombosis. With the relative risk assessment weighting scheme described (maximum possible score = 28), future studies of deep venous thrombosis prophylaxis and therapy may be stratified by the deep venous thrombosis risk factor score to ensure equality of comparison populations.

Clinical presentation

EXTENT OF THROMBUS AND SITE INVOLVEMENT

The anatomic sites of involvement must be detailed for clinical reports of deep venous thrombosis. Involvement of the following deep venous segments should be specified:

- tibial–soleal veins
- popliteal vein

- common femoral or superficial femoral vein
- iliac vein
- vena cava.

Specified superficial sites include:

- greater saphenous vein and its branches
- lesser saphenous vein and its branches
- unnamed cutaneous veins, in which case the location of the veins should be specified.

Each of the six deep and two superficial venous segments should be graded as follows and tabulated individually.

Assign grade
- 0 = patent
- 1 = subsegmental, nonocclusive thrombus
- 2 = subsegmental, occlusive thrombus
- 3 = occlusive thrombus throughout length of segment

The maximal thrombotic score for a single limb is 24. Either phlebography or duplex scanning may be used to calculate the thrombotic score.

Clinical description

Acute venous thrombosis should be described as superficial, deep, or combined.

SUPERFICIAL VENOUS THROMBOSIS

Site and extent of involvement should be specified. Tenderness, erythema, induration, or suppuration should be noted. It is essential that the patency of the deep veins be documented phlebographically or by duplex scanning in reports dealing with superficial venous thrombosis as the coexistence of deep venous thrombosis may confuse the clinical presentation and response to therapy of superficial venous thrombosis. In particular, superficial venous thrombosis involving the proximal greater saphenous vein is often associated with extension into the common femoral vein.[19]

DEEP VENOUS THROMBOSIS

The site and extent of involvement should be specified. The presence and location of pain and the extent of swelling should be noted in case reports.

Definitions

The following terms are used often enough to require uniform definition.

PHLEGMASIA ALBA DOLENS

This term indicates marked swelling of the lower extremity without associated cyanosis. It refers to a characteristic clinical picture and does not denote the existence of deep venous thrombosis at a precise site.

PHLEGMASIA CERULEA DOLENS

This term indicates massive limb swelling and cyanosis. Venous thrombosis is more extensive than in phlegmasia alba dolens and the extremity is painful. It may be associated with arterial insufficiency, compartmental compression syndrome, or venous gangrene.[20]

VENOUS GANGRENE

This refers to full-thickness skin necrosis resulting from deep venous thrombosis. Blebs or blisters represent partial thickness necrosis and as such may be regarded as early venous gangrene. Compartment syndrome(s) may coexist.

Diagnostic testing

Diagnostic tests for acute deep venous thrombosis are classified as physiologic, anatomic, or combined.

PHYSIOLOGIC TESTS

Recognized physiologic tests for the diagnosis of deep venous thrombosis include:

- continuous-wave Doppler examination with the use of flow interruption or augmentation maneuvers
- plethysmography – impedance/air/volume and strain-gauge.

These tests are valid only when performed by experienced examiners and usually only under the following conditions:

- absence of prior history of deep vein thrombosis of the same extremity;
- absence of extrinsic venous compression as may occur with pregnancy or hematoma.[21]

ANATOMIC TESTS

Contrast phlebography and ultrasound B-mode imaging combined with color-flow imaging are acceptable techniques for determining the anatomic extent of acute deep venous thrombosis. Uptake of ^{125}I-labeled fibrinogen, because of poor specificity, is not.[22]

When phlebography is used, the technique should be described in detail, specifically the use of tourniquets, head or foot table elevation, and volume and type of contrast medium. Positive phlebograms must be described as directly or indirectly positive. A directly positive test is one in which thrombus is outlined by contrast medium. Non-filling of deep vein segments without visualization of thrombus is an indirect sign of deep venous thrombosis.

B-mode image positivity requires visualization of the thrombus or absence of normal venous wall coaptation with external pressure. Color flow should be used, when available, to confirm absence of venous flow or the presence of nonoccluding thrombus.

COMBINED PHYSIOLOGIC AND ANATOMIC EVALUATION

Duplex scanning combines ultrasound image (anatomic) and Doppler flow (physiologic) data. The criteria for positivity of this test must be specified by the author. Pulse Doppler flow data are considered positive for deep venous thrombosis in the absence of a normal intraluminal venous flow signal and image evidence of thrombosis in the insonated segment as detailed above.

Treatment

The choices of treatment of deep venous thrombosis include nonoperative supportive therapy, drug treatment, and thrombectomy.

NONOPERATIVE SUPPORTIVE TREATMENT

Reports should specify use and duration of bed rest, leg elevation, and compressive therapy. If the last is used the type should be specified: bandages, inelastic devices, external pumps, elastic hosiery, etc. When describing elastic hosiery, the length of the garment (below or above knee, or waist-high), whether the garment is of gradient construction, and the manufacturer's stated amount of compression measured in mmHg should be specified.

DRUG THERAPY

Drug therapy for deep venous thrombosis includes anticoagulants, thrombolytics, and other less well-recognized medications.

Anticoagulation

Unfractionated heparin sodium and low molecular weight heparins are the usual initial anticoagulants for therapy of acute deep venous thrombosis. If unfractionated heparin sodium is used, the rate of administration, dosage and duration of therapy should be specified. The type and frequency of monitoring to determine anticoagulant effect must be reported. The usual tests for monitoring heparin anticoagulant activity include partial thromboplastin time (PTT) and activated clotting time (ACT). Whatever test is used, it should be related to the PTT to allow readers a normative reference. If the route of drug administration is other than by continuous intravenous administration, the timing of blood sampling for monitoring tests in relation to prior dose of heparin must be specified. If low molecular weight heparin is used, the molecular weight and source of the heparin must be specified, as well as the dosing schedule.

When a patient is switched from heparin to warfarin, the timing and duration of the drug overlap should be described. The dose, frequency, type of monitoring, and duration of therapy for warfarin anticoagulation must be specified. The intensity of warfarin anticoagulation ideally is expressed in terms of the international normalized ratio (INR).[23] When this is not possible, the intensity should be expressed as a prothrombin ratio (e.g. 1.5–2 × control). When the intensity of warfarin anticoagulation is expressed as a prothrombin time ratio, the test reagent used in performing the prothrombin time test should be specified.

Thrombolytic therapy

The drug, dosage, route of administration, and laboratory method of monitoring thrombolytic activity must be detailed. The frequency and results of sequential contrast phlebograms or duplex scans must be specified. A perfect result requires complete phlebographic or duplex scan determined patency and vascular laboratory determination of normal valvular competency as determined by duplex determination of valve closure times.[24]

Results of lytic therapy should be reported as the percentage of limbs experiencing total clot resolution with overall preservation of valve function. Serial objective patient outcome data regarding patency and valve function should be presented in a life-table format. Patency may be evaluated by serial phlebograms or duplex scans. Assessment of segmental valvular competence should be by duplex-derived valve closure times. Overall reflux in the limb can be evaluated with direct ambulatory venous pressure measurements, venous recovery times (VRT), or air plethysmography.[25] Because reflux may develop late,[26] separate life tables should be presented for patency and valvular competence.

Incomplete clot resolution should be reported as failure of thrombolytic therapy. Reporting outcome of thrombolytic therapy as a percentage of thrombus resolution is not acceptable. On occasion, restoration of patency in large veins, such as the vena cava or iliac veins, may be the goal of lytic therapy, and in these select cases restoration of valvular competency is irrelevant. Restoration of patency of infrainguinal veins without valvular competence should be noted.

Other drug therapy

The use of drugs other than heparin sodium, heparinoids, warfarin, or thrombolytic agents in the treatment of deep venous thrombosis should include an explanation as to why the particular agent was selected. Route of administration, dosage, duration of therapy, and the method of monitoring drug effect must also be specified.

COMPLICATIONS OF DRUG THERAPY

Complications associated with drug therapy must be detailed. General complications and complications specific to individual agents should be described and their severity indicated as mild, moderate, or severe. Deaths directly related to the agent, in-hospital deaths and deaths within 30 days of hospital discharge, must be specifically noted.

SURGICAL THERAPY

Venous thrombectomy continues to be performed occasionally for lower extremity deep venous thrombosis.[27] Reports of such procedures should provide a detailed description of the surgical technique. The same reporting requirements pertain to venous thrombectomy as to thrombolytic therapy (see above). The same method of evaluation should be used for all patients included in an individual report.

Outcome of acute deep venous thrombosis

Pulmonary embolism as a complication of deep venous thrombosis should be specifically noted, with attention to the details listed in the section 'Pulmonary embolism'. The time course for resolution of local signs, such as edema and cyanosis, should be noted if relevant. The presence of recurrent episode(s) of deep venous thrombosis should be specifically noted, together with the objective tests used to establish the diagnosis. If relevant, subsequent occurrence of the post-thrombotic syndrome should be noted with attention to the details listed in the later section, 'Chronic venous disease'. Some vascular laboratory tests may not reliably establish the presence of a new episode of deep venous thrombosis as patients may have permanent vascular laboratory abnormalities after the first episode.

Venous thrombosis prophylaxis

The term 'prophylaxis' should be used only in relation to patients who have not sustained a recent deep venous thrombosis. Many reports describe the outcome of various prophylactic measures for patients defined as being at high risk for deep venous thrombosis. Such reports should, as described in the first section, 'Risk factors', calculate a risk factor index for each patient as well as an average for the study and control groups. In addition, the following should be included in reports on the efficacy of venous thrombosis prophylaxis.

MECHANICAL METHODS OF PROPHYLAXIS

Leg exercises should be described as active or passive and type, frequency, and duration specified. For compression stockings, design (whether gradient or not), length, compression measured in mmHg, and the frequency and duration of use should be specified. Studies employing pneumatic leg compression should detail the number of individual compression chambers, the pressure and time sequence of the pumping pattern, as well as the frequency and duration of treatment.

DRUG PROPHYLAXIS

The agents, route of administration, dosage, duration, and method of monitoring drug prophylaxis should be specified. If prophylaxis is directed toward prevention of postoperative thrombosis, the timing of the initiation of prophylaxis in relation to operation as well as the type and duration of operation should be stated.

CHRONIC VENOUS DISEASE

Chronic venous disease is defined as an abnormally functioning venous system caused by venous valvular incompetence with or without associated venous outflow obstruction, which may affect the superficial venous system, the deep venous system, or both. Venous dysfunction may result from either a congenital or an acquired disorder.

The term 'post-thrombotic' may be used if the patient has experienced an objectively documented prior episode of deep venous thrombosis. The term 'post-phlebitic syndrome' should not be used because this implies the presence of an inflammatory component that is infrequently confirmed. In the absence of a clear documentation of a prior episode of deep venous thrombosis, the condition should be termed 'chronic venous disease' without additional suggestion of origin.

Physical examination: descriptive terms

VENOUS DILATION

Mild chronic venous insufficiency is signified by the occurrence of a submalleolar venous flare. Greater degrees of venous dilation are apparent by both observation and palpation. Telangiectases are defined as dilated intradermal venules less than 1 mm in size. Reticular veins are defined as dilated, nonpalpable, subdermal veins $\leq$ 4 mm in size. Varicose veins are defined as dilated, palpable, subcutaneous veins generally larger than 4 mm.

EDEMA

The presence of edema indicates more functionally advanced venous disease than the presence of venous dilation alone. In individual case reports and when otherwise applicable, the location and extent of edema should be noted and objectively documented with circumferential limb measurements.

SKIN PIGMENTATION

Pigmentation changes and other cutaneous manifestations of chronic venous disease (venous eczema, lipodermatosclerosis) are important signs of severe chronic venous disease. They should be described along with a subjective assessment of severity.

VENOUS ULCERATION

The location and measurements of any venous ulcer should be described and the presence or absence of granulation tissue noted. The presence of healed venous ulceration manifested by cutaneous scarring should be noted.

Classification of chronic venous disease: C,E,A,P system

Limbs with chronic venous disease should be classified according to clinical signs (C), etiology (E), anatomic distribution (A), and pathophysiology (P). The classification system detailed below and summarized in Table 51.1 was developed in 1994 by an international consensus conference on chronic venous disease held under the auspices of the American Venous Forum. It replaces clinical classes 0–3 outlined in the 1988 version of 'Reporting Standards in Venous Disease'. This updated method of classifying chronic venous disease is designed to provide the additional details necessary to accurately compare limbs in medical and surgical treatment trials.

Table 51.1 *C,E,A,P classification of chronic lower extremity venous disease (see text for details)*

C	Clinical signs (grade 0–6), supplemented by A for asymptomatic and S for symptomatic presentation
E	Etiologic classification (Congential, Primary, Secondary)
A	Anatomic distribution (Superficial, Deep, or Perforator, alone or in combination)
P	Pathophysiologic dysfunction (Reflux or Obstruction, alone or in combination)

CLINICAL CLASSIFICATION (C_{0-6})

Any limb with possible chronic venous disease is first placed into one of seven clinical classes (C_{0-6}) according to the objective signs of disease listed in Table 51.2.

Limbs in higher categories have more severe signs of chronic venous disease and may have some or all of the findings defining a less severe clinical category. Each limb is further characterized as asymptomatic (A), e.g. $C_{0-6,A}$, or symptomatic (S), e.g. $C_{0-6,S}$. Symptoms which may be associated with telangiectatic, reticular, or varicose veins include lower extremity aching, pain and skin irritation. Therapy may alter the clinical category of chronic venous disease. Limbs should therefore be reclassified after any form of medical or surgical treatment.

ETIOLOGIC CLASSIFICATION (E_C, E_P, OR E_S)

Venous dysfunction may be congenital, primary, or secondary. These categories are mutually exclusive.

Table 51.2 *Clinical classification of chronic lower extremity venous disease*

Class 0	No visible or palpable signs of venous disease
Class 1	Telangiectases, reticular veins, malleolar flare
Class 2	Varicose veins
Class 3	Edema without skin changes
Class 4	Skin changes ascribed to venous disease (e.g. pigmentation, venous eczema, lipodermatosclerosis)
Class 5	Skin changes as defined above with healed ulceration
Class 6	Skin changes as defined above with active ulceration

Congenital venous disorders are present at birth but may not be recognized until later. The method of diagnosis of congenital abnormalities must be described. Primary venous dysfunction is defined as venous dysfunction of unknown etiology but not of congenital origin. Secondary venous dysfunction denotes an acquired condition resulting in chronic venous disease, e.g. deep venous thrombosis (Table 51.3).

Table 51.3 *Etiologic classification of chronic lower extremity venous disease*

Congenital (E_C)	The etiology of the chronic venous disease has been present since birth
Primary (E_P)	Chronic venous disease of undetermined etiology
Secondary (E_S)	Chronic venous disease with an associated known etiology (post-thrombotic, post-traumatic, other)

ANATOMIC CLASSIFICATION ($A_{S,D,P}$)

The anatomic site(s) of the venous disease should be described as superficial (A_S), deep (A_D), or perforating (A_P) vein(s). One, two or three systems may be involved in any combination. For reports requiring greater detail, the involvement of the superficial, deep, and perforating veins may be localized using the anatomic segments listed in Table 51.4.

PATHOPHYSIOLOGIC CLASSIFICATION ($P_{R,O}$)

Clinical signs or symptoms of chronic venous disease result from reflux (P_R), obstruction (P_O), or both ($P_{R,O}$). Measurement by superficial venous cannulation of the foot venous pressure at rest in the upright position and the change in pressure on walking has historically represented the 'gold standard' for the overall objective assessment of chronic venous disease.[25] It is now recommended that reports of patients with chronic venous disease be accompanied by sufficient objective measurements of venous hemodynamics and anatomy to adequately document the individual pathophysiologic

Table 51.4 *Segmental localization of chronic lower extremity venous disease*

Segment number	
	Superficial veins (A_{S1-5})
1	Telangiectasias/reticular veins
	Greater (long) saphenous vein
2	Above knee
3	Below knee
4	Lesser (short) saphenous vein
5	Nonsaphenous
	Deep veins (A_{D6-16})
6	Inferior vena cava
	Iliac
7	Common
8	Internal
9	External
10	Pelvic: gonadal, broad ligament
	Femoral
11	Common
12	Deep
13	Superficial
14	Popliteal
15	Tibial (anterior, posterior, or peroneal)
16	Muscular (gastrocnemius, soleal, other)
	Perforating veins ($A_{P17,18}$)
17	Thigh
18	Calf

changes, reflux, and/or obstruction accompanying chronic venous disease. Phlebographic or vascular laboratory studies can objectively assess the presence of venous outflow obstruction (P_O) as well as the presence of venous reflux (P_R) in the superficial, communicating, and deep venous systems.

Ascending phlebography defines areas of obstruction, recanalization, and collateral vein formation. Descending phlebography demonstrates competency of venous valves by assessing the magnitude of contrast reflux. Comparisons of different reports of descending phlebography are facilitated by knowledge of the technical details of performance of the procedure. Accordingly, reports of descending phlebography should include details of cannulation; type, volume, and injection rate of contrast media; tilt angle of the table; and maximal timed descent of the contrast column in the deep venous system.

Assessment of maximal venous outflow (MVO) by one of various plethysmographic techniques provides objective noninvasive information on the presence and amount of venous obstruction, (P_O). Sequential examinations are helpful in following the development of venous collaterals and/or recanalization after deep venous thrombosis. Maximal venous outflow must be related to simultaneously determined venous capacitance. Pressure gradients (e.g. arm/ankle) at rest or after induced hyperemia may also permit the objective assessment of outflow obstruction.

Directional continuous-wave Doppler examinations with proximal compression or Valsalva maneuver is a qualitative test for assessing reflux (P_R), in both the superficial and deep venous systems. Because the test is qualitative and uncontrolled, its use is discouraged in modern reports concerning chronic venous disease. Venous refill time (VRT) provides a measure of overall venous reflux that can be used in the objective assessment of chronic venous disease. It can be obtained invasively with foot venous cannulation used in conjunction with ambulatory venous pressure or noninvasively with photoplethysmography. Normalization of a shortened venous refill time by application of a leg tourniquet compressing superficial veins indicates that significant venous disease is limited to the superficial venous system.

The venous filling index (VFI) as determined by air plethysmography is another quantitative method of evaluating overall venous reflux.[28] Like VRT, the test can be performed with and without tourniquets in an effort to identify significant reflux limited to the superficial veins.

Because the severity of venous dysfunction is influenced by the anatomic location of the reflux and/or obstruction,[29] it may be desirable to report the anatomic segments involved with either reflux or obstruction using the venous segments outlined in Table 51.4. Currently, duplex ultrasound with the patient upright and the limb examined non-weight bearing, in combination with proximal deflation of a venous-occluding blood pressure cuff,[25] is the best documented noninvasive method of quantifying reflux, by measuring reflux duration, in specific axial superficial or deep venous segments. Duplex is also suggested as a means of identifying reflux in individual communicating veins.

Surgical procedures

SUPERFICIAL SYSTEM INSUFFICIENCY

Valvular competence of the deep veins has an obvious relationship to both the occurrence and recurrence of superficial varicosities. Thus reports of superficial venous ligation and stripping must describe communicating and deep venous valvular competence as assessed by appropriate phlebographic or vascular laboratory testing.

DEEP VENOUS OBSTRUCTION

When various conduits are used to bypass areas of venous obstruction, a detailed description of type, extent and configuration of the bypass conduit must be provided. Procedural reports, in addition to the patients' subjective assessment of benefit, should include vascular laboratory measurements of MVO obtained preoperatively and at least 6 months postoperatively to aid in objectively assessing surgical outcome. Patency of the bypass conduit should be assessed with either duplex or phlebography and presented in a life-table format.

DEEP VENOUS VALVULAR INSUFFICIENCY

The type of procedure used to correct this defect should be categorized as follows:

- *Valvuloplasty*: include a brief technical description of the procedure and the precise location and number of valves repaired.
- *Venous segmental transposition*: specify anastomotic connection, e.g. saphenous to profunda.
- *Venous segmental transplantation*: specify donor and recipient sites, the length of the transplanted segment, and number of valves contained in the transplanted segment.

EVALUATION OF OPERATIVE RESULTS

All publications describing patients having surgical repair of deep venous insufficiency or obstruction must include vascular laboratory measurements of lower extremity venous hemodynamics before and after operation to permit objective assessment of results. The tests must include, at a minimum, an overall evaluation of venous function using venous refill time or ambulatory venous pressure, and preferably both. MVO provides helpful additional information in patients operated on for venous obstruction, while duplex assessment of valvular competence, including the operative repair, should be performed in patients operated for valvular incompetence.

An author may, at his or her discretion, report the use of new and/or non-standardized vascular laboratory tests performed in an attempt to document objectively the functional results of deep vein reconstruction, but the report of such tests does not exempt the author from reporting the requisite standardized preoperative and postoperative vascular laboratory tests of venous function. All reports of deep vein repair should report at least 6 months of postoperative vascular laboratory follow-up, and preferably 12-month follow-up since progressive deterioration of initially satisfactory surgical results has occurred with some frequency. Reports must state whether the patient regularly used postoperative elastic compression hosiery. If so, the compression, measured in mmHg, must be included. Reports should also state whether the patient used intermittent leg elevation during the day. A suggested categorization of clinical outcome is presented in Table 51.5. It is recommended that no clinical outcome grade be assigned until at least 6 months after operation.

Table 51.5 *Clinical outcome after surgery*

+3	Asymptomatic	No symptoms of chronic venous disease Improvement of VRT to normal or at least +5 seconds Improvement in AVP to normal or at least −10 mmHg
+2	Moderate improvement	Mild symptoms of chronic venous disease Improvement of VRT to normal or at least +5 seconds Improvement in AVP to normal or at least −10 mmHg
+1	Mild improvement	Clinical improvement or improvement in vascular laboratory tests (VRT or AVP)
0	Unchanged	No change clinically or by vascular laboratory
−1	Mild worsening	Worsening of symptoms of chronic venous disease or vascular laboratory tests (VRT or AVP)
−2	Significant worsening	Worsening of symptoms and worsening of vascular laboratory tests (VRT or AVP)
−3	Marked worsening	Same as −2 accompanied by either new or worsening ankle claudication

VRT = venous refill time; AVP = ambulatory venous pressure.

UPPER EXTREMITY DEEP VENOUS DISEASE

Diagnosis

The clinical diagnosis of thrombosis of the deep veins of the upper extremity and cervical veins is imprecise. Reports of axillary-subclavian or internal jugular vein thrombosis must therefore use contrast or isotope phlebography or duplex scanning to objectively establish the diagnosis.

Etiology

The author should specify the presumed etiology of the venous thrombosis. Recognized causes include: clavicular and proximal humeral fracture, either acute or with malunion or chronic malposition; central venous cannulation; injection or infusion of hypertonic or irritating solutions; or septic phlebitis. Diagnosis of the latter requires organism identification. In the absence of any of these factors, the thrombosis may be presumed idiopathic. The term 'idiopathic' as used here includes the condition termed 'effort thrombosis'. In many such idiopathic cases there is venosclerosis at the level of the head of the clavicle, which may or may not have resulted from repetitive venous compression in the region of the thoracic outlet.

Upper extremity post-thrombotic syndrome

Obstruction, not reflux, is the cause of upper extremity venous symptoms. Description should include the patient's subjective assessment of discomfort either at rest or in relation to specific activities, and should also include objective descriptions such as the presence of cyanosis and the presence and extent of limb swelling documented by circumferential limb measurements compared with the uninvolved limb. Hand edema should be specifically noted as well as any resulting functional impairment of the fingers.

Vascular laboratory

A number of vascular laboratory tests have been employed in the diagnosis of acute upper extremity venous thrombosis or documentation of upper extremity post-thrombotic syndrome. Thus far only duplex scanning for the diagnosis of upper extremity and cervical deep venous thrombosis has achieved widespread acceptance. Therefore if vascular laboratory results other than duplex are reported in the diagnosis of acute thrombosis, the author should describe in detail both the performance and results of the tests selected and include results from normal persons, as well as from the contralateral normal upper extremity.

Treatment

The same details of medical treatment should be included as described earlier in the section on 'Acute lower extremity venous thrombosis'. Reports of the results of surgical treatment for either acute axillo-subclavian vein thrombosis or upper extremity post-thrombotic syndrome should include descriptions of the postoperative phlebograms or duplex scans visualizing the area of operation. Patency of a reconstructed axillo-subclavian vein must be documented by either phlebography or duplex scanning and presented in a life-table format. Attempts to assess the efficacy of surgical therapy with only the patient's subjective assessment of benefit may be grossly inaccurate on the basis of the well-described tendency for spontaneous improvement with either of these conditions.

PULMONARY EMBOLISM

The author should state the type of pulmonary embolus being described. The most common is aseptic embolism. Less common but well-recognized pulmonary emboli include: septic pulmonary embolus, organism identification required; tumor pulmonary embolus; air pulmonary embolus; fat pulmonary embolus; and foreign body pulmonary embolus, including such items as catheters, heart valves, bullets, pellets, and caval interruption devices.

Diagnosis

The clinical manifestations of pulmonary embolism are similar to other cardiopulmonary disorders, often making a clinical diagnosis difficult or impossible. Arterial blood gas determinations and ECG changes may be suggestive, but have insufficient sensitivity and specificity to establish a firm diagnosis.[30] Reports concerning pulmonary embolism must therefore confirm the diagnosis objectively with an imaging study.

Pulmonary arteriography remains the 'gold standard' against which all other diagnostic tests must be compared. Perfusion lung scanning alone is of unacceptably low specificity to establish a diagnosis of pulmonary embolism. High probability (but not intermediate probability) ventilation–perfusion scans ($\dot{V}/\dot{P}$ scans) may be used to establish objectively the diagnosis of pulmonary embolism. A high probability scan requires an embolus sufficiently large to occlude arterial circulation to an entire pulmonary segment and requires that the patient have a normal chest x-ray film. Low-probability $\dot{V}/\dot{P}$ scans are missing one or both of these requirements and are inadequate to establish the diagnosis of pulmonary embolism. Computerized axial tomography (CT) and magnetic resonance imaging (MRI) are accurate in establishing the diagnosis of large, centrally occluding pulmonary emboli. Small or peripheral emboli are not well detected.

Classification

Pulmonary embolism has been classified anatomically and functionally. The term 'massive embolism' has traditionally required significant filling defects in two or more lobar arteries, implying greater than 40% obstruction of the pulmonary circulation. The term 'submassive embolism' defines a pulmonary embolism with obstruction of less than two lobar arteries. However, these anatomic definitions are of limited usefulness and are less accurate in predicting death than a functional definition based on hemodynamic measurements. The hemodynamic response to acute embolization is a function not only of the size of the embolus but also of coexisting cardiac and pulmonary disease and the magnitude of both the neurohumoral and vasoconstrictor response to the embolism. Serial hemodynamic measurements essential to the functional definition of pulmonary embolism include blood pressure, pulse, central venous pressure, cardiac output, pulmonary artery pressure, pulmonary capillary wedge pressure, and pulmonary vascular resistance. The presence or absence of cardiac arrest or shock should be described since these are strong predictors of death associated with pulmonary embolism. The definition of shock is not standardized and must be clearly stated along with the duration of shock. Such a definition should include standard hemodynamic alterations (pulse rate and reductions in blood pressure and cardiac output), systemic responses (based on arterial pH, mixed venous blood gas determinations, oxygen consumption, and reductions in urinary output), and the need for vasopressors and inotropic support. A classification of pulmonary embolism on the basis of clinical, anatomic and hemodynamic modifiers is given in Table 51.6.

The term 'recurrent pulmonary embolism' can be used only when either a pulmonary arteriogram or high-probability $\dot{V}/\dot{P}$ scan documents both a new and a previous embolism.

Use of the term 'chronic pulmonary embolism' requires sequential documentation of recurrent pulmonary embolism on multiple occasions over a period of months by either high-probability $\dot{V}/\dot{P}$ scans or multiple pulmonary arteriograms. Alternatively, a single pulmonary angiogram showing emboli in both lungs and obstruction of over half the pulmonary vasculature along with a classic history of exertional dyspnea progressing to severe respiratory insufficiency in the setting of documented multiple recurrent deep venous thromboses is also sufficient to establish the diagnosis of chronic pulmonary embolism syndrome. The term must not be used in the absence of such documentation.

Table 51.6 *Classification of pulmonary embolism (PE)*

Clinical class	Characteristics
0	Asymptomatic PE
1	Symptomatic PE No hemodynamic alterations < 40% pulmonary arterial circulatory obstruction
2	Symptomatic PE Minor or no hemodynamic alterations > 40% pulmonary arterial circulatory obstruction
3	PE with major hemodynamic alterations and shock regardless of degree of pulmonary arterial circulatory obstruction
4	PE with cardiac arrest regardless of degree of pulmonary arterial circulatory obstruction

Therapy for acute pulmonary embolism

Therapy for acute pulmonary embolism includes supportive measures for cardiopulmonary failure, as well as anticoagulation, thrombolysis and surgical treatment. The same details of anticoagulant treatment should be included as earlier described in the section on 'Acute lower extremity venous thrombosis'.

The surgical treatment of pulmonary embolism includes caval interruption as well as open pulmonary artery embolectomy and percutaneous suction embolectomy. Descriptions of caval interruption should specify how this was accomplished. If a percutaneous device is used, the author must specify the type of device, route of placement, final location of device, and whether placement was confirmed phlebographically.

Reports describing thrombectomy for chronic pulmonary embolism should include postoperative pulmonary function tests as well as pulmonary arteriography with measurement of pulmonary artery pressure as it is recognized that patients may display markedly improved postoperative arteriograms without improvement in pulmonary function.

Pulmonary embolism prophylaxis

Caval interruption, by whatever means, should only be described as prophylactic for patients who have not sustained a recent pulmonary embolism. The type, location, and timing of venous interruption in relation to subsequent or concomitant operations, and whether concomitant anticoagulation is used and its intensity, should be specified. The technique of device insertion should be described (i.e. operative or percutaneous) and radiographic confirmation of the localization of the device after insertion noted.

Autopsy verification of fatal pulmonary embolism

PROBABLY LETHAL PULMONARY EMBOLISM

Probably lethal pulmonary embolism consists of:

- thrombus or thrombi in the main pulmonary artery trunk and/or bifurcation, a portion of which may be in the right ventricle;
- thrombi in both right and left pulmonary arteries; thrombi in one or more contralateral lobar arteries.

POSSIBLY LETHAL PULMONARY EMBOLISM

The designation of possibly lethal pulmonary embolism requires consideration of both the extent of obstruction of the pulmonary arterial system and the patient's underlying cardiopulmonary state. A number of factors may aggravate hypoxemia and diminish the capacity of the right heart to accept an increased afterload, therefore affecting the patient's potential to survive an acute embolus. Such factors include:

- thrombus occluding the main right or left pulmonary artery;
- thrombi in two or more lobar arteries of one lung and in one or more contralateral lobar arteries;
- combination of thrombi in unilateral or bilateral lobar and/or segmental (and equivalent subsegmental) arteries equal to the above.

Consensus Committee Members

Hugh G Beebe, USA
John J Bergan, USA
David Bergqvist, Sweden
Bo Eklof, USA
Ingvar Eriksson, Sweden
Mitchel P Goldman, USA
Lazar J Greenfield, USA
Robert W Hobson, II, USA
Claude Juhan, France
Robert L Kistner, USA
Nicos Labropoulos, UK
G Mark Malouf, Australia
James O Menzoian, USA
Gregory L Moneta, USA
Kenneth A Myers, Australia
Peter Neglen, United Arab Emirates
Andrew N Nicolaides, UK
Thomas F O'Donnell, USA
Hugo Partsch, Austria
Michel Perrin, France
John M Porter, USA
Seshadri Raju, USA
Norman M Rich, USA
Graeme Richardson, Australia
Harry Schanzer, USA
Philip Coleridge Smith, UK
D Eugene Strandness, USA
David S Sumner, USA

REFERENCES

1. Kakkar VV, Howe CT, Nicolaides AN, *et al.* Deep vein thrombosis of leg. Is there a 'high risk' group? *Am J Surg* 1970; **120**: 527–30.
2. Gibbs NM (1957) Venous thrombosis of the lower limbs with particular reference to bed rest. Br. J. Surg. **45**: 209–36.
3. Warlow C, Ogston D, Douglas AS. Venous thrombosis following strokes. *Lancet* 1972; **1**: 1305–6.
4. Hartsuck JM, Greenfield U. Postoperative thromboembolism. A clinical study with ^{125}I fibrinogen and pulmonary scanning. *Arch Surg* 1973; **107**: 733–9.
5. Kakkar VV. The diagnosis of deep vein thrombosis using the ^{125}I fibrinogen test. *Arch Surg* 1972; **104**: 152–9.
6. Fejfar Z, Badger D, Crais M. Epidemiological aspects of thrombosis and vascular disease. *Thromb Diath Haemorr Suppl* 1966; **21**: 5–15.
7. Coon WW, Coller FA. Some epidemiologic considerations of thromboembolism. *Surg Gynecol Obstet* 1959; **109**: 487–501.
8. White PD.) Pulmonary embolism and heart disease. A review of twenty years of personal experience. *Am J Med Sci* 1940; **200**: 577–81.
9. Hjelmstedt A, Bergvall U. Incidence of thrombosis in patients with tibial fractures. *Acta Chir Scand* 1968; **134**: 209–18.
10. Thaler E, Lechner R. Antithrombin III deficiency and thromboembolism. *Clin Haematol* 1981; **10**: 369–90.
11. Broekmoms AW, Veltkamp JJ, Bertma RM. Congenital protein C deficiency and venous thromboembolism: a study of three Dutch families. *N Engl J Med* 1983; **309**: 340–4.
12. Comp PC, Esmon CT. Recurrent venous thromboembolism in patients with a partial deficiency of protein S. *N Engl J Med* 1984; **311**: 1525–8.
13. Much VR, Herbst KD, Rapaport SI. Thrombosis in patients with the lupus anticoagulant. *Ann Intern Med* 1980; **92**(2 pt 1): 156–9.
14. Hirsh J, McBride JA, Daric JV. Thromboembolism and increased platelet adhesiveness in post splenectomy thrombocytosis. *Aust N Z J Med* 1966; **15**: 122–8.
15. Sartwell PE, Masi AT, Arthes FG, Greene GR, Smith HE. Thromboembolism and oral contraceptives: an epidemiologic case-control study. *Am J Epidemiol* 1969; **90**: 365–80.
16. Vessey MP, Inman WHW. Speculation about mortality trends from venous thromboembolic disease in England and Wales and their relationship to the pattern of oral contraceptive usage. *Br J Obstet Gynaecol* 1973; **80**: 562–6.
17. Coon WW, Willis PW III, Keller JB. Venous thromboembolism and other venous diseases in the Tecumseh community health study. *Circulation* 1973; **48**: 839–46.
18. Nicolaides AN, Irving D. Clinical factors and the risk of deep venous thrombosis. In Nicolaides AN, ed. *Thromboembolism.* Baltimore, MD: University Park Press, 1975: 194.
19. Lohr JM, McDevitt DT, Lutter KS, *et al.* Operative management of greater saphenous thrombophlebitis involving the saphenofemoral junction. *Am J Surg* 1992; **164**: 269–75.
20. Brockman SK, Vasko JS. Phlegmasia cerulea dolens. *Surg Gynecol Obstet* 1965; **121**: 1347–56.
21. Yao JST, Flinn WR. Plethysmography. In Kempczinski RE, Yao JST, eds. *Practical Noninvasive Vascular Diagnosis.* Chicago: Yearbook Medical Publishers, 1987: 1980.
22. Hirsh J, Hull RD. Diagnosis of venous thrombosis. In Hirsh J, Hull RD, eds. *Venous Thromboembolism: Natural History, Diagnosis and Management.* Boca Raton, FL: CRC Press, 1987: 23.
23. Poller L. Laboratory control of oral anticoagulants. *Br Med J* 1987; **294**: 1184.
24. van Bemmelen PS, Bedford G, Beach K, *et al.* Quantitative segmental evaluation of venous valvular reflux with duplex ultrasound scanning. *J Vasc Surg* 1989; **10**: 425–31.
25. Plate G, Akesson H, Einarsson E, *et al.* Long-term results of venous thrombectomy combined with a temporary arterio-venous fistula. *Eur J Vasc Surg* 1990; **4**: 483–9.

26. van Bemmelen PS. Evaluation of the patient with chronic venous insufficiency: old and emerging technology. In Strandness DE Jr, van Breda A, eds. *Vascular Diseases: Surgical and Interventional Therapy,* New York: Churchill Livingstone, 1994: 941.
27. Markel A, Manzo RA, Bergelin RO, *et al.* Valvular reflux after deep vein thrombosis: incidence and time of occurrence. *J Vasc Surg* 1992; **15**: 377–82.
28. Christopoulos DG, Nicolaides AN, Szendro, *et al.* Air-plethysmography and the effect of elastic compression on venous hemodynamics of the leg. *J Vasc Surg* 1987; **5**: 148–59.
29. Hanrahan LM, Araki CT, Rodriguez AA, *et al.* Distribution of valvular incompetence in patients with venous stasis ulceration. *J Vasc Surg* 1991; **13**: 805–11.
30. Sabiston DC Jr. Pulmonary embolism. In Sabiston DC Jr, ed. *Textbook of Surgery: the Biologic Basis of Modern Surgical Practice*, 14th edn. Philadelphia: WB Saunders, 1991: 1502.

52

Classification and grading of chronic venous disease in the lower limbs: a consensus statement

PREPARED BY THE EXECUTIVE COMMITTEE, CHAIRED BY ANDREW N NICOLAIDES, OF THE AD HOC COMMITTEE,* AMERICAN VENOUS FORUM, 6TH ANNUAL MEETING, FEBRUARY 22–25, 1994, MAUI, HAWAII. ORGANIZED BY STRAUB FOUNDATION

PURPOSE OF NEW CLASSIFICATION AND GRADING

Patients with chronic venous disease have been treated for many years with different modalities of therapy, both nonsurgical and surgical. Many of these treatments have not been conclusively proven to be useful. Furthermore, the application of specific techniques to particular venous conditions has not been well established. Progress in this area is made more difficult by the lack of a common classification that allows for fair comparison between reported series.

In order to provide a complete classification that allows for scientific evaluation of the results of treatment of chronic venous disease, an international group of venous specialists was gathered under the auspices of the American Venous Forum in February 1994 to develop a new classification. The result of that meeting was the following classification which takes into account the clinical signs and symptoms, the etiology, the anatomic distribution of the pathology, and the pathophysiologic dysfunction (C,E,A,P; see Chapter 51).

It is intended that the universal acceptance and use of this classification will provide the basis for uniformity in reporting and assessing different modalities of diagnosis and treatment. This will be very important in giving further impulse to improvement of the understanding, evaluation, and treatment of chronic venous disease.

CLASSIFICATION

Chronic venous disease is an important cause of discomfort and disability and is present in a significant percentage of the population world wide. Methods to diagnose and measure severity have evolved rapidly so that accurate classification of venous disease is now possible. Standards for reporting venous disease have been based on a clinical classification developed in 1988 by a subcommittee of the Society for Vascular Surgery (SVS) and International Society for Cardiovascular Surgery (ISCVS).[1] This classification has contributed to the uniform presentation of diagnosis and results of treatment. However, advances in the knowledge of chronic venous disease have created a need to expand definitions to cover many aspects including anatomy, pathophysiology, and etiology. The aim of this document is to present a more precise classification of chronic venous dysfunction which is simple enough to encourage its universal acceptance. Acceptance of a standard classification provides a basis for uniformity in reporting and assessing different modalities of diagnosis and treatment. The classification has been developed under the following headings (see Table 51.1 on p. 514).

* This committee comprises the same members as the Consensus Committee cited on page 519. The Executive Committee comprises JJ Bergan, B Eklof, RL Kistner, GL Moneta and AN Nicolaides.

Clinical classification (C_{0-6})

The clinical classification is based on objective clinical signs of chronic venous disease (C_{0-6}) supplemented according to presentation (A) for asymptomatic (e.g. $C_{0-6,A}$) or (S) for symptomatic limbs (e.g. $C_{0-6,S}$). Symptoms include aching, pain, congestion, skin irritation, and muscle cramps as well as other complaints attributable to venous dysfunction. This clinical classification is organized in terms of ascending severity of disease.[1] Limbs in higher categories have more severe manifestations of chronic venous disease and may have some or all of the findings associated with less severe categories (Table 52.1).

Table 52.1 *Clinical classification*

Class	Signs
0	No visible or palpable signs of venous disease
1	Telangiectases or reticular veins
2	Varicose veins
3	Edema
4	Skin changes ascribed to venous disease (e.g. pigmentation, venous eczema, lipodermatosclerosis)
5	Skin changes as defined above with healed ulceration
6	Skin changes as defined above with active ulceration

Therapy may alter the clinical signs and symptoms and the limb should be reclassified after treatment.

Telangiectases are defined as dilated intradermal venules up to a diameter of approximately 1 mm and reticular veins are defined as dilated subdermal veins up to a size of about 4 mm which are not palpable. Varicose veins are palpable, dilated subcutaneous veins usually larger than 4 mm.[2] Telangiectases and reticular veins are separated from varicose veins in this classification as it is considered that the telangiectases do not lead to venous ulceration whilst the reticular veins may.[2] Both may be associated with patient symptoms.[3]

Etiologic classification (E_C, E_P or E_S)

This classification recognizes three categories of venous dysfunction: congenital, primary, and secondary. Congenital problems may be apparent at birth or be recognized later. Primary problems are neither congenital nor do they have an identifiable cause. Secondary problems are those acquired conditions that have a known pathological cause, such as thrombosis. These categories are mutually exclusive (Table 52.2).

Anatomic classification ($A_{S,D,P}$)

This classification describes the anatomic extent of venous disease whether in the superficial (A_S), deep (A_D), or perforating (A_P) veins. Disease may involve one, two, or all three systems.

Table 52.2 *Etiologic classification*

Congenital (E_C)	
Primary (E_P)	Cause undetermined
Secondary (E_S)	Cause known
	Post-thrombotic
	Post-traumatic
	Other

For those reports for which greater detail is required, the site and extent of involvement of the superficial, deep, and perforating veins may be categorized using the anatomic segments listed in Table 51.4 (p. 515).

Pathophysiologic classification ($P_{R,O}$)

Clinical signs and symptoms of venous dysfunction may be the result of reflux (P_R), obstruction (P_O), or both ($P_{R,O}$). Therefore, the simplest pathophysiologic classification of a limb would be P_R, P_O, or $P_{R,O}$.

Because the severity of venous dysfunction is determined by the location and anatomic extent of reflux and/or obstruction,[4,5] it may be desirable to report this in greater detail by using the anatomic segments listed in Table 51.4. The availability of duplex scanning allows this to be done noninvasively.[6–13] In addition, it may be appropriate to report duplex-derived severity and duration of reflux,[8,9,14] as presented later in the chapter.

Reporting of segmental obstruction can be simplified and standardized using the well-recognized major sites of occlusion,[15] caval, iliac, femoral, popliteal, and crural ($P_{O\text{-}Cav}$, $P_{O\text{-}I}$, $P_{O\text{-}F}$, $P_{O\text{-}P}$, $P_{O\text{-}C}$).

If obstruction is more extensive, this can also be reported using multiple subscripts (e.g. $P_{O\text{-}I,F,P}$). Functional obstruction is discussed later in the chapter.

SCORING OF VENOUS DYSFUNCTION

A scoring system of chronic venous dysfunction provides a numerical base for scientific comparison of limb condition and evaluation of results of treatment. This is based on three elements:

- the number of anatomic segments affected (anatomic score)
- grading of symptoms and signs (clinical score)
- disability (disability score).

Although the grading of symptoms is subjective, the grading of signs is objective. The accuracy of this scoring system needs to be tested and may be modified in the future as experience accumulates. The anatomic score is the sum of the anatomic segments, each scored as one point (see Table 51.4). The clinical score is the sum of the values assigned to the signs and symptoms listed below (Tables 52.3 and 52.4).

Table 52.3 *Clinical score*

Pain	0 = none; 1 = moderate, not requiring analgesics; 2 = severe, requiring analgesics
Edema	0 = none; 1 = mild/moderate; 2 = severe
Venous claudication	0 = none, 1 = mild/moderate, 2 = severe
Pigmentation	0 = none; 1 = localized; 2 = extensive
Lipodermatosclerosis	0 = none; 1 = localized; 2 = extensive
Ulcer: size (largest ulcer)	0 = none; 1 <2 cm diameter; 2 >2 cm diameter
Ulcer: duration	0 = none; 1 ≤3 months; 2 ≥3 months
Ulcer: recurrence	0 = none; 1 = once; 2 = more than once
Ulcer: number	0 = none; 1 = single; 2 = multiple

Table 52.4 *Disability score*

Class	Level of disability
0	Asymptomatic
1	Symptomatic, can function without support device
2	Can work 8-hour day only with support device
3	Unable to work even with support device

THE DIAGNOSTIC PROCESS

The history and physical examination are the basis for the initial evaluation of patients with suspected chronic venous disease.[16] Since valvular incompetence or obstruction form the basis for most complications, the continuous-wave Doppler can be used at the time of the initial clinical evaluation to assist in the diagnosis.[17,18] Absence or diminution of a Doppler velocity signal despite an augmentation maneuver suggests obstruction. Reflux may be detected with a Valsalva maneuver or limb compression. Because continuous-wave Doppler provides subjective information, if positive, findings should be followed by objective test.

If a patient presents with symptoms that are questionably related to venous disease, such as mild edema or aching, a noninvasive test may be required. Duplex scanning is the method of choice used to confirm or exclude the presence of venous dysfunction.[6–14] In the absence of duplex scanning, strain-gauge plethysmography,[17,19] air plethysmography,[20,21] or photoplethysmography[22,23] may be used. Because the accuracy of photoplethysmography has been challenged,[24–26] confirmation of the presence of chronic venous disease by another technique may be required if photoplethysmography is positive.

Duplex scanning has become the method of choice for testing individual veins of the superficial, deep, and perforating systems.[6–13] If the problem is confined to superficial veins, duplex scanning will determine whether this involves the greater and/or lesser saphenous veins and their tributaries. It can also detect the presence of incompetent perforating veins.[5,27,28] In addition, duplex scanning can determine the anatomy of veins in the popliteal fossa.[29–31] Also, it will detect reflux at other sites such as vulval veins or lateral thigh incompetent perforating veins. In the presence of deep venous disease, duplex scanning will determine whether the problem is due to anatomic obstruction, reflux, or both. In addition, it will provide information about the anatomic extent. Measurements to quantify reflux in individual veins by duplex scanning have been recently developed such as valve closure time,[9] venous reflux index[32] and velocity at peak reflux,[14] but experience with these is still limited.[33] Several other methods to quantify reflux are available. They include strain-gauge plethysmography,[17,19] foot volumetry[34,35] and the more recently developed air plethysmography,[20,21] which measures global reflux in ml/s. Ascending and descending phlebography should be performed when deep venous valvular reconstruction is contemplated.[36,37]

A number of tests are available to determine the functional severity of chronic obstruction. They include the arm/foot pressure differential,[38] the outflow fraction using air plethysmography[16,39] and femoral or popliteal pressure measurements during exercise.[40,41] Ascending phlebography should be performed if venous reconstruction (bypass) is being considered.

Ambulatory venous pressure is a test measuring global venous hypertension.[42,43] A high ambulatory venous pressure is associated with a high incidence of ulceration.[44]

In the presence of both obstruction and reflux, quantitative tests outlined above can be used to assess which is predominant.

REFERENCES

1. Reporting standards in venous disease. Prepared by the Subcommittee on Reporting Standards in Venous Disease, Ad Hoc Committee on Reporting Standards, Society for Vascular Surgery/North American Chapter, International Society for Cardiovascular Surgery. *J Vasc Surg* 1988; **8**: 172–81.
2. Goldman MP. *Sclerotherapy: Treatment of Varicose and Telangiectatic Leg Veins*. St Louis, MO: Mosby Year Book, 1991.
3. Weiss RA, Weiss MA. Resolution of pain associated with varicose telangiectatic leg veins after compression sclerotherapy. *J Dermatol Surg Oncol* 1990; **16**: 333–6.
4. Gooley NA, Sumner DS. Relationship of venous reflux to the site of venous valvular incompetence: implications for venous reconstructive surgery. *J Vasc Surg* 1988; **7**: 50–9.

5. Hanrahan LM, Araki CT, Rodriguez AA, *et al.* Distribution of valvular incompetence in patients with venous stasis ulceration. *J Vasc Surg* 1991; **13**: 805–12.
6. Szendro G, Nicolaides AN, Zukowski AJ, *et al.* Duplex scanning in the assessment of deep venous incompetence. *J Vasc Surg* **4**: 237–42.
7. van Bemmelen PS, Bedford G, Beach K, Strandness DE. Quantitative segmental evaluation of venous valvular reflux with duplex ultrasound scanning. *J Vasc Surg* 1989; **10**: 425–31.
8. Neglen P, Raju S. A comparison between descending phlebography and duplex Doppler investigation in the evaluation of reflux in chronic venous insufficiency: a challenge to phlebography as the gold standard. *J Vasc Surg* 1992; **16**: 687–93.
9. Welch HJ, Faliakou EC, McLaughlin RL, *et al.* Comparison of descending phlebography with quantitative photoplethysmography, air plethysmography, and duplex quantitative valve closure time in assessing deep venous reflux. *J Vasc Surg* 1992; **16**: 913–20.
10. Masuda EM, Kistner RL. Prospective comparison of duplex scanning and descending venography in the assessment of venous insufficiency. *Am J Surg* 1992; **164**: 254–9.
11. Valentin LI, Valentin WH, Mercado S, Rosado CJ. Venous reflux localisation: comparative study of venography and duplex scanning. *Phlebology* 1993; **8**: 124–7.
12. Lees TA, Lambert D. Patterns of venous reflux in limbs with skin changes associated with chronic venous insufficiency. *Br J Surg* 1993; **80**: 725–8.
13. Labropoulos N, Leon M, Nicolaides AN, *et al.* Venous reflux in patients with previous deep venous thrombosis: correlation with ulceration and other systems. *J Vasc Surg* 1994; **20**: 20–6.
14. Vasdekis SN, Clarke GH, Nicolaides AN. Quantification of venous reflux by means of duplex scanning. *J Vasc Surg* 1989; **10**: 670–7.
15. May R, Nissl R. The post-thrombotic syndrome. In May R, ed. *Surgery of the Veins of the Leg and Pelvis.* Stuttgart: Georg Thieme, 1979.
16. Nicolaides AN, Sumner DS. *Investigation of Patients with Deep Vein Thrombosis and Chronic Venous Insufficiency.* London: Med-Orion, 1991.
17. Barnes RW, Ross EA, Strandness DE Jr. Differentiation of primary from secondary varicose veins by Doppler ultrasound and strain gauge plethysmography. *Surg Gynecol Obstet* 1975; **141**: 207–11.
18. Shull KC, Nicolaides AN, Fernandes e Fernandes J, *et al.* Significance of popliteal reflux in relation to ambulatory venous pressure and ulceration. *Arch Surg* 1979; **114**: 1304–6.
19. Fernandes JF, Horner J, Needham T, Nicolaides A. Ambulatory calf volume plethysmography in the assessment of venous insufficiency. *Br J Surg* 1979; **66**: 327–30.
20. Christopoulos DG, Nicolaides AN, Szendro G, *et al.* Air-plethysmography and the effect of elastic compression on venous hemodynamics of the leg. *J Vasc Surg* 1987; **5**: 148–59.
21. Katz ML, Comerota AJ, Kerr R. Air plethysmography (APG). A new technique to evaluate patients with chronic venous insufficiency. *J Vasc Technol* 1991; **15**: 23–7.
22. Abramowitz HB, Queral LA, Flinn WR, *et al.* The use of photoplethysmography in the assessment of venous insufficiency: a comparison to venous pressure measurements. *Surgery* 1979; **86**: 434–41.
23. Nicolaides AN, Miles C. Photoplethysmography in the assessment of venous insufficiency. *J Vasc Surg* 1987; **5**: 405–12.
24. van Bemmelen PS, van Ramshorst B, Eikelboom BC. Photoplethysmography reexamined: lack of correlation with duplex scanning. *Surgery* 1992; **112**: 544–8.
25. Masser PA, De Frang RD, Gentile A, *et al.* Choice of tests for vascular laboratory evaluation of venous reflux. *J Vasc Technol* 1995, in press.
26. Bays RA, Healy DA, Atnip RG, *et al.* Validation of air plethysmography, photoplethysmography and duplex ultrasound in the evaluation of severe venous stasis. Presented at the American Venous Forum, 23–25 February 1994, Maui, Hawaii.
27. Hanrahan LM, Araki CT, Fisher JB, *et al.* Evaluation of the perforating veins of the lower extremity using high resolution duplex imaging. *J Cardiovasc Surg* 1991; **32**: 87–97.
28. Myers KA, Ziegenbein RW, Zeng GH, Matthews PG. Patterns of medial calf perforator reflux shown by duplex ultrasound scanning in 1130 legs with chronic venous disease. Presented at the American Venous Forum, 23–25 February 1994, Maui, Hawaii.
29. Hobbs JT. Errors in the differential diagnosis of incompetence of the popliteal vein and short saphenous vein by Doppler ultrasound. *J Cardiovasc Surg* 1986; **27**: 169–74.
30. Vasdekis SN, Clarke GH, Hobbs JT, Nicolaides AN. Evaluation of noninvasive and invasive methods in the assessment of short saphenous vein termination. *Br J Surg* 1989; **76**: 929–32.
31. Engel AF, Davies G, Keeman JN. Preoperative localisation of the saphenopopliteal junction with duplex scanning. *Eur J Vasc Surg* 1991; **5**: 507–9.
32. Beckwith TC, Richardson G, Sheldon M, Clarke GH. A correlation between blood flow volume and ultrasonic Doppler wave forms in the study of valve efficiency. *Phlebology* 1993; **8**: 12–16.
33. Araki CT, Back TL, Padberg FT Jr, Thompson PN, Duran WN, Hobson RW. Refinements in the ultrasonic detections of popliteal vein reflux. *J Vasc Surg* 1993; **18**: 742–8.
34. Norgren L. Functional evaluation of chronic venous insufficiency by foot volumetry. *Acta Chir Scand Suppl* 1974; **444**: 1–48.
35. Bradbury AW, Stonebridge PA, Callam MJ, *et al.* Foot volumetry and duplex ultrasonography after saphenous and subfascial perforating vein ligation for recurrent venous ulceration. *Br J Surg* 1993; **80**: 845–8.

36. Raju S, Fredericks R. Venous obstruction: an analysis of one hundred thirty-seven cases with hemodynamic, venographic, and clinical correlations. *J Vasc Surg* 1991; **14**: 305–13.
37. Kistner RL, Ferris EB, Randhawa G, Kamida C. A method of performing descending venography. *J Vasc Surg* 1986; **4**: 464–8.
38. Raju S. New approaches to the diagnosis and treatment of venous obstruction. *J Vasc Surg* 1986; **4**: 42–54.
39. Neglen P, Raju S. Detection of outflow obstruction in chronic venous insufficiency. *J Vasc Surg* 1993; **17**: 583–9.
40. Albrechtsson U, Einarsson E, Eklof B. Femoral vein pressure measurements for evaluation of venous function in patients with postthrombotic iliac veins. *Cardiovasc Interv Radiol* **4**: 43–50.
41. Perrin M. *Chronic Venous Insufficiency in the Lower Limbs.* Paris: McGraw-Hill, 1990.
42. Nicolaides AN, Zukowski AJ. The value of dynamic venous pressure measurements. *World J Surg* 1986; **10**: 919–24.
43. Welkie JF, Cornerota AJ, Katz, ML, *et al.* Hemodynamic deterioration in chronic venous disease. *J Vasc Surg* 1992; **16**: 733–40.
44. Nicolaides AN, Hussein MK, Szendro G, *et al.* The relation of venous ulceration with ambulatory venous pressure measurements. *J Vasc Surg* 1993; **17**: 414–19.

53

Critical issues in basic and clinical research of venous disease

THOMAS W WAKEFIELD, MICHAEL C DALSING, EDMUND J HARRIS JR, PETER J PAPPAS, THOMAS LYNCH AND KENNETH OURIEL

Basic research in venous disease is an area that has lagged behind basic research in arterial disease. However, venous-specific basic research has the potential to significantly advance the treatment of patients with venous disorders, ranging from the diagnosis and treatment of acute venous thrombosis to the diagnosis and treatment of chronic venous insufficiency. In this chapter, topics in basic research are addressed including:

- the bioregulatory role of thrombin in venous thrombosis (EJH);
- inflammation associated with venous thrombosis (TWW); and
- the mechanisms of dermal tissue injury in chronic venous insufficiency (PJP).

Topics in clinical research include:

- application of noninvasive diagnostic techniques in venous research (TL); and
- new treatments for chronic venous disease (MCO).

Finally, questions for future investigation are discussed.

BASIC RESEARCH

The bioregulatory role of thrombin in venous thrombosis

Venous thrombosis is far more frequent than arterial thrombosis, and venous thrombosis is more frequently clinically occult. Therefore the natural history of venous thrombosis remains incompletely defined. It is clear that patients with diagnosed venous thrombosis may develop post-thrombotic venous insufficiency, which when present is due to valvular incompetence in the majority of patients, and chronic venous occlusion in the minority. The combination of venous obstruction and valvular incompetence leads to the most severe form of chronic venous insufficiency. With the advent of venous thrombectomy, and more recently catheter-directed thrombolysis, it appears that rapid removal of thrombus decreases the incidence of valvular dysfunction and reduces the symptoms of venous insufficiency. Our understanding of the pathology of venous thrombosis and its relationship to venous wall morphological changes seen in chronic venous insufficiency is unclear.

NATURAL HISTORY OF VENOUS THROMBOSIS

In the living state, most of our knowledge of DVT resolution has come from duplex ultrasound evaluations of mostly symptomatic patients, and therefore patients who generally have been treated with systemic anticoagulation, thrombolysis, or both. True natural history data on the resolution of DVT and its effects on the venous wall are lacking. Venous duplex studies prospectively assessing the evolution of DVT have shown 50–70% of limbs with venous thrombosis develop valvular incompetence 6–9 months following acute DVT, with thickening of the previously thrombosed but subsequently recanalized venous wall. Others have identified duplex findings following recanalization of DVT that suggest future development of post-thrombotic venous insufficiency.[1] The changes suggestive of chronic damage include thickening of the vein wall, reflux, and abnormal valves. A vein wall was considered thickened when it was twice the thickness of a normal venous segment, with increased echogenicity of the damaged venous wall brighter than the normal vessel wall. Recanalized segments of deep veins demonstrate thickened walls in addition to areas of residual fibrinous thrombus. Loss of normal venous wall compliance due to this thickening may cause venous valvular insufficiency, even without damage to the valve leaflets themselves. Loss of venous wall compliance may preclude valve leaflet coaptation leading to venous reflux. Others have shown totally occluded veins more commonly develop reflux than do veins with only partial obstruction.[2]

Pathologic examination of post-thrombotic venous segments has shown thrombus organization, which appears to be acutely initiated by inflammatory cell infiltration but chronically appears to consist of smooth muscle fibrocellular proliferation. Historical evaluation of pathologic specimens from patients suffering from post-thrombotic venous insufficiency identified a fibrotic thickening of the involved venous segments. Fibrous intimal thickening was commonly found in the deep veins of the thighs of the mostly elderly patients studied in this autopsy series. The time course between acute DVT and the pathologic examination was not accurately recorded. Small fibrous strings, ridges and thickenings of the intima, visible to the naked eye, were found in most patients, whereas extensive, coarse trabeculated intimal thickenings and sclerosed lumenless veins were less frequently encountered.[3,4] In experimental thrombosis models using pig jugular vein, this thrombus organization appears quite similar morphologically to neointimal hyperplasia.[5]

We have developed a model of *in vivo* deep venous thrombosis in the rat to assess the role of venous thrombosis and outflow obstruction in recanalization and in the development of secondary venous wall morphologic changes. This work demonstrates an important temporal relationship between exposure of thrombus to the venous wall and venous wall remodeling with neointimal and myocellular proliferation. Our results suggest that the longer thrombus is exposed to the vein wall, the more vigorous and sustained is the vascular remodeling and subsequent wall thickening. Although this evidence is indirect, the differences in venous wall morphology between chronic outflow obstruction with longer thrombus exposure and temporary outflow obstruction with shorter thrombus exposure in this model are significant. This difference is even more interesting because chronic outflow obstruction induced local neovascular channel formation, whereas temporary outflow obstruction did not.[6]

THROMBIN AND DVT

It is apparent that thrombus propagation is common in acute DVT. In plasma the bulk of thrombin generation takes place after a thrombus has formed, with thrombin bound to fibrin and fibrinogen within the developing thrombus. This fibrin-bound thrombin remains biologically and functionally active within the clot, and subsequently as thrombolysis ensues and plasmin degrades the thrombus.[7,8] This clot-bound thrombin is protected from inhibition by heparin-antithrombin III but is susceptible to newer antithrombin III independent direct thrombin inhibitors such as hirudin and hirulogs.[9] Our model revealed thrombus extension both visually with vein wall dilatation and with the radiolabeled fibrinogen assay over the first 4 days following the acute thrombosis in the outflow obstruction group, whereas the temporary outflow obstruction group did not show thrombus extension. The thrombosed femoral vein enlarged initially during creation of the acute thrombosis in both groups, but the temporarily obstructed group rapidly resolved their DVT following relief of outflow obstruction. No increased radiolabeled fibrinogen was detected in the lungs of either group, so thrombus resolution was a result of thrombolysis and not embolisation.[6]

Thrombin is a multifunctional serine protease. Previously, the main function of thrombin was thought to be cleavage of circulating proteins to their bioactive forms, such as fibrinogen to fibrin and activation of protein C. More recently, thrombin has been recognized as a pluripotent stimulator of various cells. Thrombin is the most potent activator of platelets; it stimulates endothelial cells to express cellular adhesion molecules, to secrete von Willebrand factor, and to elaborate growth factors and cytokines.

Thrombin is a potent mitogen for fibroblasts and smooth muscle cells. In organ bath chambers, thrombin is a potent constrictor of vascular rings denuded of endothelium, yet a potent vasodilator of vascular rings with intact endothelium. Thrombin has been identified as a promoter of angiogenesis. Most, if not all, of these functions have recently been linked to thrombin stimulation of a membrane-bound receptor, which is activated in a novel manner. Most recently, a class of these protease-activated receptors, or PARs, has been identified.[10,11]

PROTEASE RECEPTORS

Protease-activated receptors are members of the seven transmembrane domain G protein-coupled receptor family. The amino terminal of these receptors contains a cleavage site that mimics the protease cleavage site. To date three PARs have been identified in humans: PAR-1 can be activated by thrombin and trypsin, PAR-2 is activated by trypsin and tryptase, but not thrombin, and PAR-3 is activated by thrombin alone. Receptor activation occurs when the protease binds the receptor, proteolysis occurs at the amino-terminal cleavage site by the protease, the protease is released, and the remaining tethered ligand undergoes conformational change stimulating the G-protein cascade. The receptors can also be stimulated by synthetic peptide agonists that mimic the five or six terminal amino acids exposed by proteolysis at the amino-terminus of the tethered ligand. These PAR receptors therefore contain their own agonists, the tethered ligand, which in the naive receptor state are kept quiet by a superfluous peptide tail. The protease then cleaves this peptide tail, allowing agonist stimulation by the exposed tethered ligand.[10,11]

As thrombolysis of a venous thrombus progresses, active thrombin is likely released locally. If the thrombus burden is large or there is coexisting obstruction, the thrombin can continue to act locally, either generating new fibrin and extending the thrombus, or stimulating its unique PAR receptor expressed in the venous wall and on many of the cells of the local inflammatory cell infiltrate. In this scenario, thrombin, via its receptor, would stimulate the myoproliferative response that could lead to chronic venous wall thickening. Furthermore, one thrombin molecule within the thrombus, excluded from its inhibitors, would be capable of activating many PARs. If the thrombus is not obstructing, the active thrombin would be progressively cleared with blood flow and inactivated by circulating inhibitors, with minimal chance for interaction of the thrombin locally with its receptor. Thus a small venous thrombus, or non-obstructing thrombus would not be expected to elicit myoproliferative changes and venous wall thickening. We are currently looking into the role of thrombin and PARs in our model of chronic venous thrombosis with outflow obstruction.

Inflammation associated with venous thrombosis

Inflammation occurs by the formation of venous thrombosis. Stewart initially proposed four stages for this inflammatory response.[12] First, thrombus forms in the veins, and inflammatory cells and platelets become activated within this initial thrombus. Second, further activation of neutrophils and platelets occurs, generating procoagulant and inflammatory mediators. Third, coagulation occurs on activated platelet phospholipid surfaces, speeding the rate of thrombin and fibrin generation. Finally, leukocytes and platelets layer on top of existing clot, further increasing the thrombotic/inflammatory process. Inflammation ultimately leads to the amplification of additional thrombosis, driven by both the expression of tissue factor on the surface of monocytes, and by the exposure of vein wall thrombogenic collagen after endothelial denudation, likely mediated by cathepsin G release from activated neutrophils.

VEIN WALL INFLAMMATORY RESPONSE

The above process results in leukocyte extravasation into the vein wall, migrating from both the adventitial and luminal surfaces. Using a rodent model of stasis-induced venous thrombosis by IVC ligation, we have demonstrated an active vein wall pro-inflammatory response characterized by cellular trafficking, involving early neutrophil extravasation[13] followed by monocyte/macrophage infiltration (Fig. 53.1).[14] This process occurs as early as 6 hours after thrombus formation begins. At 6 hours, an increase in all leukocyte types (except for monocytes) in the vein wall is seen. By day 2, neutrophils are the predominant cells in the thrombosed vein wall. Although inflammatory cells can be seen at the thrombus/vein wall interface, more leukocytes are recognized in the media and adventitia of the vein wall than noted at the earlier 6 hour time point. By day 6, neutrophil counts in the thrombosed vein wall fall to near baseline, while monocytes significantly rise. At day 6, the thrombus/vein wall interface is less distinct and the predominant cell type is the monocyte. FACS analysis using both rat-specific anti-neutrophil antibody and ED-1 antibody for monocytes confirms the morphometric analysis with neutrophils the predominant cell type in the vein wall at day 2. At baseline, 13% of the cells are neutrophils but by 6 hours, 63% are neutrophils and by day 2, 72% of the cells are neutrophils. By day 6, only 31% of the vein wall cells are neutrophils, whereas 24% are monocytes. MPO analysis supports both morphometric and FACS analysis with a significant increase in activity at day 2 in the thrombosed vein walls, consistent with neutrophil presence in the vein wall. By day 6, the MPO activity falls.

TUMOR NECROSIS FACTOR AND P-SELECTIN

Neutrophils, initially adherent to the endothelium, cause endothelial disruption, exposing the collagen-rich basement membrane. This leads to further thrombus propagation and is followed by leukocyte transendothelial migration and further vein injury. Factors important to leukocyte extravasation in the rodent have been identified including tumor necrosis factor (TNF), the earliest upregulated selectin (P-selectin), and the adhesion receptor intercellular adhesion molecule 1 (ICAM-1).[14,15] In a study evaluating P-selectin and TNF inhibition and their ability to reduce venous thrombosis-induced inflammation, rats were passively immunized with either neutralizing anti-TNF serum, anti-TNF serum plus anti-P-selectin antibody, anti-P-selectin antibody, control serum, or a control anti-P-selectin antibody, in groups of four rats each.[15] Antibodies or control serum were administered before IVC occlusion and then at days 2 and 4 after occlusion with the rats sacrificed at days 1–6 and day 13 after occlusion. Differences in vein wall neutrophils, monocytes, and total inflammatory cells were found on days 2, 6 and 13. TNF levels were elevated in the vein walls of the groups not given anti-TNF antibody, and TNF was not detected by ELISA in those animals treated with anti-TNF serum. The lowest vein

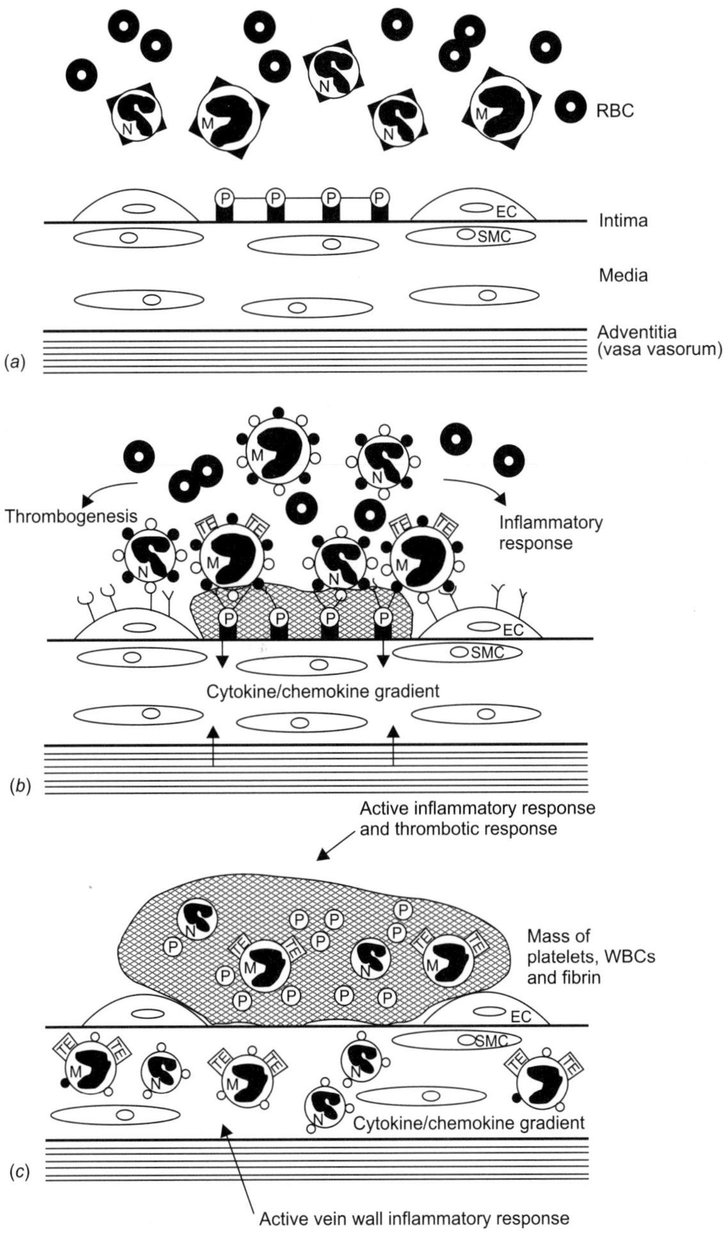

Figure 53.1 *Initially, there is little interaction between the vein wall and circulating blood. (a) At areas of injury, endothelial cell (EC) disruption results in platelet (P) adhesion to the subendothelial surface by von Willebrand factor or fibrinogen bound to the vessel wall (■). N, neutrophil; M, monocyte; RBC, red blood cell; SMC, smooth muscle cell; ▲, L-selectin. (b) With stimulation, leukocytes (neutrophils and monocytes) shed L-selectin and bind reversibly to P-selectin on endothelial cells (EC) and platelets (P) and E-selectin on ECs (both ϒ); ●, P-, E-selectin counter receptor. Monocytes express tissue factor (TF) and fibrin clot forms on the surface of activated platelets. With continued stimulation, leukocytes bind irreversibly to ICAM-1, VCAM-1 (both ϒ) and extravasate into the vein wall by a cytokine/chemokine gradient in the vein wall; ○, β_1, β_2 integrins. (c) As the process evolves, the fibrin clot matures with a mass of platelets, white blood cells (WBCs) and fibrin and an active inflammatory and thrombotic response occurs at the vein wall interface. In the vein wall itself, an active inflammatory response follows. (Reprinted with permission from Wakefield TW, Strieter RM, Prince MR, Downing LJ, Greenfield LJ. Pathogenesis of venous thrombosis: a new insight.* Cardiovasc Surg *1997;* **5**: *6–15)*

wall neutrophil count and total inflammatory count at days 2 and 6, and the lowest neutrophil count at day 13 was found in the anti-TNF plus anti-P-selectin antibody group. Monocyte influx was also inhibited at day 13 in this group. The results suggest a role for combined neutralization of TNF and P-selectin for inhibition of inflammation and emphasize the importance of these pro-inflammatory mediators in the inflammatory response to venous thrombosis.

CYTOKINES/CHEMOKINES

Cytokines/chemokines that are also upregulated in the rat vein wall include epithelial neutrophil-activating protein-78 (ENA-78), KC, macrophage inflammatory protein-2 (MIP-2), JE/monocyte chemotactic protein-1 (JE/MCP-1), macrophage inflammatory protein 1α (MIP-1α) and interleukin-6 (IL-6). Cytokine elevations were seen only under conditions of venous thrombosis in groups of four rats each.[14] Levels of ENA-78, TNF-α, IL-6, and JE/MCP-1 rose over a 6-day period, while MIP-1α peaked on day 3 after thrombus formation. Additionally, rats were passively immunized with neutralizing antibodies to cytokines and adhesion molecules in groups of three. The most effective antibody decreasing neutrophil extravasation into the vein wall was anti-TNF, whilst the most effective antibodies for decreasing monocyte/macrophage extravasation into the vein wall were anti-ICAM-1 and anti-TNF.

INTERLEUKIN-10

Although the above factors are pro-inflammatory, we have also noted that the initiation, maintenance, and eventual resolution of phlebitis is dependent on an interaction between both pro-inflammatory and anti-inflammatory cytokines. Interleukin 10 (IL-10), a naturally occurring anti-inflammatory cytokine produced by monocytes/macrophages, neutrophils, lymphocytes, mast cells and epithelial cells, has been found elevated in the vein wall in response to venous thrombosis. In the rodent stasis-induced model of IVC thrombosis, neutralization of endogenous IL-10 increased inflammation, while rIL-10 supplementation decreased inflammation in a time- and dose-related fashion.[16]

Animals received exogenous human recombinant IL-10 IV or serum albumin (SA) as control. Evaluation methods included leukocyte morphometrics and MPO analysis, with six rats per evaluation method. Animals depleted of endogenous IL-10 demonstrated statistically significantly more vein wall neutrophils and total inflammatory cells (TC) compared with the control group. Additionally, MPO analysis revealed a 36% increase compared with controls. There was an 8% increase in thrombus weight in those rats treated with antibody to IL-10. Using a specific IL-10 ELISA, IL-10 levels were decreased by 62% in those given anti-IL-10.

Recombinant IL-10 administered at 2.5 μg was found to significantly decrease vein wall total inflammatory cells, neutrophils, and monocytes. At a high dose of 40 μg, IL-10 produced a paradoxical pro-inflammatory response. In a time-dependent fashion, rIL-10 was given systemically at the most effective anti-inflammatory dose, 2.5 μg either 6 hours prior to thrombus induction (T–6), at thrombus induction (TO), or 6 hours after thrombus induction (T+6) and compared with SA control animals. An advantage to administration at TO was found, with significant differences between TO and T–6 (for neutrophils and total inflammatory cells, $P < 0.01$). This difference likely relates to the lack of detectable IL-10 in the serum 6 hours after it is administered systemically. The TO time was significantly different from SA controls for neutrophils, monocytes, and total inflammatory cells. Similarly, the T+6 time point was significantly different from SA controls for neutrophils and total inflammatory cells. Additionally, the TO time point revealed the lowest value for MPO activity, with an 8% increase at T+6 and a 14% increase at T–6.

Two additional measures of vein wall injury produced by inflammation have been measured. Vein wall permeability to Evans blue given 3 hours prior to sacrifice (VP) was used as an assessment of vein wall integrity related to inflammation. Trends in VP were noted with VP worsening by depletion of endogenous IL-10 (15% increase in VP) and VP lessening with rIL-10 supplementation, especially when given at the 2.5 μg dose at TO (8% decrease in VP). The second technique is based on magnetic resonance venography (MRV) using gadolinium (Gd). Gd is a nontoxic heavy metal chelate that extravasates into areas of inflammation, as opposed to generalized areas of edema. Gd chelates are paramagnetic heavy metals that decrease the T1 relaxation times of inflammatory foci, resulting in enhancement in areas of inflammation. Enhancement was measured and quantitated in mm^2. There was essentially no enhancement without thrombosis ($n = 6$, 1.83 ± 0.40 mm^2). In thrombosed IVCs ($n = 6$) associated with maximal inflammation (IL-10 at 40 μg), Gd enhancement was measured at 32.7 ± 6.2 mm^2, whilst in thrombosed IVCs in rats ($n = 6$) administered rIL-10 at the anti-inflammatory dose of 2.5 μg, enhancement was measured at only 14.7 ± 1.5 mm^2 ($P < 0.05$).[17] IL-10 is an important endogenous anti-inflammatory cytokine associated with venous thrombosis.

INFLAMMATION AND THROMBOSIS

Inflammation augments thrombosis. Since we had previously noted a correlation between inflammation and venous thrombosis, and IL-10 inhibits inflammation, we assessed whether IL-10 would inhibit venous thrombosis clot formation. Thrombus weight was measured with rIL-10 given at the best anti-inflammatory dose and time interval (2.5 μg at TO). Importantly, a significant 18% decrease in gross thrombus weight with rIL-10 administration compared to SA control was found ($n = 9$ each, 95 ± 6 mg versus 116 ± 7 mg; $P = 0.027$). We also noted a trend with an 8% decrease in tissue factor production with rIL-10, using flow cytometry with a mouse anti-human antibody to tissue factor known to cross-react with rat, as compared with SA control.

To further examine the mechanism of IL-10's anti-inflammatory and anti-thrombotic effect, the rodent IVC segment was transfected with an adenovirus-CMV promoter-viral IL-10 (vIL-10) construct to locally express this product. Controls included saline vehicle and the promoter (CMV or RSV)-B galactosidase (Bgal) constructs. Successful transfection was confirmed by RT-PCR for the vIL-10 cDNA and was suggested by positive X-gal staining in promoter-Bgal control rats.

A significant decrease in both total leukocyte count and neutrophil count as well as perithrombotic Gd enhancement was seen in the vIL-10 animals compared with controls ($P < 0.05$).[18] Interestingly, no significant difference in thrombus weight was found, perhaps a reflection of the balance between anti-inflammatory IL-10 and the pro-inflammatory nature of transfection. In a rat model of ARDS, IL-10 is known to decrease inflammation in part by decreasing cell adhesion molecule expression.[19] Thus, we investigated the expression of the cell adhesion molecules E- and P-selectin and ICAM-1 by immunohistochemical techniques and cell homogenate ELISA.[18] In the vIL-10 transfected rats, a reduction in the expression of all of these molecules as compared with the control promoter and saline groups was found. A trend toward lower local TNF levels was found in the vIL-10 transfected group. The thrombosed venous tissue was also analyzed for direct procoagulant properties by an amidolytic assay for active tissue factor (TF) and TF antigen by ELISA. No difference was found between any of the groups. Lastly, an *in vitro* study utilizing endothelial cells was completed to examine IL-10's effect on endothelial cell adhesion molecule expression and procoagulant properties. No significant direct effect of IL-10 on endothelial E-selectin or ICAM-1 was found nor was any effect found on the procoagulant state. Taken together, the above studies suggest that IL-10 mediates its primary effect as an anti-inflammatory molecule, perhaps by inhibiting leukocytes such as monocytes from releasing pro-inflammatory mediators that act to upregulate endothelial cell adhesion molecule expression and the procoagulant state.

PRIMATE MODEL OF VENOUS THROMBOSIS

Studies in the rat have been supplemented by evaluation of IVC thrombosis in the baboon. Leukocyte adhesion molecules, such as P-selectin, that are expressed on the surfaces of platelets and activated endothelial cells, may play an important role in the relationship between thrombosis and inflammation. Using a primate model of temporary 6-hour balloon IVC occlusion, baboons were pretreated with two different antibodies to P-selectin or saline (four per group).[20] Animals in the P-selectin antibody groups exhibited significantly less thrombus than the control animals along with a decrease in inflammation. Using an antagonist to the P-selectin receptor PS6L-1 (termed r PS6L-lg), a similar but even more striking response has been found, with thrombosis much higher in IVC segments from control animals as opposed to IVC segments from animals pretreated with the selectin antagonist.[21] These primate studies support the notion that initial leukocyte adhesion is important for thrombus formation and its amplification.

CLINICAL VENOUS THROMBOSIS

Does the same inflammatory response noted in the animal studies also occur in clinical deep venous thrombosis (DVT)? We have developed a technique to evaluate the inflammatory response noninvasively, using Gd administered during MRV. The same enhancement noted in rats and primates was seen clinically, and the presence or absence of Gd enhancement defined a DVT less than or greater than 14 days old (Fig. 53.2).[22] In addition, we have noted that vein walls demonstrate an acute increase in inflammatory cells (especially neutrophils) in phlebitic veins and positive immunohisto-

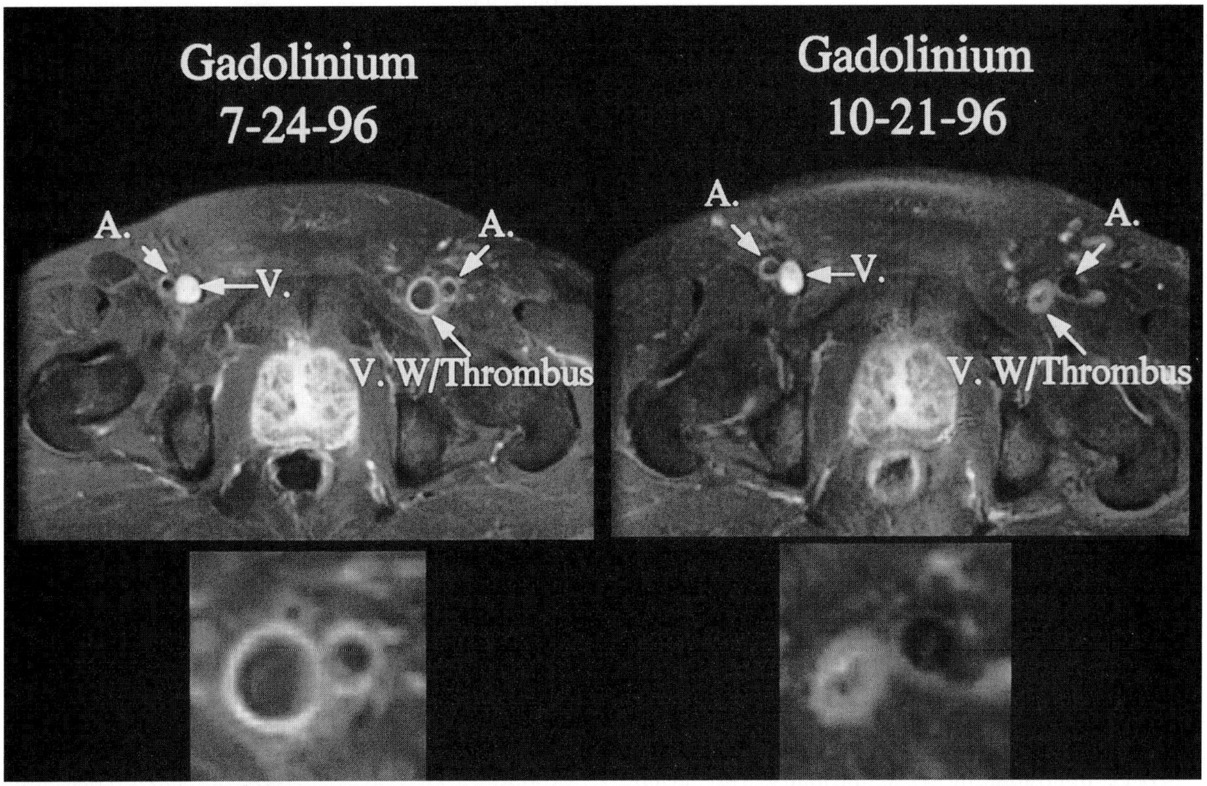

Figure 53.2 *Note that gadolinium enhancement that acutely (left) produced characteristic 'bull's-eye' sign decreased chronically (right). The vein likewise decreased in circumference. T1-weighted images after gadolinium enhancement (right and left). (Reprinted with permission from Froehlich JB, Prince MR, Greenfield LJ, Downing LJ, Shah NL, Wakefield TW. 'Bulls-eye' sign on gadolinium-enhanced magnetic resonance venography determines thrombus presence and age: a preliminary study.* J Vasc Surg *1997;* ***26****: 809–16)*

chemical staining for IL-8 and other chemokines in clinical samples. This suggests that thrombotic inflammation is similar in multiple species, including man.

Mechanisms of dermal tissue injury in chronic venous insufficiency

Injury to pelvic and infrainguinal veins from thrombus or cryptogenic etiologies results in vein wall inflammation, fibrosis and valvular reflux. Multi-segment reflux eventually causes an increase in ambulatory venous pressure. The injuries caused by venous hypertension, at the tissue level, initiate a cascade of pathologic events that manifest themselves clinically as lower extremity edema, pain, itching, skin discoloration, varicose veins, venous ulceration and in its severest form, limb loss. These clinical symptoms collectively refer to the disorder known as chronic venous insufficiency (CVI). The mechanisms regulating CVI at the tissue level are the subject of this section.

LEUKOCYTE ACTIVATION

Numerous theories on the etiology of venous ulcer development and CVI have been proposed during the twentieth century. The majority of these hypotheses are of historical interest and have been disproved. In 1988, Smith *et al.* proposed the 'leukocyte activation theory' which states that venous hypertension causes leukocytes to be trapped in the dermal microcirculation.[23] The resultant sluggish capillary blood flow leads to hypoxia, leukocyte activation, endothelial cell adhesion, diapedesis and degranulation of toxic metabolites. These metabolites subsequently cause microcirculatory damage, leading to lower extremity skin damage.

Although leukocytes have never been observed obstructing capillary flow, several investigations have demonstrated evidence of microcirculatory and leukocyte activation. Skin biopsies from CVI patients with various stages of disease have demonstrated increases in the endothelial activation markers intracellular adhesion marker-1 (ICAM-1) and vascular adhesion molecule-1 (VCAM-1) and their leukocyte ligands LFA-1 and VLA-4.[24] These studies clearly demonstrate that the dermal microcirculation of CVI patients is responding to an injury stimulus caused by persistent venous hypertension. The two best characterized stimuli are extravasated red blood cells (RBCs) and fibrinogen. Biopsies from patients with venous ulcers clearly demonstrate RBCs being forced through inter-endothelial gap junctions. Once extravasated into the interstitium, RBCs quickly begin to decay, causing leukocyte infiltration to the site of injury. RBC phagocytosis by macrophages converts hemoglobin into hemosiderin which remains deposited in the dermis of the lower extremity, resulting in skin discoloration. Similarly, persistent venous hypertension causes interstitial leakage of macromolecules like fibrinogen. Once in the interstitium, fibrinogen is a potent leukocyte chemoattractant and endothelial cell activator. Other macromolecules, like α_2-macroglobulin, have been observed in the dermal interstitium of CVI patients; however, their role and function in the disease process is unclear at the present time. Although it is clear that most of these molecules cause leukocyte attraction, their role in regulating leukocyte, endothelial, fibroblast and keratinocyte interactions is an under-investigated area of research.

LEUKOCYTE TYPE AND DISTRIBUTION

The types of leukocytes observed in the dermal microcirculation of CVI patients is controversial. Wilkinson *et al.* reported that by immunohistochemistry, T-lymphocytes and macrophages were the most commonly observed cells in patients with stasis dermatitis and lipodermatosclerosis.[25] Pappas *et al.* stratified patients according to disease classification and reported that mast cells and macrophages were the most common cells observed. No lymphocytes, plasma cells or neutrophils were observed. The exact role of mast cells in CVI pathophysiology is unknown. Mast cells and macrophages may function to regulate tissue remodeling resulting in dermal fibrosis. The mast cell enzyme chymase is a potent activator of matrix metalloproteinase-1 and 3 (collagenase and stromelysin). Chymase also causes release of latent TGF-β_1 secreted by activated endothelial cells, fibroblasts and platelets from extracellular matrices. Release and activation of TGF-β_1 initiates a cascade of events in which macrophages and fibroblasts are recruited to wound healing sites and stimulated to produce fibroblast mitogens and connective tissue proteins, respectively.

EXTRACELLULAR MATRIX (ECM) ALTERATIONS

Once leukocytes have migrated to the extracellular space, they localize around capillaries and postcapillary venules. The perivascular space is surrounded by extracellular matrix (ECM) proteins which form a perivascular 'cuff'. Adjacent to these perivascular cuffs and throughout the dermal interstitium is an intense and disorganized collagen deposition. Perivascular cuffs and the accompanying collagen deposition are the *sine qua non* of the dermal microcirculation in CVI patients. The cuff is a ring of ECM proteins consisting of collagens type I and III, fibronectin, vitronectin, laminin, tenascin and fibrin. The role of the cuff and its cell of origin is not completely understood. It has been suggested that endothelial cells of the dermal microcirculation are responsible for cuff formation.[26] The cuff was once thought to be a barrier to oxygen and nutrient diffusion; however, recent evidence suggests that cuff formation is an attempt to maintain vascular architecture in response to increased mechanical load. Although perivascular cuffs may function to preserve microcirculatory architecture, several pathologic processes may be related to cuff formation. Immunohistochemical analyses have demonstrated TGF-β_1 and α_2-macroglobulin in the interstices of perivascular cuffs. It has been suggested that these 'trapped' molecules are abnormally distributed in the dermis, leading to altered tissue remodeling and fibrosis. Cuffs may also serve as a lattice for capillary angiogenesis, explaining the capillary tortuosity and increased capillary density observed in the dermis of CVI patients.

PATHOPHYSIOLOGY OF DERMAL TISSUE FIBROSIS

Our laboratory has been interested in the mechanisms regulating dermal tissue remodeling in CVI patients. Leukocyte recruitment, ECM alterations and tissue fibrosis are characteristic of chronic inflammatory diseases caused by alterations in TGF-β_1 gene expression and protein production. To determine the role of TGF-β_1 in CVI dermal tissue alterations, biopsy specimens from the lower calf (LC) and lower thigh (LT) of CVI patients were compared with normal skin biopsies from patients without CVI.[27] The cellular location of TGF-β_1 was determined with immunohistochemistry and immunogold experiments. These experiments demonstrated increased gene expression in class 4 patients only (Fig. 53.3). Active TGF-β_1, however, was observed in class 4, 5, and 6 patients and isolated to areas with clinically active disease (LC) (Fig. 53.4). Increased protein production in the absence of increased gene expression suggested alternative mechanisms for protein production. Immunogold experiments demonstrated binding of particles to collagen fibrils, suggesting that the ECM serves as a storage source for rapid TGF-β_1 production. Immunohistochemistry demonstrated positive staining of intracellular granules in leukocytes which morphologically appeared similar to mast cells. Vimentin-positive spindle-shaped cells (fibroblasts) also stained positively for TGF-β_1, suggesting that leukocytes release TGF-β_1, resulting in fibroblast binding or autoinduction of TGF-β_1 by activated fibroblasts.

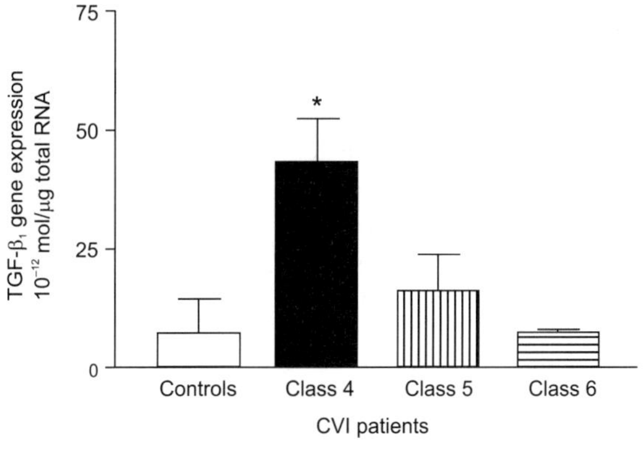

Figure 53.3 *Bar graph demonstrating increased gene expression of TGF-β_1 in class 4 patients only. Quantitative RT-PCR for TGF-β_1 mRNA from DVI skin biopsies. *Class 4 compared to controls, classes 5 and 6 (P ≤0.05).*

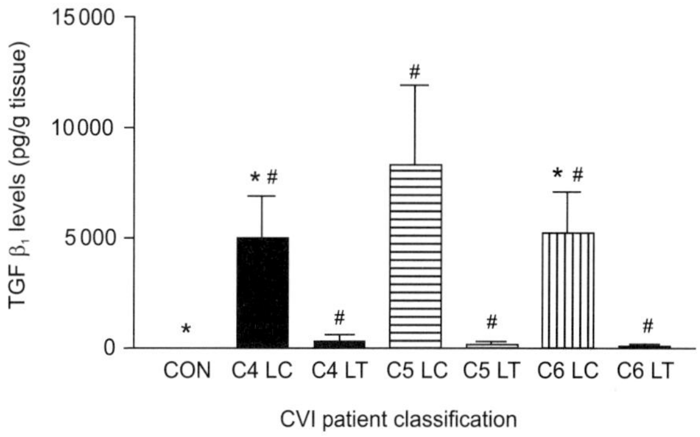

Figure 53.4 *Bar graph demonstrating increased active TGF-β_1 protein in class 4 and 6 patients in areas of clinically active disease. Bioactive TGF-β_1 protein levels from dermal skin biopsies in CVI patients. *Controls versus classes 4 and 6 (P ≤0.05). LC, lower calf; LT, lower thigh; LC VS LT biopsies within each class (p ≤ 0.02).*

DERMAL FIBROBLAST FUNCTION

Several studies have reported aberrant phenotypic behavior of fibroblasts isolated from venous ulcer edges when compared with fibroblasts obtained from ipsilateral thigh biopsies of normal skin in the same patients. Hasan *et al.* compared the ability of venous ulcer fibroblasts to produce αI procollagen mRNA and collagen after stimulation with TGF-β_1.[28] These authors were not able to demonstrate differences in αI procollagen mRNA levels after stimulation with TGF-β_1 between venous ulcer fibroblasts and normal fibroblasts (control) from ipsilateral thigh biopsies. However, collagen production was increased by 60% in a dose-dependent manner in controls whereas venous ulcer fibroblasts were unresponsive. This unresponsiveness was associated with a fourfold decrease in TGF-β_1 type II receptors. A similar investigation reported a decrease in collagen production from venous ulcer fibroblasts and similar amounts of fibronectin production when compared to normal controls.[29]

Fibroblast responsiveness to growth factors was further delineated by Stanley *et al.*[30] These investigators characterized the proliferative responses of venous ulcer fibroblasts when stimulated with basic fibroblastic growth factor (bFGF), epidermal growth factor (EGF) and interleukin 1β (IL-1β). In their initial study, they reported that venous ulcer fibroblast growth rates were markedly suppressed when stimulated with bFGF, EGF and IL-1β. They noted that normal fibroblasts appeared compact and tapered with well-defined nuclear morphologic features, whereas venous ulcer fibroblasts appeared larger, polygonal and with varied nuclear morphologic features. Venous ulcer fibroblasts appeared morphologically similar to fibroblasts undergoing cellular senescence. The authors therefore concluded that the blunted growth response of their cells was associated with cellular senescence.[30]

ROLE OF MATRIX METALLOPROTEINASES (MMPS) AND THEIR INHIBITORS IN VENOUS ULCER HEALING

The signaling event responsible for the development of a venous ulcer and the mechanisms responsible for prolonged wound healing are poorly understood. Wound healing is an orderly process that involves inflammation, re-epithelialization, matrix deposition and tissue remodeling. Tissue remodeling and matrix deposition are processes controlled by matrix metalloproteinases (MMPs) and tissue inhibitors of matrix metalloproteinases (TIMPs). In general, MMPs and TIMPs are not constitutively expressed. They are induced temporarily in response to exogenous signals such as various cytokines or growth factors, cell–matrix interactions and altered cell–cell contacts. TGF-β_1 is a potent inducer of TIMP-1 and inhibitor of MMP-1. Several studies have demonstrated that prolonged and continuous TGF-β_1 production causes tissue fibrosis by stimulating ECM production and inhibiting degradation by affecting MMP and TIMP production. Alterations in MMP and TIMP production may similarly modulate the tissue fibrosis of the lower extremity in CVI patients. In patients with active ulcers, increases in MMP activity from ulcer exudates and decreased expression of TIMP-1 in keratinocytes from venous ulcers have been reported.[31,32] These observations suggest that excessive proteolysis may be responsible for the decreased healing rates seen with venous stasis ulcers.

FUTURE INVESTIGATIONS

A paucity of information is available on the mechanisms regulating dermal fibroblast, endothelial and keratinocyte function in CVI patients. Other than fibrinogen, α_2-macroglobulin and RBCs, no other extravasated macromolecules or cells have been identified. What effects these three components have on cellular proliferation, migration, cytokine production and collagen synthesis is currently unknown. Several studies have begun focusing on fibroblast activities, as discussed above. However, no work on dermal angiogenesis and angiogenic cytokines has been performed. It is well known that capillary tortuosity and zones of hyperperfusion exist in CVI patients, yet the mechanisms regulating this event is unknown. Similarly, TGF-β_1 is the only cytokine documented to play a role in CVI stasis dermatitis and dermal fibrosis. The role of other cytokines like platelet derived growth factor-BB, basic fibroblastic growth factor and vascular endothelial growth factor are fertile areas for investigative endeavors. These cytokines are of particular interest since they are known regulators of angiogenesis, leukocyte migration and cellular mitogens. The regulation of proteases like plasmin, MMPs and TIMPs are important areas of interest due to their effect on matrix synthesis, degradation and wound healing. Finally, the least is known on keratinocyte physiology in CVI patients. What causes keratinocyte breakdown and prolongs re-epithelialization after ulcer formation continues to be a mystery. For vascular surgeons interested in research, CVI offers a multitude of under-investigated topics with a great potential for the development of new therapies. The advent of human skin equivalents and tissue engineering is one example of potential therapeutic modalities possible with currently available technology. It is our hope that this chapter will stimulate future and current investigators to include CVI in their research endeavors.

CLINICAL RESEARCH

Application of noninvasive diagnostic techniques in venous research

The clinical manifestations of venous disease can result from acute deep venous obstruction/thrombosis (DVT) or may be secondary to valvular incompetence and venous insufficiency. Noninvasive techniques used in the diagnosis and characterization of these disease processes may be broadly classified as physiologic or anatomic. The physiologic, or functional, studies provide indirect evidence of venous disease and reflect the hemodynamic or biochemical consequences of its presence. They include the venous Doppler examination and various plethysmographic techniques. More recently, biochemical assays for various markers of coagulation and thrombolysis also have been employed in screening strategies for DVT.[33–38] Anatomic studies directly demonstrate the presence of disease, localizing and quantifying the extent of venous disease and characterizing the pathological process(es) involved. ^{125}I-labeled fibrinogen uptake and scanning, radionuclide venography, platelet scintigraphy, B-mode ultrasound imaging and magnetic resonance imaging (MRI) are classified as anatomic studies. Duplex imaging combines aspects of physiologic and anatomic evaluation. Research applications incorporating these noninvasive diagnostic techniques may involve the diagnosis, treatment and natural history of acute DVT and chronic venous insufficiency, assessment prior to and following venous reconstruction and bench research investigations of acute and chronic venous disease.

ACUTE VENOUS DISEASE

At present, a lack of common standards is, by far, the greatest impediment to the use of noninvasive diagnostic methodologies in clinical research studies involving venous disease. Published research to date has dealt predominantly with the diagnosis of acute DVT and there has been very little standardization among these publications. Variables include the patient population (symptomatic, asymptomatic or mixed), the number of patients (extremities) studied, diagnostic end points and the number of venograms available for verification (all patients, only those patients having positive noninvasive studies). Recently, venographic correlation has decreased, particularly in those patients with negative noninvasive studies. In the latter cases, a follow-up examination has been used to verify the absence of morbid complications (i.e. pulmonary embolism) of DVT.

There are now an increasing number of publications assessing the diagnostic accuracy of MRI techniques. MRI[22,39–43] offers the potential for three-dimensional visualization of the deep veins without the use of iodinated contrast agents, and may provide increased sensitivity to iliac and pelvic vein obstruction. Comparison of studies evaluating MRI is complicated by the lack of uniform reporting standards. Study populations often include patients with upper and lower extremity venous disease, comparative standards may include contrast venography, duplex ultrasonography and/or clinical follow-up, and technical aspects of the imaging protocol vary considerably. Because of cost concerns, newer diagnostic modalities including MRI and adjuvant use of biochemical assays of coagulation and fibrinolysis need to be carefully assessed against well-defined standards using sound research design. Such comparative studies must be prospective evaluations of consecutive patients. The diagnostic criteria must be well defined and related to the identified clinical end points (or outcomes). Venography and duplex ultrasound imaging remain the standards for studies assessing the sensitivity and specificity of a technique relative to DVT until another standard is chosen to take their place; outcome is a legitimate end point, however, if patient management, and not diagnostic accuracy, is being assessed.

CHRONIC VENOUS DISEASE

The evaluation of chronic venous disease is also hampered by a lack of standards. Ultrasonography and plethysmographic techniques can be used to noninvasively characterize valvular function and the hemodynamic consequences of chronic venous disease. Duplex imaging has been used to assess valvular competence, to localize the level(s) of valvular insufficiency and to provide qualitative and quantitative descriptions of venous reflux. Photoplethysmography (PPG) and air plethysmography (APG) yield qualitative and quantitative descriptions of venous hemodynamics.

Before duplex imaging and plethysmographic techniques can be used to define the natural history of postphlebitic complications and chronic venous insufficiency, correlate pathophysiology and clinical symptoms, and monitor the role/efficacy of surgical and nonsurgical therapies, techniques need to be standardized. Authors generally describe the patient's position, the site(s) of examination and the method(s) of eliciting reflux; however, procedural variations in the performance and interpretation of studies are common. Patients may be examined in the standing position, with weight borne on the contralateral leg, or in a supine position at varying degrees (10–60°) of reverse Trendelenburg. Studies may assess one or more venous segments, including the common femoral, profunda femoris, superficial femoral, popliteal, posterior tibial, greater saphenous and lesser saphenous veins. Reflux may be induced by Valsalva maneuver, with or without standardization of effort, manual or automated compression and compression proximal to the ultrasonic probe, or release of compression distal to the probe. Reports providing non-quantitative data describe reflux as being present or absent. Quantitative measures include the valve closure time or duration of reflux, and the peak retrograde velocity and flow at peak reflux (mean blood velocity at peak reflux × cross-sectional area of the vein).

While noninvasive characterization of chronic venous insufficiency is appealing, an accepted 'gold standard' with which to validate such techniques is also lacking. Venography is often considered the 'gold standard', yet technical aspects of descending venography differ with respect to catheter placement, patient positioning (tilt or angle) and the volume and rate of contrast injection. In addition, the relationship between radiological and clinical standards has not been defined. Neglen and Raju[44] demonstrated no correlation between the radiographically determined grade of reflux and clinical severity determined using the criteria defined by the NA-ISCVS/SVS Ad Hoc Committee on Reporting Standards in Venous Disease.

Experimental and clinical frontiers in the care of patients with chronic venous disease

EPIDEMIOLOGY, CLASSIFICATION AND QUANTIFICATION OF VENOUS DISEASE

Research devoted to the socioeconomic impact, pathophysiologic understanding and treatment of chronic venous disease is being recognized as important by health care insurers.[45] This is true even with the knowledge that our methods of defining patients with venous disease for epidemiological study may underestimate the disease incidence. Essential to understanding its full impact in our medical community are well-designed and noninvasively evaluated patient population studies that classify the patients by the CEAP or other specialized methods for proper analysis. These studies simply do not exist. Encouraging to those concerned with chronic venous disease research, the National Institute of Health recently gathered a group of physicians together to discuss venous disease and recommend areas of focus for clinical research. In light of this renewed interest in the importance of chronic venous disease by private and governmental agencies, it appears to be an excellent time to rejuvenate our venous research endeavors.

The proper classification of patients with chronic venous disease is essential to allow comparison of treatments or even the sequelae of a particular disease state. Diagnostic methods to more clearly classify underlying pathophysiology have made some strides but are clearly still suboptimal. Even such a simple symptom as edema requires quantification.[46] Not only do we need to classify the disease but we also need to quantify the effect of treatment on the patient's existence.[47] Research is essential in this area of patient description.

CLINICAL INTERVENTION

The genesis of chronic venous disease from the ravages of acute thrombosis has been recognized for centuries. However, detailed and serial anatomic study of the acute event to determine those critical events, which may result in chronic sequelae, has only recently been possible. Acute DVT is a dynamic event with clot resolution and re-thrombosis over an extended period of time.[48] Certain hypercoagulable states may swing the pendulum from clot resolution to more significant damage. Inflammation may also play a key role in determining the aggressiveness of the early event. Prevention of acute DVT to eliminate the chronic state is a well-recognized clinical goal. This avenue of investigation seeks to define events following thrombosis that may be modified to prevent or ameliorate the chronic state. Potential clinical interventions such as prolonged anticoagulation, anti-inflammatories, and others come into perspective in the framework of this research.

Clinical treatment of chronic venous insufficiency is multifaceted and dependent on the venous system involved (deep, superficial, perforator, calf pump) and whether or not the end organ is affected (e.g. lower leg edema, ulceration, etc.). Although some controversy resolves around the treatment of isolated superficial varicose veins, the majority of current work centers around the perforator and deep veins. Exactly where perforator ligation lies in the overall picture is being actively investigated.[49] Definitive consensus will only result from a well-designed, well-funded, multicenter trial comparing varicose vein stripping alone versus the addition of perforator vein ligation. The treatment of isolated perforator incompetence in association with deep venous insufficiency is an entirely different problem also requiring study. Although limited clinical investigations have found valvuloplasty or external banding as potential answers to reflux associated with primary valvular incompetence, the number of patients so far treated are not sufficient to determine proper patient selection or true efficacy.[50] Taken together, there are likely less than a few hundred valvuloplasty operations reported in the literature. Venous insufficiency resulting from secondary causes has been investigated even less thoroughly. One of the largest series studying venous valve transplantation consists of 54 operations followed for 1–12 years.[51] A cooperative effort amongst those actively involved in the care of these patients is required to generate a study of sufficient quantity and quality to answer questions regarding the use of these operative interventions. A new avenue has emerged for those patients lacking an autogenous alternative. Basic animal experimentation has resulted in an initial clinical trial using a cryopreserved venous valve allograft transplant for the correction of venous insufficiency.[52] Clearly, before this approach can be widely advocated, long-term study is necessary. The entire topic of the surgical treatment of chronic venous disease needs extensive investigation.

BASIC SCIENCE AND END ORGAN

Evaluation of the basic science of chronic venous disease is currently interested in the study of pathologic events occurring within the diseased vein itself. Some theorize an endothelial cell injury model favorably impacted by venotrophic drug therapy.[53] Others see smooth muscle cell differentiation from a contractile to secretory phenotype as the significant factor in the development of pathophysiologic lower extremity venous dilation.[54] Precisely how these two observations interrelate is unknown. One theory suggests that endothelial damage/death may result in leukocyte activation and other events which lead to smooth muscle cell differentiation.[55] Whether venous hypertension and/or stasis cause these events or, in some way, may be a result of these structural abnormalities, is not clear. Further work may define avenues to arrest or even reverse these processes.

Stimulating the most active research yet, being the most poorly understood component of chronic venous disease, is the end-organ effect. Venous hypertension sets off a cascade of events in the lower leg which may result in mild edema or rapidly progress to large venous ulcerations, as discussed earlier. This multitude of intertwining factors, which make up this unstable wound, presents a number of potential medical interventions (e.g. b-FGF,[55], granulocyte-macrophage colony stimulating factor[56]). What is lacking is the complete picture, which makes intervention an empirical process to date.

QUESTIONS FOR FUTURE INVESTIGATIONS

Although many questions are being addressed in basic and clinical research in venous disease, others remain unanswered.

Concerning basic science, questions include:

- What events occur at the venous luminal interface to incite thrombosis?
- What are the hypercoagulable states that predispose certain individuals to thrombotic events?
- What pathophysiologic processes underlie the manifestations of the post-thrombotic syndrome in the presence and absence of a remote history of DVT?
- What are the molecular events associated with the development and perpetuation of venous ulceration?

Concerning clinical topics, questions include:

- What is the most efficient means of prophylaxis for patients at risk for DVT?
- What is the role of thrombolytic therapy, pharmacologic and mechanical, in the setting of DVT? Which agents and strategies are most efficient at removing the occluding thrombus without causing serious untoward effects?
- What is the best regimen for preventing recurrent DVT? What agent should be used (unfractionated heparin, low molecular weight heparin or warfarin), and for how long?
- What is the role of subfascial endoscopic perforator surgery (SEPS) in the treatment of post-thrombotic symptoms? Is there a role for direct venous reconstructive surgery in the form of valve repair, valve transposition or venous bypass?

Venous research is an exciting, evolving area of study. Results from basic and clinical research will better allow us to take care of our patients with venous disease.

REFERENCES

1. Markel A, Manzo RA, Bergein RO, Strandness DE. Valvular reflux after deep vein thrombosis: incidence and time of occurrence. *J Vasc Surg* 1992; **15**: 377–84.
2. Caprini JA, Arcelus JI, Hoffman KN, *et al.* Venous duplex imaging follow-up of acute symptomatic deep vein thrombosis of the leg. *J Vasc Surg* 1995; **21**: 472–6.
3. Sevitt S. The mechanisms of canalisation in deep vein thrombosis. *J Pathol* 1973; **110**: 153–65.
4. Northeast AR, Soo KS, Bobrow LG, *et al.* The tissue plasminogen activator and urokinase response in vivo during natural resolution of venous thrombus. *J Vasc Surg* 1995; **22**: 573–9.
5. Sigel B, Swami V, Can A, *et al.* Intimal hyperplasia producing thrombus organization in an experimental venous thrombosis model. *J Vasc Surg* 1994; **19**: 350–60.
6. See-Tho K, Harris EJ Jr. Thrombosis with outflow obstruction delays thrombolysis and results in chronic wall thickening of rat veins. *J Vasc Surg* 1998; **28**: 115–23.
7. Kumar R, Beguin S, Hemker HC. The influence of fibrinogen and fibrin on thrombin generation. Evidence for feedback activation of the clotting system by clot bound thrombin. *Thromb Haemost* 1994; **72**: 713–21.
8. Francis CW, Markham RE Jr, Barlow GH, Florack TM, Dobrzynski DM, Marder VJ. Thrombin activity of fibrin thrombi and soluble plasmic derivatives. *J Lab Clin Med* 1983; **102**: 220–30.
9. Weitz JI, Hudoba M, Massel D, Maraganore J, Hirsh J. Clot-bound thrombin is protected from inhibition by heparin-antithrombin III and is susceptible to inactivation by antithrombin III-independent inhibitors. *J Clin Invest* 1990; **86**: 385–91.
10. Coughlin SR. Sol Sherry lecture in thrombosis: How thrombin 'talks' to cells: molecular mechanisms and roles in vivo. *Arterioscler Thromb Vasc Biol* 1998; **18**: 514–18.
11. Molino M, Raghunath PN, Kuo A, *et al.* Differential expression of functional protease-activated receptor-2 (PAR-2) in human vascular smooth muscle cells. *Arterioscler Thromb Vasc Biol* 1998; **18**: 825–32.
12. Stewart GJ. Neutrophils and deep venous thrombosis. *Haemostasis* 1993; **23**(Suppl 1): 127–40.
13. Downing LJ, Strieter RM, Kadell AM, *et al.* Neutrophils are the initial cell type identified in deep venous thrombosis induced vein wall inflammation. *ASAIO J* 1996; **42**: M677–82.
14. Wakefield TW, Strieter RM, Wilke CA, *et al.* Venous thrombosis-associated inflammation and attenuation with neutralizing antibodies to cytokines and adhesion molecules. *Arterioscler Thromb Vasc Biol* 1995; **15**: 258–68.
15. Wakefield TW, Strieter RM, Downing LJ, *et al.* P-selectin and TNF inhibition reduce venous thrombosis inflammation. *J Surg Res* 1996; **64**: 26–31.
16. Downing LJ, Strieter RM, Kadell AM, *et al.* IL-10 regulates thrombus-induced vein wall inflammation and thrombosis. *J Immunol* 1998; **161**: 1471–6.
17. Londy FJ, Kadell AM, Wrobleski SK, Prince MR, Strieter RM, Wakefield TW. Detection of perivenous inflammation in a rat model of venous thrombosis using MRV. *J Invest Surg* 1999; **12**: 151–6.
18. Henke PK, Debrunye L, Strieter RM, *et al.* Viral IL-10 gene transfer decreases inflammation and cell adhesion molecule expression in a rat model of venous thrombosis. *J Immunol* 2000; **164**: 2131–41.
19. Mulligan MS, Jones ML, Vaporciyan AA, Howard MC, Ward PA. Protective effects of IL-4 and IL-10 against immune complex-induced lung injury. *J Immunol* 1993; **151**: 5666–74.
20. Downing LJ, Wakefield TW, Strieter RM, *et al.* Anti-P-selectin antibody decreases inflammation and thrombus formation in venous thrombosis. *J Vasc Surg* 1997; **25**: 816–28.
21. Wakefield TW, Strieter RM, Schaub R, *et al.* Venous thrombosis prophylaxis by inflammatory inhibition without anticoagulation therapy. *J Vasc Surg* 2000; **31**: 309–24.

22. Froehlich JB, Prince MR, Greenfield LJ, Downing LJ, Shah NL, Wakefield TW. 'Bull's-eye' sign on gadolinium-enhanced magnetic resonance venography determines thrombus presence and age: a preliminary study. *J Vasc Surg* 1997; **26**: 809–16.
23. Smith PD, Thomas P, Scurr JH, Dormandy JA. Causes of venous ulceration: a new hypothesis. *Br Med J* 1988; **296**: 1726–7.
24. Peschen M, Lahaye T, Hennig B, Weyl A, Simon JC, Vanscheidt W. Expression of the adhesion molecules ICAM-1, VCAM-1, LFA-1 and VLA-4 in the skin is modulated in progressing stages of chronic venous insufficiency. *Acta Dermatol Venereol* 1999; **79**: 27–32.
25. Wilkinson LS, Bunker C, Edwards JC, Scurr JH, Smith PD. Leukocytes: their role in the etiopathogenesis of skin damage in venous disease. *J Vasc Surg* 1993; **17**: 669–75.
26. Pappas PJ, DeFouw DO, Venezio LM, *et al.* Morphometric assessment of the dermal microcirculation in patients with chronic venous insufficiency. *J Vasc Surg* 1997; **26**: 784–95.
27. Pappas PJ, You R, Rameshwar P, *et al.* Dermal tissue fibrosis in patients with chronic venous insufficiency is associated with increased transforming growth factor-β_1 gene expression and protein production. *J Vasc Surg* 1999; **30**: 1129–45.
28. Hasan A, Murata H, Falabella A, *et al.* Dermal fibroblasts from venous ulcers are unresponsive to the action of transforming growth factor-beta 1. *J Dermatol Sci* 1997; **16**: 59–66.
29. Herrick SE, Ireland GW, Simon D, McCollum CN, Ferguson MW. Venous ulcer fibroblasts compared with normal fibroblasts show differences in collagen but not in fibronectin production under both normal and hypoxic conditions. *J Invest Dermatol* 1996; **106**: 187–93.
30. Stanley AC, Park H-Y, Phillips TJ, Russakovsky V, Menzoian JO. Reduced growth of dermal fibroblasts from chronic venous ulcers can be stimulated with growth factors. *J Vasc Surg* 1997; **26**: 994–1001.
31. Vaalamo M, Weckroth M, Puolakkainen P, *et al.* Patterns of matrix metalloproteinase and TIMP-1 expression in chronic and normally healing human cutaneous wounds. *Br J Dermatol* 1996; **135**: 52–9.
32. Saarialho-Kere UK, Kovacs SO, Pentland AP, Olerud JE, Welgus HG, Parks WC. Cell–matrix interactions modulate interstitial collagenase expression by human keratinocytes actively involved in wound healing. *J Clin Invest* 1993; **92**: 2858–66.
33. Jossang B, Runde I. Diagnostic value of C-reactive protein and D-dimer in deep venous thrombosis. *Tidsskr Nor Laegeforen* 1992; **112**: 1153–5.
34. Rowbotham BJ, Whitaker AN, Harrison J, Murtaugh P, Reasbeck P, Bowle EJ. Measurement of cross-linked fibrin derivatives in patients undergoing abdominal surgery: use in the diagnosis of postoperative venous thrombosis. *Blood Coagul Fibrinolysis* 1992; **3**: 25–31.
35. Bouman CS, Ypma ST, Sybesma JP. Comparison of the efficacy of D-dimer, fibrin degradation products and prothrombin fragment 1+2 in clinically suspected deep venous thrombosis. *Thromb Res* 1995; **77**: 225–34.
36. Michiels JJ. Rational diagnosis of deep vein thrombosis (RADIA DVT) in symptomatic outpatients with suspected DVT: simplification and improvement of decision rule analysis for the exclusion and diagnosis of DVT by the combined use of a simple clinical model, a rapid sensitive D-dimer test and compression ultrasonography (CUS). *Semin Thromb Hemost* 1998; **24**: 401–7.
37. Wahlander K, Tengborn L, Hellstrom M, *et al.* Comparison of various D-dimer tests for the diagnosis of deep venous thrombosis. *Blood Coagul Fibrinolysis* 1999; **10**: 121–6.
38. Legnani C, Pancani C, Palareti G, Guazzaloca G, Coccheri S. Contribution of a new, rapid, quantitative and automated method for D-dimer measurement to exclude deep vein thrombosis in symptomatic outpatients. *Blood Coagul Fibrinolysis* 1999; **10**: 69–74.
39. Carpenter JP, Holland GA, Baum RA, Owen RS, Carpenter JT, Cope C. Magnetic resonance venography for the detection of deep venous thrombosis: comparison with contrast venography and duplex Doppler ultrasonography. *J Vasc Surg* 1993; **18**: 734–41.
40. Catalano C, Pavone P, Laghi A, *et al.* Role of MR venography in the evaluation of deep venous thrombosis. *Acta Radiol* 1997; **38**: 907–12.
41. Polak JF, Fox LA. MR assessment of the extremity veins. *Semin Ultrasound CT MR* 1999; **20**: 36–46.
42. Moody AR, Pollock JG, O'Connor AR, Bagnall M. Lower-limb deep venous thrombosis: direct MR imaging of the thrombus. *Radiology* 1998; **209**: 349–55.
43. Li W, David V, Kaplan R, Edelman RR. Three-dimensional low dose gadolinium-enhanced peripheral MR venography. *J Magn Reson Imaging* 1998; **8**: 630–3.
44. Neglen P, Raju S. A comparison between descending phlebography and duplex Doppler investigation in the evaluation of reflux in chronic venous insufficiency: a challenge to phlebography as the 'gold standard'. *J Vasc Surg* 1992; **16**: 687–93.
45. Van den Oever R, Hepp B, Debbaut B, Simon I. Socio-economic impact of chronic venous insufficiency. An underestimated public health problem. *Int Angiol* 1998; **17**: 161–7.
46. Cesarone MR, Belcaro G, Nicolaides AN, *et al.* The edema tester in the evaluation of swollen limbs in venous and lymphatic disease. *Panminerva Med* 1999; **41**: 10–14.
47. Franks PJ, Bosanquet N, Brown D, Straub J, Harper DR, Ruckley CV. Perceived health in a randomized trial of treatment for chronic venous ulceration. *Eur J Vasc Endovasc Surg* 1999; **17**: 155–9.
48. Meissner MH, Caps MT, Bergelin RO, Manzo RA, Strandness DE. Early outcome after isolated calf vein thrombosis. *J Vasc Surg* 1997; **26**: 749–56.
49. Gloviczki P, Bergan JJ, Rhodes JM, *et al.* Mid-term results of endoscopic perforator vein interruption for chronic venous insufficiency: lessons learned from the North American subfascial endoscopic perforator surgery registry. *J Vasc Surg* 1999; **29**: 489–502.

50. Matsuda EM, Kistner RL. Long-term results of venous valve reconstruction: a four- to twenty-one year follow-up. *J Vasc Surg* 1994; **19**: 391–403.
51. Raju S, Fredericks RK, Neglen PN, Bass JD. Durability of venous valve reconstruction techniques for 'primary' and postthrombotic reflux. *J Vasc Surg* 1996; **23**: 357–67.
52. Dalsing MD, Raju S, Wakefield TW, Taheri S. A multi-center, phase 1 evaluation of cryopreserved venous valve allografts for the treatment of chronic deep venous insufficiency. *J Vasc Surg* 1999; **30**: 854–66.
53. Janssens D, Michiels C, Guillaume G, Cuisinier B, Louagie Y, Remacle J. Increase in circulating endothelial cells in patients with primary chronic venous insufficiency: protective effect of Ginkor Fort in a randomized double-blind, placebo-controlled clinical trial. *J Cardiovasc Pharmacol* 1999; **33**: 7–11.
54. Pappas PJ, Gwertzman GA, DeFouw DO, *et al.* Retinoblastoma protein: a molecular regulator of chronic venous insufficiency. *J Surg Res* 1998; **76**: 149–53.
55. Mendez MV, Stanley A, Phillips T, Murphy M, Menzoian JO, Park H-Y. Fibroblasts cultured from distal lower extremities in patients with venous reflux display cellular characteristics of senescence. *J Vasc Surg* 1998; **28**: 1040–50.
56. DaCosta RM, Riberio J, Ariceto C, *et al.* Randomized, double-blind, placebo-controlled, dose-ranging study of granulocyte-macrophage colony stimulating factor in patients with chronic venous leg ulcers. *Wound Repair Regen* 1999; **7**: 1–25.

Index

Abbreviations: CVD/CVI, chronic venous disease/insufficiency; DVT, deep venous thrombosis; IVC, inferior vena cava; MR, magnetic resonance; PE, pulmonary embolism; SVC, superior vena cava; VT, venous thrombosis.